Little and Falace's

DENTAL
MANAGEMENT
of the Medically Compromised Patient

TENTH EDITION **10**

Little and Falace's
DENTAL
MANAGEMENT
of the Medically Compromised Patient

A Ross Kerr, DDS, MSD
Clinical Professor
Oral & Maxillofacial Pathology, Radiology & Medicine
New York University College of Dentistry
New York, New York

Craig S. Miller, DMD, MS
Alvin L. Morris Professor of Oral Health Research
University Research Professor
Director, Nudge Unit
College of Dentistry, University of Kentucky

Nelson L. Rhodus, DMD, MPH
Morse Distinguished Professor
Diagnostic and Biological Sciences
University of Minnesota
Minneapolis, Minnesota

Eric T. Stoopler, DMD
Professor of Oral Medicine
Penn Dental Medicine
Division of Oral Medicine, Department of Oral and
  Maxillofacial Surgery
Penn Medicine
Philadelphia, Pennsylvania

Nathaniel S. Treister, DMD, DMSc
Division Chief
Division of Oral Medicine and Dentistry
Brigham and Women's Hospital
Boston, Massachusetts

ELSEVIER

Elsevier
3251 Riverport Lane
St. Louis, Missouri 63043

LITTLE AND FALACE'S DENTAL MANAGEMENT OF THE
MEDICALLY COMPROMISED PATIENT, TENTH EDITION

ISBN: 978-0-323-80945-0

Copyright © 2024 by Elsevier, Inc. All rights reserved.

Senior Content Strategist: Lauren Boyle
Content Development Manager: Danielle Frazier
Senior Content Development Specialist: Maria Broeker
Publishing Services Manager: Deepthi Unni
Senior Book Production Executive: Kamatchi Madhavan
Designer: Renee Duenow

Printed in India
Last digit is the print number: 9 8 7 6 5 4 3 2

The tenth edition is dedicated to the founding authors of this renowned text, Dr. James W. Little and Dr. Donald A. Falace, whose insight regarding the needs of dentistry made this all possible and created an appreciation of Oral Medicine.

The first edition of this textbook was published in 1980 by the two original authors, Dr. James Little and Dr. Donald Falace, both of whom were faculty members in the Department of Oral Diagnosis and Oral Medicine at the University of Kentucky College of Dentistry. It was the culmination of a long creative process that began with a multidisciplinary lecture course developed by Dr. Little. The goal of the course was to provide dental students with information and guidance that would allow them to safely provide dental care to patients with a variety of medical problems (medically compromised) that could potentially be adversely impacted by the provision of dental treatment. Lectures were provided by physicians, dentists, and other healthcare providers. Dr. Little, an oral pathologist and Chair of the Department, was the course director and primary lecturer for several years. Dr. Falace, an oral surgeon, then joined Dr. Little on faculty in 1975, and he subsequently became the course director. A large course syllabus of lecture outlines and notes had evolved over the years, and with the encouragement of students and colleagues, it was decided to use the syllabus as a basis for a textbook. C.V. Mosby was the original publisher with Darlene Cooke as the first editor. C.V. Mosby was eventually acquired by Elsevier which has continued as the publisher for all subsequent editions. Drs. Little and Falace were the sole authors through the first three editions, and then, starting with the fourth edition, Dr. Craig Miller and Dr. Nelson Rhodus joined as coauthors. In the ninth edition, Drs. Kerr, Stoopler, and Treister were invited authors, and with this tenth edition, they joined Drs. Miller and Rhodus as lead authors, with both Drs. Little and Falace retiring from contributing authorship.

Much has changed over the past four decades in medicine and dentistry resulting in a better understanding of the pathophysiology, diagnosis, therapy, and prognosis of many diseases. People are able to live relatively normal lives today with diseases that were fatal or disabling in the past. There is continuing growth of the segment of the population 65 and older, coincident with the aging of the baby boomers. In 1980, the number of Americans over the age of 65 was about 14%. Today, that figure approximates 16%, and is projected to grow to more than 21% by 2040. Contributing to these statistics is the fact that people are living longer than ever before. In 1950, the life expectancy for an individual at age 65 was about 14 years. A person who is 65 today has a life expectancy of about 20 years.

With increasing longevity comes an increase in chronic health conditions. According to 2008 CDC data, 37% of adults aged 55–64 had two or more chronic diseases, while 56% of adults aged 65 or older had two or more chronic diseases. For the 65 and older population, the most prevalent health conditions include heart disease, diabetes, cancer, stroke, and arthritis. Contributing factors for many of these health problems are obesity, poor diet, and inadequate exercise. The leading causes of death in 2019 for those over 65 were heart disease, cancer, lower respiratory disease, stroke, Alzheimer's disease, and diabetes. However, infectious disease, in the form of the COVID-19 pandemic, suddenly appeared on the scene and in 2020, was the third leading cause of death, following cancer. This phenomenon of emerging infectious diseases is likely to continue and will undoubtedly impact dental care. One can recall the tremendous impact that tuberculosis and human immunodeficiency virus infections have had on those infected, their families, and all of the health professions.

As would be expected, the use of prescription medications has increased as new therapies are developed for treating and managing diseases. While the over 65 age group constitutes about 16% of the population, they consume about one third of all prescription drugs. Almost 90% of older adults regularly take at least one prescription drug, almost 80% regularly take at least two prescription drugs, and 36% regularly take at least five prescription drugs. Prescription drugs, as well as over-the-counter medications, have the potential for producing adverse effects and drug–drug interactions. In addition to a primary care provider, patients often have specialists participating in their care, some of whom may write prescriptions. With multiple providers writing prescriptions, it is not uncommon for unintended drug–drug interactions to occur. Drug adverse effects can also include oral lesions, with cancer chemotherapy being a classic example.

It is critical that the dental health practitioner have fundamental knowledge of the many disease processes and how they relate to the provision of dental care. This includes understanding the basic pathophysiology of the disease, its effect on the various organ systems, various medical treatment modalities and their effects, drug actions, interactions and adverse effects, any possible interactions with dental treatment, and how to modify dental care. The goal of this textbook has always been, and continues to be, to provide the dental practitioner with that information in a concise and easy to use format. While not intended to be a comprehensive medical textbook, enough basic information is provided about each condition to allow a fundamental understanding of the disease and to provide an evidence-based approach to dental management recommendations.

In addition, the textbook includes several helpful appendices. Those include (A) medical emergencies, (B) an update on infection control guidelines, (C) management of common oral mucosal diseases, (D) drug–drug interactions of significance in dentistry, and (E) a listing of common herbal and alternative medications. It is our sincere hope that readers will find this text to be an invaluable addition to their professional library.

Donald A. Falace, DMD
Professor Emeritus
Oral Diagnosis and Oral Medicine
University of Kentucky College of Dentistry

Little and Falace's Dental Management of the Medically Compromised Patient welcomes its tenth edition with an expanded role for authors Dr. Ross Kerr, Dr. Eric Stoopler, and Dr. Nathaniel Treister. They join Dr. Craig Miller and Dr. Nelson Rhodus as lead authors. We are pleased that this edition utilizes the diversified oral medicine expertise of these authors, all of whom are diplomates of the American Board of Oral Medicine. Dr. A. Ross Kerr is a Clinical Professor, Oral and Maxillofacial Pathology, Radiology, and Medicine, New York University College of Dentistry; Dr. Eric T. Stoopler is a Professor of Oral Medicine and former director of the Postdoctoral Oral Medicine Program at Penn Dental Medicine and Penn Medicine; and Nathaniel Simon Treister is an Associate Surgeon and Chief, Division of Oral Medicine and Dentistry, Brigham and Women's Hospital and Dana-Farber Cancer Institute and Associate Professor of Oral Medicine, Infection and Immunity, Harvard School of Dental Medicine.

The tenth edition builds on concepts established by the original authors, Dr. Jim Little and Dr. Don Falace, that help dental practitioners identify patients with medical conditions, assess risk, and prevent adverse outcomes. The information provided is meant to help practicing dentists, practicing dental hygienists, dental graduate students in advanced education, specialty training, or medical center–based general practice residency programs, as well as dental and dental hygiene students.

This edition is designed to provide clinicians an up-to-date, concise, factual reference describing the dental management of patients with medical problems. The more common medical disorders typically encountered in a dental practice continue to be our focus. This book is not a comprehensive medical reference, but rather a book containing core information about each of the medical conditions covered to enable readers to recognize the basis for various dental management recommendations. Medical conditions and diseases are organized to provide a brief overview of the basic disease process, epidemiology, pathophysiology and complications, signs and symptoms, laboratory and diagnostic findings, and currently accepted medical treatments of each disorder. The "medical management" section continues to provide important detail on medications (i.e., dosages, side effects, and drug interactions with agents used in dentistry) and updates on new and emerging drugs used to treat patients in the contemporary healthcare setting. The medical management section is followed by a detailed explanation and recommendations for specific dental management and oral considerations. Emphasis is on providing pertinent information and an understanding of how to identify significant medical issue(s), ascertain the severity and stability of the disorder(s), and make dental management decisions that afford utmost patient health and safety.

The accumulation of evidence-based research over the years has allowed us to provide specific dental management guidelines that should benefit those who read this text. Dental management considerations are presented and summarized in a table in each chapter. The summary tables have been designed as 'checklists'; utilizing the previous A, B, C format to help clinicians understand potential issues involving anesthetics, analgesics, antibiotics, bleeding, chair position, drugs, and emergencies. These checklists are formatted for the clinician to follow the 'preoperative', 'operative,' and 'postoperative' setting considerations. In addition, we have included the "Strength of Recommendation Taxonomy (SORT)" Grade categories to indicate the level of evidence that supports the recommendations being made. This taxonomy uses **level A**—recommendation that is based on consistent and good-quality patient-oriented evidence; **level B**—recommendation that is based on inconsistent or limited-quality patient-oriented evidence; and **level C**—recommendation that is based on consensus, usual practice, opinion, disease-oriented evidence, or case series for studies of diagnosis, treatment, prevention, or screening (Ebell MH, et al. *Am Fam Physician*. Feb 1, 2004;69(3):548–556).

An important feature of the book is access to the enhanced eBook version. The enhanced version allows you to browse, search, and customize your content and make notes, highlights, or even have the content read aloud. Instructions for activating the eBook version of this title are included on the inside front cover. The Evolve Instructor Resources continue to be available at http://evolve.elsevier.com/Little/compromised/. Working with our publisher, Elsevier, it is our goal to provide more information online each year. This will allow dentists, dental hygienists, and students easy access to current information.

NEW TO THIS EDITION

As there is an ever-increasing flow of new knowledge and changing concepts in medicine, dentistry, and learning, a number of changes have been made in this tenth edition to allow for a superior learning experience. At the beginning of each chapter is a list of Key Points that provide clear statements for students and clinicians to focus attention on important objectives of each chapter. Chapter 1 presents an overview of the diagnostic risk assessment process that is used as an important framework throughout the book. Chapter 2 presents the most recent American Heart Association scientific information on the prevention of viridans group Streptococcal infective endocarditis. The most recent high blood pressure guidelines have been incorporated into Chapter 3. Chapter 8 includes new information on the use of electronic cigarettes and questionnaires that dentists may use to screen patients for tobacco use. Chapter 9 includes validated questionnaires that dentists may use to screen patients for sleep-disordered breathing and an entirely new section on the roles of the dental health care provider for patients with this disorder. Chapter 10 has been updated to include new information on the various types of hepatitis. Chapter 11 has been updated to reflect current medication regimens to manage gastrointestinal disorders and includes an entirely new section on gastroesophageal reflux disorder (GERD). Chapter 17 has updated information regarding dental implications of health issues specific to women. Chapter 22 includes an expanded section on thalassemias and up-to-date information on therapeutics to manage red blood cell disorders. Chapter 26 has been thoroughly reorganized and updated with information including novel targeted cancer therapies including immune checkpoint inhibitors and their potential impact on oral health. Psychiatric disorders have been consolidated into a single chapter (Chapter 28) and updated according to the Diagnostic and Statistical Manual of Mental Disorders, 5th Edition (DSM-5). Chapter 29 is a new and timely chapter on Substance Use Disorders that includes information valuable to the clinician. In all chapters, new color figures, boxes, and tables appear, bibliographies are provided, and we have added cases and case-based questions for better student learning and assessment.

All appendixes have been brought up to date. Specifically, Appendix A continues to serve as a quick reference guide to management of common medical emergencies. Infection control recommendations found in Appendix B contain new updates relevant to COVID-19.

Appendix C has been updated to reflect the current therapeutic regimens for a wide variety of common oral mucosal diseases. Appendix D "Drug Interactions of Significance in Dentistry" has been expanded to include information on the basic types of drug–drug interactions and the relationship between specific CYP cytochromes and drug metabolism. Appendix E has been trimmed and focuses on the primary concerns in dentistry regarding herbal and alternative medications.

The authors also are aware and are sensitive to racial and ethnic factors that may not have been appropriately presented in the epidemiology sections of past editions. In this edition, we have attempted to address this by introducing a statement in the chapters that recognizes the complexity of epidemiological associations with certain racial/ethnic populations. Accordingly, we have included sentences similar to: social, economic, and historical disparities, and differences in environment, personal behavior, and habits are factors that contribute to higher prevalence of certain diseases within select racial/ethnic populations. We will continue to listen to all persons regarding the best way to present this information to our readers.

Finally, our sincere thanks and appreciation are extended to those many individuals who have contributed their time and expertise to the writing and revision of this text. These include but are not limited to Joslyn Dumas, Maria Broeker, Lauren Boyle, and Kristin Wilhelm, our partners at Elsevier.

A. Ross Kerr
Craig S. Miller
Nelson L. Rhodus
Eric T. Stoopler
Nathaniel S. Treister

CONTENTS

1

Patient Evaluation, Risk Assessment, and the Diagnostic Process

■ KEY POINTS

- Patient evaluation and risk assessment require a standardized sequential diagnostic process of data collection. This requires obtaining the patient's chief complaint, medical history and medications, clinical and imaging examinations, review of diagnostic test results, and obtaining a medical consultation when needed.

- The diagnostic process benefits from the use of a checklist, recognizing and recording abnormalities, and formulating diagnoses.
- The treatment plan is based on the patient's findings, problems, and diagnoses. Modifications should be personalized and based on the patient's health status and the planned procedures.

The practice of dentistry continues to evolve, not only in techniques and procedures but also in the types of patients encountered. As a result of advances in medical science, people are living longer and are receiving medical treatment for disorders that were fatal only a few years ago. For example, damaged heart valves are surgically replaced, occluded coronary arteries are surgically bypassed or opened by balloons and stents, organs are transplanted, severe hypertension is medically controlled, and many types of malignancies and immune deficiencies are managed or controlled.

Dentists must be knowledgeable about a wide range of medical conditions and drug considerations. Why? Because 6 in 10 adults have a chronic disease, 4 in 10 have two or more chronic diseases, and chronic disease increases with age. Also, lifestyle choices greatly influence the development of chronic disease (Box 1.1). This is relevant because many chronic disorders or their treatments necessitate alterations in the provision of dental treatment. Failure to make appropriate treatment modifications may have serious clinical consequences.

Key to successful dental management of a medically compromised patient is a thorough evaluation of the patient followed by a thoughtful assessment of risk to determine whether a planned procedure can be safely tolerated. The fundamental question that must be addressed is whether the benefit of dental treatment outweighs the risk of a medical complication occurring either during treatment or as a result of treatment. The evaluation should follow a standardized and sequential

process beginning with a thorough review of the medical history, expanded as necessary by discussion of any relevant issues with the patient, and proceeding to identification of drugs or medications that the patient is taking (or is supposed to be taking), examining the patient for signs, symptoms, and clinical features of disease as well as obtaining vital signs, reviewing current imaging and laboratory test results, and obtaining a medical consultation if needed. The diagnostic process requires acquisition of all relevant information, then application of this information to assess the risk for problems related to specific factors identified in the evaluation. The diagnostic process benefits from the use of a checklist as summarized in Box 1.2, which illustrates the sequential nature of the assessment using an "ABC"-type format.

MEDICAL HISTORY

A medical history must be taken for every patient who is to receive dental treatment and updated annually, or more often if needed. Two basic techniques are used to obtain a medical history. The first technique consists of

BOX 1.1	Lifestyle Choices and Risks for Chronic Disease

Diet/Poor Nutrition Lack of Physical Activity
Tobacco Use Excessive Alcohol/Substance Use
Exposure to Infectious and Toxic Agents Stress

an interview of the patient (medical model), in which the interviewer questions the patient then records a narrative of the patient's verbal responses. The second technique is the use of a questionnaire that the patient fills out. The latter approach is most commonly used in dental practice and is very convenient and efficient. It is important, however, that the medical information acquired in this manner be reviewed by dialogue with the patient as appropriate to clarify and determine the significance of any finding that might impact dental treatment.

Many questionnaires are commercially available in both electronic and hard copy versions. Dentists also may develop or modify questionnaires to meet the specific needs of their individual practices. Although medical history questionnaires may differ in organization and detail, most attempt to elicit information about the same basic medical problems. The following section presents an overview of medical conditions, organized by body systems, as well as other conditions and factors of relevance, and specifies the rationale for why certain questions are asked and highlights the significance of positive responses on the questionnaire or in the interview. Detailed information concerning most of these medical problems is found in the subsequent chapters.

Cardiovascular Disease

Patients with various forms of cardiovascular disease are especially vulnerable to physical or emotional challenges that may be encountered during dental treatment.

BOX 1.2	Checklist for Patient Evaluation, Risk Assessment, and Dental Management Modification Considerations

PREOPERATIVE RISK ASSESSMENT

R: Recognize risks
- Be **aware** of adverse events that may occur in the management of a patient who has a medical condition.

P: Patient evaluation
- Review **medical history** and discuss relevant issues with the patient.
- Identify all **medications and drugs** being taken or supposed to be taken by the patient.
- **Examine** the patient for signs and symptoms of disease and obtain vital signs.
- Review or obtain recent applicable **laboratory test** results or **imaging** required to assess risk.
- Obtain a **medical consultation** if the patient has a poorly controlled or undiagnosed problem or if the patient's health status is uncertain.

A	
Antibiotics	Will the patient need antibiotics, either prophylactically or therapeutically? Is the patient currently taking an antibiotic? Is the patient at risk for infection?
Analgesics	Is the patient taking aspirin or other NSAIDs that may increase bleeding? Are analgesics indicated before the procedure, or will analgesics be needed after the procedure?
Anesthesia	Are there any potential problems or concerns associated with the use or dosage of local anesthetic or with vasoconstrictors?
Anxiety	Will the patient need a sedative or anxiolytic?

B	
Bleeding	Is abnormal hemostasis a possibility? Is the patient taking medications that can affect bleeding during or after an invasive procedure?
Breathing	Does the patient have any difficulty breathing, or is the breathing abnormally fast or slow?

Blood pressure	Is the blood pressure well controlled, or is it likely to increase or decrease during dental treatment?

C	
Capacity to tolerate care	Does the patient have sufficient functional (cardiovascular) and emotional capacity to withstand the type of dental procedure planned?

D	
Drugs	Are any drugs being taken by the patient or to be administered or prescribed by the dentist associated with relevant drug interactions, adverse effects, or allergies?
Devices	Does the patient have prosthetic or therapeutic devices that may require specific considerations in management (e.g., prosthetic heart valve, prosthetic joint, stent, pacemaker, defibrillator, arteriovenous fistula)?

E	
Equipment	Are there any potential problems associated with the use of dental equipment (e.g., X-ray machine, electrocautery, oxygen supply, ultrasonic cleaner)? Are monitoring devices such as a pulse oximeter, carbon dioxide monitor, or blood pressure measurement device indicated for use during the dental procedure?
Emergencies	Are there any medical urgencies or emergencies that might be anticipated or prevented by modifying care?

F Postoperative care	
Follow-up care	Is any follow-up care indicated? Are analgesics indicated to reduce postoperative pain? Are antibiotics indicated to reduce the risk of spreading infection? Should the patient be contacted at home to assess her or his response to treatment?

NSAID, Nonsteroidal antiinflammatory drug.

Heart Failure. Heart failure is not a disease per se but rather a clinical syndrome complex that results from an underlying cardiovascular problem such as coronary heart disease or hypertension. The underlying cause of heart failure should be identified and its potential significance assessed. Patients with untreated or symptomatic heart failure often take several medications that target the cardiovascular system. These patients who are symptomatic or poorly controlled are at increased risk for myocardial infarction (MI), arrhythmias, acute heart failure, or sudden death and generally are not candidates for elective dental treatment. Chair position may influence the ability to breathe, with some patients unable to tolerate a supine position. Vasoconstrictors should be avoided in certain circumstances, for example, if a patient has severe heart failure and in patients who take digitalis glycosides (digoxin) because the combination can precipitate arrhythmias (see Chapter 6). Stress reduction measures may be advisable.

Heart Attack. A history of a heart attack (MI) within the very recent past (i.e., within 30 days) may preclude elective dental care because during the immediate post-infarction period, patients are at increased risk for reinfarctions, arrhythmias, and heart failure. Patients may be taking medications such as antianginals, anticoagulants, adrenergic blocking agents, calcium channel blockers, antiarrhythmic agents, or digitalis. Some of these drugs may alter dental management of patients because of potential interactions with vasoconstrictors in local anesthetic, adverse side effects, or other considerations (see Chapter 4). Stress and anxiety reduction measures may be advisable.

Angina Pectoris. Brief episodes of substernal pain resulting from myocardial ischemia, commonly provoked by physical activity or emotional stress, is a common and significant symptom of coronary heart disease. Patients with angina, especially unstable or severe angina, are at increased risk for arrhythmias, MI, and sudden death. A variety of vasoactive medications, such as nitroglycerin, β-adrenergic blocking agents, and calcium channel blockers, are used to treat angina. Caution is advised with the use of vasoconstrictors. Stress and anxiety reduction measures may be appropriate. Patients with unstable or progressive angina are not candidates for elective dental care (see Chapter 4).

High Blood Pressure. Patients with hypertension (blood pressure [BP] >130/80 mm Hg) should be identified by history and the diagnosis confirmed by BP measurement. Patients with a history of hypertension should be asked if they are taking or are supposed to be taking antihypertensive medication. Failure to take medication and white coat hypertension are two causes of elevated BP commonly seen in dentistry. Current BP readings and any clinical signs and symptoms that may be associated with severe, uncontrolled hypertension, such as visual changes, dizziness, spontaneous nosebleeds, and headaches, should be noted. Caution in the use of vasoconstrictors is advised in patients who take certain antihypertensive medications such as the nonselective β-adrenergic blocking agents (see Chapter 3). The coadministration of calcium channel blockers with macrolide antibiotics (e.g., erythromycin, clarithromycin) can result in excessive hypotension. Stress and anxiety reduction measures may be appropriate. Elective dental care should be deferred for patients with severe, uncontrolled hypertension (BP of ≥180/110 mm Hg) until the condition can be brought under control because they have an increased risk of stroke.

Heart Murmur. A heart murmur is caused by turbulence of blood flow that produces vibratory sounds during the beating of the heart. Turbulence may result from physiologic (normal) factors or pathologic abnormalities of the heart valves, vessels, or both. The presence of a heart murmur may be of significance in dental patients because it may be an indication of underlying heart disease. The primary goal is to determine the nature of the heart murmur; consultation with the patient's physician often is necessary to make this determination. Previously, the American Heart Association (AHA) recommended antibiotic prophylaxis for many patients with heart murmurs caused by valvular disease (e.g., mitral valve prolapse (MVP), rheumatic heart disease) in an effort to prevent infective endocarditis. However, current AHA guidelines are less broad and recommend antibiotic prophylaxis if the underlying cardiac conditions include previous endocarditis, prosthetic heart valve, or complex congenital cyanotic heart disease for most dental procedures (see Chapter 2).

Mitral Valve Prolapse. In MVP, the leaflets of the mitral valve "prolapse," or balloon back, into the left atrium during systole. As a result, tight closure of the leaflets may not occur, which can result in leakage or backflow of blood (regurgitation) from the ventricle into the atrium. Not all patients with MVP have regurgitation, however. In past guidelines, the AHA recommended that patients with MVP with regurgitation receive antibiotic prophylaxis for invasive dental procedures to prevent infective endocarditis. However, on the basis of accumulated scientific evidence, current guidelines do not include this recommendation (see Chapter 2).

Rheumatic Fever. Rheumatic fever is an autoimmune condition that can follow an upper respiratory β-hemolytic streptococcal infection and may lead to damage of the heart valves (rheumatic heart disease). The AHA currently does not recommend antibiotic prophylaxis for patients with a history of this condition (see Chapter 2).

Congenital Heart Disease. Patients with some forms of severe congenital heart disease are at increased risk for infective endocarditis, an infection that can result in significant morbidity and mortality. The AHA recommends that patients with complex cyanotic heart disease (e.g., tetralogy of Fallot) and those who have had an incomplete surgical repair of a congenital defect, with a residual leak, receive antibiotic prophylaxis for most dental procedures. For patients with most other types of congenital heart disease, the AHA currently does not recommend antibiotic prophylaxis (see Chapter 2).

Artificial Heart Valve. A diseased valve may be replaced with artificial or prosthetic valves. Such replacement valves are associated with a high risk for development of infective endocarditis, with significant morbidity and mortality. Accordingly, the AHA recommends that all patients with a prosthetic heart valve be given prophylactic antibiotics before most dental procedures (see Chapter 2). Patients with an artificial heart valve also may be on anticoagulant medication to prevent blood clots associated with the valve. In such patients, excessive bleeding may be encountered with surgical procedures. It is therefore necessary to determine the level of anticoagulation before any invasive procedure.

Arrhythmias. Arrhythmias frequently are related to heart failure or ischemic heart disease. Stress, anxiety, physical activity, drugs, and hypoxia are elements that can precipitate arrhythmias. Vasoconstrictors in local anesthetics should be used cautiously in patients prone to arrhythmias because they may be precipitated by excessive quantities or inadvertent intravascular injections. Stress reduction measures may be appropriate. Some of these patients take antiarrhythmic drugs, which can cause orthostatic hypotension and adversely interact with vasoconstrictors. Antiarrhythmic drugs can cause adverse oral health changes. Patients with atrial fibrillation also may be taking anticoagulant or antiplatelet medications, which is associated with increased risk for excessive bleeding with surgical procedures. Patients with certain arrhythmias may require a pacemaker or a defibrillator to regulate or pace heart rhythm by artificial means. Patients with such devices do not require antibiotic prophylaxis. Caution is advised with the use of electrocautery in patients with pacemakers or defibrillators because of the possibility of intermittent electromagnetic interference with the function of these devices (see Chapter 5). Elective dental care is not recommended for patients with severe, symptomatic arrhythmias.

Coronary Artery Bypass Graft, Angioplasty, or Stent. These procedures are performed in patients with coronary heart disease to restore patency to blocked coronary arteries. One of the more common forms of cardiac surgery performed today is coronary artery bypass grafting. The grafted artery bypasses the occluded portion of the artery. These patients do not require antibiotic prophylaxis. Another method of restoring patency is by means of a balloon catheter, which is inserted into the partially blocked artery; the balloon is then inflated, which compresses the atheromatous plaque against the vessel wall. A metallic mesh stent then may be placed to aid in the maintenance of patency. After stent placement, patients often are prescribed one or more antiplatelet drugs to decrease the risk of blood clots. These patients may therefore be at increased risk for excessive bleeding with surgical procedures. Patients who have had balloon angioplasty with or without placement of a stent do not require antibiotic prophylaxis (see Chapter 4).

Hematologic Disorders

Hemophilia or Inherited Bleeding Disorder. Patients with an inherited bleeding disorder such as hemophilia A or B, or von Willebrand disease, are at risk for severe bleeding after any type of dental treatment that causes bleeding, including scaling and root planing. These patients must be identified and managed in cooperation with a physician or hematologist. Patients with severe factor deficiency may require factor replacement before invasive treatment, as well as aggressive postoperative measures to maintain hemostasis (see Chapter 25).

Blood Transfusion. Patients with a history of blood transfusions are of concern from at least two aspects. The underlying problem that necessitated a blood transfusion, such as an inherited or acquired bleeding disorder, must be identified, and alterations in the delivery of dental treatment may have to be made. These patients also may be carriers of hepatitis B or C or may have become infected with the human immunodeficiency virus (HIV) and must be identified. Laboratory screening or medical consultation may be appropriate to determine the white blood cell count or status of liver function, and, as always, standard infection control procedures are mandatory (see Chapters 10, 18, and 24).

Anemia. Anemia is associated with a significant reduction in the number of red blood cells or oxygen-carrying capacity of the red blood cells. This condition may result from an underlying pathologic process such as acute or chronic blood loss, decreased production of red blood cells, or hemolysis. Patients with some forms of anemias, such as glucose-6-phosphate dehydrogenase (G6PD) deficiency and sickle cell disease, require dental management modifications. Oral lesions, infections, delayed wound healing, and adverse responses to hypoxia all are potential matters of concern in patients who have anemia (see Chapter 22).

Leukemia and Lymphoma. Depending on the type of leukemia or lymphoma, status of the disease, white blood cell count, and type of treatment, some patients may have oral manifestations such as gingival enlargement, bleeding problems, delayed healing, or may be prone to infection. Adverse effects can result from the use of chemotherapeutic agents and may require dental management modifications (see Chapter 23).

Taking a "Blood Thinner" or the Tendency to Bleed Longer than Normal. A potentially significant problem occurs when a patient has a history of abnormal bleeding or is taking an anticoagulant or an antiplatelet drug. This is of obvious concern, especially if surgical treatment is planned. Information about an episode of unexplained bleeding should be obtained and evaluated. Many reports of abnormal bleeding are more apparent than real; additional questioning or screening laboratory tests may allow the dentist to make this distinction. Patients taking anticoagulant or antiplatelet medication need to be evaluated to determine the risk for postoperative bleeding. Many patients can be treated without alteration of their medication regimens; however, laboratory testing may help to make this determination (see Chapters 24 and 25).

Neurologic Disorders

Stroke. Disorders that predispose to stroke, such as hypertension and diabetes, must be identified so that appropriate management alterations can be made. Elective dental care should be avoided in the immediate poststroke period because of an increased risk for subsequent strokes. Vasoconstrictors should be used cautiously. Anticoagulant medications and antiplatelet medications can cause excessive bleeding. Stress and anxiety reduction measures may be necessary. Some stroke victims may have residual paralysis, speech impairment, or other physical impairments that require special dental care or oral hygiene assistance. Calcified atheromatous plaques may be seen in the carotid arteries on panoramic films; the presence of such lesions may be a risk factor for stroke and requires referral to a physician (see Chapter 27).

Epilepsy, Seizures, and Convulsions. A history of epilepsy or grand mal seizures should be identified, and the degree of seizure control should be determined. Specific triggers of seizures (e.g., odors, bright lights) should be identified and avoided. Some medications used to control seizures may affect dental treatment because of drug actions or adverse side effects. For example, gingival overgrowth is a well-recognized adverse effect of diphenylhydantoin (Dilantin). Patients may discontinue use of their anticonvulsant medication without their doctor's knowledge and thus may be susceptible to seizures during dental treatment. Verification of patients' adherence to their medication schedule is important (see Chapter 27).

Behavioral Disorders and Psychiatric Treatment. Patients with a history of a behavioral disorder or psychiatric illness as well as the nature of the problem need to be identified. This information may help explain patients' unusual or unexpected behavior, or complaints associated with atypical conditions. Additionally, some psychiatric drugs have the potential to interact adversely with vasoconstrictors in local anesthetics. Psychiatric drugs also may produce adverse oral effects such as hyposalivation or xerostomia and increased caries risk. Other adverse drug effects such as dystonia, akathisia, or tardive dyskinesia may complicate dental treatment. Patients who are excessively anxious or apprehensive about dental treatment may require stress reduction measures (see Chapter 28).

Gastrointestinal Diseases

Stomach or Intestinal Ulcers, Gastritis, and Colitis. Patients with gastric or intestinal disease should not be given drugs that are directly irritating to the gastrointestinal tract, such as aspirin or nonsteroidal antiinflammatory drugs (NSAIDs). Patients with colitis or a history of colitis may not be able to take certain antibiotics. Many antibiotics can cause a particularly severe form of colitis (i.e., pseudomembranous colitis), and older adults are more susceptible to this condition. Some drugs used to treat gastric or duodenal ulcers may cause dry mouth (see Chapter 11).

Hepatitis, Liver Disease, Jaundice, and Cirrhosis. Patients who have a history of viral hepatitis are of concern in dentistry because they may be asymptomatic carriers of the disease and can transmit it unknowingly to dental personnel or other patients. Of the several types of viral hepatitis, only hepatitis B, C, and D have carrier stages. Fortunately, laboratory tests are available to identify affected patients. Standard infection control measures are mandatory. Patients who have chronic hepatitis (B or C) may develop cirrhosis, with associated impairment of liver function or liver cancer. Impaired liver function may result in prolonged bleeding and less efficient metabolism of certain drugs, including local anesthetics and analgesics (see Chapter 10).

Respiratory Tract Disease

Allergies or Hives. Patients may be allergic to some drugs or materials used in dentistry. Common drug allergens include antibiotics and analgesics. Latex allergy also is common and in patients so affected alternative materials such as vinyl or powderless gloves and vinyl dam material should be used to prevent an adverse reaction. True allergy to amide local anesthetics is uncommon. Dentists should procure a history regarding allergy by specifically asking patients how they react to a particular substance. This information will help to distinguish a true allergy from intolerance or an adverse side effect that may have been incorrectly identified as an allergy. Symptoms and signs consistent with allergy include itching, urticaria (hives), rash, swelling, wheezing, angioedema, runny nose, and tearing eyes. Isolated signs and symptoms such as nausea, vomiting, heart palpitations, and fainting generally are not of an allergic origin but rather are manifestations of drug intolerance, adverse side effects, or psychogenic reactions (see Chapter 19).

Asthma. The type of asthma should be identified, as should the drugs taken and any precipitating factors or triggers. Stress may be a precipitating factor and should be minimized when possible. To determine the severity of the condition, it is helpful to ask whether the patient has visited the emergency department for acute treatment of asthma. A patient who uses an albuterol inhaler for treatment of acute attacks should be instructed to bring it to his or her dental appointments (see Chapter 7).

Emphysema and Chronic Bronchitis. Patients with chronic pulmonary diseases such as emphysema and chronic bronchitis must be identified. The use of medications or procedures that might further depress respiratory function or dry or irritate the airway should be avoided. Chair position may be a factor; some patients may not be able to tolerate a supine position. Use of a rubber dam may not be tolerated because of a choking or smothering feeling experienced by the patient. The use of high-flow oxygen should be avoided in patients with severe disease because it can decrease the respiratory drive (see Chapter 7). Because cigarette smoking is the most common cause of emphysema and chronic bronchitis, the dentist can assist by offering smoking cessation to the interested patient (see Chapter 8).

Contagious Respiratory Infections. Patients with a contagious respiratory infection (e.g., influenza, coronavirus [COVID-19], tuberculosis [TB]) must be identified and information about infectivity status, testing, and treatment must be sought. Dental treatment should be delayed until active disease is effectively treated. Dental providers should be familiar with the different symptoms and stages of these respiratory infections, the infection control measures required, the drugs used in chemoprophylaxis and treatment, the duration of treatment, drug side effects, and the features of disease progression, as well as the potential for comorbidities (e.g., TB occurring with HIV infection; see Chapter 7).

Sleep Apnea and Snoring. Patients with obstructive sleep apnea (OSA) are at increased risk for hypertension, MI, stroke, diabetes, and car accidents and should receive treatment for the disorder. Signs and symptoms include loud snoring, excessive daytime sleepiness, and witnessed breathing cessation during sleep. Patients who present with these symptoms should be referred to a sleep physician specialist for evaluation and then to a clinician who manages OSA. Obesity and large neck circumference are common risk factors for the disease. The gold standard for treatment is positive airway pressure; however, many patients cannot tolerate this modality. Other treatment options include use of oral appliances and upper airway surgery (see Chapter 9).

Musculoskeletal Disease

Arthritis. Many types of arthritis have been identified; the most common of these are osteoarthritis and rheumatoid arthritis. Patients with arthritis may be taking a variety of medications that could influence dental care. NSAIDs, aspirin, corticosteroids, and cytotoxic and immunosuppressive drugs are examples. Tendencies for bleeding and infection should be considered. Chair position may be a factor for physical comfort. Patients with Sjögren syndrome, which may occur with rheumatoid arthritis or independently, have a dry mouth that is often problematic. Patients with Sjögren syndrome also are at increased risk for lymphoma. Patients with arthritis may have problems with manual dexterity and oral hygiene. In addition, patients with arthritis may have involvement of the temporomandibular joints (see Chapter 20).

Prosthetic Joints. Some patients with artificial joints have been considered to be at risk for infection of the prosthesis subsequent to dental treatment. However, current evidence and guidelines do not recommend that prophylactic antibiotics be provided to these patients before any dental treatment that is likely to produce bacteremia (see Chapter 20).

Endocrine Disease

Diabetes. Patients with diabetes mellitus must be identified to determine the type of diabetes, how it is being treated, the severity of the disease, and how well controlled it is. Patients with type 1 diabetes often require insulin, whereas type 2 diabetes usually is controlled through diet, oral hypoglycemic agents, or both; however, some patients with type 2 diabetes eventually also require insulin. Those with type 1 diabetes typically have a greater number of complications and are of greater concern regarding management than are those with type 2 diabetes. Signs and symptoms suggestive of diabetes can be recognized by the dentist and include dry mouth, excessive thirst and hunger, frequent urination, weight loss, poor wound healing, and frequent infections including odontogenic infections, oral candidiasis, and periodontal disease. Long-term complications include blindness, hypertension, and kidney failure, each of which may affect dental management. Understanding the level of control of their diabetes is important. Patients with poorly controlled diabetes have altered immune function and do not manage infection well and may have demonstrate exaggerated gingival inflammation and severe periodontal disease. Patients who take insulin are at risk for episodes of hypoglycemia in the dental office if meals are skipped or if stress or infection is present (see Chapter 14).

Thyroid Disease. Patients who have uncontrolled hyperthyroidism are potentially hypersensitive to stress and the effects of α_1-adrenergic sympathomimetics, so the use of vasoconstrictors generally is contraindicated. In rare cases, infection or surgery can initiate a thyroid crisis—a serious medical emergency. These patients may be easily upset emotionally and intolerant of heat, and they may exhibit tremors. An enlarged thyroid gland and exophthalmos may be present. Patients with known hypothyroidism usually are taking a thyroid supplement; this medication regimen helps to stabilize the body's thyroid hormone level. Thyroid cancer is a common form of head and neck cancer that often is curable if detected and treated early. Thus, palpation of the thyroid gland during the head and neck examination is important to detect swelling or nodules (see Chapter 16).

Genitourinary Tract Disease

Kidney Failure. Patients with chronic kidney disease or a kidney transplant must be identified. The potential for abnormal drug metabolism, immunosuppressive drug therapy, bleeding problems, hepatitis, infection, high BP, concurrent diabetes, and heart failure must be considered in management (see Chapter 12). Certain drugs that are nephrotoxic should be avoided, and several drugs administered by dentists require dosage adjustment when kidney function is compromised. Patients on hemodialysis do not require antibiotic prophylaxis but do receive heparin, which can prolong bleeding during and after invasive procedures.

Sexually Transmitted Diseases. A variety of sexually transmitted diseases (STDs) such as syphilis, gonorrhea, herpes simplex virus (HSV), human papillomavirus (HPV), and HIV infection can have manifestations in the oral cavity because of oral–genital contact or secondary to hematogenous dissemination in the blood or immune suppression. The dentist may be the first to identify these conditions. In addition, some STDs, including HSV, HPV, HIV infection, hepatitis B and C, and syphilis, can be transmitted to the dentist through direct contact with oral lesions, infectious blood, or improperly sterilized instruments. Sexually transmitted infection with oncogenic HPV genotypes is the major cause of oropharynx cancer (see Chapters 10, 13, and 18).

Other Conditions and Factors

Tobacco and Alcohol Use. Use of tobacco products is a risk factor associated with cancer, cardiovascular disease, pulmonary disease, and periodontal disease. Excessive use of alcohol is a risk factor for periodontal disease, malignancy, heart disease and may lead to liver disease and cirrhosis. The combination of excessive alcohol and tobacco use is a significant risk factor for oral cancer. Patients who use these products should be asked about quantity of use, duration, and whether they would like to quit and should be encouraged to do so (see Chapter 8). There are many methods at the disposable of dental providers to help assist patients who want to quit use of these products.

Drug Addiction and Substance Use Disorder. Patients who have a history of injected drug use are at increased risk for infectious diseases such as hepatitis B or C, HIV, and infective endocarditis. Narcotic and sedative medications should be prescribed with caution, if at all, for these patients because of the risk of triggering a relapse. This caveat also applies to patients who are recovering alcoholics. Vasoconstrictors should be avoided in patients who are cocaine or methamphetamine users because the combination may precipitate arrhythmias, MI, or severe hypertension. Patients who take prescription narcotics or other controlled substances may engage in "doctor shopping" and drug-seeking activity (see Chapter 29).

Tumors and Cancer. Patients who have had cancer are at risk for recurrence, so they should be closely monitored by a physician and dental team. Cancer treatment regimens including chemotherapy, targeted biologic agents, immunotherapy, or radiation therapy may result in infection, gingival bleeding, oral ulcerations, dry mouth, mucositis, and impaired healing after invasive dental treatment, all of which represent significant management considerations. Patients with a history of intravenous bisphosphonate or antiangiogenic therapy for metastatic bone disease are at risk for medication-related osteonecrosis of the jaw. Invasive procedures should be performed with appropriate caution in these patients (see Chapter 26).

Therapy for Head and Neck Cancers. Patients who have had previous surgery may have severe oral functional deficits. Those with a history of radiation treatment to the head, neck, or jaw must be carefully evaluated because radiation can permanently destroy the blood supply to the jaws, leading to an increased risk for osteoradionecrosis after extraction, trauma or procedures that further compromise blood supply to the jaw. Irradiation of the head and neck causes mucositis and can irreversibly damage the salivary glands, resulting in decreased salivary flow and increased risk for dental caries. Fibrosis of masticatory muscles resulting in limited mouth opening also may occur. Chemotherapy can produce many undesirable adverse effects, most commonly a severe mucositis; however, such changes resolve after therapy is complete (see Chapter 26).

Steroids. Corticosteroids (e.g., prednisone or methylprednisolone) are used in the treatment of many inflammatory and autoimmune diseases. These drugs are important because their use can result in several adverse effects including adrenal insufficiency, which potentially can render the patient unable to mount an adequate response to the stress of an infection or invasive dental procedure such as extractions or periodontal surgery. However, in general, most routine, noninvasive dental procedures do not require administration of supplemental steroids (see Chapter 15).

Operations or Hospitalizations. A history of hospitalizations can provide a record of past serious illnesses that may have current significance. For example, a patient may have been hospitalized for cardiac catheterization for ischemic heart disease. Another example is that of a patient who is hospitalized for hepatitis C. In both instances, the patient may or may not have received medical follow-up care for the initial problem, so this aspect of the evaluation may be an effective method of identifying an underlying condition. Information about hospitalizations should include diagnosis, treatment, and complications. If a patient has undergone any operation, the reason for the procedure and any associated untoward events such as an anesthetic emergency, unusual postoperative bleeding, infection, or drug allergy should be ascertained.

Pregnancy. Women who are or may be pregnant may need special consideration in dental management. Caution typically is warranted in the administration of drugs, timing of dental treatment, and chair position. Good oral hygiene is important to maintain during pregnancy for reasons discussed in Chapter 17.

Current Physician

As part of the medical history, information should be sought regarding the identity of the patient's physician, why the patient is under medical care, diagnoses, date, and treatment received. The contact information of the patient's physician should be recorded for future reference. A patient who does not have a physician may require a more cautious approach than a patient who sees a physician regularly. This is especially true for the patient who has not seen a physician in several years, because of the possibility of the presence of undiagnosed problems. Understanding the health and health care of the patient is important for providing insight into the overall health of the patient and priorities that person assigns to health care.

Drugs, Medicines, or Pills

All drugs, medicines, and supplements that a patient takes or is supposed to be taking should be identified and investigated for actions, adverse side effects, and potential drug interactions (see Appendix D). The interviewer should specifically mention "drugs, medicines, or pills of any kind" because patients may not list injected medicines, over-the-counter drugs (e.g., aspirin), or herbal medicines (see Appendix E). The dentist should have a reliable, up-to-date, comprehensive source for drug information, which may be available in print format or through an electronic or web-based resource.

The patient's list of medications ("drug history") may provide the only clues to presence of an unreported medical disorder. The patient may believe that a particular problem is not important enough to mention or may just have omitted the information inadvertently. The patient may nevertheless report taking medication typically prescribed for a disease. For example, a patient with hypertension may fail to report a history of that problem yet may list medications used to treat hypertension. A patient with previously medically managed condition may have discontinued taking a prescribed medication owing to cost or other reasons, and questioning should uncover this possibility.

Functional Capacity

In addition to asking patients about specific diagnoses, it is important to ask screening questions regarding the ability of the patient to engage in normal physical activity (functional capacity). The ability to perform common daily tasks can be expressed in metabolic equivalents of tasks (METs), which quantify the body's use of oxygen. Thus, the patient's ability to meet MET levels as determined for specific activities reflects general physical status. A MET is a unit of oxygen consumption; 1 MET equals 3.5 mL of oxygen per kg of body weight per minute at rest. It has been shown that the risk for occurrence of a serious perioperative cardiovascular event (e.g., MI, heart failure) is increased in patients who are unable to meet a 4-MET demand during normal daily activity. Daily activities requiring 4 METs include level walking at 4 miles/hour or climbing a flight of stairs. Activities requiring greater than 10 METs include swimming and singles tennis. An exercise capacity of >10

METs indicates excellent physical conditioning. Thus, a patient who reports an inability to walk up a flight of stairs without shortness of breath, fatigue, or chest pain may be at increased risk for medical complications during dental treatment, especially when such limitation is combined with other risk factors and the patient is under stress.

PHYSICAL EXAMINATION

In addition to a medical history, each dental patient should be afforded the benefits of a simple, abbreviated physical examination to detect signs or symptoms of disease or adverse treatment outcomes. This evaluation should include assessment of general appearance, measurement of vital signs, and an examination of the head and neck.

General Appearance

Much can be learned about the patient's state of health from a purposeful but tactful visual inspection. Careful observation can lead to awareness and recognition of abnormal or unusual features or medical conditions that may exist and may influence the provision of dental care. This survey consists of an assessment of the general appearance of the patient and inspection of exposed body areas, including the skin, nails, face, eyes, nose, ears, and neck. Each visually accessible area may demonstrate peculiarities that can signal underlying systemic disease or abnormalities.

The patient's outward appearance and movement can give an indication of her or his general state of health and well-being. Examples of possible health abnormalities are a wasted, cachectic appearance; a lethargic demeanor; ill-kempt, dirty clothing and hair; body odors; a staggering or halting gait; extreme thinness or obesity; bent posture; and difficulty breathing. The dentist should remain sensitive to breath odors, which may be associated with disease such as acetone associated with diabetes, ammonia associated with renal failure, putrefaction of pulmonary infections, and alcohol odor possibly associated with alcohol use disorder or alcohol-induced liver disease.

Skin and Nails. The skin is the largest organ of the body, and dentists should inspect exposed areas of skin including the arms, head, and neck. Changes in the skin and nails frequently are associated with systemic disease. For example, cyanosis can indicate cardiac or pulmonary insufficiency, yellowing (jaundice) may be caused by liver disease, pigmentation may be associated with hormonal abnormalities, and petechiae or ecchymoses can be a sign of a blood dyscrasia or a bleeding disorder (Fig. 1.1). Alterations in the fingernails, such as clubbing (seen in cardiopulmonary insufficiency) (Fig. 1.2), white discoloration (seen in cirrhosis), yellowing (from malignancy), and splinter hemorrhages (from infective endocarditis), usually are caused by chronic disorders. The dorsal

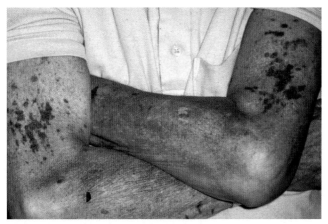

FIG 1.1 Petechiae and ecchymosis in a patient that may signal a bleeding disorder. (Courtesy of Robert Henry, DMD, Lexington, KY.)

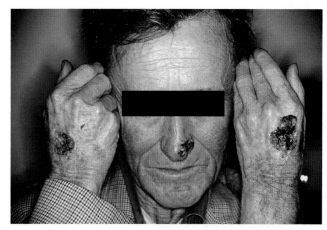

FIG 1.3 Basal cell carcinomas of the dorsum of the hands and the ala of the nose.

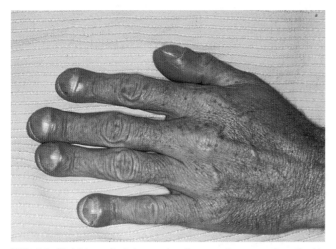

FIG 1.2 Clubbing of digits and nails may be associated with cardiopulmonary insufficiency.

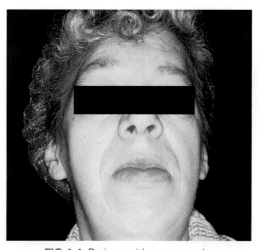

FIG 1.4 Patient with acromegaly.

surfaces of the hands are common sites for actinic keratosis and basal cell carcinomas, as are the bridge of the nose, infraorbital regions, and the ears (Fig. 1.3). A raised, darkly pigmented lesion with irregular borders may be a melanoma.

Face. The shape and symmetry of the face are abnormal in a variety of syndromes and conditions. Well-recognized examples are the coarse and enlarged features of acromegaly (Fig. 1.4), moon facies in Cushing syndrome (Fig. 1.5), and the unilateral paralysis of Bell palsy (Fig. 1.6).

Eyes. The eyes can be sensitive indicators of systemic disease and should therefore be closely inspected. Patients who wear glasses should be requested to remove them during examination of the head and neck to allow examination of the eyes and adjacent skin. Hyperthyroidism may produce a characteristic lid retraction, resulting in a wide-eyed stare (Fig. 1.7). Xanthomas of the eyelids frequently are associated with hypercholesterolemia (Fig. 1.8), as is arcus senilis in older individuals. Scleral

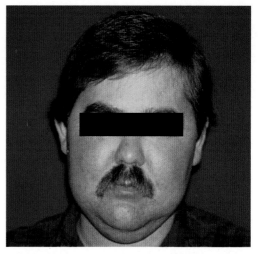

FIG 1.5 Patient who acquired cushingoid facies after several weeks of prednisone administration. (From Bricker SL, Langlais RP, Miller CS. *Oral diagnosis, oral medicine, and treatment planning.* 2nd ed. Hamilton, Ontario: BC Decker; 2002.)

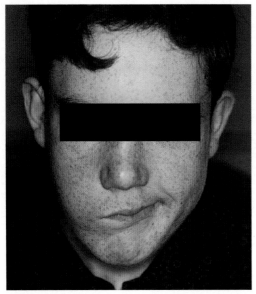

FIG 1.6 Unilateral facial paralysis in a patient with Bell palsy.

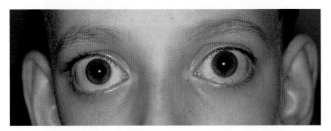

FIG 1.7 Lid retraction from hyperthyroidism.

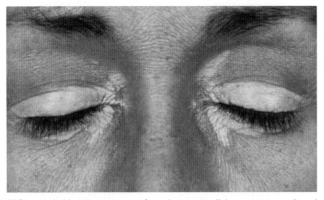

FIG 1.8 Xanthomas of the eyelids may signal hypercholesterolemia.

yellowing may be caused by liver disease. Reddening of the conjunctiva can result from sicca syndrome or allergy.

Ears. The ears should be inspected for gouty tophi in the helix and antihelix. An earlobe crease (i.e., Frank's sign) may be an indicator of coronary artery disease. Malignant or premalignant lesions (e.g., skin cancer) may be found on and around the ears (Fig. 1.9).

Neck. The neck should be inspected for enlargement, asymmetry, and structures. Lymph nodes should be evaluated for size, location, tenderness, and whether they

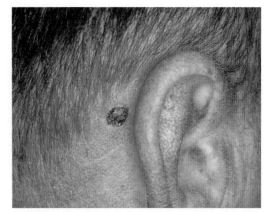

FIG 1.9 Basal cell carcinoma posterior to the ear.

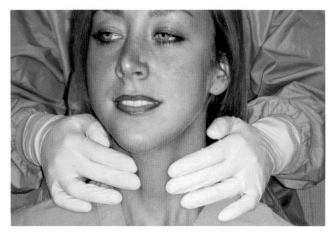

FIG 1.10 Bimanual palpation of the anterior neck.

are moveable or fixed. Bilateral palpation of the thyroid gland also should be performed (Fig. 1.10). Depending on location and consistency, enlargements in the neck may be caused by a goiter (Fig. 1.11), infection, cysts (Fig. 1.12), enlarged lymph nodes (Fig. 1.13), malignancy, or vascular deformities.

Vital Signs

Vital signs consisting of BP, pulse, respiratory rate, temperature, height, and weight should be assessed in the dental setting to best ascertain the health of the patient. Pulse oximetry and capnography also are important measures to obtain for select patients (e.g., obese, when oxygenation is a concern, those undergoing sedation). Despite their importance, vital signs are not frequently or completely recorded in private practice. Many providers do not record height, weight, oxygen saturation levels, or temperature, except when infection or systemic disease is suspected.

The benefits of vital sign measurement during an initial examination are twofold. First, the establishment of baseline normal values ensures a standard of comparison in the event of a medical emergency during treatment. If an emergency occurs, knowledge of the patient's normal values is helpful in determining the severity of the

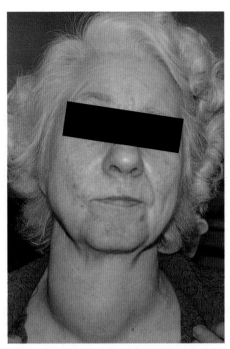

FIG 1.11 Midline neck enlargement from a goiter.

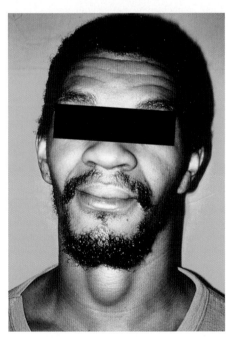

FIG 1.12 Midline neck enlargement caused by a thyroglossal duct cyst.

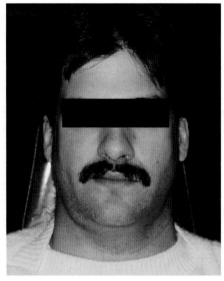

FIG 1.13 Enlarged lymph node beneath the right body of the mandible resulting from a salivary gland infection.

problem. For example, if the unexpected event is a loss of consciousness accompanied by a drop in BP to 90/50 mm Hg, the level of concern will be entirely different for a patient whose BP normally is 110/65 mm Hg from that for a patient with hypertension whose BP normally is 180/110 mm Hg. In the second instance, the patient may well be in a state of shock.

A second benefit of vital sign measurement during an examination is in screening for abnormalities, either diagnosed or undiagnosed. For example, if a person with severe, uncontrolled hypertension that was not identified received dental treatment without proper management, the potential consequences could be serious. The purpose of taking vital signs is detection of an abnormality—not diagnosis, which is the responsibility of the physician. Abnormal findings should be discussed with the patient, and if significant, the patient should be referred to a physician for further evaluation.

Pulse. The pulse rate is often determined using the electronic BP cuff, but can be determined by palpating the carotid artery at the side of the trachea (Fig. 1.14) or by palpating the radial artery on the thumb side of the wrist (Fig. 1.15). The pulse should be palpated for 1 min so that rhythm abnormalities can be detected. Use of the carotid artery for pulse determination has some advantages. First, the carotid pulse is familiar in clinical practice because of basic life support (BLS)/cardiopulmonary resuscitation (CPR) training. Second, it is reliable because it is a large, easily located, central artery that supplies the brain; therefore, in an emergency it may remain palpable when peripheral arteries in the extremities are not.

Rate. A normal heart rate for adults is typically reported to be 60 to 100 beats per minute (bpm). However, accumulating evidence suggests an ideal resting heart rate is 50−70 bpm. In fact, rates >84 increase the risk of death when hypertension or cardiovascular disease is present. A pulse rate greater than 100 bpm is called *tachycardia*; a slow pulse rate of less than 60 bpm is called *bradycardia*. An abnormal pulse rate may be a sign of CVD. The pulse rate can be influenced by anemia, anxiety, breathing, conditioning, drugs, exercise, fever, or hormone (e.g., thyroid) levels.

Rhythm. The normal pulse is a series of rhythmic beats that occur at regular intervals. When the beats occur at irregular intervals, the pulse is called *irregular*,

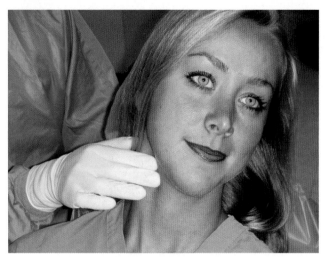

FIG 1.14 Palpation of the carotid pulse.

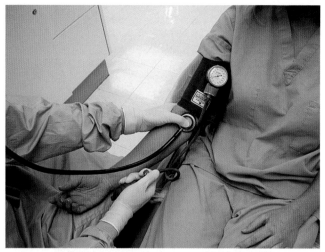

FIG 1.16 Blood pressure cuff and stethoscope in place.

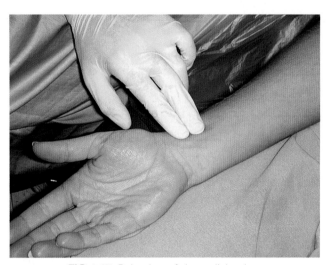

FIG 1.15 Palpation of the radial pulse.

BOX 1.3	Proper Steps in Taking Blood Pressure

1. Patient seated with feet flat on floor.
2. Patient relaxed and quiet for 5 min.
3. Patient has empty bladder, not eaten or smoked in 30 min.
4. Remove clothing from arm.
5. Use properly validated and calibrated BP measurement device.
6. Position cuff just above the elbow on bare arm at the level of their heart.
7. Use correct cuff size:
    a. 22–26 cm = small adult
    b. 27–34 cm = normal size adult
    c. 35–44 = large adult
    d. 45–52 cm = adult thigh
8. Take 2 readings separated by 1–2 min.
9. Record SBP/DBP and inform patient.

BP, blood pressure; *SBP*, systolic blood pressure, *DBP*, diastolic blood pressure.
See: https://www.heart.org/-/media/files/health-topics/high-blood-pressure/tylenol-hbp/aha_toolkit_poster_final_102618.pdf?la=en

dysrhythmic, or *arrhythmic*. To detect an arrhythmia, palpation of the pulse for 1 full minute is suggested for accuracy.

Blood Pressure. BP is determined most often by indirect measurement in the upper extremities with an automated digital BP device and less commonly using a BP cuff and stethoscope (Fig. 1.16). The cuff should be of the correct width to give an accurate recording. The bladder within the cuff ideally should encompass 80% of the circumference of the arm, with the center of the bladder positioned over the brachial artery (Box 1.3). A cuff that is too small yields falsely elevated values, and a cuff that is too large yields falsely low values. Narrower cuffs are available for use with children, and wider cuffs or thigh cuffs are available for use with obese or larger patients. As an alternative for an obese patient, a standard-size cuff can be placed on the forearm below the antecubital fossa, and the radial artery may be palpated so that only the approximate systolic pressure can be determined. The BP cuff should not be placed on the arm with an arteriovenous shunt for hemodialysis. Instruments that measure BP at the wrist or on a finger, although popular, are not recommended because of potential inaccuracies. Readers are referred to a standard physical evaluation text for information regarding the auscultation method of BP measurement, including knowledge about Korotkoff sounds, which define the BP at which beating sounds first become audible (Fig. 1.17).

In an average healthy adult, normal systolic pressure ranges between 90 and 120 mm Hg and generally increases with age. Normal diastolic pressure ranges between 60 and 80 mm Hg. Hypertension in adults is defined as BP of 130/80 mm Hg or greater (Table 1.1). It is recommended that BP be measured twice during the appointment, separated by several minutes, and the average taken as the final measurement.

Respiration. The rate and depth of respiration should be noted through careful observation of movement of the chest and abdomen during quiet breathing. The respiratory rate in a normal resting adult is approximately 12–16 breaths/min. The respiratory rate in small children is higher than that in adults. Notice should be made of patients with labored breathing, rapid breathing, or irregular breathing patterns because all may be signs of systemic problems, especially cardiopulmonary disease. A common finding in apprehensive patients is hyperventilation (rapid, prolonged, deep breathing or sighing), which may result in lowered carbon dioxide levels and may cause disturbing symptoms and signs, including perioral numbness, tingling in the fingers and toes, nausea, a "sick" feeling, and carpopedal spasms.

Oxygen Saturation. The oxygen saturation level can be determined with a simple pulse oximeter placed over the

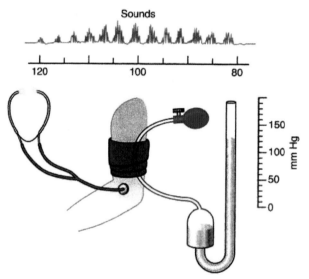

FIG 1.17 The typical sound pattern obtained when blood pressure in a normotensive adult is recorded. (From Guyton AC, Hall JE. *Textbook of medical physiology.* 11th ed. Philadelphia: Saunders; 2006.)

pad of the index finger. Levels should be ideally 98% or higher. Levels below 95% suggest respiratory compromise, and levels below 92% are suggestive of the need for supplemental oxygenation and evaluation to determine the cause of the problem.

Temperature. Temperature is important for assessing whether a patient has febrile signs or symptoms associated with an abscessed tooth, a mucosal or gingival infection, a fascial space infection, a respiratory or systemic infection. Normal oral temperature is 98.6°F (37°C) but may vary by as much as ±1°F over 24 h and usually is highest in the afternoon. Normal rectal temperature is about 1°F higher than oral, and normal axillary temperature is about 1°F lower than oral.

Height. The height of patients should be determined to help determine body mass index (BMI), as well as assessing growth and development and for conditions such as malnutrition or osteoporosis. BMI is calculated by dividing the person's weight (kilograms) by height (meter squared).

Weight. Any recent unintentional weight gain or loss should be ascertained, and BMI should be calculated to assess for malnutrition or obesity. A rapid loss of weight may be a sign of malignancy, diabetes, TB, or other wasting disease. A rapid gain in weight can be a sign of heart failure, edema, hypothyroidism, or neoplasm. Obesity, defined as a BMI of 30 or higher, is a risk factor for many health problems, including heart disease and diabetes. The World Health Organization lists four classes of obesity (Class I: BMI 30–34.9, Class II: "Severely Obese" BMI 35–39.9, Class III: "Morbidly Obese" BMI 40–49.9, Class IV: "Super Obese" BMI U 50).

Head and Neck Examination

Examination of the head and neck may vary in its comprehensiveness but should include inspection and palpation of the soft tissues of the oral cavity, maxillofacial region, and neck, as well as evaluation of cranial

TABLE 1.1	Classification of Blood Pressure (BP) in Adults and Recommendations for Follow-Up			
BP Classification	**Systolic BP (mm Hg)**		**Diastolic BP (mm Hg)**	**Recommended Follow-up**
Normal	<120	*and*	<80	Recheck in annually.
Prehypertension	120–139	*or*	80–89	Recheck in 6 months to 1 year.
Stage 1 hypertension	140–159	*or*	90–99	Confirm within 2 months.
Stage 2 hypertension	≥160	*or*	≥100	Evaluate or refer to source of care within 1 month. For patients with higher pressures (e.g., >180/110 mm Hg), evaluation and treatment referral are needed immediately or within 1 week, depending on the clinical situation and complications.

Adapted from the National Heart, Lung, and Blood Institute: *The seventh report of the Joint National Committee on Prevention, Detection, Evaluation, and Treatment of High Blood Pressure: the JNC 7 report*, Bethesda, Maryland, US Department of Health and Human Services, Public Health Service, National Institutes of Health, National Heart, Lung, and Blood Institute, August 2004, and from James PA, Oparil S, Carter BL, Cushman WC, Dennison-Himmelfarb C, Handler J, et al. *2014 evidence-based guideline for the management of high blood pressure in adults: report from the panel members appointed to the Eighth Joint National Committee (JNC 8)* [Published erratum appears in JAMA 2014; 311(17):1809], JAMA. 2014; 311(5):507–20.

nerve function. (See standard texts on physical diagnosis for additional descriptions.)

DIAGNOSTIC TESTS

Diagnostic tests can be important for evaluating a patient's health status. Whether assessing chairside, ordering laboratory tests, or referring the patient to a physician for such testing, the dentist should be familiar with indications for diagnostic testing, what the tests measure, normal reference values, and what abnormal results mean. Some tests performed chairside include blood glucose, cholesterol, respiratory capacity (spirometry), oxygen saturation, acquisition of exfoliative cells, a culture, or saliva for analysis. Common indications for clinical laboratory testing in dentistry are

- Aiding in the detection of suspected disease (e.g., diabetes, infection, bleeding disorders, malignancy)
- Screening at-risk patients for undetected disease (e.g., diabetes, HIV, chronic kidney disease, hepatitis B or C)
- Establishing normal baseline values before treatment (e.g., anticoagulant status, white blood cells, platelets)
- Assessing risk for bleeding (thrombocytopenia, international normalized ratio)

A comprehensive discussion of laboratory tests is beyond the scope of this chapter; however, Table 1.2 lists several common laboratory tests and ranges of normal values.

PHYSICIAN REFERRAL AND CONSULTATION

If there are any questions regarding the patient's general health (e.g., medical history, physical examination findings, or abnormal laboratory test results), contacting the patient's physician for consultation or referral purposes may be warranted. Requests for information should be made sending an email, fax, or a phone call, whichever is more expedient. The principal advantages of a phone call are the opportunity to obtain immediate information and the chance to ask follow-up questions. However, a physician often may be unavailable to take the call, and a nurse or receptionist must relay the response of the physician. It is imperative that the conversation be recorded in the progress notes to ensure inclusion in the permanent record. In addition, a follow-up correspondence should be sent to the physician summarizing the conversation and asking that any treatment modifications be sent to the office. These communications should be entered in the patient's chart.

Problem List and Diagnoses

After all information is collected, a problem list with diagnoses should be constructed. The problem list should be comprehensive and include final conclusions regarding abnormalities detected after assessment of the chief complaint; medical status; extraoral, neuromuscular,

TABLE 1.2 Clinical Laboratory Tests and Normal Values

Test	Reference Range
Complete blood count	
White blood cells	4500—10,000/mL
Red blood cells: male	$4.5-5.9 \times 10^6/\mu L$
Red blood cells: female	$4.5-5.1 \times 10^6/\mu L$
Platelets	150,000—350,000/μL
Hematocrit: male	41%—51%
Hematocrit: female	36%—47%
Hemoglobin: male	14—17 g/dL
Hemoglobin: female	12.—16 g/dL
Mean corpuscular volume (MCV)	80—100 μm^3
Mean corpuscular hemoglobin (MCH)	28—32 pg
Mean corpuscular hemoglobin concentration (MCHC)	32%—36%
Differential white blood cell count	Mean %
Segmented neutrophils	50—70
Bands	0—8
Eosinophils	1—4
Basophils	0—1
Lymphocytes	20—40
Monocytes	2—8
Hemostasis	
Prothrombin time (PT)	11—13 s
Activated partial thromboplastin time (aPTT)	30—40 s
Thrombin time (TT)	<20 s
International normalized ratio (INR)	<1.2
Serum chemistry	
Glucose, fasting	70—100 mg/dL
Hemoglobin A_1C (A_1C)	4.7%—6.0%
Blood urea nitrogen (BUN)	8—20 mg/dL
Cholesterol	<200 mg/dL
C-reactive protein (CRP)	<1.0 mg/dL
Creatinine	0.7—1.3 mg/dL
Bilirubin, direct—conjugated	<0.3 mg/dL
Bilirubin—Total	0.3—1.2 mg/dL
Calcium, total	9—10.5 mg/dL
Magnesium	1.5—2.4 mg/dL
Phosphorus, inorganic	3—4.5 mg/dL
Serum electrolytes	
Sodium	136—145 mEq/L
Potassium	3.5—5.0 mEq/L
Chloride	98—106 mEq/L
Bicarbonate	23—28 mmol/L
Serum enzymes	
Alkaline phosphatase (ALP)	36—150 IU/L
Alanine aminotransferase (ALT)	0—35 U/L
Aspartate aminotransferase (AST)	0—35 U/L
Amylase	0—130 U/L
Creatine kinase (CK)	30—170 U/L

From the MSD Manual Professional Version (Known as the Merck Manual in the US and Canada and the MSD Manual in the rest of the world), edited by Sandy Falk. Copyright © 2022 Merck & Co., Inc., Rahway, NJ, USA and its affiliates. All rights reserved. Available at https://www.msdmanuals.com/professional. Accessed (date).

jaw, mucosal, periodontal, and tooth-related structures. Diagnoses are recorded in the dental record, and the diagnoses dictate development of the ultimate dental management plan.

RISK ASSESSMENT

Risk assessment is recommended prior to dental treatment to minimize the development of adverse outcomes. Proper risk assessment helps guide dental management decisions, which in turn help prevent the management of an emergency or complications that possibly could have been prevented. We advocate the use of the "ABC" checklist (see Box 1.2), which provides a thoughtful and sequential assessment as to whether the patient can potentially undergo planned dental treatment in a safe manner (risk–benefit profile). One widely used method of assessing medical risk is the American Society of Anesthesiologists (ASA) Physical Classification System (Box 1.4). This system originally was developed to classify patients according to perioperative risk with general anesthesia; however, it has been adapted for outpatient medical and dental use and for all types of surgical and nonsurgical procedures regardless of the type of anesthesia used.

The implication is that as the classification level increases (ASA II through IV), so does the risk. Integrating the ASA level with other important patient and treatment factors helps to comprehensively assess risk (Table 1.3). Each factor must be carefully assessed for each patient in order to determine an accurate risk profile.

It is important to realize that risk assessment is not a cookbook exercise. Each situation requires thoughtful and individual consideration to determine whether the benefits of having dental treatment outweigh the potential risks to the patient. For example, a patient may have symptomatic heart failure, but the risk is minimal if the planned dental procedure is limited to taking radiographs (noninvasive) and the patient is not anxious or fearful. Conversely, in the same patient, the risk may be significant if the planned procedure is a full-mouth extraction (invasive) and the patient is very anxious. Therefore, the dentist must carefully weigh the physical and emotional state of the patient against the invasiveness, trauma, and pain of the planned procedure. In general, whereas noninvasive dental procedures carry lower risk, invasive/surgical procedures are associated with higher risk. In addition, the longer the procedure and the greater the blood loss, the greater the risk. Also, more risk is associated with use of conscious sedation and general anesthesia, which can affect the patient's airway, breathing, and level of oxygenation, than with local anesthesia. For each situation, the question that must be answered is whether the expected benefit of the planned dental treatment outweighs the risk of a medical complication, either occurring during treatment or arising as a result of treatment. Fortunately, in most cases, the benefit of needed dental treatment far outweighs any risk; however, in some instances, the risk can be great enough to mandate deferral of dental treatment.

Age

Age is an important component of the risk assessment. Young patients may have behavioral and cognitive issues that make it difficult to sit still or take instruction. Also, many young patients weigh less than 75 lb and accordingly need dose reduction for medications and local anesthesia. In contrast, older adults (e.g., 65 years and older) are unique in that they often have multiple comorbid conditions of variable degree, with an increased

BOX 1.4	American Society of Anesthesiologists (ASA) Physical Classifications

ASA I   Normal healthy patient. (E.g., healthy, nonsmoker, no or minimal alcohol use)

ASA II   Patient with mild systemic disease. No significant impact on daily activity; unlikely to have an impact on anesthesia and surgery. (E.g., current smoker, social alcohol drinker, pregnancy, obesity (30 < BMI <40), well-controlled diabetes mellitus or hypertension, mild lung disease)

ASA III   Patient with moderate to severe systemic disease. Substantive functional limitations to daily activity; probable impact on anesthesia and surgery. (E.g., poorly controlled diabetes mellitus or hypertension, chronic obstructive pulmonary disease, morbid obesity (BMI ≥40), active hepatitis, alcohol dependence disorder, implanted pacemaker, moderate reduction of ejection fraction, end-stage renal disease (ESRD) undergoing regularly scheduled dialysis, history (>3 months) of MI, cerebrovascular accident (CVA), transient ischemic attack (TIA), or coronary artery disease (CAD)/stents)

ASA IV   Patient with severe systemic disease that is a constant threat to life. Serious limitation of daily activity; likely major impact on anesthesia and surgery. (E.g., recent (<3 months) MI, CVA, TIA, or CAD/stents, ongoing cardiac ischemia or severe valve dysfunction, severe reduction of ejection fraction, respiratory failure requiring mechanical ventilation or mechanical circulation, sepsis, disseminated intravascular coagulation, or ESRD not undergoing regularly scheduled dialysis)

ASA V: a moribund patient not expected to survive without the operation.

ASA VI: declared brain dead whose organs are being removed for donor purposes.

TABLE 1.3	Risk Assessment Based on Patient and Treatment Factors

Patient Factors

Age

Nature, severity, control, and stability of the patient's medical condition

Capacity of the patient to respond to a physical or emotional demand

Emotional, behavioral, and cognitive status of the patient

Severity of orofacial disease and ability to heal

Treatment factors

Chair position

Drugs administered and drug interactions

Level of altered consciousness

Invasiveness (type, magnitude, amount of pain and bleeding) of the planned procedure

Duration of procedure

frequency of nonspecific signs or symptoms, frailty, cognitive impairment, physical disability, and drug management issues (metabolism, interactions, or side effects). Older adults tend to have more medical problems and therefore take more medications. In fact, half of older adults report having two or more chronic illnesses, and one-third of all prescription medications are taken by older adults. Also, this group constitutes a growing segment of the population. It is estimated that by 2030, one in five Americans will be 65 years of age or older. It is therefore important to be mindful of these realities and approach dental care in older patients with extra consideration and caution, as well as concern for proper drug selection and dosage adjustments as needed.

TREATMENT MODIFICATIONS

After it is decided to provide dental treatment (on the grounds that the expected benefits outweigh the associated risk of a medical complication), modifications may need to be made in the delivery of such treatment. Selection of the appropriate treatment modification(s) is the responsibility of the treating dentist. Treatment modifications may include the selection of a drug and amount administered (e.g., provision of antibiotic prophylaxis, anxiolytic drug for an anxious patient, or limiting the amount of vasoconstrictor in a patient who takes a nonselective beta-blocker); the adjustment of chair position; monitoring of BP, pulse, respirations or oxygen saturation; or the use of a topical hemostatic agent. Each decision regarding these modifications is based on the patient's risk for airway obstruction; bleeding; difficulty with chair position; disruptive or behavioral issues; drug dosage, metabolism, actions, or interactions; potential for emergencies; functional demand; healing issues; and infection. It is through a systematic assessment of risk and identification of potential problems that simple

modifications in the delivery of dental treatment can be made in an effort to reduce risk to the patient. It should be recognized, however, that risk is always increased when a medically compromised patient is treated and invasive procedures are performed, drugs are administered, or breathing can become altered because of dental care. The goal of this book is to provide methods to evaluate and reduce risk as much as possible, including the possibility of urgencies or emergencies that can arise in the dental office.

STRESS AND ANXIETY REDUCTION

In all patients, especially those with medical problems, stress and anxiety control are important and help to reduce risk. Establishment of good rapport and trust is of paramount importance. Allowing the patient to ask questions and encouraging frank and open discussions are equally important. Explaining what is to be done before treatment is initiated often helps put the patient at ease. Providing stress reduction (e.g., with N_2O-O_2) may be especially beneficial for patients who are anxious and those who have cardiovascular disease because oxygen is continuously administered during the procedure. Details regarding a protocol for stress reduction are found in Box 1.5; noting that intraoperative monitoring by pulse oximetry and capnography is recommended for those who are sedated with oral anxiolytic agents.

Dentists should be cognizant that injection of local anesthetic is the procedure that most patients fear; therefore, every effort should be made to avoid pain during administration. Keeping the needle and syringe out of the patient's sight until it is ready to use is important. Topical anesthetic should be applied followed by slow advancement of the needle and slow injection of the solution after aspiration. Adequate time should be allowed after injection to ensure adequate anesthesia is achieved. It is imperative to ensure profound local anesthesia to prevent intraoperative pain and reduce postoperative pain.

At the completion of the appointment, it should be determined whether postoperative pain is likely; if so, consideration may be given to administering a long-

BOX 1.5	General Stress Reduction Protocol

- Open communication with patient about concerns; provide reassurance
- Short appointments (preferably morning)
- Preoperative sedation: short-acting benzodiazepine (e.g., triazolam 0.125–0.25 mg) 1 h before the appointment and possibly the night before the appointment
- Intraoperative sedation (N_2O-O_2)
- Profound local anesthesia: use topical before injection
- Adequate operative and postoperative pain control
- Patient contacted on evening of the procedure

acting local anesthetic (e.g., bupivacaine) before the patient is dismissed. Appropriate analgesia should be prescribed. Analgesics can be started preemptively, before the procedure, and may provide enhanced effectiveness. Analgesic selection should be based on the patient's current medical conditions and potential drug–drug interactions. Nonopioids are recommended over opioids. Instructions should be provided along with a phone number to call if the patient needs to contact the dentist. Calling the patient on the evening of the appointment to see how he or she is doing is recommended.

BIBLIOGRAPHY

1. ASA Physical Status Classification System. https://www.asahq.org/standards-and-guidelines/asa-physical-status-classification-system. Accessed December 6, 2020.

2. Centers for Disease Control and Prevention. Public health and aging: trends in aging–United States and worldwide. *JAMA.* 2003;289:1371–1373.

3. Fleisher LA, Beckman JA, Brown KA, et al. ACC/AHA 2007 guidelines on perioperative cardiovascular evaluation and care for noncardiac surgery: executive summary: a report of the American College of Cardiology/American Heart Association Task Force on Practice Guidelines (Writing Committee to Revise the 2002 Guidelines on Perioperative Cardiovascular Evaluation for Noncardiac Surgery). *Circulation.* 2007;116:1971–1996.

4. Fletcher GF, Balady G, Froelicher VF, et al. Exercise standards. A statement for healthcare professionals from the American Heart Association Writing Group. *Circulation.* 1995;91:580–615.

5. Miller CS, Kaplan AL, Guest GF, et al. Documenting medication use in adult dental patients: 1987–1991. *J Am Dent Assoc.* 1992;123:40–48.

6. Myers MG. Automated office blood pressure. *Korean Circ J.* 2018;48:241–250.

7. National Heart, Lung, and Blood Institute. *The Seventh Report of the Joint National Committee on Prevention, Detection, Evaluation, and Treatment of High Blood Pressure: The JNC 7 Report.* Bethesda, Maryland: US Department of Health and Human Services, Public Health Service, National Institutes of Health, National Heart, Lung, and Blood Institute; August 2004.

8. Okin PM, Kjeldsen SE, Julius S, et al. All-cause and cardiovascular mortality in relation to changing heart rate during treatment of hypertensive patients with electrocardiographic left ventricular hypertrophy. *Eur Heart J.* 2010;31(18):2271–2279.

9. Pickering TG, Hall JE, Appel LJ, et al. Recommendations for blood pressure measurement in humans and experimental animals: Part 1: blood pressure measurement in humans: a statement for professionals from the Subcommittee of Professional and Public Education of the American Heart Association Council on High Blood Pressure Research. *Circulation.* 2005;111:697–716.

10. Roerecke M, Kaczorowski J, Myers MG. Comparing automated office blood pressure readings with other methods of blood pressure measurement for identifying patients with possible hypertension: a systematic review and meta-analysis. *JAMA Intern Med.* 179:351-362.

2

Infective Endocarditis

KEY POINTS

- Infective endocarditis (IE) is associated with significant morbidity and mortality.
- IE results when microbes enter the blood stream and colonize damaged or artificial cardiac valves.
- Viridans group streptococcal (VGS) are found in the oral cavity and can cause IE as a result of transient bacteremia from daily mouth activities and less commonly after dental procedures.
- Maintenance of good oral health and regular dental care are important to prevent VGS IE.
- The current (2021) AHA guidelines recommend antibiotic prophylaxis based on three risk factors: (1) underlying cardiac conditions, (2) dental procedure being performed, and (3) the oral microbes (i.e., VGS) mostly likely to contribute to bacteremia that causes IE.
- Dental providers must be aware of and follow the AHA guidelines for antibiotic prophylaxis in order to minimize risk of dental procedures resulting in VGS IE.
- Selection of the antibiotic agent for antibiotic prophylaxis is based on AHA guidelines and clinical judgment that includes (1) consideration for antibiotic stewardship, (2) the patient's ability to take oral medications, (3) risk of adverse outcome (e.g., allergy), and (4) recency of antibiotic use.

Infective endocarditis (IE) is a serious, life-threatening infection caused by microbes that settle on the endothelial surface of the heart or heart valves. Most often *IE* occurs in close proximity to one or more congenital or acquired cardiac defects. A similar infection that may occur in the endothelial lining of an artery, usually adjacent to a vascular defect (e.g., coarctation of the aorta) or a prosthetic device (e.g., arteriovenous shunt), is called *infective endarteritis.* Although bacteria most often cause these diseases, fungi and other microorganisms may cause such infection; thus, the designation *infective* is used in keeping with this multimicrobial origin. *Bacterial endocarditis* (BE) is a term used in the past, reflecting the fact that most cases of IE are caused by bacteria. *IE* is the currently preferred nomenclature.

IE can be classified as acute or subacute to reflect the rapidity of onset and duration of symptoms before diagnosis; however, this classification is infrequently used today. Current classification is based on the causative microorganism (e.g., streptococcal endocarditis, staphylococcal endocarditis, candidal endocarditis) and the type of valve that is infected (e.g., native valve endocarditis [NVE], prosthetic valve endocarditis [PVE]). IE also is classified according to the source of infection—that is, whether it is community acquired or hospital acquired—or whether the person is an injection drug user (IDU).

IE is a disease that is difficult to treat and has significant morbidity and mortality. Therefore, emphasis has long been directed toward prevention. Historically, various dental procedures have been reported to be a significant cause of IE, because bacterial species found in the mouth frequently have been implicated as the causative agent. Furthermore, whenever a patient is given a diagnosis of IE caused by oral flora, dental procedures performed at any point within the previous several months have been blamed for the infection. As a result, antibiotics have been administered before certain invasive dental procedures in an attempt to prevent infection. Of note, however, the effectiveness of such prophylaxis to prevent VGS IE in humans has not been substantiated based on prospective randomized trials.

EPIDEMIOLOGY

The incidence of IE varies based on the population studied, ranging from 2 to 15 cases per 100,000 person-years. It is relatively rare in the United States (about 15,000 patients each year) occurring most frequently after age 60

TABLE 2.1 Risk of Acquiring or Dying of Infective Endocarditis

Predisposing Condition or Factor	Lifetime Risk of Acquisition	If Acquired IE, Risk of Death in 5 years
	No. of Patients/100,000 Patient-Years	% of IE Admissions
General population	5	<1%
MVP without audible cardiac murmur	4.6	
MVP with audible murmur of mitral regurgitation	52	
Congenital heart lesions (i.e., aortic stenosis, bicuspid aortic valve pulmonary stenosis, ventricular septal defect, patent ductus arteriosus, coarctation of the aorta, tetralogy of Fallot)	135	8%–24%
Rheumatic (fever) heart disease	380–440	30%
Unrepaired cyanotic congenital heart disease		10%
Congenital heart disease repaired with prosthetic material		17%
Cardiac valve replacement surgery	630	19%–24%
Previous infective endocarditis	740	21%
Prosthetic valve replacement in patients with PVE	2160	>30%

MPV, Mitral valve prolapse; *PVE*, prosthetic valve endocarditis.
Data from Steckelberg JM, Wilson WR. Risk factors for infective endocarditis. *Infect Dis Clin N Am.* 1993;7:9–19; Thornhill M, Jones S, Prendergast B, et al. Quantifying infective endocarditis risk in patients with predisposing cardiac conditions. *Eur Heart J.* 2018;39:586–595; and UptoDate https://www-uptodate-com.ezproxy.uky.edu/contents/native-valve-endocarditis-epidemiology-risk-factors-and-microbiology?search=infective%20endocarditis%20epidemiology&source=search_result&selectedTitle=1~150&usage_type=default&display_rank=1.

TABLE 2.2 Predisposing Conditions Associated With Infective Endocarditis (IE)

Underlying Condition	Frequency of IE (%)
Mitral valve prolapse	25–30
Aortic valve disease	12–30
Congenital heart disease	20–37
Degenerative valve disease	1–5
Prosthetic valve	25–30
Intravenous drug abuse	5–20
No identifiable condition	25–47

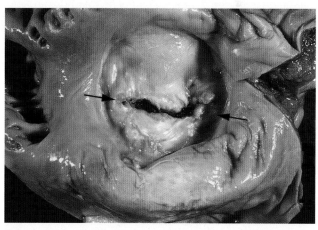

FIG. 2.1 Mitral stenosis with diffuse fibrous thickening and distortion (*arrows*) of the valve leaflets in chronic rheumatic heart disease. (From Schoen FJ, Mitchell RN. The heart. In Kumar V, et al., eds. *Robbins and Cotran Pathologic Basis of Disease.* 8th ed. Philadelphia: Saunders; 2010.)

years, in men about twice as often as women, in those with a preexisting structural cardiac abnormality and IDUs. In developed countries, the incidence has risen over the past three decades, approaching 12–15 cases per 100,000 person-years. Risk is associated with advancing age (mean age 60 years), presence of comorbidities, setting, type, and severity of a preexisting cardiac condition (Table 2.1).

About three-fourths of patients with IE have a preexisting structural cardiac abnormality (Table 2.2). Previous IE is associated with about 5% of recurrent cases. Rheumatic heart disease (RHD) (Fig. 2.1) accounts for about 5% of cases. Mitral valve prolapse (MVP) (Fig. 2.2) accounts for 25%–30% of adult cases of NVE. Aortic valve disease (either stenosis or regurgitation or both) (Fig. 2.3) accounts for 12%–30% of cases. Congenital heart disease (e.g., patent ductus arteriosus, ventricular septal defect, bicuspid aortic valve) (Fig. 2.4) is the underlying cause for IE in 10%–20% of younger adults and in 8% of older adults. Tetralogy of Fallot, the most common type of congenital cyanotic heart disease,

generally requiring extensive reconstructive surgery for survival (Fig. 2.5), accounts for fewer than 2% of cases. Risk is highest with prosthetic heart valves (Fig. 2.6), accounting for about one-third of all cases of IE.

Up to 20% of cases of IE are caused by IDU, with incidence ranging from 150 to 2000 per 100,000 person-years in this population. Of note, a predisposing cardiac condition cannot be identified in many patients who develop IE.

ETIOLOGY

IE is caused by many different microbial species including staphylococci, streptococci, enterococci, and gram-negative coccobacilli. The prevalence of these microbes in

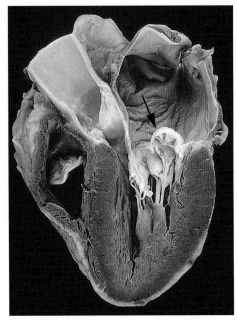

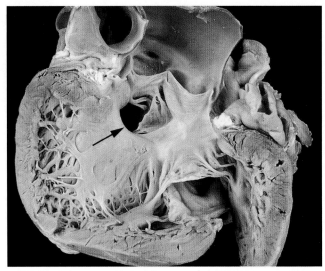

FIG. 2.4 Gross photograph of a ventricular septal defect (defect denoted by *arrow*). (Courtesy of William D. Edwards, MD, Mayo Clinic, Rochester, MN. From Schoen FJ, Mitchell RN. The heart. In Kumar V, et al., eds. *Robbins and Cotran Pathologic Basis of Disease*. 8th ed. Philadelphia: Saunders; 2010.)

FIG. 2.2 Prolapse (*arrow*) of the posterior mitral valve leaflet into the left atrium. (Courtesy William D. Edwards, MD, Mayo Clinic, Rochester, Minnesota. From Schoen FJ, Mitchell RN. The heart. In Kumar V, et al., eds. *Robbins and Cotran Pathologic Basis of Disease*. 8th ed. Philadelphia: Saunders; 2010.)

are caused by coagulase-positive *S. aureus. Staphylococcus aureus* often affects the right side of the heart (tricuspid valve), and in most cases, the cardiac valves are normal before infection. *S. aureus* also is the most common pathogen in nonvalvular cardiovascular device infections. Of note, *S. aureus* is not a normal constituent of the oral flora.

VGS (α-hemolytic streptococci), constituents of the normal oral flora and gastrointestinal (GI) tract, remain the most common cause of community-acquired NVE causing about 15%−35% of cases of IE. Infections most often involve *Streptococcus sanguis, Streptococcus oralis (mitis), Streptococcus salivarius, Streptococcus mutans,* and *Gemella morbillorum* (formerly called *Streptococcus morbillorum*). Group D streptococci, which include *Streptococcus bovis* and the enterococci (*Enterococcus faecalis*), are normal inhabitants of the GI tract and account for 5%−18% of cases of IE.

Other microbial agents that less commonly cause IE include

- Other *Streptococci* species (1%−5%)
- HACEK (*Haemophilus, Actinobacillus, Cardiobacterium, Eikenella, Kingella*) group (2%)
- Non-HACEK gram-negative bacteria (*Pseudomonas aeruginosa, Corynebacterium pseudodiphtheriticum, Listeria monocytogenes, Bacteroides fragilis*; 2%)
- Fungi (2%)
- Group A β-hemolytic streptococci (<1%)

In 5%−10% of cases, the endocarditis may be culture-negative or polymicrobial.

PATHOPHYSIOLOGY AND COMPLICATIONS

IE is the result of a series of complex interactions of several factors involving endothelium, bacteria, and the host

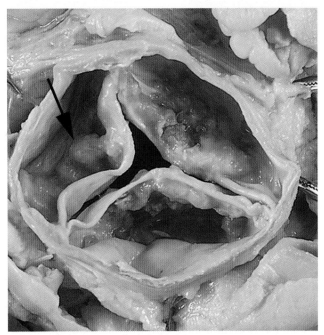

FIG. 2.3 Calcific aortic stenosis of a previously normal valve (*arrow*). Nodular masses of calcium are heaped up within the sinuses of Valsalva. (From Schoen FJ, Mitchell RN. The heart. In Kumar V, et al., eds. *Robbins and Cotran Pathologic Basis of Disease*. 8th ed. Philadelphia: Saunders; 2010.)

IE varies on the population studied. In large medical centers, Staphylococci are the most common pathogen identified in IE, accounting for 30%−35% of infections. Staphylococcal IE is associated with IDU, health care contact, and acute IE. Between 75% of staphylococcal IE

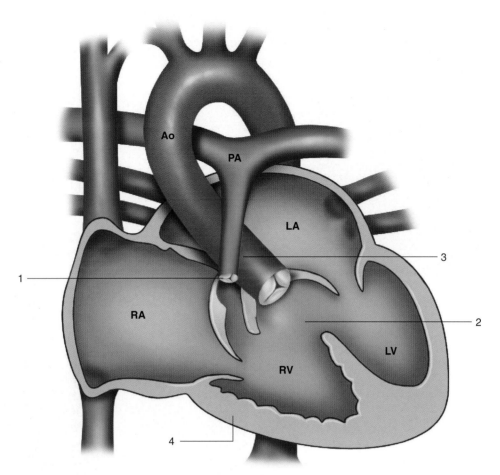

FIG. 2.5 Tetralogy of Fallot. *1,* Pulmonary stenosis. *2,* Ventricular septal defect. *3,* Overriding aorta. *4,* Right ventricular hypertrophy. *Ao,* Aorta; *LA,* left atrium; *LV,* left ventricle; *PA,* pulmonary artery; *RA,* right atrium; *RV,* right ventricle. (Redrawn from Mullins CE, Mayer DC. *Congenital Heart Disease: A Diagrammatic Atlas.* New York: Wiley-Liss; 1988.)

immune response. The sequential events leading to infection usually starts with injury or damage to an endothelial surface, most often a cardiac valve leaflet. Although IE can occur on normal endothelium, most cases begin with a damaged surface, usually in proximity to an anatomic defect or prosthesis that predispose the patient to IE (Table 2.2). The endothelial damage can result from any of a variety of events, including (i) directed flow from a high-velocity jet onto the endothelium, (ii) flow from a high- to a low-pressure chamber, or (iii) flow across a narrowed orifice at high velocity. Under these conditions, fibrin and platelets adhere to the roughened endothelial surface, where they form small clusters or masses, resulting in a condition called nonbacterial thrombotic endocarditis (NBTE) (Fig. 2.7). Bacteria that arrive during a transient bacteremia are seeded into and adhere to the mass. Platelets and fibrin are then deposited, which serves to sequester and protect the bacteria. These microbes then undergo rapid multiplication within the protection of the vegetative mass (Fig. 2.8). After the vegetative process is established, the metabolic activity and cellular division of the bacteria are diminished, which decreases the effectiveness of antibiotics. Bacteria are slowly and continually released from the

vegetations and shed into the bloodstream, resulting in a continuous bacteremia, as well as fragments of the friable vegetations that off and embolize. A variety of host immune responses to bacteria may occur. This sequence of events results in the clinical manifestations of IE.

The clinical outcome of IE depends on several factors, including

- Local destructive effects of intracardiac (valvular) lesions.
- Embolization of vegetative fragments to distant sites, resulting in infarction or infection.
- Hematogenous seeding of remote sites during continuous bacteremia.
- Antibody response to the infecting organism, with subsequent tissue injury caused by deposition of immune complexes or antibody–complement interaction with antigens deposited in tissues.

The most common complication of IE is severe valvular insufficiency that may lead to heart failure and death. Embolization of vegetation fragments often leads to complications such as stroke. Myocardial infarction

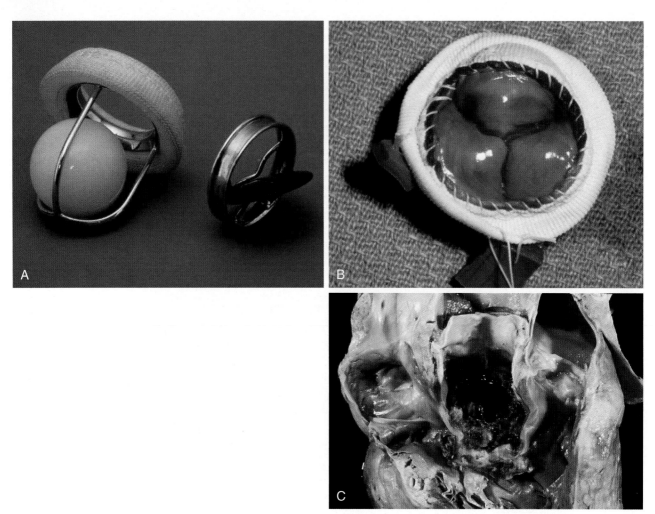

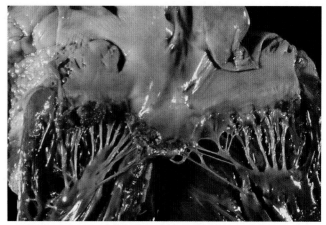

FIG. 2.6 Prosthetic cardiac valves. (**A**) Starr—Edwards caged ball mechanical valve. (**B**) Hancock porcine bioprosthetic valve. (**C**) Prosthetic valve endocarditis.

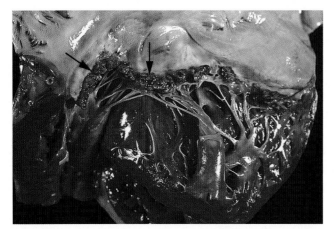

FIG. 2.7 Nonbacterial thrombotic endocarditis (*arrows*). (From Schoen FJ, Mitchell RN. The heart. In Kumar V, et al., eds. *Robbins and Cotran Pathologic Basis of Disease.* 8th ed. Philadelphia: Saunders; 2010.)

FIG. 2.8 Viridans streptococcal endocarditis of the mitral valve. (Courtesy of W. O'Conner, MD, Lexington, KY.)

(MI) can occur as the result of embolism of the coronary arteries, and distal emboli can produce peripheral metastatic abscesses. Pulmonary emboli, usually septic in nature, occur in 66%—75% of IDUs who have tricuspid valve endocarditis. Emboli also may involve other systemic organs, including the liver, spleen, and kidney, as well as abdominal mesenteric vessels. The incidence of embolic events is markedly reduced by the prompt initiation of antibiotic therapy. Renal dysfunction is common and may be due to immune complex glomerulonephritis or infarction.

obstructed prosthesis, infection uncontrollable by antibiotics alone, fungal endocarditis, and intracardiac complications with PVE.

DENTAL MANAGEMENT

Dental management continues to focus primarily on the prevention of VGS IE. Emphasis is on minimizing daily bacteremia of dental origin through good oral hygiene and providing prophylactic antibiotics when indicated.

Antibiotic Prophylaxis

Dental treatment has long been suggested as a significant cause of IE. The general theory was that in a patient with a predisposing cardiovascular disorder, IE often was caused by a bacteremia that resulted from a dental procedure and IE could be prevented through the administration of antibiotics before those procedures. On the basis of these assumptions, over the past half century, the American Heart Association (AHA) has published 11 sets of recommendations for antibiotic prophylaxis for dental patients at risk for acquiring IE (Table 2.4). These recommendations, first published in 1955 and revised every few years, varied in terms of identification of risk conditions, selection of antibiotics, and timing and route of administration of antibiotics. It is important to recognize that although these recommendations were a rational and prudent attempt to prevent life-threatening infection, they have been based largely on low-level evidence, expert opinion, and

retrospective studies in which surrogate measures of risk were used. There are no prospective, randomized controlled trials to prove the efficacy of antibiotic prophylaxis in preventing IE for a dental procedure.

Source and Frequency of Bacteremia. The primary assumption that has driven previous AHA recommendations was that dental procedures were the source of most of the bacteremias that led to IE; therefore, antibiotics given just before dental procedures would prevent IE. Although it is undisputed that many dental procedures can cause bacteremia, it also is clear that bacteremia can result from many normal daily activities such as toothbrushing, flossing, manipulation of toothpicks, use of oral water irrigation devices, and chewing (Table 2.5). Because the average person living in the United States makes fewer than two dental visits per year, it follows that the frequency of and exposure to bacteremia could be greater as a result of routine daily activities. Thus the frequency and cumulative duration of exposure to bacteremia from routine daily events over 1 year are likely much higher than those resulting from a single dental procedure. Accordingly, it seems inconsistent to recommend antibiotic prophylaxis for patients undergoing dental procedures and bacteremias, when these same patients produce similar bacteremias from routine daily activities.

Magnitude and Type of Bacteremia. Published data indicate that the magnitude of bacteremia resulting from most dental procedures is relatively low (with bacterial counts of fewer than 10^4 colony-forming units [CFU]/

TABLE 2.4 Selected Previous Iterations of American Heart Association–Recommended Antibiotic Regimens for Dental and Respiratory Tract Procedures in Adults

Year	Primary Regimen for Dental Procedures
1955	600,000 U of aqueous PCN and 600,000 U of procaine PCN in oil containing 2% aluminum monostearate administered IM 30 min before the operative procedure
1957	For 2 days before surgery, 200,000–250,000 U of PCN by mouth 4 times a day
	On day of surgery, 200,000–250,000 U by mouth 4 times a day and 600,000 U aqueous PCN with 600,000 units procaine PCN IM 30 min before surgery
	For 2 days after, 200,000–250,000 U by mouth 4 times a day
1960	Step 1: Prophylaxis 2 days before surgery with 600,000 U of procaine PCN IM on each day
	Step 2: Day of surgery: 600,000 U procaine PCN IM, supplemented by 600,000 U of crystalline PCN IM 1 h before surgical procedure
	Step 3: For 2 days after surgery: 600,000 U procaine PCN IM each day
1965	Day of procedure: Procaine PCN 600,000 U, supplemented by 600,000 U of crystalline PCN IM 1–2 h before the procedure
	For 2 days after procedure: Procaine PCN 600,000 U IM each day
1972	600,000 U of procaine PCN G with 200,000 U of crystalline PCN G IM 1 h before procedure and once daily for 2 days after the procedure
1977	Aqueous crystalline PCN G (1,000,000 U IM) mixed with procaine PCN G (600,000 U IM); give 30 min to 1 h before procedure and then give PCN V 500 mg orally every 6 h for two doses
1984	PCN V 2 g PO 1 h before procedure; then give 1 g 6 h after initial dose
1990	Amoxicillin 3 g PO 1 h before procedure; then give 1.5 g 6 h after initial dose
1997	Amoxicillin 2 g PO 1 h before procedure
2007	High-risk groups only recommended to receive AP; specified the dental procedures
2021	Clarified "high-risk" groups. Doxycycline 100 mg for adults added, clindamycin no longer recommended

AP, antibiotic prophylaxis; *IM,* intramuscular; *PCN,* penicillin; *PO,* oral.

From Wilson W, Taubert KA, Gewitz M, et al. American Heart Association Rheumatic Fever, Endocarditis, and Kawasaki Disease Committee; American Heart Association Council on Cardiovascular Disease in the Young; American Heart Association Council on Clinical Cardiology; American Heart Association Council on Interdisciplinary Working Group: Prevention of infective endocarditis: guidelines from the American Heart Association: a guideline from the American Heart Association Rheumatic Fever, Young, and the Council on Clinical Cardiology, Council on Cardiovascular Surgery and Anesthesia, and the Quality Care of Outcomes Research Interdisciplinary Working Group. *Circulation.* 2007;116(15):1736–1754.

TABLE 2.5	Reported Frequency of Bacteremia Associated With Various Dental Procedures and Oral Manipulation
Dental Procedure or Oral Manipulation	**Reported Frequency of Bacteremia (%)**
Tooth extraction	10–100
Periodontal surgery	36–88
Scaling and root planning	8–80
Teeth cleaning	≤40
Rubber dam matrix or wedge placement	9–32
Endodontic procedures	≤20
Toothbrushing and flossing	20–68
Use of wooden toothpicks	20–40
Use of water irrigation devices	7–50
Chewing food	7–51

From Wilson W, Taubert KA, Gewitz M, et al. American Heart Association Rheumatic Fever, Endocarditis, and Kawasaki Disease Committee; American Heart Association Council on Cardiovascular Disease in the Young; American Heart Association Council on Clinical Cardiology; American Heart Association Council on Interdisciplinary Working Group: Prevention of infective endocarditis: guidelines from the American Heart Association: a guideline from the American Heart Association Rheumatic Fever, Young, and the Council on Clinical Cardiology, Council on Cardiovascular Surgery and Anesthesia, and the Quality Care of Outcomes Research Interdisciplinary Working Group. *Circulation.* 2007;116(15):1736–1754.

mL) and similar to that of bacteremia resulting from normal daily activities. Levels of these bacteremias are predominantly VGS and are far less than that (10^6–10^8 CFU/mL) needed to cause experimental BE in animals. Moreover, it has been shown that in patients with poor oral hygiene, the frequency of positive blood cultures just before dental extraction was similar to that after extraction. Thus, although the infective dose required to cause IE in humans is unknown, the number of microorganisms in blood after a dental procedure or associated with daily activities is generally low, implying that cases of IE caused by oral bacteria probably result from frequent exposure to low inocula of bacteria in the bloodstream resulting from routine daily activities and not from most dental procedures. Consistent with this, studies have found that the incidence of bacteremia after toothbrushing was significantly related to poor oral hygiene and gingival bleeding. These findings imply that emphasis on maintaining good oral hygiene and eradicating dental or oral disease is key to decreasing the frequency of bacteremia produced by normal daily activities.

Efficacy of Antibiotic Prophylaxis. Antibiotic prophylaxis is administered in a single dose to limit a transient, low-magnitude exposure to a microorganism from becoming an established infection. The effectiveness of antibiotic prophylaxis given to at-risk patients before a dental procedure to prevent or reduce a bacteremia that can lead to IE is controversial. Some studies have reported that antibiotics administered before a dental procedure reduced the frequency, nature, or duration of bacteremia, although others did not. More recent retrospective studies suggest that amoxicillin therapy has a significant impact on reducing the incidence, nature, and duration of bacteria associated with dental procedures, but it does not eliminate bacteremia. However, data do not show that such a reduction caused by antibiotic therapy directly reduces the risk of or prevents VGS IE. Prospective, randomized, placebo-controlled trials have not been conducted to examine the efficacy of antibiotic prophylaxis for preventing IE in patients who undergo dental procedures, and it is highly unlikely that any such studies will ever be done because of the complex logistical, ethical, and medicolegal issues that would be involved. Nevertheless, retrospective studies suggest that prophylaxis is potentially beneficial. Studies in England based on the National Institute for Health and Care Excellence (NICE) guidelines demonstrate an increase in incidence rates after the 2008 guidelines recommended complete cessation of antibiotic prophylaxis.

Risk of Infective Endocarditis due to Dental Procedures. Risk of IE is related to the magnitude, duration and type of bacteremia, predisposition of the underlying heart condition, as well as the patient's age and host defense and immunological response. Although the absolute risk for IE caused by a dental procedure is impossible to measure precisely, available evidence estimates that if dental treatment causes 1% of all cases of IE due to VGS annually in the United States, the overall risk in the general population is as low as 1 case of IE per 14 million dental procedures. The estimated absolute risk rates for IE caused by a dental procedure in patients with underlying cardiac conditions are as follows: MVP: 1 per 1.1 million procedures; congenital heart disease: 1 per 475,000; RHD: 1 per 142,000; presence of a prosthetic cardiac valve: 1 per 114,000; and previous IE: 1 per 95,000 dental procedures.

Thus, although it has long been assumed that dental procedures may cause IE in patients with underlying cardiac risk factors and that antibiotic prophylaxis is effective, scientific proof to support these assumptions is lacking. The AHA has concluded that *"of the total number of cases of IE that occur annually, it is likely that an exceedingly small number of these cases are caused by bacteremia-producing dental procedures. Accordingly, only an extremely small number of cases of IE might be prevented by antibiotic prophylaxis, even if it were 100% effective. The vast majority of cases of IE caused by oral microflora most likely result from random bacteremias caused by routine daily activities."*

CURRENT AMERICAN HEART ASSOCIATION RECOMMENDATIONS (2021)

The AHA recommendations have evolved 11 times since 1955. The current 2021 AHA guidelines reflect minor revisions from the 2007 guidelines. The updated recommendations are based on the AHA statement: *"the preponderance of published studies suggest that there is no convincing evidence of an increase in cases of VGS IE among patients with high, low, or moderate risk of acquisition of IE or adverse outcome from VGS IE since publication of the 2007 guidelines."*

The current (2021) AHA guidelines recommend antibiotic prophylaxis based on three risk factors: (1) underlying cardiac conditions, (2) dental procedure being performed, and (3) the oral microbe(s) mostly likely to contribute to bacteremia that causes IE.

Underlying Cardiac Conditions for Which Antibiotic Prophylaxis Is Suggested

The 2021 AHA guidelines identify the underlying cardiac disorders at "greatest risk of adverse outcomes" (i.e., significant morbidity and mortality) from VGS IE, not the lifetime risk for acquiring IE as was used in past guidelines (see Table 2.1). Current AHA guidelines therefore target only those in the "highest risk" category. The four "highest risk" categories of cardiac conditions recommended for antibiotic prophylaxis to prevent adverse outcomes from VGS IE include (i) prosthetic cardiac valve or material used for cardiac valve repair or other implantable cardiac devices, (ii) previous, relapse or recurrent IE, (iii) congenital heart disease, and (iv) cardiac transplant recipients who develop cardiac valvulopathy (Box 2.1). The AHA states that emphasis on the highest risk group *"reduces uncertainties among patients and providers about who should receive prophylaxis for a dental procedure."*

Cardiac Conditions for Which Antibiotic Prophylaxis Is Not Suggested

There are several cardiac conditions that increase the lifetime risk for IE; however, these conditions (mitral valve prolapse with or without a murmur/regurgitation, RHD, bicuspid valve disease, calcified aortic stenosis, atrial or ventricular septal defect, hypertrophic cardiomyopathy, implantable pacemaker, cardiac defibrillator, and coronary artery bypass graft) are not recommended for antibiotic prophylaxis to prevent VGS IE.

Nonvalvular Cardiovascular Devices: Antibiotic Prophylaxis Is Not Suggested

The AHA reporting committee, after performing an extensive review of available data, concluded that convincing evidence does not exist suggesting that microorganisms associated with dental procedures cause infection of nonvalvular vascular devices at any time after implantation. Accordingly, the AHA does not recommend routine antibiotic prophylaxis for patients with any of these devices (Table 2.6) who undergo dental procedures.

BOX 2.1   Cardiac Conditions Associated With the Highest Risk of Adverse Outcomes From Endocarditis for Which Antibiotic Prophylaxis With Dental Procedures Is Recommended

- **Prosthetic cardiac valve or material**
  - Presence of cardiac prosthetic valve
  - Transcatheter implantation of prosthetic valves
  - Cardiac valve repair with devices, including annuloplasty, rings, or clips
  - Left ventricular assist devices or implantable heart
- **Previous, relapse, or recurrent infective endocarditis**
- **Congenital heart disease (CHD)[a]**
- Unrepaired cyanotic CHD, including palliative shunts and conduits
  - Completely repaired CHD with prosthetic material or device, whether by surgery or transcatheter during the first 6 months after the procedure[b]
  - Repaired CHD with residual defects at the site or adjacent to the site of a prosthetic patch or prosthetic device
  - Surgical or transcatheter pulmonary artery valve or conduit placement such as Melody valve and Contegra conduit
- **Cardiac transplant recipients who develop cardiac valvulopathy**

[a]Except for the conditions listed in this box, antibiotic prophylaxis is no longer recommended for any other form of CHD.
[b]Prophylaxis is recommended because endothelialization of prosthetic material occurs within 6 months after the procedure.
Note: Moderate Risk Categories, which include rheumatic fever, non-rheumatic valve disease, congenital valve anomalies, have risk for adverse outcomes from IE but are not recommended to receive antibiotic prophylaxis based on the current guidelines. Antibiotic prophylaxis is also NOT suggested for implantable electronic devices (i.e., pacemaker similar devices) septal defect closure devices when complete closure is achieved, peripheral vascular grafts and patches, including those used for hemodialysis, coronary artery stents or other vascular stents, CNS ventriculoatrial shunts, vena cava filters, and pledgets.
From Wilson W, Gewitz M, Lockhart PB, et al. *Circulation.* 2021;143(20):e963–e978.

Prophylaxis is recommended, however, for selected patients with these devices:

- Patients undergoing incision and drainage of infected tissue (abscesses)
- Patients with residual valve leak after device placement for attempted closure of leaks associated with patent ductus arteriosus, atrial septal defect, or ventricular septal defect

Intravascular Catheters: Antibiotic Prophylaxis Is Not Suggested

Concerns often arise regarding the need for antibiotic prophylaxis to prevent infection in patients with various types of IV or intraarterial catheters. Examples are listed in Table 2.7. The causative microorganisms in these infections

TABLE 2.6	Nonvalvular Cardiovascular Device–Related Infection Rates—Not Recommended for Antibiotic Prophylaxis

Type of Device	Incidence of Infection (%)
Intracardiac	
Pacemaker and implantable cardioverter defibrillator	0.13–3.2
Total artificial hearts	To be determined
Ventriculoatrial shunts	2.4–9.4
Pledgets	Rare
Patent ductus arteriosus occlusion devices	Rare
Atrial septal defect and ventriculoseptal defect closure devices	Rare
Conduits	Rare
Patches	Rare
Arterial	
Peripheral vascular stents	Rare
Peripheral vascular grafts and patches, including for hemodialysis	1.0–6
Intraaortic balloon pumps	≤5–26
Angioplasty or angiography	<1
Coronary artery stents or other vascular stents	Rare
Patches	1.8
Venous	
Vena cava filters	Rare

From Baddour LM, Bettmann MA, Bolger AF, et al. Nonvalvular cardiovascular device–related infections. *Circulation.* 2003;108:2015–2031; Özcan C, Raunsø J, Lamberts M, et al. Infective endocarditis and risk of death after cardiac implantable electronic device implantation: a nationwide cohort study. *EP Europace.* 2017;19:1007–1014.

include coagulase-negative staphylococci, *S. aureus,* enterococci, gram-negative rods, *Escherichia coli, Enterobacter* and *Candida* spp., *P. aeruginosa,* and *Klebsiella pneumoniae.* None of these, with the exception of *Candida,* are normal inhabitants of the oral cavity; thus, they do not introduce risk for infection with oral procedures. Current national guidelines do not include a recommendation for antibiotic prophylaxis for patients with any of these devices who are undergoing dental procedures.

Dental Procedures for Which Antibiotic Prophylaxis Is Recommended

A review of the published data suggests that transient VGS bacteremia may result from a dental procedure that involves manipulation of the gingival or periapical region of the teeth or perforation of the oral mucosa even in the absence of visible bleeding. Therefore, antibiotic prophylaxis is recommended only for patients with conditions listed in Box 2.1 who undergo any dental procedure that involves the manipulation of gingival tissues or the periapical region of a tooth and for those procedures that

perforate the oral mucosa. Antibiotic prophylaxis is not recommended for routine local anesthetic injections through noninfected tissue, taking of dental radiographs, placement of removable prosthodontic or orthodontic appliances, adjustment of orthodontic appliances, or the shedding of deciduous teeth and bleeding from trauma to the lips or oral mucosa (Box 2.2).

Microbe

Administration of antibiotic prophylaxis for a dental procedure is intended for the prevention of IE from VGS, not for prevention of IE caused by other microbes. The writing group for the AHA acknowledges that antibiotic prophylaxis may prevent only a small number of cases of VGS IE.

Antibiotic Prophylaxis Regimens

The current 2021 AHA guidelines provide four antibiotic prophylaxis regimens for at-risk patients. The categories are based on those who are (i) able to take oral medications, (ii) unable to take oral medication, (iii) allergic to penicillin or ampicillin and can take oral medication, and (iv) allergic to penicillin or ampicillin and unable to take oral medication (Table 2.8).

Antibiotic prophylaxis should be administered in a single dose 30–60 min before the procedure. If the antibiotic is *inadvertently* not administered before the procedure, the dosage may be administered up to 2 h after the procedure. Table 2.8 lists the recommended antibiotic regimens for use for dental procedures in patients who have an underlying cardiac condition as listed in Box 2.1. Because of the possibility of cross-allergenicity, the use of cephalosporins is *not* recommended for patients who have a history of anaphylaxis, angioedema, or urticaria (immediate-onset IgE-mediated hypersensitivity) caused by the administration of penicillin or ampicillin. Clinicians should be aware that the use of antibiotics is not without risk; their use has the potential for allergic reactions, adverse side effects, and the promotion of antibiotic resistance. In fact, the adverse effect profile demonstrated with the prophylactic use of clindamycin led to its elimination from the current AHA recommendations.

The AHA and the NICE guidelines do not recommend oral antimicrobial mouth rinses (e.g., chlorhexidine, povidone–iodine) as prophylaxis against VGS IE.

Other Considerations

Evaluation. Dentists should continue to identify from the medical history patients with cardiac conditions that increase risk for IE, such as MVP, RHD, or systemic lupus erythematosus. Patients with underlying cardiac conditions should be under the care of a physician for monitoring the status of their valvular heart disease and potential complications. The establishment and maintenance of optimal oral hygiene are critically important in these patients. Also, when treating a patient with a cardiac condition associated with an increased risk for IE,

TABLE 2.7 Catheters Used for Venous and Arterial Access

Catheter Type	Entry Site	Comments
Peripheral venous catheters (short)	Usually inserted into veins of forearm or hand	Phlebitis with prolonged use; rarely associated with bloodstream infection
Peripheral arterial catheters	Usually inserted into radial artery; can be placed in femoral, axillary, brachial, or posterior tibial arteries	Low infection risk; rarely associated with bloodstream infection
Midline catheters	Inserted through antecubital fossa into proximal basilica or cephalic veins; does not enter central veins or peripheral catheters	Anaphylactoid reactions have been reported with catheters made of elastomeric hydrogel; lower rates of phlebitis than with short peripheral catheters
Nontunneled central venous catheters	Percutaneously inserted into central veins (subclavian, internal jugular, or femoral)	Account for most catheter-related bloodstream infections
Pulmonary artery catheters	Inserted through a Teflon introducer into a central vein (subclavian, internal jugular, or femoral)	Usually heparin bonded; similar rates of bloodstream infection as central venous catheters
Peripherally inserted central venous catheters	Inserted into basilica, cephalic, or brachial veins and advanced to superior vena cava	Lower rate of infection than nontunneled central venous catheters
Tunneled central venous catheters	Implanted into subclavian, internal jugular, or femoral veins	Cuff inhibits migration of organisms into catheter tract; lower rate of infection than with nontunneled central venous catheters
Totally implantable	Tunneled beneath skin with subcutaneous port access with a needle; implanted in subclavian or internal jugular vein	Lowest risk for catheter-related bloodstream infections; improved patient self-image; no need for local catheter site care; surgery required for catheter removal
Umbilical catheters	Inserted into umbilical vein or umbilical artery	Risk for catheter-related bloodstream infection similar with use of umbilical vein and with use of artery

Adapted from O'Grady NP, Alexander M, Dellinger EP, et al. Guidelines for the prevention of intravascular catheter–related infections. Centers for Disease Control and Prevention. *MMWR Recomm Rep (Morb Mortal Wkly Rep)*. 2002;51:1–29.

the dentist should remain alert to the presence of signs or symptoms of IE (e.g., fever) and make the appropriate physician referral as indicated. This precaution applies whether or not the patient has received prophylactic antibiotics for dental procedures.

BOX 2.2 Dental Procedures in Patients With Cardiac Conditions for Which Infective Endocarditis Prophylaxis Is Recommended

- All dental procedures that involve manipulation of gingival tissue or the periapical region of teeth or perforation of the oral mucosa
- This includes all dental procedures except the following procedures and events:
  - Routine anesthetic injections through noninfected tissue
  - Taking of dental radiographs
  - Placement of removable prosthodontic or orthodontic appliances
  - Adjustment of orthodontic appliances
  - Shedding of deciduous teeth and bleeding from trauma to the lips or oral mucosa

From Wilson W, Taubert KA, Gewitz M, et al. American Heart Association Rheumatic Fever, Endocarditis, and Kawasaki Disease Committee; American Heart Association Council on Cardiovascular Disease in the Young; American Heart Association Council on Clinical Cardiology; American Heart Association Council on Interdisciplinary Working Group: Prevention of infective endocarditis: guidelines from the American Heart Association: a guideline from the American Heart Association Rheumatic Fever, Young, and the Council on Clinical Cardiology, Council on Cardiovascular Surgery and Anesthesia, and the Quality Care of Outcomes Research Interdisciplinary Working Group. *Circulation.* 2007;116(15):1736–1754.

It also is recommended that a preoperative dental evaluation be performed and necessary dental treatment be provided whenever possible before initiation of cardiac valve surgery or replacement or repair of congenital heart disease in an effort to decrease the incidence of late PVE caused by VGS.

Patients Already Taking Antibiotics. In patients who are taking penicillin or amoxicillin for eradication of an infection (e.g., sinus infection) or for long-term secondary prevention of rheumatic fever, presence of VGS that are relatively resistant to penicillin or amoxicillin is likely. Therefore, a nonpenicillin antibiotic (azithromycin, clarithromycin or doxycycline) listed in Table 2.8 should be selected for prophylaxis if treatment is necessary. Because of cross-resistance with cephalosporins, this class of antibiotics should be avoided. Current AHA recommendations are to wait for at least 10 days after completion of short-course antibiotic therapy before administration of prophylactic antibiotics for an elective dental procedure. Of note, evidence exists from prospective studies indicating that *amoxicillin-resistant VGS can persist for 24 days after a single dose of 2 g amoxicillin; thus waiting at least 24 days may have additional benefit.*

Consecutive Dental Appointments. Because of the potential for antibiotic resistance, the AHA also recommends waiting at least 10 days for the administration of antibiotic prophylaxis in a high-risk patient who is undergoing multiple sequential dental appointments. *Clinical judgment should include recognition of the benefits of using an alternative antibiotic regimen each*

TABLE 2.8   American Heart Association Antibiotic Regimens for Dental Procedures: Single Dose 30–60 min Before the Procedure

Situation	Agent	Adults	Children
Oral	Amoxicillin	2 g	50 mg/kg
Unable to take oral medication	Ampicillin or	2 g IM or IV	50 mg/kg IM or IV
	Cefazolin or ceftriaxone	1 g IM or IV	50 mg/kg IM or IV
Allergic to PCNs or ampicillin (oral)	Cephalexin[a,b] or	2 g	50 mg/kg
	Azithromycin or clarithromycin	500 mg	15 mg/kg
	Or doxycycline	100 mg	>45 kg, 100 mg <45 kg, 4.4 mg/kg
Allergic to PCNs or ampicillin and unable to take oral medication	Cefazolin or ceftriaxone[b]	1 g IM or IV	50 mg/kg IM or IV

[a]Or other first- or second-generation oral cephalosporin in equivalent adult or pediatric dosing.
[b]Cephalosporins should not be used in an individual with a history of anaphylaxis, angioedema, or urticaria with penicillin or ampicillin. Clindamycin is no longer recommended for antibiotic prophylaxis for a dental procedure. *IM*, Intramuscular; *IV*, intravenous; *PCN*, penicillin.
From Wilson W, Gewitz M, Lockhart PB, et al. American Heart Association Young Hearts Rheumatic Fever, Endocarditis, and Kawasaki Disease Committee of the Council on Lifelong Congenital Heart Disease and Heart Health in the Young; Council on Cardiovascular and Stroke Nursing and the Council on Quality of Care and Outcomes Research. Prevention of viridans group streptococcal infective endocarditis: a scientific statement from the American Heart Association. *Circulation.* 2021;143(20):e963–e978.

session, and of waiting at least 24 days between treatment sessions where antibiotic prophylaxis is being administered, when possible, to reduce the risk of antibiotic-resistant VGS strains.

Parenteral Antibiotics. The AHA states: "In patients who are receiving parenteral antimicrobial therapy for IE or other infections and require a dental procedure, the same parenteral antibiotic may be continued through the dental procedure."

Prolonged Dental Appointment. The duration of a dental appointment in relation to the effective plasma concentration of an administered antibiotic is not addressed in AHA recommendations; however, for a lengthy appointment, this may be a matter of concern. With amoxicillin, which has a half-life of approximately 80 min, the average peak plasma concentration of 4 µg/mL is reached about 2 h after oral administration of a 250-mg dose. Most of the penicillin-sensitive VGS have an MIC requirement of 0.2 µg/mL. Thus, a 2-g dose of amoxicillin should produce an acceptable MIC for at least 6 h. If a procedure lasts longer than 6 h, it may be prudent to administer an additional 2-g dose.

Clinical Judgment and Shared Decision-Making. Dental providers are responsible for being aware of the most current AHA guidelines and compliant in their use. Within this context, providers are encouraged to use clinical judgment and shared decision-making. Clinicians also should be aware of additional circumstances. Although infection of some prosthetic cardiovascular devices (e.g., implantable pacemakers/defibrillators, septal defect closure devices, peripheral vascular grafts and patches; and those used for hemodialysis and coronary and other vascular stets; central nervous system ventriculoatrial shunts, vena caval filters and pledgets) occurs, these infections are rare and most often are caused by staphylococci. Accordingly, antibiotic prophylaxis for a dental procedure in these patients is not recommended.

Also, while acknowledging that evidence is accumulating that those in the moderate risk category (i.e., rheumatic fever/heart disease, nonrheumatic valve disease, congenital valve anomalies) are at substantial risk for adverse outcomes, at present the AHA does not recommend that these groups of patients receive antibiotic prophylaxis prior to invasive dental procedures. Nevertheless, a patient or a patient's physician may request antibiotic prophylaxis when their situation falls outside current guidelines. Ultimately, the decision to administer antibiotic prophylaxis with the goal of preventing VGS IE rests with both the provider and the patient. Informing patients of their options and describing the risks and benefits (antibiotics vs. no antibiotics), including the importance of oral health, lead to better communication, informed decisions, and better outcomes.

In addition, the dentist should consult with the patient's physician to ensure that he or she is aware of the current AHA recommendations and to discuss their implementation in treatment of the patient. These conversations should be documented in the patient's progress notes.

BIBLIOGRAPHY

1. AHA. Prevention of rheumatic fever and bacterial endocarditis through control of streptococcal infection. *Circulation.* 1965;31:953–955.
2. Asi KS, Gill AS, Mahajan S. Postoperative bacteremia in periodontal flap surgery, with and without prophylactic antibiotic administration: a comparative study. *J Indian Soc Periodontol.* 2010;14(1):18–22.
3. Baddour LM, Bettmann MA, Bolger AF, et al. Nonvalvular cardiovascular device-related infections. *Circulation.* 2003;108(16):2015–2031.
4. Baddour LM, Wilson WR, Bayer AS, et al. Infective endocarditis: diagnosis, antimicrobial therapy, and

management of complications: a statement for healthcare professionals from the Committee on Rheumatic Fever, Endocarditis, and Kawasaki Disease, Council on Cardiovascular Disease in the Young, and the Councils on Clinical Cardiology, Stroke, and Cardiovascular Surgery and Anesthesia, American Heart Association: endorsed by the Infectious Diseases Society of America. *Circulation.* 2005;111(23):e394–e434.

5. Baddour LM, Bettmann MA, Bolger AF, et al. Nonvalvular cardiovascular device-related infections. *Clin Infect Dis.* 2004;38(8):1128–1130.

6. Bashore TM, Cabell C, Fowler Jr V. Update on infective endocarditis. *Curr Probl Cardiol.* 2006;31(4):274–352.

7. Beck DL, Braunwald E, AHA 2015. Increased incidence of infective endocarditis after the 2009 ESC guideline update: a nationwide study in The Netherlands. In: Goldman L, Schafer AI, eds. *Braunwald's Heart Disease: A Textbook of Cardiovascular Medicine.* Philadelphia, PA: Elsevier (Saunders); 2016:20.

8. Bor DH, Woolhandler S, Nardin R, et al. Infective endocarditis in the U.S., 1998–2009: a nationwide study. *PLoS One.* 2013;8(3):e60033.

9. Brennan MT, Kent ML, Fox PC, et al. The impact of oral disease and nonsurgical treatment on bacteremia in children. *J Am Dent Assoc.* 2007;138(1):80–85.

10. Cahill TJ, Prendergast BD. Infective endocarditis. *Lancet.* 2016;387(10021):882–893.

11. Cobe HM. Transitory bacteremia. *Oral Surg Oral Med Oral Pathol.* 1954;7(6):609–615.

12. Crasta K, Daly CG, Mitchell D, et al. Bacteraemia due to dental flossing. *J Clin Periodontol.* 2009;36(4):323–332.

13. Dajani AS, Bisno AL, Chung KJ, et al. Prevention of bacterial endocarditis. Recommendations by the American Heart Association. *JAMA.* 1990;264(22):2919–2922.

14. Dajani AS, Taubert KA, Wilson W, et al. Prevention of bacterial endocarditis: recommendations by the American Heart Association. *JAMA.* 1997;22:1794–1801.

15. Dajani AS, Taubert KA, Wilson W, et al. Prevention of bacterial endocarditis: recommendations by the American Heart Association. *J Am Dent Assoc.* 1997;128(8):1142–1151.

16. Danchin N, Duval X, Leport C. Prophylaxis of infective endocarditis: French recommendations 2002. *Heart.* 2005;91(6):715–718.

17. Dayer MJ, Chambers JB, Prendergast B, et al. NICE guidance on antibiotic prophylaxis to prevent infective endocarditis: a survey of clinicians' attitudes. *QJM.* 2013;106(3):237–243.

18. de Sa D. Epidemiological trends of infective endocarditis: a population-based study in Olmsted County. *Mayo Clin Proc.* 2010;85:422–426.

19. Durack DT. Antibiotics for prevention of endocarditis during dentistry: time to scale back? *Ann Intern Med.* 1998;129(10):829–830.

20. Felix JE, Rosen S, App GR. Detection of bacteremia after the use of an oral irrigation device in subjects with periodontitis. *J Periodontol.* 1971;42(12):785–787.

21. Durack DT. Prevention of infective endocarditis. *N Engl J Med.* 1995;332(1):38–44.

22. Durack DT, Beeson PB. Experimental bacterial endocarditis. II. Survival of a bacteria in endocardial vegetations. *Br J Exp Pathol.* 1972;53(1):50–53.

23. Durack DT, Lukes AS, Bright DK. New criteria for diagnosis of infective endocarditis: utilization of specific echocardiographic findings. Duke Endocarditis Service [see comments]. *Am J Med.* 1994;96(3):200–209.

24. Gould FK, Elliott TS, Foweraker J, et al. Guidelines for the prevention of endocarditis: report of the Working Party of the British Society for Antimicrobial Chemotherapy. *J Antimicrob Chemother.* 2006;57(6):1035–1042.

25. Guntheroth WG. How important are dental procedures as a cause of infective endocarditis? *Am J Cardiol.* 1984;54:797–801.

26. Hall G, Hedstrom SA, Heimdahl A, et al. Prophylactic administration of penicillins for endocarditis does not reduce the incidence of postextraction bacteremia. *Clin Infect Dis.* 1993;17(2):188–194.

27. Hall G, Heimdahl A, Nord CE. Effects of prophylactic administration of cefaclor on transient bacteremia after dental extraction. *Eur J Clin Microbiol Infect Dis.* 1996;15(8):646–649.

28. Hall G, Heimdahl A, Nord CE. Bacteremia after oral surgery and antibiotic prophylaxis for endocarditis. *Clin Infect Dis.* 1999;29(1):1–8; quiz 9-10.

29. Hoen B, Selton-Suty C, Lacassin F, et al. Infective endocarditis in patients with negative blood cultures: analysis of 88 cases from a one-year nationwide survey in France. *Clin Infect Dis.* 1995;20(3):501–506.

30. Hong CH, Allred R, Napenas JJ, et al. Antibiotic prophylaxis for dental procedures to prevent indwelling venous catheter-related infections. *Am J Med.* 2010;123(12):1128–1133.

31. Hussar AE. Prevention of bacterial endocarditis. *Circulation.* 1965;31:953–954.

32. Jones T. Prevention of rheumatic fever and bacterial endocarditis through control of streptococcal infections. *Circulation.* 1955;11:317–320.

33. Kang DH. Timing of surgery in infective endocarditis. *Heart.* 2015;101(22):1786–1791.

34. Karchmer AW. Infective endocarditis. In: Libby P, ed. *Braunwald's Heart Disease: A Textbook of Cardiovascular Medicine.* 8th ed. Philadelphia: Saunders; 2008:1713–1738.

35. Kaplan EL. Prevention of bacterial endocarditis. *Circulation.* 1977;56(1):139A–143A.

36. Khalil D, Hultin M, Rashid MU, et al. Oral microflora and selection of resistance after a single dose of amoxicillin. *Clin Microbiol Infect.* 2016;22(11):949.

37. Klein M, Wang A. Infective endocarditis. *J Intensive Care Med.* 2016;31(3):151–163.

38. Fowler VGJ, Bayer AS, Baddour LM. Infective endocarditis. In: Goldman L, Schafer AI, eds. *Goldman-Cecil Medicine.* 25th ed. Philadelphia, PA: Elsevier (Saunders); 2016:30.

39. Li JS, Sexton DJ, Mick N, et al. Proposed modifications to the Duke criteria for the diagnosis of infective endocarditis. *Clin Infect Dis.* 2000;30(4):633–638.

40. Lockhart PB. An analysis of bacteremias during dental extractions: a double-blind, placebo-controlled study of chlorhexidine. *Arch Intern Med.* 1996;156:513–520.

41. Lockhart PB. The risk for endocarditis in dental practice. *Periodontol 2000.* 2000;23:127–135.

42. Lockhart PB, Bahrani Mougeot FK, Saunders SE, et al. The effectiveness of antibiotic prophylaxis in preventing infective endocarditis is not easily dismissed. *Oral Surg Oral Med Oral Pathol Oral Radiol.* 2015;120(5):661–662.

43. Lockhart PB, Brennan MT, Thornhill M, et al. Poor oral hygiene is a risk factor for infective endocarditis-related bacteremia. *J Am Dent Assoc.* 2009;140:1238–1244.

44. Lockhart PB, Durack DT. Oral microflora as a cause of endocarditis and other distant site infections. *Infect Dis Clin N Am.* 1999;13(4):833–850, vi.

45. Lockhart PB, Loven B, Brennan MT, et al. The evidence base for the efficacy of antibiotic prophylaxis in dental practice. *J Am Dent Assoc.* 2007;138(4):458–475.

46. Lucas VS, Lytra V, Hassan T, et al. Comparison of lysis filtration and an automated blood culture system (BACTEC) for detection, quantification, and identification of odontogenic bacteremia in children. *J Clin Microbiol.* 2002;40(9):3416–3420.

47. Marti-Carvajal AJ, Dayer M, Conterno LO, et al. A comparison of different antibiotic regimens for the treatment of infective endocarditis. *Cochrane Database Syst Rev.* 2016;4:CD009880.

48. Mathew J, Addai T, Anand A, et al. Clinical features, site of involvement, bacteriologic findings, and outcome of infective endocarditis in intravenous drug users. *Arch Intern Med.* 1995;155(15):1641–1648.

49. Miranda WR, Connolly HM, DeSimone DC, et al. Infective endocarditis involving the pulmonary valve. *Am J Cardiol.* 2015;116(12):1928–1931.

50. Mzougeot FK, Saunders SE, Brennan MT, et al. Associations between bacteremia from oral sources and distant-site infections: tooth brushing versus single tooth extraction. *Oral Surg Oral Med Oral Pathol Oral Radiol.* 2015;119(4):430–435.

51. Muroch DR, Corey GR, Hoen B, et al. Clinical presentation, etiology, and outcome of infective endocarditits in the 21st century: the International Collaboration on Endocarditis-Prospective Cohort Study. *Arch Intern Med.* 2009;169(5):463–473.

52. Mylanakis E, Calderwood SB. Infective endocarditis in adults. *N Engl J Med.* 2001;345(18):1318–1330.

53. O'Brien MC, Pourmoghadam KK, DeCampli WM. Late postoperative prosthetic pulmonary valve endocarditis in a 13-year-old girl with repaired tetralogy of Fallot. *Tex Heart Inst J.* 2015;42(3):251–254.

54. O'Grady NP, Alexander M, Dellinger EP, et al. Guidelines for the prevention of intravascular catheter-related infections. Centers for Disease Control and Prevention. *MMWR Recomm Rep.* 2002;51(RR-10):1–29.

55. O'Leary TJ, Shafer WG, Swenson HM, et al. Possible penetration of crevicular tissue from oral hygiene procedures. I. Use of oral irrigating devices. *J Periodontol.* 1970;41(3):158–162.

56. Oliver R, Roberts GJ, Hooper L, et al. Antibiotics for the prophylaxis of bacterial endocarditis in dentistry. *Cochrane Database Syst Rev.* 2008;4:CD003813.

57. Otome O, Guy S, Tramontana A, et al. A retrospective review: significance of vegetation size in injection drug users with right-sided infective endocarditis. *Heart Lung Circ.* 2016;25(5):466–470.

58. Pallasch TJ, Slots J. Antibiotic prophylaxis and the medically compromised patient. *Periodontol 2000.* 1996;10:107–138.

59. Pang PY, Sin YK, Lim CH, et al. Surgical management of infective endocarditis: an analysis of early and late outcomes. *Eur J Cardio Thorac Surg.* 2015;47(5):826–832.

60. Pant S, Patel NJ, Deshmukh A, et al. Trends in infective endocarditis incidence, microbiology, and valve replacement in the United States from 2000 to 2011. *J Am Coll Cardiol.* 2015;65:2070.

61. Pericart L, Fauchier L, Bourguignon T, et al. Long-term outcome and valve surgery for infective endocarditis in the systematic analysis of a community study. *Ann Thorac Surg.* 2016;102(2):496–504.

62. Roberts GJ, Jaffray EC, Spratt DA, et al. Duration, prevalence and intensity of bacteraemia after dental extractions in children. *Heart.* 2006;92(9):1274–1277.

63. Round H, Kirkpatrick H, Hails C. Further investigations on bacteriological infections of the mouth. *Proc Roy Soc Med.* 1936;29:1552–1556.

64. Quan TP, Muller-Pebody B, Fawcett N, et al. Investigation of the impact of the NICE guidelines regarding antibiotic prophylaxis during invasive dental procedures on the incidence of infective endocarditis in England: an electronic health records study. *BMC Med.* 2020;18(1):84.

65. Rammelkamp CH, Catanzaro FJ, Chamovitz R, Americal Heart Association. Treatment of streptococcal infections in the general population. *Circulation.* 1957;15:154–158.

66. Revest M, Egmann G, Cattoir V, et al. HACEK endocarditis: state-of-the-art. *Expert Rev Anti Infect Ther.* 2016;14(5):523–530.

67. Richey R, Wray D, Stokes T. Prophylaxis against infective endocarditis: summary of NICE guidance. *BMJ.* 2008;336(7647):770–771.

68. Rise E, Smith JF, Bell J. Reduction of bacteremia after oral manipulations. *Arch Otolaryngol.* 1969;90:106–109.

69. Roberts GJ. Dentists are innocent! "Everyday" bacteremia is the real culprit: a review and assessment of the evidence that dental surgical procedures are a principal cause of bacterial endocarditis in children. *Pediatr Cardiol.* 1999;20(5):317–325.

70. Ross KM, Mehr JS, Greeley RD, et al. Outbreak of bacterial endocarditis associated with an oral surgery practice: New Jersey public health surveillance, 2013 to 2014. *J Am Dent Assoc.* 2018;149(3):191–201.

71. Schoenfeld M, Machhar R, Maw A. Diagnosing endocarditis in patients with *Staphylococcus aureus* bacteremia. *JAMA.* 2015;313(4):420.

72. Schlein RA, Kudlick EM, Reindorf CA, et al. Toothbrushing and transient bacteremia in patients undergoing orthodontic treatment. *Am J Orthod Dentofacial Orthop.* 1991;99(5):466–472.

73. Sconyers JR, Crawford JJ, Moriarty JD. Relationship of bacteremia to toothbrushing in patients with periodontitis. *J Am Dent Assoc.* 1973;87(3):616–622.

74. Sharara SL, Tayyar R, Kanafani ZA, et al. HACEK endocarditis: a review. *Expert Rev Anti Infect Ther.* 2016;14(6):539–545.

75. Shrestha NK, Jue J, Hussain ST, et al. Injection drug use and outcomes after surgical intervention for infective endocarditis. *Ann Thorac Surg.* 2015;100(3):875–882.

76. Shulman ST, Amren DP, Bisno AL, et al. Prevention of bacterial endocarditis. A statement for health professionals by the Committee on Rheumatic Fever and Infective Endocarditis of the Council on Cardiovascular Disease in the Young. *Circulation.* 1984;70(6):1123A–1127A.

77. Steckelberg JM, Wilson WR. Risk factors for infective endocarditis. *Infect Dis Clin N Am.* 1993;7(1):9–19.

78. Strom BL, Abrutyn E, Berlin JA, et al. Dental and cardiac risk factors for infective endocarditis: a population-based, case-control study. *Ann Intern Med.* 1998;129(10):761−769.

79. Thompson W, Sandoe JA. What does NICE have to say about antimicrobial prescribing to the dental community? *Br Dent J.* 2016;220(4):193−195.

80. Thornhill MH. Infective endocarditis: the impact of the NICE guidelines for antibiotic prophylaxis. *Dent Update.* 2012;39(1):6−10, 12.

81. Thornhill MH, Dayer, Durkin MJ, et al. Risk of adverse reactions to oral antibiotics prescribed by dentists. *J Dent Res.* 2019;98(10):1081−1087.

82. Thornhill MH, Dayer M, Lockhart PB, et al. Guidelines on prophylaxis to prevent infective endocarditis. *Br Dent J.* 2016;220(2):51−56.

83. Thornhill MH, Dayer, Lockhart PB, Prendergast B. Antibiotic prophylaxis of infective endocarditis. *Curr Infect Dis Rep.* 2017;19(2):9.

84. Thornhill MH, Dayer M, Lockhart PB, et al. A change in the NICE guidelines on antibiotic prophylaxis. *Br Dent J.* 2016;221(3):112−114.

85. Thornhill MH, Dayer JM, Jones S, et al. The effect of antibiotic prophylaxis guidelines on incidence of infective endocarditits. *Can J Cardiol.* 2016;31:1578.e9.

86. Thornhill M, Jones S, Prendergast B, et al. Quantifying infective endocarditis risk in patients with predisposing cardiac conditions. *Eur Heart J.* 2018;39:586−595.

87. Thornhill MH, Lockhart PB, Prendergast B, et al. NICE and antibiotic prophylaxis to prevent endocarditis. *Br Dent J.* 2015;218(11):619−621.

88. Tleyjeh IM, Steckelberg JM, Murad HS, et al. Temporal trends in infective endocarditis: a population-based study in Olmsted County, Minnesota. *JAMA.* 2005;293(24):3022−3028.

89. Topan A, Carstina D, Slavcovici A, et al. Assesment of the Duke criteria for the diagnosis of infective endocarditis after twenty-years. An analysis of 241 cases. *Clujul Med.* 2015;88(3):321−326.

90. Toyoda N, Chikwe J, Itagaki S, et al. Trends in infective endocarditis in California and New York State, 1998−2013. *JAMA.* 2017;317:1652.

91. van der Meer JT, Thompson J, Valkenburg HA, et al. Epidemiology of bacterial endocarditis in The Netherlands. II. Antecedent procedures and use of prophylaxis. *Arch Intern Med.* 1992;152(9):1869−1873.

92. van der Meer JT, Van Wijk W, Thompson J, et al. Efficacy of antibiotic peophylaxis for prevention of native-valve endocarditis. *Lancet.* 1992;339(8786):135−139.

93. Wallace SM, Walton BI, Kharbanda RK, et al. Mortality from infective endocarditis: clinical predictors of outcome. *Heart.* 2002;88(1):53−60.

94. Wilson W, Taubert KA, Gewitz M, et al. Prevention of infective endocarditis. Guidelines from the American Heart Association. A guideline from the American Heart Association Rheumatic Fever, Endocarditis, and Kawasaki Disease Committee, Council on Cardiovascular Disease in the Young, and the Council on Clinical Cardiology, Council on Cardiovascular Surgery and Anesthesia, and the Quality of Care and Outcomes Research Interdisciplinary Working Group. *Circulation.* 2007;115:1−17.

95. Woodman AJ, Vidic J, Newman HN, et al. Effect of repeated high dose prophylaxis with amoxicillin on the resident oral flora of adult volunteers. *J Med Microbiol.* 1985;19:15−23.

96. Yong MS, Coffey S, Prendergast BD, et al. Surgical management of tricuspid valve endocarditis in the current era: a review. *Int J Cardiol.* 2016;202:44−48.

Hypertension

KEY POINTS

- Hypertension is undiagnosed and not well controlled in many patients and often accompanied by comorbidities.
- Blood pressure (BP) should be routinely assessed in the dental office, and dental providers should assess for signs, symptoms, and comorbidities.
- BP can be elevated due to dental anxiety and pain, but can be reduced with appropriate measures.
- Routine dental care can be provided to most patients with hypertension when anxiety and pain are controlled,

and local anesthetic with 1:100,000 epinephrine is limited to two carpules or fewer.
- Dental treatment should be deferred when BP is >180/110; these patients should be referred for medical care.
- Many antihypertensive drugs are associated with hyposalivation, xerostomia, dental caries, and fungal infections.

Hypertension is an abnormal elevation in arterial pressure that can be fatal if sustained and untreated. People with hypertension may not display clinical signs or symptoms for many years but eventually can experience symptomatic damage to several target organs, including the kidneys, heart, brain, and eyes. In adults, hypertension is defined as a sustained systolic blood pressure (BP) of 130 mm Hg or greater or a sustained diastolic BP of 80 mm Hg or greater. The American Cardiology Association and the American Heart Association in 2017 defined BP in four stages: normal, elevated, stage 1, and stage 2 (Table 3.1). These stages reflect the health risks associated with BPs higher than 115/75 mm Hg, and help to encourage early interventions that could prevent adverse outcomes associated with chronic high BP such as stroke and myocardial infarction (MI).

Guidelines regarding hypertension classification, detection, diagnosis, and management in children and adolescents were revised in 2017. Current clinical practice guidelines for children and adolescents are based on the normative distribution of BP in healthy children, and are interpreted based on sex, age, and height with stage classification being based on > the 90th to 95th percentile (see Table 3.2).

Although dentists do not make the diagnosis of hypertension and direct treatment, current guidelines specifically encourage active participation of all health care professionals in the detection of hypertension and the surveillance of treatment compliance. Accordingly, dental health professionals can play a significant role in the detection and control of hypertension and may be the first to detect a patient with an elevation in BP or with symptoms of the disease. Along with detection, monitoring is equally valuable because patients who are

receiving treatment for hypertension may nevertheless fail to achieve adequate control because of poor compliance or inappropriate drug selection or dosing. An abnormal BP reading in the dental office becomes the basis for referral to, or consultation with, a physician. In addition, hypertension poses several considerations with respect to dental management, including monitoring BP during appointments, stress and anxiety reduction, prevention of drug interactions, and awareness and management of adverse drug side effects.

EPIDEMIOLOGY

Hypertension is the most common primary diagnosis in the United States, accounting for 39 million office visits annually. According to Centers for Disease Control and Prevention, at least 108 million (or 45%) adults in the United States have high blood pressure (HBP) or are taking antihypertensive medication. Thus, a typical practice population of 2000 patients will have about 900 patients who have hypertension.

Hypertension is more prevalent in men (47%) than women (43%) and varies with race and ethnicity. Social, economic, and historical determinants of health, that influence personal environment, behavior and habits, contribute to HBP being more common among non-Hispanic blacks (54%) followed by non-Hispanic whites (46%), Hispanics (36%), and non-Hispanic Asians (39%).

The prevalence of HBP increases with age, such that more than 65% of Americans aged 60 years and older have this disease. If people live long enough, more than 90% will develop hypertension. Of note, systolic BP continues to rise throughout life, but diastolic BP rises until around age 50 years and then levels off or falls; as a result,

TABLE 3.1   Classification of Blood Pressure (BP) in Adults and Recommendations for Follow-Up

BP Classification	Systolic BP (mm Hg)		Diastolic BP (mm Hg)	Recommended Follow-Up
Normal	<120	And	<80	Recheck in 2 years.
Elevated	120–129	Or	<80	Recheck in 1 year.
Hypertension				
Stage 1	130–139	Or	80–89	Confirm within 2 months.
Stage 2	≥140	Or	≥90	Evaluate or refer to source of care within 1 month. For those with higher BP (e.g., >180/110 mm Hg), evaluate and treat immediately or within 1 week, depending on the clinical situation and complications.

Note: If there is a disparity in category between the systolic and diastolic pressures, the **higher value** determines the stage.
Data from Whelton PK et al, 2017 ACC/AHA/AAPA/ABC/ACPM/AGS/APhA/ASH/ASPC/NMA/PCNA Guideline for the Prevention, Detection, Evaluation, and Management of High Blood Pressure in Adults: A Report of the American College of Cardiology/American Heart Association Task Force on Clinical Practice Guidelines, J AM Coll Cardiol. 2018 May, 71 (19)e127–e248.

TABLE 3.2   Updated Definitions of BP Categories and Stages for Children and Adolescents

For Children Aged 1–13 Years	For Children Aged > 13 Years
Normal BP: <90th percentile	Normal BP: <120/<80 mm Hg
Elevated BP: ≥90th percentile to <95th percentile or 120/80 mm Hg to <95th percentile (whichever is lower)	Elevated BP: 120/<80–129/<80 mm Hg
Stage 1 HTN: ≥95th percentile to <95th percentile + 12 mm Hg, or 130/80–139/89 mm Hg (whichever is lower)	Stage 1 HTN: 130/80–139/89 mm Hg
Stage 2 HTN: ≥95th percentile + 12 mm Hg, or ≥140/90 mm Hg (whichever is lower)	Stage 2 HTN: ≥140/90 mm Hg

BOX 3.1   Identifiable Causes of Hypertension

- Chronic kidney disease (e.g., diabetic nephropathy)
- Chronic steroid therapy and Cushing syndrome
- Coarctation of the aorta
- Drug induced or drug related (oral contraceptives, chronic NSAID use, decongestants, stimulants and weight-loss medications; cyclosporine, tacrolimus)
- Illicit drug use (methamphetamines, cocaine)
- Pheochromocytoma and other endocrine disorders (hyperthyroidism, hyperparathyroidism)
- Primary hyperaldosteronism
- Renovascular disease
- Sleep apnea

Data from the National Heart, Lung, and Blood Institute. *The Seventh Report of the Joint National Committee on Prevention, Detection, Evaluation, and Treatment of High Blood Pressure: The JNC 7 Report.* Bethesda, MD: U.S. Department of Health and Human Services, Public Health Service, National Institutes of Health, National Heart, Lung, and Blood Institute; August 2004.

after the age of 50, isolated systolic hypertension becomes the more prevalent pattern. Isolated diastolic hypertension most commonly is seen before age 50 years. Diastolic BP is a more potent cardiovascular risk factor than is systolic BP until age 50; thereafter, systolic BP is more important.

Awareness of hypertension is important to allow for early intervention and for reducing the number of deaths from coronary heart disease and stroke. For these reasons, the National High Blood Pressure Education Program was begun in 1972 and its successes have been significant. The number of people with HBP who are aware of their condition has increased over the decades from 51% to 82%, and the percentage of those receiving treatment for HBP has increased from 31% to 76%. The proportion of patients taking medication whose BP is controlled to 140/90 mm Hg is 52%; but only 24% to the level of <130/80. At present, 18% of patients with HBP remain unaware of their disease, 24% of patients with HBP are not being treated, and 76% of hypertensive patients are taking medications but not achieving adequate control of the condition (i.e., <130/80).

ETIOLOGY

About 90% of patients have no readily identifiable cause for their disease, which is referred to as primary (essential) hypertension. In the remaining 10% of patients, an underlying cause or condition may be identified; for these patients, the term *secondary hypertension* is applied. Box 3.1 is a listing of the most common identifiable causes of secondary hypertension. Risk factors for hypertension include age, race, reduced nephron number, and lifestyle factors (e.g., obesity, family history, excessive alcohol intake, high sodium diet, and physical inactivity). In children and adolescents, risk factors include obesity, heart disease, kidney disease, and sleep disorders.

PATHOPHYSIOLOGY AND COMPLICATIONS

In primary hypertension, the basic underlying defect is failure to regulate vascular resistance. The pulsating force is modified by the degree of *elasticity* of the walls of larger arteries and the *resistance* of the arteriolar bed. Control of vascular resistance is multifactorial, and abnormalities may exist in one or more areas. Mechanisms of control include neural baroreflexes and ongoing maintenance of *sympathetic vasomotor tone* and other effects mediated by neurotransmitters such as norepinephrine, extracellular fluid, and sodium stores; the renin–angiotensin–aldosterone pressor system; and locally active hormones and substances such as prostaglandins, kinins, adenosine, and hydrogen ions (H^+). In our modern culture, high salt intake appears to trigger neuromodulatory signals that activate the sympathetic nervous system, resulting in increased *renin* secretion by the kidneys. In isolated systolic hypertension, which commonly is seen in older adults, the underlying problem is one of central arterial stiffness and loss of elasticity.

Several physiologic factors may have an effect on BP. Increased *viscosity of the blood* (e.g., polycythemia) may cause an elevation in BP resulting from an increase in resistance to flow. A decrease in blood volume or tissue fluid volume (e.g., anemia, hemorrhage) reduces BP. Conversely, an increase in *blood volume or tissue fluid volume* (e.g., sodium and fluid retention) increases BP. Increases in cardiac output associated with exercise, fever, or thyrotoxicosis can increase BP. In addition, BP demonstrates a circadian variation with highest levels seen in early to mid-morning, lower levels as the day progresses, and the lowest BP at night.

A linear relationship exists between BPs at any level above normal and an increase in morbidity and mortality rates from stroke and coronary heart disease. BPs above 115 mm Hg systolic and 75 mm Hg diastolic are associated with increased risk of cardiovascular disease. It is estimated that about 15% of all BP-related deaths from coronary heart disease occur in persons with BP in the "elevated BP" range. However, the higher the BP, the greater the risk of heart attack, heart failure, stroke, and kidney disease. For every increase in BP of 20 mm Hg systolic and 10 mm Hg diastolic, the risk of death related to ischemic heart disease and stroke doubles. Poorly controlled hypertension precedes the onset of

vascular changes in the kidney, heart, brain, and retina that lead to such clinical complications as ischemic heart disease, MI, renal failure, vascular stroke, atrial fibrillation, heart failure, dementia, encephalopathy, and blindness. If the condition goes untreated, a significant number of persons die prematurely. About 50% of hypertensive patients die of coronary heart disease or congestive heart failure, about 33% of stroke, and about 10% of renal failure. Hypertension contributed to the cause of death for more than 494,000 people in the United States in 2018.

CLINICAL PRESENTATION

Signs and Symptoms

Hypertension may remain an asymptomatic disease for many years, with the only sign being an elevated BP. BP is measured with the use of a sphygmomanometer (Fig. 3.1). Pressure at the peak of ventricular contraction is the systolic pressure. Diastolic pressure represents the total resting resistance in the arterial system after passage of the pulsating force produced by contraction of the left ventricle. The difference between diastolic and systolic pressures is called pulse pressure. Mean arterial pressure is roughly defined as the sum of the diastolic pressure plus one-third the pulse pressure. Patients commonly are found to have variability in BP throughout the day and according to their environment. About 20% of patients with untreated stage 1 hypertension have what is called *white coat hypertension*, which is defined as consistently elevated BP only in the presence of a health care worker but not elsewhere. In these patients, accurate BP readings may require self-measurement at home or 24-h ambulatory monitoring. Persons with BP elevation in this setting are at lower risk for hypertensive complications than are those with sustained hypertension.

Before the age of 50 years, hypertension typically is characterized by an elevation in both diastolic and systolic pressures. Isolated diastolic hypertension, defined as a systolic BP of 130 or less and a diastolic BP of 80 or greater, is uncommon and most often is found in younger

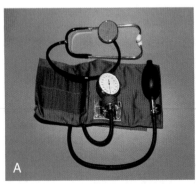
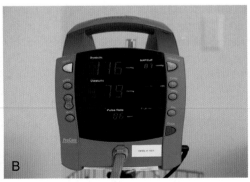
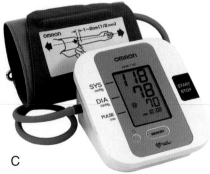

FIG. 3.1 **(A)** Standard blood pressure cuff (sphygmomanometer) and stethoscope, **(B)** and **(C)** automated blood pressure devices.

adults. Although the prognostic significance of this condition remains unclear and controversial, it appears that it may be relatively benign. Isolated systolic hypertension is defined as a systolic pressure of 130 mm Hg or higher and a diastolic BP of 80 mm Hg or less; it is the predominant form of hypertension in older adults and constitutes an important risk factor for cardiovascular disease. Occasionally, isolated systolic BP elevation is found in older children and young adults, often male. In these age groups, this form of hypertension is due to the combination of rapid growth in height and very elastic arteries.

The earliest sign of hypertension is an elevated BP reading; however, funduscopic examination of the retina may show early changes of hypertension consisting of narrowed arterioles with sclerosis. As indicated earlier, hypertension may remain an asymptomatic disease for many years, but when symptoms do occur, they can include headache, tinnitus, and dizziness. These symptoms are not specific for hypertension and may be experienced just as commonly by normotensive persons.

Late signs and symptoms are related to involvement of various target organs, including the kidneys, brain, heart, or eyes (Box 3.2). In advanced cases, blurred vision caused by retinal vessel hemorrhage, exudate, and papilledema may occur. These eye findings are indicative of accelerated malignant hypertension, a medical emergency that requires immediate intervention. Hypertensive encephalopathy is characterized by headache, irritability, alterations in consciousness, and other signs of central nervous system dysfunction. Other findings in advanced cases may include enlargement of the left ventricle with impairment of cardiac function, leading to congestive heart failure. Renal involvement can result in hematuria, proteinuria, and renal failure. Persons with hypertension may report fatigue and coldness in the legs or claudication resulting from the peripheral arterial changes that may occur in advanced hypertension. Patients with hypertension often demonstrate an accelerated cognitive decline with aging.

LABORATORY AND DIAGNOSTIC FINDINGS

The American College of Cardiology and the American Heart Association (ACC/AHA) 2017 guidelines recommend that patients who have sustained hypertension be screened through routine laboratory tests, including 12-lead electrocardiogram (ECG), complete blood count, fasting blood glucose, electrolytes, thyroid stimulating hormone, creatinine, calcium, lipid profile, and urinalysis. Results of these tests as well as the 10-year atherosclerotic cardiovascular disease risk calculator (Box 3.3) serve as baseline values that the physician uses to help guide decisions regarding therapy.

MEDICAL MANAGEMENT

Evaluation of a patient with hypertension includes a thorough medical history, a complete physical examination, and routine laboratory tests as described earlier. Additional diagnostic tests or procedures (e.g., serum aldosterone) may be performed to detect secondary causes of hypertension and to rule out target-organ damage and/or the presence of cardiovascular or renal disease. Patients found to have an identifiable cause for their hypertension should be treated for that disorder and may require a referral to a nephrologist or endocrinologist. Those without an identifiable cause are diagnosed with primary hypertension.

Classification and diagnosis of BP (see Table 3.1) are based on use of the proper technique to measure BP; i.e., an average of two or more properly measured BP readings obtained in a comfortably rested and seated patient. Measurement of BP has been traditionally achieved using the auscultatory method with a manual aneroid (with a dial) or hybrid sphygmomanometer. Electronic automated devices are now commonly used (see Fig. 3.1). In a patient who has been quietly seated for 5 min with feet flat on the floor, the appropriate sized cuff is placed around the upper arm, at the vertical height of the heart, and the cuff is

---

BOX 3.2 Signs and Symptoms of Hypertensive Disease

Early
- Elevated blood pressure readings
- Narrowing and sclerosis of retinal arterioles
- Headache, Dizziness, Tinnitus

Advanced
Eye:
- Rupture and hemorrhage of retinal arterioles
- Papilledema

Heart
- Angina pectoris, Left ventricular hypertrophy, Congestive heart failure

Kidney
- Proteinuria, Renal failure

Brain
- Dementia, Encephalopathy, Stroke

BOX 3.3 Factors Used in the ASCVD Risk Estimator

- Age
- Sex
- Systolic and Diastolic Blood Pressure
- Total Cholesterol, HDL Cholesterol, LDL Cholesterol
- History of Diabetes (Yes/No)
- Smoker (Current, Former, Never)
- On Hypertension Treatment (Yes/No)
- On a Statin (Yes/No)
- On Aspirin Therapy (Yes/No)

inflated to obtain a proper reading (see Chapter 1). Clinicians should realize that BP varies throughout the day, and accurate measurements are important for achieving the proper diagnosis and treatment.

Patients with a diagnosis of elevated BP are not usually candidates for drug therapy but rather are encouraged to adopt lifestyle modifications to decrease their risk of developing the disease. Elevated BP is not a disease but rather a designation that reflects the fact that these patients are at increased risk for the development of hypertension. Lifestyle modifications include weight management; adopting a diet rich in vegetables, fruits, and low-fat dairy products; reducing intake of foods high in cholesterol and saturated fats; decreasing sodium intake; limiting alcohol intake; quitting smoking; and engaging in daily aerobic physical activity (Box 3.4). Patients with elevated BP, as well as those with diagnosed hypertension, are strongly encouraged to follow these recommendations because lifestyle modifications have been shown to effectively reduce BP, prevent or delay the incidence of hypertension, enhance antihypertensive drug therapy, and decrease cardiovascular risk. If lifestyle modifications are found to be inadequate for achieving desired BP reduction, drug therapy is initiated.

Pharmacologic management of hypertension is guided by several publications including the 2017 ACC/AHA guideline. Because many drugs are currently available to treat patients with hypertension (Table 3.3), drug selection is determined primarily by the degree of BP reduction achieved. The 2017 ACC/AHA guidelines recommend diuretics, angiotensin-converting enzyme (ACE) inhibitors, angiotensin receptor blockers, and long-acting calcium channel blockers (LaCCBs) as first-line choices for the general nonblack population. For the general black population, a thiazide diuretic or LaCCB is recommended as initial therapy based on evidence that there may be racial/genetic factors that cause a different response to therapy. Other drugs used as secondary choices include β-blockers, α_1-adrenergic blockers, and central α_2 agonists, as well as other centrally acting drugs and direct vasodilators. Fig. 3.2 depicts the algorithm suggested by the JNC 8 for the treatment of hypertension. For early stage 1 hypertension, single-drug therapy may be effective; however, for later stage 1 and for stage 2 hypertension, two or more drug combinations are necessary. The presence of certain comorbid conditions or factors such as heart failure, previous MI, diabetes, or kidney disease may be a compelling reason to select specific drugs or classes of drugs that have been found to be beneficial in clinical trials. Of note, aggressive pharmacologic treatment of hypertension has clear benefits. In clinical trials, antihypertensive therapy resulted in an average reduction in stroke incidence of 35%–40%; MI, 20%–25%; and heart failure, greater than 50%.

Severe uncontrolled hypertension is defined as BP greater than 180/110 mm Hg (Table 3.4). When BP is greater than 180/120, the condition is called acute hypertension or hypertensive crisis. Two categories of hypertensive crisis are defined: hypertensive urgency or hypertensive emergency. A *hypertensive urgency* occurs when BP is greater than 180/120 mm Hg in the absence of progressive end-organ dysfunction. These persons may exhibit symptoms (headache, dyspnea, nosebleeds, or severe anxiety) and often are found to be noncompliant, under stress, or have an inadequate medication regimen. In contrast, a *hypertensive emergency* is characterized by a BP ≥ 180/120 mm Hg with evidence of impending or progressive target organ dysfunction (i.e., hypertensive encephalopathy, intracerebral hemorrhage, eclampsia, acute MI, left ventricular failure with pulmonary edema, or unstable angina pectoris). A hypertensive emergency can be associated with chest pain, dyspnea, change in mental status, visual disturbance, or a neurologic deficit. Early treatment is required for patients with a hypertensive emergency.

DENTAL MANAGEMENT

Medical Considerations

Identification. The first task of the dentist is to identify patients with hypertension, both diagnosed and undiagnosed. A medical history, including the diagnosis of hypertension, how it is being treated, identification of antihypertensive drugs, compliance status, presence of hypertension-associated symptoms and signs, and level of stability of the disease should be obtained. On occasion, patients may fail to report that they have been diagnosed with hypertension yet may report taking medications, including herbal medications, typically advocated to treat high BP. This may be the only way for the clinician to uncover information revealing that the patient has hypertension. Patients also may be receiving treatment for complications of hypertensive disease, such

---

BOX 3.4 **Lifestyle Modifications for Prevention and Reduction of High Blood Pressure**

- Weight loss
- DASH (Dietary Approaches to Stop Hypertension) diet: fruits, vegetables, low-fat dairy products
- Reduced intake of cholesterol-rich foods
- Reduced intake of saturated and total fats
- Reduced sodium intake to <2.4 g/day
- Regular aerobic physical activity on most days (30 min of brisk walking)
- Quit smoking
- Limited alcohol intake to no more than 1 oz/day (2 drinks for men and 1 drink for women)

Data from the National Heart, Lung, and Blood Institute. *The Seventh Report of the Joint National Committee on Prevention, Detection, Evaluation, and Treatment of High Blood Pressure: The JNC 7 Report.* Bethesda, MD: US Department of Health and Human Services, Public Health Service, National Institutes of Health, National Heart, Lung, and Blood Institute; August 2004.

TABLE 3.3   Drugs Used in the Management of Hypertension

Drug	Oral Adverse Effects	Dental Considerations
Diuretics		
Thiazide Diuretics		
Chlorothiazide (Diuril), chlorthalidone (generic), hydrochlorothiazide (HCTZ) (HydroDIURIL, Microzide), polythiazide (Renese), indapamide (Lozol), metolazone (Mykrox), metolazone (Zaroxolyn)	Dry mouth, lichenoid reactions	Orthostatic hypotension; avoid prolonged use of NSAIDs—may reduce antihypertensive effects. Vasoconstrictor interactions: none. (*Applies to all diuretics*)
Loop Diuretics		
Bumetanide (Bumex), furosemide (Lasix), torsemide (Demadex)		
Potassium-Sparing Diuretics		
Amiloride (Midamor), triamterene (Dyrenium)		
Aldosterone Receptor Blockers		
Eplerenone (Inspra), spironolactone (Aldactone)		
Combination		
Aldactazide, Dyazide		
β-Blockers (BBSs)		
Nonselective		
Propranolol (Inderal), timolol (Blocadren), nadolol (Corgard), pindolol (Visken), penbutolol (Levatol), carteolol (Cartrol)	Taste changes, lichenoid reactions	Avoid prolonged use of NSAIDs—may reduce antihypertensive effects. Vasoconstrictor interactions: nonselective—potential increase in blood pressure (use maximum of 0.036 mg of epinephrine); avoid levonordefrin
Cardioselective		
Metoprolol (Lopressor), acebutolol (Sectral), atenolol (Tenormin), betaxolol (Kerlone), bisoprolol (Zebeta)		Vasoconstrictor interactions: none
α- and β-Blockers		
Carvedilol (Coreg), labetalol (Normodyne, Trandate)	Taste changes	Orthostatic hypotension; avoid prolonged use of NSAIDs—may reduce antihypertensive effects. Vasoconstrictor interaction: Blocking both β₁- and β₂-adrenergic receptor sites has potential for adverse interaction
Angiotensin-Converting Enzyme (ACE) Inhibitors		
Benazepril (Lotensin), captopril (Capoten), enalapril (Vasotec), fosinopril (Monopril), lisinopril (Prinivil; Zestril), moexipril (Univasc), perindopril (Aceon), quinapril (Accupril), ramipril (Altace), trandolapril (Mavik),	Angioedema of lips, face, tongue; taste changes; oral burning	Orthostatic hypotension; avoid prolonged use of NSAIDs—may reduce antihypertensive effects. Vasoconstrictor interaction: none
Angiotensin Receptor Blockers (ARBSs)		
Azilsartan (Edarbi), candesartan (Atacand), eprosartan (Teveten), irbesartan (Avapro), losartan (Cozaar), olmesartan (Benicar), telmisartan (Micardis), valsartan (Diovan)	Angioedema of the lips, face, tongue	Orthostatic hypotension. Vasoconstrictor interaction: none
Calcium Channel Blockers (CCBSs)		
Amlodipine (Norvasc), Bepridil (Vascor), diltiazem (Cardizem, Cartia XT, Dilt-XR, Diltia XT, Taztia XT, Tiazac), felodipine (Plendil), isradipine (DynaCirc), nicardipine/SR (Cardene), nifedipine/PA/XL (Adalat, Nifediac, Procardia), nisoldipine (Sular), nitrendipine verapamil/SR (Calan, Isoptin, Verelan, Covera)	Gingival overgrowth, dry mouth, lichenoid eruptions (rare)	Avoid prescribing macrolide antibiotics that can raise plasma levels of CCBs resulting in hypotension and kidney damage. Vasoconstrictor interaction: none
α₁-Adrenergic Blockers		
Doxazosin (Catapres), prazosin (Minipress), terazosin (Hytrin)	Dry mouth, taste changes	Orthostatic hypotension; avoid prolonged use of NSAIDs—may reduce antihypertensive effects. Vasoconstrictor interaction: none

Continued

TABLE 3.3 Drugs Used in the Management of Hypertension—cont'd

Drug	Oral Adverse Effects	Dental Considerations
Central α₂-Adrenergic Agonists and Other Centrally Acting Drugs		
Clonidine (Catapres), methyldopa (Aldomet), reserpine (generic), guanfacine (Tenex)	Dry mouth, taste changes	Orthostatic hypotension. Vasoconstrictor interaction: none
Direct Vasodilators		
Hydralazine (Apresoline), minoxidil (Loniten)	Lupus-like oral and skin lesions, lymphadenopathy	Orthostatic hypotension; avoid prolonged use of NSAIDs—may reduce antihypertensive effects. Vasoconstrictor interaction: none

NSAID, nonsteroidal antiinflammatory drug.

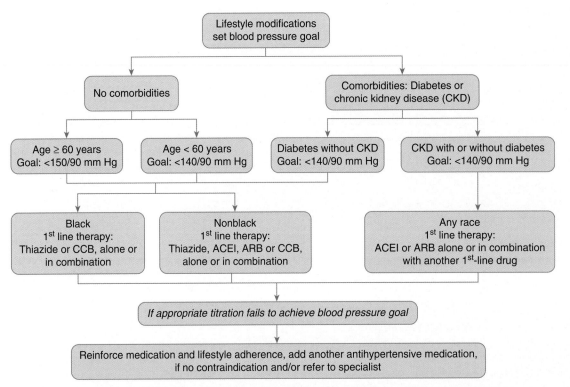

ACEI, angiotensin-converting enzyme inhibitor; ARB, angiotensin receptor blocker; CCB: calcium channel blocker; CKD: chronic kidney disease .

FIG. 3.2 Joint national committee on prevention, detection, evaluation, and treatment of high blood pressure 8 treatment recommendations and algorithm. (Adapted and created from Joint National Committee on Hypertension eighth report.)

as congestive heart failure, cerebrovascular disease, MI, renal disease, peripheral vascular disease, or diabetes mellitus. These conditions should be identified as well because they may necessitate modification of the dental management plan.

In addition to a medical history, all new patients and all recall patients should undergo BP measurement on a routine basis (see Chapter 1). More frequent BP measurements are indicated for patients who are not compliant with treatment, whose hypertension is poorly controlled, or who have comorbid conditions such as

heart failure, a previous MI, or stroke. In patients who are being treated for hypertension but have BPs above normal, the most common reason for the persistent HBP is noncompliance or inadequate treatment; they should be encouraged to return to their physician for follow-up care. A patient who has not been diagnosed with hypertension but who has an abnormally elevated BP should also be encouraged to see his or her physician. When a patient who has stage 2 BP is receiving dental treatment, consideration should be given to leaving the BP cuff on the patient's arm and periodically checking the pressure

TABLE 3.4 Expert Opinion on Management of Severe Uncontrolled Hypertension

Blood Pressure Reading (mm Hg)	Symptoms or Organ Damage	Recommendations
"Severe Uncontrolled Hypertension"		
>180/110 (diastolic <120)	No	Treatment within 1 week—not an emergency; gradually lower BP during a period of days and before surgical procedures
"Hypertensive Urgency"		
>180/120	No	Early treatment; gradually reduce BP with short-acting oral antihypertensives; hours of observation, and then follow-up visit within 1 to a few days
"Hypertensive Emergency"		
>180/120	Yes	Immediate treatment[a] (reduce BP within 1 h) with parental antihypertensives in
≥210/120	Yes or no	hospital; hours of observation, and then follow-up visit with physician within 1 to a few days

[a]Immediate treatment: blood pressure (BP) reduction (within 1 h) may require admission to an intensive care unit.
Based on Chobanian AV, Bakris GL, Black HR, et al. The seventh report of the joint national committee on prevention, detection, evaluation, and treatment of high blood pressure: the JNC 7 report. *JAMA.* 2003;289(19):2560–2572; Pak KJ, Hu T, Fee C, et al. Acute hypertension: a systematic review and appraisal of guidelines. *Ochsner J.* 2014;14(4):655–663.

during the appointment. The dentist should not make a diagnosis of hypertension but rather should inform the patient that the BP reading is elevated and that a physician should evaluate the condition.

The primary concern in dental management of a patient with hypertension is that during the course of treatment, a sudden, acute elevation in BP might occur, potentially leading to a serious outcome such as stroke or MI. Such acute elevations in BP may result from the release of endogenous catecholamines in response to stress and anxiety, from injection of exogenous catecholamines in the form of vasoconstrictors in the local anesthetic, or from absorption of a vasoconstrictor from gingival retraction cord. Other concerns include potential drug interactions between the patient's antihypertensive medications and the drugs used in dental practice and oral adverse effects that may be caused by antihypertensive medications.

Risk Assessment. Two important questions should be answered before dental treatment is provided for a patient with hypertension:

- What are the associated risks of treatment in this patient?
- At what level of BP is treatment unsafe for the patient?

The ACC/AHA have jointly published practice guidelines for the perioperative evaluation of patients with cardiovascular disease for whom noncardiac surgery of various types is planned. These guidelines provide a framework to estimate the risk for occurrence of a stroke, MI, acute heart failure, or sudden death as a result of the surgery. Oral and maxillofacial surgery and periodontal surgery both are forms of noncardiac surgery; thus, these guidelines are directly applicable. In addition, the ACC/AHA guidelines may be extrapolated and applied to

nonsurgical dental treatment, as well. In the practice guidelines, the determination of risk includes the evaluation of three factors: (1) the risk imposed by the patient's cardiovascular disease, (2) the risk imposed by the surgery or procedure, and (3) the risk imposed by the functional reserve or capacity of the patient.

The risk imposed by the presence of a specific cardiovascular condition or disease is stratified into major, intermediate, and minor risk categories (Box 3.5). Uncontrolled BP, defined as 180/110 mm Hg or greater, is classified as a minor risk condition; however, the ACC/AHA guidelines include a statement that BP should be brought under control before any surgery is performed. Of note, current guidelines recommend timely or immediate referral for patients with BP of 180/110 mm Hg or higher, depending on the presence or absence of symptoms (Table 3.5).

Risk imposed by the type of surgery (or procedure) also is stratified into high- (>5% risk), intermediate- (<5% risk), and low-risk (<1% risk) categories. In general, risk is greatest with vascular or emergency surgery, prolonged procedures, and procedures associated with excessive blood loss and general anesthesia (Box 3.6). Head and neck surgery, which may include major oral and maxillofacial procedures and extensive periodontal procedures, is classified as intermediate risk. Superficial surgical procedures, which include minor oral and periodontal surgery and nonsurgical dental procedures, are classified as low risk. Thus, it appears that the risk associated with most general, outpatient dental procedures is very low.

The third factor involved in risk assessment is determination of the ability of the patient to perform certain physical activities (functional capacity) and is defined in metabolic equivalents (METs) (see Chapter 1). Perioperative cardiac risk is increased in patients who are unable to meet a 4-MET demand during most normal daily

BOX 3.5 Clinical Predictors of Increased Perioperative Cardiovascular Risk*

Major Risk Factors (also known as "Active Cardiac Conditions")
- Unstable coronary syndromes
  - Acute or recent myocardial infarction[†] with evidence of important ischemic risk in clinical signs and symptoms or noninvasive study
  - Unstable or severe angina (Canadian class III or IV)[†‡§]
- Decompensated heart failure
- Significant arrhythmias
- Severe valvular disease

Intermediate Risk Factors
- History of ischemic heart disease
- History of compensated or previous heart failure
- History of cerebrovascular disease
- Diabetes mellitus
- Renal insufficiency

Minor Risk Factors
- Advanced age (>70 years)
- Abnormal ECG (left ventricular hypertrophy, left bundle branch block, ST-T abnormalities)
- Rhythm other than sinus rhythm
- Uncontrolled systemic hypertension (blood pressure ≥180/110 mm Hg)

*Cardiac events of MI, heart failure, or death.
[†]The American College of Cardiology National Database Library defines acute MI as occurring within 7 days, and recent MI as occurring more than 7 days but within 1 month (at or before 30 days) before the procedure.
[‡]May include "stable" angina in patients who are unusually sedentary.
[§]Data from Campeau L: Grading of angina pectoris, Circulation 54:522–523, 1976. The Canadian classification is a system of grading angina severity (grades I–IV), with grade I angina occurring only with strenuous exertion and grade IV angina occurring with any physical activity or at rest.
Note: The Revised Cardiac Risk Index is a more recent approach that assigns one point for each clinical risk factor present, with those with three or more risk factors to be considered for pharmacological heart rate control if intermediate or high risk surgery is planned.
ECG, electrocardiogram.
Data from Fleisher LA, Beckman JA, Brown KA, et al. ACC/AHA 2007 guidelines on perioperative cardiovascular evaluation and care for noncardiac surgery: a report of the American College of Cardiology/American Heart Association task force on practice guidelines. *Circulation.* 2007;116:e418–e499. Fleisher LA, Beckman JA, Brown KA, et al. 2009 ACCF/AHA focused update on perioperative beta blockade incorporated into the ACC/AHA 2007 guidelines on perioperative cardiovascular evaluation and care for noncardiac surgery. *J Am Coll Cardiol.* November 24, 2009;54(22):e13–e118.

activities, which is equivalent to climbing a flight of stairs. Thus, a patient who reports inability to climb a flight of stairs without chest pain, shortness of breath, or fatigue would be at increased risk during a procedure.

Readers should be aware of risk calculators now available to help predict the likelihood/risk of a major adverse cardiac event associated with noncardiac surgical procedures and use these as appropriate.

Recommendations

Antibiotics. For patients who have hypertension, there is little to no risk of infection beyond that of a healthy patient. Antibiotics are not indicated.

Bleeding. Hypertension rarely causes concern for bleeding after dental procedures. A patient with hypertension who has cardiovascular comorbidities, such as previous MI or stroke, may be taking daily aspirin or another antiplatelet agents (e.g., clopidogrel). Surgical procedures can be performed normally under these circumstances. If the patient is taking an anticoagulant, additional precautions are advised (see Chapters 4 and 24).

Blood Pressure. Table 3.5 provides dental management recommendations for patients with various levels of BP. In summary, patients with BPs less than 180/110 mm Hg can undergo any necessary dental treatment, both surgical and nonsurgical, with very little risk of an adverse outcome. For patients found to have asymptomatic BP of 180/110 mm Hg or greater (uncontrolled hypertension), elective dental care should be deferred, and a physician referral for evaluation and treatment within 1 week is indicated. Patients with uncontrolled BP associated with symptoms such as headache, shortness of breath, or chest pain should be referred to a physician for immediate evaluation. In patients with uncontrolled hypertension, certain problems such as pain, infection, or bleeding may necessitate urgent dental treatment. In such instances, the patient should be managed in consultation with the physician, and measures such as intraoperative BP monitoring, ECG monitoring, establishment of an intravenous line, and sedation may be used. The decision must always be made as to whether the benefit of proposed treatment outweighs the potential risks.

If treatment of a patient with upper-level stage 2 hypertension is provided, it may be advisable to leave the BP cuff on the patient's arm and to periodically check the pressure. If the BP rises above 179/109 mm Hg and attempts to lower the BP fail, then the procedure should be terminated, the patient referred to his or her physician, and the appointment rescheduled.

Capacity to Tolerate Care. After it has been determined that the patient with hypertension can be safely treated, a management plan should be developed (Box 3.7). For all patients, the dentist should make every effort to reduce as much as possible the stress and anxiety associated with dental treatment. This consideration is particularly important in patients with hypertension. A critical factor in providing an anxiety-free situation is the relationship established among the dentist, the office staff, and the patient. Patients should be encouraged to express and discuss their fears, concerns, and questions about dental treatment.

Stress management is important for patients with hypertension to lessen the chances of endogenous release of catecholamines during the dental visit (see Chapter 1). Long or stressful appointments are best avoided. Short

TABLE 3.5 Dental Management and Follow-Up Recommendations Based on Blood Pressure

Blood Pressure (mm Hg)	Stage	Dental Treatment Recommendation	Follow-Up Recommendation
≤120/80	Normal	Any required	No physician referral necessary
≥120/80 but <130/80	Elevated	Any required	Screen at least semiannually if have risk factors for HBP; encourage patient to see physician
≥130/80 but <140/90	1	Any required	Encourage patient to see physician
≥140/90 but <180/110	2	Any required; consider intraoperative monitoring of BP for stage 2 hypertension	Refer patient to physician promptly (within 1 month)
≥180/110	Severe uncontrolled	Defer elective treatment	Refer to physician as soon as possible; if patient is symptomatic, refer immediately

BOX 3.6 Cardiac Risk* Stratification for Noncardiac Surgical Procedures

High (Reported Cardiac Risk Often >5%)
- Aortic and other major vascular surgery
- Peripheral vascular surgery

Intermediate (Reported Cardiac Risk Generally <5%)
- Intraperitoneal and intrathoracic surgery
- Carotid endarterectomy
- Head and neck surgery
- Orthopedic surgery
- Prostate surgery

Low (Reported Cardiac Risk Generally <1%)
- Endoscopic procedures
- Superficial procedures
- Cataract surgery
- Breast surgery
- Ambulatory surgery

*Combined incidence of cardiac death and nonfatal MI.
Adapted from Fleisher LA, Beckman JA, Brown KA, et al. ACC/AHA 2007 guidelines on perioperative cardiovascular evaluation and care for noncardiac surgery: executive summary: a report of the American College of Cardiology/American Heart Association task force on practice guidelines (writing committee to revise the 2002 guidelines on perioperative cardiovascular evaluation for noncardiac surgery). *Circulation.* 2007;116:1971–1996.

morning appointments seem best tolerated. If the patient becomes anxious or apprehensive during the visit, the appointment may be terminated and rescheduled for another day. Anxiety can be reduced for many patients by oral premedication with a short-acting benzodiazepine such as triazolam (Halcion; Pharmacia & Upjohn, Kalamazoo, MI), taken 1 h before the start of the dental appointment. Clonidine, an α2 adrenoreceptor agonist, is also potentially useful as a sedative and as an antihypertensive. The dose of these drugs is dictated by the age and size of the patient and is determined in accordance with prescribing guidelines for the agent selected. Nitrous oxide plus oxygen for inhalation sedation is an excellent intraoperative anxiolytic for use in patients with hypertension. Care is indicated to ensure adequate oxygenation at all times, and avoiding postdiffusion hypoxia at the termination of administration, which can be associated with resultant rebound elevation in BP.

Chair. Because some antihypertensive agents, especially α-blockers, α-β-blockers, and diuretics, tend to produce orthostatic hypotension as a side effect, rapid changes in chair position during dental treatment should be avoided. This effect can be potentiated by the actions of anxiolytic and sedative drugs. Thus, when treatment has concluded for that appointment, the dental chair should be returned slowly to an upright position. After sufficient time to permit adjustment to the change in posture, the patient should be physically supported while slowly getting out of the chair to ensure that good balance and stability have been regained. A patient who experiences dizziness or lightheadedness should be directed to sit back down to allow safe recovery of equilibrium.

Drug Considerations. Ambulatory (outpatient) general anesthesia in the dental office generally is recommended only for patients whose status on the American Society of Anesthesiologists (ASA) classification is ASA I (status of a healthy, normal patient) or ASA II (presence of mild to moderate systemic disease). Some patients with severe hypertension may be excluded.

Use of Vasoconstrictors. Profound local anesthesia is critical for pain and anxiety control and is especially important for patients with hypertension or other cardiovascular disease to decrease endogenous catecholamine release. The effectiveness of local anesthesia is enhanced by the inclusion of a vasoconstrictor in the local anesthetic solution, which delays systemic absorption, increases the duration of anesthesia, and provides local hemostasis. These properties allow for enhanced quality and duration of pain control and markedly facilitate performance of the technical procedures. Thus, the advantages of including a vasoconstrictor in the local anesthetic are obvious. Concerns have emerged, however, that the use of local anesthetic with a vasoconstrictor in a patient with hypertension could result in a potentially serious spike in BP.

BOX 3.7 | Checklist for Dental Management of Patients With Hypertension[a]

PREOPERATIVE RISK ASSESSMENT

- Review medical history, determine whether hypertension exists, and discuss relevant issues with the patient.
- Identify all medications and drugs being taken or supposed to be taken by the patient.
- Examine the patient for signs and symptoms of disease and obtain vital signs (i.e., take BP correctly).
- Review recent laboratory test results or images required to assess risk.
- Confirm patient has a primary care provider and has taken antihypertensive medication today.
- Obtain a medical consultation (i.e., refer to physician) if the patient is poorly controlled or is undiagnosed.
- If BP and vital signs are well controlled, routine dental procedures can be performed without special precautions.

A

Antibiotics	Avoid the use of erythromycin and clarithromycin (not azithromycin) with CCBs because the combination can enhance hypotension.
Anesthesia	Ensure profound local anesthesia. Modest doses of local anesthetic with 1:100,000 or 1:200,000 epinephrine (e.g., one or two carpules) at a given time are of little clinical consequence in patients with BP < 180/110 mm Hg. Greater quantities may be tolerated reasonably well but with increased risk. Levonordefrin should be avoided. In patients with uncontrolled hypertension (BP ≥ 180/110 mm Hg), the use of epinephrine should be limited.
Anxiety	Patients with hypertension who are anxious or fearful are candidates for preoperative oral or intraoperative inhalation sedation (or both). Apply good stress management protocols.

B

Bleeding	Excessive bleeding caused by hypertension is possible, but unlikely.
Breathing	No issues.
BP	Monitor BP. Patients with a BP < 180/110 mm Hg may receive any necessary dental treatment. For patients with a pressure reading >180/110 mm Hg, dental

treatment should be deferred until BP is brought under control. If urgent or emergency dental treatment is required, it should be done in as limited and conservative a manner as possible.

C

Capacity to tolerate care	Patients who have hypertension <180/110 mm Hg and are asymptomatic can receive routine dental care. A BP > 180/120 mm Hg is a hypertensive emergency, which dictates provision of immediate medical care.
Chair position	Avoid rapid position changes owing to possibility of antihypertensive drug-associated orthostatic hypotension.

D

Drugs	Avoid excessive amounts of epinephrine in patients who take nonselective β-adrenergic blockers, which can potentially cause a spike in BP and appears to be dose dependent; avoid the use of epinephrine-impregnated retraction cord. Several antihypertensive drugs have reported oral manifestations.
Devices	For patients with stage 2 hypertension (BP > 140/90 mm Hg), periodic monitoring of BP during treatment may be advisable.

E

Equipment	No issues.
Emergencies	Patients with hypertension are at increased risk for cardiovascular disease; although unlikely, angina, stroke, arrhythmia, and MI should be anticipated as possible occurrences.

F

Follow-up	• After the procedure, allow patient to sit in upright position for several minutes before dismissing to avoid dizziness. • Avoid long-term (>2 weeks) use of NSAIDs because these agents may interfere with effectiveness of some antihypertensive medications. • Ensure patient is receiving regular follow-up evaluation by physician; especially for patients with stage 2 hypertension (BP ≥ 140/90 mm Hg) and those with symptoms or comorbid

[a]Strength of recommendation taxonomy (SORT) Grade: C (see Preface for further explanation).
BP, Blood pressure; *CCB*, calcium channel blocker; *MI*, myocardial infarction; *NSAID*, nonsteroidal anti-inflammatory drug.

The cardiovascular response to conventional doses of injected epinephrine, both in patients who are healthy and in those with hypertension, usually is of little clinical importance. A metaanalysis of several clinical studies determined that the mean resting venous plasma epinephrine concentration is 39 pg/mL; this is approximately doubled by the intraoral injection of a single cartridge of 2% lidocaine with 1:100,000 epinephrine. This resulting elevation in plasma epinephrine is linear and dose dependent. Although large doses of epinephrine may cause a significant rise in BP and heart rate due to its α-adrenoreceptor activity, small doses such as those contained in one or two cartridges of lidocaine with 1:100,000 epinephrine cause minimal physiologic changes (Fig. 3.3). The minimal change in BP associated with small doses of lidocaine with 1:100,000 epinephrine is due to epinephrine's separate action on vascular β2 receptors, which results in vasodilation and a decrease in diastolic pressure. Thus, mean arterial pressure is essentially unchanged, with only a minimal increase in heart rate.

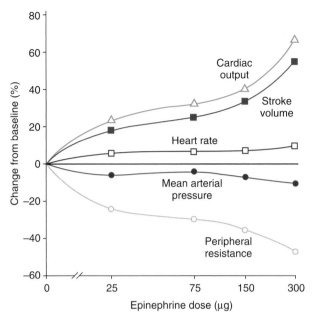

FIG. 3.3 Cardiovascular effects of epinephrine when used in regional anesthesia. (Redrawn from Jastak JT, Yagiela JA, Donaldson D. *Local Anesthesia of the Oral Cavity.* Philadelphia: Saunders; 1995.)

Several clinical investigations have evaluated changes in plasma epinephrine concentration and hemodynamic parameters in healthy patients after dental injections of 2% lidocaine with 1:100,000 epinephrine. After injection of 1.8 mL (one cartridge), plasma levels increased two- to threefold, but no significant changes were observed in heart rate or BP. With 5.4 mL of solution (three cartridges), however, plasma levels increased five- to sixfold; these changes were accompanied by significant increases in heart rate and systolic BP but with no adverse symptoms or sequelae. The critical question, then, is how a particular patient with hypertension or other cardiovascular disease will react to these dose challenges of epinephrine.

A systematic review of the literature on the cardiovascular effects of epinephrine in hypertensive dental patients concluded that although the quantity and quality of pertinent articles were problematic, the increased risk of adverse events among patients with uncontrolled hypertension was low, and the reported occurrence of adverse events associated with the use of epinephrine in local anesthetic agents was minimal. Another recent review of this subject noted an absence of adverse case reports involving epinephrine in local anesthetics and cited the numerous studies that demonstrated the safety and efficacy of these preparations.

Thus, the existing evidence indicates that use of modest doses (one or two cartridges of 2% lidocaine with 1:100,000 epinephrine) carries little clinical risk in patients with hypertension, and the benefits of its use far outweighing any potential problems. Use of more than this amount at one time may be tolerated but with

increasing risk for adverse hemodynamic changes. Levonordefrin should be avoided in patients with hypertension, however, because of its comparative excessive α_1 stimulation, and its lack of $\beta2$-adrenoceptor vasodilation. Use of epinephrine generally is not advised in patients with uncontrolled hypertension; instead elective dental care should be deferred. If urgent treatment becomes necessary, however, a decision must be made regarding the use of epinephrine, which will be dictated by the situation. A reasonable conclusion from all of the available evidence is that the benefits of use of epinephrine outweigh the increased risks, so long as modest doses (e.g., one or two carpules) are used at one time and care is taken to avoid inadvertent intravascular injection. Also, clinicians are advised to be aware of the different concentrations of epinephrine available in local anesthetics and use the appropriate concentration and dose based on the patient and procedure.

Drug Interactions. An additional concern when patients with hypertension are treated is the potential for adverse drug interactions between vasoconstrictors and antihypertensive drugs—specifically, the nonselective β-adrenergic blocking agents. The basis for concern with use of nonselective β-adrenergic blocking agents (e.g., propranolol) is that the normal compensatory vasodilatation of skeletal muscle vasculature mediated by β_2 receptors is inhibited by these drugs, and injection of epinephrine, levonordefrin, or any other pressor agent may result in uncompensated peripheral vasoconstriction because of unopposed stimulation of α_1 receptors. This vasoconstrictive effect could potentially cause a significant elevation in BP and a compensatory bradycardia. Several cases of this interaction have been reported in the literature that resulted in BPs exceeding 190/110 mm Hg and at least one death. However, the effect appears to be dose dependent, with the majority of adverse outcomes resulting when more than three carpules of local anesthetic with epinephrine were used. Adverse interactions are even less likely to occur in patients who take cardioselective β-blockers and when two carpules or less are used. Thus, the available evidence and clinical experience suggest that epinephrine in small doses of one to two cartridges containing 1:100,000 epinephrine can be used safely even in patients taking nonselective β-adrenergic-blocking agents. Indeed, a review by Brown and Rhodus concluded that adverse drug interactions between β-blockers and epinephrine were extremely unlikely; however, they noted that levonordefrin should be avoided.

Topical vasoconstrictors generally should not be used for local hemostasis in patients with hypertension. When performing crown and bridge procedures for patients with hypertension, the dentist should avoid using gingival retraction cord that contains epinephrine because this material contains highly concentrated epinephrine, which can be quickly absorbed through abraided gingival sulcus tissues, resulting in tachycardia and elevated BP. Alternative gingival hemostatic agents with minimal cardiovascular effects include products that contain 12%–20% ferric sulfate (Astringent, Ultradent Products, Inc., South Jordan, UT), or 25% aluminum chloride (ViscoStat, Ultradent Products, Inc., South Jordan, UT). Clinicians can also soak untreated retraction cord with tetrahydrozoline (Visine; Pfizer Inc., New York, NY), oxymetazoline (Afrin; Schering-Plough, Summit, NJ), or phenylephrine (Neo-Synephrine; Bayer, Morristown, NJ) to control gingival bleeding in these patients.

A few additional drug interactions should be considered. Erythromycin and clarithromycin can exacerbate the hypotensive effect of CCBs and result in acute kidney injury. Thus, this interaction should be avoided. Anxiolytics and sedatives may be used for patients who take antihypertensive medications; however, the usual dosage may need to be reduced, especially in older adults. Prolonged use of nonsteroidal antiinflammatory drugs (NSAIDs) should be avoided in patients who have hypertension and take antihypertensive drugs. Prolonged NSAIDs use is associated with decreased efficacy of antihypertensive drugs and increased risk for MI and stroke in this population. This risk is likely due to NSAIDs' inhibition of cyclooxygenase and reduced prostaglandin I2 production concurrent with an imbalance in prothrombotic platelet thromboxane A2 production. The use of NSAIDs for a few days in these patients, however, does not significantly affect cardiovascular status.

Oral Manifestations. Oral complications have not been associated with hypertension itself. The development of facial palsy has been described in the occasional patient with malignant hypertension. Excessive bleeding after surgical procedures or trauma has been reported in patients with severe hypertension; however, such bleeding in this patient population is uncommon. Patients who take antihypertensive drugs, especially diuretics, may experience hyposalivation and complain of dry mouth. Mercurial diuretics may cause oral lesions with an allergic or toxic basis. Lichenoid reactions have been reported with thiazides, methyldopa, propranolol, and labetalol. ACE inhibitors may cause neutropenia, resulting in delayed healing or gingival bleeding. Angioedema, a persistent cough, and oral burning sensations are associated with ACE inhibitor use. CCBs can cause gingival overgrowth, with highest prevalence occurring with nifedipine (Fig. 3.4; see also Table 3.3).

BIBLIOGRAPHY

1. Whelton PK, Carey RM, Aronow WS, et al. 2017 ACC/AHA/AAPA/ABC/ACPM/AGS/APhA/ASH/ASPC/NMA/PCNA guideline for the prevention, detection, evaluation, and management of high blood pressure in adults: a report of the American College of Cardiology/American Heart Association Task Force on Clinical Practice Guidelines, *Hypertension.* 2018; 71(6):e13–e115.
2. Bader JD, Bonito AJ, Shugars DA. A systematic review of cardiovascular effects of epinephrine on hypertensive dental patients. *Oral Surg Oral Med Oral Pathol Oral Radiol Endod.* 2002;93(6):647–653.
3. Barengo NC, Kastarinen M, Antikainen R, et al. The effects of awareness, treatment and control of hypertension on cardiovascular and all-cause mortality in a community-based population. *J Hum Hypertens.* 2009;23(12):808–816.
4. Bolivar JJ. Essential hypertension: an approach to its etiology and neurogenic pathophysiology. *Int J Hypertens.* 2013;2013:547809.
5. Bowles WH, Tardy SJ, Vahadi A. Evaluation of new gingival retraction agents. *J Dent Res.* 1991;70(11):1447–1449.
6. Brown RS, Farquharson AA, Sam FE, et al. A retrospective evaluation of 56 patients with oral burning and limited clinical findings. *Gen Dent.* 2006;54(4):267–271; quiz 72, 89–90.
7. Brown RS, Rhodus NL. Epinephrine and local anesthesia revisited. *Oral Surg Oral Med Oral Pathol Oral Radiol Endod.* 2005;100(4):401–408.
8. Burt VL, Whelton P, Roccella EJ, et al. Prevalence of hypertension in the US adult population. Results from the Third National Health and Nutrition Examination Survey, 1988–1991. *Hypertension.* 1995;25(3):305–313.
9. Centers for Disease Control and Prevention (CDC). *Hypertension. FastStats;* 2022. http://www.cdc.gov/nchs/fastats/hypertension.htm. Accessed August 20, 2022.
10. Centers for Disease Control and Prevention (CDC). *Hypertension Cascade: Hypertension Prevalence, Treatment and Control Estimates Among US Adults Aged 18 Years and Older Applying the Criteria from the American College of Cardiology and American Heart Association's 2017 Hypertension Guideline—NHANES 2013–2016 external icon.* Atlanta, GA: US Department of Health and Human Services; 2019.
11. Centers for Disease Control and Prevention. *Underlying Cause of Death, 1999–2018. CDC WONDER Online Database.* Atlanta, GA: Centers for Disease Control and Prevention; 2018. http://wonder.cdc.gov/ucd-icd10.html. Accessed March 12, 2020.

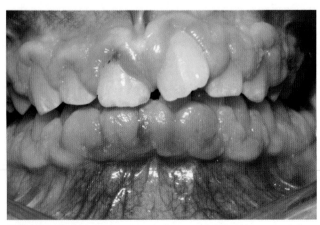

FIG. 3.4 Gingival overgrowth in a patient taking a calcium channel blocker. (Courtesy of Dr. Terry Wright.)

12. Chen L, Yang G. Recent advances in circadian rhythms in cardiovascular system. *Front Pharmacol*. 2015;6:71.

13. Cioffi GA, Chernow B, Glahn RP, et al. The hemodynamic and plasma catecholamine responses to routine restorative dental care. *J Am Dent Assoc*. 1985;111(1):67–70.

14. Chernow B, Balestrieri F, Ferguson CD, et al. Local dental anesthesia with epinephrine. Minimal effects on the sympathetic nervous system or on hemodynamic variables. *Arch Intern Med*. 1983;143(11):2141–2143.

15. Chobanian AV, Bakris GL, Black HR, et al. The seventh report of the joint national committee on prevention, detection, evaluation, and treatment of high blood pressure: the JNC 7 report. *JAMA*. 2003;289(19):2560–2572.

16. Dasgupta K, Quinn RR, Zarnke KB, et al. The 2014 Canadian hypertension education program recommendations for blood pressure measurement, diagnosis, assessment of risk, prevention, and treatment of hypertension. *Can J Cardiol*. 2014;30(5):485–501.

17. Fleisher LA, Beckman JA, Brown KA, et al. ACC/AHA 2007 guidelines on perioperative cardiovascular evaluation and care for noncardiac surgery: executive summary: a report of the American College of Cardiology/American Heart Association task force on practice guidelines (writing committee to revise the 2002 guidelines on perioperative cardiovascular evaluation for noncardiac surgery): developed in Collaboration with the American society of echocardiography, American society of nuclear cardiology, heart rhythm society, society of cardiovascular anesthesiologists, society for cardiovascular angiography and interventions, society for vascular medicine and biology, and society for vascular surgery. *Circulation*. 2007;116(17):1971–1996.

18. Fleisher LA, Fleischmann KE, Auerbach AD, et al. ACC/AHA guideline on perioperative cardiovascular evaluation and management of patients undergoing noncardiac surgery. *J Am Coll Cardiol*. 2014;64(22):e77–e137.

19. Flynn JT, Kaelber DC, Baker-Smith CM, et al. Clinical practice guideline for screening and management of high blood pressure in children and adolescents. *Pediatrics*. 2017;140(3):e20171904.

20. Foster CA, Aston SJ. Propranolol-epinephrine interaction: a potential disaster. *Plast Reconstr Surg*. 1983;72(1):74–78.

21. Franklin SS, Jacobs MJ, Wong ND, et al. Predominance of isolated systolic hypertension among middle-aged and elderly US hypertensives: analysis based on National Health and Nutrition Examination Survey (NHANES) III. *Hypertension*. 2001;37(3):869–874.

22. Franklin SS. Hypertension in older people: part 1. *J Clin Hypertens (Greenwich)*. 2006;8(6):444–449.

23. Gandhi S, Fleet JL, Bailey DG, et al. Calcium-channel blocker-clarithromycin drug interactions and acute kidney injury. *JAMA*. 2013;310(23):2544–2553.

24. Hatch CL, Chernow B, Terezhalmy GT, et al. Plasma catecholamine and hemodynamic responses to the placement of epinephrine-impregnated gingival retraction cord. *Oral Surg Oral Med Oral Pathol*. 1984;58(5):540–544.

25. Hersh EV, Giannakopoulos H. Beta-adrenergic blocking agents and dental vasoconstrictors. *Dent Clin N Am*. 2010;54(4):687–696.

26. Houben H, Thien T, van't Laar A. Effect of low-dose epinephrine infusion on hemodynamics after selective and nonselective beta-blockade in hypertension. *Clin Pharmacol Ther*. 1982;31(6):685–690.

27. James PA, Oparil S, Carter BL, et al. 2014 evidence-based guideline for the management of high blood pressure in adults: report from the panel members appointed to the Eighth Joint National Committee (JNC 8). *JAMA*. 2014;311(5):507–520.

28. Knapp JF, Fiori T. Oral hemorrhage associated with periodontal surgery and hypertensive crisis. *J Am Dent Assoc*. 1984;108(1):49–51.

29. Kram J, Bourne HR, Melmon KL, et al. Letter: propranolol. *Ann Intern Med*. 1974;80(2):282.

30. Kung H-C, Xu J. *Hypertension-related Mortality in the United States, 2000–2013*. 2015:193. NCHS Data Brief.

31. Lee TH, Marcantonio ER, Mangione CM, et al. Derivation and prospective validation of a simple index for prediction of cardiac risk of major noncardiac surgery. *Circulation*. 1999;100:1043–1049.

32. Lewington S, Clarke R, Qizilbash N, et al. Age-specific relevance of usual blood pressure to vascular mortality: a meta-analysis of individual data for one million adults in 61 prospective studies. *Lancet*. 2002;360(9349):1903–1913.

33. Livada R, Shiloah J. Calcium channel blocker-induced gingival enlargement. *J Hum Hypertens*. 2014;28(1):10–14.

34. Mito RS, Yagiela JA. Hypertensive response to levonordefrin in a patient receiving propranolol: report of case. *J Am Dent Assoc*. 1988;116(1):55–57.

35. Miura K, Daviglus ML, Dyer AR, et al. Relationship of blood pressure to 25-year mortality due to coronary heart disease, cardiovascular diseases, and all causes in young adult men: the Chicago Heart Association Detection Project in Industry. *Arch Intern Med*. 2001;161(12):1501–1508.

36. National High Blood Pressure Education Program Working Group on High Blood Pressure in C, Adolescents. The fourth report on the diagnosis, evaluation, and treatment of high blood pressure in children and adolescents. *Pediatrics*. 2004;114(2 suppl 4th report):555–576.

37. Nwankwo T, Yoon SS, Burt V, et al. Hypertension among adults in the United States: National Health and Nutrition Examination Survey, 2011–2012. *NCHS Data Brief*. 2013;133:1–8.

38. Oates JA, FitzGerald GA, Branch RA, et al. Clinical implications of prostaglandin and thromboxane A2 formation (1). *N Engl J Med*. 1988;319(11):689–698.

39. Pak KJ, Hu T, Fee C, et al. Acute hypertension: a systematic review and appraisal of guidelines. *Ochsner J*. 2014;14(4):655–663.

40. Pickering TG. Isolated diastolic hypertension. *J Clin Hypertens (Greenwich)*. 2003;5(6):411–413.

41. Pickering TG, Hall JE, Appel LJ, et al. Recommendations for blood pressure measurement in humans and experimental animals: part 1: blood pressure measurement in humans: a statement for professionals from the Subcommittee of Professional and Public Education of the American Heart Association Council on High Blood Pressure Research. *Circulation*. 2005;111(5):697–716.

42. Reeves RA, Boer WH, DeLeve L, et al. Nonselective beta-blockade enhances pressor responsiveness to epinephrine, norepinephrine, and angiotensin II in normal man. *Clin Pharmacol Ther*. 1984;35(4):461–466.

43. Reinprecht F, Elmstahl S, Janzon L, et al. Hypertension and changes of cognitive function in 81-year-old men: a 13-year follow-up of the population study "Men born in 1914", Sweden. *J Hypertens*. 2003;21(1):57–66.

44. Schonberger RB, Fontes ML, Selzer A. *Anesthesia for Patients with Hypertension. UptoDate*; 2022. https://www.uptodate.com/contents/anesthesia-for-patients-with-hypertension. Accessed August 20, 2022.

45. Sheridan S, Pignone M, Donahue K. Screening for high blood pressure: a review of the evidence for the U.S. Preventive Services Task Force. *Am J Prev Med*. 2003;25(2):151–158.

46. Tai S, Mascaro M, Goldstein NA. Angioedema: a review of 367 episodes presenting to three tertiary care hospitals. *Ann Otol Rhinol Laryngol*. 2010;119(12):836–841.

47. Tolas AG, Pflug AE, Halter JB. Arterial plasma epinephrine concentrations and hemodynamic responses after dental injection of local anesthetic with epinephrine. *J Am Dent Assoc*. 1982;104(1):41–43.

48. Tomek M, Nandoskar A, Chapman N, et al. Facial nerve palsy in the setting of malignant hypertension: a link not to be missed. *QJM*. 2015;108(2):145–146.

49. Turnbull F. Blood Pressure Lowering Treatment Trialists C. Effects of different blood-pressure-lowering regimens on major cardiovascular events: results of prospectively-designed overviews of randomised trials. *Lancet*. 2003;362(9395):1527–1535.

50. Victor R. *Arterial hypertension. Goldman-Cecil Medicine.* 25th ed. Philadelphia: Saunders; 2016:381–397.

51. Victor R, Kaplan A. Systemic hypertension: mechanisms and diagnosis. In: Libby P, ed. *Braunwald's Heart Disease: A Textbook of Cardiovascular Medicine.* 8th ed. Philadelphia: Saunders; 2008:1027–1048.

52. Weber MA, Schiffrin EL, White WB, et al. Clinical practice guidelines for the management of hypertension in the community a statement by the American Society of Hypertension and the International Society of Hypertension. *J Hypertens*. 2014;32(1):3–15.

53. Whelton PK, Carey RM, Aronow WS, et al. 2017 ACC/AHA/AAPA/ABC/ACPM/AGS/APhA/ASH/ASPC/NMA/PCNA guideline for the prevention, detection, evaluation, and management of high blood pressure in adults external icon. *Hypertension*. 2018;71(19):e13–e115.

54. Wright JM, Musini VM. First-line drugs for hypertension. *Cochrane Database Syst Rev*. 2009;3:CD001841.

55. Xie X, Atkins E, Lv J, et al. Effects of intensive blood pressure lowering on cardiovascular and renal outcomes: updated systematic review and meta-analysis. *Lancet*. 2016;387(10017):435–443.

Ischemic Heart Disease

Coronary atherosclerotic heart disease is the leading health problem in the United States and the world. Atherosclerosis is the buildup of lipid plaque in the walls of arteries. The atherosclerotic process results in a narrowed arterial lumen with diminished blood flow and oxygen supply. Atherosclerosis is the most common underlying cause of coronary heart disease (angina and myocardial infarction [MI]), cerebrovascular disease (stroke), and peripheral vascular disease (intermittent claudication).

Symptomatic coronary atherosclerotic heart disease often is referred to as ischemic heart disease. Ischemic symptoms are the result of oxygen deprivation secondary to reduced blood flow to a portion of the myocardium. Other conditions such as embolism, coronary ostial stenosis, coronary artery spasm, and congenital abnormalities also may cause ischemic heart disease. Dental practitioners should be aware that these patients are at risk for angina, MI, stroke, or peripheral artery disease.

EPIDEMIOLOGY

More than 85 million Americans ($\approx$25% of the population) have some form of cardiovascular disease, with about 18.2 million having coronary artery disease (CAD). Cardiovascular atherosclerotic disease begins early in life, and autopsy studies have shown that one in six American teenagers already has pathologic intimal thickening of the coronary arteries. The incidence and prevalence of ischemic heart disease increase with age; its symptoms and complications typically manifest in midlife, and more than half of those affected are older than 59 years of age.

Cardiovascular diseases continue to be the leading cause of death in the United States, accounting for about 29% of all deaths. CAD accounts for the majority of cardiac arrests, 13% of deaths in the United States, and is the leading cause of death after age 65 years. CAD is responsible for 805,000 new or recurrent heart attacks annually, of which more than 40% are fatal. Of the 805,000 Americans who have a heart attack each year, it is a first heart attack for 605,000 and a recurrent heart attack in the remaining 200,000. About 356,000 adults have a sudden cardiac arrest in the United States each year and nearly 90% of these events are fatal. Men are at higher risk than women for having a heart attack or fatal CAD, and black men are at highest risk. In the United States the average age at first heart attack is reported to be 65.6 years for men and 72.0 years for women.

The average dental practice with 2000 patients is expected to include at least 100 patients with ischemic heart disease.

ETIOLOGY

Coronary atherosclerosis is the result of inflammation and cholesterol buildup in the intimal layer of the arterial wall. This disease is related to a variety of risk factors; several of these are associated with behavior (Table 4.1).

Age, Sex, and Race. Before the age of 75 years, the risk of coronary atherosclerosis is greater for men than for

TABLE 4.1 Risk Factors for Coronary Atherosclerosis

Modifiable (Lifestyle Choices)	Not Modifiable
Hypertension, cigarette smoking	Older age
Physical inactivity	Male gender
Diet rich in simple sugars and starches	Family history of cardiovascular disease
Obesity, insulin resistance, diabetes mellitus	
Hyperlipidemia	Genetic hyperlipidemia
Mental stress, depression	
Infections and systemic inflammation	

women. MI and sudden death are rare in premenopausal women; however, after menopause the incidence rises in women. Clinical manifestations of coronary atherosclerosis are more common among men of nonwhite populations (e.g., African Americans, Native Americans, Hispanics, Latinos), which relates to social, economic, and historical disparities and differences in environment, personal behavior, and habits.

Genetics. Studies have confirmed that a paternal history, sibling history, or history in both parents of coronary atherosclerotic heart disease increases the risk for development of the disease at a younger age than typical for those without such a history.

Diet. Elevation in serum lipid levels is a major risk factor for atherosclerosis. Increased levels of small dense low-density lipoprotein (LDL) cholesterol and its subparticle (β-lipoprotein levels, ApoB) pose the greatest risk for coronary atherosclerosis, whereas increased levels of high-density lipoprotein (HDL) cholesterol have been shown to reduce risk. Persons with elevated triglyceride also have increased risk for the disease. Obesity and a diet rich in simple sugars and starches with high glycemic index (e.g., processed foods), red meat, and trans fats enhance the risk of developing CAD.

High blood pressure (HBP). HBP is one of the most significant risk factors for coronary atherosclerotic heart disease. In general, systolic blood pressure (SBP) is more strongly related to the incidence of cardiovascular disease than is diastolic blood pressure (DBP), especially in older adults. SBP rises throughout life, and DBP tends to level off or decrease after the age of 50 years. Most epidemiologic studies, however, recognize the importance of both DBP and SBP in the assessment of cardiovascular risk. It has been shown that morbidity and mortality increase linearly with blood pressures greater than 115/75 mm Hg. In the Framingham Study, SBP of 130–139 mm Hg and DBP of 85–89 mm Hg was associated with a risk of cardiovascular disease double that for lower pressures.

Smoking. Cigarette smoking is the single most important modifiable risk factor for coronary heart disease (see Chapter 8). Multiple prospective studies have clearly documented that, compared with nonsmokers, persons who smoke 20 or more cigarettes daily have a two- to fourfold increase in CAD. This increased risk appears to be proportionate to the number of cigarettes smoked per day, with habit cessation having well-documented benefits. In a study of 113,752 women and 88,496 men, smokers who quit by age 34 years gained 10 years of life, those quitting between 35 and 44 years gained 9 years, and those 45–54 years gained 6 years of life, on average, compared with those who continued to smoke. Pipe and cigar smoking apparently convey minor risk for development of heart disease.

Diabetes. Patients with diabetes mellitus have a greater incidence of CAD and more extensive lesions. In diabetics CAD develops at an earlier age than that typical for persons who do not have diabetes. Almost 88 million Americans have some degree of abnormal glucose tolerance (prediabetes)—a condition that along with obesity markedly increases the risk for type 2 diabetes and premature atherosclerosis (see Chapter 14). Patients with diabetes have two- to eightfold higher rates of future cardiovascular events compared with age-matched and ethnically matched nondiabetic patients. Three-fourths of all deaths among patients with diabetes result from CAD. Compared with unaffected persons, patients with diabetes have a greater degree of atherosclerosis in the major arteries and in the microvascular circulation. Although hyperglycemia is associated with microvascular disease, insulin resistance itself promotes atherosclerosis even before it produces frank diabetes, and available data corroborate the role of insulin resistance as an independent risk factor for atherothrombosis. *Metabolic syndrome* is the term used to describe a cluster of pathologic findings consisting of obesity, insulin resistance, low HDL cholesterol, elevated triglycerides, and hypertension, all of which are risk factors for atherosclerosis. The recognized importance of this clinical syndrome as a setting for the development of atherosclerosis reflects a synergistic effect of the multiple risk factors. The prevalence of metabolic syndrome among adults in the United States is estimated to be about 34%, which increases with age from about 19.5% in 20–39 years to 48.6% of those 60 years or older.

Inflammation. Inflammation is a known risk factor for cardiovascular disease and acute coronary events; known drivers of inflammation are microbial infections and inflammatory diseases including periodontal disease. Studies have shown that persons with chronic periodontal disease have two to three times the risk of having a heart attack, stroke, or other serious cardiovascular event as those who do not have periodontal disease. Although the causal mechanism has not been fully demonstrated, chronic periodontal disease appears to contribute by allowing periodontal pathogens to (i) enter the circulation and induce systemic inflammation, (ii) promote atheroma formation, (iii) translocate and enter atherothrombotic lesions, and (iv) impair vascular endothelial function (i.e., arterial stiffness).

No single risk factor is responsible for the development of coronary atherosclerosis, but many factors act synergistically. Evidence suggests that lifestyle modification of risk factors that can be controlled, such as cigarette smoking, hypertension, obesity, sedentary activity, hyperlipidemia, diabetes, and oral health, can reduce or modify the clinical effects of the disease.

PATHOPHYSIOLOGY AND COMPLICATIONS

Atherosclerosis is an inflammatory disorder of the cellular lining of the arteries, with inflammation playing a fundamental role at all stages of the disease. The formation of atheromatous plaques involves several steps. The first step involves an inflammatory repair response of the injured arterial intima. Chronic injury to the arterial endothelium is common and results from both physiologic and pathologic processes. Physiologic injury often occurs as the result of disturbed blood flow at bending points or bifurcations (branch points) in the artery. Endothelial injury or dysfunction also may be caused by hypercholesterolemia, oxidative stress, glycation end products in diabetes, irritants in tobacco smoke, circulating vasoactive amines, immune complexes, and infection.

Atheroma formation is initiated by adherence of *monocytes* to an area of injured or altered endothelium. Monocytes usually do not adhere to intact endothelium; however, triggers of atherosclerosis such as a high-saturated-fat diet, smoking, hypertension, hyperglycemia, obesity, and insulin resistance initiate the expression of adhesion molecules by the endothelial cells, thus promoting attachment. The attached monocytes then migrate into the intima of the vessel and become *macrophages*. Lipids derived from plasma LDLs enter through damaged endothelium, forming extracellular deposits or small pools. Macrophages then engulf lipid molecules to become foam cells, which are characteristic features of the fatty streak. Foam cells are highly inflammatory, and when joined by T lymphocytes, together they produce a variety of inflammatory cytokines, which promote the migration and proliferation of smooth muscle cells and collagen to surround the foam cells, thereby forming a fibrous covering or cap. The arrival of the smooth muscle cells triggers a coalescence of the foam cells and small extracellular pools of lipid into a larger pool or lipid core. The T lymphocytes secrete cytokines that inhibit the further production of collagen, along with myeloperoxidase produced by the white blood cells, possibly lead to weakening and thinning of the fibrous cap and rendering it susceptible to rupture. With erosion or rupture of the plaque surface, tissue factor comes into contact with blood, and a thrombus is subsequently formed (Fig. 4.1).

Plaques may grow and proliferate outwardly, away from the lumen of the artery, or inwardly, into the lumen. With inward proliferation, the size of the lumen is

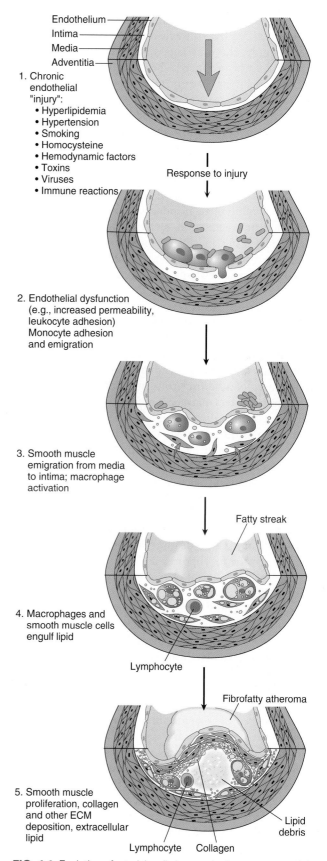

FIG. 4.1 Evolution of arterial wall changes in the response to injury hypothesis. *ECM,* extracellular matrix. (From Schoen FJ. Blood vessels. In: Kumar V, et al., eds. *Robbins and Cotran Pathologic Basis of Disease.* 8th ed. Philadelphia: Saunders; 2010.)

progressively reduced (stenosis). Thus, blood flow may be chronically decreased, and when the demand for oxygen exceeds supply, the outcome is ischemic pain. Ischemic symptoms may be produced when occlusion reaches 75% of the cross-sectional area of the artery (Fig. 4.2). However, in most instances of an acute coronary event, the vessels are less than 50% occluded by plaque growth.

Acute coronary syndromes (ACSs, e.g., unstable angina [UA], MI) are caused most often by physical disruption or fracture of the vulnerable atheromatous plaque. In plaque rupture, the fibrous cap tears, allowing arterial blood to enter the lipid core, where contact with tissue factor and collagen induces platelet adhesion and aggregation and activation of the coagulation cascade. These events result in clot or thrombus formation and sudden expansion of the lesion. Blood flow through the affected artery may become compromised or completely blocked.

Atherosclerosis usually is a focal disease that commonly occurs in certain areas or regions of arteries while sparing others. Those affected include the brain, heart, aorta, and peripheral arteries (Fig. 4.3). The proximal left anterior descending coronary artery is a common area of atherosclerotic involvement. The lumen of an affected artery may be circumferentially narrowed evenly or eccentrically, depending on the location and extent of the plaque; collateral circulation may develop to compensate for diminished blood flow. For lesions that produce symptoms, flow-limiting intact plaques typically precipitate symptoms such as chest pain (angina) when oxygen need exceeds demand, as during physical activity. However, plaque rupture produces an acute or unstable clinical picture with signs and symptoms such as angina at rest, MI, or sudden death. Not all plaques have the same propensity to rupture, and risk depends on the physical and biochemical characteristics of the plaque as well as level of systemic inflammation.

Intraarterial complications of coronary atherosclerosis consist of luminal narrowing, intramural hemorrhage, thrombosis, embolism, and aneurysm. Intramural hemorrhage, which results from weakening of the intimal tissues, may lead to thrombosis. A thrombus, once formed, may become encapsulated and may undergo fibrous organization and recanalization.

If the degree of ischemia that results from coronary atherosclerosis is significant and the oxygen deficit is prolonged, the area of myocardium supplied by that vessel may undergo necrosis. Reduced blood flow may result from thrombosis of the affected artery, a hypotensive episode, an increased demand for blood, or emotional stress. The infarct, or area of necrosis, may be subendocardial or transmural, the latter involving the entire thickness of the myocardium (Fig. 4.4). A significant clot in a coronary artery that leads to oxygen insufficiency or infarct can trigger ventricular fibrillation, a significant electrical conduction arrhythmia (see Chapter 5).

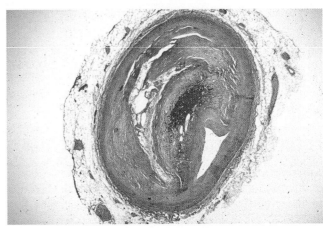

FIG. 4.2 Photomicrograph of a cross section of a coronary artery with severe stenosis and narrowing. (Courtesy of W. O'Conner, MD, Lexington, KY.)

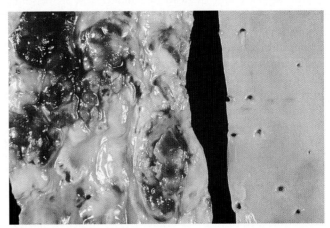

FIG. 4.3 The segment of aorta on the *left* demonstrates advanced atheromatous plaques, and the specimen on the *right* side is unaffected. (Courtesy of W. O'Conner, MD, Lexington, KY.)

Complications of MI include weakened heart muscle, resulting in congestive heart failure, postinfarction angina, infarct extension, cardiogenic shock, pericarditis, and arrhythmias. Features of congestive heart failure include fatigue, dyspnea, orthopnea, paroxysmal nocturnal dyspnea, edema, hemoptysis, fatigue, weakness, and cyanosis (see Chapter 6). Causes of death in patients who have had an acute MI include ventricular fibrillation, cardiac standstill, congestive heart failure, embolism, and rupture of the heart wall or septum.

CLINICAL PRESENTATION

Symptoms

Chest pain due to ischemic myocardial pain is the most important symptom of CAD. This condition, known as *angina pectoris* or *angina*, results from an imbalance between the supply of oxygen-rich blood and the oxygen

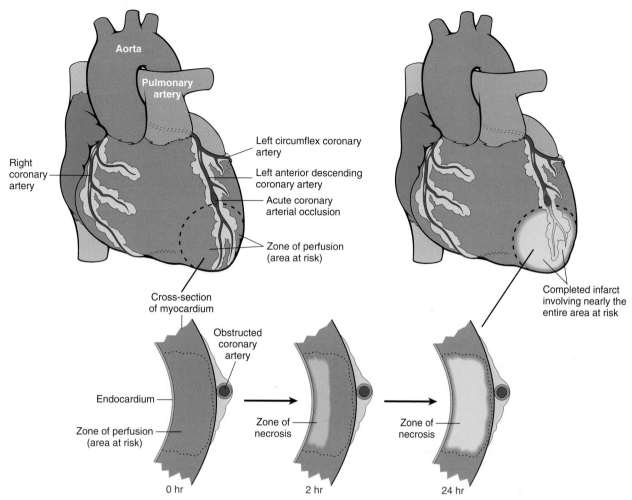

FIG. 4.4 Progression of myocardial necrosis after coronary artery occlusion. (From Schoen FJ, Mitchell, RN. The heart. In: Kumar V, et al., eds. *Robbins and Cotran Pathologic Basis of Disease.* 8th ed. Philadelphia: Saunders; 2010.)

demand of the muscle. Atherosclerotic narrowing of the coronary arteries is an important cause of this imbalance.

Angina pectoris is described as a sensation of aching, heavy, squeezing pressure, or tightness in the midchest region that may radiate into the shoulder, left or right arm, neck, or lower jaw. In rare cases, it may be present in only one of these distant sites, and the patient is free of central chest pain. The pain is of brief duration, lasting 5−15 min if the provoking stimulus is stopped or for a shorter time if nitroglycerin is used.

Angina is defined in terms of its pattern of symptom stability. *Stable angina* is pain that is predictably reproducible, unchanging, and consistent over time. The pain typically is precipitated not only by exertion such as walking or climbing stairs but also may occur with eating or stress; it is relieved by cessation of the precipitating activity, by rest, or with the use of nitroglycerin. Unstable angina (*UA*) is defined as new-onset pain, pain that is increasing in frequency, increasing in intensity, precipitated by less effort than before, or occurring at rest. This pain is not readily relieved by nitroglycerin. The key

feature is the changing character (increasing intensity) or pattern of the pain. Patients with stable angina have a relatively good prognosis. Patients with UA are at increased risk of an acute MI and have a poorer prognosis. A relatively uncommon form of angina, Prinzmetal variant angina, occurs at rest and is caused by focal spasm of a coronary artery, usually with varied amounts of atherosclerosis. Angina also may occur in persons with normal coronary vessels due to vaso-occlusive spasms. ACS describes a continuum of myocardial ischemia that ranges from UA at one end to non−ST segment MI at the other. Differentiation requires characterization of the symptoms along with diagnostic and laboratory testing. In patients with CAD, the severity and duration of chest pain helps distinguish UA from an acute MI. During an acute MI, the pain usually is more severe and lasts longer than 15 min but has the same general character as that described for stable angina. Its location is the same as for the brief pain that results from temporary myocardial ischemia, and it may radiate in the same pattern into the shoulder, left or right arm, neck, or lower jaw and teeth.

Use of vasodilators or cessation of activity does not relieve the pain caused by infarction. Neither brief nor prolonged pain resulting from myocardial ischemia is aggravated by deep breathing. Of interest, women and men report different symptoms of MI, with fewer women experiencing chest pain but more often experiencing fatigue, dyspnea, and gastrointestinal complaints (e.g., heartburn).

Predominant symptoms and signs that most often precede sudden death include chest pain, cough, shortness of breath, diaphoresis, dizziness, fainting, fatigue, and palpitations (tachycardia). However, about 25% of patients have no symptoms before onset of the arrest.

Palpitations of the heart (disagreeable awareness of the heartbeat) may be present in patients with CAD with normal or abnormal rhythm. The complaint is not directly related to the seriousness of the underlying cardiac problem. Syncope, a transient loss of consciousness resulting from inadequate cerebral blood flow, also may occur in patients with coronary atherosclerotic heart disease.

Signs

Clinical signs of CAD are few, and the patient's clinical appearance may be entirely normal. Most clinical signs relate to other underlying cardiovascular disease or conditions such as congestive heart failure. Conditions such as corneal arcus and xanthoma of the skin are related to hyperlipidemia and hypercholesterolemia. Blood pressure may become elevated, and abnormalities in the rate and/or rhythm of the pulse may occur. Diminished peripheral pulses in the lower extremities may be noted, along with bruits in the carotid arteries. Panoramic radiographs of the jaws may demonstrate carotid calcifications, which are visible in the areas of vertebrae C3 and C4. These calcifications are risk markers of sustaining an adverse vascular event (MI, stroke) in the future. Retinal changes are common in hypertensive disease and diabetes mellitus. When advanced CAD is associated with congestive heart failure, signs can include fatigue, distention of neck veins, peripheral edema, cyanosis, ascites, and enlarged liver.

LABORATORY AND DIAGNOSTIC FINDINGS

Blood tests are used in the evaluation of atherosclerosis and ischemic heart disease, and to screen for abnormalities that may contribute to or worsen the disease. Tests include a complete blood count to rule out anemia, thyroid function tests to exclude hyperthyroidism, renal function tests to exclude renal insufficiency, lipid screening for hypercholesterolemia, and glucose screening for diabetes. Serum risk markers of atherosclerosis include elevated levels of C-reactive protein (CRP), fibrinogen (procoagulant), plasminogen activator inhibitor (thrombolytic), and apolipoprotein B (ApoB). Other diagnostic modalities that are specific for coronary heart disease include resting electrocardiogram (ECG), chest computed tomography, exercise stress testing,

ambulatory (Holter) electrocardiography, stress thallium-201 perfusion scintigraphy, exercise echocardiography, ambulatory ventricular function monitoring, and cardiac catheterization and coronary angiography.

The diagnosis of acute MI and determination of the extent of the infarction is based primarily on serum cardiac enzyme determinations, physical examination findings (symptoms of ischemia), and diagnostic test (ECG and echocardiogram) abnormalities (Box 4.1). Cardiac serum biomarkers of acute MI include troponin I, troponin T, creatine kinase isoenzyme (CK-MB), and myoglobin. Troponins and CK-MB are enzymes released only when cell death (infarction) or injury occurs. Troponins are proteins derived from the breakdown of myocardial sarcomeres. Troponin assays are the most sensitive and specific in differentiating cardiac muscle damage from trauma to skeletal muscle or other organs and are virtually absent in the plasma of normal persons and are found only after cardiac injury. Troponins are first detectable 2–4 h after the onset of an acute MI; they are maximally sensitive at 8–12 h, peak at 10–24 h, and persist for 5–14 days.

CK-MB is another enzymatic marker of cardiac cell injury with characteristics similar to those of the troponins; however, CK-MB is also found after injury to skeletal muscle and other tissues. Despite this relative lack of specificity, elevated levels of CK-MB are considered to be the result of an MI when criteria in Box 4.1 are met. CK-MB is detectable within 4 h after infarction; it reaches peak values at 12–24 h and persists for 2–4 days. In most cardiac centers, troponin assay has replaced CK-MB determination as the diagnostic test of choice for MI because of its sensitivity and specificity and as a result of cost issues. In any case, definitive diagnosis

---

BOX 4.1 **Diagnosis of Myocardial Infarction**

Detection of a rise and/or fall of cardiac biomarker values (preferably cardiac troponin) with at least one value above the 99 percentile upper reference limit and with at least one of the following:
- Symptoms of ischemia[a]
- ECG abnormality:
  - New or presumed new significant ST segment T-wave changes or new left bundle branch block
  - Development of pathological Q waves on ECG
- Evidence of myocardial injury:
  - Imaging evidence of a new loss of viable myocardium or new regional wall motion abnormality
- Identification of an intracoronary thrombus by angiography or autopsy.

[a]Note a review of over 430,000 patients with confirmed acute MI from the National Registry of Myocardial Infarction 2, one-third had no chest pain on presentation to the hospital based on Canto JG, Shlipak MG, Rogers WJ, et al. Prevalence, clinical characteristics, and mortality among patients with myocardial infarction presenting without chest pain. *JAMA.* 2000;283:3223.

of MI requires serial serum testing (every 2—8 h) over a few days. Testing for levels of B-natriuretic peptide, which is produced largely by the left ventricle, aids in determining the extent of ventricular damage and the prognosis of heart failure.

The extent of involvement of an acute MI is reflected in the ECG. Elevation of the ST segment (STEMI) is seen in cases with more complete obstruction, profound ischemia, and a larger area of necrosis. In contrast, the ST segment is not elevated (NSTEMI) in cases with only partial obstruction to blood flow and limited myocardial necrosis.

MEDICAL MANAGEMENT

Physicians are encouraged to enter patient and laboratory data into a cardiovascular (e.g., Framingham) risk score calculator (Fig. 4.5). These calculators help determine the long-term risk (e.g., 10-year risk) for CAD, which help guide medical treatment decisions.

Angina Pectoris

Medical management of a patient with chronic stable angina consists of an array of interventions as shown in (Box 4.2). Management may include general lifestyle

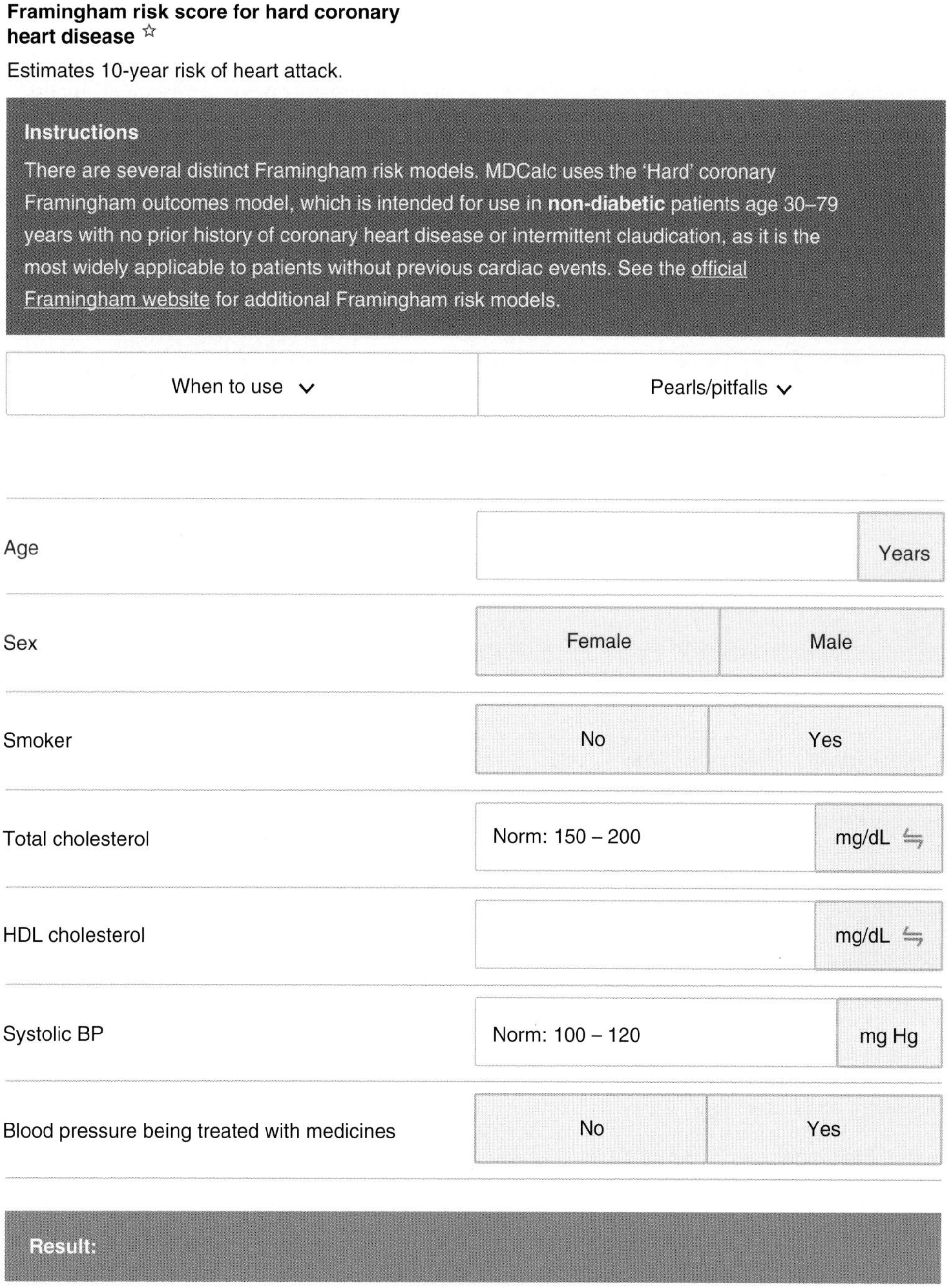

Framingham risk score for hard coronary heart disease ☆

Estimates 10-year risk of heart attack.

Instructions

There are several distinct Framingham risk models. MDCalc uses the 'Hard' coronary Framingham outcomes model, which is intended for use in **non-diabetic** patients age 30–79 years with no prior history of coronary heart disease or intermittent claudication, as it is the most widely applicable to patients without previous cardiac events. See the official Framingham website for additional Framingham risk models.

When to use ⌄	Pearls/pitfalls ⌄

Age	Years
Sex	Female / Male
Smoker	No / Yes
Total cholesterol	Norm: 150 – 200 · mg/dL ⇆
HDL cholesterol	mg/dL ⇆
Systolic BP	Norm: 100 – 120 · mg Hg
Blood pressure being treated with medicines	No / Yes

Result:

FIG. 4.5 Framingham risk score for hard coronary heart disease. (From MD+Calc, © 2005—2022. All rights reserved. https://www.mdcalc.com/framingham-risk-score-hard-coronary-heart-disease.)

BOX 4.2 **Medical Management of Patients With Stable Angina Pectoris**

- Identification and treatment of associated diseases that can precipitate or worsen angina (anemia, obesity, hyperthyroidism, sleep apnea)
- Reduction in risk factors for cardiovascular disease (hypertension, smoking, hyperlipidemia)
- Behavioral modification and lifestyle intervention (weight loss, exercise)
- Pharmacologic management
  - Nitrates
  - Beta-blockers
  - Calcium channel blockers
  - Antiplatelet agents
- Revascularization
  - Percutaneous transluminal coronary angioplasty with stenting
  - Coronary artery bypass grafting

---

measures such as an exercise program; weight control; restriction of salt, cholesterol, and saturated fatty acids; cessation of smoking; and control of exacerbating conditions such as anemia, hypertension, and hyperthyroidism. Patients who have significant angina are encouraged to avoid long hours of work, take rest periods during the working day, obtain adequate rest at night, use mild sedatives, employ stress reduction measures, and, in some cases, change their occupation or retire. Patients should avoid known precipitating factors that may bring on cardiac pain, such as cold weather, hot and humid weather, big meals, emotional upset, cigarette smoking, and certain drugs and stimulants (e.g., amphetamines, caffeine, ephedrine, cyclamates, alcohol).

Drug therapy consists of nitrates (nitroglycerin or long-acting nitrates), antiplatelet agents, statins, β-adrenergic blockers, calcium channel blockers (CCBs), and angiotensin-converting enzyme (ACE) inhibitors (Table 4.2). Nitrates are a cornerstone of the

---

TABLE 4.2 **Drugs Used in the Management of Angina**

Drug	Oral Adverse Effects	Dental Considerations
Nitrates		
Isosorbide dinitrate (Dilatrate-SR, Isonate, Isorbid, Isordil, Isotrate, Sorbitrate), isosorbide 5-mononitrate (Imdur, Ismo, Monoket), nitroglycerin (Minitran, Nitro-Dur, Nitrolingual, Nitro-Bid, Nitrek, Nitrol, Nitromist, Nitrostat, Nitro-Tab, Nitro-Time)	Dry mouth	Dizziness, orthostatic hypotension, headache Vasoconstrictor interactions: none
Beta-Blockers **Nonselective: Blockade of β_1 and β_2 Receptors**		
Carteolol (Cartrol), nadolol (Corgard), penbutolol (Levatol), pindolol (Visken), propranolol/LA (Inderal), sotalol (Betapace), timolol (Blocadren)	Taste changes, lichenoid reactions	Dizziness, orthostatic hypotension Vasoconstrictor interactions: increase in BP possible with sympathomimetics, limit use (maximum, 0.036 mg epinephrine; 0.20 mg levonordefrin)
Cardioselective: Blockade of β_1 Receptors Only		
Acebutolol (Sectral), Atenolol (Tenormin), Bisoprolol (Zebeta)[a], Metoprolol/XL (Lopressor), Nebivolol (Bystolic)		Vasoconstrictor interactions: minimal effect with sympathomimetics; normal use
Alpha- and Beta-Blockers		
Carvedilol (Coreg), Labetalol (Normodyne, Trandate)	Taste changes	Dizziness, orthostatic hypotension
Calcium Channel Blockers		
Amlodipine (Norvasc), Bepridil (Vascor), diltiazem (Cardizem, Cartia XT, Dilt-XR, Diltia XT, Taztia XT, Tiazac), felodipine (Plendil), isradipine (DynaCirc), nicardipine/SR (Cardene), nifedipine/PA/XL (Adalat, Nifediac, Procardia), nisoldipine (Sular), nitrendipine verapamil/SR (Calan, Isoptin, Verelan, Covera)	Gingival overgrowth, dry mouth, lichenoid eruptions (rare)	None Vasoconstrictor interactions: none Avoid prescribing macrolide antibiotics
Platelet Aggregation Inhibitors		
Aspirin	None	Increased bleeding, but not clinically significant with daily doses ≤325 mg. Vasoconstrictor interactions: none
Platelet Aggregation (P2Y12 Receptor) Inhibitors		
Clopidogrel (Plavix), Prasugrel (Effient), Ticagrelor (Brilinta)	None	Increased bleeding time. Vasoconstrictor interactions: none

[a]β_1 selective with low affinity for β_2.
BP, blood pressure.

pharmacologic management of angina. By action of vasodilation, they decrease cardiac load, resulting in decreased oxygen demand and hypotension. Nitrates also may alleviate coronary artery spasm. Nitroglycerin may be used acutely for the relief of anginal pain and prophylactically to prevent angina. Nitrates comes in a variety of forms, including tablets, lingual sprays, ointments, and transdermal patches. Nitroglycerin tablets are placed and dissolved under the tongue; the spray can be administered beneath the tongue or onto the oral mucosa. Nitrates are taken orally to prevent anginal symptoms and are supplied in tablet form, as a topical ointment or as long-acting transdermal nitrate patches that are applied to the skin. Nitrates are used to reduce symptoms of angina, but they do not slow, alter, or reverse the progression of CAD.

Beta-blockers, which are effective in the treatment of many patients with angina, compete with catecholamines for β-adrenergic receptor sites, resulting in decreased heart rate and myocardial contractility and reducing myocardial oxygen demand. There are nonselective β-blockers that block the β_1 and β_2 receptors, and cardioselective β-blockers that preferentially block the β_1 receptors. Nonselective β-blockers may cause unwanted effects, such as increasing the tone of vascular smooth muscle and causing both vasoconstriction of peripheral vessels and contraction of bronchial smooth muscle. Thus, nonselective β-blockers are not prescribed for patients with a history of asthma.

CCBs are effective in the treatment of chronic stable angina when given alone or in combination with β-blockers and nitrates. These drugs decrease intracellular calcium, resulting in vasodilation of coronary, peripheral, and pulmonary vasculature, along with decreased myocardial contractility and heart rate.

The statins inhibit 3-hydroxy-3-methylglutaryl—coenzyme A reductase (HMG-CoA) in the liver, thereby leading to enhanced expression of the LDL receptors that capture blood cholesterol. They are used to lower LDL cholesterol and increase HDL cholesterol and have been shown to decrease the risk for a major coronary event and the risk of death. Statins also are antiinflammatory.

ACE inhibitors are indicated for use in patients with CAD who also have diabetes, left ventricular dysfunction, or hypertension. The benefit of these agents appears to be primarily due to their antihypertensive effects. Angiotensin receptor blockers (ARBs) are used in patients who are intolerant to ACE inhibitors.

Antiplatelet therapy with aspirin is another cornerstone of treatment in patients with angina. Regular use of aspirin in patients with stable angina is associated with a significant reduction in fatal events, and in patients with UA, aspirin decreases the chances of fatal and nonfatal MI. Aspirin, in daily doses of 75—325 mg, is recommended for all patients with acute and chronic ischemic heart disease, regardless of the presence or absence of symptoms. Other oral antiplatelets (i.e., clopidogrel,

prasugrel, and ticagrelor) are used in place of, and often in combination with, aspirin (dual antiplatelet therapy) in patients who have ACS, after stent placement to prevent stent thrombosis, and after an acute MI.

Revascularization is an option for patients with stable or UA. Available procedures for revascularization include percutaneous transluminal coronary angioplasty, stents, and coronary artery bypass grafting. Percutaneous transluminal coronary angioplasty, also known as balloon angioplasty, involves the use of a small, inflatable balloon catheter over a thin guidewire that is threaded through the occluded segment of the artery. Once in place, the balloon is inflated and compresses the plaque and thrombus against the arterial wall, with consequent enlargement of the lumen of the vessel (Fig. 4.6). Widening of the lumen results in an immediate increase in blood flow and provides symptomatic relief for ischemia.

One method of decreasing the occurrence of restenosis with percutaneous transluminal coronary angioplasty involves the use of a thin, expandable, metallic mesh stent positioned by the balloon and expanded against the plaque and vessel wall, then left in place. The stent functions as a permanent scaffold to help maintain vessel patency (Fig. 4.7). The use of stents has decreased the incidence of restenosis to 3%—10% within 9 months; however, it has not prevented restenosis from occurring.

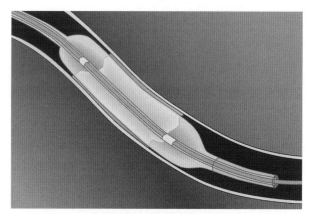

FIG. 4.6 Balloon angioplasty catheter. (From Teirstein PS. Percutaneous coronary interventions. In: Goldman L, Ausiello D, eds. *Cecil Textbook of Medicine*. 23rd ed. Philadelphia: Saunders; 2008.)

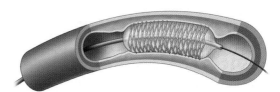

FIG. 4.7 Expandable metallic stent. The stent is left in place after deflation and withdrawal of the balloon catheter.

Restenosis is associated with a return of symptoms, and is more common in patients with diabetes.

Currently, two types of stents are used: bare metal and drug eluting. The bare metal stents maintain mechanical patency; however, they do not prevent endothelial proliferation that results in restenosis. Drug-eluting stents are coated with antiproliferative agents (e.g., sirolimus, everolimus) to control restenosis. Drug-eluting stents carry an increased risk for thrombosis for up to 1 year; therefore these patients require long-term use of dual antiplatelet drugs.

Other non–balloon angioplasty methods are rotational atherectomy and the use of lasers. With percutaneous intervention, a successful outcome is achieved in more than 95% of patients, with very few complications.

Coronary artery bypass graft (CABG) surgery is an effective means of controlling symptoms in the management of UA; it can improve the long-term survival rate in certain subsets of patients. It also is effective in controlling symptoms in patients whose pain persists despite medical control. With CABG, a segment of artery or vein is harvested or released from a donor site; it is then grafted to the affected segment of coronary artery, thus bypassing the area of occlusion (Fig. 4.8). Two primary

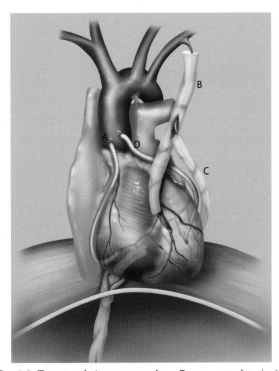

FIG. 4.8 Types of bypass grafts. Bypass grafts include reversed saphenous vein graft from aorta to right coronary artery (**A**), in situ left internal mammary artery graft to anterior descending coronary artery (**B**), Y graft of right internal mammary artery from left internal mammary artery to circumflex coronary artery (**C**), radial artery graft from the aorta to the circumflex coronary artery (**D**), and in situ gastroepiploic graft to the posterior descending branch of the right coronary artery (**E**). (Adapted from Lytle BW. Surgical treatment of coronary artery disease. In: Goldman L, Ausiello D, eds. *Cecil Textbook of Medicine*. 23rd ed. Philadelphia: Saunders; 2008.)

graft donor sites are used: the saphenous vein from the leg and the internal mammary artery from the chest. Of the two, the internal mammary artery graft is sturdier and much less susceptible to graft atherosclerosis and occlusion than are vein grafts. Within 10 years postoperatively, 30% of saphenous vein grafts become occluded, but internal mammary artery grafts are much more resistant to occlusion. The arterial grafts are preferred for first bypass procedures when possible. Reoperation is difficult because of surgical site scarring and the limited supply of graft donor material. The perioperative mortality rate for primary elective CABG procedures is less than 1%.

Myocardial Infarction

Patients who experience an acute MI should receive emergency treatment and should be hospitalized as soon as possible (Box 4.3). If the condition involves sudden cardiac arrest and loss of consciousness, basic life support should be provided that involves properly patient positioning, keeping the blood pumping and the airway open, and air exchange to the lungs (see Appendix A). Early administration of oxygen, nitrates, and aspirin is recommended. Oxygen is provided by nasal cannula to enhance oxygen saturation of the blood (to >90%) and keep the heart workload at a minimum level; nitrates are provided to reduce cardiac preload; and 81–325 mg of aspirin is chewed and swallowed by the conscious patient, which decreases platelet aggregation and limits

---

BOX 4.3 **Medical Management of Patients With Acute Myocardial Infarction**

- Rapid hospitalization and determination of ST segment changes
- Aspirin administration
- Early thrombolytic therapy (for patients with ST segment elevation only)
  - Reteplase or Tenecteplase > Alteplase
- Early revascularization
  - Thrombolysis (for patients with ST segment elevation only)
  - Percutaneous transluminal coronary angioplasty with stenting
  - Coronary artery bypass grafting
- Pharmacologic therapy
  - Antiplatelet drugs (aspirin, clopidogrel, or glycoprotein IIb/IIIa inhibitors: Abciximab [ReoPro], Tirofiban [Aggastat])
  - Anticoagulants (unfractionated heparin, low-molecular-weight heparin)
  - Nitrates
  - β-Adrenergic blockers
  - Calcium channel blockers
  - Angiotensin-converting enzyme inhibitors
  - Lipid-lowering drugs
  - Morphine (STMEI)
  - Sedative-hypnotics
- Oxygen (when O_2 saturation < 92%)

thrombus formation. Use of an automated external defibrillator may also be required if a shockable rhythm is identified.

The basic management goal of the medical team is to relieve the ischemia and pain, minimize the size of the infarction, and prevent death from lethal arrhythmias. The size and extent of the infarct are critical determinants of the outcome. Definitive treatment for patients with acute MI depends on the extent of ischemia as reflected on the ECG, which shows the presence or absence of STEMI (Fig. 4.9). An MI without ST segment elevation (non-STEMI) is caused by partial blockage of coronary blood flow. An MI with ST segment elevation (STEMI) is caused by complete blockage of coronary blood flow and more profound ischemia involving a relatively large area of myocardium. This distinction is clinically important because early fibrinolytic therapy improves outcomes in STEMI but not in non-STEMI. Also, morphine use for pain relief is recommended for STEMI; however, use of morphine in non-STEMI patients is associated with increased mortality rate, thus has limited indications for use in non-STEMI patients.

Management of acute MI targets early recanalization with percutaneous coronary intervention (PCI) or fibrinolytic therapy for an STEMI. The greatest benefit is realized when patients receive fibrinolytic drugs as soon as possible, i.e., within the first 3 h after infarction, and current guidelines recommend that PCI be provided

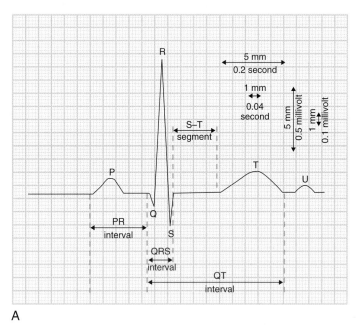

A

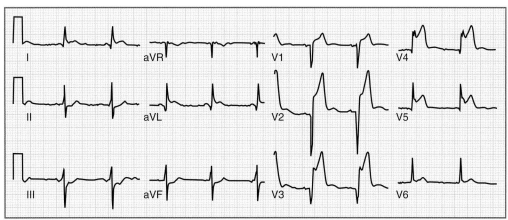

B

FIG. 4.9 A) Waves and intervals on a normal electrocardiogram (ECG). The ST segment characteristically lies only very slightly above the baseline tracing. **(B)** Electrocardiographic tracing shows an acute anterior/lateral myocardial infarction. ST segment elevation is evident in leads I, aVL, and V₁ to V₆. ((**A**) From Ganz L, Curtiss E. Electrocardiography. In: Goldman L, Ausiello D, eds. *Cecil Textbook of Medicine*. 23rd ed. Philadelphia: Saunders; 2008. (**B**) Courtesy Dr. Thomas Evans. From Anderson JL. ST-elevation acute myocardial infarction and complications of myocardial infarction. In: Goldman L, Ausiello D, eds. *Cecil Textbook of Medicine*. 23rd ed. Philadelphia: Saunders; 2008.)

within 90 min of first medical contact. Early use of fibrinolytic drugs helps decrease the extent of necrosis and myocardial damage and dramatically improve outcome and prognosis. Fibrinolytic (or thrombolytic) drugs used in the treatment of acute MI include third-generation agents: reteplase (recombinant plasminogen activator [r-PA]) or tenecteplase (tissue plasminogen activator [t-PA]), which have generally replaced second-generation agent alteplase (t-PA) and first-generation streptokinase (SK). For most patients with STEMI, the preferred method for revascularization is percutaneous coronary angioplasty. In patients with STEMI, non-STEMI, or UA (ACS), anticoagulation often is effected with unfractionated heparin or low-molecular-weight heparin (LMWH); in addition, glycoprotein IIa/IIIb inhibitors (abciximab, eptifibatide, tirofiban) are administered intravenously for their antiplatelet effects. General pharmacologic measures for patients with acute MI include the use of sedatives and anxiolytic medications, nitrates, beta-blockers, CCBs, ACE inhibitors, lipid-lowering agents, oxygen if needed, along with bedrest. Dual antiplatelet therapy (aspirin in daily doses of 75–325 mg plus either clopidogrel, prasugrel, or ticagrelor) is used for ACS to reduce risk of morbidity and mortality. Alternatively, anticoagulants (LMWH, factor Xa inhibitors, or direct oral anticoagulants) may be used.

The development of an arrhythmia in a patient who has had an acute MI constitutes an emergency that must be treated aggressively with antiarrhythmic drugs. During the first several weeks after an infarction, the conduction system of the heart may be unstable, and patients are prone to serious arrhythmias and reinfarction. A pacemaker may be used in patients who have severe myocardial damage and resultant heart failure.

DENTAL MANAGEMENT

Medical Considerations

Identification. Any patient whose condition remains undiagnosed but has cardinal clinical or radiographic signs or symptoms of ischemic heart disease should be referred to a physician for diagnosis and treatment. The dentist must be able to distinguish a patient who has stable versus UA versus MI. In the former, the chest pain characteristically demonstrates a consistent, recurring, and unchanging pattern brought on by exertion or stress that typically subsides within 5–15 min with rest or use of nitroglycerin. UA causes a worsening chest pain with a pattern of increasing severity, frequency, or duration. If pain is unremitting after 15 min, an MI should be assumed. Laboratory testing and diagnostic imaging are helpful in identifying those who have varying severity of ischemic heart disease.

Risk Assessment. Assessment of risk for the dental management of patients with ischemic heart disease involves three determinants:

1. Severity of the disease
2. Stability and cardiopulmonary reserve of the patient (i.e., the ability to tolerate dental care)
3. Type and magnitude of the dental procedure

All must be factored into a dental management plan so that a rational and safe decision can be made to determine whether a patient can safely tolerate a planned procedure. The American College of Cardiology (ACC) and the American Heart Association (AHA) have published risk stratification guidelines for patients with various types of heart disease who are undergoing noncardiac surgical procedures. These guidelines provide a framework for determination of associated risk for surgical as well as for nonsurgical dental procedures (Boxes 4.4 and 4.5). For example, recent MI (within the past 7–30 days) and UA are classified as clinical predictors of major risk for perioperative complications. By contrast, a past history of ischemic heart disease (i.e., stable [mild] angina and past history of MI) is considered one of the intermediate risk factors for perioperative complications. Accordingly, a past history of ischemic heart disease with no other clinical risk factors, as shown in Box 4.4, is unlikely to be associated with significant risk for an adverse event during dental procedures.

The type and magnitude of the planned procedure are important considerations. Procedures that are performed with the patient under general anesthesia and have the potential for significant blood and fluid loss with resultant adverse hemodynamic effects pose the "highest risk." At the "intermediate cardiac risk" category are extensive oral and maxillofacial surgical procedures and extensive periodontal surgical procedures (see "head and neck procedures" Box 4.5), with a 1%–5% risk. Minor oral surgery and periodontal surgery fall within the low-risk, "superficial surgery" or "ambulatory surgery" category, with less than 1% risk. Although not included in the list, nonsurgical dental procedures are likely to carry even less of a risk, considering that local anesthesia is used, minimal blood loss is anticipated, and procedures typically are of short duration.

The final element included in the AHA/ACC Guidelines is the ability of the patient to perform basic physical tasks. The energy expended in performing these tasks is measured in metabolic equivalents of tasks (METs), which is a measure of oxygen consumption. Studies have shown that a person who cannot perform at a minimum of a 4-MET level is at increased risk for a cardiovascular event. Climbing a flight of stairs requires a 4-MET effort; thus, a person who cannot climb a flight of stairs without chest pain or shortness of breath is at increased risk.

These medical risk stratification guidelines should be applied in the context of the planned dental procedures. For example, a patient with UA or recent MI (within 30 days) is assigned to the major cardiac risk category. It

BOX 4.4   Clinical Predictors of Increased Perioperative Cardiovascular Risk

Major Clinical Risk Factors (or "Active Cardiac Conditions")
- Unstable coronary syndromes
  - Acute or recent MI[a] associated with important ischemic risk as indicated by clinical signs and symptoms or by noninvasive study
  - Unstable or severe angina (Canadian class III or IV)[b,c]
- Decompensated heart failure (NYHA class 4: worsening or new-onset heart failure)
- Significant arrhythmias
  - High-grade AV block
  - Mobitz type 2 AV block
  - Third-degree AV block
  - Symptomatic ventricular arrhythmias in the presence of underlying heart disease
  - Supraventricular arrhythmias with uncontrolled ventricular rate
  - Symptomatic bradycardia
  - Newly recognized ventricular tachycardia
- Severe valvular disease
  - Severe aortic stenosis
  - Symptomatic mitral stenosis

Intermediate Clinical Risk Factors
- History of ischemic heart disease
- History of compensated or previous heart failure
- History of cerebrovascular disease
- Diabetes mellitus
- Renal insufficiency

Minor Clinical Risk Factors
- Advanced age (>70 years)
- Abnormal ECG (left ventricular hypertrophy, left bundle branch block, ST–T wave abnormalities)
- Rhythm other than sinus (e.g., atrial fibrillation)
- Uncontrolled systemic hypertension (≥180/110 mm Hg)

[a]The American College of Cardiology National Database Library defines acute myocardial infarction (MI) as occurring within 7 days, and recent MI as occurring after 7 days but within 1 month (at or before 30 days) before the procedure.
[b]May include "stable" angina in patients who are unusually sedentary.
[c]Data from Campeau L. Grading of angina pectoris. *Circulation.* 1976;54:522–523. The Canadian classification is a system of grading angina severity (grades I to IV), with grade I angina occurring only with strenuous exertion and grade IV angina occurring with any physical activity or at rest.
AV, atrioventricular; *ECG,* electrocardiogram; *NYHA,* New York Heart Association.
Note: The Revised Cardiac Risk Index is a more recent approach that assigns one point for each clinical risk factor present, with those with three or more risk factors to be considered for pharmacological heart rate control if intermediate or high risk surgery is planned.
Data from Fleisher LA, Beckman JA, Brown KA, et al. ACC/AHA 2007 guidelines on perioperative cardiovascular evaluation and care for noncardiac surgery: executive summary: a report of the American College of Cardiology/American Heart Association task force on practice guidelines. *Circulation.* 2007;116:1971–1996.

BOX 4.5   Cardiac Risk[a] Stratification for Noncardiac Surgical Procedures

High (Reported Cardiac Risk Often >5%)
- Aortic and other major vascular surgery

Intermediate (Reported Cardiac Risk Generally <5%)
- Intraperitoneal and intrathoracic surgery
- Carotid endarterectomy
- Head and neck surgery
- Orthopedic surgery
- Prostate surgery

Low (Reported Cardiac Risk Generally <1%)
- Endoscopic procedures
- Superficial procedures
- Cataract surgery
- Breast surgery
- Ambulatory surgery

[a]Combined incidence of cardiac death and nonfatal myocardial infarction.).
Adapted from Fleisher LA, Beckman JA, Brown KA, et al. ACC/AHA 2007 guidelines on perioperative cardiovascular evaluation and care for noncardiac surgery: executive summary: a report of the American College of Cardiology/American Heart Association task force on practice guidelines. *Circulation.* 2007;116:1971–1996.

---

also is likely that this person would have difficulty climbing a flight of stairs. By contrast, if the planned dental procedure is limited to routine clinical examination with radiographs (extremely low-risk category), and the patient is stable and not anxious, the risk for an adverse occurrence is minimal; thus, alterations in the dental management approach would be unnecessary. If, however, a patient with stable angina or a past history of MI (intermediate-risk category) with minimal cardiac reserve is scheduled for multiple extractions and implant placement (low- to intermediate-risk category), the risk for an adverse perioperative event is more significant, and a more complex dental management plan may be required. Also, dentists should be aware that patients who have ischemic heart disease who have comorbidities such as concurrent valvulopathology, low ejection fraction (<50%) or a significant arrhythmia are at higher risk for major adverse outcomes when invasive procedures are performed.

Clinicians should be aware of, and utilize as needed, risk calculators that are available to help predict the likelihood of a major adverse cardiac event (MACE) associated with noncardiac surgical procedures (see https://www.mdcalc.com/heart-score-major-cardiac-events).

Recommendations. Based on the assessment of medical risk, the type of planned dental procedure, and the stability and anxiety level of the patient, general management strategies for patients with stable angina or a past history of MI without ischemic symptoms (intermediate risk category) and no other risk factors should include the following: short appointments in the morning, comfortable chair position, reduced stress environment with consideration for oral sedation or nitrous oxide–oxygen sedation, pretreatment vital signs, availability of nitroglycerin, profound local anesthesia, limited amount of vasoconstrictor, avoidance of epinephrine-impregnated retraction cord, and effective postoperative pain control (Box 4.6).

For patients with symptoms of UA or those who have had an MI within the past 30 days (major risk category), elective care should be postponed (Box 4.7). If treatment becomes necessary, it should be performed as conservatively as possible and directed primarily toward pain relief, infection control, or the control of bleeding, as appropriate. Consultation with the physician is advised.

Additional management recommendations may include establishing and maintaining an intravenous line, continuously monitoring the ECG and vital signs, using a pulse oximeter, and administering nitroglycerin prophylactically just before the initiation of treatment. These measures may require that the patient be treated in a special patient care facility or hospital dental clinic.

Antibiotics. Antibiotic prophylaxis is not recommended for the patient who has coronary heart disease, a coronary artery stent, or undergone a CABG procedure.

BOX 4.6	Checklist for Dental Management of Patients With Stable (Mild) Angina or Past History of Myocardial Infarction More Than 30 Days, Without Ischemic Symptoms[a]

PREOPERATIVE RISK ASSESSMENT

- Review medical history, determine whether (i) patient has active cardiac conditions or clinical risk factors, (ii) functional capacity, (iii) risk level of surgery, and discuss relevant issues with the patient.
- Identify all medications and drugs being taken or supposed to be taken by the patient.
- Examine the patient for signs and symptoms of disease and obtain vital signs.
- Review recent laboratory test results or images required to assess risk.
- Confirm patient has a primary care provider and has taken cardiac medication(s) today.
- Obtain a medical consultation (i.e., refer to physician) if the patient is poorly controlled or is undiagnosed.
- If vital signs indicate well control, routine dental procedures can be performed without special precautions.

A

Antibiotics	No issues. Patients with ischemic heart disease, coronary artery stents, or CABG surgery do *not* require antibiotic prophylaxis.
Analgesics	See F—Follow-up.
Anesthesia	Ensure profound local anesthesia. Avoid use of excessive amounts of epinephrine; limit to 2 carpules of 1:100,000 epinephrine at a time (within 30–45 min); greater quantities may be tolerated well but increase risk.
Anxiety	Use stress reduction protocol (see Chapter 1). Consider the use of preoperative oral sedation (short-acting benzodiazepine) 1 h before procedure, as well as using N_2O–O_2 inhalational sedation intraoperatively.

B

Bleeding	If the patient is taking aspirin or other antiplatelet medication, anticipate some increased bleeding, but modification of drug regimen is not required.
Breathing	No issues.

Blood pressure	Monitor BP during procedure. Use a pulse oximeter if oral sedation is used or if the patient becomes symptomatic.

C

Capacity to tolerate care	Patients who have stable angina that is relieved by nitrates can receive routine dental care. Have nitroglycerin available.
Chair position	Ensure a comfortable chair position and avoid rapid position changes.

D

Drugs	Use of excessive amounts of epinephrine with nonselective beta-blockers can potentially cause a spike in blood pressure and appears to be dose dependent; avoid the use of epinephrine-impregnated retraction cord.
Devices	Patients who have coronary artery stents do not require antibiotic prophylaxis.

E

Equipment	Consider taking preoperative vital signs and the use of a pulse oximeter if oral sedation is used or if the patient becomes symptomatic.
Emergencies	Precipitation of an angina attack, MI, arrhythmia, or cardiac arrest is possible. Have nitroglycerin readily available as well as oxygen. Be prepared to perform basic life support (activate EMS, provide CPR, use AED, if needed).

F

Follow-up	• Ensure adequate postoperative pain control to reduce risk of cardiac event. • Contact patients who have had invasive procedures between 24 and 72 h to ensure that the postoperative course proceeds without complications. • Ensure that patient is maintaining regular follow-up visits with his or her physicians.

[a]Strength of recommendation taxonomy (SORT) Grade: C (see Preface for further explanation).
AED, automated external defibrillator; *CABG*, coronary artery bypass graft; *CPR*, cardiopulmonary resuscitation; *EMSs*, emergency medical services; *MI*, myocardial infarction.

BOX 4.7	Checklist for Dental Management of Patients With Unstable Angina or History of Recent Myocardial Infarction (Within Past 30 Days)[a]

PREOPERATIVE RISK ASSESSMENT
- Be aware that there is higher risk for cardiac arrest in these patients; appropriate precautions are advised.
- Special precautions:
  - Avoid elective dental care.
- If care becomes necessary,
  - follow thorough risk assessment as listed in Box 4.6.
  - consult with a physician to develop a treatment plan.
  - best treated in a hospital dental clinic or special care facility.

A

Antibiotics	No issues. Patients with coronary artery stents or CABG surgery do not require antibiotic prophylaxis.
Analgesics	Ensure adequate postoperative pain control. Avoid NSAIDs.
Anesthesia	Avoid use of vasoconstrictor if possible. If vasoconstrictor is needed, limit to 2 carpules of 1:100,000 epinephrine at a time (within 30–45 min); greater quantities may be tolerated but increase risk. May need to discuss use with physician.
Anxiety	Use stress reduction protocol (see Chapter 1). Consider use of preoperative oral sedation (short-acting benzodiazepine) 1 h before procedure, as well as using N_2O-O_2 inhalational sedation intraoperatively.

B

Bleeding	If patient is taking aspirin or other antiplatelet medication, anticipate some excessive bleeding, but modification of drug regimen is not required.
Breathing	No issues.
Blood pressure	Continuous monitoring of blood pressure, pulse and oxygen saturation is recommended.

C

Capacity to tolerate care	Defer care if patient has unstable angina; refer to physician. Defer care of patient who has a history of MI that occurred <1 month or if the patient has chest pain–related symptoms.
Chair position	If urgent care is required, ensure a comfortable chair position and avoid rapid position changes.

D

Drugs	Consider administering prophylactic nitroglycerin just before procedure. Provide continuous oxygen by nasal cannula or nasal mask. Use of excessive amounts of epinephrine with nonselective beta-blockers can potentially cause a spike in blood pressure and appears to be dose-dependent; avoid the use of epinephrine-impregnated retraction cord.
Devices	Patients who have coronary artery stents do not require antibiotic prophylaxis.

E

Equipment	Recommended management includes placement of IV line, continuous ECG monitoring, ongoing monitoring of vital signs, and use of a pulse oximeter.
Emergencies	Precipitation of an angina attack, MI, arrhythmia, or cardiac arrest is possible. Have nitroglycerin readily available as well as oxygen. Be prepared to perform basic life support (activate EMS, provide CPR, use AED, if needed).

F

Follow-up	As delineated in Box 4.6

[a]Strength of recommendation taxonomy (SORT) Grade: C (see Preface for further explanation).
AED, automated external defibrillator; *CABG*, coronary artery bypass graft; *CPR*, cardiopulmonary resuscitation; *ECG*, electrocardiogram; *EMSs*, emergency medical services; *IV*, intravenous; *MI*, myocardial infarction; *NSAIDs*, nonsteroid anti-inflammatory drugs.

Bleeding. Patients who take daily aspirin or other antiplatelet agents (Table 4.2) can expect some increase in surgical and postoperative bleeding, but this can be controlled with local measures. Discontinuation of these agents before dental treatment is not necessary and can increase the risk of thrombosis, MI, or death. Patients who are taking warfarin for anticoagulation can safely undergo dental or surgical procedures, provided that the international normalized ratio (INR) is 3.5 or less (see Chapter 24). The INR results should be performed within 24–72 h within the scheduled invasive procedure depending on the level of INR stability.

Capacity to Tolerate Care. The ability to tolerate care is determined based on the presence, severity, and stability of ischemic symptoms, as well as the proximity of the most recent ACS event. Patients who have stable angina pose an intermediate cardiac risk and can receive routine dental care when attention to minimize risk is provided. In contrast, patients who have UA should be considered to be at major cardiac risk and are not candidates for elective dental care. Asking the patient if the chest pain occurs at rest or during sleep, a particularly ominous sign, is helpful in distinguishing this condition.

Patients who have had an MI in the past may or may not have ischemic symptoms. For an asymptomatic patient with no other risk factors, the risk for an adverse event is minimal, especially 1 month or more after the MI. If, however, symptoms such as chest pain, shortness of breath, dizziness, or fatigue are present, or the MI was less than 1 month ago, then the patient falls in the major risk category, and elective dental care should be deferred and medical consultation obtained. Likewise, a patient who has a history of MI in association with other clinical risk factors (e.g., valvulopathy, heart failure, arrhythmia) is at increased risk for an adverse event, and medical consultation should be obtained before elective dental care.

Chair. The clinician should ensure a comfortable chair position and avoid rapid position changes. A rapid change in chair position can cause hypotension and a change in hemodynamics that can potentially affect the heart and blood pressure, especially in patients who take nitrates and antihypertensive medications.

Drug Considerations. Nonsteroidal antiinflammatory drugs (NSAIDs) (except for aspirin) should be avoided in patients with hypertension and CAD, especially those whose cardiac history includes an MI. Use of NSAIDs in patients with previous MI has been shown to increase the risk for a subsequent MI, even after only 7 days of NSAID administration, with the exception of naproxen. Whether shorter duration of use decreases the risk is not clear, but this correlation seems likely. Thus, we recommend that NSAIDs be used with caution, if at all, in patients who have had a previous MI and that if an NSAID is used, naproxen be the drug of choice, administered for less than 7 days.

The use of vasoconstrictors in local anesthetics poses potential problems for patients with ischemic heart disease because of the possibility of precipitating cardiac tachycardias, arrhythmias, and increases in blood pressure. Local anesthetics without vasoconstrictors may be used as needed. If a vasoconstrictor is necessary, patients with intermediate clinical risk factors and those taking nonselective beta-blockers can safely be given up to 0.036 mg of epinephrine (two cartridges containing 1:100,000 epinephrine) at one appointment; intravascular injections are to be avoided. Greater quantities of vasoconstrictor may be tolerated, but increasing quantities increase the risk of adverse cardiovascular effects. In the majority of patients, modest quantities of vasoconstrictors (two cartridges containing 1:100,000 epinephrine) have been shown to be safe even in high-risk patients when accompanied by oxygen, sedation, nitroglycerin, and excellent pain control measures. However and of note, in patients taking nonselective beta-blockers (e.g., propranolol, sotalol, timolol; see Table 4.2), injections of sympathomimetic drugs such as epinephrine or levonordefrin may result in elevation of blood pressure; therefore, caution is indicated in use of these agents.

For patients at all levels of cardiac risk, the use of gingival retraction cord impregnated with epinephrine should be avoided because of the rapid absorption of a high concentration of epinephrine and the potential for adverse cardiovascular effects. Alternatives that can be used to provide gingival effects equivalent to those of epinephrine without adverse cardiovascular effects include: a paste containing 15% aluminum chloride (Traxodent, Premier Dental Products), viscous 20% ferrous sulfate (Viscostat, Ultradent Products Inc.), or aqueous 12.7% iron (Astrigedent, Ultradent Products Inc.).

Drug Interactions. Many patients who have ischemic heart disease take cholesterol-lowering medications, such as simvastatin (Lipitor). Concurrent use of macrolide antibiotics has been shown to increase the plasma level of statin drugs (i.e., HMG-CoA reductase inhibitors) and increases the risk of rhabdomyolysis (myalgia and muscle weakness). Certain macrolide antibiotics also can increase the plasma level of CCBs, resulting in severe hypotension and acute kidney injury. Thus, a dentist should not prescribe erythromycin or clarithromycin to patients who take either HMG-CoA reductase inhibitors (e.g., simvastatin, atorvastatin, pravastatin) or CCBs (see Table 4.2). In summary, dentists are responsible for checking drug–drug interactions for any medication they prescribe (e.g., the antiplatelet drug clopidogrel has many drug interactions).

ORAL MANIFESTATIONS

Coronary atherosclerotic heart disease does not directly induce oral lesions or oral complications. However, carotid calcifications can be detected on panoramic images in about one-third of patients who have atherosclerosis (Fig. 4.10). Also, an association between ischemic heart disease and periodontal disease, poor oral health (e.g., chronic apical periodontitis), and tooth loss has been documented. Drugs used in the treatment of ischemic heart disease may produce oral changes such as dry mouth, taste aberrations, lichenoid eruptions, and oral ulcerations. CCBs can induce gingival overgrowth when plaque control is less than optimal and is more prominent at anterior interproximal sites. In rare cases, patients with angina or ACS may experience pain referred to the neck, shoulder, lower jaw, or teeth. The

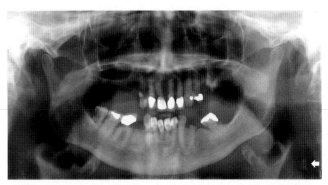

FIG. 4.10 Calcification of the left carotid artery as indicated by the *arrow.*

pattern of onset of pain with physical activity and its disappearance with rest usually serves as a diagnostic clue as to its cardiac origin.

BIBLIOGRAPHY

1. Ambrose JA, Martinez EE. A new paradigm for plaque stabilization. *Circulation*. 2002;105(16):2000–2004.

2. Anderson JL, Adams CD, Antman EM, et al. 2012 ACCF/ AHA focused update incorporated into the ACCF/AHA 2007 guidelines for the management of patients with unstable angina/non-ST-elevation myocardial infarction: a report of the American College of Cardiology Foundation/ American Heart Association task force on practice guidelines. *J Am Coll Cardiol*. 2013;61(23):e179–e347.

3. American Heart Association. *AHA Releases Latest Statistics on Sudden Cardiac Arrest*; 2018. https://www.sca-aware.org/ sca-news/aha-releases-latest-statistics-on-sudden-cardiac-arrest. Accessed October 5, 2019.

4. Baddour LM, Bettmann MA, Bolger AF, et al. Nonvalvular cardiovascular device-related infections. *Circulation*. 2003;108(16):2015–2031.

5. Bavry AA, Khaliq A, Gong Y, et al. Harmful effects of NSAIDs among patients with hypertension and coronary artery disease. *Am J Med*. 2011;124(7):614–620.

6. Beck JD, Eke P, Heiss G, et al. Periodontal disease and coronary heart disease: a reappraisal of the exposure. *Circulation*. 2005;112(1):19–24.

7. Bowles WH, Tardy SJ, Vahadi A. Evaluation of new gingival retraction agents. *J Dent Res*. 1991;70(11):1447–1449.

8. Brennan MT, Wynn RL, Miller CS. Aspirin and bleeding in dentistry: an update and recommendations. *Oral Surg Oral Med Oral Pathol Oral Radiol Endod*. 2007;104(3):316–323.

9. Canto JG, Goldberg RJ, Hand MM, et al. Symptom presentation of women with acute coronary syndromes: myth vs reality. *Arch Intern Med*. 2007;167(22):2405–2413.

10. Canto JG, Shlipak MG, Rogers WJ, et al. Prevalence, clinical characteristics, and mortality among patients with myocardial infarction presenting without chest pain. *JAMA*. 2000;283:3223.

11. Caplan DJ. Chronic apical periodontitis is more common in subjects with coronary artery disease. *J Evid Base Dent Pract*. 2014;14(3):149–150.

12. Centers for Disease Control and Prevention. Heart Disease Facts; 2021. Available at: http://www.cdc.gov/HeartDisease/facts.htm. Accessed February 8, 2021.

13. Campeau L. Grading of angina pectoris. *Circulation*. 1976;54:522–523.

14. Chen ZY, Chiang CH, Huang CC, et al. The association of tooth scaling and decreased cardiovascular disease: a nationwide population-based study. *Am J Med*. 2012;125(6):568–575.

15. Chen TT, D'Aiuto FD, Yeh YC, et al. Risk of myocardial infarction and ischemic stroke after dental treatments. *J Dent Res*. 2019;98(2):157–163.

16. Chobanian AV, Bakris GL, Black HR, et al. The seventh report of the joint national committee on prevention, detection, evaluation, and treatment of high blood pressure: the JNC 7 report. *JAMA*. 2003;289(19):2560–2572.

17. Chow CK, Islam S, Bautista L, et al. Parental history and myocardial infarction risk across the world: the INTER-HEART Study. *J Am Coll Cardiol*. 2011;57(5):619–627.

18. Cintron G, Medina R, Reyes AA, et al. Cardiovascular effects and safety of dental anesthesia and dental interventions in patients with recent uncomplicated myocardial infarction. *Arch Intern Med*. 1986;146(11):2203–2204.

19. Danesh-Sani SH, Danesh-Sani SA, Zia R, et al. Incidence of craniofacial pain of cardiac origin: results from a prospective multicentre study. *Aust Dent J*. 2012;57(3):355–358.

20. Elter JR, Hinderliter AL, Offenbacher S, et al. The effects of periodontal therapy on vascular endothelial function: a pilot trial. *Am Heart J*. 2006;151(1):47.

21. Findler M, Galili D, Meidan Z, et al. Dental treatment in very high risk patients with active ischemic heart disease. *Oral Surg Oral Med Oral Pathol*. 1993;76(3):298–300.

22. Fleisher LA, Beckman JA, Brown KA, et al. ACC/AHA 2007 guidelines on perioperative cardiovascular evaluation and care for noncardiac surgery: executive summary: a report of the American College of Cardiology/American Heart Association task force on practice guidelines (writing committee to revise the 2002 guidelines on perioperative cardiovascular evaluation for noncardiac surgery): developed in collaboration with the American Society of Echocardiography, American Society of Nuclear Cardiology, heart rhythm society, society of cardiovascular anesthesiologists, society for cardiovascular angiography and interventions, society for vascular medicine and biology, and society for vascular surgery. *Circulation*. 2007;116(17):1971–1996.

23. Fleisher LA, Fleischmann KE, Auerbach AD, et al. ACC/ AHA guideline on perioperative cardiovascular evaluation and management of patients undergoing noncardiac surgery. *J Am Coll Cardiol*. 2014;64(22):e77–e137.

24. Friedlander AH. Atheromas on panoramic radiographs often denote stenotic lesions and portend adverse vascular events. *Oral Surg Oral Med Oral Pathol Oral Radiol Endod*. 2007;104(4):451–452. author reply 52-4.

25. Friedlander AH, Cohen SN. Panoramic radiographic atheromas portend adverse vascular events. *Oral Surg Oral Med Oral Pathol Oral Radiol Endod*. 2007;103(6):830–835.

26. Gandhi S, Fleet JL, Bailey DG, et al. Calcium-channel blocker-clarithromycin drug interactions and acute kidney injury. *JAMA*. 2013;310(23):2544–2553.

27. Garrett BE, Dube SR, Trosclair A, et al. Cigarette smoking—United States, 1965–2008. *MMWR Surveill Summ*. 2011;60(suppl):109–113.

28. Grines CL, Bonow RO, Casey Jr DE, et al. Prevention of premature discontinuation of dual antiplatelet therapy in patients with coronary artery stents: a science advisory from the American Heart Association, American College of Cardiology, society for cardiovascular angiography and interventions, American College of Surgeons, and American Dental Association, with representation from the American College of Physicians. *J Am Coll Cardiol*. 2007;49(6):734–739.

29. Gu K, Cowie CC, Harris MI. Mortality in adults with and without diabetes in a national cohort of the U.S. population, 1971–1993. *Diabetes Care*. 1998;21(7):1138–1145.

30. Jha P, Ramasundarahettige C, Landsman V, et al. 21st-century hazards of smoking and benefits of cessation in the United States. *N Engl J Med.* 2013;368(4):341–350.

31. Hirode G, Wong RJ. Trends in the prevalence of metabolic syndrome. *JAMA.* 2020;323(24):2526–2528.

32. Holmlund A, Holm G, Lind L. Number of teeth as a predictor of cardiovascular mortality in a cohort of 7,674 subjects followed for 12 years. *J Periodontol.* 2010;81(6):870–876.

33. Howard BV, Rodriguez BL, Bennett PH, et al. Prevention conference VI: diabetes and cardiovascular disease: writing group I: epidemiology. *Circulation.* 2002;105(18):e132–e137.

34. Libby P. Inflammation and cardiovascular disease mechanisms. *Am J Clin Nutr.* 2006;83(2):456S–460S.

35. Husted SE, Ohman EM. Pharmacological and emerging therapies in the treatment of chronic angina. *Lancet.* 2015;386(9994):691–701.

36. Kreiner M, Alvarez R, Waldenstrom A, et al. Craniofacial pain of cardiac origin is associated with inferior wall ischemia. *J Oral Facial Pain Headache.* 2014;28(4):317–321.

37. Kushner FG, Hand M, Smith Jr SC, et al. 2009 focused updates: ACC/AHA guidelines for the management of patients with ST-elevation myocardial infarction (updating the 2004 guideline and 2007 focused update) and ACC/AHA/SCAI guidelines on percutaneous coronary intervention (updating the 2005 guideline and 2007 focused update): a report of the American College of Cardiology Foundation/American Heart Association task force on practice guidelines. *Circulation.* 2009;120(22):2271–2306.

38. Kwong JC, Schwartz KL, Campitelli MA, et al. Acute myocardial infarction after laboratory-confirmed influenza infection. *N Engl J Med.* 2018;378:345–353.

39. Lam OL, Zhang W, Samaranayake LP, et al. A systematic review of the effectiveness of oral health promotion activities among patients with cardiovascular disease. *Int J Cardiol.* 2011;151(3):261–267.

40. Lewandrowski KB. Cardiac markers of myocardial necrosis: a history and discussion of milestones and emerging new trends. *Clin Lab Med.* 2014;34(1):31–41 (xi).

41. Libby P, Theroux P. Pathophysiology of coronary artery disease. *Circulation.* 2005;111(25):3481–3488.

42. Lloyd-Jones D. Epidemiology of cardiovascular disease. In: Goldman L, Schafer A, eds. *Goldman-Cecil Medicine.* Philadelphia: Saunders/Elsevier; 2016:257–262.

43. Mozaffarian D, Benjamin EJ, Go AS, et al. Heart disease and stroke statistics-2016 update: a report from the American Heart Association. *Circulation.* 2016;133(4):e38–e360.

44. Lockhart PB, Bolger AF, Papapanou PN, et al. Periodontal disease and atherosclerotic vascular disease: does the evidence support an independent association?: a scientific statement from the American Heart Association. *Circulation.* 2012;125(20):2520–2544.

45. Murabito JM, Pencina MJ, Nam BH, et al. Sibling cardiovascular disease as a risk factor for cardiovascular disease in middle-aged adults. *JAMA.* 2005;294(24):3117–3123.

46. Mazzarelli J, Hollenberg S. Acute coronary syndromes. In: Vincent J-L, Abraham E, Moore F, et al., eds. *Textbook of Critical Care.* Philadelphia: Saunders/Elsevier; 2011:548–558.

47. Kong MH, Fonarow GC, Peterson ED, et al. Systematic review of the incidence of sudden cardiac death in the United States. *J Am Coll Cardiol.* 2011;57(7):794–801.

48. Meine TJ, Roe MT, Chen AY, et al. Association of intravenous morphine use and outcomes in acute coronary syndromes: results from the CRUSADE Quality Improvement Initiative. *Am Heart J.* 2005;149(6):1043–1049.

49. Minassian C, D'Aiuto F, Hingorani AD, et al. Invasive dental treatment and risk for vascular events: a self-controlled case series. *Ann Intern Med.* 2010;153(8):499–506.

50. Niwa H, Sato Y, Matsuura H. Safety of dental treatment in patients with previously diagnosed acute myocardial infarction or unstable angina pectoris. *Oral Surg Oral Med Oral Pathol Oral Radiol Endod.* 2000;89(1):35–41.

51. Olsen AM, Fosbol EL, Lindhardsen J, et al. Long-term cardiovascular risk of nonsteroidal anti-inflammatory drug use according to time passed after first-time myocardial infarction: a nationwide cohort study. *Circulation.* 2012;126(16):1955–1963.

52. Omar WA, Kumbhani DJ. The current literature on bioabsorbable stents: a review. *Curr Athreroscler Rep.* 2019;21(12):54.

53. Rafferty B, Jönsson D, Kalachilkov S, et al. Impact of monocytic cells on recovery of uncultivable bacteria from atherosclerotic lesions. *J Intern Med.* 2011;270(3):273–280.

54. Reddy K, Khaliq A, Henning RJ. Recent advances in the diagnosis and treatment of acute myocardial infarction. *World J Cardiol.* 2015;7(5):243–276.

55. Sanz M, Del Castillo AM, Jepsen S, et al. Periodontitis and vardiovascular diseases: consensus report. *J Clin Periodontol.* 2002;47(3):268–288.

56. Schenkein HA, Loos BG. Inflammatory medhanisms linking periodontal diseases to cardiovascular diseases. *J Clin Periodontol.* 2013;40(014):S51–S69. Suppl 14.

57. Schjerning Olsen AM, Fosbol EL, Lindhardsen J, et al. Duration of treatment with nonsteroidal anti-inflammatory drugs and impact on risk of death and recurrent myocardial infarction in patients with prior myocardial infarction: a nationwide cohort study. *Circulation.* 2011;123(20):2226–2235.

58. Sesso HD, Lee IM, Gaziano JM, et al. Maternal and paternal history of myocardial infarction and risk of cardiovascular disease in men and women. *Circulation.* 2001;104(4):393–398.

59. Skaar D, O'Connor H, Lunos S, et al. Dental procedures and risk of experiencing a second vascular event in a Medicare population. *J Am Dent Assoc.* 2012;143(11):1190–1198.

60. Slocum C, Kramer C, Genco CA. Immune dysregulation mediated by the oral microbiome: potential link to chronic inflammation and atherosclerosis. *J Intern Med.* 2016;280(1):114–128.

61. Smith MM, Barbara DW, Mauermann WJ, et al. Morbidity and mortality associated with dental extraction before cardiac operation. *Ann Thorac Surg.* 2014;97(3):838–844.

62. StatPearls. https://www.ncbi.nlm.nih.gov/books/NBK532966/#:~:text=In%20the%20proper%20clinical%20setting,be%20helpful%20in%20some%20situations. Accessed January 3, 2021.

63. Teeuw WJ, Slot DE, Susanto H, et al. Treatment of periodontitis improves the atherosclerotic profile: a systematic review and meta-analysis. *J Clin Periodontol*. 2014;41(1):70–79.

64. Teirstein P, Lytle B. Interventional and surgical treatment of coronary artery diseas. In: Goldman L, Schafer AI, eds. *Goldman-Cecil Medicine*. Philadelphia: Saunders/Elsevier; 2016:456–461.

65. Thompson PD, Clarkson P, Karas RH. Statin-associated myopathy. *JAMA*. 2003;289(13):1681–1690.

66. Tuzcu EM, Kapadia SR, Tutar E, et al. High prevalence of coronary atherosclerosis in asymptomatic teenagers and young adults: evidence from intravascular ultrasound. *Circulation*. 2001;103(22):2705–2710.

67. Udell JA, Steg PG, Scirica BM, et al. Metabolic syndrome, diabetes mellitus, or both and cardiovascular risk in outpatients with or at risk for atherothrombosis. *Eur J Prev Cardiol*. 2014;21(12):1531–1540.

68. Vasan RS, Larson MG, Leip EP, et al. Impact of high-normal blood pressure on the risk of cardiovascular disease. *N Engl J Med*. 2001;345(18):1291–1297.

69. Virmani R, Robinowitz M, Geer JC, et al. Coronary artery atherosclerosis revisited in Korean war combat casualties. *Arch Pathol Lab Med*. 1987;111(10):972–976.

70. Wahl MJ. Myths of dental surgery in patients receiving anticoagulant therapy. *J Am Dent Assoc*. 2000;131(1):77–81.

Cardiac Arrhythmias

Cardiac arrhythmia refers to any variation in the normal heartbeat and includes disturbances in rhythm, rate, or the conduction pattern of the heart. Cardiac arrhythmias are present in a significant percentage of the population, many of whom will seek dental treatment. Some arrhythmias are of little clinical concern for either the patient or the dentist; however, others can produce symptoms such as anxiety, and loss of consciousness due to abnormal hemodynamics, and a few may be life-threatening. Dental practitioners should be aware that patients with significant arrhythmias are at risk for fatal cardiac arrhythmias, which can be precipitated by strong emotion, various drugs, or the performance of dental procedures.

EPIDEMIOLOGY

Cardiac arrhythmias are relatively common in the general population, and their prevalence increases with age. They more frequently occur in older adults, people with a long history of smoking or alcohol use, patients with underlying ischemic heart disease, structural heart disease, congestive heart failure, diabetes, or sleep apnea, and those taking certain drugs. In the United States, arrhythmias occur in 5%–15% of the population and are present in about 35% of people older than 65 years of age. In studies of patients treated in dental and other health care settings, about 4% of the detected cardiac arrhythmias have been serious and potentially life-threatening. Arrhythmias contribute to approximately 300,000 sudden deaths annually and constitute the underlying or contributing cause in over 450,000 cases. The most common type of persistent arrhythmia is atrial fibrillation (AF). AF affects about 2% of the adult population (i.e., more than 2.7 million people) and the majority are older than 60 years of age. AF contributes to about 158,000 deaths each year. A dental practice of 2000 adults can expect to have about 300 patients to have some type of cardiac arrhythmia.

ETIOLOGY

Cardiac contractions are controlled by a complex system of specialized excitatory and conductive neuronal circuitry (Fig. 5.1). The normal pattern of sequential depolarization involves the structures of the heart in the following order: (1) sinoatrial (SA) node, (2) atrioventricular (AV) node, (3) bundle of His, (4) right and left bundle branches, and finally (5) subendocardial Purkinje network. The electrocardiogram (ECG) is a recording of this electrical activity. The primary anatomic pacemaker for the heart is the SA node, a small (~1 cm) crescent-shaped structure that is located at the junction of the superior vena cava and the right atrium. The SA node regulates the functions of the atria and is responsible for production of the P wave (atrial depolarization) on the ECG (Fig. 5.2). The ends of the sinus nodal fibers connect with atrial muscle fibers. The generated action potential travels along the muscle fibers (internodal pathways) and eventually arrives at and excites the AV node, which serves to regulate the entry of atrial impulses into the ventricles. It also slows the conduction rate of impulses generated within the SA node. From the AV node, impulses travel along the AV bundle (His bundle) within the

formed by repolarization of the ventricles. Repolarization of the atria occurs at about the same time as depolarization of the ventricles and thus is usually obscured by the QRS wave.

Normal cardiac function depends on cellular automaticity (impulse formation), conductivity, excitability, and contractility. Disorders in automaticity and conductivity constitute the underlying cause of the vast majority of cardiac arrhythmias. Under normal conditions, the SA node is responsible for impulse formation, resulting in a sinus rhythm with a normal rate of 60–100 beats/min. However, other cells or groups of cells also are capable of generating impulses (ectopic pacemakers), and under certain conditions, these impulses may emerge outside of the normal conduction system. After a normal impulse is generated (depolarization), cells of the SA node need time for recovery and repolarization and are said to be refractory; during this time, they cannot conduct an impulse. Disturbances causing complete refractoriness result in a block, and those inducing partial refractoriness result in delay of conductivity.

Disorders of conductivity (block or delay) paradoxically may lead to rapid cardiac rhythm through the mechanisms of reentry. Reentry arrhythmias occur when accessory or ectopic pacemakers reexcite previously depolarized fibers before they would become depolarized in the normal sequential impulse pathway, typically producing tachyarrhythmias. The type of arrhythmia

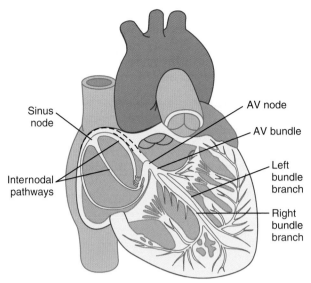

FIG. 5.1 The electrical conduction system of the heart. *AV,* atrioventricular. (From Hall JE. *Guyton and Hall: Textbook of Medical Physiology.* 13th ed. St. Louis; Elsevier; 2016.)

ventricular septum, which divides into right and left bundle branches. The bundle branches then terminate in the small Purkinje fibers, which course throughout the ventricles and become continuous with cardiac muscle fibers. Simultaneous depolarization of the ventricles produces the QRS complex on ECG. The T wave is

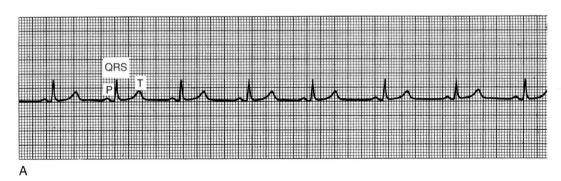

A

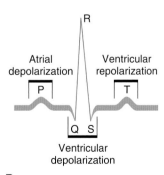

B

FIG. 5.2 **A**) Electrocardiographic (ECG) tracing of the cardiac cycle. (**B**) Normal ECG deflections. The normal ECG consists of a P wave, representing atrial depolarization; a QRS complex, representing ventricular depolarization; and a T wave, representing rapid repolarization of the ventricles. ((**A**) From Goldberger AL, Goldberger E. *Clinical Electrocardiography: A Simplified Approach.* 4th ed. St. Louis; Mosby; 1990. (**B**) From Pagana KD, Pagana TJ. *Mosby's Manual of Diagnostic and Laboratory Tests.* 4th ed. St. Louis: Mosby; 2010.)

may suggest the nature of its cause. For example, paroxysmal atrial tachycardia with block suggests digitalis toxicity. However, many cardiac arrhythmias are not specific for a given cause. In such cases, a careful search is undertaken to identify the cause of the arrhythmia. The most common causes of arrhythmias include primary cardiovascular disorders, pulmonary disorders (e.g., embolism, hypoxia), autonomic disorders, systemic disorders (e.g., thyroid disease), drug-related adverse effects, and electrolyte imbalances. Cardiac arrhythmias also are associated with many systemic diseases (Table 5.1) and various drugs or other substances, including foods (Table 5.2).

PATHOPHYSIOLOGY AND COMPLICATIONS

The outcome of an arrhythmia often depends on the nature of the arrhythmia and the physical condition of the patient. For example, a young healthy person with paroxysmal atrial tachycardia may have minimal symptoms, but an older adult who has heart disease with the same arrhythmia is at risk for developing altered hemodynamics (e.g., shock), congestive heart failure, or myocardial ischemia. Furthermore, evidence suggests that patients with certain types of cardiac arrhythmias (e.g., AF) are susceptible to ischemic events within the dental office.

Arrhythmias are classified by site of origin (Box 5.1). Any arrhythmia that arises above the bifurcation of the bundle of His into right and left bundle branches is classified as supraventricular. Supraventricular cardiac arrhythmias may be broadly categorized into tachyarrhythmias and bradyarrhythmias. Brief descriptions of some of the more common arrhythmias are provided.

TABLE 5.2 Drugs and Foods that Can Induce Cardiac Arrhythmias

Cardiac Arrhythmia	Precipitating Drugs and Food Substances
Bradycardia	Digitalis
	Morphine
	Beta-blockers
	Calcium channel blockers
Tachycardia	Amphetamines
	Atropine
	Epinephrine
	Nicotine
	Ephedrine
	Caffeine
Premature atrial beats	Alcohol
	Nicotine
	Tricyclic antidepressants
	Caffeine
Ventricular extrasystoles	Digitalis
	Alcohol
	Epinephrine
	Amphetamines
Ventricular tachycardia	Digitalis
	Quinidine
	Procainamide
	Potassium
	Sympathetic amines

TABLE 5.1 Cardiac Arrhythmias Associated With Various Systemic Diseases

Arrhythmia	Associated Systemic Conditions
Sinus bradycardia	Infectious diseases, hypothermia, myxedema, obstructive jaundice, increased intracranial pressure, MI
Atrial extrasystoles	Congestive heart failure, coronary insufficiency, MI
Sinoatrial block	Rheumatic heart disease, MI, acute infection
Sinus tachycardia	Febrile illness, infection, anemia, hyperthyroidism
Atrial tachycardia	Obstructive lung disease, pneumonia, MI
Atrial flutter	Ischemic heart disease, mitral stenosis, MI, open heart surgery
Atrial fibrillation	MI, mitral stenosis, ischemic heart disease, thyrotoxicosis, hypertension
Atrioventricular block	Rheumatic heart disease, ischemic heart disease, myocardial infarction, hyperthyroidism, Hodgkin disease, myeloma, open heart surgery
Ventricular extrasystole	Ischemic heart disease, congestive heart failure, MVP
Ventricular tachycardia	MVP, MI, coronary atherosclerotic heart disease
Ventricular fibrillation	Blunt cardiac trauma, MVP, anaphylaxis, cardiac surgery, rheumatic heart disease, cardiomyopathy, coronary atherosclerotic heart disease

MI, myocardial infarction; *MVP,* mitral valve prolapse.

BOX 5.1 Classification of Common Cardiac Arrhythmias

Supraventricular Arrhythmias
- Sinus nodal disturbances
  - Sinus arrhythmia
  - Sinus tachycardia
  - Sinus bradycardia
- Disturbances of atrial rhythm
  - Premature atrial complexes
  - Atrial flutter
  - Atrial fibrillation
  - Atrial tachycardias
- Tachycardias involving the AV junction
  - Preexcitation syndrome (Wolff–Parkinson–White)
- Heart block
  - Atrioventricular (AV) block or complete AV block

Ventricular Arrhythmias
- Premature ventricular complexes
- Ventricular tachycardia
- Ventricular fibrillation

Disorders of Repolarization
- Long QT syndrome

Supraventricular Arrhythmias

Sinus Nodal Disturbances

- **Sinus arrhythmia.** Sinus arrhythmia is characterized by a prolonged sinus cycle length (i.e., length of the P-P interval—normally 120 ms). In the *respiratory* type of sinus arrhythmia, heart rate increases with inhalation and decreases with exhalation. It is seen predominantly in young individuals and reflects variations in parasympathetic and sympathetic signals to the heart and is considered a normal event. *Nonrespiratory* sinus arrhythmia is unrelated to respiratory effort and is seen in digitalis intoxication.

- **Sinus tachycardia.** *Tachycardia* in an adult is defined as a heart rate greater than 100 beats/min, with otherwise normal findings on the ECG. The rate usually is between 100 and 180 beats/min. This condition most often is a physiologic response to exercise, anxiety, stress, or emotion, which triggers increased sympathetic tone. Pathophysiologic causes include fever, hypotension, hypoxia, infection, anemia, hyperthyroidism, and heart failure. Drugs that may cause sinus tachycardia include atropine, epinephrine, alcohol, nicotine, and caffeine.

- **Sinus bradycardia.** *Bradycardia* is defined as a heart rate less than 60 beats/min, with an otherwise normal ECG tracing. It often coexists with a sinus arrhythmia. It is relatively common among well-conditioned athletes and healthy young adults and decreases in prevalence with advancing age. Pathophysiologic causes of bradycardia include intracranial tumor, increased intracranial pressure, myxedema, hypothermia, and gram-negative sepsis. Bradycardia may occur during vomiting and vasovagal syncope and as the result of carotid sinus stimulation. Drugs that may cause bradycardia include lithium, amiodarone, beta-blockers, clonidine, and calcium channel blockers.

Disturbances of Atrial Rhythm

- **Atrial premature beats (APBs).** Impulses arising from ectopic foci anywhere in the atrium may result in APBs. APBs, also known as premature atrial complexes or contractions, occur frequently in otherwise healthy people but often occur during infection, inflammation, or myocardial ischemia. APBs produce a sensation of a skipped beat or palpitations and may be provoked by smoking, lack of sleep, excessive caffeine, or alcohol. They are common in persons older than 60 years of age and in conditions associated with dysfunction of the atria such as heart failure.

- **Atrial flutter.** Atrial flutter is characterized by a rapid, regular atrial rate of 250–350 beats/min. It is rare in healthy persons; occurs in about 0.15% of older adults; and most often occurs in association with septal defects, pulmonary emboli, obstructive lung disease, mitral or tricuspid valve stenosis or regurgitation, or chronic ventricular failure. Atrial flutter also may be noted in patients with hyperthyroidism, alcoholism, or pericarditis.

- **Atrial fibrillation.** AF is the most common sustained arrhythmia in adults, and its prevalence is strongly associated with age and hypertension. AF is characterized by rapid, disorganized, and ineffective atrial contractions that occur at a rate of 350–600 beats/min. The ventricular response is highly irregular. The atria do not contract effectively, thereby promoting the formation of intraarterial clots, along with consequent embolism and stroke. The development of AF is associated with hypertension, valvular heart disease, left atrial enlargement, diabetes, heart failure, stroke, and heavy alcohol use, as well as with advanced age. It may occur intermittently or may be chronic. Symptoms are variable and depend on underlying cardiac status, ventricular rate, and loss of atrial contraction. Complications of AF include increased risk of thromboembolism and stroke (causing one in seven strokes).

- **Atrial tachycardias.** Any tachycardia arising above the AV junction for which the ECG shows a P-wave configuration different from that for sinus rhythm is called *atrial tachycardia*. Atrial tachycardia is characterized by an atrial rate between 150 and 200 beats/min and may result from enhanced normal automaticity, abnormal automaticity, triggered activity, or reentry. It commonly is seen in patients with coronary artery disease, myocardial infarction (MI), cor pulmonale (right ventricular hypertrophy and pulmonary hypertension), or digitalis intoxication.

Tachycardias Involving the Atrioventricular Junction

- **Preexcitation syndrome** (e.g., Wolff–Parkinson–White syndrome). The atria and ventricles are electrically insulated from each other by fibrous tissue that forms the anatomic AV junction. Normally, impulses are transmitted from atria to ventricles across this electrical bridge; however, in some persons, additional electrical bridges connect the atria and ventricles, bypassing the normal pathways and forming the basis for preexcitation syndromes such as Wolff–Parkinson–White syndrome. The basic defect in this disorder involves premature activation (preexcitation) of the ventricles by way of an accessory AV pathway that allows the normal SA-AV pathway to be bypassed. This accessory pathway allows rapid conduction and short refractoriness, with impulses passed rapidly between atria and ventricles, and it provides a route for reentrant (backflow) tachyarrhythmias. Resultant paroxysmal tachycardia is characterized by a normal QRS complex, a regular rhythm, and ventricular rates of 150–250 beats/min, along with sudden onset and termination. Wolff–Parkinson–White syndrome is found in all age groups but is more prevalent among men and decreases with age. For most patients with recurrent tachycardia, the prognosis is good, but sudden death occurs rarely, at a frequency of 0.1%.

Heart Block

- **AV block.** Heart block is a disturbance of impulse conduction that may be permanent or transient, depending on the underlying anatomic or functional impairment. AV block occurs when the atrial impulse is conducted with delay or is not conducted at all to the ventricles at a time when the AV junction is not physiologically refractory. Conduction delay may occur at the AV node, within the His-Purkinje system (bundle branches), or at both sites. Conduction impairment in heart block is classified by severity, with the various forms divided into three categories (first-, second-, or third-degree [complete] block). During first-degree heart block, conduction time is prolonged, but all impulses are conducted. Second-degree heart block occurs in two forms: Mobitz type I (Wenckebach) and type II. Mobitz I heart block is characterized by progressive lengthening of conduction time resulting in a nonconducted P wave. Type II second-degree heart block denotes occasional or repetitive sudden block of conduction of an impulse without previous lengthening of conduction time. When no impulses are conducted, complete or third-degree block is present. AV block may be caused by a multitude of conditions such as surgery, electrolyte disturbance, myoendocarditis, tumor, myxedema, rheumatoid nodules, Chagas disease,[1] calcific aortic stenosis, polymyositis, and amyloidosis. In children, the most common cause is congenital. Drugs (e.g., digitalis, propranolol, potassium, quinidine) also may cause AV heart block. Symptoms increase in severity with increasing degree of block, with first-degree and Mobitz I block being asymptomatic and Mobitz II and third-degree block requiring a permanent pacemaker.

Ventricular Arrhythmias

- **Premature ventricular complexes (PVCs).** PVCs (or contractions) are very common arrhythmias that are characterized by the premature occurrence of an abnormally shaped QRS complex (ventricular contraction) followed by a pause. PVCs may occur alone, as bigeminy (every other beat is a PVC), as trigeminy (every third beat is a PVC), or with higher periodicity. The combination of two consecutive PVCs is called a couplet; three or more in a row at a rate of 100 beats/min are referred to as ventricular tachycardia (VT). PVCs may be provoked by a variety of medications; electrolyte imbalance; tension states; and excessive use of tobacco, caffeine, and alcohol. The prevalence of PVCs increases with age; they are associated with male gender and are associated with low serum potassium concentration and heart failure. In patients without structural heart disease, PVCs have no prognostic significance and no impact on longevity

or limitation of activity. Among patients with previous MI, valvular heart disease, or heart failure, frequent PVCs are associated with an increased risk of death.
- **Ventricular tachycardia (VT).** The occurrence of three or more ectopic ventricular beats (PVCs) at a rate of 100 or more per minute is defined as VT. This disorder may be sustained or episodic. Sustained VT that persists for 30 s or longer may require termination because of hemodynamic instability. VT can quickly degenerate into ventricular fibrillation (VF). A variant of VT called torsades de pointes is characterized by QRS complexes of changing amplitude that appear to twist around the isoelectrical line; this rhythm occurs at rates of 200–250 beats/min. VT almost always occurs in patients with heart disease, most commonly ischemic heart disease and cardiomyopathy. Certain drugs such as digitalis, sympathetic amines (epinephrine), potassium, quinidine, and procainamide may induce VT.
- **Ventricular flutter and fibrillation.** Ventricular flutter and VF are lethal arrhythmias characterized by chaotic, disorganized electrical activity that results in failure of sequential cardiac contraction and inability to maintain cardiac output. The distinction between flutter and fibrillation can be difficult and is of academic interest only; therefore, the two can be discussed together. If these disorders are not rapidly treated within 3–5 min, death will ensue. VF occurs most commonly as a sequela of ischemic heart disease.

Disorders of Repolarization

- **Long QT syndrome.** Long QT syndrome is a disorder of the conduction system in which the recharging of the heart during repolarization (i.e., the QT interval) is delayed. It is caused by a genetic mutation in myocardial ion channels and by certain drugs or may be the result of a stroke. The condition can lead to fast, chaotic heartbeats, which can trigger unexplained syncope, a seizure, or sudden death.

CLINICAL PRESENTATION

Signs and Symptoms

Arrhythmias may be symptomatic or asymptomatic; however, symptoms alone cannot determine the seriousness of an arrhythmia. Whereas some arrhythmias such as PVCs may be highly symptomatic yet are not associated with an adverse outcome, some patients with AF have no symptoms at all but may be at significant risk for stroke. Signs and symptoms most commonly associated with cardiac arrhythmias are listed in Box 5.2.

LABORATORY AND DIAGNOSTIC FINDINGS

The 12-lead ECG is the primary tool used in the identification and diagnosis of cardiac arrhythmias. Additional

---

1. Chagas disease, also known as American trypanosomiasis, is a tropical acute and chronic parasitic disease of the Americas caused by the flagellate protozoan *Trypanosoma cruzi* usually transmitted by an insect bite.

BOX 5.2 Signs and Symptoms of Cardiac Arrhythmias

Signs
- Irregular heart beat
  - Slow heart rate (<60 beats/min)
  - Fast heart rate (>100 beats/min)
  - Irregular rhythm

Symptoms
- Anxiety, palpitations, fatigue
- Dizziness, feeling faint, syncope, angina
- Congestive heart failure
  - Shortness of breath
  - Orthopnea
  - Peripheral edema
- Tinnitus, visual changes

tests that may be used include ambulatory ECG (Holter) for 24–48 h, event recording, mobile continuous outpatient cardiac telemetry, exercise or stress testing, baroreceptor reflex sensitivity testing, body surface mapping, and upright tilt-table testing. Electrode catheter techniques (insertable cardiac monitor) allow for intracavitary recordings of the specialized conducting systems, which aid greatly in the diagnosis of arrhythmias.

MEDICAL MANAGEMENT

Management of cardiac arrhythmias involves medications, cardioversion, pacemakers, implanted cardioverter-defibrillators (ICDs), radiofrequency catheter ablation, and surgery. Patients with asymptomatic arrhythmias usually do not require therapy; those with symptomatic arrhythmias typically are treated first with medications based on symptoms, type of arrhythmia, and underlying heart condition. Patients who do not respond to medications or who are at risk for sudden death may be treated by cardioversion, ablation, or implanted pacemaker or ICD. Surgery may be necessary for the treatment of patients with certain arrhythmias. Emergency cardioversion is indicated for any tachyarrhythmias that compromise hemodynamics or are life-threatening (e.g., cardiac arrest).

Antiarrhythmic Drugs

Generally, molecular targets for antiarrhythmic drugs involve the channels within cellular membranes (cardiac myocytes) through which ions are diffused rapidly. Antiarrhythmic drugs are therefore classified on the basis of their effect on sodium, potassium, or calcium channels and whether they block beta receptors (Table 5.3). Class I drugs work by blocking primarily the fast sodium channels which results in membrane-stabilizing effects (similar to local anesthetics). Class II drugs are β-adrenergic-blocking agents. Class III drugs prolong the duration of

the cardiac action potential and enhance refractoriness through their effects on blocking potassium channels. Class IV drugs are slow calcium channel blockers, which are used primarily for supraventricular tachycardias. Class V drugs have variable mechanism. Although this classification scheme implies a single action for each class, the reality is that they typically have multiple sites of action across different classification categories. For example, procainamide blocks both sodium and potassium channels, and amiodarone blocks sodium, potassium, and calcium channels.

Many of the antiarrhythmic drugs have very narrow therapeutic ranges, so optimum blood levels that are within acceptable range may be difficult to achieve. Thus, undermedicated patients may be at increased risk for an adverse event during dental treatment; conversely, in those who are overmedicated, drug toxicity is a possibility.

Oral Anticoagulant Therapy

Patients who have AF are at increased risk for stroke and thromboembolism. To reduce this risk, the American Heart Association (AHA) recommends oral anticoagulant (OAC) therapy. The AHA guidelines to provide OAC are based on the CHA2DS2-VASc score (Table 5.4). For a score of 2 or greater, OAC is recommended. Four OACs are available for use: warfarin sodium (Coumadin; Bristol-Myers Squibb, Princeton, NJ) or one of the more recently approved direct oral anticoagulant (DOAC) drugs, such as an antithrombin drug dabigatran (Pradaxa, Boehringer Ingelheim, Ridgefield, CT), or one of the direct factor Xa inhibitors: rivaroxaban (Xarelto; Janssen Pharmaceuticals, Beerse, Belgium), apixaban (Eliquis; Bristol-Myers Squibb), or edoxaban (Savaysa; Dalichi Sankyo Co, Tokyo). Warfarin is less expensive and can be used for both valvular and nonvalvular AF, whereas DOACs are approved by the US Food and Drug Administration only for nonvalvular AF. When warfarin is used in OAC therapy, the dosage is adjusted to have the international normalized ratio (INR) between 2.0 and 3.0. Although the DOACs are more expensive, they have a better efficacy and safety profile (i.e., cause less major bleeding) compared with warfarin when used at recommended doses. Dosage adjustments of DOACs are required when creatinine clearance is < 95 mL/min and in frail older adults. Because the pharmacologic profiles of DOACs are predictable after oral use, routine coagulation testing for patients on DOACs is not required; however, use of warfarin requires routine coagulation testing to ensure the INR is within the therapeutic range.

Implanted Permanent Pacemakers. More than 2.9 million people in North America have received implanted pacemakers, and more than 70% are in persons 65 years or older. A permanent, implanted pacemaker consists of a lithium battery–powered generator implanted subcutaneously in the left infraclavicular area that produces an

TABLE 5.3 Drugs Used to Treat Arrhythmias

Drug	Oral Adverse Effects	Dental Considerations
Class Iª: Fast Sodium Channel Blockers		
IA—Quinidine	Bitter taste, dry mouth, petechiae, gingival bleeding	Syncope, hypotension, nausea, vomiting, thrombocytopenia
IA—Procainamide	Bitter taste, oral ulcerations, xerostomia	Worsening of arrhythmias, lupus-like syndrome, rash, myalgia, fever, agranulocytosis
IA—Disopyramide (Norpace)	Dry mouth	Urinary hesitancy, constipation
IB—Mexiletine (Mexitil)	Dry mouth	Tremor, dizziness, diplopia, nausea, vomiting
IB—Lidocaine		Hypotension, seizure
IC—Propafenone (Rythmol)	Taste aberration, dry mouth	Worsening of arrhythmias, dizziness, nausea, vomiting
IC—Flecainide (Tambocor)	Metallic taste	Worsening of arrhythmias, confusion, irritability
Class II: Beta-Blockers (Partial List)		
Propranolol (Inderal)—nonselective beta-blocker	Taste changes; lichenoid reactions	Hypotension, bradycardia, fatigue; avoid long-term use of NSAIDs. Vasoconstrictor interactions: nonselective—potential increase in blood pressure (use maximum of 0.036 mg of epinephrine); avoid levonordefrin
Also: Acebutolol, atenolol, bisoprolol, esmolol, metoprolol, timolol		Vasoconstrictor interactions: none
Class III: Potassium Channel Blockers		
Amiodarone (Cordarone)	Taste (bitter) change	May cause bradycardia when lidocaine is given as a local anesthetic. Regular blood test to rule out organ toxicity, which can appear as interstitial pneumonitis, hyper- or hypothyroidism, elevated liver enzymes, bluish skin discoloration
Sotalol (Betapace)—nonselective beta-blocker	Taste changes; lichenoid reactions	Hypotension, bradycardia, torsades de pointes, fatigue; avoid long-term use of NSAIDs. Vasoconstrictor interactions: nonselective—potential increase in blood pressure (use maximum of 0.036 mg of epinephrine); avoid levonordefrin
Dofetilide	Angioedema	Headache, dizziness
Ibutilide		Headache, bradycardia, hypotension
Class IV: Slow Calcium Channel Blockers		
Verapamil (Calan)	Gingival overgrowth	Hypotension, bradycardia
Diltiazem	Gingival overgrowth	Hypotension, bradycardia, headache
Class V: Variable Mechanism		
Adenosine	Metallic taste, burning sensation	Hypotension, hyperventilation, bradycardia
Digoxin (Lanoxin)	Hypersalivation (toxicity)	Precipitation of arrhythmias, toxicity (headache, nausea, vomiting, altered color perception, malaise). Vasoconstrictor interactions: increased risk for arrhythmias; avoid if possible

ªClass I drugs are subdivided based on kinetics of the sodium channel effects: 1A intermediate kinetics, 1B fast kinetics, 1C slow kinetics.
NSAID, nonsteroidal antiinflammatory drug.

electrical impulse that is transmitted by a lead inserted into the heart through the subclavian vein to an electrode in contact with endocardial or myocardial tissue (Fig. 5.3). The leads may be either unipolar (stimulating only one chamber) or, more commonly, bipolar (stimulating two chambers). With a bipolar pacemaker, one lead usually is inserted into the right atrium, and the second lead is positioned within the right ventricle.

Pacemakers are capable of very specific individualized pacing programs or modes, depending on the individual's needs. A classification code is used to describe the various pacing modes of a pacemaker unit, which include the chamber that is paced, the chamber that is sensed, inhibitory or tracking function capability, rate modulation capability, and capability for antitachycardia pacing (ATP) or the delivery of a shock. Most pacemakers are of the demand variety, which can detect the patient's natural heartbeat and prevent competitive pacemaker firing; they are rate adaptive. Current units contain pacing circuits that allow for programming, memory, and telemetry. In general, pacemakers are indicated to treat bradycardias in patients with acquired AV block, congenital AV block, chronic bifascicular and trifascicular block, AV block associated with acute MI, sinus node dysfunction, hypersensitive carotid sinus and neurocardiogenic syncope, and certain forms of cardiomyopathy. They also are

TABLE 5.4 CHA₂ DS₂—VASc Score

Letter	Points	Description
C	1	**C**ongestive heart failure: moderate to severe systolic left ventricular dysfunction
H	1	**H**ypertension history
A₂	2	**A**ge > 75 years
D	1	**D**iabetes mellitus
S₂	2	**S**troke/transient ischemic attack (TIA)/thromboembolism history
V	1	**V**ascular disease: history of myocardial infarction, complex aortic plaque, or peripheral artery disease
A	1	**A**ge 65—74 years
Sc	1	Sex category (female)

Oral anticoagulation is recommended for those with a score of >2, and OAC or aspirin may be considered for a score of 1.

Dual-chamber pacemaker device

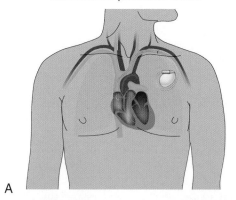

A

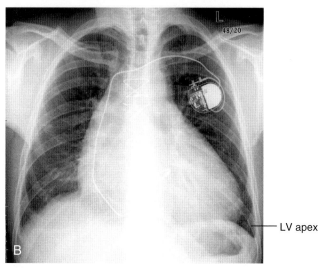

B

— LV apex

FIG. 5.3 A) The site of implantation of a permanent pacemaker (note: can be inserted in the left or right intraclavicular chest wall). **(B)** A chest radiograph showing a pacemaker in a patient. *LV*, left ventricular. ((**A**) Courtesy of Matt Hazzard, University of Kentucky. (**B**) From Bonow RO, et al., eds. *Braunwald's Heart Disease: A Textbook of Cardiovascular Medicine.* 9th ed. Philadelphia: Saunders; 2012.)

indicated for the prevention and termination of certain tachyarrhythmias.

Complications are infrequent but have been reported as a result of pacemaker placement. These include pneumothorax, perforation of the atrium or ventricle, subsequent dislodgment of the leads, infection, and erosion of the pacemaker pocket (i.e., the anatomic site where the pacemaker resides). Infective endocarditis rarely may occur; however, antibiotic prophylaxis for dental treatment is not recommended.

Implantable Cardioverter-Defibrillators

An ICD is a device that is similar to a pacemaker and is implanted in the same way as for a pacemaker. ICDs are capable not only of delivering a shock but also of providing ATP and ventricular bradycardia pacing. Most ICDs have a single lead that is inserted into the right ventricle and function by continuously monitoring a patient's cardiac rate and delivering ATP or a shock when the rate exceeds a predetermined cutoff point, such as in VT or VF. ATP has the advantage of terminating a rhythm disturbance without delivering a shock. ICDs generally are larger than pacemakers, and their batteries do not last as long as those of a pacemaker, the life span of ICDs being 5—10 years. Antibiotic prophylaxis for dental treatment in patients with these devices is not recommended.

Electromagnetic Interference. Electromagnetic interference (EMI) from nonintrinsic electrical activity can temporarily interfere with the function of a pacemaker or ICD. The pacemaker or ICD senses these extraneous signals and misinterprets them, which may cause rate alterations, sensing abnormalities, asynchronous pacing, noise reversion, or reprogramming. Numerous sources of EMI are present in daily life, industry, and medical and dental settings (see Box 5.3). The effects of EMI on pacemakers and ICDs vary with the shielding placed by different manufacturers, intensity of the electromagnetic field, frequency of the spectrum of the signal, distance and positioning of the device relative to the source, electrode configuration, nonprogrammable device characteristics, programmed settings, and patient characteristics. Electrical and magnetic fields are reduced inversely with the square of the distance from the source. Of note, current models contain improved shielding and algorithms (i.e., noise reversion mode) that reduce EMI better than older models.

Studies suggest that most dental devices (i.e., ultrasonic bath cleaners; ultrasonic scaling devices; and battery-operated curing lights, amalgamators, electrical pulp testers and apex locators, handpieces, electric toothbrushes, microwave ovens, and X-ray units) do not cause significant interference with the sensing and pacing of pacemakers and ICDs. This probably reflects the increased internal shielding provided in the newer pacemakers and ICDs. However, caution in the use of

---

BOX 5.3   Sources of Potential Electromagnetic Interference for Pacemakers and Implanted Cardioverter-Defibrillators

Daily Living
- Cell phones, portable headphones, metal detectors
- High-voltage power lines
- Household appliances (e.g., electric razors)

Industrial
- Arc welders, induction furnaces

Medical
- Magnetic resonance imaging scanners
- Electrosurgery, therapeutic diathermy
- Neurostimulators, defibrillators
- Transcutaneous electrical nerve stimulation (TENS) units
- Radiofrequency catheter ablation
- Therapeutic ionizing radiotherapy
- Lithotripsy

Dental
- Electrosurgery

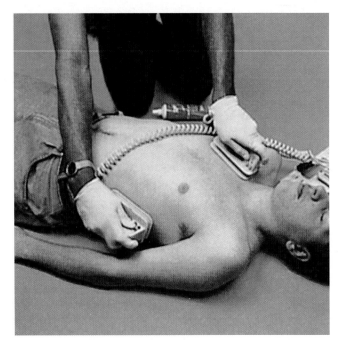

FIG. 5.4 Cardioversion/defibrillation paddles in place on a patient. (From Sanders MJ. *Mosby's Paramedic Textbook.* 3rd ed. St. Louis: Mosby; 2005.)

electrosurgery units is still recommended because these units showed EMI in medical settings and in vitro, and in vivo studies with dental electrosurgery devices have yet to be performed.

Radiofrequency Catheter Ablation. Radiofrequency catheter ablation is a technique whereby a catheter (electrode) is introduced percutaneously into a vein and is threaded into the heart. The catheter is positioned in contact with the area determined by electrophysiologic testing to be the anatomic source of an arrhythmia. Radiofrequency energy is then delivered through the electrode catheter whose tip is in contact with the target cardiac tissue. This results in resistive heating of the tissue, producing irreversible tissue destruction of an area 5–6 mm in diameter and 2–3 mm deep, destroying the ectopic pacemaker activity. This technique can eliminate a variety of supraventricular and VTs that previously required long-term pharmacologic treatment for suppression or surgery for cure.

Surgery

Surgery is another therapeutic approach used to treat patients with tachycardia. Direct surgical approaches designed to interrupt accessory pathways consist of tissue resection and ablation. In addition to direct surgical approaches, indirect approaches such as aneurysmectomy, coronary artery bypass grafting, or relief of valvular regurgitation or stenosis may be useful in selected patients.

Cardioversion and Defibrillation

Transthoracic delivery of an electric shock can be performed electively (cardioversion) to terminate persistent or refractory arrhythmias or on an emergency basis (defibrillation) to terminate a lethal arrhythmia. Direct current defibrillators deliver an electrical charge by way of two paddles (electrodes) placed on the chest wall. One electrode is placed on the left chest over the region of the apex, and the other is placed on the right side of the chest just to the right of the sternum and below the clavicle (Fig. 5.4). The shock terminates arrhythmias caused by reentry by simultaneously depolarizing large portions of the atria and ventricles, thereby causing reentry circuits to disappear momentarily. Defibrillation usually is instantaneous and cardiac pumping resumes within a few seconds. It may have to be repeated if defibrillation is unsuccessful (i.e., if a regular heartbeat is not occurring). The most common arrhythmias treated by cardioversion/defibrillation are VF, VT, AF, and atrial flutter. Treatment of patients with VF is always emergent. Treatment of patients with VT may be elective or emergent, depending on the patient's hemodynamic status. Treatment of those with atrial flutter and AF usually is elective.

Several types of automated external defibrillators (AEDs) are available for use in dental offices for emergency defibrillation. An AED should be considered for inclusion in the dentist's emergency medical kit. The use of AEDs is taught as part of basic and advanced cardiopulmonary resuscitation courses, and familiarity with these devices and their application among laypersons is encouraged by public health agencies. AEDs are commonly found in public areas, are simple and easy to use, and their use is a critical part of successful resuscitation for a victim of cardiac arrest.

DENTAL MANAGEMENT

Medical Considerations

Identification. Identification of patients with a history of an arrhythmia, those with an undiagnosed arrhythmia, and those prone to developing a cardiac rhythm disturbance is the first step in risk assessment and in avoiding an untoward event (Box 5.4). This process is accomplished by obtaining a thorough medical history, including a pertinent review of systems, and taking and evaluating vital signs (pulse rate and rhythm, blood pressure, respiratory rate). In the review of systems, patients should be asked about the presence of signs or symptoms related to the cardiovascular and pulmonary systems. Patients who report palpitations, dizziness, chest pain, shortness of breath, or syncope may have a cardiac arrhythmia or other cardiovascular disease and should be evaluated by a physician. Patients with an irregular pulse/cardiac rhythm (even without symptoms) also may require consultation with the physician to determine its significance. Patients with an existing arrhythmia, diagnosed or undiagnosed, are at increased risk for adverse events in the dental environment. In addition, patients at risk for developing an arrhythmia may be in danger in the dental office if they are not identified and measures are not taken to minimize situations that can precipitate an arrhythmia. Other patients may have their arrhythmias under control with the use of drugs or a pacemaker but require special consideration when receiving dental treatment. The keys to successful dental management of patients prone to developing a cardiac arrhythmia and those with an existing arrhythmia are identification and prevention. Even under the best of circumstances, however, a patient may develop a cardiac arrhythmia that requires immediate emergency measures.

Risk Assessment. Patients with a known history of arrhythmia should be interviewed carefully to ascertain the type of arrhythmia (if known), how it is being treated, medications being taken, presence of a pacemaker or defibrillator, effects on their activity, and stability of their disease. Because the classification and diagnosis of arrhythmia can be complex, patients often do not know the specific diagnosis that has been assigned to their disorder; thus, the physician must be relied on to provide this information. It is important to identify any known triggers, such as stress, anxiety, or medications. The presence of other heart, thyroid, kidney, or chronic pulmonary disease also should be determined because such disorders may be a cause of, or contributor to, the arrhythmia and may necessitate additional changes in dental management. If any questions or uncertainties arise, a medical consultation should be sought regarding the patient's diagnosis and current status and to aid the dentist in assessing risk for precipitating or aggravating a cardiac arrhythmia, stroke, or MI during or in relation to dental treatment.

Risk assessment requires determining the type and severity of arrhythmia, stability of the patient, and potential risk involved in providing dental treatment to a patient with a history of arrhythmia. This often requires consultation with the patient's physician. The American College of Cardiology (ACC) and the AHA have published guidelines that can help make this determination. These guidelines are intended for use by physicians who are evaluating patients with cardiovascular disease to determine whether they can safely undergo surgical procedures. They also may be applied to the provision of dental care and may be of significant value to the dentist in making a determination of risk.

Box 5.5 is based on these ACC/AHA guidelines and provides an estimate of the risk that a serious event (acute MI, unstable angina, or sudden death) may occur during noncardiac surgery in patients with various arrhythmias. Patients with a significant arrhythmia (i.e., high-grade AV block, symptomatic ventricular arrhythmias in the presence of cardiovascular disease, and supraventricular arrhythmias with an uncontrolled ventricular rate) that are untreated or inadequately managed are at major risk for complications and are not candidates for elective dental care. Dental care should be deferred until a consultation with the physician has occurred. The presence of other types of arrhythmias carries significantly less risk. The presence of pathologic Q waves (marker of a previous MI) is a clinical predictor of intermediate risk for perioperative complications; other ECG abnormalities, including left ventricular hypertrophy, left bundle branch block, and ST-T wave abnormalities, as well as any rhythm other than sinus rhythm, are associated with minor perioperative risk. Patients with these types of arrhythmias can undergo elective dental treatment with only minimally increased risk for an adverse event.

BOX 5.4 Identifying Patients With Cardiac Arrhythmias

Patients with cardiac arrhythmias may be identified by
- Assessing the medical history[a]
  - Type of arrhythmia
  - Frequency of occurrence and severity
  - How treated
  - Presence of pacemaker or defibrillator
  - Level of control or stability
- Understanding risk for arrhythmia is increased in the presence of other cardiovascular or pulmonary disease
- Identifying the patient who does not report an arrhythmia but may be taking one or more of the antiarrhythmic drugs
- Pertinent review of systems—asking about the presence of symptoms that could be caused by arrhythmias (palpitations, dizziness, chest pain, shortness of breath, syncope)
- Obtaining vital signs suggestive of arrhythmia (rapid pulse rate, slow pulse rate, irregular pulse)
- Referring patient to physician if signs or symptoms are present that are suggestive of a cardiac arrhythmia or other cardiovascular disease

[a]Consultation with the patient's physician may be required to obtain or verify this information.

BOX 5.5   Perioperative Risk and Dental Treatment for Patients With Cardiac Arrhythmias

Arrhythmias Associated With Major Perioperative Risk
- High-grade AV block
- Symptomatic ventricular arrhythmias in the presence of underlying heart disease
- Supraventricular arrhythmias with uncontrolled ventricular rate
  Dental management: Avoid elective dental care.

Arrhythmias Associated With Intermediate Perioperative Risk
- Abnormal Q waves on ECG (marker of previous myocardial infarction)
  Dental management: Elective dental care is appropriate.

Arrhythmias Associated With Minor Perioperative Risk
- ECG abnormalities consistent with
  - Left ventricular hypertrophy
  - Left bundle branch block
  - ST-T wave abnormalities
  - Any rhythm other than sinus (e.g., atrial fibrillation)
  Dental management: Elective dental care is appropriate.

AV, atrioventricular; *ECG,* electrocardiogram.
Data from Fleisher LA, Beckman JA, Brown KA, et al. ACC/AHA 2007 guidelines on perioperative cardiovascular evaluation and care for noncardiac surgery: a report of the American College of Cardiology/American Heart Association task force on practice guidelines (writing committee to revise the 2002 guidelines on perioperative cardiovascular evaluation for noncardiac surgery). *Circulation.* 2007;116:e418–e499.

BOX 5.6   Cardiac Risk Stratification for Noncardiac Surgical Procedures

High (Reported Cardiac Risk Often >5%)
- Emergent major operations, particularly in older adults
- Aortic and other major vascular surgery
- Peripheral vascular surgery
- Anticipated prolonged surgical procedures associated with large fluid shifts and/or blood loss

Intermediate (Reported Cardiac Risk Generally <5%)
- Carotid endarterectomy
- Head and neck surgery
- Intraperitoneal and intrathoracic surgery
- Orthopedic surgery
- Prostate surgery

Low (Reported Cardiac Risk Generally <1%)
- Endoscopic procedures
- Superficial procedures
- Cataract surgery
- Breast surgery

Data from Fleisher LA, Beckman JA, Brown KA, et al. ACC/AHA 2007 guidelines on perioperative cardiovascular evaluation and care for noncardiac surgery: a report of the American College of Cardiology/American Heart Association task force on practice guidelines (writing committee to revise the 2002 guidelines on perioperative cardiovascular evaluation for noncardiac surgery. *Circulation.* 2007;116:e418–e499.

The type and magnitude of the planned dental procedure also must be considered in determination of perioperative risk. Box 5.6 provides an estimate of cardiac risk for specific surgical procedures in patients with cardiovascular disease. Although dental procedures are not specifically listed, they would be included in the low-risk category, associated with less than a 1% chance of an adverse perioperative event. Nonsurgical dental procedures are likely to pose even less risk than that for surgical procedures. More extensive oral and maxillofacial surgical procedures, and perhaps some of the more extensive periodontal surgical procedures, would be classified in the intermediate cardiac risk category under "head and neck procedures," with a risk of less than 5%. Procedures associated with the highest risk (>5%) include emergency major surgery in elderly persons, aortic or vascular surgery, and peripheral vascular surgery. These procedures are performed with the patient under general anesthesia and carry the potential for significant blood and fluid loss with resultant adverse hemodynamic effects. Therefore, the vast majority of dental procedures, whether surgical or nonsurgical, are associated with low to very low risk for an adverse event in patients with arrhythmias and other cardiovascular diseases.

Recommendations (see Box 5.7)

Antibiotics: Infection Risk. Patients who have cardiac arrhythmias, pacemakers, or ICDs are not at risk for infective endocarditis related to dental procedures; thus, antibiotic prophylaxis is not indicated.

Appointment Scheduling. A patient who is susceptible to cardiac arrhythmias can receive virtually any indicated dental procedure after the arrhythmia has been identified and the appropriate recommendations mentioned here are followed. Complex dental procedures and multiple extractions should be scheduled over several appointments to avoid overstressing the patient and to limit the amount of drugs required for pain control.

Bleeding: Warfarin (Coumadin). Patients with AF often are taking warfarin to prevent thrombus formation, embolism, and stroke; thus, they are at risk for increased bleeding. The usual target range for anticoagulation in patients with AF is an INR between 2 and 3 times the normal value. Studies have shown that minor oral surgery, such as simple extractions, can be performed without altering or stopping the warfarin regimen, provided that the INR is between 2.0 and 3.5. Management recommendations include the use of local measures such as placing of gelatin sponges, oxidized cellulose, or chitosan hemostatic products in extraction sockets, suturing, gauze sponges for pressure pack, or stents during the surgery and the topical use of tranexamic acid or

BOX 5.7 | Checklist for Dental Management Considerations in Patients With Cardiac Arrhythmia[a]

PREOPERATIVE RISK ASSESSMENT

- Review medical history, determine whether arrhythmia exists, ascertain the cause and nature of the arrhythmia, and discuss relevant issues with the patient.
- Identify all medications and drugs being taken or supposed to be taken by the patient.
- Examine the patient for signs and symptoms of disease and obtain vital signs.
- Review recent laboratory test results or images required to assess risk.
- Confirm patient has a primary care provider and has taken medications today.
- Obtain a medical consultation if the patient's heart condition is poorly controlled or is undiagnosed.
- If arrhythmia and vital signs are well controlled, routine dental procedures can be performed with attention to the following precautions.

A

Analgesics	Provide good postoperative analgesia to minimize pain and associated stress.
Antibiotics	Based on current AHA guidelines, patients with pacemakers or ICDs do *not* require antibiotic prophylaxis. Some antibiotics (e.g., metronidazole, extended-spectrum penicillins) are known to increase the INR in patients on warfarin (Coumadin); caution in their use is advised.
Anesthesia	Ensure profound local anesthesia. Epinephrine-containing local anesthetic can be used with minimal risk if the dose is limited to 0.036 mg epinephrine (two capsules containing 1:100,000 concentration). Higher doses may be tolerated, but the risk of complications increases with dose. Avoid the use of epinephrine in retraction cord.
Anxiety	Use anxiety reduction techniques (see Chapter 1) to reduce catecholamine levels, as needed: • Provide preoperative sedation (short-acting benzodiazepine the night before and/or 1 h before the appointment). • Administer intraoperative sedation (nitrous oxide–oxygen).

B

Bleeding	In patients taking warfarin: • Review current INR laboratory test results (lab laboratory should be performed within 24–72 h of the surgical procedure); confirm that the patient is taking warfarin regularly and has consistent INR within therapeutic range. • If INR is within the therapeutic range (2.0–3.5), dental treatment, including minor oral surgery, can be performed without stopping or altering the warfarin regimen. In patients taking DOAC: • Minor oral surgery, typically can be performed without stopping or altering the DOAC regimen. • Consult with physician regarding planned dental procedure if major surgery is required, patient's coagulation status is uncertain, drug compliance is an issue, or the patient is frail. • Ensure that the patient has normal renal function. In patients taking warfarin, DOAC, or another anticoagulant or antiplatelet: • Use local hemostatic measures and products, including gelatin sponge, oxidized cellulose, or chitosan products in sockets, suturing, gauze pressure packs, and preoperative stents. Tranexamic acid or ε-aminocaproic acid can be used as mouth rinse or to soak gauze for placement at the bleeding site.
Blood pressure/vital sign monitoring	Obtain pretreatment vital signs and monitor pulse and blood pressure throughout stressful and invasive procedures.

C

Capacity to tolerate care	Determine functional capacity (e.g., METs) relative to the presence of an arrhythmia.
Chair position	Ensure comfortable chair position. Raise the chair slowly, and in case of slow heart rate or hypotension, stabilize the patient in an upright position before dismissing.

D

Devices	Pacemakers and ICDs may experience electromagnetic interference with electrosurgery devices; thus, avoid electrosurgery. Other electrical dental devices are not associated with interference of pacemaker activity.
Drugs	Avoid excessive amounts of epinephrine in patients who take nonselective β-adrenergic blockers, which can potentially cause a spike in BP and appears to be dose dependent. In patients taking digoxin, watch for signs or symptoms of toxicity (e.g., hypersalivation, visual changes) and avoid epinephrine and levonordefrin. See Table 5.3 for additional drug considerations.

E

Emergencies and urgent care	Have an emergency medical kit readily available. For a high-risk patient who requires urgent care, consider treating in a special care clinic or hospital

---

BOX 5.7   Checklist for Dental Management Considerations in Patients With Cardiac Arrhythmia[a]—cont'd

where a defibrillator can be used if needed. After consulting with physician, provide limited care only for pain control, treatment of acute infection, or control of bleeding, as appropriate. The following measures may be used as needed:

- Placement of intravenous line
- Sedation
- Monitoring with BP, ECG, pulse oximetry, capnography

F

| Follow-up | • After the procedure, allow patient to sit in upright position for several minutes before dismissing to avoid dizziness.
• Patients who have had invasive procedures should be contacted between 24 and 72 h to ensure that the postoperative course proceeds without complications.
• Ensure patient is receiving regular follow-up evaluation by physician; especially for patients with symptoms or poorly controlled arrhythmia. |

[a]Strength of recommendation taxonomy (SORT) Grade: C (see Preface for further explanation).
BP, blood pressure; *DOAC*, direct oral anticoagulant; *ECG*, electrocardiogram; *HF*, heart failure; *ICD*, implantable cardioverter-defibrillator; *INR*, international normalized ratio; *METs*, metabolic equivalents.

ε-aminocaproic acid as a mouth rinse or to soak sponges postoperatively.

Bleeding: Direct Oral Anticoagulants. Patients who have AF may be taking one of the DOACs to prevent clot formation, embolism, and stroke. These agents (i.e., dabigatran, apixaban, betrixaban, edoxaban, and rivaroxaban) have a better efficacy and safety profile (i.e., cause less major bleeding) than warfarin when used at recommended doses. Evidence available to date suggest that DOACs are not predicted to cause major bleeding during and after invasive dental procedures. However, patients who receive higher doses and those who have kidney function impairment are at increased risk for major bleeding. Accordingly, dentists are advised to limit the number of extractions performed at one appointment, monitor kidney function, and use good local hemostatic procedures for patients taking these drugs. If extractions of four or more teeth or surgical extractions are planned (major surgery), withholding the DOAC the night before surgery and resuming the drug the day after surgery, based on approval of the physician, has been performed with minimal complications. Reversal agents (idarucizumab, Praxbind, Boehringer Ingelheim; recombinant coagulation factor Xa, Andexxa, Portola Pharmaceuticals) are available to be administered in a hospital setting, if an emergency arises.

Capacity to Tolerate Care. Stress associated with dental treatment or use of excessive amounts of injected epinephrine may lead to life-threatening cardiac arrhythmias in susceptible dental patients. Patients with significant arrhythmias and those with cardiac comorbidities also may have difficulty adapting to stressful dental situations. Thus, the dentist must provide stress reduction strategies based on the level of medical risk, type of planned dental procedure, and stability and anxiety level of the patient. Stress reduction strategies for patients with arrhythmias of low to intermediate risk may include the following: (1) establishing good rapport, (2) scheduling short appointments in the morning before daily fatigue, (3) ensuring comfortable chair position, (4) pretreatment assessment of vital signs, (5) preoperative oral sedation, (6) intraoperative use of nitrous oxide–oxygen sedation, (7) ensuring profound local anesthesia, and (8) providing effective postoperative pain control (see Chapter 1). On occasion, it may be necessary to provide urgent dental care to a patient with a significant arrhythmia. If treatment is necessary, it should be performed as conservatively as possible and should be directed primarily toward pain relief, infection control, or control of bleeding. Consultation with the patient's physician is advised. The patient may be required to be treated in a special care clinic or hospital dental clinic in order to establish and maintain an intravenous line, provide continuously monitoring of the ECG, vital signs, and oxygen saturation.

Drug Considerations

Use of Vasoconstrictors. The use of vasoconstrictors in local anesthetics poses potential problems for patients with arrhythmias because of the possibility of precipitating cardiac tachycardia or another arrhythmia. However, profound anesthesia is important for limiting the pain response and the upregulation of sympathetic tone that can stimulate an arrhythmia. Hence, local anesthetic without vasoconstrictor is recommended when possible.

When using a local anesthetic with vasoconstrictor, patients in the low- to intermediate-risk category and those taking nonselective beta-blockers can safely be given up to 0.036 mg of epinephrine (two cartridges containing 1:100,000 epinephrine); intravascular injections should be avoided. Greater quantities of vasoconstrictor may well be tolerated, but increasing quantities are associated with increased risk for adverse cardiovascular effects. Vasoconstrictors should be avoided in patients taking digoxin because of the potential for inducing arrhythmias. For patients at major risk for arrhythmias, the use of vasoconstrictors should be avoided, but if their use is considered essential, it should be discussed with the physician. Studies have shown that modest amounts of vasoconstrictor can be used safely in high-risk cardiac patients when accompanied by oxygen, sedation, nitroglycerin, and excellent pain control measures.

For patients at all levels of cardiac risk, the use of gingival retraction cord impregnated with epinephrine should be avoided because of the rapid absorption of a high concentration of epinephrine and the potential for adverse cardiovascular effects. Alternatives that can be used to provide gingival effects equivalent to those of epinephrine without adverse cardiovascular effects include: a paste containing 15% aluminum chloride (Traxodent, Premier Dental Products), viscous 20% ferrous sulfate (Viscostat, Ultradent Products Inc.), or aqueous 12.7% iron (Astrigedent, Ultradent Products Inc.).

Digoxin Toxicity. Because the therapeutic range for digoxin is very narrow, toxicity can easily occur. This is a special concern in older adults and in those who have hypothyroidism, renal insufficiency, dehydration, hypokalemia, hypomagnesemia, or hypocalcemia. Patients with electrolyte disturbances generally are more susceptible to digoxin toxicity. Signs of toxicity include hypersalivation, nausea, vomiting, headache, drowsiness, visual distortions, with objects appearing yellow or green, and ventricular premature beats. The dentist should be alert to these changes and refer the patient reporting such changes to the physician.

Drug Interactions. There are drug interactions to consider in addition to avoiding the epinephrine–digoxin drug–drug interaction. Macrolide antibiotics can cause cardiac arrhythmias and should be avoided in patients who have QT prolongation or bradycardia or who concurrently use class IA and class III antiarrhythmia drugs.

Devices: Pacemakers and Implanted Cardioverter-Defibrillators and Electromagnetic Interference. The risk of encountering significant EMI with a pacemaker in the dental office is low. Box 5.3 lists potential sources of EMI. In the dental setting, electrosurgery should not be used on or around a patient with a pacemaker or ICD until further studies are performed (Box 5.7).

Oral Manifestations

Oral complications found in patients with arrhythmias are those that occur primarily as a result of adverse effects of medications used to control arrhythmia. Table 5.3 lists oral manifestations that can occur with use of antiarrhythmic drugs. Also, AF is associated with the thromboembolism, which on rare occasions has resulted in ischemia of the tongue.

BIBLIOGRAPHY

1. Aframian DJ, Lalla RV, Peterson DE. Management of dental patients taking common hemostasis-altering medications. *Oral Surg Oral Med Oral Pathol Oral Radiol Endod.* 2007;103(suppl):S45 e1–S45 e11.
2. Albert RK, Schuller JL, Network CCR. Macrolide antibiotics and the risk of cardiac arrhythmias. *Am J Respir Crit Care Med.* 2014;189(10):1173–1180.
3. Baddour LM, Bettmann MA, Bolger AF, et al. Nonvalvular cardiovascular device-related infections. *Circulation.* 2003;108(16):2015–2031.
4. Baddour LM, Epstein AE, Erickson CC, et al. Update on cardiovascular implantable electronic device infections and their management: a scientific statement from the American Heart Association. *Circulation.* 2010;121(3):458–477.
5. Dajani AS, Taubert KA, Wilson W, et al. Prevention of bacterial endocarditis: recommendations by the American Heart Association. *J Am Dent Assoc.* 1997;128(8):1142–1151.
6. Barnes BJ, Hollands JM. Drug-induced arrhythmias. *Crit Care Med.* 2010;38(6 suppl):S188–S197.
7. Blinder D, Manor Y, Shemesh J, et al. Electrocardiographic changes in cardiac patients having dental extractions under a local anesthetic containing a vasopressor. *J Oral Maxillofac Surg.* 1998;56(12):1399–1402. discussion 402-3.
8. Blinder D, Shemesh J, Taicher S. Electrocardiographic changes in cardiac patients undergoing dental extractions under local anesthesia. *J Oral Maxillofac Surg.* 1996;54(2):162–165. discussion 65-6.
9. Bowles WH, Tardy SJ, Vahadi A. Evaluation of new gingival retraction agents. *J Dent Res.* 1991;70(11):1447–1449.
10. Brand HS, Entjes ML, Nieuw Amerongen AV, et al. Interference of electrical dental equipment with implantable cardioverter-defibrillators. *Br Dent J.* 2007;203(10):577–579.
11. Brand HS, van der Hoeff EV, Schrama TA, et al. Electromagnetic interference of electrical dental equipment with cardiac pacemakers. *Ned Tijdschr Tandheelkd.* 2007;114(9):373–376.
12. Cairns JA, Connolly S, McMurtry S, et al. Canadian Cardiovascular Society atrial fibrillation guidelines 2010: prevention of stroke and systemic thromboembolism in atrial fibrillation and flutter. *Can J Cardiol.* 2011;27(1):74–90.
13. Cintron G, Medina R, Reyes AA, et al. Cardiovascular effects and safety of dental anesthesia and dental interventions in patients with recent uncomplicated myocardial infarction. *Arch Intern Med.* 1986;146(11):2203–2204.
14. Cheng JW, Barillari G. Non-vitamin K antagonist oral anticoagulants in cardiovascular disease management: evidence and unanswered questions. *J Clin Pharm Ther.* 2014;39(2):118–135.
15. Chow GV, Marine JE, Fleg JL. Epidemiology of arrhythmias and conduction disorders in older adults. *Clin Geriatr Med.* 2012;28(4):539–553.
16. Colilla S, Crow A, Petkun W, Singer DE, Simon T, Liu X. Estimates of current and future incidence and prevalence of atrial fibrillation in the U.S. adult population. *Am J Cardiol.* October 15, 2013;112(8):1142–1147.
17. Culic V, Eterovic D, Miric D, et al. Triggering of ventricular tachycardia by meteorologic and emotional stress: protective effect of beta-blockers and anxiolytics in men and elderly. *Am J Epidemiol.* 2004;160(11):1047–1058.
18. Dukes JW, Dewland TA, Vittinghoff E, et al. Ventricular ectopy as a predictor of heart failure and death. *J Am Coll Cardiol.* 2015;66(2):101–109.
19. Elayi CS, Lusher S, Meeks Nyquist JL, et al. Interference between dental electrical devices and pacemakers or defibrillators: results from a prospective clinical study. *J Am Dent Assoc.* 2015;146(2):121–128.

20. Fleisher LA, Beckman JA, Brown KA, et al. ACC/AHA 2007 guidelines on perioperative cardiovascular evaluation and care for noncardiac surgery: a report of the American College of Cardiology/American Heart Association task force on practice guidelines (writing committee to revise the 2002 guidelines on perioperative cardiovascular evaluation for noncardiac surgery): developed in collaboration with the American society of echocardiography, American society of nuclear cardiology, heart rhythm society, society of cardiovascular anesthesiologists, society for cardiovascular angiography and interventions, society for vascular medicine and biology, and society for vascular surgery. *Circulation*. 2007;116(17):e418–e499.

21. Fleisher LA, Fleischmann KE, Auerbach AD, et al. ACC/AHA guideline on perioperative cardiovascular evaluation and management of patients undergoing noncardiac surgery. *J Am Coll Cardiol*. 2014;64(22):e77–e137.

22. Frommeyer G, Eckardt L. Drug-induced proarrhythmia: risk factors and electrophysiological mechanisms. *Nat Rev Cardiol*. 2016;13(1):36–47.

23. Fuster V, Ryden LE, Cannom DS, et al. ACC/AHA/ESC 2006 guidelines for the management of patients with atrial fibrillation: a report of the American College of Cardiology/American Heart Association task force on practice guidelines and the European society of cardiology committee for practice guidelines (writing committee to revise the 2001 guidelines for the management of patients with atrial fibrillation): developed in collaboration with the European heart rhythm association and the heart rhythm society. *Circulation*. 2006;114(7):e257–e354.

24. Garofalo RR, Ede EN, Dorn SO, et al. Effect of electronic apex locators on cardiac pacemaker function. *J Endod*. 2002;28(12):831–833.

25. Garan H. Ventricular arrhythmias. In: Goldman L, Schafer A, eds. *Goldman-Cecil Textbook of Medicine*. Philadelphia: Saunders/Elsevier; 2016.

26. Go AS, Hylek EM, Phillips KA, et al. Prevalence of diagnosed atrial fibrillation in adults: national implications for rhythm management and stroke prevention: the AnTicoagulation and Risk Factors in Atrial Fibrillation (ATRIA) Study. *JAMA*. May 9, 2001;285(18):2370–2375.

27. Goldenberg I, Moss AJ. Long QT syndrome. *J Am Coll Cardiol*. 2008;51(24):2291–2300.

28. Greenspon AJ, Patel JD, Lau E, et al. Trends in permanent pacemaker implantation in the United States from 1993 to 2009: increasing complexity of patients and procedures. *J Am Coll Cardiol*. 2012;60(16):1540–1545.

29. Gregoratos G, Abrams J, Epstein AE, et al. ACC/AHA/NASPE 2002 guideline update for implantation of cardiac pacemakers and antiarrhythmia devices: summary article. A report of the American College of Cardiology/American Heart Association task force on practice guidelines (ACC/AHA/NASPE committee to update the 1998 pacemaker guidelines). *J Cardiovasc Electrophysiol*. 2002;13(11):1183–1199.

30. Guize L, Thomas F, Bean K, et al. Atrial fibrillation: prevalence, risk factors and mortality in a large French population with 15 years of follow-up. *Bull Acad Natl Med*. 2007;191(4–5):791–803. discussion 03-5.

31. Hall JE. *Guyton and Hall: Textbook of Medical Physiology*. 13th ed. St. Louis: Elsevier; 2016.

32. Hersh EV, Giannakopoulos H. Beta-adrenergic blocking agents and dental vasoconstrictors. *Dent Clin N Am*. 2010;54(4):687–696.

33. Hirsh J, Guyatt G, Albers GW, et al. Antithrombotic and thrombolytic therapy: American College of Chest Physicians evidence-based clinical practice guidelines (8th edition). *Chest*. 2008;133(6 suppl):110S–112S.

34. Humphries R, Cameron M. Lingual-artery thromboembolism. *N Eng J Med*. 2021;385:65.

35. Jafri SM. Periprocedural thromboprophylaxis in patients receiving chronic anticoagulation therapy. *Am Heart J*. 2004;147(1):3–15.

36. January CT, Wann LS, Alpert JS, et al. 2014 AHA/ACC/HRS guideline for the management of patients with atrial fibrillation: a report of the American College of Cardiology/American Heart Association task force on practice guidelines and the heart rhythm society. *J Am Coll Cardiol*. 2014;64(21):e1–e76.

37. Jeske AH, Suchko GD, Affairs ADACoS, Division of S, Journal of the American Dental A. Lack of a scientific basis for routine discontinuation of oral anticoagulation therapy before dental treatment. *J Am Dent Assoc*. 2003;134(11):1492–1497.

38. Kanji S, MacLean RD. Cardiac glycoside toxicity: more than 200 years and counting. *Crit Care Clin*. 2012;28(4):527–535.

39. Kyprianou K, Pericleous A, Stavrou A, et al. Surgical perspectives in the management of atrial fibrillation. *World J Cardiol*. 2016;8(1):41–56.

40. Lampert R, Joska T, Burg MM, et al. Emotional and physical precipitants of ventricular arrhythmia. *Circulation*. 2002;106(14):1800–1805.

41. Little JW, Simmons MS, Rhodus NL, et al. Dental patient reaction to electrocardiogram screening. *Oral Surg Oral Med Oral Pathol*. 1990;70(4):433–439.

42. Miller J, Zipes D. Diagnosis of cardiac arrhythmias. In: Mann D, Zipes D, Libby M, et al., eds. *Braunwald's Heart Disease: A Textbook of Cardiovascular Medicine*. Philadelphia: Saunders/Elsevier; 2015.

43. Matsuura H. The systemic management of cardiovascular risk patients in dentistry. *Anesth Pain Control Dent*. 1993;2(1):49–61.

44. Mauprivez C, Khonsari RH, Razouk O, et al. Management of dental extraction in patients undergoing anticoagulant oral direct treatment: a pilot study. *Oral Surg Oral Med Oral Pathol Oral Radiol*. 2016;122(5):e146–e155.

45. Mazzini MJ, Monahan KM. Pharmacotherapy for atrial arrhythmias: present and future. *Heart Rhythm*. 2008;5(6 suppl):S26–S31.

46. Miller CS, Leonelli FM, Latham E. Selective interference with pacemaker activity by electrical dental devices. *Oral Surg Oral Med Oral Pathol Oral Radiol Endod*. 1998;85(1):33–36.

47. Misiri J, Kusumoto F, Goldschlager N. Electromagnetic interference and implanted cardiac devices: the nonmedical environment (part I). *Clin Cardiol*. 2012;35(5):276–280.

48. Montebugnoli L, Prati C. Circulatory dynamics during dental extractions in normal, cardiac and transplant patients. *J Am Dent Assoc*. 2002;133(4):468–472.

49. Morais J, De Caterina R. Stroke prevention in atrial fibrillation: a clinical perspective on trials of the novel oral anticoagulants. *Cardiovasc Drugs Ther*. 2016;30(2):201–214.

50. Mozaffarian D, Benjamin EJ, Go AS, et al. Executive summary: heart disease and stroke statistics-2016 update: a report from the American Heart Association. *Circulation*. 2016;133(4):447–454.

51. Nijjer SS, Sohaib SM, Whinnett ZI, et al. Diagnosis of supraventricular tachycardias. *Br J Hosp Med (Lond)*. 2014;75(2):C22–C25.

52. Niu Y, Chen Y, Li W, Xie R, Deng X. Electromagnetic interference effect of dental equipment on cardiac implantable electrical devices: a systematic review. *Pacing Clin Electrophysiol*. December 2020;43(12):1588–1598.

53. Novo S, Barbagallo M, Abrignani MG, et al. Increased prevalence of cardiac arrhythmias and transient episodes of myocardial ischemia in hypertensives with left ventricular hypertrophy but without clinical history of coronary heart disease. *Am J Hypertens*. 1997;10(8):843–851.

54. Prineas RJ, Le A, Soliman EZ, et al. United States national prevalence of electrocardiographic abnormalities in black and white middle-age (45- to 64-year) and older (>/=65-year) adults (from the reasons for geographic and racial differences in stroke study). *Am J Cardiol*. 2012;109(8):1223–1228.

55. Patel NJ, Deshmukh A, Pant S, et al. Contemporary trends of hospitalization for atrial fibrillation in the United States, 2000 through 2010: implications for healthcare planning. *Circulation*. 2014;129(23):2371–2379.

56. Pineo G, Hull RD. Coumarin therapy in thrombosis. *Hematol Oncol Clin North Am*. 2003;17(1):201–216 (viii).

57. Pinski SL, Trohman RG. Interference in implanted cardiac devices, part II. *Pacing Clin Electrophysiol*. 2002;25(10):1496–1509.

58. Prystowsky EN, Padanilam BJ, Fogel RI. Treatment of atrial fibrillation. *JAMA*. 2015;314(3):278–288.

59. Rochford C, Seldin RD. Review and management of the dental patient with Long QT syndrome (LQTS). *Anesth Prog*. 2009;56(2):42–48.

60. Roedig JJ, Shah J, Elayi CS, et al. Interference of cardiac pacemaker and implantable cardioverter-defibrillator activity during electronic dental device use. *J Am Dent Assoc*. 2010;141(5):521–526.

61. Romond KK, Miller CS, Henry RG. Dental management considerations for a patient taking dabigatran etexilate: a case report. *Oral Surg Oral Med Oral Pathol Oral Radiol*. 2013;116(3):e191–e195.

62. Rubino RT, Dawson 3rd DR, Kryscio RJ, Al-Sabbah M, Miller CS. Postoperative bleeding associated with antiplatelet and anticoagulant drugs: a retrospective study. *Oral Surg Oral Med Oral Pathol Oral Radiol*. September 2019;128(3):243–249.

63. Simmons MS, Little JW, Rhodus NL, et al. Screening dentists for risk factors associated with cardiovascular disease. *Gen Dent*. 1994;42(5):440–445.

64. Smith MM, Barbara DW, Mauermann WJ, et al. Morbidity and mortality associated with dental extraction before cardiac operation. *Ann Thorac Surg*. 2014;97(3):838–844.

65. Taira CA, Opezzo JA, Mayer MA, et al. Cardiovascular drugs inducing QT prolongation: facts and evidence. *Curr Drug Saf*. 2010;5(1):65–72.

66. van Ryn J, Stangier J, Haertter S, et al. Dabigatran etexilate—a novel, reversible, oral direct thrombin inhibitor: interpretation of coagulation assays and reversal of anticoagulant activity. *Thromb Haemost*. 2010;103(6):1116–1127.

67. Wahl MJ. Myths of dental surgery in patients receiving anticoagulant therapy. *J Am Dent Assoc*. 2000;131(1):77–81.

68. Wiber D. Electrophysiologic interventional procedures and surgery. I. In: Goldman L, Schafer A, eds. *Goldman-Cecil Textbook of Medicine*. 25th ed. Philadelphia: Saunders; 2016.

69. Wilson BL, Broberg C, Baumgartner JC, et al. Safety of electronic apex locators and pulp testers in patients with implanted cardiac pacemakers or cardioverter/defibrillators. *J Endod*. 2006;32(9):847–852.

70. Zambon A, Polo Friz H, Contiero P, et al. Effect of macrolide and fluoroquinolone antibacterials on the risk of ventricular arrhythmia and cardiac arrest: an observational study in Italy using case-control, case-crossover and case-time-control designs. *Drug Saf*. 2009;32(2):159–167.

71. Zipes DP. Antiarrhythmic therapy in 2014: contemporary approaches to treating arrhythmias. *Nat Rev Cardiol*. 2015;12(2):68–69.

6

Heart Failure (Congestive Heart Failure)

KEY POINTS

- Heart failure (HF) is common and may be undiagnosed or poorly controlled, thus clinicians must assess for signs, symptoms, and comorbidities.
- Deterioration in cardiac output, known as decompensated HF, is associated with clinical signs and symptoms that are readily recognizable and include dyspnea, lightheadedness, fatigue, and exertion during limited physical activity.
- Dyspnea at rest and/or use of potent loop diuretics are features of severe HF.
- Dental providers should screen a patient's functional capacity by inquiring about the patient's ability to walk up a flight of steps without being out of breath.
- Dental providers must be cognizant of and avoid potential drug–drug interactions in patients who have HF.
- Clinicians should be aware that advancing age, low ejection fraction, and low blood pressure are associated with increased mortality in patients who have HF.
- Dental providers should ensure that patients who have HF are evaluated on a regular basis by their primary care physician or cardiologist to ensure that their cardiac condition is well controlled.

Heart failure (HF) is a condition with a primary abnormality of the heart that impairs the ability of the ventricle(s) to fill with or eject blood. It is defined by the Heart Failure Society of America as a clinical syndrome caused by a structural and/or functional cardiac abnormality and corroborated by elevated natriuretic peptide levels and/or objective evidence of pulmonary or systemic congestion. It is a condition mostly of the elderly and a major public health problem that is growing in both incidence and prevalence in the United States. The disorder is the primary reason for nearly 15 million office visits and more than 6 million hospital days each year. The number of HF deaths has increased steadily despite advances in treatment, in part due to increasing numbers of patients with HF who are of advancing age and have precursor conditions such as hypertension, dyslipidemia, diabetes, obesity, and cardiac arrhythmias, as well as longer-term survival of people with ischemic heart disease. Dental practitioners should be aware that patients with untreated or poorly managed HF are at high risk for myocardial infarction (MI), cardiac arrest, and cerebrovascular accident.

EPIDEMIOLOGY

HF is primarily a condition of older adults and is associated with several cardiac predisposing conditions. There are about 6 million persons currently diagnosed with HF in the United States with 700,000 new cases and nearly 300,000 deaths per year. HF is progressive with about 8 per 1000 men/women age 50–59 years affected, rising to about 70 per 1000 men/women by age 80 years or older. The incidence HF continues to increase primarily because of advances in medical technology that helps preserve and maintain life after cardiovascular events. Accordingly, more Medicare dollars are spent on the diagnosis and treatment of HF than any other diagnosis. A dental practice serving 2000 patients would expect to treat approximately 15–20 individuals with HF.

Etiology

Heart failure is caused by the inability of the heart to function efficiently as a pump, which results in either an inadequate emptying of the ventricles during systole or an incomplete filling of the ventricles during diastole. This in turn results in a decrease in cardiac output with an inadequate volume of blood being supplied to the tissues or in a backup of blood, causing systemic congestion. HF may involve one or both ventricles, and can result from acute injury to the heart (e.g., MI) or more commonly from a chronic process such as from hypertension or cardiomyopathy.

The most common underlying causes of HF in the United States are coronary heart disease (secondary to atherosclerosis), hypertension, cardiomyopathy, and valvular heart disease, with coronary heart disease and myocardial necrosis damage accounting for 60%–75% of cases. The second most common cause of HF, accounting for about one-fourth of all cases, is dilated cardiomyopathy (DCM). DCM is a syndrome characterized by cardiac enlargement with impaired systolic function of one or both ventricles, often accompanied by signs and symptoms of HF. About half of all cases of DCM have no identifiable cause and are therefore considered idiopathic. Known causes of cardiomyopathy include alcohol abuse, hereditary cardiomyopathies, and viral infections. Although hypertension is often not a primary cause of HF, it is a major contributor to HF with more than 75% of HF patients having a long-standing history of hypertension. Valvular heart disease used to be a more significant cause of HF; however, with the rates of rheumatic heart disease and congenital heart disease declining in the United States, there has been a subsequent decline in HF resulting from valvular disease. Also, type 2 diabetes mellitus is associated with several biochemical and physiological changes that increase the risk for HF.

Most of the acquired disorders that lead to HF result in initial failure of the left ventricle brought on by an increased workload or disease of the heart muscle. Left ventricular heart failure (LVHF) often is followed by failure of the right ventricle. In adults, left ventricular involvement is almost always present even if the manifestations are primarily those of right ventricular dysfunction (fluid retention without dyspnea or rales). By the time most patients are evaluated for medical treatment, failure of both sides of the heart usually has occurred.

The determination of left ventricular failure is often based upon a finding of an abnormal *ejection fraction* (*EF*), which is the percentage of blood ejected from the left ventricle during systole. Normal values for EF at rest vary between 55% and 70% (Fig. 6.1). An LVEF of 41%–49% is considered "mildly reduced" and often is used as a threshold to diagnose left ventricular failure. The outstanding symptom of left ventricular failure is dyspnea, which results from the accumulation or congestion of blood in the pulmonary vessels, thus the term *congestive* HF. Acute pulmonary edema is often the result of left ventricular failure. Left-sided HF is the most common cause of right-sided HF, because LVHF leads to pulmonary hypertension, which increases the work of the right ventricle pumping against increased pressure. The outcomes of right ventricular failure are systemic venous congestion and peripheral edema (Figs. 6.2 and 6.3). Failure of the right side of the heart alone is uncommon. The most common cause of pure right-sided HF is emphysema.

PATHOPHYSIOLOGY AND COMPLICATIONS

Heart failure is a symptom complex that impairs the ability of the ventricle to fill with or eject blood and is characterized by signs and symptoms of intravascular and interstitial volume overload and/or manifestations of inadequate tissue perfusion (see Fig. 6.2). The underlying pathophysiology of HF generally involves one or more processes: (1) impaired myocardial contractility (systolic dysfunction, commonly characterized as reduced LVEF);

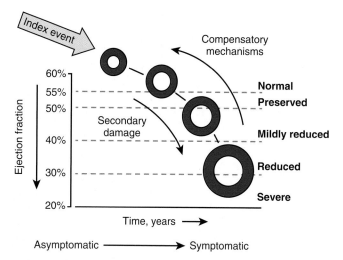

FIG. 6.1 Progression of heart failure with depression of ejection fraction. Heart failure begins with a decline in the heart's pumping capacity at which time several compensatory mechanisms are activated. For a time, these compensatory mechanisms can keep the heart functioning, but over time, because of increasing myocardial damage and secondary damage from other end organs, the heart's function (and ejection fraction) deteriorate. Normal ejection fraction is 55% −70%; 50%−54% is considered preserved; 40%−49% is considered mildly reduced, 30%−39% is considered reduced, and <30% is considered to be severe dysfunction.

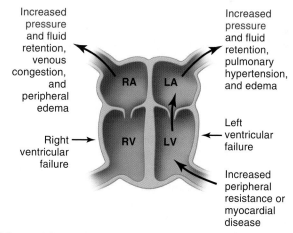

FIG. 6.2 Effects of right- and left-sided heart failure. *LA,* left atrium; *LV,* left ventricle; *RA,* right atrium; *RV,* right ventricle.

(2) increased ventricular stiffness or impaired myocardial relaxation (diastolic dysfunction, which is commonly associated with a relatively normal LVEF); (3) a variety of other cardiac abnormalities, including obstructive or regurgitant valvular disease, intracardiac shunting, or disorders of heart rate or rhythm; or (4) states in which the heart is unable to compensate for increased peripheral blood flow or metabolic requirements (see Fig. 6.3).

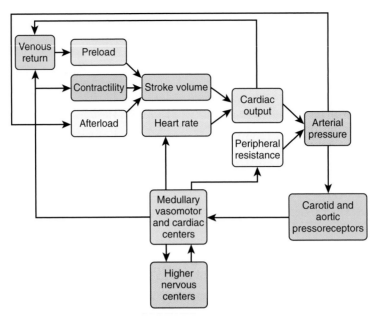

FIG. 6.3 Interactions in the intact circulation of preload, contractility, and afterload in producing stroke volume. Stroke volume combined with heart rate determines cardiac output, which, when combined with peripheral vascular resistance, determines arterial pressure for tissue perfusion. The characteristics of the arterial system also contribute to afterload, an increase in which reduces stroke volume. The interaction of these components with carotid and aortic arch baroreceptors provides a feedback mechanism to higher medullary and vasomotor cardiac center and to higher levels in the central nervous system to effect a modulating influence on heart rate, peripheral vascular resistance, venous return, and contractility. (From Starling MR. Physiology of myocardial contraction. In: Colucci WS, Braunwald E, eds. *Atlas of Heart Failure: Cardiac Function and Dysfunction*. 3rd ed. Philadelphia: Current Medicine; 2002, pp 19–35.)

Heart failure can affect the left or right side of the heart. Left ventricular failure (left-sided) leads to dilation and hypertrophy of the ventricle as it attempts to compensate for its inability to keep up with the workload. Venous pressure and myocardial tone increase along with the increase in blood volume. The net effect is diastolic dilation, which increases the force and volume of the subsequent systolic contraction. When right-sided ventricular enlargement occurs as a result of a lung disorder (e.g., emphysema) that produces pulmonary hypertension, the condition is called *cor pulmonale*.

Signs and symptoms of HF appear when the heart no longer functions properly as a pump. As the cardiac output falls, there is an increasing disproportion between the required hemodynamic load and the capacity of the heart to handle the load. With decreasing cardiac output, HF causes activation of neurohumoral systems to maintain perfusion. The physiological changes involved stimulate sympathetic tone and thus activate the renin—angiotensin system and production of vasoactive substances. Effects of these responses include increased heart rate and myocardial contractility, increased peripheral resistance, sodium and water retention, redistribution of blood flow to the heart and brain, and an increased efficiency of oxygen utilization by the tissues.

In 2021, the Heart Failure Society of America revised the classification of HF. This classification provides four stages of HF that reflect the fact that the disease is progressive and whose outcome can be modified by early identification and treatment (Box 6.1). Stages A and B denote patients with risk factors that predispose to the development HF, such as coronary artery disease, hypertension, and diabetes but who have not yet developed any symptoms of HF.

The difference between stages A and B is that in stage A, "at-risk for HF" patients do not demonstrate left ventricular hypertrophy (LVH), dysfunction or signs or symptoms; but those in stage B, "pre-HF," do have structural changes or dysfunction (structural heart disease) or elevated natriuretic peptide levels. Stage C denotes patients with past or current symptoms of HF associated with underlying structural heart disease (the bulk of patients), and stage D designates patients with "advanced HF" who have severe symptoms, often display recurrent or complicated hospitalization despite guideline-directed medical therapy and may require specialized advanced treatment, mechanical circulatory support, or end-of-life care. This classification system complements the older New York Heart Association (NYHA) classification system (Box 6.1), which is based on symptoms only.

BOX 6.1   Heart Failure Classifications

Heart Failure Society of America

Stage A: "At-risk for HF"—Patients at risk for HF who have not yet developed structural heart, no signs/symptoms.

Stage B: "Pre-HF"—Patients with structural heart disease or abnormal cardiac function or elevated natriuretic peptide levels, who are without current or prior signs/symptoms of HF.

Stage C: "HF"—Patients with current or prior symptoms and/or signs of HF caused by a structural and/or functional cardiac abnormality.

Stage D: "Advanced HF"—Patients with severe symptoms and/or signs of HF at rest, recurrent hospitalizations despite guideline-directed management and therapy (GDMT), refractory or intolerant to GDMT, requiring advanced therapies such as consideration for transplant, mechanical circulatory support, or palliative care.

New York Heart Association Classification

Class I: No limitation of physical activity. No dyspnea, fatigue, or palpitations with ordinary physical activity.

Class II: Slight limitation of physical activity. Patients experience fatigue, palpitations, and dyspnea with ordinary physical activity but are comfortable at rest.

Class III: Marked limitation of activity. Less than ordinary physical activity results in symptoms, but patients are comfortable at rest.

Class IV: Symptoms are present with the patient at rest, and any physical exertion exacerbates the symptoms.

*Bozkurt B, Coats AJS, Tsutsui J, et al. Universal definition and classification of heart failure: a report of the heart failure society of America, heart failure association of the European society of cardiology, Japanese heart failure society and writing committee of the universal definition of heart failure. *J Card Fail.* March 1, 2021; S1071-9164(21)00050-6.
https://doi.org/10.1016/j.cardfail.2021.01.022 Endorsed by Canadian heart failure society, heart failure association of India, the cardiac society of Australia and New Zealand, and the Chinese heart failure association. *Eur J Heart Fail.* 2021; 23(3):252–380.

BOX 6.2   Symptoms of Heart Failure

Dyspnea (perceived shortness of breath)

Fatigue and weakness

Orthopnea (dyspnea in recumbent position)

Paroxysmal nocturnal dyspnea (dyspnea awakening patient from sleep)

Acute pulmonary edema (cough or progressive dyspnea)

Exercise intolerance (inability to climb a flight of stairs)

Fatigue (especially muscular)

Dependent edema (swelling of feet and ankles after standing or walking)

Report of weight gain or increased abdominal girth (fluid accumulation; ascites)

Right upper quadrant pain (liver congestion)

Anorexia, nausea, vomiting, constipation (bowel edema)

Hyperventilation followed by apnea during sleep (Cheyne–Stokes respiration)

BOX 6.3   Signs of Heart Failure

Physical Appearance
- Cyanosis
- Clubbing of fingers
- Distended neck veins
- Peripheral edema
- Weight gain
- Unexplained weight loss (advanced HF)

Breathing/Respiration
- Rapid, shallow breathing
- Cheyne–Stokes respiration (hyperventilation alternating with apnea)
- Inspiratory rales (crackles) and pulmonary congestion

Cardiac (Rate or Rhythm)
- Heart murmur
- Increased heart rate
- Gallop rhythm
- Elevated jugular venous pressure
- Low pulse pressure
- Pulsus alternans (alternating strong and weak beats)
- Enlargement of cardiac silhouette on chest radiograph

Liver
- Enlarged tender liver
- Jaundice, ascites

Clinically the condition is described as either *compensated* or *decompensated* HF. In *compensated* HF, cardiac output and symptoms are stable, and most overt features (i.e., fluid retention and edema) are absent. Symptomatic HF is termed *decompensated* HF and refers to the presence of signs and symptoms and a deterioration of cardiac output.

HF is a progressive disease, characterized by multiple relapses and poor prognosis. Symptoms worsen over time because of ongoing deterioration of cardiac structure and function. Of patients who survive an acute onset of HF, only 35% of men and 50% of women are alive after 5 years. HF also predisposes the patient to ischemic stroke, the risk for which is twice as high as normal. The prognosis is better if the underlying cause can be treated. In people diagnosed with HF, sudden death occurs six to nine times the rate of the general population.

CLINICAL PRESENTATION

The symptoms and signs of HF (Boxes 6.2 and 6.3) reflect respective ventricular dysfunction and the side of heart damage. Left ventricular failure (left-sided) produces pulmonary vascular congestion with resulting pulmonary edema, dyspnea and orthopnea. The dyspnea is accompanied by lightheadedness or fatigue and usually is present with exertion or physical activity. Right-sided HF commonly presents with systemic venous congestion (distended neck veins, peripheral edema, and liver congestion).

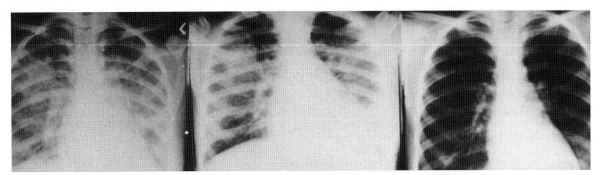

FIG. 6.4 Serial chest radiographs demonstrating the resolution of pulmonary edema (*left* to *right*). Note the enlargement of the cardiac silhouette. (Courtesy of J. Noonan, MD, Lexington, KY.)

The primary manifestations of HF is dyspnea. Dyspnea can occur during activity or at rest; the latter being a sign of severe HF. Orthopnea is positional dyspnea that is precipitated or worsened by the patient assuming a recumbent or semirecumbent position. Most patients with mild to moderate HF do not exhibit orthopnea when treated adequately. Paroxysmal nocturnal dyspnea (PND) is an attack of sudden, severe shortness of breath that awakens the patient from sleep, usually within 1−3 h after the patient goes to bed, and resolves within 10−30 min after the patient arises. The occurrence of PND is uncommon. Both orthopnea and PND are indicators of HF and are caused by increased venous return encouraged by the recumbent position with resulting increase in pulmonary venous pressure and alveolar edema. Central regulation of respiration also may be impaired in patients with advanced HF, resulting in alternating cycles of rapid, deep breathing (hyperventilation) with periods of central apnea, called *Cheyne−Stokes respiration.* PND is a common clinical feature associated with Cheyne−Stokes respiration in patients with HF.

Exercise intolerance is a hallmark symptom of HF (e.g., inability to climb a flight of stairs) and is caused by a combination of dyspnea and reduced blood and oxygen supply to the skeletal muscles. Fatigue (especially muscle fatigue) is a common, nonspecific symptom of HF. The pulmonary examination of patients with HF can be unremarkable; however, pulmonary congestion (rales or crackles), representing alveolar fluid and pulmonary effusions, is a hallmark sign of HF. The chest radiograph may reveal enlargement and displacement of the cardiac silhouette or abnormalities of the pulmonary vasculature (Fig. 6.4). Right ventricular failure results in systemic venous congestion and peripheral edema. Evidence of systemic venous congestion may be detected by low BP, the presence of distended neck veins (Fig. 6.5), a large tender liver, peripheral edema (Fig. 6.6), and ascites (Fig. 6.7). The retention of fluid results in weight gain and may increase body girth because of accumulation of fluid in the peritoneal cavity. On occasion, patients with chronic HF may have clubbing of the fingers (Fig. 6.8), cool extremities, and other features of poor perfusion.

The cardiac examination will usually reveal evidence of the underlying cardiac abnormality, as well as

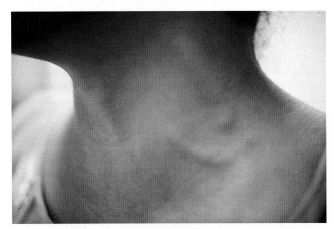

FIG. 6.5 Distended jugular vein in a patient with heart failure.

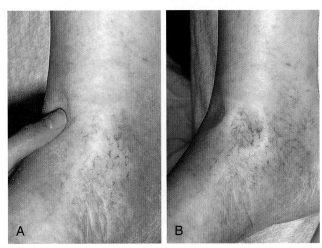

FIG. 6.6 (**A**) and (**B**) Pitting edema in a patient with heart failure. A depression ("pit") remains in the edematous tissue for some minutes after firm fingertip pressure is applied. (From Forbes, CD, Jackson, WF. *Color Atlas and Text of Clinical Medicine.* Edinburgh: Mosby; 2004.)

compensatory or degenerative changes in cardiac structure. Auscultation often reveals a laterally displaced apical impulse caused by LVH. A murmur of mitral regurgitation may be heard as well as an S_3 or S_4 gallop. Pulsus alternans, a regular rhythm with alternating strong and weak ventricular contractions, is pathognomonic of left ventricular failure that carries a poor prognosis with

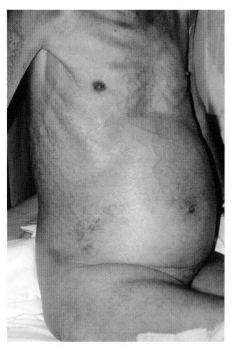

FIG. 6.7 Ascites. (Courtesy of P. Akers, MD, Evanston, IL.)

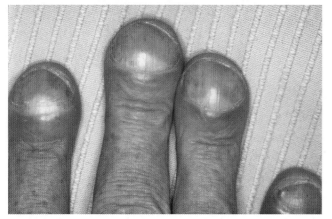

FIG. 6.8 Clubbing of the fingers in a patient with congestive heart failure.

patients who have HF. Another simple indictor of HF is increased pulse rate (tachycardia). Tachycardia is an indicator of increased myocardial oxygen demand, coronary blood flow, and overall myocardial performance. Tachycardia and atrial fibrillation are common in patients with HF and are known to increase adverse outcomes in these patients.

LABORATORY AND DIAGNOSTIC FINDINGS

The diagnosis of HF is based on the presence of clinical signs (fluid retention/hypoperfusion) and symptoms, and evidence of cardiac dysfunction and impaired functional capacity. A variety of specialized tests are used to diagnose and monitor HF, depending on the cause. Among

these are chest radiography, electrocardiography, echocardiography, radionuclide angiography or ventriculography, cardiovascular magnetic resonance, single-photon or positron emission computed tomography myocardial perfusion imaging, exercise stress test, ambulatory electrocardiography (Holter) monitoring, and cardiac catheterization. Measurement of systolic EF by one of the above imaging techniques is helpful in the determination of the efficacy of cardiac function and therefore the level of HF (see Fig. 6.1).

Normal, healthy cardiac function results in an EF of approximately 60%. However, with damage to the myocardium, the efficacy of cardiac function diminishes, and evidence of HF begins around 50%. Compensatory mechanisms and medical management will delay further HF until there is advanced myocardial damage. Reduced function is associated with an EF < 40% and severe HF occurs when the EF is below 30% (see Fig. 6.1).

HF often is associated with a decline in renal function, hyponatremia, hypoalbuminemia, and hepatic congestion. The main serum biomarker is natriuretic peptide (BNP or proBNP). An elevated BNP helps differentiate dyspnea of cardiac origin versus pulmonary origin, and helps determine the severity and prognosis of HF and response to therapy. Other routine blood tests include a complete blood count, renal and liver function testing, and measurements of electrolytes, blood glucose, lipids, and thyroid function.

MEDICAL MANAGEMENT

The medical management of patients with HF is complex and generally applied in a graduated approach, depending on the stage of the disease (see Box 6.1). Management for stages A and B begins with risk reduction and includes the identification and treatment of underlying medical problems, including controlling hypertension, atherosclerotic disease, diabetes, obesity, and metabolic syndrome (abdominal obesity, elevated blood glucose, dyslipidemia, hypertension). Fig. 6.9 illustrates the therapeutic decision-making process and drug therapy algorithm recommended according to the stage of HF. In addition, behavioral modification is promoted and includes smoking cessation, weight loss for obese patients, reduction of risk factors for cardiovascular disease, mild aerobic exercise, adequate rest, and avoidance of alcohol and illicit drugs. Drug therapy also may be indicated for the treatment of vascular disease or diabetes in stage A, as well as for ventricular dysfunction for stage B.

For stage C, all measures from stage A and B apply in addition to salt restriction and drug therapy (Table 6.1). Drug therapy is recommended to begin with angiotensin-converting enzyme inhibitors (ACEI). These drugs prevent the ACE enzyme from producing angiotensin II, which results in vasodilation. ACEI are quite effective in reducing mortality. Angiotensin receptor blockers (ARBs) are for patients who are ACEI intolerant. ARBs interfere

At Risk for Heart Failure   **Heart Failure**

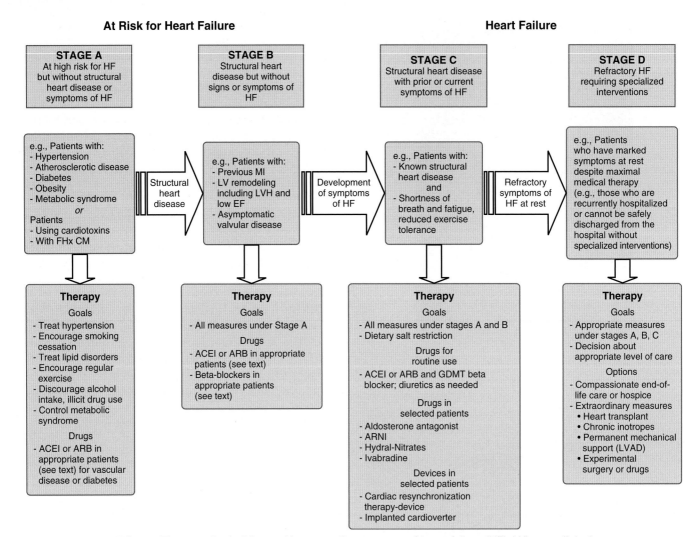

FIG. 6.9 Therapeutic decision-making according to stage of heart failure (HF). When a clinical diagnosis of HF is established, fluid retention should be treated before the patient starts an angiotensin-converting enzyme (ACE) inhibitor (or an angiotensin receptor blocker [ARB]) if the patient is intolerant to ACE inhibitors. Drug selection is based on ejection fraction, blood pressure, heart rate, kidney function, electrocardiogram findings, and race. In certain patients, device therapy may be necessary in addition to pharmacologic therapy. *ACEI,* angiotensin-converting enzyme inhibitor; *ARB,* angiotensin receptor-blocker; *ARNI,* angiotensin receptor-neprilysin inhibitor; *CM,* Cardiomyopathy; *EF,* ejection fraction; *FHx,* family history; *LV,* left ventricular; *LVAD,* left ventricular assist device; *LVH,* left ventricular hypertrophy; *MI,* myocardial infarction. (Adapted from *Circulation.* 2014;112:1825–1852 and from *Journal of the American College of Cardiology.* 2017;70(6):776–803.)

with the action of angiotensin II, also resulting in vaso-dilatation similar to ACEI. A newer approach combines an ARB (valsartan) with a neprilysin inhibitor (sacubitril), the latter serving to inhibit the enzyme neprilysin from breaking down peptides that lower BP. This class of drugs, known as (ARNI), are used in patients with chronic HF to further help reduce morbidity and mortality. However, ACEI are to be avoided in combination with an ARNI. Diuretics are typically prescribed to control fluid retention along with an ACEI/ARB/ARNI and are generally used with patients in Stage C (see Fig. 6.9). This combination approach helps reduce the

need for large doses of diuretics as well as some of the adverse metabolic effects of the diuretics. Several types of diuretics are used, including thiazide diuretics, potassium-sparing diuretics, and loop diuretics. Diuretics are used for three purposes: they are the only drugs that can adequately control fluid retention, they produce more rapid symptomatic relief than other drugs, and they modulate other drugs used to treat HF. Although diuretics are effective in decreasing the signs and symptoms of fluid retention, they cannot maintain the clinical stability of patients with HF when used alone. Spironolactone, a potassium-sparing diuretic, also blocks the

TABLE 6.1   Drugs Used for the Treatment of Heart Failure

Drug	Oral Adverse Effects	Dental Considerations
Thiazide Diuretics		
Chlorothiazide (Diuril), chlorthalidone (Thalitone), hydrochlorothiazide (HCTZ), indapamide (Lozol), metolazone (Mykrox)	Dry mouth; lichenoid reactions	Orthostatic hypotension. Vasoconstrictor interactions: none
Potassium-Sparing Diuretics		
Amiloride (Midamor), spironolactone (Aldactone), triamterene (Dyrenium)	Dry mouth	Orthostatic hypotension. Vasoconstrictor interactions: none
Loop Diuretics		
Bumetanide (Bumex), furosemide (Lasix), torsemide (Demadex)	Dry mouth	Orthostatic hypotension. Vasoconstrictor interactions: none
ACE Inhibitors (ACEIs)		
Benazepril (Lotensin), captopril (Capoten), enalapril (Vasotec), fosinopril (Monopril), lisinopril (Prinivil), moexipril (Univasc), perindopril (Coversyl), quinapril (Accupril), ramipril (Altace), trandolapril (Mavik)	Angioedema of the lip, face, or tongue; taste changes; burning mouth; lichenoid reactions	Cough, orthostatic hypotension; avoid use of NSAIDs. Vasoconstrictor interactions: none
Angiotensin Receptor Blockers (ARBs)		
Candesartan (Atacand), eprosartan (Teveten), irbesartan (Avapro), losartan (Cozaar), olmesartan (Benicar), telmisartan (Micardis), valsartan (Diovan)		Orthostatic hypotension. Vasoconstrictor interactions: none
Angiotensin Receptor-Neprilysin Inhibitors (ARNIs)		
Sacubitril-valsartan (Entresto)		Cough, dizziness, lightheadedness, orthostatic hypotension
Hyperpolarization-Activate Cyclic Nucleotide Gated (HCN) Channel Blocker		
Ivabradine (Corlanor)		Bradycardia, orthostatic hypotension, visual changes, angioedema
Aldosterone Inhibitors		
Eplerenone (Inspra), spironolactone (Aldactone)		Orthostatic hypotension. Vasoconstrictor interactions: none
Beta-Blockers		
Acebutolol (Sectral) (CS), atenolol (Tenormin) (CS), betaxolol (Kerlone) (CS), bisoprolol (Zebeta) (CS), carteolol (Cartrol) (NS), carvedilol (Coreg) (NS/α blocker), labetalol (Normodyne) (CS), metoprolol (Lopressor) (CS), nadolol (Corgard) (NS), penbutolol (Levatol) (NS), pindolol (Visken) (NS), propranolol (Inderal) (NS), timolol (Blocadren) (NS)	Lichenoid reactions	Orthostatic hypotension; avoid use of NSAIDs Possible increase in BP is possible with NS beta-blockers; cautious use of vasoconstrictors is recommended (maximum, 0.036 mg of epinephrine; 0.20 mg of levonordefrin) With CS beta-blockers, use vasoconstrictors normally
Digitalis		
Digoxin (Lanoxin)	Increased gag reflex; hypersalivation (sign of toxicity)	Increased risk for arrhythmias; avoid vasoconstrictors if possible
Vasodilators		
Hydralazine (Apresoline), isosorbide dinitrate (Isordil)	Lupus-like oral lesions, lymphadenopathy, dry mouth	Orthostatic hypotension. Vasoconstrictor interactions: none

ACE, angiotensin-converting enzyme; *BP*, blood pressure; *CS*, cardioselective; *NS*, nonselective; *NSAID*, nonsteroidal antiinflammatory drug.

action of aldosterone (aldosterone antagonist) and when used in patients with Stage D symptoms has been shown to reduce the risk of death by 25%–30%. Other than spironolactone, the diuretics do not influence the natural history of chronic HF.

The β-adrenergic blockers are used in combination with the ACE inhibitors, and (i.e., bisoprolol, carvedilol, and metoprolol) can help reduce the risk of death or hospitalization for HF by 30%–40%.

Digitalis glycosides have been used in the treatment for HF for many years, with digoxin being the most commonly prescribed. However, with the advent of the ACE inhibitors and ARBs, digoxin use has declined. Digoxin has not been shown to decrease either the risk of death or of hospitalization, unlike the ACE inhibitors and beta-blockers. Digoxin is, however, effective in alleviating symptoms; therefore, it is principally used to treat residual symptoms not controlled by other drugs. A significant problem with digitalis glycosides is their narrow therapeutic range and the resulting toxicity that easily can occur (Box 6.4).

Other drugs used to treat patients with HF unresponsive, or in addition, to ACEI, ARB, ARNI, or β-adrenergic blockers include direct-acting vasodilators (hydralazine, isosorbide dinitrate) and a newer medication (ivabradine, Corlanor) that slows down the heart's pacemaker cells. Combination hydralazine–isosorbide dinitrate has shown particular efficacy in patients with significantly reduced EFs. Ivabradine is for patients with poor EF, a resting heart rate of >70 and those who can't use a β-blockers or are on the maximum dose of a β-blocker. In selected patients, other nonpharmacologic measures may be indicated, including biventricular pacing or the use of an implantable defibrillator.

For all patients with HF, drugs that are known to worsen the clinical status should be avoided. These include nonsteroidal antiinflammatory drugs (NSAIDs), most antiarrhythmic drugs, and calcium channel blockers. NSAIDs are avoided because they can cause sodium retention, vasoconstriction, and can reduce the effectiveness and increase the toxicity of ACEIs.

As with many conditions, a large degree of success of medical therapy depends on patient compliance with treatment recommendations. Unfortunately, compliance with treatment recommendations is often suboptimal. Because many of these patients are treated with a plethora of drugs, it is important to monitor and encourage their compliance. However, a study has demonstrated that even after telemonitoring and multiple verbal reminders, the overall impact on improving outcomes in HF was not significant. In patients with severe refractory HF (stage D), and drug therapy is found to be inadequate, mechanical and surgical intervention may be provided. These measures can include intraaortic balloon counterpulsation, left ventricular assist device (LVAD), and heart transplantation. These assist systems include second- and third-generation devices such as the Heart-Mate II (Thoratec; Pleasanton, CA), Jarvik 2000 (Jarvik Heart Inc; New York, NY), DeBakey LVAD (MicroMed Technology; Houston, TX), and HeartWare HVAD (Medtronic; Minneapolis, MN). These devices may require anticoagulation so dental providers should inquire as to the medications these patients take, and LVADs are similar to an extended heart valve; therefore, antibiotic prophylaxis is recommended (see Chapter 2).

Implantable cardioverter-defibrillator (ICD) therapy has demonstrated benefits in treating HF patients in Stages C and D. When cardiac resynchronization therapy is added to ICD, the mortality and morbidity in patients with HF are improved. The final measure is end-of-life care with hospice. Improvements in continuous-flow LVADs have demonstrated significant improvements in survival of patients with HF as well as quality of life and functional capacity.

DENTAL MANAGEMENT

Identification. Identification of patients with a history of HF, those with undiagnosed HF, or those prone to developing HF is the first step in risk assessment and avoiding an untoward event. As HF is a symptom complex that is the end result of an underlying disease such as coronary heart disease, hypertension, or cardiomyopathy, the cause of HF must be identified and steps taken for appropriate dental management. Identification is accomplished by obtaining a thorough medical history, including a pertinent review of systems, and measuring the vital signs (pulse rate and rhythm, blood pressure [BP], respiratory rate). All medications being taken should be identified as well. In a review of systems, patients should be asked about the presence of clinical signs or symptoms related to the cardiovascular and pulmonary systems. Patients reporting shortness of breath, orthopnea, PND, fatigue, or exercise intolerance may have HF or other cardiovascular disease.

Patients with advanced HF may deteriorate suddenly. Features of more advanced HF include symptoms associated with *decompensated* HF (Stages C and D, see Box 6.1), escalating doses of diuretics, use of more potent loop diuretics, poor functional capacity (i.e., inability to climb a flight of stairs without shortness of breath or fatigue), frequent use of nitroglycerin.

BOX 6.4	**Clinical Manifestations of Digitalis Toxicity**

Headache, nausea, vomiting
Hypersalivation
Altered vision and color perception
Fatigue, malaise, drowsiness
Arrhythmias (tachycardias or bradycardias)

Risk Assessment. The dentist must make a determination of the risk involved in providing dental treatment to a patient with HF and decide if the benefits of treatment outweigh the risk. This often requires consultation with the patient's physician/cardiologist to determine the patient's physical status, laboratory test results, level of control, compliance with medications and recommendations, and overall stability. The ACC and the AHA have published guidelines that can help to make this determination. These guidelines are intended for use by physicians who are evaluating patients with cardiovascular disease to determine if they can safely undergo surgical procedures. They also can be applied to the provision of dental care and be of significant value to the dentist in making a determination of risk.

The guidelines suggest that patients with *decompensated* HF are at major risk for occurrence of a serious event (acute MI, unstable angina, or sudden death) during treatment. Thus, patients with symptoms of HF (*decompensated*; NYHA class II, III, or IV/Stage D; Box 6.1) generally are not candidates for elective dental care, and treatment should be deferred until medical consultation can be obtained (Box 6.5). Patients who have a history of HF but who are asymptomatic (*compensated*; Stage A and B) constitute an intermediate risk for a serious event occurring. With good functional capacity and reserve (i.e., can climb a flight of stairs; see Chapter 1), however, they can generally undergo any required treatment with little likelihood of problems. Thus, patients who are Stage A and B can receive routine outpatient dental care. However, the dentist should be aware that even these HF patients with Stage A and B should not be considered "mild" because they indeed could become decompensated during dental treatment. Many patients who are Stage C may undergo routine treatment in an outpatient setting after approval by their physician. However, it is important to realize that even the patient who has compensated HF may become decompensated during a dental procedure. The most common reason for this happening is failure to take their medications properly. Therefore, the dentist must be aware, monitor them closely, inquire about medication compliance, and be prepared for an emergency.

Stage C patients with reduced EF and all Stage D patients are better suited for treatment in a special care facility such as a hospital dental clinic with continuous monitoring. Clinicians should be aware that advancing age, low EF, and low BP are associated with increased mortality in this patient population. Moreover, patients who have HF as well as patients discussed in Chapters 2–5 on an occasion may require cardiac surgery. A study by Smith et al. indicated a significantly higher risk of serious adverse outcomes of patients undergoing elective heart surgery if they had a tooth extracted within 30 days of the surgery. A total of 3% of those patients died, and another 8% had serious adverse events. Therefore, caution should be exercised in performing extractions in dental patients before cardiac surgery.

Recommendations (see Box 6.5)

In general, patients with HF who are under good medical management can receive any indicated dental treatment as long as the dental management plans deal effectively with the problems presented by the HF, its underlying cause, and the effects of medications. Patients with symptomatic HF present a definite challenge that mandates specific management considerations.

Antibiotics. There is no need for antibiotic prophylaxis unless there is an underlying prosthetic heart valve or other cardiac conditions (refer to AHA guidelines). LVADs are similar to an extended heart valve; therefore, antibiotic prophylaxis are recommended (see Chapter 2).

Anxiety. Recommendations for management include short, stress-free appointments. Untreated or poorly controlled patients may appear very anxious and stressed and possibly progress to a serious arrhythmia or cardiac arrest. It may be necessary to use anxiety and stress reduction techniques.

Analgesics. Clinicians should provide good postoperative pain control but avoid NSAIDs. NSAIDs should be avoided because they can exacerbate symptoms of HF.

Bleeding. Excessive bleeding may occur in patients who are taking anticoagulants (e.g., warfarin) or antiplatelets (e.g., clopidogrel, prasugrel, ticagrelor). An INR should be obtained at least 72 h before an invasive procedure for those taking warfarin, and invasive procedures should be postponed if the INR is >3.5.

Blood Pressure. Monitor BP before and during the procedure, because BP may significantly increase or decrease in poorly controlled patients. If the BP drops below 100/60 mm Hg and the patient is unresponsive to fluid replacement and vasopressive measures, seek immediate medical attention.

Chair Position. Patients with HF may not tolerate a supine chair position because of pulmonary edema and need a semisupine or upright chair position. If the patient is hypotensive and syncopal because of cardiac stress and pulmonary congestion, he or she may not tolerate a supine position; thus tilt the chair slightly upwards in these instances.

Consultation. If under good medical management, the dental treatment plan is unaffected. However, consultation with the patient's physician to establish the level of control (e.g., EF) is recommended.

Drug Considerations. Before administering medications to patients who have HF, drug–drug interactions should be checked and avoided. Patients with HF are typically on many medications.

Anesthesia. It is important to administer good anesthesia to reduce stress and cardiac crisis. For patients who are Stages C or D, vasoconstrictors should be limited to a

BOX 6.5	Checklist for Dental Management of Patients With Heart Failure[a]

PREOPERATIVE RISK ASSESSMENT (SEE BOX 1.1)
- Evaluate and determine whether HF exists. Review medical history and discuss relevant issues with the patient.
- Identify all medications and drugs being taken or supposed to be taken by the patient.
- Examine the patient for signs and symptoms of disease and obtain vital signs.
- Review or obtain recent laboratory test results or images required to assess risk.
- Confirm patient has a primary care provider/cardiologist and has taken medications today.
- Obtain a medical consultation if the patient is poorly controlled or if the condition is undiagnosed or if the cause or nature of HF is uncertain.
- If vital signs indicate well control, routine dental procedures can be performed without special precautions.

A

Antibiotics	There is no need for antibiotic prophylaxis unless there is an underlying prosthetic heart valve/LVAD or other cardiac conditions (refer to AHA guidelines: Box 2.1 and Table 2.6).
Anesthesia	It is important to administer good anesthesia to reduce stress and risk for cardiac crisis. Epinephrine (1 : 100,000 and no more than 2 carpules) in local anesthetics is generally no problem, but patients should be monitored closely. Clinicians should provide good postoperative pain control. General anesthesia should be avoided.
Analgesics	See "F" (Follow-up care)
Anxiety	Untreated or poorly controlled patients may appear anxious or stressed, which could precipitate a cardiac crisis. It is important to control the heart rate. It may be necessary to use anxiety and stress reduction techniques (see Chapter 1).

B

Bleeding	Excessive bleeding may occur as a result of invasive procedures in patients who are taking anticoagulants (warfarin) or antiplatelets (clopidogrel, prasugrel, ticagrelor). INR should be obtained if the patient is taking warfarin. Hemostatic methods should be used in these patients.
Blood pressure (BP)	Monitor BP because it may significantly increase or decrease in poorly controlled patients. Monitor BP and blood loss throughout procedure. If BP drops below 100/60 mm Hg and

the patient is unresponsive to fluid replacement and vasopressive measures, seek immediate medical attention.

C

Chair position	If hypotensive and syncopal because of cardiac stress and pulmonary congestion, the patient may not tolerate a supine position.
Consultation	Patients with HF who have cardiac-related symptoms or signs should receive consultation with their physician to establish the level of control (e.g., ejection fraction) and need for medical treatment.

D

Devices	These patients may have pacemakers, implanted defibrillators, LVADs, or prosthetic valves. Those with LVADs or prosthetic heart valves should receive antibiotic prophylaxis prior to an invasive dental procedure.
Drugs	These patients are typically taking many medications (see Table 6.1). Be aware of adverse effects and potential drug interactions. The use of epinephrine or other pressor amines in gingival retraction cords (or to control bleeding) must be avoided.

E

Equipment	BP and pulse oximetry monitoring may be necessary for patients in Stage C/D (III/IV) when invasive procedures are performed.
Emergencies	Patients undergoing a cardiac crisis may progress to cardiac arrest and need to be treated as a medical emergency, and 911 may need to be called. If the patient is ambulatory and stable, he or she should seek urgent medical care. Ongoing vital signs must be monitored and CPR initiated; if necessary, transport the patient to emergency medical facilities.

POSTOPERATIVE CARE

F

Follow-up	• After the procedure, allow patient to sit in upright position for several minutes before dismissing to avoid dizziness. • Ensure adequate postoperative pain control to reduce risk of cardiac event. • In the postoperative phase, avoid NSAIDs, which can exacerbate HF. • Ensure patient is receiving regular follow-up evaluation by physician.

[a]Strength of recommendation taxonomy (SORT) Grade: C (see Preface for further explanation).
AHA, American Heart Association; *CPR*, cardiopulmonary resuscitation; *HF*, heart failure; *LVAD*, left ventricular assist device; *NSAID*, nonsteroidal anti-inflammatory drug.

maximum of 0.036 mg of epinephrine (i.e., two cartridges of 2% lidocaine with 1:100,000 epinephrine), taking care to avoid inadvertent intravascular injection. Epinephrine-impregnated gingival retraction cord should be avoided.

Nitrous oxide plus oxygen sedation can be used if adequate O_2 flow (at least 30%) is maintained. Supplemental low-flow oxygen alone also may be used. General anesthesia should be avoided in patients with HF.

For patients taking a digitalis glycoside (digoxin), epinephrine should be avoided, if possible, because the combination can potentially precipitate arrhythmias. Patients should be observed for signs of digitalis toxicity, such as hypersalivation. If toxicity is suspected, patients should promptly be referred to their physician.

Devices. Patients who have HF may have pacemakers, implanted defibrillators, LVADs, or prosthetic valves in which case national guidelines should be followed (see Chapters 2 and 5). There is little evidence that electromagnetic interference from dental instruments is a problem, but it should be considered. Patients with LVADs have priority for heart transplantation, and dental care should be limited to urgent treatment until the patient is more stable, and coordinated with the patient's cardiology team.

Equipment. BP and pulse oximetry monitoring may be necessary.

Emergencies. Patients undergoing a cardiac crisis may progress to cardiac arrest and need to be treated as a medical emergency, in which case 911 should be called, vital signs are monitored and cardiopulmonary resuscitation is initiated and performed.

ORAL MANIFESTATIONS AND COMPLICATIONS

There are no oral manifestations related to HF per se; however, many of the drugs used to manage HF can cause dry mouth and oral lesions (see Table 6.1). Digitalis may exaggerate the patient's gag reflex and can cause hypersalivation when serum levels exceed therapeutic dose.

BIBLIOGRAPHY

1. Agha SA, Kalogeropoulos AP, Shih J, et al. Echocardiography and risk prediction in advanced heart failure: incremental value over clinical markers. *J Card Fail.* 2009;15(7):586−592.
2. Alattar FT, Imran N, Debari VA, et al. Fractional excretion of sodium predicts worsening renal function in acute decompensated heart failure. *Exp Clin Cardiol.* 2010;15(3):e65−e69.
3. Ambrosy AP, Braunwald E, Morrow DA, et al. Angiotensin receptor-neprilysin inhibition based on history of heart failure and use of renin-angiotensin system antagonists. *J Am Coll Cardiol.* 2020 1;76(9):1034−1048.
4. Bozkurt B, Coats AJS, Tsitsio J, et al. Universal definition and classification of heart failure: a report of the Heart Failure Society of America, Heart Failure Association of the European Society of Cardiology, Japanese Heart Failure Society and Writing Committee of the Universal Definition of Heart Failure: endorsed by Canadian Heart Failure Society, Heart Failure Association of India, the Cardiac Society of Australia and New Zealand, and the Chinese Heart Failure Association. *Eur J Heart Fail.* 2021;23(3):352−380. https://doi.org/10.1002/ejhf.2115.
5. Chaundry S, Mattera J, Curtis JP, et al. Telemonitoring in patients with heart failure. *N Engl J Med.* 2010;363(24):2301−2311.
6. Conrado VC, Andrade J, de Angelis GA, et al. Cardiovascular effects of local anesthesia with vasoconstrictor during dental extraction in coronary patients. *Arq Bras Cardiol.* 2007;88(5):507−513.
7. Feldmann C, Chatterjee A, Haverich A, et al. Left ventricular assist devices—a state of the art review. *Adv Exp Med Biol.* 2018;1067:287−294.
8. Findler MD, Findler M, Rudis E. Dental treatment of a patient with an implanted left ventricular assist device: expanding the frontiers. *Oral Surg Oral Med Oral Pathol Oral Radiol Endod.* 2011;111:e1−e4.
9. Fonarrow GC, Albet NM, Curtis AB, et al. Improving evidence-based care for heart failure. *Circulation.* 2010;122:585−595.
10. Friedlander AH, Yoshikawa TT, Chang DS, et al. Atrial fibrillation: pathogenesis, medical-surgical management and dental implications. *J Am Dent Assoc.* 2009;140(2):167−177; quiz 248.
11. Herman WW, Ferguson HW. Dental care for patients with heart failure: an update. *J Am Dent Assoc.* 2010;141(7):845−853.
12. Hollenberg SM, Stevenson LW, Ahmad T, et al. 2019 ACC expert consensus decision pathway on risk assessment, management, and clinical trajectory of patients hospitalized with heart failure: a report of the American College of Cardiology Solution Set Oversight Committee. *J Am Coll Cardiol.* 2019;74(15):1966−2011.
13. Horsley L. American Heart Association update of heart failure guidelines. *Am Fam Physician.* 2011;81(5):654−665.
14. House AA. Pharmacological therapy of cardiorenal syndromes and heart failure. *Contrib Nephrol.* 2010;164:164−172.
15. Jackson SL, Tong X, King RJ, Loustalot F, Hong Y, Ritchey MD. National burden of heart failure events in the United States, 2006 to 2014. *Circulation.* 2018;11(12):e004873.
16. Jessup M. Defining success in heart failure: the end-point mess. *Circulation.* 2010;121(18):1977−1980.
17. Kalogeropoulos A, Georgiopoulou V, Kritchevsky SB. Epidemiology of incident heart failure. *Arch Intern Med.* 2009;169(7):708−714.
18. Katsanos AH. Heart failure and the risk of ischemic stroke recurrence: a systematic review and meta-analysis. *J Neurol Sci.* 2016;361:172−178.
19. Khalaf KI, Taegtmeyer H. Insulin sensitizers and heart failure: an engine flooded with fuel. *Curr Hypertens Rep.* 2010;12(6):399−401.
20. Leung AA, Eurich DT, Lamb DA, et al. Risk of heart failure in patients with recent-onset type 2 diabetes: population-based cohort study. *J Card Fail.* 2009;15(2):152−157.

21. Loyaga-Rendon RY, Acharya D, Pamboukian SV, et al. Duration of heart failure is an important predictor of outcomes after mechanical circulatory support. *Circ Heart Fail.* 2015;8(5):953−959.

22. Maggioni AP, Anker SD. Are hospitalized or ambulatory patients with heart failure treated in accordance with the European Society for Cardiology guidelines? *Eur J Heart Fail.* 2013;15:1173−1189.

23. Massie B, Goldman L, Schafer AI, eds. *Cecil Textbook of Medicine.* 24th ed. Philadelphia, PA, USA: Elsevier; 2012:608−622. ISBN 978-1-4377-1604-7 (Chapter 58, 59).

24. McMurray JJV. Angiotensin-neprilysin inhibition versus enalapril in heart failure. *N Engl J Med.* 2014;371(11): 993−1005.

25. McMurray JJV, Packer M, Desai AS. Dual angiotensin receptor and neprilysin inhibition as an alternative to ACEI in person with chronic systolic heart failure. *Eur J Heart Fail.* 2013;15:1062−1069.

26. Metra M, Zacà V, Parati G, et al. Heart Failure Study Group of the Italian Society of Cardiology. Cardiovascular and noncardiovascular comorbidities in patients with chronic heart failure. *J Cardiovasc Med (Hagerstown).* 2011;12(2):76−84.

27. Mosalpuria K, Agarwal SK, Yaemsiri, et al. Outpatient management of heart failure in the United States, 2006−2008. *Texas Heart J.* 2014;41(3):253−261.

28. Owen TE, Hodge D, Herges RM, et al. Trends in prevalence and outcome of heart failure with preserved ejection fraction. *N Engl J Med.* 2006;355(3):251−262.

29. Pocock SJ, Ariti CA, McMurra JJV, et al. Predicting survival in heart failure: a risk score based on 39 372 patients from 30 studies. *Eur Heart J.* May 2013;34(19): 1404−1413.

30. Sacks CA, Jarcho JA, Curfman GD. Paradigm shifts in heart failure—a timeline. *N Engl J Med.* 2014;371(11): 989−991.

31. Shaaya G, Al-Khazaali A, Arora R. Heart rate as a biomarker in heart failure: role of heart rate lowering agents. *Am J Therapeut.* 2017;24(5):e532−e539.

32. Smith MM, Barbara DW, Mauermann WJ, et al. Morbidity and mortality associated with dental extraction before cardiac operation. *Ann Thorac Surg.* 2014;97:838−844.

33. Sochalski J, Jaarsma T, Krumholtz HM, et al. What works in chronic care management: the case of heart failure. *Health Aff.* 2009;28(1):179−189. https://doi.org/10.1377/hlthaff.28.1.179.

34. Stevenson LW, Zile M, Bennett TD, et al. Chronic ambulatory intracardiac pressures and future heart failure events. *Circ Heart Fail.* 2010;3(5):580−587.

35. Tang A, Wells G, Talajuc M, et al. Cardiac resynchronization therapy for mild-to-moderate heart failure. *N Engl J Med.* 2010;363(25):2385−2392.

36. Travessa AM, Menezes Falcao LF. Treatment of heart failure with reduced ejection-fraction-recent developments. *Am J Therapeut.* 2016;23(2):531−549.

37. Uhlig K, Balk EM, Earley A, et al. Assessment on implantable defibrillators and the evidence for primary prevention of sudden cardiac death. *A Report from the Agency for Healthcare Research and Quality.* Rockville, MD; 2014.

38. Ungprasert P. Nonsteroidal anti-inflammatory drugs and the risk for heart failure. *Eur J Intern Med.* 2015;22(6): 763−774.

39. Waterworth S, Gott M. Decision making among older people with advanced heart failure as they transition to dependency and death. *Curr Opin Support Palliat Care.* 2010;18(4):266−272.

40. Xie W, Zheng F, Song X, et al. Renin-angiotensin-aldosterone system blockers for heart failure with reduced ejection fraction or left ventricular dysfunction: network meta-analysis. *Int J Cardiol.* 2016;205:65−71.

41. Yancy CW, Jessup M, Bozkurt B, et al. 2013 ACCF/AHA guidelines for the management of heart failure. *J Am Coll Cardiol.* 2013;62(10):147−239.

42. Yancy CW, Jessup M, Bozkurt B, et al. 2017 ACC/AHA/HFSA focused update of the 2013 ACCF/AHA guideline for the management of heart failure. *J Am Coll Cardiol.* 2017;70(6):776−803.

7

Pulmonary Disease

KEY POINTS

- Pulmonary disease may be undiagnosed or not well controlled in many patients.
- Signs and symptoms of pulmonary disease should be assessed for routinely in the dental office.
- Dental practitioners should be aware that pulmonary diseases pose several dental management considerations including

- risk for acute and chronic airway and breathing issues,
- risk for acute respiratory distress and arrest,
- risk of infectious disease spread,
- oral manifestations including oral ulcers, candidiasis, and gingivitis

CHRONIC OBSTRUCTIVE PULMONARY DISEASE

Chronic obstructive pulmonary disease (COPD) is a general term for pulmonary disorders characterized by chronic airflow limitation from the lungs that is not fully reversible. COPD encompasses two main diseases: chronic bronchitis and emphysema. *Chronic bronchitis* is defined as a condition associated with chronic inflammation of the bronchi that produces excessive tracheobronchial mucus production (at the bronchial level) and a persistent cough with sputum for at least 3 months in at least two consecutive years in a patient in whom other causes of productive chronic cough have been excluded. *Emphysema* is defined as a permanent enlargement of the air spaces in the lung (e.g., distal to the terminal bronchioles) that is accompanied by destruction of the air space (alveolar) walls. These conditions are related, often represent the progression of disease, and may have overlapping symptoms, making differentiation difficult. COPD is disabling, second only to arthritis as the leading cause of long-term disability and functional impairment. COPD currently is diagnosed on the basis of the presence of cough, sputum production, and dyspnea together with an abnormal measurement of lung function.

Epidemiology

COPD is the third leading cause of death and affects approximately 5% of adults, with about 70% of cases occurring in people older than 45.

Prevalence, incidence, and hospitalization rates increase with age. Although age-adjusted death rates for COPD declined in the United States among men from 1999 (57.0 per 100,000) to 2014 (44.3 per 100,000), death rates have not changed significantly among women (35.3 per 100,000 in 1999 and 35.6 per 100,000 in 2014). Based on the current prevalence, the average dental practice of 2000 patients is estimated to have about 100 patients who have a diagnosis of COPD.

Etiology

Tobacco smoking is the most important cause of COPD and accounts for 85%−90% of COPD-related deaths in both men and women. Despite the increased risk, only about one in five chronic smokers develops COPD. In addition to cigarette smoking, long-term exposure to occupational and environmental pollutants, and the absence or deficiency of α_1-antitrypsin are factors that contribute to COPD.

Pathophysiology and Complications

Chronic exposure to cigarette smoke induces pathophysiologic responses of the airways and lung tissue. Chronic bronchitis affects both the large and small airways, with obstructive changes in the small airways due to narrowing, scarring, increased sputum production, mucous plugging, and collapse of peripheral airways resulting from the loss of surfactant (Fig. 7.1). Obstruction is present on both inspiration and expiration.

Emphysematous changes develop as chronic smoke inhalation continually injures lung parenchyma. Damaged alveolar epithelium stimulates the release of inflammatory mediators that destroy the alveolar walls, resulting in enlarged air spaces distal to the terminal

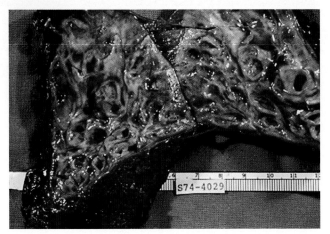

FIG 7.1 Gross pathologic specimen shows lung changes (thickened bronchial walls, narrowing of small airways) caused by chronic bronchitis. (Courtesy of McLay RN. *Wells: Tulane gross pathology tutorial.* New Orleans, LA: Tulane University School of Medicine; 1997.)

bronchioles and loss of elastic recoil of the lungs (Fig. 7.2). Obstruction is caused by the collapse of these unsupported and enlarged air spaces.

COPD is generally a chronic and progressive disease. Up to 20% of patients develop progressive dyspnea and hypercapnia to the point of severe debilitation. Recurrent pulmonary infections with *Haemophilus influenzae*, *Moraxella catarrhalis*, and *Streptococcus pneumoniae* are common with bronchitis. Pulmonary hypertension can develop and lead to *cor pulmonale* (right-sided heart failure). Patients with emphysema are at risk for developing thoracic bullae and pneumothorax. Poor quality of sleep secondary to nocturnal hypoxemia is common with COPD.

Clinical Presentation

The onset phase of COPD is insidious. Symptoms develop slowly, and many patients are unaware of the emerging condition. Key indicators are a chronic cough with sputum production and dyspnea that is persistent

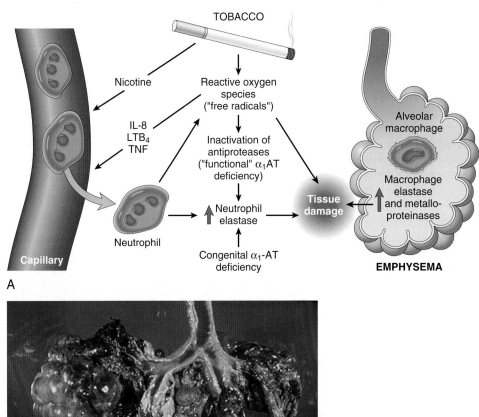

FIG 7.2 A, Pathogenesis of emphysema involving imbalance in proteases and antiproteases that results in tissue damage and collapse of alveoli. **B**, Gross pathologic specimen of an emphysemic lung. α_1-AT, antitrypsin; IL-8, interleukin-8; LTB_4, leukotriene B_4; *TNF*, tumor necrosis factor. (**A**, From Kumar V, Abbas A, Fausto N, eds. *Robbins & Cotran pathologic basis of disease.* 8th ed. Philadelphia: Saunders; 2010 and **B**, Courtesy of McLay RN, et al. *Tulane gross pathology tutorial.* New Orleans, LA: Tulane University School of Medicine; 1997.)

and progressive or worsens with exercise. As the disease progresses, weight loss and decreased exercise capacity also are seen. Comorbid conditions include cardiovascular disease, respiratory infections, and osteoporosis.

Individuals with chronic bronchitis are characterized as sedentary, overweight, cyanotic, edematous, and breathless; accordingly, they have been described as "blue bloaters." In contrast, individuals diagnosed with emphysema are described as "pink puffers" because they present with enlarged chest walls (i.e., "barrel-chested" appearance), weight loss with disease progression, severe exertional dyspnea with a mild nonproductive cough, lack of cyanosis, and pursing of the lips with efforts to forcibly exhale air from the lungs. Many individuals with COPD may exhibit features of both diseases (Box 7.1).

BOX 7.1	Predominant Findings in Patients With Chronic Obstructive Pulmonary Disease
History	Exposure to risk factors, reduced exercise capacity
Clinical	Cough, sputum production, exertional dyspnea
Laboratory	Spirometry revealing airflow limitation, blood gas abnormalities
Imaging	Chest radiography or computed tomography scan revealing prominent bronchovascular markings or evidence of hyperinflation

- *Features of chronic bronchitis*: onset at the age of approximately 50 years, overweight, chronic productive cough, copious mucopurulent sputum, mild dyspnea, frequent respiratory infections, elevated PCO_2, decreased PO_2 (hypoxia), cor pulmonale, chest radiograph showing prominent blood vessels and large heart
- *Features of emphysema*: onset at the age of approximately 60 years, thin physique, barrel chested, seldom coughing, scanty sputum, severe dyspnea, few respiratory infections, normal PCO_2, decreased PO_2, chest radiograph showing hyperinflation and small heart

Laboratory and Diagnostic Findings

Diagnosing COPD in its early stages can be difficult, but the possibility should be considered in any patient who experiences unusual dyspnea and demonstrates chronic cough in the context of exposure to risk factors, especially cigarette smoke. A 6-minute walk distance test can help screen for compromised respiratory function and reduced oxygen uptake; however, the key diagnostic procedures for COPD involve measures of expiratory airflow. Forced vital capacity (FVC) and forced expiratory volume in 1 second (FEV_1) are determined by spirometry, a simple objective test that measures the amount of air a person can breathe out (Fig. 7.3). A diagnosis of COPD is made when patients have pulmonary symptoms and FEV_1 less than 70% of predicted volume (FVC) in the absence of any other pulmonary disease. The four stages of COPD are shown in Box 7.2.

Arterial blood gas measurement and chest radiographs contribute to the diagnosis. Patients with chronic bronchitis have an elevated partial pressure of carbon dioxide (PCO_2) and decreased partial pressure of oxygen (PO_2) (as measured by arterial blood gases), leading to

BOX 7.2	Stages of Chronic Obstructive Pulmonary Disease

Stage I—mild COPD: defined by an FEV_1/FVC ratio of <70% and an FEV_1 of ≥80% of that predicted and sometimes chronic cough and sputum production

Stage II—moderate COPD: worsening airflow limitation and FEV_1/FVC <70% and FEV_1 of 50% to <80% predicted, with shortness of breath typically developing on exertion

Stage III—severe COPD: FEV_1/FVC <70% and FEV_1 of 30% to <50% predicted, with further worsening of airflow limitation and exacerbations that impact a patient's quality of life

Stage IV—very severe COPD: FEV_1/FVC <70%; FEV_1 <30% predicted, with chronic respiratory failure and exacerbations that may be life threatening

COPD, Chronic obstructive pulmonary disease; *FEV_1*, forced expiratory volume in 1 second; *FVC*, forced vital capacity.

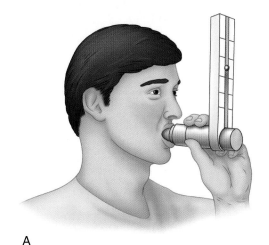 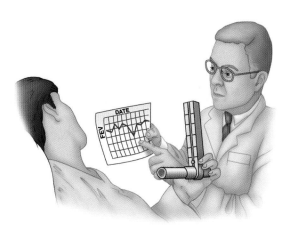

FIG 7.3 A, Measure of forced expiratory volume by spirometry. **B**, Discussion of daily spirometry results with the physician.

secondary erythrocytosis, an elevated hematocrit value, and compensated respiratory acidosis. Patients with emphysema have a relatively normal PCO_2 and a decreased PO_2 that help maintain normal hemoglobin saturation, thus avoiding erythrocytosis. Total lung capacity and residual volume are markedly increased. The ventilatory drive of hypoxia also is reduced in both types of COPD.

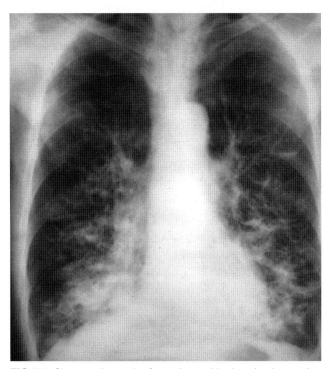

FIG 7.4 Chest radiograph of a patient with chronic obstructive pulmonary disease showing prominent vascular markings (consistent with chronic bronchitis).

Chest radiographs and computed tomography scans assist in classifying COPD and identifying comorbid conditions. In chronic bronchitis, typical radiographic abnormalities consist of increased bronchovascular markings at the base of the lungs (Fig. 7.4). In emphysema, radiographic images demonstrate persistent and marked overdistention of the lungs, flattening of the diaphragm, and emphysematous bullae.

Medical Management

Although COPD is irreversible, treatment can control symptoms and slow disease progression. Management strategies target severity of symptoms and risk of future exacerbations include smoking cessation, avoidance of pulmonary irritants, influenza and pneumococcal vaccinations, and use of short- and long-acting bronchodilators, corticosteroids, and other agents. Other recommended measures include improving exercise tolerance, good nutrition, and adequate hydration.

Inhaled bronchodilators serve as the cornerstone of pharmacologic management and are recommended in a stepwise manner (Fig. 7.5). The primary inhaled agents are short- and long-acting anticholinergics (e.g., ipratropium, tiotropium) that reduce glandular mucus and relax smooth muscle by blocking acetylcholine at the muscarinic receptors, and short- and long-acting β_2-adrenergic bronchodilators that relax smooth muscle by increasing cyclic adenosine monophosphate levels. Combining bronchodilators can lead to pronounced benefits, because they work by different mechanisms (Table 7.1). Inhaled corticosteroids are added to the regimen for symptomatic patients at stage III or above who have repeated exacerbations. Phosphodiesterase inhibitors are alternative agents used. Theophylline, a methylxanthine nonselective

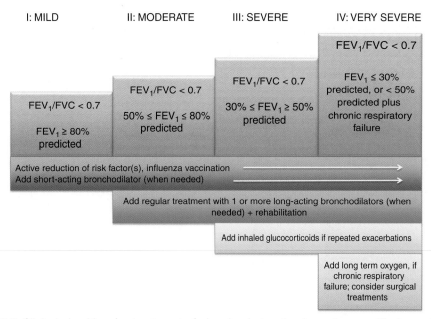

FIG 7.5 Clinical algorithm for treatment of chronic obstructive lung disease. (Redrawn from Global Initiative for Chronic Obstructive Lung Disease: *Pocket Guide to COPD diagnosis, management and prevention, a guide for health care professionals*; 2010. http://fitsweb.uchc.edu/student/selectives/jkoliani/GOLD_Pocket_2010Mar31.pdf.)

TABLE 7.1 Drugs Used in Outpatient Management of Chronic Obstructive Pulmonary Disease (COPD) and Asthma

Drug	Trade Name	Dental Considerations
Antiinflammatory drugs		
Corticosteroids—inhaled		
Beclomethasone dipropionate	Vanceril, Beclovent	Not intended for acute asthma attacks; may contribute to the development of oral candidiasis if used improperly or excessively
Budesonide	Pulmicort	
Ciclesonide		
Dexamethasone	Decadron	
Flunisolide	AeroBid	
Fluticasone propionate	Flonase	
Mometasone		
Triamcinolone acetonide	Azmacort	
Corticosteroids combination with long-acting β₂-selective agonist inhalers		
Formoterol—budesonide	Symbicort	Not intended for acute asthma attacks; may contribute to the development of oral candidiasis if used improperly or excessively
Salmeterol—fluticasone	Advair HFA inhaler	
Formoterol—mometasone	Dulera	
Corticosteroids—systemic		
Prednisone	Deltasone or generic	Not intended for acute asthma attacks; possible adrenal suppression, cushingoid features, and osteoporosis with long-term use
Prednisolone	Delta-Cortef	
Methylprednisolone	Solu-Medrol	
Antileukotrienes		
5-Lipoxygenase inhibitor		Not intended for acute asthma attacks
Zileuton	Zyflo	
Leukotriene Receptor Antagonists		
Montelukast	Singulair	
Zafirlukast	Accolate	
Nonsteroidal—Chromones		
Cromolyn sodium	Intal inhaler	Not intended for acute asthma attacks
Nedocromil	Tilade inhaler	
β-adrenergic bronchodilators		
Fast-acting nonselective β—agonist inhalers		
Epinephrine[a]	Primatene Mist, Bronkaid (available in parenteral form also)	For use during acute asthma attacks
Ephedrine[b]	Eted II	
Intermediate-acting nonselective β-agonist inhalers (3–6 hours)		
Isoproterenol[c]	Isuprel	Not best choice for use during acute asthma attacks
Isoetharine	Bronkosol	
Metaproterenol[d]	Alupent, Metaprel, others	
β₂-selective agonist inhalers (4–6 hours)		
Albuterol[c]	Proventil, Ventolin	For use during acute asthma attacks
Bitolterol mesylate	Tornalate	
Fenoterol	Berotec	
Levalbuterol	Xopenex	
Pirbuterol	Maxair, Maxair Autohaler	
Terbutaline[c]	Brethaire, Bricanyl	
Long-acting β₂-selective agonist inhalers (>12 hours)		
Indacaterol	Arcapta Neohaler	For COPD; not indicated for asthma
Salmeterol (slow onset, long duration)	Serevent	Not intended for acute asthma attacks
Formoterol (rapid onset, long duration)	Foradil	

Continued

TABLE 7.1 Drugs Used in Outpatient Management of Chronic Obstructive Pulmonary Disease (COPD) and Asthma—cont'd

Drug	Trade Name	Dental Considerations
Combination β₂-selective agonist inhalers plus anticholinergic in one inhaler		
Fenoterol—ipratropium	Duovent	Paradoxical bronchospasm, dry mouth, throat irritation
Albuterol (Salbutamol)—ipratropium	Combivent	Headache, dizziness, dry mouth
Short acting muscarinic antagonists (sama)/anticholinergic bronchodilators		
Aclidinium bromide	Tudorza Pressair	Not intended for acute asthma attacks; generally
Ipratropium bromide	Atrovent	used in combination with other antiasthma
Tiotropium (long acting)	Spiriva	drugs or for COPD; can cause headache
Phosphodiesterase (PD) inhibitors		
Theophylline (nonselective)	Theo-Dur	Adverse drug interaction with erythromycin and azithromycin; serum drug levels should be monitored for toxicity
Roflumilast (selective PD-4)	Daxas, Daliresp	Adverse effects of headache, coughing may
Cilomilast (selective PD-4)	Ariflo	affect diagnostic workup and treatment
Anti-IgE		
Omalizumab	Xolair	Dizziness, muscle aches

^aInhalation and parenteral.
ᵃInhalation and parenteral.
ᵇOral and parenteral.
ᶜInhalation, oral, and parenteral.
ᵈInhalation and oral. Some combination drugs are formoterol + budesonide propionate (Symbicort) and salmeterol + fluticasone propionate (Advair).
Injectable α₁-proteinase inhibitor formulations (Aralast, Prolastin, Zemaira) are available for treatment of emphysema caused by inherited α₁-antitrypsin deficiency. *COPD,* Chronic obstructive pulmonary disease.

phosphodiesterase inhibitor, relaxes bronchial smooth muscle cells but has a limited role in COPD management because of its narrow therapeutic range and likelihood of adverse effects (especially in older adults). When used, theophylline is administered as a slow-release formulation. More recently, phosphodiesterase-4—selective inhibitors (e.g., roflumilast, cilomilast) are being used to reduce exacerbations in patients with more advanced COPD.

Antibiotics are used for pulmonary infections, and low-flow supplemental O_2 (2 L/min) is recommended when the patient's PO_2 is 88% or less. Other important treatment options include pulmonary rehabilitation, screening for comorbid conditions, and continual monitoring for disease progression.

Dental Management
Prevention of Potential Problems

Identification. Most patients with COPD have a history of smoking tobacco and may present with a cough, exertional dyspnea, or a change in skin color. Recognition of these features should stimulate the dentist to refer these patients to a physician for care. Dental health care providers can also encourage smokers to quit through several available resources and mechanisms (see Chapter 8).

Risk Assessment. Before initiating dental care, clinicians should assess the severity of the patient's respiratory

disease and the degree to which it is controlled. A patient who displays shortness of breath at rest, a productive cough, upper respiratory infection (URI), or an oxygen saturation (O_2 sat) level less than 91% (as determined by pulse oximetry) is unstable.

Recommendations

Airway and Breathing. If the patient is stable (O_2 sat >95%) and breathing is adequate (no dyspnea), efforts should be directed toward the avoidance of anything that could further depress respiration (Box 7.3). Pulse oximetry monitoring is recommended. Humidified low-flow O_2—generally at a rate of 2–3 L/min—may be provided and should be considered for use when the oxygen saturation level is less than 95%. The patient may be using their own oxygen; if so, they should bring and use it during the dental procedure. If the O_2 sat is less than 91% or there is dyspnea or an URI present, then the patient is considered unstable, and the appointment should be rescheduled and an appropriate medical referral made.

Capacity to Tolerate Care. Dental care can be provided to patients with stages I to III COPD but should be avoided in patients who have stage IV (very severe) COPD. Of note, patients with COPD often have coexisting hypertension and coronary heart disease and a higher risk of heart failure, arrhythmia, and MI. If coexisting cardiovascular disease is present, stress

BOX 7.3	Checklist for Dental Management for Patients With Chronic Obstructive Pulmonary Disease (COPD)[1]

PREOPERATIVE RISK ASSESSMENT
- Evaluate and determine severity of COPD.
- Confirm patient has a primary care provider and has taken medication(s) today.
- Obtain medical consultation if the condition is poorly controlled (e.g., dyspnea, coughing, or frequent upper respiratory infections) or undiagnosed.
- Review history and clinical findings for concurrent heart disease.
- Determine predisposing or exacerbating factors.
- Remind patient to bring their rescue inhaler to appointment.
- Encourage current smokers to stop smoking.

A

Analgesics	No issues.
Antibiotics	Avoid erythromycin, macrolide antibiotics, and ciprofloxacin in patients taking theophylline.
Anesthesia	Avoid outpatient general anesthesia.
Anxiety	Avoid nitrous oxide—oxygen inhalation sedation in patients with severe (stage 3 or worse) COPD. Consider low-dose oral diazepam or another benzodiazepine.

B

Bleeding	No issues.
Blood pressure	Patients with COPD can have cardiovascular comorbidity. Assess blood pressure.

C

Chair position	Semisupine or upright chair position may be better for treatment in these patients.

D

Devices	Avoid use of rubber dam in patients with severe disease. Use pulse oximetry to monitor oxygen saturation. Spirometry readings are helpful in determining level of control.
Drugs	Avoid use of barbiturates and narcotics, which can depress respiration. Avoid use of antihistamines and anticholinergic drugs because they can further dry mucosal secretions.

E

Equipment	Monitor oxygen saturation with pulse oximeter during sedation and invasive procedures. Use low-flow (2—3 L/min) supplemental O_2 when oxygen saturation drops below 95%; it may become necessary when oxygen saturation drops below 91%.
Emergencies	No issues.

F

Follow-up	Contact patient, post-op to determine whether they are experiencing any respiratory difficulty. In smokers, at each follow-up appointment, encourage the patient to quit smoking and examine the oral cavity for lesions that may be related to smoking.

[1]Strength of Recommendation Taxonomy (SORT) Grade: C (see Preface for further explanation).

reduction measures should be implemented, and vital sign monitoring is advised (see Chapters 3 and 4). Supplemental oxygen should be provided as described earlier.

Chair Position. Patients who have stages III or IV COPD should be placed more upright in chair position for treatment, rather than in the supine position. The more upright chair position (e.g., semisupine) helps prevent orthopnea and a feeling of respiratory discomfort.

Drug Considerations. The use of bilateral mandibular blocks or bilateral palatal blocks can cause an unpleasant airway constriction sensation in some patients. This sensation may be amplified with a rubber dam or when medications are administered that dry mucous secretions. Humidified low-flow O_2 can be provided to alleviate the unpleasant airway feeling produced by nerve blocks, use of a rubber dam, and/or medications.

If sedative medication is required, low-dose oral diazepam (Valium) or triazolam (Halcion) may be used. Nitrous oxide—oxygen inhalation sedation can be used with caution in patients with mild to moderate (stage I or II) chronic bronchitis, but is contraindicated in patients with stage III or IV COPD because the nitrous oxide may accumulate in air spaces of the diseased lung. Flow rates should be reduced to no greater than 3 L/min, and the clinician should anticipate induction and recovery times with nitrous oxide approximately twice as long as those in healthy patients. Narcotics and barbiturates should be avoided because of their respiratory depressant properties. Anticholinergics and antihistamines generally should be used with caution in patients with COPD because of their drying properties and the resultant increase in mucus tenacity.

Macrolide antibiotics (e.g., erythromycin, azithromycin) and ciprofloxacin hydrochloride should be avoided in patients taking theophylline because these antibiotics can reduce the metabolism of theophylline, resulting in theophylline toxicity. Outpatient general anesthesia is contraindicated for most patients with COPD.

Oral Complications and Manifestations. Patients with COPD who are smokers are at risk for developing oral leukoplakia and are at an increased risk for developing head and neck squamous cell carcinoma.

ASTHMA

Asthma is a chronic inflammatory disease of the airways characterized by reversible episodes of increased airway hyperresponsiveness, which results in recurrent episodes of dyspnea, coughing, and wheezing. The bronchiolar lung tissue of patients with asthma is particularly sensitive to a variety of stimuli. Overt attacks (flare-ups) may be provoked by allergens, URI, exercise, cold air, certain medications (salicylates, nonsteroidal antiinflammatory drugs [NSAIDs], cholinergic drugs, and β-adrenergic blocking drugs), chemicals, smoke, and highly emotional states such as anxiety and stress.

Epidemiology

Asthma affects 300 million persons worldwide and accounts for 1 of every 250 deaths worldwide. In the United States, its prevalence has more than doubled since the 1960s, from about 2% to 8% (affecting 25 million people). Asthma is a disease primarily of adults, with 7.7% of adults (almost 20 million) affected. Approximately six million children have asthma. Females have higher rates of asthma than males and there is an association with a higher body mass index. Patients with asthma in the United States make more than two million visits to emergency departments (EDs) annually, and more than 3500 asthma-related deaths occur annually. The average dental practice of 2000 patients is estimated to include at least 100 patients who have asthma.

Etiology

Asthma is a multifactorial and heterogeneous disease whose development requires interaction between the environment and genetic susceptibility, with clinical manifestations resulting from dysfunction of the airway epithelium, smooth muscle, immune cells, and neuronal elements. Many factors may exacerbate asthma. These are grouped into one of four categories based on pathophysiology: extrinsic (allergic or atopic), intrinsic (idiosyncratic, nonallergic, or nonatopic), drug induced, and exercise induced. From a management perspective, the type of trigger is more important than the category.

Allergic or *extrinsic asthma* is the most common form and accounts for approximately 35% of all adult cases. It is an exaggerated inflammatory response that is triggered by inhaled seasonal allergens such as pollens, dust, house mites, and animal danders. Allergic asthma usually is seen in children and young adults. In these patients, a dose—response relationship exists between allergen exposure and immunoglobulin E (IgE)—mediated sensitization, positive skin testing to various allergens, and associated family history of allergic disease. Inflammatory responses are mediated primarily by type 2 helper T (T_H2) cells, which secrete interleukins and stimulate B cells to produce IgE (Fig. 7.6). During an attack, allergens interact with IgE antibodies affixed to mast cells, basophils, and eosinophils along the tracheobronchial tree. The complex of antigen with antibody causes leukocytes to degranulate and secrete vasoactive autocoids and cytokines such as bradykinins, histamine, leukotrienes, and prostaglandins. Histamine and leukotrienes cause smooth muscle contraction

(bronchoconstriction) and increased vascular permeability, and they attract eosinophils into the airway. The release of platelet-activating factor sustains bronchial hyperresponsiveness. Release of E-selectin and endothelial cell adhesion molecules, neutrophil chemotactic factor, and eosinophilic chemotactic factor of anaphylaxis is responsible for recruitment of leukocytes (neutrophils and eosinophils) to the airway wall, which increases tissue edema and mucus secretion. T lymphocytes prolong the inflammatory response (late-phase response), and imbalances in matrix metalloproteinases and tissue inhibitor metalloproteinases may contribute to fibrotic changes.

Intrinsic asthma accounts for about 30% of asthma cases and seldom is associated with a family history of allergy or with a known cause. Patients usually are nonresponsive to skin testing and demonstrate normal IgE levels. This form of asthma generally is seen in middle-aged adults, and its onset is associated with endogenous factors such as emotional stress (implicated in at least 50% of affected persons), gastroesophageal acid reflux, or vagally mediated responses.

Ingestion of certain drugs (e.g., aspirin, NSAIDs, beta-blockers, angiotensin-converting enzyme inhibitors) and some food substances (e.g., nuts, shellfish, strawberries, milk, tartrazine food dye yellow color no. 5) can trigger asthma. Aspirin causes bronchoconstriction in about 10% of patients with asthma, and sensitivity to aspirin occurs in 30%—40% of people with asthma who have pansinusitis and nasal polyps (the so-called "triad asthmaticus"). The ability of aspirin to block the cyclooxygenase pathway causes a buildup of arachidonic acid and leukotrienes mediated by the lipoxygenase pathway which results in bronchial spasm.

Metabisulfite preservatives of foods and drugs (specifically in local anesthetics containing epinephrine) may cause wheezing when metabolic levels of the enzyme sulfite oxidase are low. Sulfur dioxide is produced in the absence of sulfite oxidase. The buildup of sulfur dioxide in the bronchial tree precipitates an acute asthma attack.

Exercise-induced asthma is stimulated by exertional activity. Although the pathogenesis of this form of asthma is unknown, thermal changes during inhalation of cold air provoke mucosal irritation and airway hyperactivity. Children and young adults are more severely affected because of their high level of physical activity.

Infectious asthma is a term previously used to describe persons who developed asthma because of the inflammatory response to bronchial infection. Now it is recognized that several respiratory viral infections during infancy and childhood can result in the development of asthma. Also, causative agents of respiratory infections (bacteria, dermatologic fungi *Trichophyton* spp., and *Mycoplasma* organisms) can exacerbate asthma. Treatment of the respiratory infection generally improves control of bronchospasm and constriction.

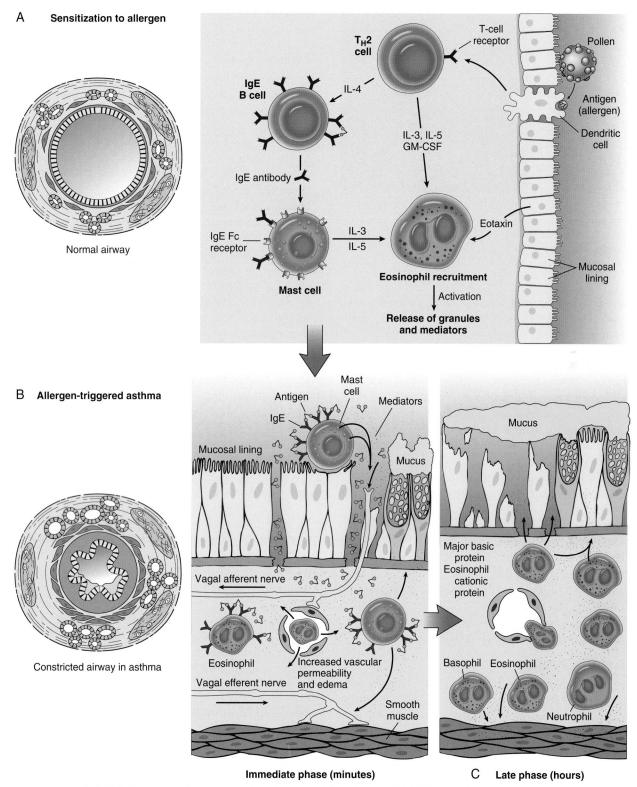

FIG 7.6 Processes involved in allergic (extrinsic) asthma. *GM-CSF*, Granulocyte-macrophage colony-stimulating factor; *IL*, interleukin. (From Kumar V, Abbas A, Fausto N, eds. *Robbins & Cotran pathologic basis of disease*. 8th ed, Philadelphia: Saunders; 2010.)

Pathophysiology and Complications

In asthma, obstruction of airflow occurs as the result of bronchial smooth muscle spasm, inflammation of bronchial mucosa, mucus hypersecretion, and sputum plugging (Fig. 7.7). Histologic findings include inflammation and airway remodeling and appear as (1) thickening of the basement membrane (from collagen deposition) of the bronchial epithelium, (2) edema, (3)

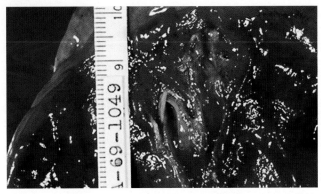

FIG 7.7 Section of a lung with the bronchioles occluded by mucous plugs. (Courtesy McLay RN et al. *Tulane gross pathology tutorial.* New Orleans, LA: Tulane University School of Medicine; 1997.)

mucous gland hypertrophy and goblet cell hyperplasia, (4) hypertrophy of the bronchial wall muscle, (5) accumulation of mast cell and inflammatory cell infiltrate, (6) epithelial cell damage and detachment, and (7) blood vessel proliferation and dilation. These changes contribute to decreased diameter of the airway, increased airway resistance, and difficulty in expiration.

Most patients can expect a reasonably good prognosis, especially those in whom the disease develops during childhood. In many young children, the condition resolves spontaneously after puberty. In a small percentage of patients, both young and old, the condition can progress to COPD, and respiratory failure, or status asthmaticus, the most serious manifestation of asthma, may occur.

Status asthmaticus is a particularly severe and prolonged asthmatic attack (one lasting longer than 24 hours) that is refractory to usual therapy. Signs include increased and progressive dyspnea, jugular venous pulsation, cyanosis, and pulsus paradoxus (a fall in systolic pressure with inspiration). Status asthmaticus often is associated with a respiratory infection and can lead to exhaustion, severe dehydration, peripheral vascular collapse, and death.

Clinical Presentation

Asthma is a disease of episodic attacks of airway hyperresponsiveness. For reasons that are unclear, flare-ups often occur at night or on waking, but they also may follow or accompany exposure to an allergen, exercise, respiratory infection, or emotional upset and excitement. Typical symptoms and signs of asthma consist of wheezing, reversible episodes of breathlessness (dyspnea), cough, chest tightness, and flushing. Onset is sudden, with peak symptoms occurring within 10–15 minutes. Inadequate treatment results in ED visits for about 25% of patients. Respirations become difficult and are accompanied by expiratory wheezing. Tachypnea and prolonged expiration are characteristic. Termination of an attack is often accompanied by a productive cough with thick, stringy mucus. Episodes usually are self-limiting, although severe attacks may necessitate medical assistance.

Laboratory and Diagnostic Findings

Experienced clinical judgment and recognition of the signs and symptoms are essential because laboratory tests for asthma are relatively nonspecific, and no single test is diagnostic. Commonly ordered tests include 6-minute walk test, spirometry before and after administration of a short-acting bronchodilator, chest radiographs (to detect hyperinflation), skin testing (for specific allergens), bronchial provocation (by histamine or methacholine chloride challenge) testing, sputum smear examination and cell counts (to detect neutrophilia or eosinophilia), arterial blood gas determination, and antibody-based enzyme-linked immunosorbent assay (ELISA) for measurement of environmental allergen exposure. Spirometry (Fig. 7.3) is widely applied in diagnosing asthma because by definition, the associated airflow obstruction must be episodic and at least partially reversible. Reversibility is demonstrated by an increase in pulmonary function (i.e., FEV_1) of 12% or greater from baseline after therapy or after inhalation of a short-acting bronchodilator. Also, a recent drop in FEV_1 can be interpreted as a predictive of an asthma attack (see Fig. 7.3), and a drop of more than 10% during exercise fulfills the diagnosis of exercise-induced asthma.

Classification. Patients with chronic asthma are clinically classified as mild, moderate, or severe, based on age, frequency of symptoms, impairment of lung function, and risk of attacks (Box 7.4). Persons older than 12 years of age are classified as mild persistent asthma when they have symptoms more than twice per week but not daily and an FEV_1 greater than 85%. Symptoms generally last less than 1 hour. Patients with moderate asthma have FEV_1 greater than 60% but less than 80% and daily symptoms that affect sleep and activity level and, on occasion, require occasional emergency care. Asthma is classified as severe when patients have less than 60% FEV_1, which results in symptoms throughout the day that limit normal activity. Attacks are frequent or continuous, occur at night, and result in emergency hospitalization.

Medical Management

The goals of asthma therapy are to limit exposure to triggering agents, allow normal activities, restore and maintain normal pulmonary function, minimize the frequency and severity of attacks, control symptoms, and avoid adverse effects of medications. These goals are best accomplished by educating patients and involving them in the prevention or elimination of precipitating factors (e.g., smoking cessation) and comorbid conditions (rhinosinusitis, obesity) that confound management, establishment of a plan for regular self-monitoring, and provision of regular follow-up care. Specifically, it is recommended that a written education and action plan be given to each patient, with appropriate

BOX 7.4	Classification of Asthma and Recommended Drug Management (12 Years and Older)[1]

INTERMITTENT

Symptoms ≤2 per week; brief exacerbations; asymptomatic between exacerbations; nocturnal symptoms <2 per month; FEV_1 >80% of predicted; FEV_1/FVC ratio >85% (normal)	Short-acting β_2-agonist as needed

Mild persistent

Symptoms >2 per week but not daily; nocturnal symptoms 3–4 per month (limited exercise tolerance; rare ED visits); FEV_1 >80% of predicted; FEV_1/FVC >85% (normal 8–19 years), 80% (20–39 years), 75% (40 –59 years), 70% (60–80 years)	Low-dose inhaled corticosteroids or other antiinflammatory drug as needed; short-acting β_2-agonist as needed

Moderate persistent

Daily symptoms; daily use of inhaled short-acting β-agonist; exacerbations that may affect activity and sleep; nocturnal symptoms >1 time per week but not nightly (occasional ED visits); FEV_1 60%–80% of predicted; FEV1/FVC reduced 5%	Low- or medium-dose inhaled corticosteroids + long-acting bronchodilator as needed; short-acting β_2-agonist as needed

Severe persistent

Symptoms throughout the day; frequent (often 7 times a week) exacerbations and nocturnal asthma symptoms; exercise intolerance; FEV_1 <60%; $FEV_1/$ FVC reduced >5% (often resulting in hospitalization)	High-dose inhaled corticosteroids + long-acting bronchodilator or montelukast + oral corticosteroid as needed; short-acting β_2-agonist as needed

[1]There are differences in the criteria based on ages 0–4 years, 5–11 years, and older than 12 years.

ED, Emergency department; *FEV_1*, forced expiratory volume in 1 second; *FVC*, forced vital capacity.

Adapted from National Heart, Lung, and Blood Institute. *Asthma care quick reference: diagnosing and managing asthma.* http://www.nhlbi.nih.gov/health-pro/guidelines/current/asthma-guidelines/quick-reference-html.

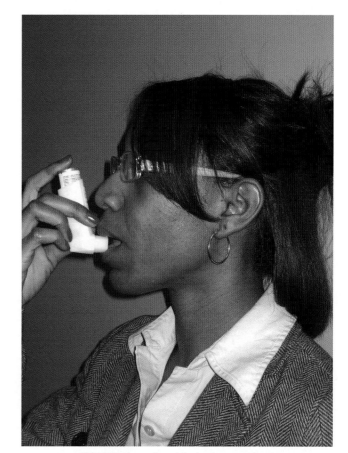

FIG 7.8 Use of an inhaler by a patient.

support and instructions for its use. Inexpensive peak expiratory flow meters should be used regularly at home and levels recorded daily in diaries. For patients with known allergies, the importance of avoidance of allergens to prevent attacks should be underscored. Unfortunately, poor control of asthma often is related to low socioeconomic status (e.g., the patient cannot afford medication), increased anxiety, poor compliance, and unfavorable home environment.

Antiasthmatic drug selection is based on the type and severity of asthma and whether the drug is to be used for long-term control or quick relief (see Table 7.1). Current guidelines for the long-term management and prophylaxis of persistent asthma recommend a "stepwise" approach with the use of inhaled antiinflammatory agents as first-line drugs and addition of β-adrenergic agonists as secondary agents when antiinflammatory drugs are inadequate alone. Combination therapy may include mast cell stabilizers (cromolyn and nedocromil), immunomodulators (e.g., omalizumab), short-acting muscarinic antagonists (SAMA, also known as anticholinergics; e.g., tiotropium), and theophylline.

Inhaled corticosteroids are the most effective therapy for the treatment of persistent asthma. Onset of action is after 2 hours, and peak effects occur 6 hours later. Use of systemic steroids is reserved for asthma unresponsive to inhaled corticosteroids and bronchodilators and for use during the recovery phase of a severe acute attack. Agents such as omalizumab (Xolair) that block IgE (monoclonal antibody against human IgE) are used for additive therapy in patients with severe persistent asthma who have allergy triggers.

For relief of acute asthma attacks, inhaled short-acting β_2-adrenergic agonists are the drugs of choice because of their rapid (within 5 minutes) bronchodilatory and smooth muscle relaxation properties (Fig. 7.8).

Exercise-induced asthma can be prevented with use of both β_2-adrenergic agonists (and cromolyn sodium when taken 30 minutes before initiation of physical activity). Cromolyn and nedocromil decrease airway hyper-responsiveness by stabilizing the membrane of mast cells and interfering with chloride channel function so that mediators are not released when challenged by exercise or cold air. Theophylline is a mild to moderate bronchodilator and can be used as an alternative (see Table 7.1).

Dental Management

Identification and Prevention. The primary goal in dental management of patients with asthma is to prevent an acute asthma attack (Box 7.5).

Risk Assessment. The dentist, through a good history, should be able to determine the severity and stability of disease. Questions should be asked that ascertain adherence to medication use, the type of asthma (e.g., allergic

vs. nonallergic), precipitating factors, timing, frequency and severity of attacks, how attacks usually are managed, and whether the patient has received emergency treatment for an acute attack (see Box 7.4).

The stability of the disease can be assessed during the interview component of the history and by clinical examination, as well as understanding the regularity of physician visits and the results of laboratory measures. Features such as symptoms 2 or more days per week, use of a short-acting β_2-agonist more than 2 days a week, increased respiratory rate (>50% above normal), FEV_1 that has fallen more than 10% or to below 80% of peak FEV_1, an eosinophil count that is elevated to above 50/mm^3, poor drug use compliance, and one or more ED visits within the previous 3 months suggest inadequate treatment and poor disease control. Also, the use of more

---

BOX 7.5	Checklist for Dental Management of Patients With Asthma[1]

PREOPERATIVE RISK ASSESSMENT
- Evaluate and identify asthma as a medically confirmed or likely diagnosis along with its severity and type.
- Determine predisposing or exacerbating factors.
- Remind patient to bring their rescue inhaler to appointment.
- Obtain medical consultation if asthma is poorly controlled (as indicated by wheezing or coughing or a recent hospitalization) or is undiagnosed or if the diagnosis is uncertain.
- Encourage current smokers to stop smoking.

A

Analgesics	No issues.
Antibiotics	Avoid erythromycin, macrolide antibiotics, and ciprofloxacin in patients taking theophylline.
Anesthesia	Clinicians may elect to avoid solutions containing epinephrine or levonordefrin because of sulfite preservative.
Anxiety	Provide a stress-free environment through establishment of rapport and openness to reduce risk of anxiety-induced asthma attack. If sedation is required, use of nitrous oxide–oxygen inhalation sedation or small doses of oral diazepam (or both) is recommended.
Allergy	Asthmatics with nasal polyps are increased risk for allergy to aspirin. Avoid aspirin use.

B

Bleeding	No issues.
Blood pressure	Monitor blood pressure during asthma attacks to observe for the development of status asthmaticus.

C

Chair position	Semisupine or upright chair position for treatment may be better tolerated than supine due to orthopnea.

D

Devices	Instruct patients to bring their current medication inhalers to every appointment; use prophylactically in moderate to severe disease. Obtain spirometry reading to determine level of control. May consider the use of pulse oximetry to monitor oxygen saturation during long or invasive dental procedures.
Drugs	Avoid precipitating odorants and drugs (aspirin). Avoid use of barbiturates and narcotics, which can depress respiration and release histamine, respectively.

E

Equipment	Use low-flow (2–3 L/min) supplemental O_2 when oxygen saturation drops below 95%; supplemental O_2 also may become necessary when oxygen saturation drops below 91%.
Emergencies	Recognize the signs and symptoms of a severe or worsening asthma attack, including inability to finish sentences with one breath, ineffectiveness of bronchodilators to relieve dyspnea, recent drop in FEV_1 as determined by spirometry, tachypnea with respiratory rate of 25 ≥breaths/min, tachycardia with heart rate of ≥110 beats/min, diaphoresis, accessory muscle usage, and paradoxical pulse. Administer fast-acting bronchodilator, oxygen, and, if needed, subcutaneous epinephrine (1:1000) in a dose of 0.3–0.5 mL. Activate EMS; repeat administration of fast-acting bronchodilator every 20 minutes until EMS personnel arrive.

F

Follow-up	Contact patient, post-op to determine whether they are experiencing any exacerbation. Ensure that patient is receiving adequate medical follow-up care on a routine basis.

[1]Strength of Recommendation Taxonomy (SORT) Grade: C (see Preface for further explanation).
EMS, Emergency medical system; *FEV*, forced expiratory volume in 1 second.

than 1.5 canisters of a β-agonist inhaler per month (>200 inhalations per month) or doubling of monthly use indicates high risk for a severe asthma attack.

For severe and unstable asthma, consultation with the patient's physician is advised and routine dental treatment should be postponed.

Recommendations

Appointment, Airway, and Breathing. Modifications during the preoperative and operative phases of dental management of a patient with asthma can minimize the likelihood of an attack. Patients who have nocturnal asthma should be scheduled for late-morning appointments, when attacks are less likely. Use of operatory odorants (e.g., methyl methacrylate) should be reduced before the patient is treated. Patients should be instructed to regularly use their medications, to bring their inhalers (bronchodilators) to each appointment, and to inform the dentist at the earliest sign or symptom of an asthma attack. Prophylactic bronchodilator use at the beginning of the appointment may help prevent an asthma attack. Alternatively, patients may be advised to bring their spirometer and daily expiratory record to the office. The dentist may request that the patient exhale into the spirometer and record the expired volume. A significant drop in lung function (to below 80% of peak FEV_1 or a greater than 10% drop from previously recorded values) indicates that prophylactic use of the inhaler or referral to a physician is needed. The use of a pulse oximeter may be valuable for determining the patient's oxygen saturation level. In healthy patients, this value remains between 97% and 100%; a drop to 91% or below indicates poor oxygen exchange and the need for intervention.

Capacity to Tolerate Care. Because anxiety and stress may be precipitating factors in asthma attacks, dental staff members should identify patients who are anxious and attempt to reduce stress. Preoperative and intraoperative sedation may be desirable. If sedation is required, nitrous oxide–oxygen inhalation is best as it is not a respiratory depressant, nor is it an irritant to the tracheobronchial tree. Oral premedication may be accomplished with small doses of a short-acting benzodiazepine. Reasonable alternatives with children are hydroxyzine (Vistaril) for its antihistamine and sedative properties, and ketamine, which causes bronchodilation.

Drug Considerations. Barbiturates and narcotics, particularly meperidine, are histamine-releasing drugs that can provoke an attack and thus should be avoided. Outpatient general anesthesia generally is contraindicated for patients with asthma.

Selection of local anesthetic may require adjustment because those containing sulfites may cause allergic-type reactions in susceptible individuals. Sulfite preservatives are found in local anesthetic solutions that contain epinephrine or levonordefrin. The dentist should discuss with the patient any past responses to local anesthetics and allergy to sulfites and should consult with the physician on this issue. As an alternative, local anesthetics without a vasoconstrictor may be used in at-risk patients.

Administration of aspirin-containing medication or other NSAIDs to patients with asthma is not advisable because aspirin ingestion is associated with the precipitation of asthma attacks in a small percentage of patients. Likewise, barbiturates and narcotics are best not used because they also may precipitate an asthma attack. Patients who are taking theophylline preparations should not be given macrolide antibiotics (i.e., erythromycin and azithromycin) or ciprofloxacin because these agents can increase serum levels of theophylline.

Emergency (Asthma Attack). An acute asthma attack requires immediate recognition and therapy (Box 7.5). A short-acting β2-adrenergic agonist inhaler should be administered at the first sign of an attack. With a severe asthma attack, use of subcutaneous injections of epinephrine (0.3–0.5 mL, 1:1000) or inhalation of epinephrine (Primatene Mist) is the most potent and fastest acting method for relieving the bronchial constriction. Supportive treatment includes providing positive-flow oxygenation, repeating bronchodilator doses as necessary every 20 minutes, monitoring vital signs (including oxygen saturation, which should reach 90% or higher), and activating the emergency medical system, if indicated.

Oral Complications and Manifestations

The medications taken by patients who have asthma may contribute to oral disease. For example, β2-agonist inhalers reduce salivary flow by 20%–35% and are associated with increased prevalence of gingivitis and caries in patients with moderate to severe asthma. Gastroesophageal acid reflux is common in patients with asthma and is exacerbated by the use of β-agonists and theophylline. This reflux can contribute to erosion of enamel. Oral candidiasis occurs in approximately 5% of patients who use inhalation steroids for long periods at high dose or frequency. However, development of this condition is rare if a "spacer" or aerosol-holding chamber is used and the mouth is rinsed with water after each use. Candidiasis readily responds to local (i.e., nystatin, clotrimazole) or systemic (fluconazole) antifungal therapy. Patients should receive instructions on the proper use of their inhaler and the need for oral rinsing.

TUBERCULOSIS

There are many communicable respiratory diseases that patients may bring into the dental office. Tuberculosis, or TB, caused *Mycobacterium tuberculosis* is used as an example for this chapter. TB represents a major global health problem that is responsible for illness and deaths in large segments of the world's population. The disease is spread by inhalation of infected droplets of *M. tuberculosis*. A prolonged period of replication of

M. tuberculosis leads to an inflammatory and granulo-matous response in the host, with consequent development of classic pulmonary and systemic symptoms. Although *M. tuberculosis* is by far the most common causative agent in this human infection, other species of mycobacteria occasionally infect humans, such as *M. avium complex*, *M. kansasii*, *M. abscessus*, *M. xenopi*, *M. bovis*, *M. africanum*, *M. microti*, and *M. canetti*. These mycobacterial species may cause systemic diseases (manifesting as pulmonary lymphadenitis, cutaneous, or disseminated) that are referred to as mycobacterioses.

Epidemiology

Tuberculosis has a worldwide incidence of approximately 10 million, and the World Health Organization (WHO) estimates that one-third of the world population—representing over two billion people—is infected. This disease kills more adults worldwide each year than does any other single pathogen. In contrast, the occurrence of TB in the United States steadily decreased during the past century and has dropped at a rate of 5% per year over the past 50 years. Tuberculosis continues to occur in almost every US state and affects about 4% of the population (12 million people), with more than half of new US cases occurring in foreign-born persons who migrate or travel to the country.

Although the rate of infection for the United States as a whole is low, there are populations at higher risk, including racial and ethnic minorities, the urban poor, people living in congregate facilities (community dwellings, prisons, and shelters), and patients who have acquired immunodeficiency syndrome, who have rates several times the national average (Box 7.6). Efforts to reduce the spread of TB in the United States include improved sanitation and hygiene measures and the use of effective antituberculosis drugs. Complicating factors include failure to complete the course of therapy (in ~20% of patients) and the development of multidrug-resistant TB (MDR-TB).

Etiology

In most cases of human TB, the causative agent is *M. tuberculosis*, an acid-fast, nonmotile, intracellular rod that is an obligate aerobe. As an aerobe, this organism exists best in an atmosphere of high oxygen tension; therefore, it most commonly infects the lung.

M. tuberculosis typically is transmitted by way of infected airborne droplets of mucus or saliva that are forcefully expelled from the lungs, most commonly through coughing but also by sneezing and during talking. Transmission by ingestion (e.g., of contaminated milk) occurs but is rare because of the use of pasteurized milk. A secondary mode of transmission—by ingestion—is possible when a patient coughs up infected sputum, thereby potentially inoculating oral tissues.

The number of organisms inhaled and the level of immunocompetency largely determine whether an

---

BOX 7.6   Groups at High Risk for Tuberculosis (TB)

- Close contacts of persons who have TB
- Skin test converters (within the past 2 years)
- Residents and employees of high-risk congregate settings (correctional facilities, nursing homes, mental institutions, homeless shelters, health care facilities)
- Recent immigrants and foreign-born persons (and migrant workers) from countries that have a high TB incidence or prevalence
- Persons who visit areas with a high prevalence of active TB, especially if visits are frequent or prolonged
- Populations defined as having increased incidence of latent *Mycobacterium tuberculosis* infection: medically underserved persons, those with low incomes, persons who abuse drugs or alcohol
- Infants, children, and adolescents exposed to persons who are at increased risk for latent *M. tuberculosis* infection or active TB or who have a positive result on tuberculin skin testing

Adapted from Mazurek GH, Jereb J, Vernon A, et al. Updated guidelines for using interferon gamma release assays to detect *Mycobacterium tuberculosis* infection—United States, 2010. *MMWR Recomm Rep.* 2010;59(RR-5):1–25.

---

exposed person will contract the disease. The interval from infection to development of active TB is widely variable, ranging from a few weeks to decades. Most cases of TB result from reactivation of a dormant tubercle; only 5%–10% of cases arise de novo at the time of the initial infection.

Pathophysiology and Complications

Tuberculosis can involve virtually any organ of the body, although the lungs are the most common site of infection. The typical infection begins with inhalation of infected droplets which enter the alveoli where bacteria are engulfed by macrophages. Replication occurs within alveolar macrophages and spread of infection occurs locally to regional (hilar) lymph nodes. The term *Ghon complex* is used when the infection involves a primary granulomatous lung lesion and an infected hilar lymph node. If the infection is not controlled locally, distant dissemination through the bloodstream may occur. Approximately 2–8 weeks after onset, delayed hypersensitivity to the bacteria develops resulting in a positive tuberculin skin test. Subsequently, a chronic granulomatous inflammatory reaction develops that involves activated epithelioid macrophages and formation of granulomas. These natural host defenses usually control and contain the primary pulmonary TB infection, resulting in latent TB infection (LTBI). If not contained, the nidus of infection (granuloma) may become a productive tubercle with central necrosis and caseation. Cavitation may occur (Fig. 7.9), resulting in the dumping of organisms into the airway for further dissemination into other lung tissue or the exhaled air.

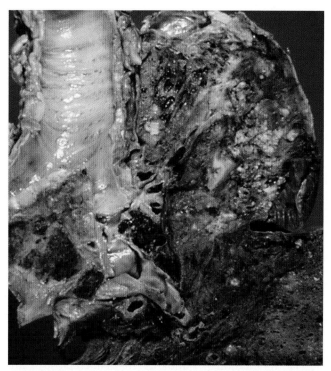

FIG 7.9 Gross specimen of a tuberculous lung, demonstrating caseating granulomas and cavitation. (Courtesy of Powell R. Lexington, KY.)

Limitation and local containment of infection is influenced by a variety of factors, including host resistance, host immune capabilities, and virulence of the mycobacterium. After the infection has been successfully interrupted, the lesion heals spontaneously and then undergoes inspissation, hardening, encapsulation, and calcification. Although the lesion "heals," some bacteria may remain dormant. If infection is not interrupted, dissemination of bacilli may occur through the lung parenchyma, resulting in extensive pulmonary lesions and lymphohematogenous spread. Widespread infection with multiple organ involvement is called *miliary TB*. Secondary or reinfection TB represents relapse of a previous infection and is usually confined to the lungs with cavitation common. Reasons for relapse include inadequate treatment of the primary infection and underlying disease risk factors.

Some of the more common sequelae of TB include progressive primary TB, cavitary disease, pleurisy and pleural effusion, meningitis, and disseminated or miliary TB. Isolated organ involvement other than that of the lung may occur, with the pericardium, peritoneum, kidneys, adrenal glands, and bone (known as Pott disease when occurring in the spine) commonly affected. Factors that increase the risk of a poor clinical outcome are listed in Box 7.7.

Risk of progression from LTBI to TB is largely a function of the immune status of the host, with a rate of reactivation of about 5% over a person's lifetime. Approximately 5%–10% of persons who develop TB die of the disease.

Clinical Presentation

Primary infection with *M. tuberculosis* in about 90% of patients' results in few manifestations other than a positive result on tuberculin skin/laboratory test and characteristic radiographic changes. Nonspecific symptoms include cough, lassitude and malaise, anorexia, unexplained weight loss, night sweats, and fever. Fever is common in the evening or during the night and is accompanied by profuse sweating.

Manifestations of extrapulmonary disease occur in about 10%–20% of cases and may include localized lymphadenopathy (scrofula) with the development of sinus tracts, back pain over the affected spine, gastrointestinal disturbances (intestinal), dysuria and hematuria (renal), heart failure, and neurologic deficits.

Laboratory and Diagnostic Findings

Laboratory tests are directed toward determining whether the patient has active infection or LTBI. Active infection is considered when there is a positive acid-fast bacillus sputum smear, symptoms are present (cough, fever, weight loss, night sweats), and characteristic chest radiographic changes are observed. The definitive diagnosis of TB is based on culture or direct molecular tests (e.g., nucleic acid amplification) that identify *M. tuberculosis* or other mycobacterial species from body fluids and tissues, usually sputum. Cultures are accompanied by antimicrobial susceptibility testing for all isolates of *M. tuberculosis* due to risk of drug-resistant TB.

Radiographic findings in active progressive primary TB include patchy or lobular infiltrates with cavitation and hilar adenopathy. Healed primary lesions leave a calcified peripheral nodule associated with a calcified hilar lymph node (Ghon complex).

LTBI can be diagnosed using either the tuberculin (Mantoux) skin test (tuberculin skin test [TST]) or the interferon-gamma release assay (IGRA). The TST is 95% sensitive and 95% specific for determining whether the patient has been infected with *M. tuberculosis*. This test is of limited utility in immunocompromised persons and during the first 6–8 weeks after primary infection because of false-negative results. Also, up to 25% of people with active TB have false-negative skin test results. Individuals who had the BCG (Bacillus Calmette–Guérin) vaccine may show as false positive as well.

The TST is administered by intradermal injection of 0.1 mL of purified protein derivative (PPD), which contains 5 units of tuberculin (culture extract from *M. tuberculosis*), on the volar or dorsal surface of the forearm. The test measures the delayed hypersensitivity response by evidence of induration noted 48–72 hours later. The size of the induration determines whether the results are read as negative (induration size <5 mm) or positive (with 10 and 15 mm used as cut points), interpreted in light of the presence of risk factors, abnormalities on the chest radiographs, and risk of disease progression (Table 7.2). Induration of 15 mm or greater is considered positive evidence of TB in all persons tested. A positive result on PPD testing necessitates a physical examination, a radiographic evaluation, and, if necessary, sputum culture to rule out active disease.

IGRAs are performed on fresh whole blood as an alternative to the TST. IGRAs are commercially available in the United States as QuantiFERON-TB Gold-in-Tube test or T-SPOT TB test. These tests measure the person's immune reactivity to white blood cells infected with *M. tuberculosis*, which release interferon-γ when mixed with antigens from the mycobacteria. These assays are advantageous because they can detect recent infections, results are available within 24 hours, and previous bacille Calmette-Guérin (BCG) vaccination does not cause a false-positive result. Similar to the TST, however, they cannot discriminate active from latent infection.

Medical Management

Treatment protocols for TB are directed toward whether the patient has LTBI or active TB. Most persons who have LTBI (i.e., those with inactive disease) are not candidates for treatment, unless they are considered at high risk for disease progression (see Box 7.7). The standard regimen for those with LTBI designated as high risk for disease progression is isoniazid (INH), 300 mg daily for 9 months (10 mg/kg for 9 months in children). Alternatively, a 6-month course with INH, a 12-dose once-weekly (3-month) regimen of INH and rifapentine, or a 4-month regimen of rifampin can be used. Although these regimens usually prevent the occurrence of active disease, the treated person retains hypersensitivity to PPD, so skin tests and IGRA will continue to give positive results.

The International Standards for Tuberculosis Care (ISTC) and the American Thoracic Society/CDC recommendations for effective chemotherapy for active TB include:

Early and accurate diagnosis should be established; prompt initiation of effective treatment, standardized treatment regimens that involve multiple drug use; treatment and response to treatment should be monitored to ensure full course of therapy is taken; patient education and compliance; and appropriate public health measures. Of particular concern are patient compliance and completion of therapy, as well as exposure of personal contacts, who may be at risk for the disease.

The ISTC and CDC currently recommend that all patients receive at least a four-drug, initial phase regimen of INH, rifampin, ethambutol, and pyrazinamide can have both preemptive and treatment regimens. The four-drug regimen is given for 2 months, and a sputum specimen is collected to determine response to therapy. If the specimen

TABLE 7.2 Significance of Positive Results on Purified Protein Derivative Testing		
GROUPS AT RISK FOR PROGRESSION TO ACTIVE TB DISEASE, STRATIFIED BY INDURATION SIZE		
Positive IGRA Result or a TST Reaction of ≥5 mm	**Positive IGRA Result or TST Induration ≥10 mm**	**TST Induration ≥15 mm**
• HIV-infected persons • Recent contacts of a TB case • Persons with fibrotic changes on chest radiographs consistent with old TB • Persons who are immunosuppressed for other reasons (e.g., taking the equivalent of >15 mg/day of prednisone for 1 month or longer; taking TNF-α antagonists)	• Children younger than <5 years of age and children and adolescents exposed to adults in high-risk categories • Recent immigrants (<5 years) from high prevalence countries • Injection drug users • Residents and employees of high-risk congregate settings • Mycobacteriology laboratory personnel	All persons in this category are considered to have TB (despite absence of risk factors for TB)

HIV, Human immunodeficiency virus; *IGRA*, interferon-gamma release assay; *TB*, tuberculosis; *TNF-α*, tumor necrosis factor-α; *TST*, tuberculin skin test.

is negative for *M. tuberculosis*, INH and rifampin are given daily or twice weekly for the next 4 months, for a total of 6 months of therapy. If, however, at 2 months, the sputum is positive, cavitational pulmonary TB is present, or the initial phase of treatment did not include pyrazinamide, then the continuation phase of INH and rifampin—rifamycin should be extended for three additional months, for a total of 7 months (Box 7.8).

After the initiation of chemotherapy, reversal of infectiousness depends on proper drug selection and patient compliance. Within 3–6 months, approximately 90% of patients become noninfectious, and their sputum cultures convert to negative. Patients are allowed to return to normal public contact on the basis of reversal of infectiousness and continued chemotherapy.

Because of its contagiousness and the problem of noncompliance with treatment regimens, protection measures have been introduced to control the spread of disease. Public health measures include screening close contacts for the disease, hospitalizing patients with potentially infectious TB, and treating infected patients in isolation rooms with negative air pressure. In addition, "directly observed therapy" and text reminders are used to ensure that infected patients take the appropriate medicine at the appropriate time for the duration of therapy.

MDR-TB, defined by the WHO as resistant to two first-line antituberculosis drugs, is a threatening feature of the disease affecting about 5% of patients globally with a mortality rate of up to 40%. Ninety percent of drug-resistant cases occur in HIV-infected persons and in many countries where TB is endemic. Management of MDR-TB follows a specific protocol and is provided in a hospital using directly observed therapy (see Box 7.8).

Dental Management

Identification. Many patients with infectious disease, including TB, cannot be clinically or historically identified; therefore, all patients should be treated as though they are potentially infectious, and the CDC's standard precautions for infection control should be strictly followed. The CDC guidelines for infection control and the prevention of transmission of TB in health care facilities should be followed in patients who have a known diagnosis of TB (see Appendix B). The CDC places most dental facilities in the low-risk category for potential occupational exposure to TB, and recommends that each dental facility have a written TB control protocol that includes instrument reprocessing and operatory cleanup, as well as protocols for identifying, managing, and referring patients with active TB and educating and training staff (Box 7.9). The CDC also recommends baseline and periodic PPD screening of dental care workers.

Risk Assessment. Of primary concern is identification of patients infected with TB based on potential infectivity status (symptomatic) and risk for spread of infection. The four infectivity categories are (1) active TB, (2) a history of TB, (3) a positive tuberculin test or IGRA, and (4) signs or symptoms suggestive of TB (Box 7.10).

Patients With Clinically Active Sputum-Positive Tuberculosis. Care for patients with recently diagnosed, clinically active TB and positive sputum cultures should be limited to urgent procedures and rendered in a hospital setting with appropriate isolation, sterilization (mask, gloves, gown), and special engineering control (ventilation) systems and filtration masks (i.e., N95). A rubber dam and high-speed suction should be used to minimize aerosolization of oropharyngeal microbes. Following adequate medical therapy and after receiving confirmation from the physician that he or she is noninfectious and lacks any complicating factors, the patient may be treated routinely on an outpatient basis without special precautions (Box 7.11). For greater detail, please see http://www.cdc.gov/mmwr/pdf/rr/rr5417.pdf.

Patients With a Past History of Tuberculosis. Fortunately, relapse is rare among patients who have received adequate treatment for the initial infection. This is not the case, however, in patients who have received inadequate treatment and in those who are immunosuppressed. Regardless of what type of treatment was received, any person with a history of TB requires an initial careful workup to investigate infectivity status before any dental treatment is contemplated. The dentist should obtain a medical history, including diagnosis and dates and type of treatment. Treatment duration of less than 18 months if treatment was provided more than two decades ago, or

---

BOX 7.8	Common Drug Regimens for the Treatment of Tuberculosis (TB)

DRUG-SUSCEPTIBLE TB
- Four-drug, *initial phase* regimen (isoniazid + rifampin + ethambutol + pyrazinamide) for 2 months.
- Then two-drug, *continuation phase* therapy (isoniazid and rifampin) for 4 months (18 weeks) or for 7 months if patients (1) have cavitary pulmonary tuberculosis caused by drug-susceptible organisms and whose sputum culture obtained at the time of completion of 2 months of treatment is positive; (2) whose initial phase of treatment did not include pyrazinamide; and (3) patients being treated with once-weekly INH and rifapentine and whose sputum culture obtained at the time of completion of the initial phase is positive.

CONFIRMED MULTIDRUG-RESISTANT TB[1]
- Five-agent regimen: pyrazinamide + a fluoroquinolone, an injectable drug—(amikacin or kanamycin), ethionamide, and either cycloserine or para-aminosalicylic acid—to which the organism is susceptible, continued for at least 8 months up to 20 months. Treatment regimens are individualized in accordance with several factors, including resistance pattern, extent of disease, and presence of comorbid conditions.

[1]*Multidrug-resistant TB* is defined as TB resistant to therapy with isoniazid (INH) and rifampin.
Data from Treatment of tuberculosis. *MMWR Recomm Rep.* 2003;52 (RR11):1–77 and Guidelines for the programmatic management of drug-resistant tuberculosis: 2011 update. World Health Organization, Geneva, 2011.

BOX 7.9	Centers for Disease Control and Prevention Guidelines: Tuberculosis (TB) Precautions for Use in Outpatient Dental Settings

ADMINISTRATIVE CONTROLS
- Assign responsibility for managing TB infection control program.
- Conduct annual risk assessments.
- Develop written TB infection control policies for promptly identifying and isolating patients with suspected or confirmed TB for medical evaluation or urgent treatment.
- Ensure dental health care personnel are educated regarding the signs and symptoms of TB.
- Instruct patient to cover mouth when coughing and to wear a surgical mask.
- Screen newly hired personnel for latent TB infection and disease.
- Postpone urgent dental treatment if TB is suspected or active.

ENVIRONMENTAL CONTROLS
- Use airborne infection isolation room to provide urgent treatment to patients with suspected or confirmed TB.
- Use high-efficiency particulate air filters or UV-germicidal irradiation in settings with a high volume of patients with suspected or confirmed TB.
- Cover and clean and disinfect exposed patient area surfaces.
- Sterilize patient care items.

RESPIRATORY PROTECTION CONTROLS
- Use respiratory protection (at least an N95 filtering face piece [disposable], N99 or N100 respirators) for exposed personnel when they are providing urgent dental treatment to patients with suspected or confirmed TB.
- Instruct TB patients to cover their mouth when coughing and to wear a surgical mask.

UV, Ultraviolet.

Data from Jensen PA, Lambert LA, Iademarco MF, Ridzon R. CDC: Guidelines for preventing the transmission of *Mycobacterium tuberculosis* in health-care settings, 2005. *MMWR Recomm Rep.* 2005;54(RR-17):1–142.

less than 9 months if treatment was given before the year 2000, requires consultation with the physician to assess adequacy of the regimen used. Patients should provide a history of periodic physical examinations and chest radiographs to check for evidence of reactivation of the disease. Further consultation with the physician is advisable to verify the patient's current status. Patients who are found to be free of active disease and are not immunosuppressed may be treated with the use of standard precautions.

Patients With a Positive Tuberculin Test or Positive IGRA. A person with a positive result on skin testing for TB or IGRA should be viewed as having been infected with mycobacteria. The patient should provide a history of being evaluated by a physician for active disease by physical examination and chest radiography. In the absence of clinically active disease, such patients have LTBI and are not considered infectious. A regimen of prophylactic INH is typically administered for 9 months if they are considered to be at risk for disease progression

BOX 7.10	Principles of Dental Management for Patients With a History of Tuberculosis

ACTIVE SPUTUM-POSITIVE TUBERCULOSIS
- Consult with a physician before treatment.
- Perform urgent care only; palliate urgent problems with medication if contained facility in a hospital environment is not available.
- Perform urgent care that requires the use of a handpiece (in patients older than 6 years) only in a hospital setting with isolation, sterilization (gloves, mask, gown), and special respiratory protection.
- Treat those less than 6 years of age as a normal patient (noninfectious after consultation with physician to verify status).
- Treat patients who consistently produce negative sputum as normal (noninfectious—verify with physician).

TUBERCULOSIS HISTORY SPECIFICS
- Approach with caution; obtain thorough history of disease and its treatment duration, with appropriate review of systems.
- Obtain verification of periodic chest radiographs and physical examination to rule out reactivation or relapse.
- Consult with physician and postpone treatment with identification of any of the following:
  - Questionable adequacy of treatment time
  - Lack of appropriate medical follow-up evaluation since recovery
  - Sign or symptom of relapse
- Treat as for normal patient if present status is "free of clinically active disease."

RECENT CONVERSION TO POSITIVE TUBERCULIN SKIN TEST
- Verify evaluation by physician to rule out active disease.
- Verify completion of drug therapy.
- Treat as normal patient.

SIGNS OR SYMPTOMS SUGGESTIVE OF TUBERCULOSIS
- Refer to a physician and postpone treatment.
- Treat as for a patient with sputum-positive status if treatment is necessary.

BOX 7.11	General Guidelines[85] for Determining When a Patient With Pulmonary Tuberculosis (TB) Has Become Noninfectious During Therapy

- Likelihood of multidrug-resistant TB has been determined to be negligible.
- Patient has received standard multidrug anti-TB therapy for 2–3 weeks.
- Patient has demonstrated compliance with standard multidrug anti-TB treatment.
- Patient exhibits clinical improvement.
- Results of AFB testing on three consecutive sputum smears are negative.
- All close contacts of the patient have been identified; evaluated; advised; and, if indicated, started on treatment for latent TB infection.

AFB, Acid-fast bacilli.

(see Box 7.7). These patients may be treated in a normal manner with the use of standard precautions.

Patients With Signs or Symptoms Suggestive of TB. Any time a patient demonstrates unexplained, persistent signs or symptoms that may be suggestive of TB or has a positive result on skin testing or positive IGRA and has not been given follow-up medical care, dental care should not be rendered, and the patient should be referred to a physician for evaluation. If a health care provider is exposed to TB, the provider should be evaluated for TB infection and treated promptly if indicated.

Recommendations

Airway and Breathing. There are no issues with breathing and contagiousness in patients with LTBI; however, those with active TB have compromised pulmonary function and are infectious. Thus, these patients should not be treated in a dental setting until their condition is medically managed.

Bleeding. INH and rifampin can lower the platelet count and increase the risk of bleeding. A complete blood count should be obtained when an invasive procedure is planned for these patients.

Capacity to Tolerate Care. An active TB patient can tolerate dental care after receiving (1) appropriate anti-TB chemotherapy for at least 2–3 weeks and (2) confirmation is received from the physician that the patient is noninfectious and lacks any complicating factors (see Box 7.11).

Drug Considerations. Several anti-TB drugs have notable adverse effects and drug interactions in which dentists should be knowledgeable. Isoniazid (INH), rifampin (Rifadin), and pyrazinamide (Rifater) therapy may cause hepatotoxicity and elevations in serum aminotransferases (Table 7.3). When serum aminotransferases are elevated in patients taking INH, acetaminophen-containing medications should be avoided because of the increased potential for hepatotoxicity. Additional precautions regarding liver dysfunction, including drug dosage reductions, are discussed in Chapter 10.

Rifampin induces cytochrome P-450 enzymes. As a result, the use of rifampin can lower plasma levels of oral contraceptives, diazepam (Valium), midazolam (Versed), clarithromycin (Biaxin), ketoconazole (Nizoral), itraconazole (Sporanox), and fluconazole (Diflucan). In addition, rifampin can cause leukopenia, hemolytic anemia (jaundice), and thrombocytopenia, resulting in an increased incidence of infection, delayed healing, and gingival bleeding. Streptomycin and aspirin can adversely interact and cause ototoxicity.

Oral Complications and Manifestations

Tuberculosis manifests infrequently in the oral cavity. The classic mucosal lesion is a painful, deep, irregular ulcer on the dorsum of the tongue although other mucosal sites may be affected. Extension into the jaws can result in osteomyelitis. The cervical and submandibular lymph nodes may become infected with TB and

---

TABLE 7.3 Dental Treatment Considerations With Antituberculosis Drugs

Drug (Trade Name)	Adverse Effects	Dental Considerations
Isoniazid (INH) (Laniazid, Nydrazid, Tubizid)	Hepatotoxicity; elevation in serum amino-transferase activity in 10%—20% of patients[a]; rash, fever, peripheral neuropathy	Avoid acetaminophen Increases the concentrations of other drugs (e.g., diazepam)
Rifampin (Rifadin, Rimactane), Rifabutin, Rifapentine	Hepatotoxicity; GI disturbances, flulike symptoms, thrombocytopenia, rash; turns urine red-orange	Increases the incidence of infection, delayed healing, gingival bleeding; bidirectional interaction that decreases serum levels of diazepam, triazolam, erythromycin, clarithromycin (Biaxin), ketoconazole (Nizoral), itraconazole (Sporanox), fluconazole (Diflucan), and oral contraceptives
Pyrazinamide (generic)	Arthralgias, rash (photoallergy), hyperuri-cemia, GI disturbances, arthralgias, and hepatitis	—
Ethambutol (Myambutol)	Decreased red-green color discrimination; reduced visual acuity; optic neuritis (rare)	—
Ethionamide (Trecator-SC)	—	—
Streptomycin (generic)	Ototoxicity, vestibular disturbances, infrequent renal toxicity, perioral numbness	Avoid concurrent use of aspirin
Amikacin (Amikin), kanamycin (Kantrex), capreomycin (Capastat)	Nephrotoxicity and ototoxicity	Avoid concurrent use of aspirin
Cycloserine	Neurotoxicity and hypersensitivity, vitamin deficiency	—
Aminosalicylic acid (Sodium P.A.S., Teebacin)	GI disturbances	—

[a]Greater risk of liver damage in persons older than 35 years of age; vitamin B$_6$ (pyridoxine) is recommended to counteract the potential for adverse effects of INH.

GI, Gastrointestinal.

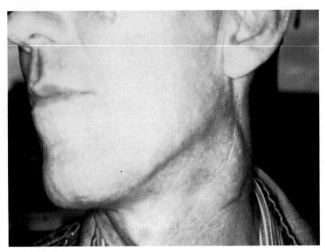

FIG 7.10 Tuberculosis of the cervical lymph nodes.

become enlarged and painful (Fig. 7.10), and abscesses may form with subsequent drainage.

Biopsy in addition to culture can be diagnostic if acid-fast bacilli are found. Resolution of the infectious oral lesion may result from treatment of TB with antituberculosis drugs.

Occupational Safety and Health Association

Policy mandates that employers (including dentists) provide a safe, healthful workplace and permit inspection for occupational exposure to TB in health care facilities when complaints are received from public sector employees.

Since 1997, OSHA has mandated a specific policy regarding the risk of TB transmission based on CDC guidelines. Current policy can be viewed at http://www.osha.gov/SLTC/tuberculosis/index.html, which requires that dentists prepare a written exposure control plan, provide baseline skin test results and medical history, make medical management available after an exposure incident, provide medical removal protection if necessary, provide information and training to employees with exposure potential, comply with record-keeping requirements, and document any occupationally related tuberculosis infection. In addition, if respirators are deemed necessary to protect the health of an employee, the employer is required to establish and implement a written respiratory protection program. Periodic medical surveillance and respiratory protection are not required if the dental facility does not admit or treat patients with active TB, has not had a confirmed case of infectious TB within the past year, and is located in a county in which cases of active TB have not been reported within the previous 2 years. By contrast, stricter guidelines (i.e., isolation rooms for patients with suspected or confirmed infectious TB and use of ventilation equipment) are provided for instances in which employees may have been exposed to the exhaled air of a person with suspected or confirmed TB or were exposed to a high-hazard procedure performed on a person who may have TB that

has the potential to generate aerosols containing potentially infectious respiratory secretions. OSHA requires use of personal protective equipment to reduce employee exposure to hazards. To familiarize themselves with their legal responsibilities, dentists should visit OSHA's website at https://www.osha.gov/pls/oshaweb/owasrch.search_form?p_doc_type=STANDARDS&p_toc_level=0&p_keyvalue=.

BIBLIOGRAPHY

1. American Lung Association. *Trends in COPD (Chronic Bronchitis and Emphysema): Morbidity and Mortality.* http://www.lung.org/assets/documents/research/copd-trend-report.pdf. Accessed January 10, 2021.
2. Centers for Disease Control and Prevention. Asthma—United States. *MMWR Morb Mortal Wkly Rep*; 2018. https://www.cdc.gov/asthma/default.htm. Accessed January 10, 2021.
3. Centers for Disease Control and Prevention. Deaths from chronic obstructive pulmonary disease—United States. *MMWR Morb Mortal Wkly Rep*; 2018 Accessed January 10, 2021 https://www.cdc.gov/copd/basics-about.html.
4. Centers for Disease Control and Prevention. *Current TB Guidelines—United States*; 2020. https://www.cdc.gov/tb/publications/guidelines/default.htm. Accessed January 10, 2021.
5. Centers for Disease Control and Prevention. *Current Infection Control Guidelines—United States*; 2020. https://www.cdc.gov/tb/publications/guidelines/infectioncontrol.htm. Accessed January 10, 2021.
6. Centers for Disease Control and Prevention. *Current treatment for TB.* http://www.cdc.gov/tb/topic/treatment/tbdisease.htm. Accessed January 10, 2021.
7. Centers for Disease Control and Prevention. *TB Elimination: Extensively Drug-Resistant Tuberculosis.* http://www.cdc.gov/tb/publications/factsheets/drtb/xdrtb.pdf. Accessed January 10, 2021.
8. Data and Statistics. *COPD. National Center for Chronic Disease Prevention and Health Promotion, Division of Population Health.* https://www.cdc.gov/copd/data.html. Accessed January 10, 2021.
9. Global Initiative for Chronic Obstructive Lung Disease. *Global Strategy for the Diagnosis, Management and Prevention of Chronic Obstructive Lung Disease*; 2016. Available from: http://www.goldcopd.org/uploads/users/files/WatermarkedGlobal Strategy 2016(1).pdf. Accessed January 10, 2021.
10. Hanioka T, Ojima M, Tanaka H, et al. Intensive smoking-cessation intervention in the dental setting. *J Dent Res.* 2010;89(1):66–70.
11. Harrison's™ Principles of Internal Medicine, 20th edition. Jameson, Fauci, Kasper, et al. Copyright © 2018. McGraw-Hill Publishers. Volume 1 eBook ISBN 978-1-259-64400-9; MHID 1-259-64400-6; Volume 2 eBook ISBN 978-1-259-64402-3; MHID 1-259-64402-2.
12. National Heart Lung and Blood Institute. *Guidelines for the Diagnosis and Management of Asthma (EPR-3).* Available from: http://www.nhlbi.nih.gov/health-pro/guidelines/current/asthma-guidelines. Accessed January 10, 2021.

Smoking and Tobacco Use Cessation

- Dental patients who are smokers or otherwise use tobacco are at risk for the development of a number of health risks and problems, including periodontal disease, leukoplakia, and squamous cell carcinoma.

- Dentists can play a valuable role in promoting tobacco cessation programs.

EPIDEMIOLOGY

It is estimated that approximately 13.7% (34.2 million) of adults older than the age of 18 years in the United States are current smokers, down from over 20% in 2005. Thus, in a dental practice of 2000 patients, it can be expected that approximately 400 patients will be smokers, although this will vary by region of the country. Over the past few decades, the percentage of daily smokers who smoked more than 25 cigarettes per day (i.e., heavy smokers) has decreased steadily (Fig. 8.1). This trend is encouraging, however smoking continues to be a serious public health issue.

The prevalence of current cigarette smoking varies substantially across population subgroups. Social disparities in smoking prevalence are impacted by social, economic, and historical factors, as well as differences in environment, personal behavior, and habits. Current smoking rates are higher among men (23.5%) than women (17.9%). Among racial/ethnic populations, smoking rates vary considerably. Smoking is least prevalent among adults with higher levels of education. Smoking prevalence is higher among adults who live below the poverty level and prevalence also varies significantly by state and area, ranging from 9.0% in Utah to 25.2% in Kentucky and West Virginia, with a trend toward higher rates in southern states (Fig. 8.2).

The use of smokeless tobacco became a national public health issue in the early to mid-1980s, when tobacco companies aggressively marketed their products by targeting young people. This practice has recently shifted to vaping (i.e., the use of e-cigarettes).

The US Public Health Service estimates a total annual cost of $50 billion for the treatment of patients with smoking-related disease in addition to another $50 billion in lost wages and productivity.

PATHOPHYSIOLOGY AND COMPLICATIONS

Smoking is a learned or conditioned behavior that is reinforced by nicotine. Cigarettes (including e-cigarettes) promote this conditioning because they allow precise dosing that can be repeated as often as necessary to avoid discomfort and produce maximal desired effects. In addition, smoking behavior is reinforced by and associated with common daily events such as awakening, eating, and socializing.

Nicotine is a highly addictive drug that has been equated with heroin, cocaine, and amphetamine in terms of addiction potential and its effects on brain neurochemistry. Nicotine targets the *nucleus accumbens* in the brain. The addictive and behavioral effects of nicotine are complex and are due primarily to its effects on dopaminergic pathways. The physiologic and behavioral effects of nicotine include increased heart rate, increased cardiac output, increased blood pressure, appetite suppression, a sense of euphoria, improved task performance, and reduced anxiety. Tolerance develops with repeated exposure so that it takes more and more nicotine to produce the same level of effect.

Nicotine is absorbed through the mucosal lining of the nose and mouth and by inhalation in the lungs. A cigarette is a very efficient delivery system for the inhalation of nicotine, with rapid distribution throughout the body, reaching the brain in as little as 10 s. Mucosal absorption from smokeless tobacco is slower, but the effects are more sustained. Nicotine that is swallowed is not well absorbed in the stomach because of the acidic environment.

The effects of nicotine gradually diminish over 30–120 min; this produces withdrawal effects that may include agitation, restlessness, anxiety, difficulty concentrating, insomnia, hunger, and a craving for cigarettes. The elimination half-life of nicotine is about 2 h.

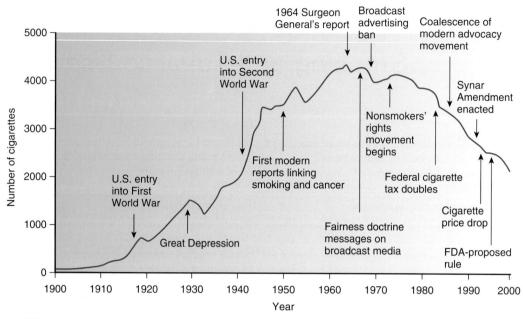

FIG 8.1 Decline of cigarette smoking in the United States over the period from 1900 to 2000. *FDA*, Food and Drug Administration.

Map of Current Cigarette Use Among Adults

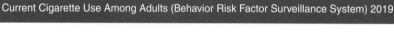

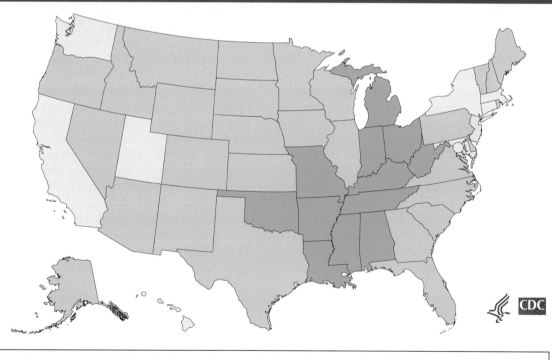

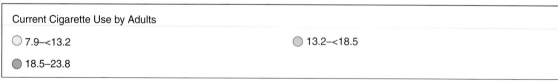

FIG 8.2 Cigarette use among adults in the United States in 2019. (From Centers for Disease Control and Prevention, State Tobacco Activities Tracking and Evaluation (STATE) System. Oct 2021.)

However, nicotine can accumulate with repeated exposure to cigarettes throughout the day, with effects persisting for hours.

A typical smoker will take 10 puffs of every cigarette over a period of about 5 min that the cigarette is lit. Each cigarette delivers about 1 mg of nicotine. Thus, a person who smokes about 1½ packs (30 cigarettes) a day gets 300 hits of nicotine to the brain every day, each one within 10 s after a puff. This repeated reinforcement is a strong contributor to the highly addictive nature of nicotine.

Tobacco companies have long promoted smoking aimed at youth. Ninety percent of adult tobacco users took up the habit by age 18, and 99% by age 26. The CDC currently estimates that 31.2% of high school students use tobacco in some form (Fig. 8.3). Nicotine is uniquely dangerous to youth because the developing child's brain does not fully develop until around age 26. Moreover, using nicotine in adolescence can harm attention, learning, mood, and impulse control and may also increase risk for future addiction to other drugs. Therefore, dentistry should be sending preventive messages at an earlier age during regular oral health maintenance visits.

Cigarette smoking is a major risk factor for stroke, myocardial infarction, peripheral vascular disease, aortic aneurysm, and sudden death. It is the leading cause of lung disease, including chronic obstructive pulmonary disease, pneumonia, and lung cancer. It is also strongly linked to cancers of the mouth, esophagus, stomach, pancreas, cervix, kidney, colon, and bladder. Other effects include premature skin aging and an increased risk for cataracts. Cigar and pipe smokers are subject to similar addictive and general health risks as are cigarette smokers, although pipe and cigar users typically do not inhale.

E-cigarettes

In recent years, many people have engaged in the use of E-cigarettes or switching from tobacco products. E-cigarettes are electronic devices that heat a liquid and produce an aerosol, or mix of small particles in the air. E-cigarettes come in many shapes and sizes. Most have a battery, a heating element, and a place to hold a liquid. Some e-cigarettes look like regular cigarettes, cigars, or pipes. Some look like USB flash drives, pens, and other everyday items. Larger devices such as tank systems, or

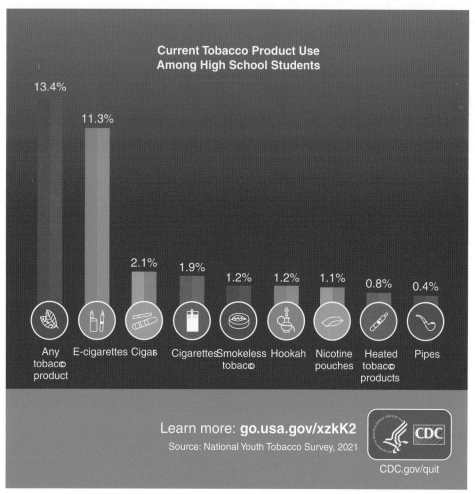

FIG 8.3 Tobacco use by youth in the United States in 2021. (From Centers for Disease Control and Prevention. National Youth Tobacco Survey 2021. *Smoking & Tobacco Use.* March 2022.)

"mods," do not look like other tobacco products. E-cigarettes are known by many different names. They are sometimes called "e-cigs," "e-hookahs," "mods," "vape pens," "vapes," "tank systems," and "electronic nicotine delivery systems (ENDS)." Using an e-cigarette is sometimes called "vaping."

JUUL is a popular brand of e-cigarette that is shaped like a USB flash drive. Unfortunately, approximately two-thirds of JUUL users aged 15—24 do not know that JUUL always contains nicotine. According to the manufacturer, a single JUUL pod contains as much nicotine as a pack of 20 regular cigarettes. UUL is one of a few e-cigarettes that use nicotine salts, which allow particularly high levels of nicotine to be inhaled more easily and with less irritation than the free-base nicotine that has traditionally been used in tobacco products, including e-cigarettes Other companies that sell e-cigarettes that look like USB flash drives include the MarkTen Elite, and the PAX Era, a marijuana delivery device that looks like JUUL.

E-cigarette aerosol can contain harmful and potentially harmful substances, including nicotine; ultrafine particles that can be inhaled deep into the lungs; flavorings such as diacetyl, a chemical linked to a serious lung disease; volatile organic compounds; and cancer-causing chemicals and heavy metals such as nickel, tin, and lead. Some of the ingredients in e-cigarette aerosol also could be harmful to the lungs in the long term and await long-term studies.

MEDICAL MANAGEMENT

Interventions for Smoking Cessation

Health care professionals must be vigilant in identifying patients who use tobacco with the goals of encouraging them to stop smoking and assisting them in their efforts. Studies indicate that 70% of smokers want to quit smoking. However, many do not succeed. Tobacco dependence is a chronic condition that often requires repeated attempts at intervention. Smokers typically fail multiple attempts to quit before they achieve success.

People who quit smoking live longer than those who continue to smoke because of avoiding the development of smoking-related fatal diseases. The extent to which a smoker's risk is reduced by quitting depends on several factors, including number of years as a smoker, number of cigarettes smoked per day, and presence or absence of disease at the time of quitting. Box 8.1 lists short- and long-term benefits of smoking cessation.

Numerous ways have been devised to encourage and assist the cessation of smoking and tobacco use. Public health measures include raising awareness of the dangers of smoking and tobacco use by airing public service television or radio ads, age restrictions on buying products, increasing the price of cigarettes and other tobacco products, taxing their use, and banning smoking in public places. Individual methods of smoking cessation include

BOX 8.1	Benefits of Quitting Smoking According to the US Surgeon General

- 20 min after quitting: Your heart rate drops (US Surgeon General's Report, 1988, pp. 39, 202).
- 12 h after quitting: Carbon monoxide level in your blood drops to normal (US Surgeon General's Report, 1988, p. 202).
- 2 weeks to 3 months after quitting: Your circulation improves, and your lung function increases (US Surgeon General's Report, 1990, pp. 193, 194, 196, 285, 323).
- 1—9 months after quitting: Coughing and shortness of breath decrease; cilia (tiny hairlike structures that move mucus out of the lungs) regain normal function in the lungs, increasing the ability to handle mucus, clean the lungs, and reduce the risk of infection (US Surgeon General's Report, 1990, pp. 285—287, 304).
- 1 year after quitting: The excess risk of coronary heart disease is half that of a smoker (US Surgeon General's Report, 1990, p. vi).
- 5 years after quitting: Your stroke risk is reduced to that of a nonsmoker 5—15 years after quitting (US Surgeon General's Report, 1990, p. vi).
- 10 years after quitting: The lung cancer death rate is about half that of a continuing smoker. Risks of cancer of the mouth, throat, esophagus, bladder, cervix, and pancreas decrease (US Surgeon General's Report, 1990, pp. vi, 131, 148, 152, 155, 164, 166).
- 15 years after quitting: The risk of coronary heart disease is that of a nonsmoker (US Surgeon General's Report, 1990, p. vi).

Quitting helps to stop the damaging effects of tobacco on your appearance, including the following:
- Premature wrinkling of the skin
- Bad breath
- Stained teeth
- Gum disease
- Bad-smelling clothes and hair
- Yellow fingernails
- Food tastes better
- Sense of smell returns to normal
- Ordinary activities (e.g., climbing stairs, light housework) no longer leave you out of breath

the use of telephone quit lines, nicotine replacement therapy (NRT), and medications, along with individual or group counseling. Overall success rates are low with high rates of relapse. The 1-year success rate for stopping "cold turkey" is about 5%. The use of telephone quit lines or brief counseling roughly doubles one's chance of success, as does the use of any of the NRT products. The 1-year success rate with bupropion is about 23%. Varenicline appears to be as effective as bupropion. NRT combined with bupropion improves the success rate to about 36%. In general, the chance for success increases when more than one option is used, which can include counseling combined with NRT or medication.

Health care providers should ask their patients about smoking or tobacco use at each appointment, advise current users to quit, and assist those who express an interest in quitting. Clinical Practice Guidelines for Treating Tobacco Use and Dependence, published by the US Department of Health and Human Services, Public Health Service, is intended to aid health care professionals in helping their patients to quit smoking. These guidelines are based on the **5 As**, which include *asking* patients about their tobacco use, *advising* those who use tobacco to quit, *assessing* the willingness of patients to make a quit attempt, *assisting* in the quit attempt, and *arranging* for follow-up. However, most dentists and physicians are unaware of this potentially helpful resource. Reasons most often cited by dentists for not incorporating smoking cessation services into their practices include time involved, lack of training, lack of adequate reimbursement, lack of knowledge of available referral sources, and lack of patient education materials. In view of the poor outcomes of the 5 As, a suggested alternative approach is to *ask*, *advise*, and *then refer* (to an internal resource, an external resource, or a telephone quit line). This approach requires practitioners to be familiar with available referral sources.

DENTAL MANAGEMENT

Dental health professionals should ask every patient about their use of tobacco. This can be easily accomplished by inclusion of tobacco use questions on the medical or dental history followed by a brief interview. For patients who are current tobacco users, additional questions, including the type of tobacco product used, the frequency of use, and the length of time the product has been used, should be asked. During the oral mucosal and oropharyngeal examination, mucosal changes associated with tobacco use should be noted, and the patient should be advised of their presence and the association with tobacco use. Patients who use smokeless tobacco should be asked where they hold the tobacco in their mouth, and special attention should be paid to examination of that area. Any oral changes or systemic diseases that are present that may be related to tobacco use should be discussed and can be used as motivation to quit smoking. Patients should then be asked whether they have ever considered quitting and whether they would like to quit. They should be made aware that you support and encourage their quitting to improve their overall health and that you will assist them in their efforts to quit.

If a patient does not wish to quit, the health care provider is encouraged to point out the benefits of quitting as a potential method of motivating the patient. If there is resistance to intervention, the topic should be dropped and the patient not badgered. It is generally counterproductive to pursue the issue with a non-interested patient. However, patients can be told that, if

at any time they would like to quit, you would be happy to speak with them about it. If a patient indicates that he or she wishes to quit, the practitioner has several options:

- Help to coordinate a program for the patient or designate another individual (auxiliary) in the office to perform that function.
- Prescribe smoking cessation medications for the patient.
- Refer the patient to an outside smoking cessation program.
- Refer the patient to his or her primary care physician.
- Refer the patient to a counseling source, such as a telephone help line.

Depending on how involved the practitioner wishes to become, the following sections describe many options and resources that are available to assist patients in the effort to quit smoking.

Patient Education Literature

It is recommended that practitioners have patient education and motivational materials available for patients to read to encourage and support tobacco use cessation. Posters can be placed on the walls of the waiting room and treatment areas. Brochures may be kept in the waiting room and in treatment areas to be given to patients who express a desire to quit. Patient education materials are readily available from sources such as the American Cancer Society, the National Cancer Institute, and the US Surgeon General. These can be ordered by phone or through their websites (Box 8.2). Brochures or handouts may be used to provide telephone quit line numbers or for referral to local smoking cessation programs or support groups. Practitioners also may wish to develop their own patient education materials.

BOX 8.2 | Resources for Support Material

TELEPHONE HELP AND QUIT LINES
- 800-QUITNOW (US Department of Health and Human Services national quit line)
- 877-44-U-QUIT (National Cancer Institute dedicated quit smoking line)
- 877-YES-QUIT (American Cancer Society quit line)
- 800-4-CANCER (Cancer Information Service of the National Cancer Institute)

HELPFUL WEBSITES
- www.surgeongeneral.gov/tobacco
- www.smokefree.gov
- www.nlm.nih.gov/medlineplus/smokingcessation.html
- www.cancer.gov/cancertopics/pdq/prevention/control-of-tobacco-use/HealthProfessional
- www.cdc.gov/tobacco
- www.cancer.org/docroot/PED/content/PED_10_13X_Guide_for_Quitting_Smoking.asp

Fagerström Test

The Fagerström Test for Nicotine Dependence (Fig. 8.4) is a standard instrument for assessing the intensity of physical addiction to nicotine. The test was designed to provide an ordinal measure of nicotine dependence related to cigarette smoking. It contains six items that evaluate the quantity of cigarette consumption, the compulsion to use, and dependence. In scoring the Fagerström Test for Nicotine Dependence, yes/no items are scored from 0 to 1 and multiple-choice items are scored from 0 to 3. The items are summed to yield a total score of 0–10. The higher the total Fagerström score, the more intense is the patient's physical dependence on nicotine. In the clinic, the Fagerström test may be used by the dentist to document indications for referring a patient for further treatment.

NIDA Clinical Trials Network

Fagerström Test for Nicotine Dependence (FND)

Segment: _ _

Visit Number: _ _

Date of Assessment: (mm/dd/yyyy)   _ _ / _ _ / _ _ _ _

Do you currently smoke cigarettes?

☐ No   ☐ Yes

If "yes," read each question below. For each question, enter the answer choice which best describes you response.

1. **How soon after you wake up do you smoke your first cigarette?**

   ☐ Within 5 minutes   ☐ 31 to 60 minutes

   ☐ 6 to 30 minutes   ☐ After 60 minutes

2. **Do you find it difficult to refrain from smoking in places where it is forbidden** (e.g., in church, at the library, in the cinema)**?**

   ☐ No   ☐ Yes

3. **Which cigarette would you hate most to give up?**

   ☐ The first one in the morning   ☐ Any other

4. **How many cigarettes per day do you smoke?**

   ☐ 10 or less   ☐ 21 to 30

   ☐ 11 to 20   ☐ 31 or more

5. **Do you smoke more frequently during the first hours after waking than during the rest of the day?**

   ☐ No   ☐ Yes

6. **Do you smoke when you are so ill that you are in bed most of the day?**

   ☐ No   ☐ Yes

Comments:

Heatherton TF, Kozlowski LT Frecker RC (1991). The Fagerström Test for Nicotine Dependence: A revision of the Fagerström Tolerance Questionnaire. British Jornal of Addiction 86:1119

-27.

FIG 8.4 The Fagerström Test for Nicotine Dependence (FND). (From Heatherton TF, Kozlowski LT, Frecker RC. The Fagerström Test for Nicotine Dependence: A revision of the Fagerstrom Tolerance Questionnaire. *Br J Addiction.* 1991;86:1119.)

Counseling

Even brief counseling, such as occurs when a health care professional routinely asks about smoking and encourages quitting, has been shown to increase quit success rates. Telephone counseling help lines (quit lines) have become widely available and have been shown to double success rates over those reported with quitting "cold turkey." Help lines are available on national, regional, and state levels (see Box 8.2). Help lines provide the opportunity for the patient to speak to a counselor and can provide support for patients, regardless of whether they are considering quitting, attempting to quit, have successfully quit, or have relapsed. Group counseling can be especially effective by providing the social support and encouragement of the group. Counseling typically consists of both cognitive and behavioral therapies. Cognitive therapy attempts to change the way a patient thinks about smoking, and behavioral therapy attempts to help smokers avoid situations that might trigger the desire to smoke. Evidence has shown that the more intensive the counseling, the better the success rate and that when counseling is combined with other forms of therapy, such as NRT or pharmacotherapy, it is even more effective. Local, regional, and state health departments are additional sources for smoking cessation counseling.

Nicotine Replacement Therapy

The rationale for NRT is to replace cigarettes or smokeless tobacco with a source of nicotine that does not have the tars and carbon monoxide of tobacco and then to gradually reduce the use of that replacement product to (ideally) the point of abstinence. To prevent withdrawal symptoms, a smoker must maintain a baseline blood level of nicotine of about 15–18 ng/mL. A cigarette rapidly increases nicotine blood levels to 35–40 ng/mL, producing the "hit" or "rush" that a smoker experiences when smoking; this level then gradually returns to baseline within about 25–30 min. NRT attempts to provide a blood level that is adequate to prevent withdrawal symptoms without producing the "hit" or "rush" caused by the cigarette. The patient then gradually learns to accept progressively lower and lower blood nicotine levels. Five distinct nicotine replacement products are available (transdermal patch, gum, lozenge, inhaler, nasal spray) that differ in cost, route of delivery, and efficiency of delivery of nicotine (Table 8.1).

All of the NRT products have been approved by the US Food and Drug Administration (FDA) for smoking cessation. They all appear to be effective when included as part of a program of smoking cessation, and they generally double the chances of success over quitting "cold turkey." Selection of an NRT product should depend on the number of cigarettes smoked per day, its potential adverse effects, and patient preference. Generally, the more dependent the patient is on nicotine, the higher the required beginning doses will be and the greater the need to titrate nicotine levels. For very dependent smokers, the combination of a patch with a shorter acting method such as gum, lozenge, or nasal spray may be indicated.

Non—Nicotine Replacement Therapy Pharmacotherapy

Bupropion SR (Zyban) is an FDA-approved atypical antidepressant that is thought to affect the dopaminergic or noradrenergic pathways (or both) involved in nicotine addiction. Bupropion is effective when used alone or in combination with an NRT product, counseling, or both. An attractive feature of bupropion is that it may prevent weight gain, which is a common adverse effect of smoking cessation. It is contraindicated in patients with seizure disorders and in those who might be prone to seizures. Varenicline (Chantix) is an $\alpha_4\beta_2$ nicotinic receptor partial agonist that stimulates dopamine and blocks nicotinic receptors, thus preventing the reward and reinforcement associated with smoking. This medication is started 3 days before the quit date and is taken for 12 weeks, and appears to be as effective as bupropion. Reports of depression and suicidal ideation have reported, resulting in a change in product labeling (Table 8.2).

Additional treatment strategies with less proven efficacy include the use of monoamine oxidase inhibitors, selective serotonin reuptake inhibitors, opioid receptor antagonists, bromocriptine, antianxiety drugs, nicotinic receptor antagonists, glucose tablets, and alternative and complementary therapies.

ORAL MANIFESTATIONS AND COMPLICATIONS

Tobacco use contributes to a number of oral diseases including halitosis, leukoplakia, squamous cell carcinoma, stomatitis, sialometaplasia, and periodontal disease (Figs. 8.5–8.12).

Reports from the US Surgeon General and others conclude that cigarette smoking is the main cause of cancer mortality in the United States, contributing to an estimated 30% of all cancer deaths and substantially to cancers of the head and neck (Fig. 8.5). Tobacco use also

TABLE 8.1   Nicotine Replacement Products

Product	How Supplied	How Used	Adverse Effects	Advantages and Disadvantages
Nicotine Transdermal Patches (OTC)				
Nicoderm CQ Nicorette Nicotrol, generic	Nicoderm CQ: 7, 14, 21 mg Nicorette: 5, 10, 15 mg Nicotrol: 5, 10, 15 mg	Start with patches of highest concentration; then use patches of progressively lower concentration over a 6- to 12-week period	Skin irritation, insomnia	Slow onset; takes 6—8 h to reach peak blood level; cannot be readily titrated
Nicotine Gum (OTC)				
Nicorette, generic	Available in strengths of 2 and 4 mg	Not to be chewed as normal gum; should be chewed slightly and then "parked" in the vestibule; repeat the chew—park sequence every 30 min; nicotine is absorbed through the mucosa; do not eat or drink for 15 min before using or while using; start with 8—24 pieces/day and gradually reduce over several weeks; maximum, 24/day	Mucosal irritation; indigestion	Quicker delivery than patch but not as quick as lozenge; produces less of a "rush" than is produced by cigarettes or lozenges
Nicotine Lozenges (OTC)				
Commit	Available in strengths of 2 and 4 mg	Strength required is determined by time to first cigarette in the morning; the lozenge is "parked" and moistened and allowed to dissolve in the mouth; start with 9—20/day and use progressively fewer per day over a 12-week period; do not eat or drink for 15 min before using or while using; maximum, 20/day	Gingival and throat irritation; indigestion	Peak blood levels in 20—30 min; 25% higher blood levels than gum; can be titrated as needed; very efficient; produces less of a rush than is caused by cigarettes but more of a rush than is produced by gum
Nicotine Nasal Spray (Prescription)				
Nicotrol NS	Supplied in a pump nasal spray bottle	One dose is a spray into each nostril; maximum of 40 doses per day is progressively decreased over 10—12 weeks	Nose and throat irritation	Fastest delivery system; provides the rush of cigarettes
Nicotine Inhaler (Prescription)				
Nicotrol inhaler	Supplied as plastic cartridges; each cartridge provides 4 mg of nicotine (only 2 mg is absorbed)	Each inhaler contains 400 puffs; 80 puffs are equal to 1 cigarette; maximum, 16 cartridges/day; gradually decreased usage over several months	Mouth and throat irritation	Inefficient delivery system; expensive

OTC, Over the counter.

TABLE 8.2   Non—Nicotine Replacement Therapy Pharmacotherapeutic Agents

Drug	Dosage	Adverse Effects	Precautions/Advantages
Bupropion SR (Zyban)	150 mg daily for 3 days; then 150 mg twice a day for 2—3 months; begin 1—2 weeks before quit date, and continue for at least 2—3 months	Dry mouth, insomnia	Contraindicated in patients with history of seizures or at risk for seizures; may prevent weight gain
Varenicline (Chantix)	Starting 1 week before quit date, 0.5 mg daily for 3 days; then 0.5 mg twice a day for 4 days; then 1.0 mg twice daily for 12 weeks	Nausea, insomnia, flatulence, headache; may cause mood changes, including depression and suicidal ideation	No clinically relevant drug interactions have been identified; may cause taste disturbance

NRT, Nicotine replacement therapy.

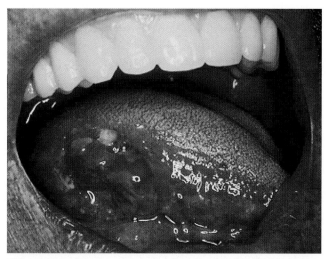

FIG 8.5 Squamous cell carcinoma of the tongue in a heavy cigarette smoker.

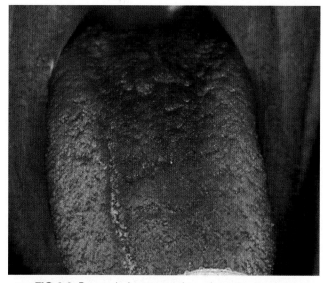

FIG 8.8 Brown hairy tongue in a cigarette smoker.

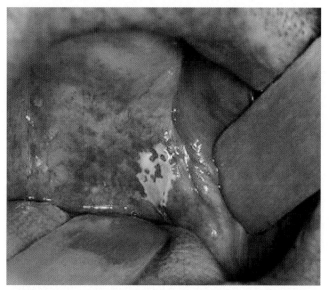

FIG 8.6 Leukoplakia of the palate in a cigarette smoker.

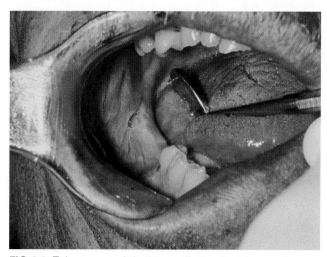

FIG 8.9 Tobacco pouch in the vestibule of a tobacco chewer.

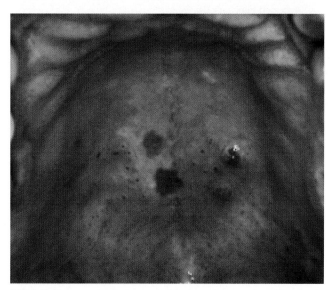

FIG 8.7 Severe nicotine stomatitis in a pipe smoker. Smoker's melanosis evident along the palatal vault.

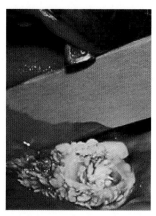

FIG 8.10 Verrucous carcinoma in a snuff user.

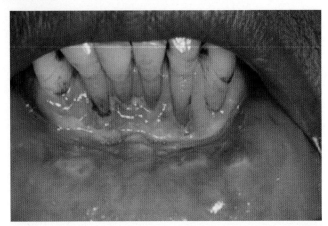

FIG 8.11 Gingival recession and leukoplakia in the area where snuff is held.

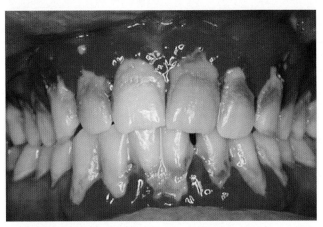

FIG 8.12 Necrotizing ulcerative gingivitis in a cigarette smoker.

increases the high risk for developing recurrences of oral cancer as well as second primary oral and pharyngeal cancers.

Benzo[a]pyrene, one of the most potent of these carcinogens, binds to nucleoproteins and is mutagenic as well as carcinogenic. Tobacco use (both smoking and smokeless) also has been shown to increase periodontal disease, impair wound healing in the oral cavity, and perhaps contribute to localized alveolitis (dry socket) and increase the risk for implant failure.

Other adverse effects of smokeless tobacco aside from oral cancer include leukoplakia (Fig. 8.6), nicotine stomatitis (Fig. 8.7), smoker's melanosis, hairy tongue (Fig. 8.8), smokeless tobacco keratosis/pouch (Fig. 8.9), verrucous carcinoma (Fig. 8.10), gingival recession (see Fig. 8.11), periodontitis, necrotizing ulcerative gingivitis (Fig. 8.12), and halitosis. Smokeless tobacco increases the risk of failure of intraosseous implants and the risk of dry socket, and it impairs wound healing following extractions. The sense of taste and smell is diminished as well.

BIBLIOGRAPHY

1. Primack BA, et al. Initiation of traditional cigarette smoking after electronic cigarette use among tobacco-Naive US young adults. *Am J Med*. 2017;131(4):443.e1.
2. CDC. National Cancer Institute. *State Tobacco Activities Tracking and Evaluation (STAT) System*. Bethesda, MD: U.S. Department of Health and Human Services, National Cancer Institute; 2017. ww.cdc.gov/mmwr/preview/mmwrhtml/mm6346a4.htm?s_cid=mm6347a4_w. Accessed February 08, 2021.
3. CDC. *National Cancer Institute National Youth Tobacco Survey (2019) US FDA and CDC*. https://www.cdc.gov/tobacco/data_statistics/fact_sheets/youth_data/tobacco_use/index.htm. Accessed February 08, 2021.
4. CDC. *Severe Lung Disease form Tobacoo Use*. Atlanta, GA: U.S. Department of Health and Human Services. CDC; 2019; 2018. https://www.cdc.gov/tobacco/basic_information/e-cigarettes/severe-lung-disease.html. Accessed February 08, 2021.
5. CDC. *National Cancer Institute. Smokeless Tobacco and Public Health: A Global Perspective*. Bethesda, MD: U.S. Department of Health and Human Services, National Cancer Institute; 2014. www.cdc.gov/mmwr/preview/mmwrhtml/mm6419a6.htm?s_cid=mm6419a6_e. Accessed February 08, 2021.
6. CDC. *Best Practices for Comprehensive Control Programs—2018*. Atlanta, GA: U.S. Department of Health and Human Services. CDC; 2019. www.cdc.gov/tobacco/standcommunity/bestpractices/pdfs/2014/comprehensive.pdfs. Accessed February 08, 2021.
7. Creamer MR, Wang TW, Babb S, et al. Tobacco product use and cessation indicators among adults- U.S. 2018. *MMWR (Morb Mortal Wkly Rep)*. 2019;68(45):1013–1019. Accessed February 08, 2021.
8. Kandel ER, et al. A molecular basis for nicotine as a gateway drug. *N Engl J Med*. 2014;317(10):932–943.
9. National Institute on Drug Abuse. *Electronic Cigarettes (E-cigarettes)*. www.drugabuse.gov/publications/drugfacts/electronic-cigarettes-e-cigarettes. Accessed February 08, 2021.
10. U.S. Department of Health and Human Services. *The Health Consequences of Smoking—50 Years of Progress: A Report of the Surgeon General*. Washington, DC: U.S. Department of Health and Human Services, CDC; 2014. http://surgeongeneral.gov/libarary/reports/50yearsofprogress/full-report.pdf. Accessed February 08, 2021.

9

Sleep Disordered Breathing

KEY POINTS

- Snoring and obstructive sleep apnea (OSA) are common sleep-related breathing disorders (SRBDs).
- SRBDs are associated with systemic comorbidities such as hypertension, stroke, obesity, and metabolic syndrome.
- Management of SRBDs consists of behavioral modifications, oral/medical devices, and surgical interventions.

- Dentists can potentially identify signs and symptoms of undiagnosed SRBDs and refer to physicians for appropriate evaluation and management.
- Common orofacial findings associated with SRBDs include tooth wear, treatment-related salivary disturbances, temporomandibular disorders (TMDs), and headache.

SNORING AND OBSTRUCTIVE SLEEP APNEA

DEFINITION

Sleep-related breathing disorders (SRBDs) constitute a spectrum of clinical entities with variations in sleep structure, respiration, and blood oxygen saturation. The spectrum ranges from intermittent snoring to obesity-hypoventilation syndrome (formerly called Pickwickian syndrome), which is characterized by severe obesity, daytime hypoventilation, and sleep-disordered breathing (Fig. 9.1). Upper airway resistance syndrome is a clinical entity midway between snoring and obstructive sleep apnea (OSA) characterized by snoring, variable complaints of daytime sleepiness, and fragmentation of sleep. Snoring and OSA are the most common SRBDs and will be the focus of this chapter.

All SRBDs are caused by upper airway obstruction of variable degree, leading to resistance to airflow during respiration. Attempts to breathe continue despite the obstruction. A related disorder, central sleep apnea, is the cessation of breathing that is caused by disruption of central nervous system (CNS) ventilatory drive; this type of apnea usually is associated with an underlying medical problem such as heart failure and is not caused by obstruction, so it is not included in this chapter.

Snoring may occur alone or may be caused by a more significant airway impairment. Snoring is the result of vibration of the soft tissues of the upper airway, primarily during inspiration. Primary snoring is sometimes referred to as simple snoring or benign snoring. It occurs as an independent entity and is not associated with disrupted sleep or complaints of daytime sleepiness and occurs without abnormal ventilation. Findings on an overnight sleep study, or polysomnogram (PSG), are normal.

To appreciate the consequences of SRBDs, it is necessary to understand the aspects of normal sleep. Normal sleep patterns vary with age but are nevertheless similar across patient groups; thus, for illustrative purposes, the sleep of young adults is discussed here. Normal sleep occurs in two phases: non—rapid eye movement (NREM) sleep and rapid eye movement (REM) sleep (Table 9.1). This chapter uses the traditional terminology and definitions on which most descriptive and experimental research has been based since the 1960s.

The phases of sleep are characterized by distinctive patterns on the electroencephalogram (EEG), as well as by the presence or absence of eye movements. NREM sleep occurs in three (or four) classical stages and generally is characterized by synchronous and increasingly high-amplitude, lower frequency brain waves, mental inactivity, and physiologic stability (Fig. 9.2). Stage 1 NREM is a brief, transitional stage that lasts only a few minutes between wakefulness and sleep and from which the person can be easily aroused. Stage 2 NREM is the initial stage of true sleep, from which arousal is more difficult. The appearance of EEG waves called *sleep spindles,* or *K-complexes,* identifies this stage, which typically lasts 10—25 min. Stage 3 is characterized by the appearance on the EEG of high-voltage, high-amplitude slow waves that last for a few minutes and then undergo transition into stage 4, with more frequent and higher amplitude slow waves. This stage lasts for 20—40 min. Stages 3 and 4 often are combined, and this combination is referred to as slow-wave sleep. Updated terminology by the American Academy of Sleep Medicine refers to Stage 1 NREM as N1, Stage 2 NREM as N2 and the sum of NREM Stage 3 and 4 as N3.

After a period of NREM sleep, entry into REM sleep occurs and is characterized by asynchronous, low-amplitude, high-frequency brain waves, an active brain,

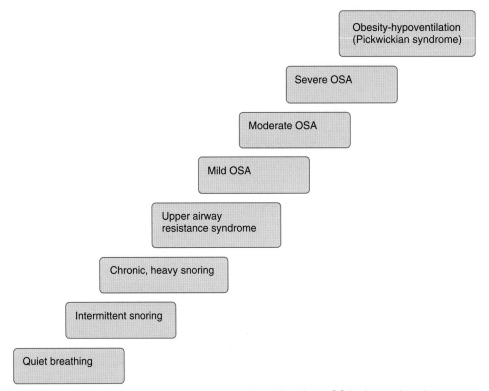

FIG. 9.1 Clinical spectrum of sleep-related breathing disorders. *OSA,* obstructive sleep apnea. (Redrawn from Phillips B, Naughton MT. *Fast Facts: Obstructive Sleep Apnea.* Oxford: Health Press Limited; 2004.)

physiologic instability, and muscular inactivity. A key feature is the presence of periodic rapid movement of the eyes with low-voltage EEG waves resembling those typical of wakefulness (Fig. 9.3). Variations in blood pressure, heart rate, and respiration occur, along with general muscle atonia and poikilothermia. Dreaming also occurs during REM sleep. Sleep normally is entered through NREM sleep and progresses to REM. Over the course of a night, sleep cycles between NREM and REM sleep, with each complete cycle (NREM + REM)

averaging about 90 min. Depending on the length of the sleep period, the sleeper typically passes through four to six cycles per night. The length of time in each stage varies, with NREM predominating in the earlier part of the night and REM predominating in the later part of the

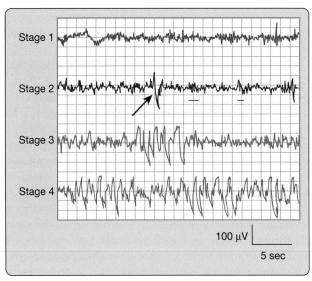

FIG. 9.2 Electroencephalographic tracings of the four classical non–rapid eye movement sleep stages. (From Sullivan SS, Carskadon MA, Dement WC, Jackson CL. Normal human sleep: an overview. In: Kryger MH, Roth T, Goldstein CA, Dement WC, eds. *Principles and Practice of Sleep Medicine.* 7th ed. Philadelphia: Elsevier; 2022.)

TABLE 9.1	**Percentage of Time Spent in the Various Stages of Sleep for Normal, Healthy Young Adults**
Stage Plus EEG Characteristics	**Percent of Sleep (%)**
Relaxed wakefulness	<5
Non–rapid eye movement sleep (NREM)	
Stage 1: transitional; easy arousal	2–5
Stage 2: sleep onset; K-complexes (sleep spindles)	45–55
Stage 3: high-voltage, high-amplitude slow waves	3–8
Stage 4: increased numbers of high-voltage slow waves	10–15
Rapid eye movement sleep (REM)	20–25
Associated with desynchronized brain waves on EEG, muscle atonia, bursts of rapid eye movement	

EEG, electroencephalogram.

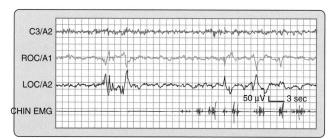

FIG. 9.3 Phasic events in human rapid eye movement (REM) sleep. C3/A2 is an electrooculographic (EOG) lead. ROC/A1 is a lead from the outer canthus of the right eye, and LOC/A2 is another lead from the outer canthus of the left eye. Note the several bursts of activity in the eye lead tracings. (From Sullivan SS, Carskadon MA, Dement WC, Jackson CL. Normal human sleep: an overview. In: Kryger MH, Roth T, Goldstein CA, Dement WC, eds. *Principles and Practice of Sleep Medicine.* 7th ed. Philadelphia: Elsevier; 2022.)

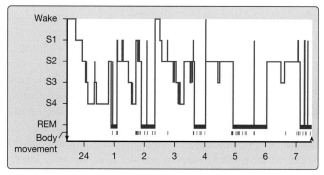

FIG. 9.4 Histogram showing progression of sleep stages across a single night in a normal, healthy, young adult volunteer. *REM*, rapid eye movement. (From Sullivan SS, Carskadon MA, Dement WC, Jackson CL. Normal human sleep: an overview. In: Kryger MH, Roth T, Goldstein CA Dement WC, eds. *Principles and Practice of Sleep Medicine.* 7th ed. Philadelphia: Saunders; 2022.)

night (Fig. 9.4). It is difficult to define a "normal" length of sleep because of multiple variables, including age, environment, circadian rhythm, and medication effects; however, most young adults report that they sleep an average of 7.5 h per weeknight and 8.5 h on weekend nights.

To gain the restorative benefits of sleep, it is necessary to progress through the normal stages of sleep. Whereas NREM sleep provides *physical* restoration, REM sleep provides *psychic* restoration. If such restoration does not occur because of sleep disruption or sleep fragmentation, cognitive and physiologic disturbances will result. Across the spectrum of SRBDs, different physiologic outcomes may be seen. With primary snoring, the degree of airway resistance is such that vibration of the parapharyngeal soft tissues is the only result. No sleep fragmentation or disruption occurs, and no other impairment of airflow or oxygenation is noted. Primary snoring has no significant adverse health effects, but may be a risk factor for type 2 diabetes, hypertension, carotid atherosclerosis, and stroke.

With *OSA*, increasing resistance to airflow occurs as a result of partial (hypopnea) collapse or complete (apnea) collapse of the airway with the cessation of breathing despite continuing efforts to breathe. Depending on the degree and duration of the collapse, hypoxia, anoxia, and hypercarbia may occur. These changes lead to CNS arousal and transition to a lighter stage of sleep (stage 1 or 2), stimulating partial awakening, relief of the obstruction, and resumption of breathing. Depending on the frequency and duration of arousals during the night, sleep can be fragmented (Fig. 9.5). Sleep quality is poor, and the restorative benefits of sleep are not achieved, leading to a variety of cognitive and physiologic abnormalities.

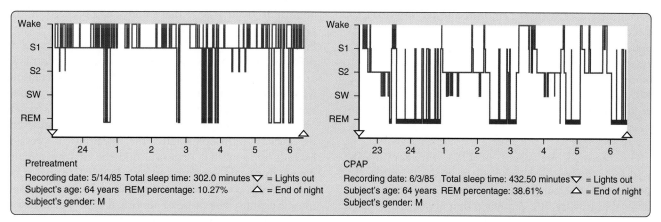

FIG. 9.5 These sleep histograms show sleep study data for a 64-year-old male patient with obstructive sleep apnea syndrome. The *left graph* shows the sleep pattern before treatment. Note the absence of slow-wave sleep (SWS), the preponderance of stage 1 (S1), and the very frequent disruptions. The *right graph* shows the sleep pattern in this patient during the second night of treatment with continuous positive airway pressure (CPAP). Note that sleep is much deeper (with more SWS) and more consolidated, and rapid eye movement (REM) sleep in particular is abnormally increased. The pretreatment REM percentage of sleep was only 10% versus nearly 40% with treatment. (From Sullivan SS, Carskadon MA, Dement WC, Jackson CL. Normal human sleep: an overview. In: Kryger MH, Roth T, Goldtein CA, Dement WC, eds. *Principles and Practice of Sleep Medicine.* 7th ed. Philadelphia: Elsevier; 2022.)

Neurocognitive effects of OSA include sleepiness, decreased alertness, irritability, poor concentration, lack of libido, and memory loss. These deficits can lead to poor job performance, marital discord, interpersonal conflicts, and driving impairment. It has been estimated that approximately 30% of fatal motor vehicle accidents involve drowsy drivers.

In addition to neurocognitive impairment, OSA is associated with numerous cardiovascular effects, including hypertension, stroke, congestive heart failure, myocardial infarction, pulmonary hypertension, and cardiac arrhythmia. OSA, which is now recognized as one of the treatable causes of hypertension, also has been shown to significantly increase the risk of stroke and death. Patients with OSA have two- to fourfold greater odds of experiencing complex arrhythmias over those without the sleep disorder. It also is thought that treatment of OSA may increase the survival rate among patients with heart failure. In addition, a relationship between OSA, obesity, and metabolic syndrome has been noted. An independent relationship among sleep apnea, glucose intolerance, and insulin resistance may lead to type 2 diabetes. Overall, the mortality rate from all causes is significantly increased among people with untreated OSA and is proportional to the severity.

EPIDEMIOLOGY

Snoring is extremely common in both genders and in all age groups. It is reported to occur in nearly 50% of the adult population, with a higher prevalence among men. Estimates of its prevalence vary widely because detection methods rely heavily on subjective reports by bed partners or parents. Reported prevalence rates for snoring range between 5% and 86% in men and between 2% and 57% in women. Evidence suggests that the frequency of snoring increases with age until about age 60 years, at which time a decrease occurs. In children, snoring is common, with a reported prevalence of 10%. When present in children, snoring is often associated with enlarged tonsils and adenoids, as well as obesity. Snoring also has been reported to increase markedly during pregnancy. In a typical dental practice of 2000 adult patients, approximately 1000 patients will report a history of snoring.

The reported prevalence of OSA varies primarily because of differences in assessment methods and in the number of abnormal respiratory events per hour used to define abnormality. It is estimated that about 2%–4% of the adult population 30–60 years of age is affected by OSA. Different rates of occurrence have been reported for males and for females, with males affected more often. Variation among racial groups may be due to historical, socioeconomic, genetic or dietary differences that has led to African Americans, Hispanics, and Asian Americans having a somewhat higher prevalence of OSA than whites. About 3% of children are affected with OSA, with the highest prevalence reported between the ages of 2 and 5 years. In a typical dental practice of 2000 adult patients, approximately 100 patients will report a diagnosis of OSA.

Etiology and Pathophysiology

The underlying defect in SRBDs is an anatomically narrowed upper airway combined with pharyngeal dilator muscle collapsibility. The exact pathogenesis, however, is not well understood. Depending on the extent of narrowing, increased resistance to airflow may be clinically expressed as vibration of soft tissues (snoring), reduced ventilation (hypopnea), or complete obstruction (apnea).

Anatomic narrowing may occur at any site in the upper airway from the nasal cavity to the larynx. Within the nasal cavity, septal deviation and enlarged turbinates may cause narrowing. In the nasopharynx, hypertrophic adenoids and tonsils, an elongated soft palate, and an elongated and edematous uvula may be the cause. In the oropharynx, narrowing may be caused by an enlarged tongue, retrognathia, excessive lymphoid tissue, palatine tonsils, or redundant parapharyngeal folds. The most common sites of airway narrowing or closure during sleep are the retropalatal and retroglossal regions. Most patients with OSA have more than one site of narrowing. It also has been demonstrated that the volume of the upper airway soft tissue structures (i.e., tongue, lateral pharyngeal walls, soft palate, parapharyngeal fat pads) is significantly greater in patients with OSA than in normal control participants. Factors that contribute to enlargement of the upper airway soft tissues in apneic patients include obesity, edema secondary to negative pressures, vibration trauma of the uvula, male gender, and possibly genetics.

In addition to anatomic narrowing of the airway, an abnormal degree of collapsibility is observed in the pharyngeal dilator muscles surrounding the airway. Patency of the airway depends on a balance between air pressure within the airway and pressure outside of the airway exerted by the parapharyngeal musculature. Muscles that surround the airway receive phasic activation during inspiration and tend to promote a patent pharyngeal lumen by dilating the airway and stiffening the airway walls. Normally, the intraluminal pressure exceeds the external pressure, and the airway remains patent during inhalation and exhalation. Normal function requires coordinated timing and activity of opposing muscle groups. The cause of abnormal pharyngeal airway collapse is complex, involving both dynamic and static factors. These factors may include tissue volume, changes in the adhesive character of mucosal surfaces, changes in neck and jaw posture, decreased tracheal tug, effects of gravity, autonomic and catecholamine dysfunction, and decreased intraluminal pressure resulting from increased upstream resistance in the nasal cavity or pharynx.

CLINICAL PRESENTATION

Signs and Symptoms

The signs and symptoms of SRBDs are those most often described by the bed partner or parent of a patient; they include snoring, snorting, gasping, and breath holding. Snoring is very common and is the most common symptom in patients with OSA. However, most people who snore do not have OSA, but almost all patients with OSA snore.

Snoring may be very loud and disruptive to other members of the household. When snoring is the only complaint, the problem most often is primary snoring. Snoring accompanied by snorting, choking, gasping, or a complete cessation of breathing is likely to be a sign of OSA. Of note, however, definitive diagnosis of SRBDs cannot be made only on the basis of clinical signs and symptoms.

Complaints of excessive daytime sleepiness are common in patients with OSA but are not specific, and the problem may be multifactorial. A general screening tool for sleep disorders is the Global Sleep Assessment Questionnaire, comprised of 11 items regarding symptom frequency (never, sometimes, usually, always) during the preceding 4 weeks. The 11 items cover mood, life activities, and medical issues as they relate to sleep, along with symptoms associated with insomnia, OSA, restless legs syndrome/periodic limb movement, and parasomnias (Table 9.2). Another commonly used subjective measure of sleepiness is the Epworth Sleepiness Scale (Fig. 9.6). This assessment tool has been validated in clinical studies and correlates with objective measures of sleepiness. It is composed of eight questions or situations in which patients are asked how likely they are to fall asleep. Each question is answered on a scale of 0–3, with 0 meaning no likelihood of falling asleep and 3 indicating 100% likelihood of falling asleep in that situation. The maximum possible score is 24. A score greater than 10 is indicative of significant daytime sleepiness but is not specific for SRBDs. Other complaints that may be associated with OSA are nocturia or enuresis, mood changes, memory or learning difficulties, erectile dysfunction, morning headache, and dry mouth noted upon awakening.

Obesity is common among patients with OSA and increases the risk of OSA several fold. Approximately 70% of patients with OSA are obese. One measure of obesity is the body mass index (BMI), which is calculated by dividing weight in kilograms by the height in meters squared. Adults with BMIs greater than 25 are considered overweight, and those with BMIs over 30 are considered to be obese. Of interest, however, is that neck circumference has been found to be more closely related to severity of OSA than is BMI. A neck circumference greater than 17 inches (43 cm) in men and greater than 16 inches (41 cm) in women is predictive of OSA. The STOP-BANG Questionnaire is a validated tool for

TABLE 9.2 Global Sleep Assessment Questionnaire (GSAQ)	
Did you have difficulty falling asleep, staying asleep, or did you feel poorly rested in the morning?	Never Sometimes Usually Always
Did you fall asleep unintentionally or did you have to fight to stay awake during the day?	Never Sometimes Usually Always
Did sleep difficulties or daytime sleepiness interfere with your daily activities?	Never Sometimes Usually Always
Did work or other activities prevent you from getting enough sleep?	Never Sometimes Usually Always
Did you snore loudly?	Never Sometimes Usually Always
Did you hold your breath, have breathing pauses, or stop breathing in your sleep?	Never Sometimes Usually Always
Did you have restless or "crawling" feelings in your legs at night that went away if you moved your legs?	Never Sometimes Usually Always
Did you have repeated rhythmic leg jerks or leg twitches during your sleep?	Never Sometimes Usually Always
Did you have nightmares, or did you scream, walk, punch, or kick in your sleep?	Never Sometimes Usually Always
Did the following things disturb you in your sleep: pain, other physical symptoms, worries, medications, or other (specify)?	Never Sometimes Usually Always
Did you feel sad or anxious?	Never Sometimes Usually Always

Adapted from Klingman KJ, Jungquist CR, Perlis ML. Questionnaires that screen for multiple sleep disorders. *Sleep Med Rev.* 2017;32:37–44.

assessing OSA risk (Box 9.1). This is an 8-item assessment of snoring, daytime tiredness, stoppage of breathing while sleeping, hypertension, BMI, age, neck circumference, and gender. A score of 3 or greater correlates with a high risk of OSA.

LABORATORY AND DIAGNOSTIC FINDINGS

Definitive diagnosis of an SRBD is made by PSG, in which the patient's brain waves, breathing, and other physiologic parameters are recorded during sleep. As noted earlier, a PSG is an overnight sleep study that is often performed in a laboratory setting. During the performance of a standard laboratory-based PSG, a technician who is present throughout the night records the activities of the patient during sleep. Multiple physiologic parameters are monitored and recorded on a computer. The components of a PSG typically include EEG to monitor brain waves, electrooculogram to monitor eye movements, electromyogram to monitor jaw muscle activity and leg movements, electrocardiogram to monitor heart rate and rhythm, pulse oximetry to monitor blood oxygen saturation, nasal thermistor monitoring of nasal airflow and CO_2 levels, and use of chest and abdominal strain gauges to track breathing efforts.

After recording sensors are attached, the patient is allowed to go to sleep. Most contemporary sleep

THE EPWORTH SLEEPINESS SCALE

Name: _____

Today's date: _____   Your age (years): _____

Your sex (male = M; female = F): _____

How likely are you to doze off or fall asleep in the following situations, in contrast to feeling just tired? This refers to your usual way of life in recent times. Even if you have not done some of these things recently try to work out how they would have affected you. Use the following scale to choose the *most appropriate number* for each situation:

0 = would *never* doze
1 = *slight* chance of dozing
2 = *moderate* chance of dozing
3 = *high* chance of dozing

Situation	Chance of dozing
Sitting and reading	_____
Watching TV	_____
Sitting, inactive in a public place (e.g., a theater or a meeting)	_____
As a passenger in a car for an hour without a break	_____
Lying down to rest in the afternoon when circumstances permit	_____
Sitting and talking to someone	_____
Sitting quietly after a lunch without alcohol	_____
In a car, while stopped for a few minutes in the traffic	_____

Thank you for your cooperation

FIG. 9.6 Epworth sleepiness scale. (Redrawn from Johns MW. A new method for measuring daytime sleepiness: the Epworth sleepiness scale. *Sleep.* 1991;14:540–545.)

laboratories have sleeping rooms that resemble a normal bedroom. In addition to the sensors attached to the patient, an infrared camera often is used to enable the technician to watch patient movements, such as leg movements or sleep walking, or to relate sleeping position to periods of disturbed breathing. A microphone is present in the room to record snoring or other sounds such as tooth grinding or sleep talking.

A typical PSG study encompasses the entire night and usually is sufficient to make a diagnosis despite obvious questions about the "normality" of the night's sleep in such an environment. Often, a diagnosis can be made early in the course of the night, and a trial of therapy with positive airway pressure (PAP) will be attempted. This is called a *split-night study*. If trial PAP therapy is not possible during the initial PSG, a second sleep study may be necessary to assess the effects of PAP. A computer recording of the entire night is produced (Fig. 9.7); this tracing is scrutinized and interpreted by a qualified

physician trained in sleep medicine, who then makes a diagnosis and recommends treatment.

Evidence suggests that home-based sleep apnea testing (HSAT) followed by treatment in the home leads to equivalent outcomes for patients with uncomplicated OSA. Although HSAT does not include EEG, it records oximetry, airflow, and chest movement with easily self-applied monitors. Advantages of HSAT include lower cost, more rapid initiation of treatment, and broader access to care.

Quantification of OSA severity is expressed by means of the *apnea-hypopnea index* (AHI) or the *respiratory disturbance index* (RDI). These two indices commonly are used interchangeably; however, there is a technical difference between the two. The AHI is scored by adding all of the apneic episodes together with all of the hypopneic episodes that occurred during the night and then dividing this total by the number of hours slept. The result is expressed as the average number of respiratory events per

BOX 9.1 STOP-BANG Questionnaire

1. Snoring
   Do you snore loudly (louder than talking or loud enough to be heard through closed doors)?
   Yes No
2. Tired
   Do you often feel tired, fatigued, or sleepy during daytime?
   Yes No
3. Observed
   Has anyone observed you stop breathing during your sleep?
   Yes No
4. Blood pressure
   Do you have or are you being treated for high blood pressure?
   Yes No
5. BMI
   BMI more than 35 kg/m^2?
   Yes No
6. Age
   Age over 50 yr old?
   Yes No
7. Neck circumference
   Neck circumference greater than 40 cm?
   Yes No
8. Gender
   Gender male?
   Yes No
   High risk of OSA: answering yes to three or more items
   Low risk of OSA: answering yes to less than three items

Adapted from Chung F, Yegneswaran B, Liao P, et al. STOP questionnaire: a tool to screen patients for obstructive sleep apnea. *Anesthesiology.* 2008;108:812–821.

hour. To calculate the RDI, respiratory effort–related arousals (RERAs) are added to the apneas and hypopneas. It is important to define these terms for use in characterizing the various sleep disorders. According to the American Academy of Sleep Medicine, an *apnea* (apneic episode) is defined as the cessation or near-complete cessation (>90% reduction) of airflow for a minimum of 10 s. *Hypopnea* is an episode of greater than 30% reduction in amplitude in thoracoabdominal movement or airflow from baseline, with a greater than 3% oxygen desaturation. *RERAs* are episodes that include a clear drop in respiratory airflow, increased respiratory effort, and a brief change in sleep state (arousal) but do not meet the criteria for an apnea or a hypopnea.

A diagnosis of OSA is made if the AHI or RDI is greater than 5/hour and symptoms of excessive daytime sleepiness, witnessed nocturnal apneas, or awakening with choking, breath holding, or gasping are noted. In quantifying the severity of OSA, some disagreement has been expressed; however, a commonly used classification defines an AHI of 0–5/hour as normal, 5–15/hour as mild, 15–30/hour as moderate, and greater than 30/hour as severe. Along with the AHI, the lowest point (nadir) of oxygen desaturation is reported. Primary snoring is associated with completely normal findings on the PSG,

with no complaint of excessive sleepiness in the presence of snoring.

Other aspects of the PSG that may be reported are total time spent in the various sleep stages, AHI for various sleep stages, and AHI for various sleep positions. In addition, a sleep histogram, which is a graph of the sleep pattern during the entire night that depicts cycling into and out of the various sleep stages, may be provided. Other tests that may be used include the *multiple sleep latency test*, which assesses the ability to fall asleep, and the *maintenance of wakefulness test*, which assesses the ability to stay awake.

Medical Management

The decision of when and how to treat SRBDs depends on the diagnosis and the severity of the disorder. Treatment of primary snoring is elective and essentially is a personal decision commonly motivated by the effects of snoring on a spouse or bed partner. Of interest, snoring rarely disturbs the snorer. Parents of a child who snores often seek treatment out of concern for the health of the child. Simple snoring can progress, evolving into OSA over time, most often caused by weight gain or aging (or both). Patients who are given a diagnosis of OSA require treatment, not only to alleviate snoring and sleepiness but also to prevent or treat the numerous adverse health effects associated with the disease. Even mild sleep apnea is associated with significant morbidity and mortality, which increases with severity. Treatment of OSA involves three different approaches: behavioral modification, medical devices (e.g., PAP, oral appliances), and surgery.

Behavioral Modification

Several measures may help decrease or eliminate the signs or symptoms of SRBDs. Weight loss is one of the most effective measures that can be instituted; however, it may not result in normalization alone. Even modest weight loss can result in significant improvement. Furthermore, independent of body habitus, regular aerobic exercise has been shown to be of clinical benefit in patients with OSA. For patients with obstruction in the nasal cavity, nasal dilator strips may be helpful to physically open the nasal passages, as may the use of nasal decongestants, topical corticosteroids, or both. Nasal expiratory positive airway pressure valves have been developed recently with limited use, which consist of two small, disposable, one-way valves placed over each nostril with adhesive tape. The goal of these devices is to utilize the patient's own breathing to generate a small positive end-expiratory pressure, however, this may be challenging to achieve in patients with nasal obstruction. Many patients with OSA have positional apnea, with apneas occurring more frequently or with greater severity in the supine position. For patients with position-dependent apnea, measures to prevent sleeping in a supine position may be helpful and include sewing a tennis ball into a pocket on the back of the pajamas, using a backpack-type device, or placement

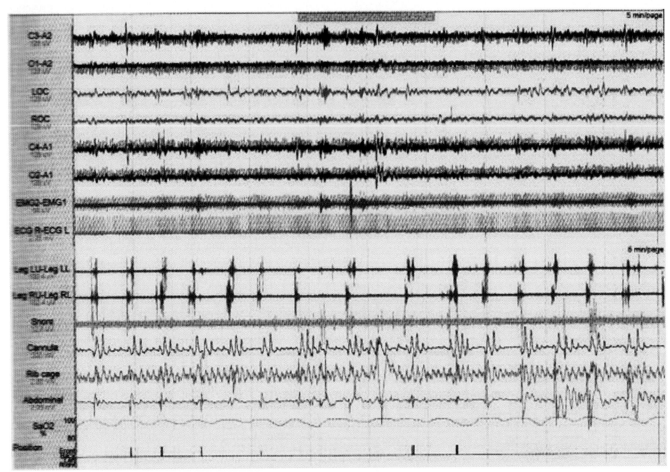

FIG. 9.7 A 5-minute epoch of a polysomnogram. *C3-A2, O1-A2, C4-A1,* and *O2-A1* are electroencephalographic leads used to determine sleep stages. *LOC* and *ROC* designate eyelid leads at left and right outer canthi, respectively, for recording rapid eye movement. *EMG* tracing is an electromyogram of the chin used to record jaw movement. *ECG* tracing is an electrocardiogram that records heart rate and rhythm. *Leg LU* and *Leg RU* designate leads for recording leg movements. *Snore* tracing tracks the subject's snoring. *Cannula* designates measurement of nasal airflow pressure. *Rib cage* tracing is a recording of rib cage movement. *Abdominal* tracing is a recording of abdominal movement. *Sao$_2$* is blood oxygen saturation. *Position* tracing is a recording of body position. (From Phillips B, Naughton M. *Fast Facts: Obstructive Sleep Apnea.* Oxford; Health Press Limited; 2004.)

of pillows to maintain a side-sleeping posture. Alcohol, sedatives, or muscle relaxants near bedtime should be avoided. Patients who smoke should be encouraged to quit smoking, although the relationship between smoking and OSA remains unclear.

Medical Devices

Positive Airway Pressure. The "gold standard" of treatment for OSA is the delivery of PAP to the patient's airway during sleep. This is accomplished with the use of an air compressor that is connected by tubing to a nasal or full-face mask attached to the patient's face (Fig. 9.8). Room air is delivered under pressure to the patient's airway, where it acts in effect as a pneumatic stent, producing positive intraluminal pressure along the

entire pharyngeal airway, thereby maintaining patency. The air can be heated and humidified.

An advantage of PAP is that it relieves obstruction at all levels of the airway. Delivery of PAP may be accomplished using one of three modalities:

1. Continuous positive airway pressure (CPAP)
2. Bilevel positive airway pressure (BiPAP or BPAP)
3. Auto-adjusting positive airway pressure (APAP)

CPAP provides air continuously throughout inspiration and exhalation at a single, set pressure, expressed in cm H$_2$O. BiPAP consists of two set pressures, with use of a higher pressure during inhalation and a lower pressure setting for during exhalation. With APAP, pressures vary

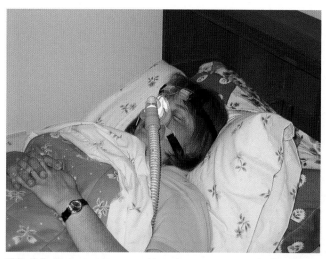

FIG. 9.8 Patient using a positive airway pressure device with a nasal mask. (Courtesy of June Sorrenson, CRT, Lexington, KY.)

continuously according to what is sensed to be required at a particular moment to maintain airway patency. CPAP is most often titrated to an effective level during a PSG in the sleep laboratory, either as part of a split-night study or during a subsequent full-night study. Pressures typically are started at 3–5 cm H_2O and are gradually titrated upward until all manifestations of OSA are eliminated. With CPAP, typical treatment pressures range between 5 and 15 cm H_2O.

Current evidence indicates that PAP eliminates respiratory disturbances and reduces AHI compared with placebo, conservative management, or positional therapy. PAP also improves stage 3 and 4 sleep and decreases EEG arousals versus placebo. It significantly improves sleep architecture and sleep fragmentation, but these effects are not always consistent. In addition, daytime sleepiness may be decreased and neurobehavioral performance, psychological functioning, and quality of life may be improved.

The impact on cardiovascular risk is unclear; however, there appears to be a trend toward reduction of risk. Compliance with PAP has long been a problem, with only about 50% of patients who try it able to tolerate it. Of those who are able to use PAP, the average patient uses it for only about 4–5 h per night and for only about five nights per week. Adverse effects with PAP are common and include mask leaks, skin ulceration or irritation under the mask, epistaxis, rhinorrhea, nasal congestion, sinus congestion, dry eyes, conjunctivitis, ear pain, and claustrophobia.

Oral Appliances. Oral appliances offer an attractive alternative for the management of SRBDs (1) as a primary treatment option, (2) in patients who are unable to tolerate the use of PAP, or (3) in patients who refuse to use PAP. Oral appliances exert their effects by mechanically increasing the volume of the upper airway in the retropalatal and retroglossal areas, as has been confirmed by imaging and physiologic monitoring. These areas of the oropharynx are the most common sites of obstruction in patients with OSA. Oral appliances are associated with increased airway size in *both* the retropalatal and retroglossal regions, with increases occurring not only anteroposteriorly but in the lateral dimension as well.

The two basic types of oral appliances are (1) mandibular advancement devices (MADs), which engage the mandible and reposition it (and indirectly, the tongue) in an anterior or forward position (Fig. 9.9), and (2) tongue-retaining devices (TRDs), which directly engage the tongue and hold it in a forward position (Fig. 9.10). Many different types of OAs are available to treat snoring and OSA; however, not all have been approved by the U.S. Food and Drug Administration for specific use in the treatment of OSA.

MADs are the type of oral appliance most commonly used to treat patients with SRBDs. They are typically custom made of acrylic resin and are composed of two pieces (biblock) that cover the upper and lower dental arches (similar to retainers or athletic mouth guards) and are connected together in such a way as to reposition and hold the mandible in a forward position. The parts may be fused together into a single (monoblock), nonadjustable appliance, or they may be connected in such a way as to allow some degree of mandibular movement and adjustability (titratability) between the two pieces. Several over-the-counter, so-called "boil and bite" appliances are available in drug stores and on the Internet; however, they tend to be unsatisfactory and are not recommended.

TRDs are made of silicone in the shape of a bulb or cavity with wings that fit outside the mouth or between the teeth and lips. The tongue is stuck into the bulb, which is then squeezed and released, producing a suction that holds the tongue forward in the bulb. see (Fig. 9.10) TRDs generally provide treatment effects similar to those achieved with MADs; however, they are not tolerated as well as are MADs. Also available is a hybrid type of tongue displacement appliance that fits over one or both arches and depresses the tongue and guides it forward without moving the mandible.

When compared with PAP, MADs are not as effective in treating OSA, especially the more severe cases, but about two-thirds of patients benefit from using oral appliances, with either complete or partial success. They are generally well tolerated, and patients tend to prefer MADs compared with wearing PAP devices; however, adverse effects are common. Fortunately, most such effects are minor and transient and resolve quickly on removal of the device. Common problems include temporomandibular joint (TMJ) pain, muscular pain, tooth pain, hypersalivation, TMJ sounds, dry mouth, gum irritation, and occlusal changes. Infrequently, a patient may develop jaw pain severe enough that may prevent use of the device.

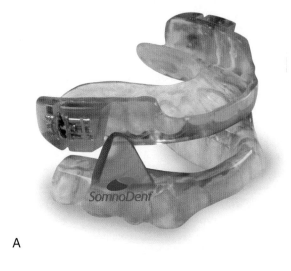

A

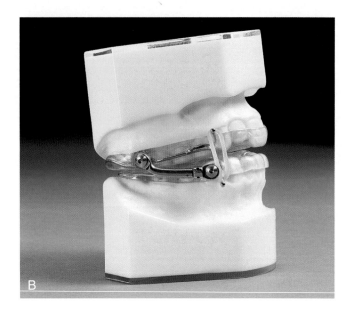

B

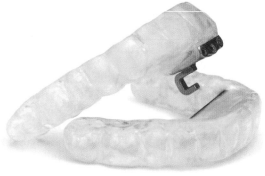

C

FIG. 9.9 Examples of oral appliances used for the treatment of obstructive sleep apnea. **(A)** SomnoDent MAS (Mandibular Advancement Splint). **(B)** Modified Herbst appliance. **(C)** TAP-T (Thornton Adjustable Positioner). ((**A**) Courtesy of Somnomed, Inc., Denton, TX. **(B)** Courtesy of Great Lakes Orthodontics, Tonawanda, NY. **(C)** Courtesy Airway Management, Inc., Dallas, TX.)

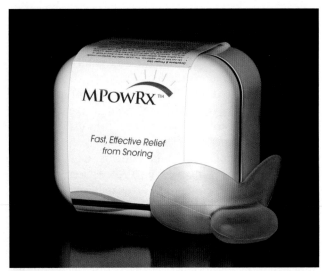

FIG. 9.10 Example of oral appliance used for the treatment of obstructive sleep apnea. MPowRX tongue retainer.

The American Academy of Sleep Medicine has published practice parameters and clinical guidelines for the use of OAs in the treatment of snoring and OSA. They recommend that a qualified dentist use a custom-made titratable appliance over a noncustom appliance with regular oversight or follow-up to survey for side effects or dental changes. Furthermore, it is recommended that the sleep physician perform follow-up sleep testing to confirm treatment efficacy. Use of an oral appliance is recommended for the following categories of patients:

- Patients with primary snoring
- Patients with mild to moderate OSA who prefer OAs to CPAP, who do not respond to CPAP, who are not appropriate candidates for CPAP, or who do not obtain adequate relief with CPAP or behavioral measures
- Patients with severe OSA in whom an initial trial of CPAP has failed to correct the problem

Also of note, upper airway surgery may supersede the use of oral appliances in patients for whom such operations are predicted to be highly effective.

Oral pressure therapy is a novel approach to nonsurgical management of OSA. This device is intended to "suck" the uvula and soft palate anteriorly in order to increase the size of the retro-palatal airway and stabilize the tongue.

Surgical Approaches

A variety of surgical procedures have been advocated to treat OSA, including tracheostomy, tonsillectomy, adenoidectomy, nasal septoplasty, turbinate reduction, uvulopalatopharyngoplasty (UPPP), laser-assisted uvulopalatoplasty (LAUP), radiofrequency volumetric tissue reduction (RVTR), pillar implants, genioglossus advancement–hyoid myotomy and suspension (GAHMS), tongue base reduction, maxillary and mandibular advancement osteotomy (MMO), and bariatric surgery. Hypoglossal nerve stimulation is a newer surgical procedure that increases pharyngeal dilator muscle tone during sleep. Some of these procedures achieve relatively modest success rates when performed alone, such as UPPP, while others, such as MMO or performance of a combination of procedures, typically result in much higher success rates. Tracheostomy, which bypasses all obstruction in the entire upper airway, is almost uniformly effective in curing OSA. Its use is limited, however, in that it is unacceptable to most patients but may be used for the occasional patient with very severe OSA who is intolerant of CPAP and who requires urgent treatment. Another predictably successful procedure is the removal of adenoids and tonsils in children.

Because upper airway surgery is invasive and irreversible, efforts must be made to identify the site(s) of obstruction to determine which surgical approach should be used and to avoid unnecessary or ineffective surgery. A number of imaging techniques and laboratory modalities, including cephalometrics, computed tomography scanning, nasopharyngoscopy, and measurements of regional pharyngeal pressure, flow, and resistance have been used for this purpose. A phased approach to surgery, beginning with less aggressive procedures and advancing to more aggressive interventions when the response to initial treatment is inadequate, is often advocated.

Complications and adverse effects of upper airway surgery vary with the procedure. For example, UPPP may result in velopharyngeal insufficiency, velopharyngeal stenosis, voice changes, postoperative bleeding, postoperative airway obstruction, and death. MMO and GAHMS may result in lip, cheek, or chin paresthesia or anesthesia, as well as tooth injury, postoperative bleeding, postoperative airway obstruction, and changes in facial appearance.

Because obesity is a major risk factor for OSA, bariatric surgery has become a more commonly accepted treatment for patients with severe obesity. Morbid or severe obesity is defined as a BMI of 40 or greater. Surgically induced weight loss results in significant relief of clinical signs and symptoms associated with obesity-related OSA.

DENTAL HEALTH CARE PROVIDERS AND SRBDS

Dental professionals can play an important role in reducing the public health care burden of undiagnosed SRBDs. The dental team should be aware of SRBDs, the potential health risks associated with SRBDs and role in referring patients with suspected SRBDs to appropriate medical providers for evaluation and management. Dentists should inquire about general sleep habits, sleep quality, and potential disturbances to sleep. Patients with SRBDs may have orofacial complaints associated with the condition itself or its treatment. These include tooth

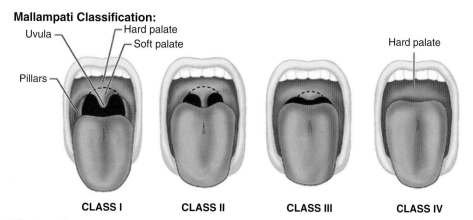

FIG. 9.11 The Mallampati score. Class I: Full view of the soft palate; Class II: Full view of the uvula; Class II: View of only the base of the uvula; Class IV: No view of the soft palate. (From Steven M. Green and Mark G. Roback, 2019. Is the Mallampati Score Useful for Emergency Department Airway Management or Procedural Sedation? Pain Management and Sedation, 74(2), PP.251–259.)

pain and mobility, temporomandibular disorders (TMDs [e.g., TMJ and/or myofascial muscle pain]) and headache commonly related to sleep bruxism in patients with SRBDs. Xerostomia may be a result of PAP device use while hypersalivation is often associated with OAs. Thorough clinical examination of the head, neck, and oral cavity for patients with a suspected SRBD can potentially identify these comorbidities as previously described. In addition, inspection of the visible oropharyngeal region may reveal uvular and/or tonsillar enlargement often associated with SRBDs. The Mallampati Score, commonly used by anesthesiologists, evaluates tongue position relative to oropharyngeal structures and may be used as a risk assessment tool for OSA. It is graded on a scale of I–IV with the risk of OSA increasing with a higher score (Fig. 9.11).

Dental health care providers may identify signs of sleep bruxism that may impact SRBDs. Sleep bruxism is a repetitive jaw-muscle activity characterized by clenching or grinding of the teeth and/or by bracing or thrusting of the mandible that occurs during sleep. Orofacial signs of sleep bruxism may include tooth wear/fractures, masseter hypertrophy, tongue indentation, and linea alba. Treatment of sleep bruxism is dependent on the severity of negative consequences for the patient. Management of sleep bruxism by dental and medical providers is multifactorial, including use of pharmacologic agents, occlusal stabilization appliances, and/or behavioral medicine techniques. The American Academy of Dental Sleep Medicine recommends only qualified dentists (i.e., those who meet specific educational and clinical requirements) manage SRBD patients with OAs in collaboration with physicians.

BIBLIOGRAPHY

1. Addy N, Bennett K, Blanton A, et al. Policy statement on a dentist's role in treating sleep-related breathing disorders. *J Dent Sleep Med.* 2018;5:25–26.
2. Araghi MH, Chen YF, Jagielski A, et al. Effectiveness of lifestyle interventions on obstructive sleep apnea (OSA): systematic review and meta-analysis. *Sleep.* 2013;36:1553–1562, 1562a-1562e.
3. Balasubramaniam R, Paesani D, Koyano K, et al. Sleep bruxism. In: Farah CS, Balasubramaniam R, McCullough MJ, eds. *Contemporary Oral Medicine.* 1st ed. New York: Springer International Publishing; 2019: 2267–2301.
4. Berry RB, Budhiraja R, Gottlieb D, et al. Rules for scoring respiratory events in sleep: update of the 2007 AASM manual for the scoring of sleep and associated events. Deliberations of the sleep apnea definitions task force of the American academy of sleep medicine. *J Clin Sleep Med.* 2012;8:597–619.
5. Bisogni V, Pengo M, Maiolino G, et al. The sympathetic nervous system and catecholamines metabolism in obstructive sleep apnoea. *J Thorac Dis.* 2016;8:243–254.
6. Sullivan S, Carskadon M, Dement W, Jackson C. Normal human sleep: an overview. In: Kryger MH, Roth T, Goldstein C, Dement W, eds. *Principles and Practice of Sleep Medicine.* 7th ed. Philadelphia: Elsevier; 2022:16–26.e4.
7. Chang SJ, Chae KY. Obstructive sleep apnea syndrome in children: epidemiology, pathophysiology, diagnosis and sequelae. *Korean J Pediatr.* 2010;53:863–871.
8. Chobanian AV, Bakris GL, Black HR, et al. The seventh report of the joint national committee on prevention, detection, evaluation, and treatment of high blood pressure: the JNC 7 report. *JAMA.* 2003;289:2560–2572.
9. Chung F, Abdullah HR, Liao P. STOP questionnaire: a tool to screen patients for obstructive sleep apnea. *Anesthesiology.* 2008;108:812–821.
10. Davies RJ, Ali NJ, Stradling JR. Neck circumference and other clinical features in the diagnosis of the obstructive sleep apnoea syndrome. *Thorax.* 1992;47:101–105.
11. de Almeida FR, Lowe AA, Tsuiki S, et al. Long-term compliance and side effects of oral appliances used for the treatment of snoring and obstructive sleep apnea syndrome. *J Clin Sleep Med.* 2005;1:143–152.
12. Deane SA, Cistulli PA, Ng AT, et al. Comparison of mandibular advancement splint and tongue stabilizing device in obstructive sleep apnea: a randomized controlled trial. *Sleep.* 2009;32:648–653.
13. Deary V, Ellis JG, Wilson JA, et al. Simple snoring: not quite so simple after all? *Sleep Med Rev.* 2014;18: 453–462.
14. Ferguson KA, Cartwright R, Rogers R, et al. Oral appliances for snoring and obstructive sleep apnea: a review. *Sleep.* 2006;29:244–262.
15. Gay P, Weaver T, Loube D, et al. Evaluation of positive airway pressure treatment for sleep related breathing disorders in adults. *Sleep.* 2006;29:381–401.
16. Genta PR, Edwards BA, Sands SA, et al. Tube law of the pharyngeal airway in sleeping patients with obstructive sleep apnea. *Sleep.* 2016;39:337–343.
17. Gottlieb DJ, Punjabi NM. Diagnosis and management of obstructive sleep apnea: a review. *JAMA.* 2020;323: 1389–1400.
18. Gupta R, Pandi-Perumal SR, Almeneessier AS, et al. Hypersomnolence and traffic safety. *Sleep Med Clin.* 2017;12:489–499.
19. Guo J, Sun Y, Xue LJ, et al. Effect of CPAP therapy on cardiovascular events and mortality in patients with obstructive sleep apnea: a meta-analysis. *Sleep Breath.* 2016;20:965–974.
20. Haines KL, Nelson LG, Gonzalez R, et al. Objective evidence that bariatric surgery improves obesity-related obstructive sleep apnea. *Surgery.* 2007;141:354–358.
21. Hillman D, Vanderveken O, Malhotra A, et al. Sleep medicine. In: Farah CS, Balasubramaniam R, McCullough MJ, eds. *Contemporary Oral Medicine.* 1st ed. New York: Springer International Publishing; 2019:2241–2265.
22. Javaheri S, Wexler L. Prevalence and treatment of breathing disorders during sleep in patients with heart failure. *Curr Treat Options Cardiovasc Med.* 2005;7:295–306.
23. Johns MW. Daytime sleepiness, snoring, and obstructive sleep apnea. The epworth sleepiness scale. *Chest.* 1993;103:30–36.

24. Katz I, Stradling J, Slutsky AS, et al. Do patients with obstructive sleep apnea have thick necks? *Am Rev Respir Dis.* 1990;141:1228–1231.

25. Klingman KJ, Jungquist CR, Perlis ML. Questionnaires that screen for multiple sleep disorders. *Sleep Med Rev.* 2017;32:37–44.

26. Levine M, Bennett KM, Cantwell MK, et al. Dental sleep medicine standards for screening, treating and managing adults with sleep-related breathing disorders. *J Dent Sleep Med.* 2018;5:61–68.

27. Lindberg E, Taube A, Janson C, et al. A 10-year follow-up of snoring in men. *Chest.* 1998;114:1048–1055.

28. Lobbezoo F, de Vries N, de Lange J, et al. A Further Introduction to dental sleep medicine. *Nat Sci Sleep.* 2020;12:1173–1179.

29. Lyons-Coleman M, Bates C, Barber S. Obstructive sleep apnoea and the role of the dental team. *Br Dent J.* 2020;228:681–685.

30. Maurer JT. Update on surgical treatments for sleep apnea. *Swiss Med Wkly.* 2009;139(43–44):624–629.

31. Mehra R, Benjamin EJ, Shahar E, et al. Association of nocturnal arrhythmias with sleep-disordered breathing: the sleep heart health study. *Am J Respir Crit Care Med.* 2006;173:910–916.

32. Mokhlesi B. Obesity hypoventilation syndrome: a state-of-the-art review. *Respir Care.* 2010;55:1347–1362; discussion 1363-1345.

33. Naughton MT. Epidemiology of central sleep apnoea in heart failure. *Int J Cardiol.* 2016;206(suppl):S4–S7.

34. Ng DK, Chow PY, Chan CH, et al. An update on childhood snoring. *ActaPaediatr.* 2006;95:1029–1035.

35. Ng JH, Yow M. Oral appliances in the management of obstructive sleep apnea. *Sleep Med Clin.* 2020;15:241–250.

36. Nuckton TJ, Glidden DV, Browner WS, et al. Physical examination: mallampati score as an independent predictor of obstructive sleep apnea. *Sleep.* 2006;29:903–908.

37. Patel SR. Obstructive sleep apnea. *Ann Intern Med.* 2019;171:ITC81–ITC96.

38. Patil SP, Schneider H, Schwartz AR, et al. Adult obstructive sleep apnea: pathophysiology and diagnosis. *Chest.* 2007;132:325–337.

39. Peppard PE, Young T. Exercise and sleep-disordered breathing: an association independent of body habitus. *Sleep.* 2004;27:480–484.

40. Pien GW, Fife D, Pack AI, et al. Changes in symptoms of sleep-disordered breathing during pregnancy. *Sleep.* 2005;28:1299–1305.

41. Punjabi NM, Shahar E, Redline S, et al. Sleep-disordered breathing, glucose intolerance, and insulin resistance: the sleep heart health study. *Am J Epidemiol.* 2004;160:521–530.

42. Rama AN, Tekwani SH, Kushida CA. Sites of obstruction in obstructive sleep apnea. *Chest.* 2002;122:1139–1147.

43. Ramar K, Dort LC, Katz SG, et al. Clinical practice guideline for the treatment of obstructive sleep apnea and snoring with oral appliance therapy: an update for 2015. *J Clin Sleep Med.* 2015;11:773–827.

44. Ravesloot MJ, van Maanen JP, Dun L, et al. The undervalued potential of positional therapy in position-dependent snoring and obstructive sleep apnea—a review of the literature. *Sleep Breath.* 2013;17:39–49.

45. Resta O, Foschino-Barbaro MP, Legari G, et al. Sleep-related breathing disorders, loud snoring and excessive daytime sleepiness in obese subjects. *Int J Obes Relat Metab Disord.* 2001;25:669–675.

46. Ryan CF, Love LL, Peat D, et al. Mandibular advancement oral appliance therapy for obstructive sleep apnoea: effect on awake calibre of the velopharynx. *Thorax.* 1999;54:972–977.

47. Schwab RJ, Pasirstein M, Pierson R, et al. Identification of upper airway anatomic risk factors for obstructive sleep apnea with volumetric magnetic resonance imaging. *Am J Respir Crit Care Med.* 2003;168:522–530.

48. Series F. Upper airway muscles awake and asleep. *Sleep Med Rev.* 2002;6:229–242.

49. Silber MH, Ancoli-Israel S, Bonnet MH, et al. The visual scoring of sleep in adults. *J Clin Sleep Med.* 2007;3:121–131.

50. Singh GD, Keropian B, Pillar G. Effects of the full breath solution appliance for the treatment of obstructive sleep apnea: a preliminary study. *Cranio.* 2009;27:109–117.

51. Sutherland K, Vanderveken OM, Tsuda H, et al. Oral appliance treatment for obstructive sleep apnea: an update. *J Clin Sleep Med.* 2014;10:215–227.

52. Centers for Disease Control and Prevention (CDC). Unhealthy sleep-related behaviors—12 states, 2009. *MMWR Morb Mortal Wkly Rep.* 2011;60:233–238.

53. Yaggi HK, Concato J, Kernan WN, et al. Obstructive sleep apnea as a risk factor for stroke and death. *N Engl J Med.* 2005;353:2034–2041.

54. Young T, Finn L, Peppard PE, et al. Sleep disordered breathing and mortality: eighteen-year follow-up of the Wisconsin sleep cohort. *Sleep.* 2008;31:1071–1078.

55. Young T, Palta M, Dempsey J, et al. The occurrence of sleep-disordered breathing among middle-aged adults. *N Engl J Med.* 1993;328:1230–1235.

56. Young T, Peppard PE, Gottlieb DJ. Epidemiology of obstructive sleep apnea: a population health perspective. *Am J Respir Crit Care Med.* 2002;165:1217–1239.

57. Youngstedt SD, Goff EE, Reynolds AM, et al. Has adult sleep duration declined over the last 50+ years? *Sleep Med Rev.* 2016;28:69–85.

10

Liver Disease

Hepatitis, defined as inflammation of the liver, may result from infectious or other causes. The most common cause of infectious hepatitis is viral hepatitis; other causes include infectious mononucleosis, secondary syphilis, and tuberculosis. Noninfectious hepatitis can result from excessive or prolonged use of toxic substances, including drugs (i.e., acetaminophen, halothane, ketoconazole, methyldopa, and methotrexate) or, more commonly, alcohol. Because the several types of hepatitis have various degrees of impact on dental treatment, each is discussed separately in subsequent sections.

Viral hepatitis is a collective term describing liver inflammation or hepatitis caused by a group of at least five different viruses. Three of these viruses, hepatitis A virus (HAV), hepatitis B virus (HBV), and hepatitis C virus (HCV), cause most cases of viral hepatitis in the United States.

Unlike HAV hepatitis, infections by HBV and HCV are blood-borne and often persist for years, resulting in ongoing (chronic) but usually asymptomatic liver inflammation and, in some cases, scarring (cirrhosis) that leads to liver failure, liver cancer, or both. Chronic hepatitis is a major cause of liver cancer and chronic liver disease globally and in the United States.

EPIDEMIOLOGY

Acute viral hepatitis is a common disease that affects 0.5%–1.0% of persons in the United States with approximately 80,000 new cases each year. Approximately 15,000 people in the United States die each year of cirrhosis caused by viral hepatitis. The annual incidence of acute hepatitis has been decreasing steadily since 1990, largely because of the administration of hepatitis A and B vaccines and decrease in high-risk behaviors. Worldwide, almost 600 million persons are living with chronic viral hepatitis, nearly 400 million infected with HBV and approximately 200 million infected with HCV.

In the United States, chronic viral hepatitis occurs in approximately 4.5 million Americans. The vast majority (~75%) are not aware they are infected. In the absence of appropriate treatment, liver cirrhosis will develop in 15%–40% of infected persons. Chronic hepatitis causes considerable morbidity. Globally, an estimated 80% of primary liver cancer and 60% of liver cirrhosis are caused by chronic viral hepatitis, and about one million deaths from viral hepatitis occur each year. Liver cancer is the fourth leading cause of death from cancer worldwide and the third leading cause among men.

ETIOLOGY

The clinical manifestations of the five types of viral hepatitis are quite similar, and the diseases can be distinguished from each other only by serologic assays. The five known causes of acute hepatitis are hepatitis virus types A (HAV), B (HBV), C (HCV), D or delta (HDV), and E

TABLE 10.1 Most Common Agents of Acute Viral Hepatitis, With Associated Characteristics

Hepatitis Virus	Size (nm)	Genome	Spread[a]	Incubation Period (Days)	Fatality Rate (%)	Chronicity Rate (%)	Antibody	Diagnosis[b,c]
A (HAV)	27	RNA	Fecal–oral	15–45; mean, 25	1	None	Anti-HAV	Anti-HAV IgG
B (HBV)	45	DNA	Parenteral	30–180; mean, 75	1	2–7	Anti-HBs	HBsAg (infectious)
								Anti-HBsAg (recovery)
								Anti-HBc (acute, persistently infected nonprotective)
								HBeAg (infectious)
								Anti-HBeAg (clearing/ cleared infection)
			Sexual				Anti-HBc	
							Anti-HBe	
C (HCV)	60	RNA	Parenteral	15–150; mean, 50	<0.1	50–85	Anti-HCV	Anti-HCV (previous infection)
								HCV RNA (infectivity)
D (delta) (HDV)	40	RNA	Parenteral	30–150	2–10	2–7	Anti-HDV	Anti-HDV
								HD-Ag
			Sexual			50		
E (HEV)	32	RNA	Fecal–oral	30–60	1	None	Anti-HEV	Anti-HEV

HBc, Hepatitis B core; *HBeAg*, hepatitis B e antigen; *HBsAg*, hepatitis B surface antigen; *HCC*, hepatocellular carcinoma; *IgG*, immunoglobulin G.

The US Food and Drug Administration requires that all donated whole blood, transfusable components, and plasma for human blood use in the United States be subjected to serologic testing for syphilis, HBsAg, anti-HBc, anti-HCV, and anti-HIV. The current incidence of posttransfusion hepatitis B is approximately 0.002% per transfusion recipient.

A small number of cases of transmission of HAV through clotting factor concentrates also have been reported.

(HEV) (see Table 10.1). Hepatitis A and hepatitis E are spread largely by the *fecal–oral* route, often occurring in outbreaks associated with poor sanitary conditions, and, while highly contagious, cause self-limited infection. Hepatitis B, hepatitis C, and hepatitis D are spread largely by *parenteral* routes and less commonly by intimate or sexual exposure, and are capable of contributing to chronic infection and, ultimately, to cirrhosis and hepatocellular carcinoma.

PATHOPHYSIOLOGY AND COMPLICATIONS

The pathogenesis of the liver injury in viral hepatitis is not well understood. None of the five primary agents seems to be directly cytopathic, at least at levels of replication found during typical acute and chronic hepatitis. The timing and histologic appearance of hepatocyte injury in viral hepatitis suggest that immune responses, particularly cytotoxic T-cell responses, may be the major effectors of injury. Proinflammatory cytokines, natural killer cell activity, and antibody-dependent cellular cytotoxicity also may play modulating roles in cell injury and inflammation during acute hepatitis virus infection. Recovery from hepatitis virus infection usually is accompanied by the appearance of rising titers of antibody against viral envelope antigens, such as anti-HAV, anti-HBs, anti-HCV-E1 and anti-HCV-E2, and anti-HEV; these antibodies may provide at least partial immunity to reinfection.

CLINICAL PRESENTATION

The course of acute hepatitis is highly variable and ranges in severity from a transient, asymptomatic infection to severe or fulminant disease. The *acute infection* may be self-limited with complete resolution, run a relapsing course, or lead to chronic infection. In a typical course, the *incubation period* typically ranges from 2 to 4 weeks

Chronic Carrier State	Complications[d] of the Liver	Associated Clinical Syndromes	IMMUNIZATION	
			Passive	Active
No	Rare		Immune globulin (0.02 mg/kg)	Harivax, vaqta, Twinrix
Yes—90% risk of becoming carrier if infected as neonate; 25%—50% risk if infected as infant; 5%—10% risk if infected as adult	Yes—increased risk of cirrhosis and HCC after 25—30 years of infection	Yes	Hepatitis B immune globulin (HBIg) (0.06 mg/kg)	Recombivax, Engerix,[e] Twinrix
Yes—risk of becoming carrier is 80%—90%	Yes—10-fold increased risk of liver cirrhosis within 20 years; 1%—5% of carriers develop HCC by 20 years, risk of HCC with chronic HCV infection exceeds risk with chronic HBV infection	Yes	Not available	None (difficult development because of the many genotypes)
Yes—carrier state in 20%—70%	Yes		Not available	Yes—protected with Recombivax, engerix[e], and Twinrix
No	Rare morbidity and mortality except in pregnant women		Not available	Genentech has applied for vaccine patent

[a]With parenteral and sexual modes of transmission: Risk groups include intravenous drug users, health care workers, hemodialysis patients, persons of low socioeconomic status, sexual and household contacts of infected persons, persons with multiple sex partners, and patients with a history of transfusion before 1991.

[b]Diagnostic markers of viral hepatitis include elevation of aspartate aminotransferase, alanine aminotransferase, γ-glutamyl transferase, and white blood cell count and prolongation of prothrombin time.

[c]*Preicteric phase:* anorexia, nausea, vomiting, fatigue, myalgia, malaise, fever. *Icterus:* jaundice, discolored stool, dark urine, hepatosplenomegaly, bleeding disorder. *Serum sickness–like features:* arthralgia, rash, angioedema (seen in 5%—10% of patients).

[d]Risk for complications and severe liver disease increases with coinfection with HBV and HCV and with chronic alcohol consumption.

[e]Immunization is recommended for dental personnel.

Data from Centers for Disease Control and Prevention. Hepatitis A among persons with hemophilia who received clotting factor concentrate—United States, September–December 1995. *MMWR Morb Mortal Wkly Rep* 1996;45:29–32.

with HAV and HEV but up to 20 weeks with HBV and HCV (see Table 10.1). Early acute infection is characterized by detectable virus in the blood, normal serum aminotransferase and bilirubin levels, and antibodies not yet detected.

The *preicteric phase* of illness is marked by the onset of nonspecific symptoms such as fatigue, nausea, loss of appetite, and vague right upper quadrant pain. Virus-specific antibody first appears during this phase. The preicteric phase typically lasts 3—10 days but may be of longer duration and even constitute the entire course of illness in patients with subclinical or anicteric forms of acute hepatitis. Viral titers generally are highest at this point, and serum aminotransferase levels start to increase.

The onset of production of dark urine marks the *icteric phase* of illness, during which jaundice appears and symptoms of fatigue and nausea worsen. Typically, acute

viral hepatitis rarely is diagnosed correctly before the onset of jaundice. If jaundice is severe, stool color lightens, often in association with pruritus. Other manifestations may include anorexia, dysgeusia, and weight loss. Physical examination usually shows jaundice and hepatic tenderness. In more severe cases, hepatomegaly and splenomegaly are present. Serum bilirubin levels (total and direct) rise, and aminotransferase levels generally are higher than 10 times the upper limit of normal, at least at onset. During the symptomatic icteric phase, levels of hepatitis virus begin to decrease in serum and liver.

The duration of clinical illness is variable, typically lasting 1—3 weeks. Recovery is first manifested by return of appetite and is accompanied by resolution of serum bilirubin and aminotransferase elevations and clearance of virus. *Convalescence* can be prolonged, requiring weeks before full energy and stamina return to the patient.

Neutralizing antibodies usually appear during the icteric phase and rise to high levels during convalescence.

Complications of acute viral hepatitis include chronic infection, fulminant hepatic failure, relapsing or cholestatic hepatitis, and extrahepatic syndromes. *Chronic hepatitis*, generally defined as illness of at least 6 months' duration, develops in approximately 2%–7% of adults with hepatitis B and in 50%–85% of adults with hepatitis C. Hepatitis B, C, and D infections are said to be chronic if viremia persists for more than 6 months, but chronicity can be suspected if viremia persists for 3 months after the onset of symptoms.

Acute liver failure or fulminant hepatitis occurs in 1%–2% of patients with symptomatic acute hepatitis. The disease is called *fulminant* when evidence of hepatic encephalopathy appears; however, the initial symptoms (changes in personality, aggressive behavior, or abnormal sleep patterns) may be subtle or misunderstood. The most reliable prognostic factor in acute hepatic failure is the degree of prolongation of the prothrombin time; other prognosticators include worsening jaundice, ascites, and decreased liver size. Serum aminotransferase levels and viral titers have little prognostic value and often decrease with worsening hepatic failure. Some patients develop a cholestatic pattern of illness consisting of prolonged and fluctuating jaundice and pruritus. Patients may experience one or more clinical relapses and may feel relatively well despite marked jaundice.

LABORATORY AND DIAGNOSTIC FINDINGS

While high levels of virus are detectable in the stool during the early course of the disease, serologic test findings are used to make the diagnosis of acute viral hepatitis (see Table 10.2). Liver biopsy is infrequently recommended unless the diagnosis remains unclear and a therapeutic decision is needed. If biopsy is required, viral antigens can be detected in infected hepatocytes, and the histologic pattern is characterized by widespread parenchymal inflammation and spotty necrosis. Inflammatory cells are predominantly lymphocytes, macrophages, and histiocytes. Fibrosis is absent. There are no reliably distinctive anatomic features in the liver that separate the five viral forms of acute hepatitis from each other.

HEPATITIS A

Hepatitis A virus is a small RNA virus that belongs to the family Picornaviridae (genus *Hepatovirus*). The viral genome is 7.5 kilobases (kb) in length and has a single large open reading frame that encodes a polyprotein with structural and nonstructural components. This virus is highly contagious and is spread largely by the fecal–oral route, especially when sanitary conditions are poor.

Epidemiology

Hepatitis A has been decreasing in frequency in the United States with about 6000 cases per year. It is an

TABLE 10.2	Serologic Diagnosis of Acute Hepatitis	
Diagnosis	Screening Assays	Supplemental Assays
Hepatitis A	IgM anti-HAV	None needed
Hepatitis B	HBsAg, IgM anti-HBc	HBeAg, anti-HBe, HBV DNA
Hepatitis C	Anti-HCV by EIA	HCV RNA by PCR assay; anti-HCV by immunoblot analysis
Hepatitis D	HBsAg	Anti-HDV
Hepatitis E	History	Anti-HEV, HEV RNA
Mononucleosis	History, WBC differential counts	Heterophile antibody
Drug-induced hepatitis	History	

EIA, Enzyme immunoassay; *HAV*, hepatitis A virus; *HBc*, hepatitis B core; *HBeAg*, hepatitis B e antigen; *HBsAg*, hepatitis B surface antigen; *HBV*, hepatitis B virus; *HCV*, hepatitis C virus; *HDV*, hepatitis D virus; *HEV*, hepatitis E virus; *IgM*, immunoglobulin M; *PCR*, polymerase chain reaction; *WBC*, white blood cell.

important cause of acute liver disease worldwide with more than 300,000 cases per year.

Pathophysiology and Complications

Hepatitis A virus replicates largely in the liver and is assembled in the hepatocyte cytoplasm as a 27-nm particle with a single RNA genome and an outer capsid protein (HAVAg). The virus is secreted into bile and, to a lesser extent, serum. The highest titers of HAV are found in stool (10^6 to 10^{10} genomes per gram) during the incubation period and early symptomatic phase of illness.

Clinical Presentation

The clinical course of typical acute hepatitis A (Fig. 10.1) begins with an incubation period that usually is

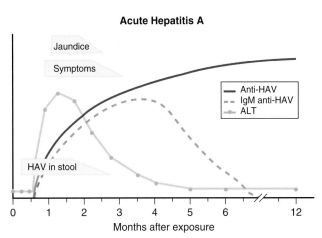

FIG 10.1 Serologic course of acute hepatitis A. *ALT*, Alanine aminotransferase; *HAV*, hepatitis A virus. (From Goldman L, Ausiello D, eds. *CECIL Textbook of Medicine.* 23rd ed. Philadelphia: Saunders; 2008.)

15–45 days in duration (mean, 25 days). The course is usually self-limiting and generally includes symptoms of nausea, vomiting, anorexia, fever, malaise, and abdominal pain. Jaundice occurs in 70% of adults infected with HAV but in smaller proportions of children. Hepatitis A is invariably a self-limiting infection, although severe and fulminant cases of hepatitis A can occur, particularly in older adults and in patients with preexisting chronic liver disease. Hepatitis A is the most common cause of relapsing cholestatic hepatitis.

Laboratory and Diagnostic Findings

The diagnosis of acute hepatitis A is made by detection of IgM anti-HAV in the serum of a patient with the clinical and biochemical features (i.e., elevated serum aminotransferase levels) of acute hepatitis. IgM-specific anti-HAV persists for 4–12 months. Serum IgG antibodies to HAV (anti-HAV [IgG antibody]) appear after IgM, early in the convalescent phase, and remain detectable for decades. Testing for total anti-HAV is not helpful in diagnosis but is used to assess immunity to hepatitis A.

Medical Management

Hepatitis A infection is usually self-limiting, and treatment consists of supportive care, including bed rest and good nutrition. Measures to prevent spread to contacts are to be implemented, and include good hygiene practices and administration of the vaccine or immune globulin.

A safe and effective HAV vaccine is available and recommended for all children 1 year of age and older and for persons at increased risk for acquiring hepatitis A, including travelers to endemic areas of the world (i.e., parts of Africa and Asia), men who have sex with men, injection drug users, and individuals experiencing homelessness. HAV vaccine also is recommended for all patients with chronic liver disease and recipients of pooled plasma products, such as patients with hemophilia. Two formulations of HAV vaccine are available in the United States; both consist of inactivated hepatitis A antigen purified from cell culture. Havrix (GlaxoSmithKline, Philadelphia, PA) is recommended to be given as two injections 6–12 months apart in an adult dose of 1440 enzyme-linked immunosorbent assay (ELISA) units (1.0 mL) and in a pediatric (2–18 years of age) dose of 720 ELISA units (0.5 mL). Vaqta (Merck, West Point, PA) is recommended to be given as two injections 6–18 months apart in an adult dose of 50 U (1.0 mL) and in a pediatric dose (1–18 years) of 25 U (0.5 mL). A combination HAV–HBV vaccine (Twinrix) (GlaxoSmithKline) also is available; this preparation is recommended for adults who require vaccination against hepatitis A and hepatitis B and is given in a three-injection schedule at 0, 1, and 6 months after exposure. HAV vaccines have an excellent safety record, with serious complications occurring in fewer than 0.1% of recipients. Seroconversion rates after HAV vaccine are greater than 95% but are lower among patients with chronic liver disease, human immunodeficiency virus (HIV) infection, and other conditions of immunocompromise.

HEPATITIS B

Hepatitis B virus is a double-shelled, enveloped DNA virus belonging to the family Hepadnaviridae (genus *Orthohepadnavirus*). The viral genome consists of partially double-stranded DNA, is 3.2 kb in length, and possesses four partially overlapping open reading frames that encode the genes for HBsAg (S gene), HBcAg (C gene), HBV polymerase (P gene), and a small protein, HBxAg, that seems to have transactivating functions (X gene). This virus can be transmitted easily and is spread predominantly by the parenteral route or by intimate personal contact.

Epidemiology

Approximately 350 million people are infected with HBV worldwide. In the United States, hepatitis B is the most common cause of acute hepatitis with approximately 4000 new cases of HBV per year accounting for approximately 1700 deaths (and ≈1.3 million cases of chronic HBV infection). The incidence of HBV has remained stable in the United States for the past decade (Fig. 10.2). Investigations of the source of infection reveal that most adult cases are caused by sexual or parenteral contact. Maternal–infant spread of hepatitis B is another important mode of transmission not only in endemic areas of the world but also in the United States among immigrants from these endemic areas.

Pathophysiology and Complications

Hepatitis B virus replicates predominantly in hepatocytes. The clinical course of hepatitis B with serologic markers is depicted in Fig. 10.3. During both acute and chronic infection, large amounts of HBsAg are detectable in serum. Chronic hepatitis B virus infection develops in approximately 5%–10% of adults with hepatitis B and a small percentage of these patients develop cases of fulminant hepatitis or liver cancer.

Clinical Presentation

The typical course of acute, self-limited hepatitis B begins with an incubation period of 30–150 days (mean, 75 days). During the incubation period, HBsAg, HBeAg, and HBV DNA (see Fig. 10.3) become detectable in serum and rise to high titers, with the virus reaching titers of 10^8 to 10^{11} virions/mL. By onset of symptoms, anti-HBc rises and serum aminotransferase levels are elevated. Jaundice appears in one-third of adults with hepatitis B and in a lesser proportion of children. Generally, HBV DNA and HBeAg begin to fall at the onset of illness and may be undetectable at the time of peak clinical illness. During recovery, HBsAg becomes

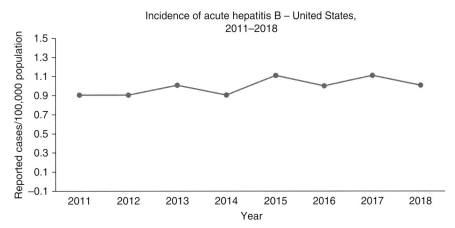

FIG 10.2 Stable incidence of Hepatitis B in the United States (From Centers for Disease Control and Prevention. Surveillance for acute viral hepatitis—United States; 2018. https://www.cdc.gov/hepatitis/statistics/2017surveillance/index.htm. Accessed February 08, 2021.)

undetectable, and anti-HBs appears, which is several weeks to months after loss of HBsAg. Anti-HBs is a long-lasting antibody that indicates immunity.

The risk of chronic hepatitis B infection is high if infected as an infant or child (~90%) but develops in about 2%–7% of adults infected with HBV. Also, chronic HBV infection occurs more commonly in men and in immunosuppressed persons. Chronic hepatitis B infection is the third or fourth most common cause of cirrhosis in the United States (depending on the year data are collected) and is an important cause of liver cancer.

Laboratory and Diagnostic Findings

The diagnosis of acute hepatitis B can be made on the basis of detecting HBsAg in the serum of a patient with the clinical and biochemical features of acute hepatitis. HBsAg also may be present as a result of chronic hepatitis

B or the carrier state. Testing for IgM anti-HBc (IgG antibody) is therefore helpful because this antibody arises early and is lost within 6–12 months of the onset of illness. Testing for HBeAg, anti-HBe, HBV DNA, and anti-HBs generally is not helpful in the diagnosis of hepatitis B but may be valuable in assessing prognosis. Persons who remain HBV DNA or HBeAg positive (or both) at 6 weeks after the onset of symptoms are likely to be developing chronic hepatitis B. Loss of HBeAg or HBV DNA is a favorable serologic finding, and loss of HBsAg plus the development of anti-HBs denotes recovery.

Medical Management

The use of therapy with direct antiviral agents for acute hepatitis B is effective. Regimens of interferon alfa and lamivudine are established therapies for chronic hepatitis B as are other antiviral agents (Tables 10.3A and B). Typically, acute hepatitis B is treated with lamivudine (100 mg/day until the disease has resolved and results of HBsAg testing have become negative) for patients with signs or symptoms of fulminant liver disease (rising prothrombin time, severe jaundice), particularly if high levels of HBV DNA are present. Management of patients with acute hepatitis B also should focus on avoidance of further hepatic injury and prophylaxis of contacts. Patients should be monitored by repeat testing for HBsAg and alanine aminotransferase levels 3–6 months later to determine whether chronic hepatitis B has developed.

Vaccination against HBV is recommended for all newborns, children, and adolescents, as well as adults at risk for acquiring HBV, including those listed in Box 10.1. Two formulations of HBV vaccine are available in the United States; both are made by recombinant techniques using cloned HBV *S* gene expressed in *Saccharomyces cerevisiae*. For adults, the recommended regimen is three injections of 1.0 mL (20 μg of Energix-B [GlaxoSmithKline] or 10 μg of Recombivax HB [Merck]) given intramuscularly in the deltoid muscle at 0, 1, and 6 months. Prevaccination screening for anti-HBs is not

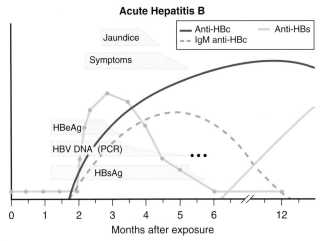

FIG 10.3 Serologic course of acute hepatitis B. *HBc*, Hepatitis B core; *HBeAg*, hepatitis B e antigen; *HBs*, hepatitis B surface; *HBsAg*, hepatitis B surface antigen; *HBV*, hepatitis B virus; *PCR*, polymerase chain reaction. (From Goldman L, Ausiello D, eds. *CECIL Textbook of Medicine.* 23rd ed. Philadelphia: Saunders; 2008.)

TABLE 10.3A Recommended Therapeutic Regimens for HCV

Regimen	Genotype	Pills Per Day	Duration (week)	Comments
Genotype-Specific Treatment Regimens				
Elbasvir/grazoprevir (Zepatier)	la, lb, 4	1	12–16	Resistance testing recommended before use in genotype la
Ledipasvir/sofosbuvir (Harvoni)	la, lb, 4, 5, 6	1	8–24	
Paritaprevir/ritonavir/ombitasvir + dasabuvir (Holkira Pak)	1, lb	4	8–24	Ribavirin must be added for genotype la
Paritaprevir/ritonavir/ombitasvir (Technivie)	4	2	12	Ribavirin must be added
Sofosbuvir + daclatasvir (Sovaldi + Daklinza)	la, lb, 3	2	12–24	
Pan-Genotypic Regimens				
Glecaprevir/pibrentasvir (Maviret)	1–6	3	8–16	
Sofosbuvir/velpatasvir (epclusa)	1–6	1	12	
Sofosbuvir/velpatasvir/voxilaprevir (vosevi)	1–6	1	12	Approved only for direct-acting antiviral agent failures

Data from Dhawan VK et al. Hepatitis C Treatment & Management; Updated Oct 07, 2019. Medscape http://emedicine.medscape.com/article/177792-treatment#d13.

TABLE 10.3B Recommended Regimens and Durations (Weeks) for Patients With Compensated Cirrhosis Who Have Never Been Treated, According to HCV Genotype[a]

Regimen	HCV GENOTYPE la	lb	2	3	4	5	6
Ledipasvir/sofosbuvir (Harvoni)	12 week ± ribavirin[b]	12 week	NR	+ Ribavirin 12 week	12 week	12 week	12 week
Elbasvir/grazoprevir (Zepatier)	12–16 week ± ribavirin[b]	12 week	NR	+ Sofosbuvir × 12 week	12 week	NR	NR
Paritaprevir/ritonavir/ombitasvir + dasabuvir (Holkira Pak)	+ RBV 12 week	12 week	NR	NR	Paritaprevir/ritonavir/ ombitasvir + ribavirin 12 week	NR	NR
Sofosbuvir + daclatasvir (Sovaldi + Daklinza)	24 week	24 week	24 week	24 week ± Ribavirin	NR	NR	NR
Sofosbuvir/velpatasvir (epclusa)	12 week	12 week	12 week	12 week ± ribavirin[c]	12 week	12 week	12 week
Glecaprevir/pibrentasvir (Maviret)	12 week	12 week	12 week	12 week	12 week	12 week	12 week
Sofosbuvir/velpatasvir/voxilaprevir (vosevi)	NR	NR	NR	NR	NR	NR	NR

[a]Where indicated, to be dosed according to weight: < 75 kg: 1000 mg daily; > 75 kg: 1200 mg daily See Appendix A for reference supporting recommendations.

[b]Resistance testing suggested for people with genotype la infection with compensated cirrhosis before treatment with ledipasvir/sofosbuvir or elbasvir/grazoprevir. If resistance to nonstructural 5A (NS5 A) inhibitors is present, treatment should be extended to 16 weeks with the addition of weight-based ribavirin.

[c]Resistance testing suggested for people with genotype 3 infection with compensated cirrhosis before treatment with sofosbuvir/velpatasvir. If resistance to NS5 A inhibitors is present, addition of weight-based ribavirin may be considered

Open in a separate window.

Note: HCV, hepatitis C virus; NR, not recommended; RBV, ribavirin.

Data from Dhawan VK et al. Hepatitis C Treatment & Management; Updated Oct 07, 2019. Medscape http://emedicine.medscape.com/article/177792-treatment#d13.

recommended except for adults in high-risk groups (e.g., persons born in endemic countries, injection drug users, men who have sex with men, and HIV-infected persons). Postvaccination testing for anti-HBs to document seroconversion is not recommended routinely except in persons whose subsequent clinical management depends on knowledge of their immune status, particularly health care and public safety workers. At present, booster doses are not recommended, but they may be appropriate for persons at high risk if titers of anti-HBs fall below what is considered protective (10 IU/mL).

Hepatitis B immune globulin (HBIg) provides immediate, short-term protection against hepatitis B infection. It contains large amounts of hepatitis B antibodies taken from donated human blood. Postexposure prophylaxis with HBIG is recommended for persons with percutaneous exposure to a patient with hepatitis B, and at birth for infants born to infected mothers. A single dose of HBIG (0.5 mL in newborns of infected mothers and 0.06 mL/kg in other settings and in adults) should be given as soon as possible after exposure, and HBV vaccination should be started immediately.

HEPATITIS C

Hepatitis C virus is an RNA virus that belongs to the family Flaviviridae (genus *Hepacivirus*). It circulates as a double-shelled enveloped virus, 50–60 nm in diameter. The genome is a positive-stranded RNA molecule approximately 9.6 kb in length. HCV contains a single large open reading frame encoding a large polyprotein that is posttranslationally modified into three structural and several nonstructural polypeptides. The structural proteins include two highly variable envelope antigens, E1 and E2, and the relatively conserved nucleocapsid protein C.

HCV can be transmitted easily and is spread predominantly by the parenteral route. The virus can cause a serious liver infection, permanent liver complications, and liver cancer. There is presently no vaccine for hepatitis C. For all these reasons, hepatitis C is a significant infectious condition of concern to dental health care professionals.

Epidemiology

Although only 3600 cases of hepatitis C were reported to the CDC, it is estimated that approximately 40,000 persons per year in the United States were infected in 2019 representing an incidence of 0.8 per 100,000 people. Approximately 85% of people infected with hepatitis C virus develop chronic hepatitis C in the United States resulting in over three million people in the United States having chronic HCV infection.

At highest risk for contracting this disease are persons with multiple parenteral exposures. Sexual transmission of hepatitis C is uncommon (<1% per year of exposure). Maternal–infant spread occurs in approximately 5% of cases, usually in infants whose mothers have high levels of HCV RNA in serum and have experienced a protracted delivery or early rupture of membranes. Other potential sources of HCV are needlestick accidents and either contamination or inadequate sterilization of reusable needles and syringes (more than 60% of cases are attributable to injection drug use while approximately 15%–20% to sexual exposure).

Pathophysiology and Complications

HCV replicates largely in the liver and is detectable in serum in titers of 10^5 to 10^7 virions/mL during acute and chronic infection. Chronic HCV infection typically follows a progressive course extending over many years and can ultimately result in chronic liver disease, liver failure, hepatocellular carcinoma, and the need for liver transplantation. Hepatitis C also increases the risk of chronic kidney disease (CKD, see Chapter 12). The major complication of acute hepatitis C is the development of chronic hepatitis, which occurs in up to 85% of cases. Complications include the development of immune complex phenomena and cryoglobulinemia, though these complications are more typical of chronic disease. Fulminant hepatitis resulting from HCV is rare.

Clinical Presentation

The clinical course of acute hepatitis C (Fig. 10.4) begins with an incubation period that ranges from 15 to 120 days (mean, 50 days). During the incubation period, often within 1–2 weeks of exposure, HCV RNA can be detected by sensitive assays such as those based on reverse transcriptase–polymerase chain reaction (PCR). HCV RNA persists until well into the clinical course of disease. Antibody to HCV (anti-HCV) arises late in the course of acute hepatitis C and may not be present at the time of onset of symptoms and serum aminotransferase

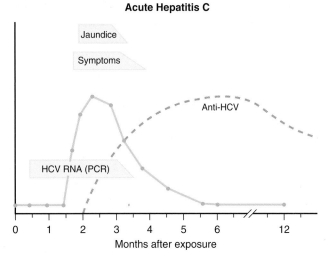

FIG 10.4 Serologic course of acute hepatitis C. *HCV,* Hepatitis C virus; *PCR,* polymerase chain reaction. (From Goldman L, Ausiello D, eds. *CECIL Textbook of Medicine.* 23rd ed. Philadelphia: Saunders; 2008.)

elevations. If the hepatitis is self-limited, HCV RNA soon becomes undetectable in serum; in this situation, titers of anti-HCV generally are modest and eventually may fall to undetectable levels.

Laboratory and Diagnostic Findings

The diagnosis of acute hepatitis C generally is based on detection of anti-HCV in serum in a patient with the clinical and biochemical features of acute hepatitis. The diagnostic criteria for hepatitis C is detailed in Table 10.4, and the clinical course and serologic markers are depicted in Fig. 10.4. In some patients detectable

TABLE 10.4	Laboratory Criteria for the Diagnosis of Hepatitis C

One or More of the Following Three Criteria:
- Antibodies to HCV (anti-HCV) screening test positive with a signal-to-cutoff ratio predictive of a true positive as determined for the particular assay as defined by the CDC (signal to cut-off ratios: http://www.cdc.gov/hepatitis/HCV/LabTesting.htm)[a] *or*
- HCV RIBA positive *or*
- NAT for HCV RNA positive (including qualitative, quantitative, or genotype testing)

And, If Done, Meets the Following Two Criteria:
- Absence of IgM antibody to HAV (if done) (IgM anti-HAV) *and*
- Absence of IgM anti-HBc (if done)

[a]A documented negative HCV antibody laboratory test result followed within 6 months by a positive test result (as described in the laboratory criteria for diagnosis) does not require an acute clinical presentation to meet the surveillance case definition.
CDC, Centers for Disease Control and Prevention; *HAV,* hepatitis A virus; *HCV,* hepatitis C virus; *NAT,* nucleic acid test; *RIBA,* recombinant immunoblot assay.
Laboratory Criteria for the Diagnosis of HCV; 2015. http://www.cdc.gov/hepatitis/HCV/Labtesting.htm.

levels of anti-HCV do not develop until weeks or months after the onset of illness. In these cases, retesting for anti-HCV during convalescence or direct tests for HCV RNA are necessary to determine the diagnosis of acute hepatitis C.

Chronic infection is marked by detectable levels of HCV RNA and elevated aminotransferase levels, often in a fluctuating pattern. In some instances, aminotransferase levels become normal despite persistence of viremia.

Coinfection with HCV may occur with HBV. There are four serologic profiles seen in coinfection with both HBC and HCV: codominant, HCV dominant, HBV dominant, and neither replicative. These subtypes influence the clinical course, complications of infection, and treatment decisions (Table 10.5).

Medical Management

At present, there are no means of prevention of hepatitis C other than avoidance of high-risk behaviors and appropriate use of standard precautions. There is no vaccine. Injection drug use is currently the most common cause of newly acquired cases of hepatitis C.

Accidental needlestick exposure is perhaps the most frequent issue in transmission. At present, neither immune globulin nor preemptive therapy with antiviral agents or interferon is recommended in this situation. Monitoring by means of determination of aminotransferase levels and HCV RNA and anti-HCV testing (at baseline and again at 1 and 6 months after exposure) is appropriate. This approach allows for early intervention and treatment (Table 10.4).

A new infection with HCV does not always require treatment, as the immune response in some people will clear the infection. However, when HCV infection becomes chronic, treatment is necessary. The goal of hepatitis C treatment is cure. WHO's updated 2018 guidelines recommend therapy with pan-genotypic direct-acting antivirals (DAAs). DAAs can cure most persons with HCV infection, and treatment duration is short (usually 12–24 weeks), depending on the absence or presence of cirrhosis. WHO recommends treating all persons with chronic HCV infection over the age of 12 with pan-genotypic DAAs (see Tables 10.3A and B). Several combinations of antiviral agents (i.e., sofosbuvir and velpatasvir or ledipasvir; grazoprevir plus elbasvir) have demonstrated good viral control (Tables 10.3A and B). However, pan-genotypic DAAs remain expensive in many high- and upper-middle-income countries. Treatment with peginterferon alfa and ribavirin has been shown to be beneficial in chronic hepatitis C (Tables 10.3A and B). Approximately 90% of patients with acute hepatitis C treated with peginterferon with or without ribavirin for 24 weeks experience resolution of disease and sustained loss of HCV RNA. Boceprevir added to standard therapy with peginterferon–ribavirin has shown significant response to therapy in previously

TABLE 10.5 Serologic Patterns in Coinfection[a]

Codominant	HCV Dominant		HBV Dominant	Neither Replicative
	HCV/Occult HBV	HCV/Overt HBV		
+++ HCV RNA	+++ HCV RNA	+++ HCV RNA	+++ HCV RNA	+++ HCV RNA
++ HBV DNA	− HBV DNA	+ HBV DNA	+++ HBV DNA	− HBV DNA
+ Anti-HC V Ab	+ Anti-HC V Ab	+ Anti-HC V Ab	+ Anti-HC V Ab	+ Anti-HC V Ab
± HBsAg	− HBsAg	+ HBsAg	+ HBsAg	+ HBsAg
+ Anti-HBc	± Anti-HBc	+ Anti-HBc	+ Anti-HBc	+ Anti-HBc
+ Anti-HBs	± Anti-HBs	+ Anti-HBs	+ Anti-HBs	+ Anti-HBs

[a]There are four serologic profiles seen in coinfection with both HBC and HCV: codominant, HCV dominant, HBV dominant and neither replicative.

Abbreviations: *Ab*, antibody; *HBc*, hepatitis B core protein; *HBs*, hepatitis B surface protein; *HBsAg*, hepatitis B surface antigen; *HBV*, hepatitis B virus; *HCV*, hepatitis B virus.

Data from Dhawan VK et al. Hepatitis C Treatment & Management; Updated Oct 07, 2019. Medscape http://emedicine.medscape.com/article/177792-treatment#d13.

untreated adults with HCV infection. HCV genotyping is also helping guide therapy with the most effective agents.

HEPATITIS D

Hepatitis delta virus (HDV) is a unique RNA virus that requires HBV for replication. The viral genome is a short, 1.7-kb circular single-stranded molecule of RNA that has a single open reading frame and a highly conserved, nontranslated region that resembles the self-replicating element of viroids. HDV infects hepatocytes but requires HBV to do so. Hepatitis D tends to be more severe than hepatitis B alone and is more likely to lead to fulminant hepatitis and to cause severe chronic hepatitis and ultimately cirrhosis when a super- or coinfection.

Epidemiology

People at greatest risk are chronic carriers of hepatitis B and persons who have repeated parenteral exposures. In the United States, 50% of the chronically HBV-infected IDUs in 2010 in Baltimore, MD, had anti-HD and an 8% prevalence of anti-HD was found in 499 HBsAg carriers in northern California. In this study, HDV-positive patients had higher rates of cirrhosis than those with HBV monoinfection. Superinfection with HDV (i.e., when HDV occurs after the HBV infection) is more frequent than coinfection and is far more likely to lead to chronic delta hepatitis.

Pathophysiology and Complications

HDV is spread like HBV, that is, by parenteral exposure. Direct parenteral inoculation is the most efficient way of transmission in HBsAg-positive hosts. Infectivity titration studies in chimpanzees showed that the virus could be passaged to HBsAg-positive animals with HDV-positive serum diluted as much as 10^{-11}-fold. In contrast to HBV, vertical transmission from mother to offspring, homosexual promiscuity, or nosocomial exposure seem to be inconspicuous risk factors for the transmission of HDV.

HDV is pathogenic. Clinical studies from all continents have shown that HDV infection aggravates the natural history of the underlying HBV infection. Hepatitis D is considered the most severe form of viral hepatitis in humans, accelerating progression to cirrhosis and leading to early decompensation of liver function compared with HBV monoinfection. In Greece, Samoa, and the Far East, HDV is associated with benign clinical conditions or normal liver function, suggesting that disease expression may vary, possibly related to different HDV genotypes.

Clinical Presentation

Delta hepatitis occurs in two clinical patterns termed *coinfection* and *superinfection*. Delta coinfection is the simultaneous occurrence of acute HDV and acute HBV infections. Acute delta superinfection is the occurrence of acute HDV infection in a person with chronic hepatitis B or the HBsAg carrier state. Clinically and serologically, coinfection resembles acute hepatitis B but may manifest a second elevation in aminotransferase levels associated with the period of delta virus replication. Superinfection is the HDV infection of an individual chronically infected with HBV. This pattern of infection causes a severe acute hepatitis that may be self-limited but that in most cases (up to 80%) progresses to chronicity.

Laboratory and Diagnostic Findings

The diagnosis of acute delta coinfection is made in patients with clinical features of acute hepatitis when HBsAg, anti-HDV, and IgM anti-HBc are present in serum. Immunoassays for anti-HDV are commercially available and reliable, although the antibody may appear late during the illness. In patients suspected of having delta hepatitis, repeat testing for anti-HDV during convalescence is appropriate.

The diagnosis of superinfection is made in a patient with clinical features of acute hepatitis who has HBsAg and anti-HDV but no IgM anti-HBc in serum. Other tests that are helpful in making the diagnosis of ongoing HDV infection are determinations of serum HDV RNA (detectable by PCR assay) and HDV antigen (detectable by immunoblot analysis). Delta antigen is detectable in liver biopsy specimens with immunohistochemical staining.

Medical Management

Delta hepatitis can be prevented by preventing hepatitis B, through hepatitis B vaccination, which is especially important in areas of the world where delta hepatitis is endemic (regions of Africa and Asia). There are no means of prevention of delta hepatitis in a person who is already an HBsAg carrier; in this situation, avoidance of further exposure is important. There are no specific therapies available for acute delta hepatitis.

HEPATITIS E

Hepatitis E virus is a small nonenveloped RNA virus with a size of 27–34 nm. HEV is classified as a Hepevirus in the Hepeviridae family.

The hepatitis E virus is mainly transmitted through drinking water contaminated with fecal matter. Symptoms include jaundice, lack of appetite, and nausea. In rare cases, it may progress to acute liver failure. Hepatitis E usually resolves on its own within four to 6 weeks. Treatment focuses on supportive care, rehydration, and rest.

Epidemiology

Hepatitis E is responsible for epidemic and endemic forms of non-A, non-B hepatitis that occur in less developed areas of the world. While there are less than 20,000 cases per year in the United States, there are an estimated 20 million HEV infections worldwide every year, leading to an estimated 3.3 million symptomatic cases of hepatitis E. Hepatitis E is endemic in Africa, Asia, and Mexico.

Pathophysiology and Complications

Hepatitis E infection is transmitted in regions with limited access to essential water, sanitation, hygiene, and health services. In these areas, the disease occurs both as outbreaks and as sporadic cases. The outbreaks usually follow periods of fecal contamination of drinking water supplies. Several outbreaks have occurred in areas of conflict and humanitarian emergencies such as war zones and camps for refugees or internally displaced populations, where sanitation and safe water supply pose special challenges.

Pregnant women are at greater risk for experiencing severe illness, including fulminant hepatitis and death.

Clinical Presentation

The clinical course of hepatitis E resembles that of other forms of hepatitis (fever, fatigue, gastrointestinal symptoms). The incubation period is 15–60 days (mean,

35 days). The disease frequently is cholestatic, with prominence of bilirubin and alkaline phosphatase elevations.

Laboratory and Diagnostic Findings

The diagnosis of hepatitis E should be considered in a patient with acute hepatitis who has recently traveled to an endemic area, particularly if tests for other forms of hepatitis are negative. Detection of anti-HEV, particularly of the IgM subclass, or HEV RNA is sufficient to make the diagnosis.

Medical Management

There are no known means of prevention or treatment of hepatitis E. Travelers (particularly pregnant women) to areas of the world where hepatitis E is endemic should be cautioned regarding drinking water and uncooked food. Infected patients are advised to get rest, adequate nutrition, and avoid alcohol and hepatotoxic drugs.

The diagnostic approach to the patient with clinical features of acute hepatitis begins with a careful history for risk factors and possible exposure; for medication use, including herbal and over-the-counter drugs; and for alcohol use. The onset and progression of symptoms may give clues to the presence of other causes of liver or biliary tract disease, such as alcohol abuse or gallstones. Laboratory findings involving ALT, AST, ALT:AST ratio, and alkaline phosphatase levels are used to help differentiate HEV infection from obstructive jaundice or alcoholic liver disease (Table 10.2).

HEPATITIS NON–A-E

Cases of acute hepatitis that appear to be viral in etiology but cannot be attributed to any known virus are called *hepatitis non–A-E*. Based on serologic surveys of cases of acute hepatitis in Western countries, *hepatitis non–A-E* appears to occur in up to 20% of cases. Various candidate viruses have been reported in association with this disease, but none has been clearly linked to the clinical entity. The clinical features of non–A-E hepatitis are similar to those of recognized forms of acute hepatitis. In most cases of non–A-E hepatitis, no clear source of exposure can be identified. The absence of typical risk factors for viral hepatitis suggests that in some instances, non–A-E hepatitis may be due to nonviral causes, such as an autoimmune process, environmental exposure, or drugs.

Non–A-E hepatitis is a diagnosis of exclusion. There are no means of treatment or prevention of this infection. The syndrome of non–A-E hepatitis is associated with the complications of acute liver failure and aplastic anemia. It is a more common cause of fulminant hepatic failure than both hepatitis A and hepatitis B combined and often accounts for 30%–40% of cases. Chronic hepatitis develops in approximately one-third of patients with non–A-E hepatitis, and cirrhosis ultimately develops in a small percentage.

DENTAL MANAGEMENT

Treatment Considerations in Specific Patient Groups

The identification of potential or actual carriers of HBV, HCV, and HDV is problematic because in most instances, carriers cannot be identified by history. Therefore, all patients with a history of viral hepatitis must be managed as though they were potentially infectious (see Box 10.1).

The recommendations for infection control practice in dentistry published by the CDC and the American Dental Association have become the standard of care to prevent cross-infection in dental practice (see Appendix B). These organizations strongly recommend that all dental health care workers who provide patient care receive vaccination against HBV and implement standard precautions during the care of all dental patients. In addition, Occupational Safety and Health Administration (OSHA) standards require employers to offer hepatitis B vaccine for free to employees occupationally exposed to blood or other potentially infectious materials.

Patients With Active Hepatitis. No dental treatment other than urgent care should be rendered for a patient with active hepatitis unless the patient has attained clinical and biochemical recovery (Box 10.2). Urgent care should be provided only in an isolated operatory with strict adherence to standard precautions (see Appendix B). Aerosols should be minimized, and drugs that are metabolized in the liver should be avoided as much as possible (Box 10.3) (Fig. 10.5). If surgery is necessary, a preoperative prothrombin time and bleeding time should be obtained, and abnormal results discussed with the physician. The dentist should refer patients who have acute hepatitis for medical diagnosis and treatment.

Patients With a History of Hepatitis. Most carriers of HBV, HCV, and HDV are unaware that they have had hepatitis due to mild subclinical infections. Thus, the only practical method of protection from exposure to potential infection associated with providing dental care for persons with undiagnosed hepatitis or with other undetected infectious diseases is to adopt a strict program of clinical asepsis for all patients (see Appendix B).

Patients at High Risk for Hepatitis B Virus or Hepatitis C Virus Infection. Several groups are at unusually high risk for HBV and HCV infection (see Box 10.1). Screening for HBsAg and anti-HCV is recommended in persons who fit into one or more of these categories unless they are already known to be seropositive. Even if a patient is found to be a carrier, no modifications in treatment approach theoretically would be necessary. Information derived from such screening may nevertheless be of benefit in certain situations. If a patient is found to be a

carrier, this knowledge could be of extreme importance for the modification of lifestyle. In addition, the patient might have undetected chronic active hepatitis, which could lead to bleeding complications or drug metabolism problems. Finally, if an accidental needlestick or puncture wound occurs during treatment and the dentist is not vaccinated (or antibody titer status is unknown), knowing whether the patient was HBsAg or HCV positive would be of extreme importance in determining the need for HBIG, vaccination, and follow-up medical care.

Patients Who Are Hepatitis Carriers. If a patient is found to be a hepatitis B carrier (HBsAg positive) or has a history of hepatitis C, standard precautions (see Appendix B) must be followed to prevent transmission of infection. In addition, some hepatitis carriers may have chronic active hepatitis, leading to compromised liver function and interference with hemostasis and drug metabolism. Physician consultation and laboratory screening of liver function are advised to determine current status and future risks.

Patients With Signs or Symptoms of Hepatitis. Any patient who has signs or symptoms suggestive of hepatitis should not receive elective dental treatment but instead should be referred immediately to a physician (see Box 10.2). Emergency dental care can be provided using an isolated operatory and minimizing aerosol production.

Drug Administration

No special drug considerations are needed for a patient who has completely recovered from viral hepatitis. If the patient has chronic active hepatitis, however, or is a carrier of HBsAg or HCV and has impaired liver function, the dosage for drugs metabolized by the liver should be decreased or such drugs avoided if possible, as advised by the patient's physician (see Box 10.3). As a guideline, drugs metabolized in the liver should be considered for diminished dosage when one or more of the following factors are present: (1) elevation of aminotransferase levels to greater than four times normal; (2) elevation of serum bilirubin above 35 mM/L or 2 mg/dL; (3) serum albumin levels less than 35 g/L; and (4) signs of ascites, encephalopathy, and malnutrition; which are components of the Child-Pugh classification and the Model of End-Stage Liver Disease (MELD) scoring system (see Table 10.6). Many drugs commonly used in dentistry are metabolized principally by the liver, but in other than the most severe cases of hepatic disease, these drugs can be used, although in limited amounts (see Box 10.3).

Treatment Planning Modifications

Treatment planning modifications are not required for patients who have recovered from hepatitis.

Oral Manifestations and Complications. Patients with chronic hepatitis and significant liver damage (or cirrhosis) are at risk for abnormal bleeding (see Chapter 24). This can be due to numerous factors including abnormal synthesis of blood clotting factors, abnormal

BOX 10.2	Checklist for Dental Management of Patients With Patients With Liver Disease[1]

PREOPERATIVE RISK ASSESSMENT
- Evaluation is directed at determining the nature, severity, control, and stability of disease.
- Review recent laboratory test results (AST, ALT, bilirubin, aPTT, bleeding time, CBC with differential) to assess risk.
- Confirm patient has a primary care provider and is stable.
- Determine comorbid conditions (hypertension, renal disease, spleen disorder).
- Obtain a medical consultation (i.e., refer to physician) if the patient is poorly controlled or is undiagnosed.

A

Analgesics	NSAIDs, including aspirin, and acetaminophen, as well as codeine and meperidine, should be avoided or their use very limited in persons who have end-stage liver disease.
Antibiotics	Antibiotic prophylaxis is not recommended; however, patients who have severe liver disease may be more susceptible to infection. Selection of antibiotic agent is based on risk and severity of dental infection. Avoid use of metronidazole and vancomycin.
Anesthesia	Higher doses may be required to achieve adequate anesthesia in presence of alcoholic liver disease. Knowledge of current liver function is important to establish proper dosages. Epinephrine (1 : 100,000, in a dose of no more than 2 carpules) in local anesthetics generally is not associated with any problems, but patients should be monitored closely.
Anxiety	Use anxiety and stress reduction techniques as needed but avoid benzodiazepines.
Allergy	No issues.

B

Breathing	No issues.
Bleeding	Excessive bleeding may occur in patients with end-stage liver disease. Most such patients will have reductions in coagulation factors and thrombocytopenia, so they are at greater risk for postsurgical bleeding; they may need vitamin K or platelet or clotting factor replacement (or both).
Blood pressure	Monitor blood pressure because it may be significantly increased with portal hypertension in patients with end-stage liver disease.

Blood tests	HBsAg testing for HBV status as well as anti-HBs and anti-HCV testing as indicated by history and exposure.

C

Chair position	No issues.
Consultation	When the patient is under good medical management, the dental treatment plan is unaffected. However, consultation with the patient's physician to establish the level of chronic liver disease and control (CBC, ALT/AST) and to identify bleeding tendencies (PT, BT) and altered drug metabolism is recommended as part of the management program.
	Elective treatment should be delayed for patients with any form of active hepatitis.

D

Devices	No issues.
Drugs	Because many medications are metabolized in the liver, certain drugs may need to be avoided or reduced in dosage. Limit or avoid use of acetaminophen, aspirin, ibuprofen, codeine, meperidine, diazepam, barbiturates, metronidazole, and vancomycin. Refer to a good drug reference. The use of epinephrine or other pressor amines (in gingival retraction cord or to control bleeding) must be limited, especially if portal hypertension is present.

E

Equipment	No issues.
Emergencies and urgent care	For patients with severe liver disease who require urgent care, consider treating in a special care clinic or hospital. When emergency dental treatment is necessary in patients with active hepatitis, isolation may be necessary. After consulting with a physician, provide limited care only for pain control, treatment of acute infection, or control of bleeding until condition improves.

Postoperative Care F	
Follow-up	It is important to follow-up with the patient postoperatively to be certain that there are no complications.

[1]Strength of Recommendation Taxonomy (SORT) Grade: C (see Preface for further explanation).
ALT, Alanine aminotransferase; *AST*, aspartate aminotransferase; *BT*, bleeding time; *CBC*, complete blood count; *HBsAg*, hepatitis B surface antigen; *HBV*, hepatitis B virus; *HCV*, hepatitis C virus; *NSAID*, nonsteroidal antiinflammatory drug; *PT*, prothrombin time.

polymerization of fibrin, inadequate fibrin stabilization, excessive fibrinolysis, or thrombocytopenia associated with splenomegaly that accompanies chronic liver disease. Before any surgery is undertaken, a platelet count should be performed to determine whether platelet replacement may be required before surgery and bleeding risk should be assessed and discussed when needed with the patient's physician (see Chapter 24).

TRANSMISSION AND POSTEXPOSURE PROTOCOLS FOR HEALTH CARE WORKERS

There is little to no risk for transmission of HAV, HEV, and non—A-E hepatitis viruses to a dental health care worker from occupational exposure. By contrast, risk for transmission of HBV is well recognized after occupational exposure to infected blood or body fluids. HCV is

BOX 10.3 Dental Drugs Metabolized Primarily by the Liver

Local Anesthetics[1]
Lidocaine (Xylocaine)
Mepivacaine (Carbocaine)
Prilocaine (Citanest)
Bupivacaine (Marcaine)

Analgesics
Aspirin[2]
Acetaminophen (Tylenol, Datril)[3]
Codeine[3]
Meperidine (Demerol)[3]
Ibuprofen (Motrin)[2]

Sedatives
Diazepam (Valium)[3]
Barbiturates[3]

Antibiotics
Ampicillin
Tetracycline
Metronidazole[4]
Vancomycin[4]

[1]Most of these agents appear to be safe for use in patients with liver disease when given in appropriate amounts.
[2]Limit dose or avoid if severe liver disease (acute hepatitis and cirrhosis) or hemostatic abnormalities are present.
[3]Limit dose or avoid if severe liver disease (acute hepatitis and cirrhosis) or encephalopathy is present, or if taken with alcohol.
[4]Avoid if severe liver disease (acute hepatitis and cirrhosis) is present.

less infectious and less efficient in transmission than HBV. The risk of contracting HBV infection after percutaneous or other sharps injury in health care workers involving exposure to contaminated blood is reported to range from 6% to 30%. By contrast, the seroconversion rate for accidental blood exposure to HCV is between 2% and 8%. Seroconversion is related to the amount and depth of blood exposure.

To reduce the risk of transmission of hepatitis viruses, the CDC has published postexposure protocols for percutaneous or permucosal exposures to blood (Table 10.7). Implementation of the protocol is dependent on the virus present in the source person and the vaccination status of the exposed person (e.g., a dental health care worker).

The CDC guidelines for exposures involving HBV outline protocols for both vaccinated and unvaccinated persons. For example, a vaccinated health care worker who sustains a needlestick or puncture wound contaminated with blood from a patient known to be HBsAg positive should be tested for an adequate titer of anti-HBs, if those levels are unknown. If the levels are inadequate, the worker should immediately receive an injection of HBIG and a vaccine booster dose. If the antibody titer is adequate, nothing further is required. If an unvaccinated person sustains an inadvertent percutaneous or permucosal exposure to hepatitis B, immediate administration of HBIG and initiation of the vaccine are recommended.

Although no postexposure protocol or vaccine is available yet for HCV infection, current CDC guidelines include the following recommendations: (1) the source person should receive baseline testing for anti-HCV, (2) the exposed person should receive baseline and follow-up testing at 6 months for anti-HCV and liver enzyme activity, (3) anti-HCV enzyme immunoassay positive results should be confirmed by recombinant immunoblot assay (RIBA), (4) postexposure prophylaxis with immunoglobulin or antiviral agents should be avoided, and (5) health care workers should be educated regarding the risk and prevention of bloodborne infections.

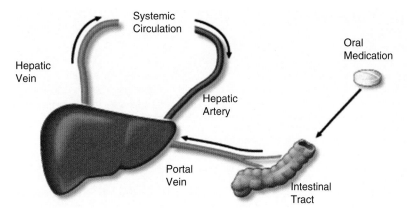

FIG 10.5 First-pass metabolism of orally ingested medications. The drug enters the liver via the portal vein, becomes bioavailable after metabolism in the liver into active metabolites, and then enters systemic circulation via the hepatic vein. In patients with liver disease, impaired hepatic function, reduced hepatic blood flow, and portosystemic shunting reduce first-pass metabolism, thereby increasing the proportion of drug that is bioavailable and increasing the risk for toxicity. (From Rakoski M, Goyal P, Spencer-Safier M, Weissmean J, Mohr G, Volk M. Pain management in patients with cirrhosis. *Clin Liv Dis*. July 26, 2018;11(6):135–140.)

TABLE 10.6   The Two Most Commonly Used Scoring Systems in Grading Cirrhosis

1. Child-Pugh-Turcotte (CPT) Score (Range, 5–15)

Parameter	Points Ascribed		
	1	**2**	**3**
Ascites	None	Grade 1–2 (or easy to treat)	Grade 3–4 (or refractory)
Hepatic encephalopathy	None	Grade 1–2 (or induced by a precipitant)	Grade 3–4 (or spontaneous)
Bilirubin (mg/dL)	<2	2–3	>3
Albumin (g/dL)	>3.5	2.8–3.5	<2.8
Prothrombin time (seconds > control) *or*	<4	4–6	>6
INR	<1.7	1.7–2.3	>2.3

CPT Classification

Child A: score of 5–6; Child B: score of 7–9; Child C: score of 10–15

2. Model of End-Stage Liver Disease (Meld) Score (Range, 6–40)

Score = [0.957 × ln creatine (mg/dL) + 0.378 × ln bilirubin (mg/dL) + 1.12 × ln INR + 0.643] × 10. Score <10, 10–14, >14 may correspond to CTP class A, B, C. Patients with child class C cirrhosis and MELD scores> 14 are generally not considered candidates for surgery.

INR, International normalized ratio; *In*, natural logarithm.

EXPOSURE CONTROL PLAN

With respect to hepatitis viruses, OSHA mandates that all employers maintain an exposure control plan and protect their employees from the hazards of bloodborne pathogens by using standard precautions and providing the following as a minimum: (1) hepatitis B vaccinations to employees, (2) postexposure evaluation and follow-up, (3) recordkeeping for exposure data, (4) generic bloodborne pathogens training, and (5) personal protective equipment made available at no cost. All dentists should be familiar with OSHA's compliance directive

"Enforcement Procedures for the Occupational Exposure to Bloodborne Pathogens" (CPL 02-02-069; available at: http://www.osha.gov/pls/oshaweb/owadisp.show_document?p_table=DIRECTIVES&p_id=257).

ALCOHOLIC LIVER DISEASE

Definition

Excessive alcohol consumption causes alcoholic liver disease and ultimately cirrhosis of the liver and worsens other

TABLE 10.7   Recommendations for Management After Accidental Exposure to Blood of a Person Infected With Hepatitis Virus

Infectivity Status of Source Person	Unvaccinated HCW	Vaccinated HCW,[a] Known Responder	Vaccinated HCW, Known Nonreceptor	Vaccinated HCW, Response Unknown
HBsAg positive	1 dose of HBIG (0.06 mL/kg IM) as soon as possible (preferably within 24 h) + initiate hepatitis B vaccine	No treatment	Administer one dose of HBIG + hepatitis B vaccine *or* two doses of HBIG, with second dose 1 month after the first	Test exposed worked for anti-HBsAg; with inadequate response (<10 mU/mL), one dose of HBIG + hepatitis B vaccine booster dose
HBsAg negative	Initiate hepatitis B vaccine series	No treatment	No treatment	No treatment
If unknown, not tested	Initiate hepatitis B vaccine series	No treatment	If known high-risk source, consider treating as for HBsAg-positive source	Test exposed[b] worked for anti-HBsAg; with inadequate response, initiate revaccination

[a]Exposed worker vaccinated against hepatitis B virus.

[b]After a percutaneous or permucosal exposure, the blood of the source person (and of the exposed person) should be tested for HBsAg, anti-hepatitis C virus (HCV), and human immunodeficiency virus antibody. Testing should be done in accordance with state laws and where appropriate pretest and posttest counseling are available. Currently, no treatment is available or recommended for occupational postexposure to HCV, hepatitis E virus, and non–A-E hepatitis viruses.

Also, current data suggest that a hepatitis A virus (HAV) percutaneous or permucosal exposure in an occupational setting is unlikely to result in transmission of HAV. Unvaccinated persons (younger than 2 years of age) recently exposed to HAV are advised to receive a single 0.02-mL/kg intramuscular (IM) injection of immune globulin according to the Advisory Committee on Immunization Practices recommendations.

HBIG, Hepatitis B immune globulin; *HBsAg*, hepatitis B surface antigen; *HCW*, health care worker.

(a) Data from Centers for Disease Control and Prevention. Immunization of health-care workers: recommendations of the Advisory Committee on Immunization Practices (ACIP) and the Hospital Infection Control Practices Advisory Committee (HICPAC). *MMWR Recomm Rep.* 1997;46(RR-18):1–42. (b) Data from Centers for Disease Control. Recommendations for follow-up of health-care workers after occupational exposure to hepatitis C virus. *MMWR Morb Mortal Wkly Rep.* 1997;46:603–606; Data from Centers for Disease Control and Prevention. Prevention of hepatitis A through active or passive immunization: recommendation of the Advisory Committee on Immunization Practices. *MMWR Recomm Rep.* 1999;48[RR-12]:1–31.

liver disorders such as viral hepatitis. Alcohol is hepatotoxic and its metabolite, acetyl aldehyde, is fibrinogenic. The quantity and the duration of alcohol ingestion required to produce cirrhosis are not clear. However, the typical alcoholic with cirrhosis has a history of at least 10 years of daily consumption of a pint or more of whiskey, several quarts of wine, or an equivalent amount of beer. A relationship exists between excessive alcohol ingestion and liver dysfunction, leading to end-stage liver disease or cirrhosis. Also implicated in the pathogenesis of alcoholic liver disease are *cytokines*. Alcohol-induced influx of endotoxin (lipopolysaccharides) from the gut into the portal circulation can activate Kupffer cells, leading to enhanced chemokine release. Chemokines, in turn, directly and indirectly damage liver hepatocytes. Curiously, only 10%−15% of heavy alcohol users ever develop cirrhosis, a fact probably explained by hereditary, nutrition, and biochemical differences among individuals.

Untreated alcohol abuse leads to significant morbidity and mortality rates. Current figures indicate that more than 100,000 persons die annually in the United States as a consequence of alcohol abuse, and more than 20% of all hospital admissions are alcohol related. Cirrhosis is a sequela of alcohol abuse and the 10th leading cause of death among adults in the United States. In addition, ethanol alone or with other drugs such as benzodiazepines probably is responsible for more toxic overdose deaths than those attributable to any other agent.

Pathophysiology and Complications

Alcohol has a deleterious effect on neural development, the corticotropin-releasing hormone system, metabolism of neurotransmitters, and the function of neurotransmitter receptors. As a result, the acetylcholine and dopaminergic systems are impaired, causing sensory and motor disturbances (e.g., peripheral neuropathies). Prolonged abuse of alcohol contributes to malnutrition (folic acid deficiency), anemia, and decreased immune function. Increased mortality rates have been noted for men who consume more than three drinks daily.

The pathologic effects of alcohol on the liver are expressed as one of three disease entities. These conditions may exist alone but commonly appear in combination. The earliest change seen in alcoholic liver disease is so-called *fatty liver*, characterized by presence of a fatty infiltrate. The hepatocytes become engorged with fatty lobules and distended, with enlargement of the entire liver. No other structural changes usually are noted. This condition may emerge after only moderate usage of alcohol for a brief time; however, it is considered completely reversible.

A second and more serious form of alcoholic liver disease is *alcoholic hepatitis*. This diffuse inflammatory condition of the liver is characterized by destructive cellular changes, some of which may be irreversible. The irreversible changes can lead to necrosis. Nutritional factors may play a significant role in the progression of

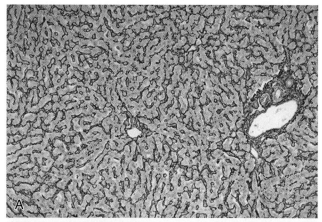

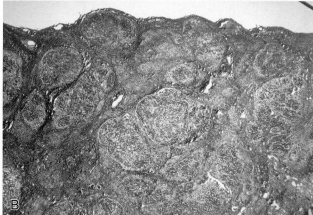

FIG 10.6 Photomicrographs showing liver architecture. **A,** Normal liver. **B,** Liver in alcoholic cirrhosis. (**A**, From Klatt EC. *In Robbins & Cotran Atlas of Pathology*. 2nd ed. Philadelphia: Saunders; 2010. **B**, From Kumar V, Abbas AK, Mitchell RN, et al. eds. *Robbins Basic Pathology*. 8th ed. Philadelphia: Saunders; 2007.)

this disease. For the most part, alcoholic hepatitis is considered a reversible condition; however, it can be fatal if damage is severe.

The third and most serious form of alcoholic liver disease is *cirrhosis,* which generally is considered an irreversible condition characterized by progressive fibrosis and abnormal regeneration of liver architecture in response to chronic injury or insult (i.e., prolonged and heavy use of ethanol) (Fig. 10.6). Cirrhosis results in the progressive deterioration of the metabolic and excretory functions of the liver, ultimately leading to hepatic failure. Hepatic failure is manifested by a myriad of health problems. Some of the more important of these are esophagitis, gastritis, and pancreatitis, which contribute to generalized malnutrition, weight loss, protein deficiency (including coagulation factors), impairment of urea synthesis and glucose metabolism, endocrine disturbances, encephalopathy, renal failure, portal hypertension, and jaundice. Accompanying portal hypertension is the development of ascites and esophageal varices (Fig. 10.7). In some patients with cirrhosis, blood from bleeding ulcers and esophageal varices is

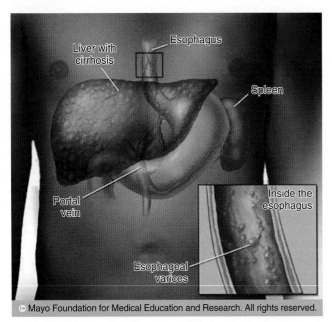

FIG 10.7 Esophageal varices from an alcoholic patient.

incompletely metabolized to ammonia, which travels to the brain and contributes to encephalopathy. In addition, chronic large consumption of ethanol can result in dementia and psychosis (Wernicke and Korsakoff syndromes), cerebellar degeneration, upper alimentary tract cancer and liver cancer, and hematopoietic changes.

Classically, severe alcoholic steatohepatitis is characterized by the sudden development of tender hepatomegaly, jaundice, and fever in a person who has been drinking heavily. Often, the illness is associated with a flulike prodrome that includes malaise, anorexia, and weakness. These symptoms sometimes prompt reduced alcohol ingestion, which in turn may precipitate an alcohol withdrawal syndrome (see Chapter 29). Some affected persons require hospitalization because of decompensated liver disease or associated conditions such as alcohol withdrawal syndrome, GI bleeding, infection, or pancreatitis. Although most people gradually recover during early abstinence, others deteriorate despite abstinence and aggressive management of their associated problems.

Bleeding tendencies are a significant feature in advanced liver disease. The basis for the diathesis is in part a deficiency of coagulation factors, especially the prothrombin group (factors II, VII, IX, and X). These factors all rely on vitamin K as a precursor for production (see Chapter 24). Vitamin K is absorbed from the large intestine and stored in the liver, where it is converted into an enzymatic cofactor for the carboxylation of prothrombin complex proteins. Widespread hepatocellular destruction as seen in cirrhosis decreases the liver's storage and capacity for conversion of vitamin K, leading to deficiencies of the prothrombin-dependent coagulation factors. In addition, thrombocytopenia may be caused by hypersplenism secondary to portal hypertension and

bone marrow depression. Anemia and leukopenia also may result from toxic effects of alcohol on the bone marrow and nutritional deficiencies. Accelerated fibrinolysis also is seen.

The combination of hemorrhagic tendencies and severe portal hypertension, which causes thrombocytopenia as a consequence of sequestration of platelets in the spleen, sets the stage for episodes of GI bleeding, epistaxis, ecchymoses, or ruptured esophageal varices. Most patients with advanced cirrhosis die of complications of hepatic coma, often precipitated by massive hemorrhage from esophageal varices or intercurrent infection.

Ethanol abuse predisposes the person to infection by several mechanisms. The liver's resident cell population in patients with alcoholism is exposed to high concentrations of ethanol. The Kupffer cells, representing more than 80% of tissue macrophages in the body, become impaired with continued bathing of the liver sinusoids in alcohol. Alcohol-induced impairment of Kupffer cell function and T-cell responses results in increased risk of infection. Although cirrhosis generally is considered to be an end-stage condition, some evidence suggests that at least partial reversibility of the process is possible with complete and permanent removal of the offending agent during the early phase of cirrhosis.

Clinical Presentation

The behavioral and physiologic effects of alcohol depend on the amount of intake, its rate of increase in plasma, concomitant use of other drugs or concurrent medical problems, and the past experience with alcohol. Chronic heavy alcohol intake can result in clinically significant cognitive impairment (even when the affected person is sober) or distress. Alcoholic blackouts may be a feature. In some patients, alcohol-induced dementia and severe personality changes develop.

Clinically, with the possible exception of enlargement, no visible manifestations of a fatty liver are present, and the diagnosis usually is made incidentally in conjunction

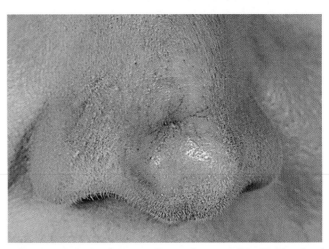

FIG 10.8 Spider angioma. (From Swartz MH. *Textbook of Physical Diagnosis*. 6th ed. Philadelphia: Saunders; 2010.)

with evaluation for another illness. The clinical presentation of alcoholic hepatitis often is nonspecific and may include features such as nausea, vomiting, anorexia, malaise, weight loss, and fever. More specific findings include hepatomegaly, splenomegaly, jaundice, ascites, ankle edema, and spider angiomas. With advancing disease, encephalopathy and hepatic coma may ensue, ending in death.

Alcoholic cirrhosis may remain asymptomatic for many years until sufficient destruction of the liver parenchyma has occurred to produce clinical evidence of hepatic failure. Ascites, spider angiomas (Fig. 10.8), ankle edema, and jaundice may be the earliest manifestations, but frequently hemorrhage from esophageal varices is the initial sign. The hemorrhagic episode may herald rapid progression to hepatic encephalopathy, coma, and death. Other, less specific signs of alcoholic liver disease include anemia, purpura, ecchymoses, gingival bleeding, palmar erythema, nail changes, and parotid gland enlargement (known as sialadenosis).

Laboratory Findings

Laboratory findings in alcoholic liver disease range in significance from minimal abnormalities caused by a fatty liver to manifestations of alcoholic hepatitis and cirrhosis. Liver abnormalities cause elevations of bilirubin, alkaline phosphatase, AST, ALT, GGT, amylase, uric acid, triglyceride, and cholesterol levels. Leukopenia (or leukocytosis) or anemia often is present.

Folate deficiency may also occur. Folic acid is a type of B vitamin which enhances the number of healthy red blood cells (vitamin deficiency anemia). Symptoms include fatigue and mouth sores.

A simple blood screen for alcoholism can be performed using a sequential Mult-Analyzer-20 and CBC with differential. Elevated blood levels of GGT and mean corpuscular volume are highly suggestive of alcoholism, and an AST-to-ALT ratio of at least 2 is 90% predictive of alcoholic liver disease. The carbohydrate-deficient transferrin test also is used to screen for and monitor clinical status in alcohol dependency.

Alcoholic liver disease leads to deficiencies of clotting factors reflected as elevations in the prothrombin time and partial thromboplastin time. Thrombocytopenia may be present owing to hepatosplenomegaly, causing a decreased platelet count. Increased fibrinolytic activity may be evidenced by a prolonged thrombin time or a decreased euglobulin clot lysis time (see Chapter 24).

Medical Management

The best management for alcoholic liver disease is total abstinence. Significant improvement in alcoholic fatty degeneration of hepatic cells can be seen 18 months after abstinence. However, this is often difficult to achieve. Treatment of patients with alcoholism consists of three basic steps. The first and second steps consist of identification and intervention, respectively. A thorough physical examination is performed to evaluate organ systems that could be impaired. This assessment includes a search for evidence of liver failure, GI bleeding, cardiac arrhythmia, and glucose or electrolyte imbalance. Hemorrhage from esophageal varices and hepatic encephalopathy require immediate treatment. Ascites mandates measures to control fluids and electrolytes, alcoholic hepatitis is treated often with glucocorticoids; infection or sepsis is managed with antimicrobial agents. Vitamin B and folate supplementation may be necessary.

The third step is to manage the central nervous system (CNS) depression caused by the rapid removal of ethanol. Administration of a benzodiazepine, such as diazepam or chlordiazepoxide, with gradual decrease in serum levels of the drug occurring over a 3- to 5-day period, alleviates alcohol withdrawal symptoms. Use of beta-blockers, clonidine, and carbamazepine are more recent additions to the pharmacotherapeutic management of withdrawal.

After treatment of withdrawal is complete, the patient is educated about the disease of alcoholism. The education program should include teaching family members and friends to stop protecting the patient from the problems caused by alcohol. Attempts are made to help the patient with alcoholism achieve and maintain a high level of motivation toward abstinence. Other interventions are aimed at helping the patient readjust to life without alcohol and reestablish a functional lifestyle. The drug disulfiram has been used for some patients during alcohol rehabilitation. Disulfiram inhibits aldehyde dehydrogenase, causing accumulation of acetaldehyde blood levels and thus sweating, nausea, vomiting, and diarrhea when taken with ethanol. Naltrexone (an opioid antagonist) and acamprosate (an inhibitor of the γ-aminobutyric acid [GABA] system) may be used to decrease the amount of alcohol consumed or shorten the period during which alcohol is used in cases of relapse (Table 10.8). Untreated disease that progresses to cirrhosis requires alcohol withdrawal and management of any complications that arise. End-stage cirrhosis cannot be reversed and is remedied only by liver transplantation (see Chapter 21).

Recently, some new concepts for the treatment of chronic cirrhosis have emerged. Because the main pathology associated with cirrhosis is decreased blood supply, fibrosis, and scarring of the liver parenchyma, investigators are successfully using angiogenic agents to essentially grow new blood vessels to supply liver tissue and decrease the damage from cirrhosis.

Dental Management

The dental patient with significant liver disease should be managed carefully (see Box 10.2). A CBC with differential and determinations of AST and ALT, bleeding time, thrombin time, and prothrombin time are needed to identify the patient for potential problems. Abnormal laboratory values, on a background of suggestive findings from the clinical examination or a positive history,

TABLE 10.8   Summary of Opioid Pharmacokinetics in Cirrhosis, Including Management Recommendations

Drug[a]	No Liver Disease (t1/2 in hours)[b]	Cirrhosis (t1/2 in hours)[d]	Recommended Starting Dosage in Advanced Liver Disease	Important Considerations
Tramadol IR	5.1	13.3	50mgql2hj	Use with caution in patients taking SSRIs or TCAs. Avoid in patients with seizure history.
Hydrocodone IR	3.8	n/a	5 mg q6h	Common form contains 325 mg acetaminophen per tablet. Limit is 6 tablets day.
Oxycodone IR	3.4	13.9	5 mg q6h	Has variable onset and analgesic efficacy.
Morphine IR[c]	3.3	5.5	5 mg q6h (elixir form)c	Avoid in renal failure.
Hydromoiphone	2.5	n/a	1–2.5 mg q6h	Consider first choice opioid in patients with renal failure.
Methadone	19	35d		Not recommended unless used as part of addiction program. Avoid in severe liver disease.
Codeine	2.9	n/a	15mgq6h	Avoid use, if possible.

[a]Opioid-tolerant individuals will require careful uptitration of dosages. Dosages represent general guidelines and should be individualized.
[b]$t_{1/2}$ by Child Pugh class: Class A = 3.4 h, Class B = 4.3 h, Class C = 4.5 h.
[c]Morphine IR in 5-mg increments is available only in elixir form. If tablet form is desired, the smallest dosage is 15 mg. Splitting tablets is not recommended.
[d]$t_{1/2}$ by Child Pugh class: Class A = 11.3 h, Class B = 13.0 h, Class C = 35.5 h.
Abbreviations: *n/a*, not available.
From Wehrer M. Pain management considerations in Cirrhosis. *US Pharm.* 2015;40(12):HS5-HS11.

constitute the basis for referral to a physician for definitive diagnosis and treatment. A patient with untreated alcoholic liver disease is not a candidate for elective, outpatient dental care and should be referred to a physician. After good medical management has been instituted and the patient is stable, dental care may be provided after consultation with the physician.

If a patient provides a history of alcoholic liver disease or alcohol abuse, the physician should be consulted to verify the patient's current status; medications; laboratory values; and contraindications to medications, surgery, or other treatment. When a patient has not been seen by a physician within the past several months, screening laboratory tests should be ordered, including a CBC with differential and determinations of AST and ALT, platelet count, thrombin time, and prothrombin time before invasive procedures are undertaken.

Antibiotics. Patients with chronic liver disease may be susceptible to infection, but there is rarely a need for antibiotic prophylaxis. However, there is risk for infection or spread of infection in the patient who has alcoholic liver disease. Risk increases with surgical procedures or trauma, which can cause bacteremias. These oral microorganisms introduced into the blood circulation may not be efficiently eliminated by the reticuloendothelial system owing to impaired cellular function. The need for antibiotic prophylaxis is not well studied, nor well justified. Of greater concern is the risk for spread of a preexisting infection, because bacterial infections are more serious and sometimes fatal in patients with liver disease. To identify patients likely to respond poorly to invasive procedures

and infections, the clinician should consider using one of the assessment formulas for staging liver disease (i.e., Child-Pugh or MELD classification scheme) (Table 10.6) as well as identifying whether a history of bacterial infections (e.g., spontaneous bacterial peritonitis, pneumonia, bacteremia) exist. Consultation with the patient's physician regarding the use of antibiotics should be considered for persons with moderate to severe disease (Child-Pugh class B or C—characterized by ascites, encephalopathy, elevated bilirubin levels, or increase in systolic blood pressure). Antibiotics should be provided when infection is present and unlikely to resolve without such treatment.

Some antibiotics may be contraindicated, or their dose may require adjustment. There may be some issues with analgesics as well (see Box 10.3).

Bleeding. Precautionary measures to minimize the risk for bleeding (see Chapter 24), including a prothrombin time test that is particularly sensitive to deficiency of factor VII, are indicated. Bleeding diatheses should be managed in conjunction with the physician and may entail use of local hemostatic agents, fresh-frozen plasma, vitamin K, platelets, and antifibrinolytic agents. Hemostatic measures are particularly important when major invasive or traumatic procedures are performed in a patient who has been assigned an American Society of Anesthesiologists category of III or higher and exhibits signs of jaundice, ascites, or clubbing of the fingers or with alcoholic liver disease of Child-Pugh class B or C or MELD grade of moderate-severe (see Table 10.6).

Capacity to Tolerate Care

Drug Considerations. An area of concern in patients with liver disease is the unpredictable metabolism of drugs. This concern is twofold. In mild to moderate alcoholic liver disease, significant enzyme induction is likely to have occurred, leading to an increased tolerance of local anesthetics, sedative and hypnotic drugs, and general anesthesia. Thus, larger-than-normal doses of these medications may be required to obtain the desired effects. In contrast, with more advanced liver destruction, drug metabolism may be markedly diminished, potentially leading to an increased or unexpected effect.

Several factors should be taken into consideration prior to starting any pain regimen in patients with cirrhosis. Factors to consider include potential for overuse/abuse, severity of hepatic and renal impairment, and presence of hepatic encephalopathy. In patients with cirrhosis, choice of analgesic and dosing regimen should be highly individualized and side effects carefully monitored. There is a common misconception regarding the use of acetaminophen in patients with cirrhosis, resulting in recommendations that these patients should *never* take acetaminophen. It is true that when ingested in large amounts (doses greater than 10–15 g), acetaminophen can cause severe hepatic necrosis and fulminant hepatic failure. Moreover, nearly half of all acetaminophen overdoses are unintentional, in part due to lack of knowledge that many over-the-counter and prescription medications contain acetaminophen. However, if taken in appropriate doses (i.e., not exceed 2 g total dose per day), acetaminophen is one of the safest analgesics for patients with cirrhosis. Patients should be educated about over-the-counter and prescription medications that may also contain acetaminophen.

NSAIDs should be avoided in all patients with cirrhosis. Due to prostaglandin inhibition and increased bioavailability among patients with cirrhosis, nonsteroidal antiinflammatory drugs (NSAIDs) can precipitate acute renal failure and gastrointestinal bleeding. NSAIDs also increase the risk for thrombocytopenia, which can further increase the risk for variceal and nonvariceal gastrointestinal bleeding. Finally, NSAIDs promote sodium retention, thereby worsening ascites and edema. Topical NSAIDs can be considered; however, further studies are needed to elucidate their safety profile in patients with cirrhosis.

The dentist should exercise caution in use of the drugs listed in Box 10.3 when treating patients with chronic alcoholism. The dose may need to be adjusted (e.g., half the regular adult dose may be appropriate if cirrhosis or alcoholic hepatitis is present), or a specific agent or class of drugs may be contraindicated as advised by the patient's physician. Again, the presence of more than one of the following findings is suggestive that drug metabolism will be impaired: aminotransferase levels elevated to higher than four times normal; serum bilirubin level elevated above 35 mM/L (2 mg/dL); serum albumin level less than 35 g/L; and signs of ascites, encephalopathy, or malnutrition (see Table 10.4).

Treatment Planning Modifications. The treatment plan for the patient who uses alcohol should be based on the degree of neglect and extent of caries and periodontal disease, the risk for oral cancer, and the patient's interest in and ability to care for their oral health. When dental care is provided, the dentist should be aware that liver enzyme induction and CNS effects of alcohol in patients with alcoholism can require use of increased amounts of local anesthetic or additional anxiolytic procedures.

Oral Complications and Manifestations. Poor hygiene and neglect (as evidenced by caries) are prominent oral manifestations of chronic alcoholism. In addition, a variety of other abnormalities may be found (Box 10.4). Nutritional deficiencies can result in glossitis and loss of

---

BOX 10.4   Features Suggestive of Advanced Alcoholic Liver Disease

Systemic complications
Traumatic or unexplained injuries (driving under the influence, bruises, cuts, scars, broken teeth)
Attention and memory deficits
Encephalopathy
Slurred speech
Spider angiomas
Jaundice (sclerae, mucosa)
Peripheral edema (edematous puffy face, ankle edema)
Ascites
Palmar erythema, white nails or transverse pale band on nails
Ecchymoses, petechiae, or prolonged bleeding
Failure to fulfill role obligations at work, school, home (e.g., missed dental appointments)
Increased levels of bilirubin >35 mg/mL, aminotransferases (>4× normal), alkaline phosphatase, and γ-glutamyl transpeptidase; increased mean corpuscular volume and decreased serum albumin (<35 mg/mL)

Oral Complications
Poor oral hygiene
Oral neglect: caries, gingivitis, periodontitis
Glossitis
Angular or labial cheilosis
Candidiasis
Gingival bleeding
Oral cancer
Petechiae
Ecchymoses
Jaundiced mucosa
Parotid gland enlargement
Alcohol (sweet musty) breath odor
Impaired healing
Bruxism
Dental attrition
Xerostomia

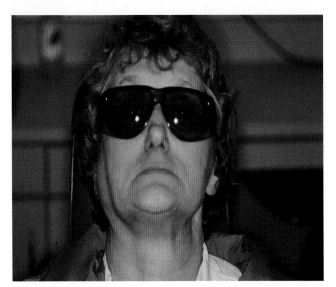

FIG 10.9 Painless enlargement of the parotid glands associated with alcoholism.

tongue papillae, along with angular or labial cheilitis, which may be complicated by concomitant candidal infection. Vitamin K deficiency, disordered hemostasis, portal hypertension, and splenomegaly (causing thrombocytopenia) can result in spontaneous gingival bleeding and mucosal ecchymoses and petechiae.

A bilateral, painless hypertrophy of the parotid glands, termed *sialadenosis*, is a frequent finding in patients with cirrhosis (Fig. 10.9). In sialadenosis, the parotid ducts remain patent and produce clear salivary flow.

Alcohol abuse and tobacco use are strong risk factors for the development of oral squamous cell carcinoma, and as with all patients, the dentist must be aggressive in the detection of unexplained or suspicious soft tissue lesions (especially leukoplakia, erythroplakia, or ulceration) in patients with chronic alcoholism. Sites with a marked predilection for development of oral squamous cell carcinoma include the lateral border of the tongue and the floor of the mouth (see Chapter 26).

NONALCOHOLIC FATTY LIVER DISEASE

Nonalcoholic fatty liver disease (NAFLD) is a very common disorder and refers to a group of conditions where there is accumulation of excess fat in the liver of people who drink little or no alcohol. NAFLD is a nonserious condition in which fat accumulates in the liver cells, hence the name "fatty liver." Although having fat in the liver is not normal, by itself it probably does not damage the liver. A small group of people with NAFLD may have a more serious condition named nonalcoholic steatohepatitis (NASH). In NASH, fat accumulation is associated with liver cell inflammation and different degrees of scarring. NASH is a potentially serious condition that may lead to severe liver scarring and cirrhosis. Cirrhosis occurs when the liver sustains substantial

damage, and the liver cells are gradually replaced by scar tissue, which results in the inability of the liver to work properly. Some patients who develop cirrhosis may eventually require a liver transplant (surgery to remove the damaged liver and replace it with a "new" liver).

Epidemiology and Risk Factors

NAFLD affects 80%−90% of obese adults, 90% of those with hyperlipidemia, and 30%−50% of patients with diabetes. It occurs in about 1 in 5 adults and 1 in 10 children in the United States. Obesity is thought to be the most common cause of fatty infiltration of the liver. Some experts estimate that about two-thirds of obese adults and half of obese children may have fatty liver. About 2 to 5% of adult Americans and up to 20% of those who are obese may suffer from the more severe condition NASH. The number of children who have NASH is not known. The presence of type 2 diabetes and other conditions associated with insulin resistance, such as polycystic ovarian syndrome are known risk factors for the development of fatty liver and NASH.

Etiology of NAFLD/NASH

NAFLD is part of the metabolic syndrome characterized by diabetes, or prediabetes (insulin resistance), being overweight or obese, elevated blood lipids such as cholesterol and triglycerides, as well as high blood pressure. Not all patients have all the manifestations of the metabolic syndrome. Less is known about what causes NASH to develop. Researchers are focusing on several factors that may contribute to the development of NASH. These include

- Oxidative stress (imbalance between prooxidant and antioxidant chemicals that lead to liver cell damage)
- Production and release of toxic inflammatory proteins (cytokines) by the patient's own inflammatory cells, liver cells, or fat cells
- Liver cell necrosis or death, called apoptosis
- Adipose tissue (fat tissue) inflammation and infiltration by white blood cells
- Gut microbiota (intestinal bacteria) which may play a role in liver inflammation

Clinical Presentation

The majority of individuals with NAFLD have no symptoms and a normal examination. Affected children may exhibit symptoms such as abdominal pain, which may be in the center or the right upper part of the abdomen, and sometimes fatigue. On physical examination, the liver might be slightly enlarged and some children may have patchy, dark discoloration of the skin present (acanthosis nigricans) most commonly over the neck and the under arm area.

Screening/Diagnosis

People with risk factors for fatty liver are often overweight or obese, and can have diabetes, or high levels of triglycerides/cholesterol in their blood. People with these risk factors should have their liver tests checked at least once per year. Those who are found to have elevated liver tests or possible fat in their liver on an abdominal ultrasound, or other imaging study, should be evaluated for possible fatty liver in addition to other causes of elevated liver tests. Once fat is identified in the liver, other causes of liver fat such as drinking too much alcohol, certain medications, and other liver diseases must be checked for before making a diagnosis of fatty liver.

The next step is to determine whether the patient with fatty liver has only fat within their liver (also called steatosis), where scarring of the liver is rare or nonalcoholic steatohepatitis (NASH). The most accurate way to determine this is to perform a liver biopsy, a procedure where a small needle is inserted through the skin after numbing medicine is given to obtain a small piece of the liver for examination under a microscope. A pathologist then interprets the biopsy sample and determines whether NASH is present and, if so, whether any liver damage or scarring has taken place. There are a growing number of alternatives to liver biopsy that can also provide much of the same information without requiring needle insertion into the liver. These include measuring liver stiffness and fat content of the liver with elastography testing through the use of a specialized ultrasound (Fibroscan) or MRI scan. Special blood tests or a combination of routine blood tests can also be used to evaluate for possible liver scarring in patients with NAFLD. Because none of these tests are perfect, patients with fatty liver are advised to discuss the risks and benefits of these tests with their doctor to decide which tests are best in their situation. In general, it is most beneficial to do a combination of tests to see if they all point to the same degree of fat in the liver and liver scarring.

Medical Management

In addition to good control of diabetes and high cholesterol/triglycerides when present, the most effective treatment for fatty liver, either NAFLD or NASH, involves behavioral changes including weight loss, increasing exercise, eating a balanced diet, and avoiding alcohol. Various diets can lead to a reduction in liver fat, as long as there is a decrease in calories eaten in a day compared to a person's daily required calories to maintain their current weight, with a goal of 500 fewer calories daily. Weight loss through exercise, medication, or weight loss procedure or surgery are available treatment approaches. While there are currently no US Food and Drug Administration (FDA)-approved medications for treatment of NASH specifically, several are being studied and medicines to improve liver scarring in patients with NASH and fibrosis may soon become available.

If inflammation from NASH continues for years, an extensive amount of liver scar tissue can form which eventually leads to liver cirrhosis (severe scarring of the liver that can be permanent). Patients who develop cirrhosis related to NASH are at risk for two major developments: hepatocellular carcinoma (liver cancer) and/or end-stage liver disease. Developing either complication of cirrhosis significantly impacts life expectancy, but certain patients can be cured by undergoing a liver transplant if they are evaluated and found to be a good candidate. For this reason, patients with NASH cirrhosis should see a GI or liver specialist regularly who will monitor their liver function and screen them for liver cancer with periodic liver ultrasounds or other scans, in addition to monitoring for other complications.

HEPATOCELLULAR CARCINOMA

Hepatocellular carcinoma (HCC) is potentially the terminal outcome of any of the chronic liver disorders. HCC is the most common primary liver malignancy and is a leading cause of cancer-related death worldwide. In the United States, approximately 35,000 cases of HCC occur each year and is the ninth leading cause of cancer deaths (approximately 25,000 per year; see Chapter 26). Despite advances in prevention techniques, screening, and new technologies in both diagnosis and treatment, incidence and mortality continue to rise. Cirrhosis remains the most important risk factor for the development of HCC regardless of etiology. Hepatitis B and C are independent risk factors for the development of cirrhosis. Alcohol consumption remains an important additional risk factor in the United States as alcohol abuse is five times higher than hepatitis C. Diagnosis is confirmed without pathologic confirmation. Screening includes both radiologic tests, such as ultrasound, computerized tomography, and magnetic resonance imaging, and serological markers such as α-fetoprotein at 6-month intervals.

Multiple treatment modalities exist; however, only orthotopic liver transplantation (OLT) or surgical resection is curative. OLT is available for patients who meet or are downstaged into the Milan or University of San Francisco criteria. Additional treatment modalities include transarterial chemoembolization, radiofrequency ablation, microwave ablation, percutaneous ethanol injection, cryoablation, radiation therapy, systemic chemotherapy, and molecularly targeted therapies. Selection of a treatment modality is based on tumor size, location, extrahepatic spread, and underlying liver function. HCC is an aggressive cancer that occurs in the setting of cirrhosis and commonly presents in advanced stages. HCC can be prevented if there are appropriate measures taken, including hepatitis B virus vaccination, universal screening of blood products, use of safe injection practices, treatment and education of alcoholics and intravenous drug users, and initiation of antiviral therapy. Continued improvement in both surgical and nonsurgical approaches has demonstrated significant benefits in overall survival. While OLT remains the only curative surgical procedure, the shortage of available organs precludes this therapy for many patients with HCC (see Chapter 26).

BIBLIOGRAPHY

1. Centers for Disease Control and Prevention. *Surveillance for Acute Viral Hepatitis—United States*; 2018. https://www.cdc.gov/hepatitis/statistics/2017surveillance/index.htm. Accessed February 08, 2021.

2. Centers for Disease Control and Prevention (CDC). Update: prevention of hepatitis A after exposure to hepatitis A virus and in international travelers. Updated recommendations of the Advisory Committee on Immunization Practices (ACIP). *MMWR Morb Mortal Wkly Rep.* 2007;56:1080–1084.

3. Centers for Disease Control and Prevention. *Hepatitis B Information for Health Professionals.* https://www.cdc.gov/hepatitis/hbv/hbvfaq.htm#overview. Accessed February 08, 2021.

4. *CDC Guidelines for Infection Control in Dental Health-Care Settings*; 2003. http://www.cdc.gov/oralhealth/infectioncontrol/#socialMediaShareContainer. Accessed February 08, 2021.

5. Cohen JI, Nagy LE. Pathogenesis of alcoholic liver disease: interactions between parenchymal and non-parenchymal cells. *J Dig Dis.* 2011;12:3–9.

6. *Current Treatment Options for Viral Hepatitis:* Medscape. http://emedicine.medscape.com/article/177792-treatment. Accessed February 08, 2021.

7. Dhawan VK, Anand BS. *Hepatitis C Treatment & Management with Viekira pak (Ombitasvir, Paritaprevir, Ritonavir).* http://www.hepatitisfoundation.org/HEPATITIS/Hepatitis-overview.html?gclid=CJL03aKl1MkCFYMDaQod7NkLfw. Accessed February 08, 2021.

8. Durham DP, Scrip LA, Brucec RD, et al. The impact of enhanced screening and treatment on hepatitis C in the U.S. *Clin Infect Dis.* 2016;62(3):298–304.

9. Fassio E. Hepatitis C and hepatocellular carcinoma. *Ann Hepatol.* 2010;9(suppl):119–122.

10. Firriolo FJ. Dental management of patients with end-stage liver disease. *Dent Clin.* 2006;50:563–590. vii.

11. Foster GR, Afdahl SK, Robets SK, et al. Sofosbuvir and velpatasvir for HCV genotype 2 and 3 infection. *N Engl J Med.* 2015;373(27):2608–2613.

12. Gex L, Bernard C, Spahr L. Child-pugh, MELD and maddrey scores. *Rev Med Suisse.* 2010;6:1803–1804, 1806–1808.

13. Ghany M, Hoofnagle JH. Approach to the patient with liver disease. In: Jameson J, Fauci A, Kasper D, et al. *Harrison's Principles of Internal Medicine.* 20th ed. Copyright © 2018. McGraw- Hill Publishers. vol. 1 eBook ISBN 978-1-259-64400-9; MHID 1-259-64400-6; vol. 2 eBook ISBN 978-1-259-64402-3; MHID 1-259-64402-2.

14. Golla K, Epstein JB, Cabay RJ. Liver disease: current perspectives on medical and dental management. *Oral Surg Oral Med Oral Pathol Oral Radiol Endod.* 2004;98:516–521.

15. Hung CH, Hu TH, Lu SN, et al. Tenofovir versus entecavir in treatment of chronic hepatitis B virus with severe acute exacerbation. *Antimicrob Agents Chemother.* 2015;59(6):3168–3173.

16. OSHA'S Compliance Directive "Enforcement Procedures for The Occupational Exposure to Bloodborne Pathogens" (CPL 02-02-069). Available at: http://www.osha.gov/pls/oshaweb/owadisp.show_document?p_table=DIRECTIVES&p_id=257. Accessed February 08, 2021.

17. Poordad F, McCone Jr J, Bacon BR, et al. SPRINT-2 Investigators. Boceprevir for untreated chronic HCV genotype 1 infection. *N Engl J Med.* 2011;364:1195–1204.

18. Roth D. Grazoprevir plus elbasvir in treatment-naive and treatment-experienced patients with hepatitis C virus genotype 1 infection and stage 4-5 chronic kidney disease (the C-SURFER study): a combination phase 3 study. *Lancet.* 2015;386(10003):1537–1545.

19. Simmons B. Long-term treatment outcomes of patient infected with hepC virus. *Clin Infect.* 2015;61(5):730–740.

Gastrointestinal Diseases

Gastrointestinal (GI) diseases such as gastroesophageal reflux disease (GERD), peptic ulcer disease (PUD), inflammatory bowel disease (IBD), and pseudomembranous colitis are common and may affect the delivery of dental care. These diseases are of clinical importance, and dental practitioners must (1) be cognizant of the patient's condition, (2) monitor for symptoms indicative of initial disease or relapse, and (3) be aware of drugs that interact with GI medications or that may aggravate these conditions. In addition, oral manifestations of GI diseases are common, so the dentist must be familiar with oral patterns of systemic disease.

GASTROESOPHAGEAL REFLUX DISEASE

GERD involves dysfunction of the lower esophageal sphincter and is characterized by a spectrum of clinical features, including heartburn, regurgitation, and dysphagia.

EPIDEMIOLOGY

Global prevalence of GERD in adults is approximately 13% with higher than average rates in South Asia, the Americas, and Europe. Prevalence is age dependent, and a recent meta-analysis reported 17% of adults aged 50 or older with the condition. Pooled analysis demonstrates a higher global prevalence of GERD in women. An average dental practice of 2000 adult patients would expect to treat about 300 patients with GERD.

ETIOLOGY

Obesity is associated with increased risk of developing GERD attributed to increased intraabdominal pressure, higher gradient of abdominal to thoracic pressure, and increased production of bile and pancreatic enzymes. Tobacco is an established risk factor for GERD, as it may prolong esophageal acid clearance time and reduce lower esophageal sphincter pressure. Genetic predisposition is a known risk factor for this disease; however, no single specific risk chromosome has been identified. Both impairment of salivary secretion, which compromises the protective mechanism of saliva to clear reflux acid from the esophagus and highly acidic carbonated beverages, which alters intraesophageal pH, can contribute to GERD development.

PATHOPHYSIOLOGY AND COMPLICATIONS

GERD is associated with several factors and physiological changes. Transient relaxation of the lower esophageal sphincter is a normal physiologic response to gastric distention that facilitates belching. Frequent and prolonged relaxations can contribute to development of GERD (Fig. 11.1). The most common hernia is the "sliding" type where a portion of the proximal stomach herniates through the diaphragm and is located in the thoracic cavity. This common anatomical configuration facilitates GERD by increasing the angulation between the gastroesophageal junction and gastric fundus, reducing valve function. GERD symptoms may not be as pronounced with the less common "rolling" hernia, where the entire stomach or a part of it (e.g., antrum) herniates into the thorax, adjacent and toward the left side of the intact gastroesophageal junction. In addition, abnormalities with esophageal peristalsis results in prolonged exposure of the esophageal epithelium to gastroduodenal contents contributing to a spectrum of esophageal injuries.

Esophagitis, stricture, Barrett esophagus (BE), and esophageal adenocarcinoma (EA) are complications of

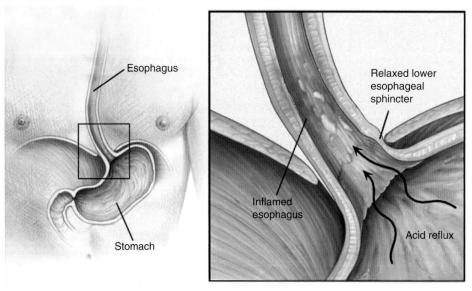

FIG. 11.1 Gastroesophageal reflux disease. ((GERD). © From Mayo Foundation for Medical Education and Research All rights reserved. https://www.mayoclinic.org/diseases-conditions/gerd/symptoms-causes/syc-20361940.)

GERD. Esophagitis occurs in up to 25% of patients with GERD and is the most common complication of this disease. Chronic acidic exposure to the esophagus can result in fibrotic scarring (stricture), further compromising physiologic function. The most severe complications of GERD are development of BE with the associated risk of EA. BE is endoscopically recognized by tongues of salmon-colored mucosa extending proximally from the gastroesophageal junction or histopathologically by columnar-lined intestinal metaplasia of the distal esophagus. Men older than age 60 who have GERD are considered high risk for BE, which is considered the precursor to EA, especially in the presence of dysplasia. Unfortunately, the incidence of EA has increased precipitously in the last 40 years with a global incidence of 0.7 cases per 100,000 person-years with less than 20% of patients surviving 5 years.

CLINICAL PRESENTATION

The signs and symptoms of GERD are shown in Table 11.1.

LABORATORY AND DIAGNOSTIC FINDINGS

For individuals with signs and symptoms of typical GERD elicited through patient history and physical examination, laboratory testing is not indicated. A positive response to proton-pump inhibitor (PPI) therapy confirms the diagnosis. Endoscopy, esophageal manometry, and esophageal pH monitoring is warranted if the patient does not respond to PPI treatment and/or if atypical (i.e., extraesophageal) symptoms suggest other etiologies. A flexible endoscope can visualize inflammatory changes to the

esophageal mucosa and obtain tissue samples to detect histological changes (Fig. 11.2). Esophageal manometry measures the coordination and force of esophageal muscle contractures that may be compromised in patients with GERD. Esophageal pH monitoring utilizes a probe to assess esophageal acidity from regurgitated stomach contents (<4 indicates recent activity) over a 24–96 h period.

MEDICAL MANAGEMENT

Lifestyle modifications can reduce GERD symptoms and include weight management for obese patients and tobacco cessation for smokers. Avoidance of triggers (e.g., chocolate, spicy food, and alcohol) and refraining from late meals helps to reduce symptoms of GERD. Chewing sugarless gum, which increases salivary flow, can be beneficial. Antisecretory drugs, such as PPIs, are the main medications used to manage GERD and promote healing of erosive esophagitis (Table 11.2). Clinical guidelines advocate an initial treatment period of a once daily PPI at standard dose for 4 weeks for patients with typical GERD symptoms and 8 weeks for healing of

TABLE 11.1	Clinical Presentation of Gastroesophageal Reflux Disease	
Typical Features	**Atypical (i.e., Extraesophageal) Features**
Heartburn	Chronic cough
Regurgitation	Laryngitis
Dysphagia	Hoarseness
Chest pain	Asthma

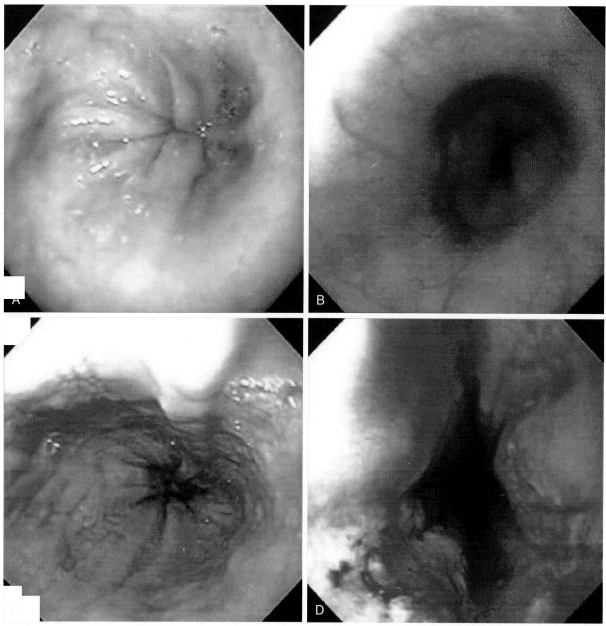

FIG. 11.2 Endoscopic findings in GERD. (**A**) normal esophageal mucosa. (**B**) mild erythema. (**C**) moderate thickening and erythema of the mucosa. (**D**) severe erosive disease. (From Harb R, Thomas D. Conjugated hyperbilirubinemia screening and treatment in older infants and children. Pediatr Rev Am Acad Pediatr. 2007;28:83–91.)

endoscopy-verified erosive esophagitis. Patients with typical GERD unresponsive to initial therapy may increase to twice-daily PPI dosing and may warrant further investigation based on clinical response. Long-term consequences of PPI treatment remain uncertain. Patients who do not respond to PPIs may be prescribed histamine$_2$ receptor antagonists, which reduces gastric acid production, as alternative therapy. Antacids (e.g., magnesium hydroxide) neutralize stomach acids and are used for symptomatic relief. Management of GERD complications include combination PPI therapy and endoscopic balloon dilatation for strictures and continuous PPI therapy and endoscopic removal of affected mucosa for BE.

Management of early EA consists of eradication of neoplastic tissue through endoscopic resection and ablation. Advanced and/or metastatic EA typically requires neoadjuvant chemoradiotherapy.

Patients with GERD refractory to medical therapy may require surgical intervention to manage the disease. Laparoscopic fundoplication, which enhances the esophagogastric junction's ability to prevent reflux into the esophagus, is the most commonly performed surgical procedure. While this procedure is effective in managing GERD, up to 20% of patients experience side effects from the procedure, such as dysphagia, bloating, vomiting, and difficulty belching.

TABLE 11.2   Antisecretory Drugs

Class	Drug	Trade Name	Dental Considerations
Proton-pump inhibitors (PPIs)	Omeprazole	Prilosec, Zegarid	PPIs can reduce absorption of ampicillin, ketoconazole, and itraconazole; may increase the concentration of benzodiazepines, warfarin, and phenytoin. Dental providers should check drug interaction resources before prescribing antiinfective drugs in these patients. Can be associated with vitamin B_{12} deficiency.
	Lansoprazole	Prevacid	
	Pantoprazole	Protonix	
	Rabeprazole	Aciphex	
	Esomeprazole	Nexium	
	Dexlansoprazole	Dexilant	
Histamine H_2 receptor antagonists	Cimetidine	Tagamet	Delayed liver metabolism of benzodiazepines; reversible joint symptoms with preexisting arthritis.
	Ranitidine	Zantac	—
	Famotidine	Pepcid	Anorexia, dry mouth
	Nizatidine	Axid	Potentially increased serum salicylate levels with concurrent aspirin use
Prostaglandins[a]	Misoprostol	Cytotec	Diarrhea, cramps

[a]Not a first-line drug for treating patients with peptic ulcer disease (PUD). Used in the prevention of PUD and in users of nonsteroidal antiinflammatory drugs.

DENTAL MANAGEMENT

Risk Assessment

The dental provider must identify GERD symptoms through a careful history taken before initiation of dental treatment because many GI diseases, although chronic and recurrent, remain undetected for long periods. If GI symptoms are suggestive of active disease, a medical referral is needed. When the patient is medically stable, the dentist should update current medications in the dental record, including the type and dosage, and should follow physician guidelines. Furthermore, periodic physician visits should be encouraged to afford early diagnosis and cancer screenings for at-risk patients.

It is important for the dentist to establish the severity and stability of a patient with a known history of GERD. Severe disease or poor control is evident by ongoing pain, recent physician visits, or hospitalization in which medical treatment has not remedied the condition or signs of dental erosion.

Prevention and Management Recommendations

Capacity to Tolerate Care. Routine dental treatment can be provided to patients with GERD; however, the decision should be based on patient comfort, convenience, and severity of disease. Patients with active GERD symptoms may benefit from dental chair positioning at a 45° angle to minimize gastric retrograde flow while undergoing dental treatment.

Drug Considerations. Of primary importance are the impact and interactions of certain drugs prescribed to patients with GERD. Acid-blocking drugs, such as cimetidine, decrease the metabolism of certain dentally prescribed drugs (i.e., diazepam, lidocaine, tricyclic antidepressants) and enhance the duration of action of these medications (Table 11.2). Under such circumstances, dosing of these drugs may require adjustment. Antacids also impair the absorption of tetracycline, erythromycin, oral iron, and fluoride, thereby preventing attainment of optimal blood levels of these drugs. To mitigate this problem, antibiotics and dietary supplements should be taken 2 h before or 2 h after antacids are ingested.

Oral Manifestations

Dental erosion is associated with GERD and typically correlates with severity of symptoms (Fig. 11.3). Chemical dissolution of enamel may be evident on palatal and lingual surfaces of teeth and can lead to exposed dentin, thermal sensitivity, and pulpal damage. Dental management recommendations include proper medical care of GERD and topical fluoride application with custom occlusive trays as well as restoration of tooth structure as indicated. Patients with GERD can also experience mucosal atrophy/erythema, dysgeusia, halitosis, and glossodynia.

PEPTIC ULCER DISEASE

A peptic ulcer is a well-defined break in the mucosa (at least 0.5 mm in diameter) of the stomach and/or

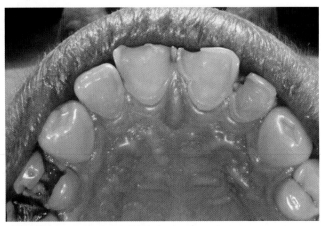

FIG. 11.3 Destruction of palatal enamel of maxillary incisors in a patient with persistent regurgitation.

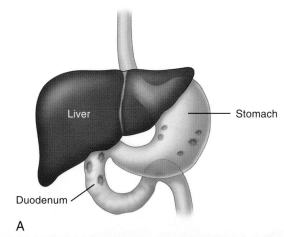

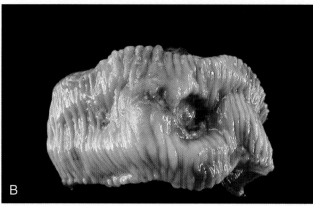

FIG. 11.4 **(A)** Location of peptic ulceration *(Shaded Areas).* *Darker-stippled areas* are higher-risk sites. **(B)** Peptic ulcer of the duodenum. (**(B)** From Kumar V, Abbas A, Fausto N, editors. *Robbins & Cotran Pathologic Basis of Disease,* 7th ed. Philadelphia, PA: Saunders; 2005. Courtesy of Robin Foss, University of Florida–Gainesville.)

duodenum that results from chronic acid or pepsin secretions and the destructive effects of and host response to *Helicobacter pylori* (Fig. 11.4).

EPIDEMIOLOGY

PUD is common affecting up to 15% of the population in industrialized countries. Duodenal ulcers are more common than stomach (gastric) ulcers and current estimates suggest 500,000 new cases of PUD are diagnosed annually in the United States. The incidence of peptic ulceration peaked between 1900 and 1950 and progressively decreased thereafter. The decline in northern Europe and the United States may be the result of decreased cigarette and aspirin consumption, increased use of vegetable cooking oils (a rich source of raw materials for synthesis of prostaglandins, which have cytoprotective properties), and better sanitation leading to fewer *H. pylori* infections. The first portion of the duodenum is most commonly affected with chronic and focal distribution of ulceration; only about 10% of patients have multiple ulcers.

About two-thirds of persons with ulcers are men, and prevalence of peptic ulceration is associated with increasing age. First-degree relatives have a threefold greater risk of developing PUD. A higher prevalence is seen among patients with hyperparathyroidism and hypersecretory states (e.g., renal dialysis, Zollinger–Ellison syndrome, mastocytosis). The disease is rare in children, with only 1 in 2500 pediatric hospital admissions attributable to peptic ulceration. When a peptic ulcer is diagnosed in a child younger than 10 years of age, the condition most often is associated with an underlying systemic illness, such as severe burn injury or other major trauma. Most deaths resulting from PUD occur in patients older than 65 years of age. An average dental practice of 2000 adult patients would expect to treat about 100 patients with PUD.

ETIOLOGY

Peptic ulcers result when the balance between aggressive factors that are potentially destructive to the GI mucosa and defensive factors that usually are protective of the mucosa is disrupted (Fig. 11.5). The primary aggressive factor is *H. pylori* (formerly *Campylobacter pylori*); this bacterium is associated with more approximately 70% of duodenal and gastric ulcers in the United States. Use of nonsteroidal antiinflammatory drugs (NSAIDs) is the second most common cause of PUD. Other risk factors include advanced age, psychological and physical stress, acid hypersecretion, cigarette smoking, use of certain drugs (Table 11.3), and major comorbid disease.

H. pylori is a microaerophilic, gram-negative, spiral-shaped motile bacillus with four to six flagella that is known to reside in the antral mucosa. The organism is an adherent but noninvasive bacterium that resides at the interface between the surface of the gastric epithelium and the overlying mucous gel. It produces a potent urease that hydrolyzes urea to ammonia and carbon dioxide. This urease may protect bacteria from the immediate acidic environment by increasing local pH while damaging mucosa through generation of its by-product, ammonia. Upregulation of cyclooxygenase-2 (COX-2), chemotaxis of neutrophils, and the cellular immune response are involved in the local tissue damage that subsequently occurs.

Humans are the only known hosts of *H. pylori*. The overall prevalence of *H. pylori* infection in the United States is approximately 30%, with those born before 1950 having a higher infection rate. *H. pylori* can persist in the stomach indefinitely, and infection with the bacterium remains clinically silent in most affected persons. The rate of *H. pylori* acquisition is higher in developing than in developed countries. In developing countries, 80% of the population carries the bacterium by the age of 20 years, but in the United States, only 10% of 20-year-old individuals are infected. The prevalence of infection in the United States among African Americans and Hispanics is twice

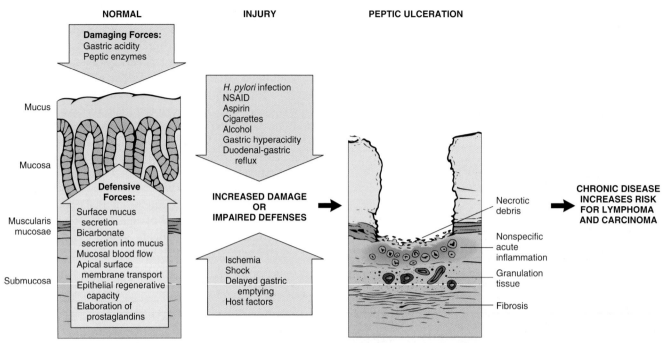

FIG. 11.5 Complex interplay of aggressive and defensive factors involved in the formation of peptic ulcer disease. *NSAID,* Nonsteroidal antiinflammatory drug. (Modified from Kumar V, Abbas A, Fausto N, editors. *Robbins & Cotran Pathologic Basis of Disease,* 7th ed. Philadelphia, PA: Saunders; 2005.)

that for whites. Infection is correlated with lower socioeconomic status and less education. Approximately 15% of infected persons go on to develop PUD, suggesting that other physiologic and psychological (stress) factors are required for presentation of this disease.

Use of NSAIDs is an etiologic factor in approximately 30% of cases of peptic ulcer. These drugs directly damage mucosa, reduce mucosal prostaglandin production, and inhibit mucus secretion. Ulcers caused by NSAIDs are located more often in the stomach than in the duodenum. Risk factors with NSAID use include advancing age, high-dose NSAIDs, multiple NSAIDs, and concomitant use of alcohol, corticosteroids, anticoagulants, or aspirin.

H. pylori–negative, non-NSAID ulcer disease accounts for the remainder of cases and occurs more often in older adults with chronic medical conditions, such as pulmonary or renal disease. Causative agents implicated include viral infections (e.g., cytomegalovirus) and medications (e.g., bisphosphonates, immunosuppressants),

which are associated with development of esophageal and gastric ulcers.

PATHOPHYSIOLOGY AND COMPLICATIONS

Ulcer formation is the result of a complex interplay of aggressive and defensive factors (see Fig. 11.5). Resistance to acidic breakdown normally is maintained by the mucosa, mucus and prostaglandin production, blood flow, bicarbonate secretion, and ion carrier exchange. Additional resistance is gained from the actions of antibacterial proteins such as lysozyme, lactoferrin, interferon, and α-defensin, or cryptdin.

Under normal circumstances, food stimulates gastrin release, gastrin stimulates histamine release by enterochromaffin-like cells in the stomach, and parietal cells secrete hydrogen ions and chloride ions (hydrochloric acid). Vagal nerve stimulation, caffeine, and histamine also are stimulants of parietal cell secretion of hydrochloric acid. Physical and emotional stress; obsessive-compulsive behavior; parasitic infections; and drugs such as caffeine, high-dose corticosteroids, and phenylbutazone enhance hypersecretion of stomach acid. Alcohol and NSAIDs are directly injurious to gastric mucosa. Alcohol alters cell permeability and can cause cell death. NSAIDs and aspirin disrupt mucosal resistance by impairing prostaglandin production and denaturing mucous glycoproteins. Smoking tobacco and family history are risk factors independent of gastric acid secretion for PUD. Tobacco smoke, similar to other aggressive factors, can affect gastric mucosa by reducing levels of

TABLE 11.3	Drugs That Increase the Risk of Peptic Ulcer Disease
Drug	**Frequency**
NSAIDs, aspirin	Very common
Anticoagulants	Less common
Amphetamines, crack cocaine	Less common
Corticosteroids, mycophenolate	Less common
Oral bisphosphonates	Less common
Serotonin reuptake inhibitors	Less common

NSAID, Nonsteroidal antiinflammatory drug.

nitric oxide, which is important for stimulating mucus secretion and maintaining mucosal blood flow.

H. pylori is strongly associated with PUD; however, the mechanism whereby effect of *H. pylori* on the GI tract is determined by interplay of microbial (e.g., toxins) and host factors (e.g., innate immune response). *H. pylori* causes inflammation of the gastric mucosa by producing virulence factors (e.g., gamma-glutamyl transpeptidase) and proteases that induce mucosal damage. There may be a genetic predisposition to acquire *H. pylori* with individual variability in mucosal and systemic humoral response, resulting in epithelial cell injury, which ultimately leads to ulcer formation.

Complications associated with PUD vary with the degree of destruction of the GI epithelium and supporting tissues. Superficial ulcers are characterized by the presence of necrotic debris, fibrin and subjacent inflammatory infiltrate, granulation tissue, and fibrosis. Ulcers that penetrate through the fibrotic tissue into the muscularis layer (muscularis mucosae) can perforate into the peritoneal cavity (peritonitis) or into the head of the pancreas. Arteries or veins in the muscularis layer may be eroded by ulcers (bleeding ulcer), giving rise to acute hemorrhage, anemia, and potential shock. Untreated ulcers often heal by fibrosis, which can lead to pyloric stenosis, gastric outlet obstruction, dehydration, and alkalosis. Complications are more common in older adults and those with comorbid liver, kidney, and malignant disease. Approximately 5% of those with duodenal ulcers die annually because of such complications. *H. pylori* is associated with the development of gastric mucosa–associated lymphoid tissue lymphoma and gastric cancer. Ulcers of the greater curvature of the stomach have a greater propensity for malignant degeneration than do those of the duodenum. Eradication of *H. pylori* helps to halt the progression of atrophic gastritis and thus reduces the risk of malignant transformation.

CLINICAL PRESENTATION

The signs and symptoms of PUD are shown in Table 11.4.

TABLE 11.4	Clinical Presentation of Peptic Ulcer Disease
Duodenal Ulcers	**Gastric Ulcers**
May be asymptomatic	May be asymptomatic
Localized, recurrent epigastric pain (primarily nocturnal)	Localized, recurrent epigastric pain (postprandial)
Hunger sensation	Nausea/Vomiting
Ingestion of food, milk, or antacids rapidly reduces pain	Weight loss
Changing symptoms may indicate worsening of condition:	
• Increased discomfort, loss of antacid relief, or pain radiating to the back, protracted vomiting, melena	

LABORATORY AND DIAGNOSTIC FINDINGS

A peptic ulcer is diagnosed primarily by fiberoptic endoscopic biopsy and laboratory testing for *H. pylori*. During endoscopy, a biopsy of the marginal mucosa adjacent to the ulcer is performed to confirm the diagnosis and rule out malignancy. A rapid urease test is then performed to detect the bacterial product urease in the mucosal biopsy specimen. Microscopic analysis of biopsied tissue prepared with Giemsa, acridine orange, and Warthin–Starry stains is effective in the microscopic detection of *H. pylori* (Fig. 11.6). Culture of the organism is reserved for cases in which antimicrobial resistance is suspected because the technique is tedious, difficult, and no more sensitive than routine histologic analysis.

Nonendoscopic laboratory tests include urea breath tests (UBTs) and, less commonly, stool antigen tests. A UBT is a highly sensitive, noninvasive test that involves the ingestion of urea labeled with carbon-13 (^{13}C) or carbon-14 (^{14}C). Degradation of urea by the bacillus releases ^{13}C or ^{14}C in expired carbon dioxide. These tests are advantageous because they indirectly measure the presence of *H. pylori* before treatment and its eradication after treatment. Upper GI imaging is infrequently performed because it lacks the sensitivity of biopsy. A low red blood count may occur in persons with a GI bleed.

MEDICAL MANAGEMENT

Most patients with PUD suffer for several weeks before going to a doctor for treatment. If the peptic ulcer is confined and uncomplicated and *H. pylori* is not present, an antisecretory drug, such as a PPI, is administered for 10–14 days; treatment is for 4 or more weeks if complications occur. If the patient is infected with *H. pylori*, inhibitors of gastric acid secretion and at least two antimicrobial agents are recommended. Various treatment

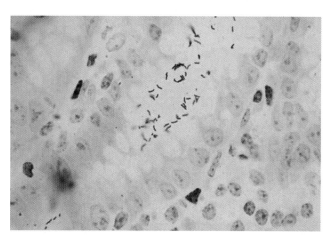

FIG. 11.6 *Helicobacter pylori* organisms *(dark rods)* evident in the lumen of the intestine. (Warthin–Starry Stain). (Courtesy of Eun Lee, Lexington, KY.)

BOX 11.1 Medical Management of Peptic Ulcer Disease

	Drug Combinations	Regimen	Recommended Duration
Triple therapy	PPI plus amoxicillin[a] plus clarithromycin	Double dose[b] of PPI every 12 h 1000 mg amoxicillin every 12 h 500 mg clarithromycin every 12 h	14 days
Quadruple non–bismuth-based concomitant therapy	PPI plus amoxicillin plus clarithromycin plus metronidazole	Standard dose of PPI every 12 h 1000 mg amoxicillin every 12 h 500 mg clarithromycin every 12 h 500 mg metronidazole every 12 h	14 days
Bismuth-based quadruple therapy	PPI plus bismuth subcitrate plus tetracycline plus metronidazole	Standard dose of PPI every 12 h 120 mg bismuth subcitrate every 6 h 500 mg tetracycline every 6 h 500 mg metronidazole every 8 h	14 days
Fluoroquinolone-based triple therapy[c]	PPI plus amoxicillin plus levofloxacin with or without bismuth	Standard dose of PPI every 12 h 1000 mg amoxicillin every 12 h 500 mg levofloxacin every 24 h 240 mg bismuth every 12 h	14 days
Rifabutin-based triple therapy[d]	PPI plus amoxicillin plus rifabutin	Standard dose of PPI every 12 h 1000 mg amoxicillin every 12 h 150 mg rifabutin every 12 h	10 days

[a]Use metronidazole if patients have penicillin allergy.
[b]Double doses: omeprazole 40 mg, lansoprazole 60 mg, rabeprazole 40 mg, esomeprazole 40 mg.
[c]Used as rescue regimen; bismuth-based therapy can be added to these drugs (for fluoroquinolone-based quadruple therapy).
[d]To be used when at least three recommended options have failed and if H pylori susceptibility testing is not available.
Other regimens used in the treatment of *Helicobacter pylori* combine different antibiotics with similar results (e.g., triple therapy could combine a proton pump inhibitor [PPI] plus amoxicillin plus metronidazole or PPI plus metronidazole plus clarithromycin). Sequential quadruple therapy consists of a 5-day dual therapy with a PPI and amoxicillin followed by a 5-day triple therapy with a PPI plus clarithromycin plus tinidazole or metronidazole. Hybrid quadruple therapies combine 10–14 days of dual therapy with PPI and amoxicillin with 7 days of treatment with clarithromycin and metronidazole at the end (or start, for reverse therapy).
From Lanas A, Chan FKL. Peptic ulcer disease. Lancet. 2017;390(10094):613–624.

regimens are used, which vary by country and prevalence of *H. pylori* antibiotic resistance (Box 11.1).

The conventional "triple" regimen is effective in eradicating *H. pylori* in more than 90% of treated patients. Quadruple therapy is used in areas where high prevalence of antimicrobial resistance occurs. Eradication of *H. pylori* with antibiotic treatment reduces the rate of recurrence of peptic ulceration by 85%–100%. Reemergence of an ulcer usually is traced to the persistence of *H. pylori* after treatment because of inappropriate drug choice, discontinuance of drug therapy, lack of behavior modification, or bacterial resistance.

In all patients who undergo peptic ulcer therapy, ulcerogenic factors (e.g., use of alcohol, aspirin or other NSAIDs, and corticosteroids; consumption of foods that aggravate symptoms and stimulate gastric acid secretion; persistent stress) should be eliminated to accelerate healing and limit relapses. Patients benefit from smoking cessation, as perforation rates are higher in smokers, and continued smoking results in a higher relapse rate after treatment and lower rates of eradication of *H. pylori*. When *H. pylori* is successfully eradicated, cigarette smoking does not appear to increase the risk of recurrence.

Surgery is reserved primarily for complications of PUD such as significant bleeding (when unresponsive to coagulant endoscopic procedures), perforation, and gastric outlet obstruction. On occasions when PUD is associated with hyperparathyroidism and parathyroid adenoma, surgical removal of the affected gland is the treatment of choice. Resolution of GI disease occurs after abnormal endocrine function is terminated.

DENTAL MANAGEMENT
Risk Assessment

The dental provider must identify intestinal symptoms through a careful history taken before dental treatment is initiated because many GI diseases, although they are chronic and recurrent, remain undetected for long periods. This history includes a careful review of medications (e.g., aspirin and other NSAIDs, oral anticoagulants) and level of alcohol consumption that may result in GI bleeding. If GI symptoms are suggestive of active disease, a medical referral is needed. When the patient is medically stable, the dentist should update current medications in the dental record, including the type and dosage, and should follow physician guidelines. Furthermore, periodic physician visits should be encouraged to afford early diagnosis and cancer screenings for at-risk patients.

It is important for the dentist to establish the severity and stability of a patient with a known history of PUD. Severe disease or poor control is evident by ongoing pain, blood in the stool, anemia, or recent physician visits or hospitalization in which medical treatment has not remedied the condition.

Prevention and Management Recommendations

Antibiotics: Infection Risk. Antibiotics used during PUD therapy would likely keep most dental infections in check. However, the selection of antibiotics for dental issues may need alteration based on the antibiotics used recently in the treatment of PUD.

Bleeding. Bleeding from oral tissues is not an issue with PUD. In contrast, GI bleeding associated with PUD can be of major concern and lead to significant complications (e.g., anemia) that can delay dental treatment.

Capacity to Tolerate Care. Routine dental treatment may be provided during medical therapy for peptic ulceration; however, the decision should be based on patient comfort, convenience, and severity of disease. A patient with ongoing signs and symptoms of active PUD is not a candidate for elective dental care.

Drug Considerations. Of primary importance are the impact and interactions of certain drugs prescribed to patients with PUD (Box 11.2). In general, the dentist should avoid prescribing aspirin, aspirin-containing compounds, and other NSAIDs to patients with a history of PUD because of the irritative effects of these drugs on the GI epithelium. Acetaminophen and compounded acetaminophen products are recommended instead. If NSAIDs are used, a COX-2–selective inhibitor (e.g., celecoxib [Celebrex]) given in combination with a PPI or misoprostol (Cytotec), $200 \, \mu g$ four times per day—a prostaglandin E_1 analogue—is advised for short-term use to reduce the risk of GI bleeding. Analgesic selection should be based on patient risk factors (previous GI bleeding; advanced age, use of alcohol, anticoagulants, or steroids) and the lowest dose for the shortest period to achieve the desired effect. Histamine H_2 receptor antagonists and sucralfate are not beneficial selections because they do not appear to protect patients from NSAID-induced complications.

Acid-blocking drugs, such as cimetidine, decrease the metabolism of certain dentally prescribed drugs (i.e., diazepam, lidocaine, tricyclic antidepressants) and enhance the duration of action of these medications. Under such circumstances, dosing of anesthetics, benzodiazepines, and antidepressants that are metabolized in the liver may require adjustment. Antacids also impair the absorption of tetracycline, doxycycline, erythromycin, oral iron, and fluoride, thereby preventing attainment of optimal blood levels of these drugs. To mitigate this problem, antibiotics and dietary supplements should be taken 2 h before or 2 h after antacids are ingested.

Oral Manifestations

H. pylori is found in dental plaque and may serve as a reservoir of infection and reinfection along the alimentary tract. Good oral hygiene measures and periodic scaling and prophylaxis may be useful in reducing the spread of this organism. The need for rigorous hygiene measures should be explained to the patient and consideration given to laboratory detection of oral organisms in patients who have a history of PUD and are symptomatic or are experiencing recurrences.

The use of systemic antibiotics for PUD may result in *fungal overgrowth* (candidiasis) in the oral cavity. The dentist should be alert to identifying oral fungal infections, including median rhomboid glossitis, in these patients (Fig. 11.7). A course of antifungal agents (see Appendix C) should be prescribed to resolve the fungal infection.

Vascular malformations of the lip and *erosion of the enamel* are two less common oral manifestations of PUD. The former have been reported to range in size from a small macule (microcherry) to a large venous pool, and they typically occur in older men with PUD. Enamel erosion is the result of persistent regurgitation of gastric juices into the mouth when pyloric stenosis occurs (Fig. 11.3). The finding of such erosion combined with a history of reflux indicates that the patient must be evaluated by a physician.

Medications taken by patients for the treatment of PUD can produce oral manifestations. PPIs can alter taste perception. Cimetidine and ranitidine may have a toxic effect on bone marrow; infrequently, they cause anemia, agranulocytosis, or thrombocytopenia. Mucosal ulcerations may be a sign of agranulocytosis, anemia may manifest as mucosal pallor, and thrombocytopenia as gingival bleeding or petechiae. Xerostomia has been associated with the use of famotidine and anticholinergic drugs, such as propantheline (Pro-Banthine). A chronic dry mouth renders the patient susceptible to bacterial infection (caries and periodontal disease) and fungal disease (candidiasis). Erythema multiforme has been associated with the use of cimetidine, ranitidine, omeprazole, and lansoprazole.

INFLAMMATORY BOWEL DISEASE

IBD is a term encompassing two idiopathic diseases of the GI tract: ulcerative colitis and Crohn's disease. The main distinction between the two diseases are the site and extent of tissue involvement; thus, it is logical to consider these clinical entities together. *Ulcerative colitis* is a mucosal disease that is limited to the large intestine and rectum. In contrast, *Crohn's disease* is a transmural process (involving the entire thickness of the bowel wall) that may produce "patchy" ulcerations at any point along the alimentary canal from the mouth to the anus but most commonly involves the distal ileum and proximal colon.

BOX 11.2 | Checklist for Dental Management of Patients With Gastrointestinal Diseases

PREOPERATIVE RISK ASSESSMENT

R: Recognize Risks
- Be **aware** of adverse events that may occur in the management of a patient who has a medical condition.

P: Patient Evaluation
- Review **medical history** and discuss relevant issues with the patient.
- Identify all **medications and drugs** being taken or supposed to be taken by the patient.
- **Examine** the patient for signs and symptoms of disease and obtain vital signs.
- Review or obtain recent **laboratory test** results or **images** required to assess risk.
- Obtain a **medical consultation** if the patient has a poorly controlled or undiagnosed problem or if the patient's health status is uncertain.

A

Analgesics	Avoid prescribing aspirin, aspirin-containing compounds, and other NSAIDs for patients with a history of PUD or IBD. Use acetaminophen-containing products or celecoxib (Celebrex) in combination with a PPI or misoprostol (Cytotec).
Antibiotics	Selection of antibiotics for oral infections may be influenced by recent use of antibiotics for PUD; certain drugs can increase the risk of intestinal flare-up in patients with IBD. Avoid long-term use of antibiotics, especially in older and debilitated persons, to minimize the risk of pseudomembranous colitis. Monitor for signs or symptoms (diarrhea, GI distress) suggestive of pseudomembranous colitis or disease worsening. Contact patient's physician if GI symptoms worsen while patient is on antibiotics so that alternative therapies can be initiated.
Anesthesia	No issues.
Anxiety	Intraoperative sedation can be provided by an oral, inhalation, or intravenous route.

B

Bleeding	Concurrent use of acid-blocking drugs and PPIs with warfarin (Coumadin) can enhance blood levels of the anticoagulant. Obtain CBC if medication profile increases patient risk for anemia, leukopenia, thrombocytopenia, or bleeding.
Blood pressure and vital sign monitoring	Obtain pretreatment vital signs.

C

Capacity to tolerate care	Patients with active, symptomatic disease may defer elective dental treatment until condition(s) are stable.
Chair position	Chair position should be based on patient comfort relative to the GI disorder or comorbidities.

D

Devices	No issues.
Drugs	Lower doses of diazepam, lidocaine, or TCAs may be required if the patient is taking acid-blocking drugs, such as cimetidine, which decreases the metabolism of some dentally prescribed drugs and enhances the duration of action of these medications. PPIs may reduce absorption of select antibiotics and antifungals. Monitor effects of immunosuppressant medications. If patient has recently taken corticosteroids, dosage modification generally is not needed; however, the clinician should evaluate the need for supplemental steroids as indicated by health status, level of anxiety or fear, presence of infection, and invasiveness of the dental procedure.

E

Equipment	No issues.
Emergencies and urgent care	No issues.

F

Follow-up care	Schedule appointments during periods of remission. Be flexible in scheduling appointments; disease flare-ups can be unpredictable. Shorter appointments may be necessary. Increased risk for medical complications could affect scheduling—for example: • PUD is more likely in patients older than 65 years of age and those with previous history of ulcer complications; prolonged use of NSAIDs; and concomitant use of anticoagulants, corticosteroids, or bisphosphonates. • IBD flare-ups are more likely when the patient is reporting symptoms and has a fever. • Pseudomembranous colitis is more likely in patients older than 65 years of age and those with history of recent hospitalization or taking broad-spectrum antibiotics (clindamycin, cephalosporins, ampicillin) or multiple antibiotics or with HIV-seropositive status associated with immune suppression. • Patients with persistent *Helicobacter pylori* are at increased risk for MALT lymphoma; patients with Crohn's disease or ulcerative colitis are at increased risk for colon cancer. Routine physician evaluation of these patients is advised.

CBC, Complete blood count; *GI*, gastrointestinal; *IBD*, inflammatory bowel disease; *MALT*, gastric mucosa–associated lymphoid tissue; *NSAID*, nonsteroidal antiinflammatory drug; *PPI*, proton pump inhibitor; *PUD*, peptic ulcer disease; *TCA*, tricyclic antidepressant.

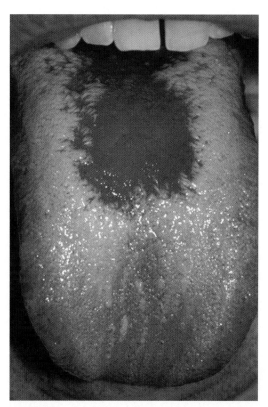

FIG. 11.7 Median rhomboid glossitis caused by antibiotic use.

EPIDEMIOLOGY

The incidence and prevalence of IBD vary widely by race and geographic location, with occurrences being higher among Jews and whites than in blacks. Also, IBD prevalence is considerably higher in the United States and northern and western Europe than in Africa and Asia, although the incidence is rising in Asia. Fifteen to 25 new cases of IBD per 100,000 people are diagnosed annually in the United States, Australia, and Europe. Currently there are more than three million people in the United States with IBD. Peak age at onset is 20–40 years; however, a second incidence peak for Crohn's disease has been noted between the seventh and ninth decades of life. Children can develop IBD with patients <18 years of age comprising approximately 25% of all IBD patients. Crohn's disease and ulcerative colitis affect men and women equally. A 10-fold increased risk of disease in first-degree relatives of patients strongly suggests that genetic factors are involved. Environment factors also are contributory: Crohn's disease occurs more often in smokers, but smoking protects against ulcerative colitis. In the average general dentistry practice with 2000 adult patients, approximately 15 adults are estimated to have IBD.

ETIOLOGY

Ulcerative colitis and Crohn's disease are inflammatory diseases of unknown cause and more than 200 genetic susceptibility genes have been identified in these conditions, including those that affect intracellular pathways recognizing microbial products (e.g., *NOD2)*; the autophagy pathway (e.g., *ATG16L1)*; genes regulating epithelial barrier function (e.g., *ECM1)*; and pathways regulating innate and adaptive immunity (e.g., *interleukin-23R* and *interleukin-10*). The disruption of homeostasis between commensal microbiota, intestinal epithelial cells and immune cells in response to environmental factors in genetically susceptible persons, results in a chronic state of dysregulated inflammation that is IBD. No specific enteric microbe has been determined to be responsible for inducing the proinflammatory responses observed in IBD; however, microbial diversity is reduced in patients with active IBD.

PATHOPHYSIOLOGY AND COMPLICATIONS

Both ulcerative colitis and Crohn's disease are the result of a dysregulated innate immune response to commensal bacteria that triggers a complex inflammatory cascade mediated by T-helper cells (e.g., T_h17) and proinflammatory cytokines (e.g., tumor necrosis factor, interleukins, Janus kinase).

Ulcerative Colitis

Ulcerative colitis is an inflammatory disease that targets the large intestine characterized by remissions and exacerbations. It starts in the colon and rectum region and may spread proximally to involve the entire large intestine. Persistent disease causes epithelial erosions and hemorrhage, pseudopolyp formation, crypt abscesses, and submucosal fibrosis. Chronic deposition of fibrous tissue may lead to fibrotic shortening, thickening, and narrowing of the colon.

Ulcerative colitis usually is a lifelong disease, and progression to its more severe forms predisposes affected persons to toxic dilatation (toxic megacolon) and dysplastic changes (predisposing patients to carcinoma) of the intestine. *Toxic megacolon* is the result of disease extension through deep muscular layers. The colon dilates because of weakening of the wall and intestinal perforation then becomes likely. Associated fever, electrolyte imbalance, and volume depletion are reported. Having ulcerative colitis increases the risk of colon cancer (i.e., 1.5–2 times higher than in the general population). Risk of malignant transformation is approximately 2% after 10 years, 8% after 20 years, and 18% after 30 years of disease.

Crohn's Disease

Crohn's disease is a chronic, relapsing idiopathic disease that is characterized by segmental distribution of intestinal mucosal ulcers (so-called "skip lesions") interrupted by normal-appearing mucosa. Although the distal ileum and the proximal colon are affected most frequently, any portion of the bowel may be involved. In gross specimens, the intestine displays sharply noncontinuous regions of thickened bowel wall, irregular glandular openings, mucosal fissuring, ulcerations, erosions, and benign strictures (Fig. 11.8). With chronic disease, the intestinal mucosa takes on a nodular or "cobblestone" appearance as a result of dense inflammatory infiltrates and submucosal thickening. Transmural involvement of the intestinal wall and noncaseating epithelioid granulomas of the intestine and mesenteric lymph nodes are classic features of the disease. As a result, the mesentery thickens and fixes the intestine in one position. Mesenteric fat tissue contributes numerous immune-regulating adipokines that influence the disease process.

Crohn's disease is further characterized by defects in mucosal immunity and in the mucosal barrier that result in increased intestinal permeability, increased adherence of bacteria, and decreased expression of defensins. The clinical course in Crohn's disease consists of remissions and relapses; relapses are more common in persons who smoke tobacco. Unremitting disease is complicated by small bowel stenosis and fistula formation. Most patients who have Crohn's disease require at least one operation for their condition. Long-standing colonic Crohn's

disease increases the risk for the development of colorectal cancer.

CLINICAL PRESENTATION

The signs and symptoms of IBD are shown in Table 11.5.

Ulcerative Colitis

It is important to note that many patients with ulcerative colitis undergo long periods of remission, however, fewer than 5% remain symptom-free over a 10-year period and about 50% experience a relapse in any given year.

Crohn's Disease

Three major patterns of Crohn's disease are recognized: (1) disease of the ileum and cecum, (2) disease confined to the small intestine, and (3) disease confined to the colon. Variability in symptoms and the episodic pattern contribute to the average 1–2 year delay in diagnosis from onset of symptoms. Intestinal complications are common, as 70%–80% of patients require surgery within their lifetime. Extraintestinal manifestations occur in about 33% of patients.

LABORATORY AND DIAGNOSTIC FINDINGS

The diagnosis of IBD is based primarily on clinical findings, results of endoscopy and biopsy, and observations on histopathologic examination of intestinal mucosa. Abdominal radiographic imaging, including computed tomography and magnetic resonance enterography, and stool examinations also may provide supportive evidence.

Endoscopic and histopathologic evaluation of ulcerative colitis shows friable, granular, erythematous, and eroded mucosa of the colon, with regions of edema and chronic inflammation. Histopathologic findings include epithelial necrosis, edema, vascular congestion, distorted

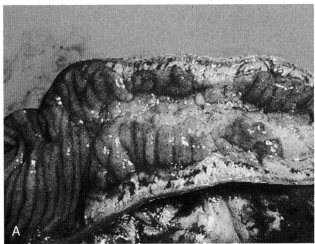

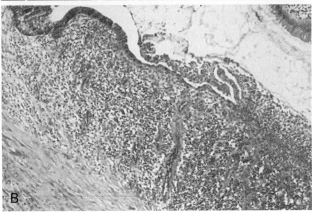

FIG. 11.8 (A) Crohn's disease that exhibits ulceration of the intestinal mucosa. **(B)** Low-power micrograph showing ulcerated intestinal mucosa of Crohn's disease with dense inflammatory infiltrate. ((**A**) From Allison MC, Dhillon AP, Lewis WG, et al. *Inflammatory Bowel Disease*, London: Mosby; 1998.)

TABLE 11.5	Clinical Presentation of Inflammatory Bowel Disease	
Ulcerative Colitis	**Crohn's Disease**
Abdominal cramps	Right lower quadrant abdominal pain or cramping
Diarrhea attacks (may be bloody)	Recurrent or persistent diarrhea (without blood)
Rectal bleeding	Intestinal complications include transmural fibrosis, intestinal fissuring, and formation of fistulas or abscesses
Malabsorption may lead to dehydration, fatigue, weight loss, and/or fever	Malabsorption may lead to dehydration, fatigue, weight loss and/or fever
Extraintestinal manifestations may include arthritis, erythema nodosum, pyoderma gangrenosum, and iritis/uveitis	Extraintestinal manifestations may include peripheral arthritis, erythema nodosum, aphthous, uveitis, episcleritis, and hepatic complications

cryptic architecture, and monocellular infiltration. The histological hallmark of Crohn's disease is the epithelioid granuloma, which is seen in only about 15% of mucosal biopsies but in up to 70% of cases in surgical specimens. Chronic focal, patchy, discontinuous, and transmural inflammatory infiltrate, goblet cell preservation, transmural lymphoid aggregates, and pyloric gland metaplasia are common findings of Crohn's disease. Blood tests in IBD may show anemia (deficiencies of iron, folate, or vitamin B_{12}) caused by malabsorption, decreased levels of serum total protein and albumin (as a result of malabsorption), inflammatory activity (evidenced as elevated erythrocyte sedimentation rate and increased C-reactive protein titer), and an elevated platelet or leukocyte count in conjunction with a negative microbial stool sample. Anti–*Saccharomyces cerevisiae* (yeast) antibodies are elevated in 40%–70% of patients who have Crohn's disease but in fewer than 15% of those with ulcerative colitis.

MEDICAL MANAGEMENT

Ulcerative colitis and Crohn's disease can be managed by an array of drugs but not cured (Table 11.6). Drugs containing 5-ASA remain the mainstay of treatment for ulcerative colitis and play a small role in management of Crohn's disease. These drugs are covalently bound to 5-ASA, which is released when cleaved by colonic bacteria. The released 5-ASA delivers local antiinflammatory effects within the intestine. Sulfasalazine is not well delivered past the proximal bowel, therefore, controlled-release oral formulations of 5-ASA that dissolve in the distal ileum and colon are used.

Corticosteroids often are combined with sulfasalazine to induce remission in patients who are experiencing flare-ups. Steroids are not prescribed for maintenance therapy because several adverse effects are associated with long-term use. When severe attacks produce abdominal tenderness, dehydration, fever, vomiting, and severe bloody diarrhea, the patient should be hospitalized and parenteral corticosteroids administered. When a satisfactory response is achieved, oral steroids are substituted for parenteral steroids, and the dosage is gradually reduced until the drug is no longer needed.

Immunomodulators are used in patients who have active disease that is unresponsive to corticosteroids and in corticosteroid-dependent patients to reduce the

TABLE 11.6   Common Medications Used to Treat Inflammatory Bowel Disease

Class	Drug	Trade Name	Dental Considerations
Aminosalicylates **(5-aminosalicylic acid derivatives)**	Sulfasalazine	Azulfidine	Serious complications include agranulocytosis, nephrotoxicity, and hepatotoxicity. Dental providers should consider evaluation of CBC with differential, renal function and liver function tests. Stomatitis is a rare complication.
	Mesalamine[a]	Pentasa	Serious complications include cytopenias, nephritis, hepatitis, Steven–Johnson syndrome. Dental providers should consider evaluation of CBC with differential, renal function and liver function tests.
	Olsalazine[a]	Dipentum	Serious complications include thrombocytopenia, nephritis, and hepatitis. Dental providers should consider evaluation of CBC with differential, renal function and liver function tests. Stomatitis is a rare complication.
	Balsalazisde[a]	Colazal	Serious complications include thrombocytopenia, nephritis, and hepatitis. Dental providers should consider evaluation of CBC with differential, renal function and liver function tests. Stomatitis is an uncommon complication.
Corticosteroids	Prednisone	Deltasone	See Chapter 15 for dental considerations.
	Hydrocortisone	Cortef	
	Budesonide	Entocort EC	
Immunomodulators	Azathioprine	Imuran	Myelosuppression, hepatotoxicity, increased risk of lymphoma. Dental providers should consider evaluation of CBC with differential and liver function tests.
	6-Mercaptopurine	Purixan	Same as azathioprine.
	Methotrexate	Otrexup	Cytotoxicity, hepatotoxicity. Dental providers should consider evaluation of CBC with differential and liver function tests. Stomatitis is an uncommon complication.
	Cyclosporine	Sandimmune	Nephrotoxicity, hepatotoxicity, increased risk of infection/lymphoma. Dental providers should consider evaluation of CBC with differential, renal function and liver function tests. Gingival hypertrophy is a complication.
Antibiotic	Metronidazole	Flagyl	Hepatotoxicity. Dental providers should consider evaluation of liver function tests.
Biologics	Infliximab[b]	Remicade	Cytopenias, hepatotoxicity, increased risk of infection, reactivation of hepatitis B infection, lymphoma (rare), progressive multifocal leukoencephalopathy (natalizumab specific). Dental providers should consider evaluation of CBC with differential, liver function tests and hepatitis B serologies.
	Adalimumab[b]	Humira	
	Certolizumab[b]	Cimzia	
	Natalizumab[c]	Tysabri	

[a]Controlled-release formulations.
[b]Tumor necrosis factor-alpha inhibitor.
[c]Novel biologic agent.

amount of steroid needed and to limit dose-dependent adverse effects of steroids. They may be given for years; however, their use is limited by their toxicity (flu-like symptoms, leukopenia, pancreatitis, hepatitis, and life-threatening infections); thus, white blood cell count and liver function tests must be monitored routinely. Bone marrow and hematopoietic stem cell transplantation has been associated with permanent remission.

Several biologics are used to manage IBD and their use is generally reserved for severe disease (more than one relapse per year) that is refractory to other drugs and for maintenance of remission. These drugs are expensive and require either slow intravenous (IV) infusion generally performed at 8-week intervals or subcutaneous injections every 2–4 weeks. Greater efficacy and a lower rate of side effects occur when biologics are given in combination with other antiinflammatory and immunomodulator drugs.

Antibiotics have been used for treatment of active Crohn's disease (e.g., abscesses) and to maintain remission. They also are used after surgery when toxic colitis develops or when fever and leukocytosis are present. Additional medications such as opioids, cromolyn sodium, and supplemental iron sometimes are used for their different effects, as required: antidiarrheal, anti–mast cell release, and treatment of anemia, respectively.

Surgery is recommended for severe cases of IBD that do not respond to corticosteroids and to manage serious complications (e.g., massive hemorrhage, obstruction, perforation, toxic megacolon, carcinomatous transformation). Total proctocolectomy with ileostomy is the standard but infrequent treatment for intractable ulcerative colitis. Over 50% of patients with Crohn's disease require some form of surgery and 30% have recurrent disease, thus necessitating additional resections.

DENTAL MANAGEMENT

Identification and Risk Assessment

The dentist should identify those with GI signs and symptoms and refer to a physician for further evaluation. The dentist should also evaluate the patient with IBD to determine the severity and stability of the condition. The severity of disease can be assessed by taking the patient's temperature and by reviewing the patient's symptoms to ascertain the number of diarrheal bowel movements occurring per day and whether blood is present in the stool. Patients who have less than four bowel movements per day with little or no blood, no fever, few symptoms, and a sedimentation rate below 20 mm/h are considered to have mild disease and can receive dental care in the dentist's office. Patients with moderate disease (i.e., between mild and severe) or severe disease—the latter defined as having six or more bowel movements per day with blood, fever, anemia, and a sedimentation rate

higher than 30 mm/hr—should defer elective dental care and be referred to their physicians.

Recommendations

Antibiotics: Risk of Infection. The majority of patients who have IBD are at low risk for infection; however, immune suppressed patients are at increased risk of infection. Another concern to the dentist is the administration of antibiotics in this population. Some antibiotics can promote overgrowth of *Clostridium difficile,* leading to symptomatic flares and diarrhea (see next section). Clindamycin and penicillins have documented association with pseudomembranous colitis. Dentists who prescribe antibiotics are encouraged to minimize the use of clindamycin, if possible, and should advise the patient to report a symptomatic flare (diarrhea) so that the physician can be alerted to check for C. *difficile,* with consequent modification of therapy as appropriate.

Appointments. The severity, clinical course, and prognosis of IBD are highly variable and can have an impact on routine dental care. Most patients with IBD experience intermittent attacks, with asymptomatic remissions between attacks. Patients often require physical rest and emotional support throughout the disease because anxiety and depression may be severe. Only urgent dental care is advised during acute exacerbations of GI disease. Elective dental procedures should be scheduled during periods of remission when complications are absent and a feeling of well-being has returned. Flexibility in appointment scheduling may be required because of the unpredictability of the disease.

Bleeding. Bleeding generally is not an issue with these patients unless a flare-up is accompanied by thrombocytopenia or one or more of the drugs causing immune suppression taken by the patient cause thrombocytopenia. When elective surgical procedures are scheduled for patients with IBD who take sulfasalazine, the dentist should review preoperatively the patient's systemic health and obtain a complete blood count with differential and coagulation studies. This preoperative assessment can be important because in addition to the immunosuppressive effects of IBD medications, sulfasalazine is associated with pulmonary, nephrotic, and hematologic abnormalities (i.e., a variety of anemias, leukopenia, and thrombocytopenia).

Capacity to Tolerate Care. The use of steroids by a patient with IBD can be of clinical concern because corticosteroids can suppress adrenal function and reduce the ability of the patient to withstand stress. Current guidelines recommend that the patient take the usual daily dose of corticosteroids before the dental appointment and that the dentist provide adequate pain and anxiety control (see Chapter 15). Supplemental corticosteroids may be required in rare circumstances if the patient's health is poor, infection is present, the patient is fearful, and surgery is being performed.

Drug Considerations. Patients with IBD are likely to be taking antiinflammatory drugs, corticosteroids, or immunomodulators, which can have an impact on dental care. The use of antiinflammatory drugs and the involvement of the intestinal tract suggest that aspirin and other NSAIDs are to be avoided. Acetaminophen may be used alone or in combination with opioids. Alternatively, cotherapy with a COX-2 inhibitor (celecoxib) and a PPI can provide pain relief and simultaneous protection of the GI mucosa. A careful drug history should be obtained to avoid prescribing additional opioids to patients who take these medications to manage their intestinal pain (see Box 11.2).

Immunomodulators (azathioprine and 6-mercaptopurine) are associated with the development of pancytopenia in approximately 5% of patients. In addition, a thorough head and neck examination should be performed in patients who take these medications because of their increased risk for lymphoma and infection (e.g., infectious mononucleosis, reactivation of latent tuberculosis, recurrent herpes). The presence of fever without an obvious causative illness in this select patient population mandates prompt referral to the physician.

Oral Manifestations

Several oral manifestations have been associated with IBD. Aphthous-like lesions occur in up to 20% of patients with ulcerative colitis (Fig. 11.9). Oral lesions erupt generally during GI flare-ups. The ulcers are mildly painful and may be of the major or minor variety. They typically are located on the alveolar, labial, and buccal mucosa, as well as the soft palate, uvula, and retromolar trigone, and they may be difficult to distinguish from aphthous lesions.

Pyostomatitis vegetans also can affect patients with ulcerative colitis and may aid in the diagnosis. This form of stomatitis produces raised papillary, vegetative projections or pustules on an erythematous base of the labial mucosa, gingiva, and palate (Fig. 11.10). The tongue rarely is involved. Without treatment, the initial

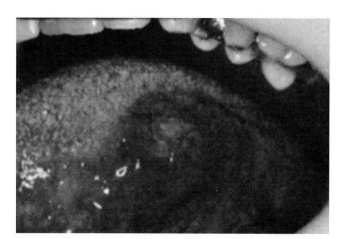

FIG. 11.9 Oral ulceration associated with ulcerative colitis. (From Allison MC, Dhillon AP, Lewis WG, et al. *Inflammatory Bowel Disease,* London: Mosby; 1998.)

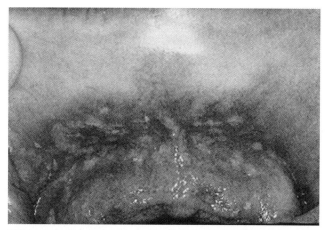

FIG. 11.10 *Pyostomatitis vegetans.* Pustular raised lesions of palate in a patient with ulcerative colitis. (From Allison MC, Dhillon AP, Lewis WG, et al. *Inflammatory Bowel Disease,* London: Mosby; 1998.)

erythematous appearance worsens, with eventual degeneration into an ulcerative and suppurative mass. Treatment of both the aphthous-like lesions and *Pyostomatitis vegetans* requires medical control of the colitis. Oral lesions that persist after antiinflammatory drug therapy typically respond to repeated topical steroid applications. The vegetative growths can be eradicated by surgical means.

Unique oral manifestations of Crohn's disease occur in approximately 20% of patients and may precede the diagnosis of GI disease by several years. Features include atypical mucosal ulcerations and diffuse swelling of the lips and cheeks (orofacial granulomatosis). Oral ulcers appear as linear mucosal ulcers with hyperplastic margins or papulonodular "cobblestone" proliferations of the mucosa, often in the buccal vestibule and on the soft palate. Oral lesions are intermittent but chronically present. They become symptomatic when intestinal disease is exacerbated. Similar to the oral lesions associated with ulcerative colitis, oral ulcerations of Crohn's disease resolve when the GI state is medically controlled. Topical steroids are beneficial during symptomatic phases.

Use of sulfasalazine has been associated with toxic effects on bone marrow, resulting in anemia, agranulocytosis, or thrombocytopenia, which can manifest as a bald tongue, oral infection, or bleeding, respectively. Corticosteroid use can result in osteopenia, which may involve the alveolar bone. Additional information on the oral management of these abnormalities is found in Appendix C.

PSEUDOMEMBRANOUS COLITIS

Pseudomembranous colitis is a severe and sometimes fatal form of colitis that results from the overgrowth of *C. difficile* in the large colon. Overgrowth results from the loss of competitive anaerobic gut bacteria, most commonly with use of broad-spectrum antibiotics, but it also can result from heavy metal intoxication, sepsis, and organ failure. The causative organism, *C. difficile*, produces and releases potent enterotoxins that induce colitis and diarrhea. Rarely, other pathogenic microbes may cause pseudomembranous colitis.

EPIDEMIOLOGY

Pseudomembranous colitis is the most common nosocomial infection of the GI tract. The incidence is about 50 cases per 100,000 persons in the United States and is rising. The reported incidence varies with the type and frequency of antibiotic exposure. No gender predilection exists; however, the disease is most common in older adults, patients in hospitals and nursing homes, those who receive tube feeding, and those who have suppressed immune systems. Infants and young children rarely are affected.

ETIOLOGY

C. difficile, the causative agent in 90%–99% of pseudomembranous colitis cases, is a gram-positive, spore-forming anaerobic rod that has been found in sand, soil, and feces. Spores may survive on contaminated surfaces for months and are relatively resistant to many disinfectants. *C. difficile* colonizes the gut in 2%–5% of asymptomatic adults, 15% of hospitalized patient with 2-week stays in the hospital, and 50% of patients with stays >4 weeks. The risk of disease increases in areas where spores are inhaled (e.g., hospitals, farm yards) and when broad-spectrum antibiotics are in prolonged use. Risk also increases with increasing age, obesity, concurrent irritable bowel disease, and use of PPIs. The most frequently offending antimicrobial agents are broad-spectrum agents and those that target anaerobic flora of the colon. The highest risk is associated with clindamycin (2%–20% of usage) or ampicillin or amoxicillin (5%–9% of usage) and third-generation cephalosporins (<2% of usage). Macrolides, penicillins, trimethoprim–sulfamethoxazole (Bactrim, Septra), and tetracycline are involved less frequently, and aminoglycosides, antifungal agents, metronidazole, and vancomycin are rarely causative. In general, oral antibiotics are more often causative than parenteral antibiotics.

PATHOPHYSIOLOGY AND COMPLICATIONS

As commensal intestinal bacteria are eliminated, *C. difficile* overgrows and produces enzymes that mediate tissue degradation, as well as three toxins, A, B, and a binary toxin that bind to intestinal mucosal cells, resulting in cytoskeletal disaggregation and altered vascular permeability, respectively. As cells (enterocytes) die, fluid is lost, and microscopic and macroscopic pseudomembranes form in the distal colon. Mild disease is characterized by patchy distribution; severe disease manifests

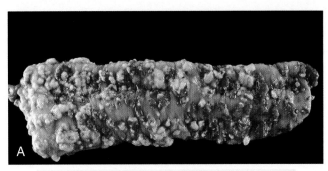
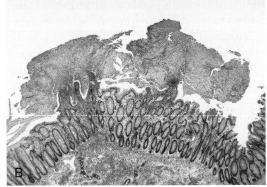

FIG. 11.11 Pseudomembranous colitis from *clostridium difficile* infection. (**A**) Gross photograph showing plaques of yellow fibrin and inflammatory debris adhering to a reddened colonic mucosa. (**B**) Low-power micrograph showing superficial erosion of the mucosa and adherent pseudomembrane of fibrin, mucus, and inflammatory debris. (From Kumar V, et al. *Robbins & Cotran Pathologic Basis of Disease*, 8th ed. Philadelphia, PA: Saunders; 2010.)

with large, coalescent plaques and extensive denuded areas (Fig. 11.11). Complications include recurrences, perforation, toxic megacolon, and death.

CLINICAL PRESENTATION

The signs and symptoms of pseudomembranous colitis is shown in Table 11.7.

LABORATORY AND DIAGNOSTIC FINDINGS

Pseudomembranous colitis is associated with leukocytosis, leukocyte-laden stools, and a stool sample positive for *C. difficile* or one of its toxins, as determined by tissue culture assay or enzyme immunoassay. Colonic

TABLE 11.7	Clinical Presentation of Pseudomembranous Colitis

Diarrhea (can develop 1 day to 8 weeks after drug administration)
Watery, loose stool (mild disease)
Bloody diarrhea accompanied by abdominal pain, cramping, fever (severe disease)
Complications
- Severe dehydration, metabolic acidosis, hypotension, peritonitis, toxic megacolon

yellow-white pseudomembranes that are 5−10 mm in diameter often are visible on colonoscopy or sigmoidoscopy. Histopathologic findings include epithelial necrosis; distended goblet cells; leukocyte infiltration of the lamina propria; and pseudomembranous plaques consisting of inflammatory cells, mucin, fibrin, and sloughed mucosal cells.

MEDICAL MANAGEMENT

First-line treatment of pseudomembranous colitis involves discontinuing use of the offending antimicrobial agent along with introducing an antibiotic that will eradicate the toxin-producing *C. difficile*. In patients with mild disease, cessation of the offending antibiotic is all that may be needed. In moderate disease, oral metronidazole (Flagyl) (500 mg three times a day for 10−14 days) is recommended. Vancomycin (125−500 mg four times a day for 10−14 days) is recommended for patients whose disease is severe or unresponsive to metronidazole. However, *C. difficile* spores can survive treatment, and relapse occurs in more than 20% of patients. Hydration and IV fluids are provided to correct electrolyte and fluid imbalances. Recurrences are managed with vancomycin, fidaxomicin, or rifaximin, with or without probiotics or alternatively with fecal bacteriotherapy.

DENTAL MANAGEMENT RECOMMENDATIONS

Antibiotics

The practitioner should be cognizant that the use of certain systemic antibiotics—especially clindamycin, ampicillin, and cephalosporins—is associated with a higher risk of pseudomembranous colitis in older, debilitated patients and in those with a previous history of pseudomembranous colitis (see Box 11.2). The risk increases with higher doses, longer duration of administration, and greater number of antimicrobials used. The decision to use an antibiotic and the duration of use should be based on sound clinical judgment that these drugs are necessary and should not be prescribed haphazardly.

Appointment

Elective dental care should be delayed until after pseudomembranous colitis has resolved.

Oral Manifestations

The use of systemic antibiotics for the treatment of patients with pseudomembranous colitis can result in fungal overgrowth (candidiasis) in the oral cavity (see Fig. 11.7). Metronidazole can cause peripheral neuropathy, nausea, and a metallic taste.

BIBLIOGRAPHY

1. Ahsberg K, Ye W, Lu Y, et al. Hospitalisation of and mortality from bleeding peptic ulcer in Sweden: a nationwide time-trend analysis. *Aliment Pharmacol Ther.* 2011;33:578−584.
2. Alsop BR, Sharma P. Esophageal cancer. *Gastroenterol Clin N Am.* 2016;45:399−412.
3. Annaloro C, Onida F, Lambertenghi Deliliers G. Autologous hematopoietic stem cell transplantation in autoimmune diseases. *Expet Rev Hematol.* 2009;2:699−715.
4. Batra A, Zeitz M, Siegmund B. Adipokine signaling in inflammatory bowel disease. *Inflamm Bowel Dis.* 2009;15:1897−1905.
5. Benchimol EI, Fortinsky KJ, Gozdyra P, et al. Epidemiology of pediatric inflammatory bowel disease: a systematic review of international trends. *Inflamm Bowel Dis.* 2011;17:423−439.
6. Borody TJ, George LL, Brandl S, et al. Smoking does not contribute to duodenal ulcer relapse after *Helicobacter pylori* eradication. *Am J Gastroenterol.* 1992;87:1390−1393.
7. Borum ML. Peptic-ulcer disease in the elderly. *Clin Geriatr Med.* 1999;15:457−471.
8. Centers for Disease Control and Prevention. Inflammatory Bowel Disease (IBD): Data and Statistics. Available at: https://www.cdc.gov/ibd/data-statistics.htm. Accessed January 31, 2021.
9. Chan FK, Wong VW, Suen BY, et al. Combination of a cyclo-oxygenase-2 inhibitor and a proton-pump inhibitor for prevention of recurrent ulcer bleeding in patients at very high risk: a double-blind, randomised trial. *Lancet.* 2007;369:1621−1626.
10. Chang J. Pathophysiology of inflammatory bowel diseases. *N Engl J Med.* 2020;383:2652−2664.
11. Chandan JS, Thomas T. The impact of inflammatory bowel disease on oral health. *Br Dent J.* 2017;222:549−553.
12. Cohen SH, Gerding DN, Johnson S, et al. Clinical practice guidelines for *Clostridium difficile* infection in adults: 2010 update by the society for healthcare epidemiology of America (SHEA) and the infectious diseases society of America (IDSA). *Infect Control Hosp Epidemiol.* 2010;31:431−455.
13. Colombel JF, Vernier-Massouille G, Cortot A, et al. [Epidemiology and risk factors of inflammatory bowel diseases]. *Bull Acad Natl Med.* 2007;191:1105−1118; discussion 18-23.
14. Colombel JF, Sandborn WJ, Reinisch W, et al. Infliximab, azathioprine, or combination therapy for Crohn's disease. *N Engl J Med.* 2010;362:1383−1395.
15. Danese S. New therapies for inflammatory bowel disease: from the bench to the bedside. *Gut.* 2012;61:918−932.
16. Del Valle J. Peptic ulcer disease and related disorders. In: Jameson J, Fauci A, Kasper D, Hauser S, Longo D, Loscalzo J, eds. *Harrison's Principles of Internal Medicine,* 20e. New York, NY: McGraw Hill; 2018:1−49.
17. Drumm B, Rhoads JM, Stringer DA, et al. Peptic ulcer disease in children: etiology, clinical findings, and clinical course. *Pediatrics.* 1988;82:410−414.
18. Ehsanullah RS, Page MC, Tildesley G, et al. Prevention of gastroduodenal damage induced by non-steroidal anti-inflammatory drugs: controlled trial of ranitidine. *BMJ.* 1988;297:1017−1021.

19. Forbes GM, Glaser ME, Cullen DJ, et al. Duodenal ulcer treated with *Helicobacter pylori* eradication: seven-year follow-up. *Lancet.* 1994;343:258–260.

20. Friedman S, Blumberg RS. Inflammatory bowel disease. In: Jameson J, Fauci A, Kasper D, Hauser S, Longo D, Loscalzo J, eds. *Harrison's Principles of Internal Medicine.* 20e. New York, NY: McGraw Hill; 2018:1–39.

21. Gajendran M, Loganathan P, Catinella AP, et al. A comprehensive review and update on Crohn's disease. *Dis Mon.* 2018;64:20–57.

22. Gajendran M, Loganathan P, Jimenez G, et al. A comprehensive review and update on ulcerative colitis. *Dis Mon.* 2019;65:100851.

23. Gerding D, Johnson S. *Clostridium difficile* infection, including pseudomembranous colitis. In: Jameson J, Fauci A, Kasper D, Hauser S, Longo D, Loscalzo J, eds. *Harrison's Principles of Internal Medicine.* 20e. New York, NY: McGraw Hill; 2018:1–10.

24. Gius JA, Boyle DE, Castle DD, et al. Vascular formations of the lip and peptic ulcer. *JAMA.* 1963;183:725–729.

25. Gklavas A, Dellaportas D, Papaconstantinou I. Risk factors for postoperative recurrence of Crohn's disease with emphasis on surgical predictors. *Ann Gastroenterol.* 2017;30:598–612.

26. Graham DY. *Helicobacter pylori* infection in the pathogenesis of duodenal ulcer and gastric cancer: a model. *Gastroenterology.* 1997;113:1983–1991.

27. Hollander D, Tarnawski A. Is there a role for dietary essential fatty acids in gastroduodenal mucosal protection? *J Clin Gastroenterol.* 1991;13(suppl 1):S72–S74.

28. Huang JQ, Sridhar S, Hunt RH. Role of *Helicobacter pylori* infection and non-steroidal anti-inflammatory drugs in peptic-ulcer disease: a meta-analysis. *Lancet.* 2002;359:14–22.

29. Jacobsen BA, Fallingborg J, Rasmussen HH, et al. Increase in incidence and prevalence of inflammatory bowel disease in northern Denmark: a population-based study, 1978–2002. *Eur J Gastroenterol Hepatol.* 2006;18:601–606.

30. Kahrilas PJ, Hirano I. Diseases of the esophagus. In: Jameson J, Fauci A, Kasper D, Hauser S, Longo D, Loscalzo J, eds. *Harrison's Principles of Internal Medicine,* 20e. New York, NY: McGraw Hill; 2018:1–21.

31. Kashyap A, Forman SJ. Autologous bone marrow transplantation for non-Hodgkin's lymphoma resulting in long-term remission of coincidental Crohn's disease. *Br J Haematol.* 1998;103:651–652.

32. Katz JA. Management of inflammatory bowel disease in adults. *J Dig Dis.* 2007;8:65–71.

33. Kavitt R, Lipowska AM, Anyane-Yeboa A, et al. Diagnosis and treatment of peptic ulcer disease. *Am J Med.* 2019;132:447–456.

34. Kikendall JW, Evaul J, Johnson LF. Effect of cigarette smoking on gastrointestinal physiology and non-neoplastic digestive disease. *J Clin Gastroenterol.* 1984;6:65–79.

35. Kociolek LK, Gerding DN. Breakthroughs in the treatment and prevention of *Clostridium difficile* infection. *Nat Rev Gastroenterol Hepatol.* 2016;13:150–160.

36. Kornbluth A, Sachar DB. Practice parameters committee of the American college of gastroenterology. Ulcerative colitis practice guidelines in adults: American college of gastroenterology, practice parameters committee. *Am J Gastroenterol.* 2010;105:501–523; quiz 524.

37. Kuipers E, Blaser M. Acid peptic disease. In: Goldman L, Schafer A, eds. *Goldman-Cecil Medicine.* Philadelphia, PA: Saunders/Elsevier; 2016:908–918.

38. Lakatos PL, Lakatos L. Risk for colorectal cancer in ulcerative colitis: changes, causes and management strategies. *World J Gastroenterol.* 2008;14:3937–3947.

39. Lanas A, Chan FKL. Peptic ulcer disease. *Lancet.* 2017;390:613–624.

40. Leoci C, Ierardi E, Chiloiro M, et al. Incidence and risk factors of duodenal ulcer. A retrospective cohort study. *J Clin Gastroenterol.* 1995;20:104–109.

41. Leontiadis GI, Molloy-Bland M, Moayyedi P, et al. Effect of comorbidity on mortality in patients with peptic ulcer bleeding: systematic review and meta-analysis. *Am J Gastroenterol.* 2013;108:331–345; quiz 46.

42. Levenstein S, Rosenstock S, Jacobsen RK, et al. Psychological stress increases risk for peptic ulcer, regardless of *Helicobacter pylori* infection or use of nonsteroidal anti-inflammatory drugs. *Clin Gastroenterol Hepatol.* 2015;13:498–506.e1.

43. Lichtenstein G. Inflammatory bowel disease. In: Goldman L, Schafer A, eds. *Goldman-Cecil Medicine.* Philadelphia, PA: Saunders/Elsevier; 2016:935–943.

44. Lourenco SV, Hussein TP, Bologna SB, et al. Oral manifestations of inflammatory bowel disease: a review based on the observation of six cases. *J Eur Acad Dermatol Venereol.* 2010;24:204–207.

45. Maity P, Biswas K, Roy S, et al. Smoking and the pathogenesis of gastroduodenal ulcer—recent mechanistic update. *Mol Cell Biochem.* 2003;253:329–338.

46. Malaty HM, Evans DG, Evans Jr DJ, et al. *Helicobacter pylori* in Hispanics: comparison with blacks and whites of similar age and socioeconomic class. *Gastroenterology.* 1992;103:813–816.

47. Maret-Ouda J, Markar SR, Lagergren J. Gastroesophageal reflux disease: a review. *JAMA.* 2020;324:2536–2547.

48. Marshall BJ, Warren JR. Unidentified curved bacilli in the stomach of patients with gastritis and peptic ulceration. *Lancet.* 1984;1:1311–1315.

49. McFarland LV. Renewed interest in a difficult disease: clostridium difficile infections—epidemiology and current treatment strategies. *Curr Opin Gastroenterol.* 2009;25:24–35.

50. McQuade K. Peptic ulcer disease. In: Papadakis M, et al., eds. *Current Medical Diagnosis and Treatment 2021.* 60th ed. New York, NY: McGraw Hill; 2021:1–13.

51. Mittal R, Vaezi MF. Esophageal motility disorders and gastroesophageal reflux disease. *N Engl J Med.* 2020;383:1961–1972.

52. Modi A, Siris ES, Steve Fan CP, et al. Gastrointestinal events among patients initiating osteoporosis therapy: a retrospective administrative claims database analysis. *Clin Therapeut.* 2015;37:1228–1234.

53. Muzyka BC. Gastrointestinal disease. In: Patton LL, Glick M, eds. *The ADA Practical Guide to Patients with Medical Conditions.* 2nd ed. Hoboken, NJ: John Wiley and Sons; 2016:135–151.

54. Nguyen AM, el-Zaatari FA, Graham DY, et al. *Helicobacter pylori* in the oral cavity. A critical review of the literature. *Oral Surg Oral Med Oral Pathol Oral Radiol Endod.* 1995;79:705–709.

55. Ozturk E, Yeşilova Z, Ilgan S, et al. A new, practical, low-dose 14C-urea breath test for the diagnosis of *Helicobacter pylori* infection: clinical validation and comparison with the standard method. *Eur J Nucl Med Mol Imag.* 2003;30:1457–1462.

56. Salen P, Stankewicz HA. Pseudomembranous colitis. In: *StatPearls [Internet].* Treasure Island, FL: StatPearls Publishing; August 10, 2020, 2020 Jan–.

57. Salkind AR. *Clostridium difficile:* an update for the primary care clinician. *South Med J.* 2010;103:896–902.

58. Shaheen NJ, Hansen RA, Morgan DR, et al. The burden of gastrointestinal and liver diseases, 2006. *Am J Gastroenterol.* 2006;101:2128–2138.

59. Shames B, Krajden S, Fuksa M, et al. Evidence for the occurrence of the same strain of *Campylobacter pylori* in the stomach and dental plaque. *J Clin Microbiol.* 1989;27:2849–2850.

60. Siegel MA, Solomon LW, Mejia LM. Diseases of the gastrointestinal tract. In: Glick M, ed. *Burket's Oral Medicine.* 12th ed. Shelton, CT: People's Medical Publishing House; 2015:389–410.

61. Sonnenberg A, Everhart JE. The prevalence of self-reported peptic ulcer in the United States. *Am J Publ Health.* 1996;86:200–205.

62. Surawicz CM. Antibiotic-associated diarrhea and pseudomembranous colitis: are they less common with poorly absorbed antimicrobials? *Chemotherapy.* 2005;51(suppl 1):81–89.

63. Take S, Mizuno M, Ishiki K, et al. Baseline gastric mucosal atrophy is a risk factor associated with the development of gastric cancer after *Helicobacter pylori* eradication therapy in patients with peptic ulcer diseases. *J Gastroenterol.* 2007;42(suppl 17):21–27.

64. Tan CX, Brand HS, de Boer NK, et al. Gastrointestinal diseases and their oro-dental manifestations: Part 1: Crohn's disease. *Br Dent J.* 2016;221:794–799.

65. Tan CX, Brand HS, de Boer NK, et al. Gastrointestinal diseases and their oro-dental manifestations: Part 2: ulcerative colitis. *Br Dent J.* 2017;222:53–57.

66. Thornhill MH, Dayer MJ, Prendergast B, et al. Incidence and nature of adverse reactions to antibiotics used as endocarditis prophylaxis. *J Antimicrob Chemother.* 2015;70:2382–2388.

67. Torres J, Mehandru S, Colombel JF, et al. Crohn's disease. *Lancet.* 2017;389:1741–1755.

68. Ungara R, Mehandru S, Allen PB, et al. Ulcerative colitis. *Lancet.* 2017;389:1756–1770.

69. Vassallo A, Tran MC, Goldstein EJ. *Clostridium difficile:* improving the prevention paradigm in healthcare settings. *Expert Rev Anti Infect Ther.* 2014;12:1087–1102.

70. Veauthier B, Hornecker JR. Crohn's disease: diagnosis and management. *Am Fam Physician.* 2018;98:661–669.

71. Wilson J, Hair C, Knight R, et al. High incidence of inflammatory bowel disease in Australia: a prospective population-based Australian incidence study. *Inflamm Bowel Dis.* 2010;16:1550–1556.

72. Xia B, Xia HH, Ma CW, et al. Trends in the prevalence of peptic ulcer disease and *Helicobacter pylori* infection in family physician-referred uninvestigated dyspeptic patients in Hong Kong. *Aliment Pharmacol Ther.* 2005;22:243–249.

73. Yuan Y, Padol IT, Hunt RH. Peptic ulcer disease today. *Nat Clin Pract Gastroenterol Hepatol.* 2006;3:80–89.

74. Zagari RM, Eusebi LH, Rabitti S, et al. Prevalence of upper gastrointestinal endoscopic findings in the community: a systematic review of studies in unselected samples of subjects. *J Gastroenterol Hepatol.* 2016;31:1527–1538.

75. Zhou L, Lin S, Ding S, et al. Relationship of *Helicobacter pylori* eradication with gastric cancer and gastric mucosal histological changes: a 10-year follow-up study. *Chin Med J.* 2014;127:1454–1458.

76. Zucca E, Bertoni F, Roggero E, et al. Molecular analysis of the progression from *Helicobacter pylori*-associated chronic gastritis to mucosa-associated lymphoid-tissue lymphoma of the stomach. *N Engl J Med.* 1998;338:804–810.

77. Zullo A, Hassan C, Campo SM, et al. Bleeding peptic ulcer in the elderly: risk factors and prevention strategies. *Drugs Aging.* 2007;24:815–828.

12

Chronic Kidney Disease and Dialysis

KEY POINTS

- Chronic kidney disease (CKD) is a worldwide problem that continues to increase in prevalence.
- CKD is often a "silent disease" until it enters late stage.
- CKD is associated with serious comorbidities, most commonly hypertension and diabetes.
- The dentist needs to recognize the clinical status of these patients and be familiar with their laboratory test results to prevent possible adverse outcomes and provide proper dental management.
- Progressive kidney disease can result in reduced renal function and lead to kidney failure with effects on multiple organ systems. Potential manifestations include anemia, abnormal bleeding, electrolyte and fluid imbalance, hypertension, drug intolerance, and mineral bone abnormalities that can affect the delivery of dental care.
- Patients who have severe and progressive disease may require artificial filtration of the blood through dialysis or kidney transplantation, which can impact patient's immune response, oral health, and bleeding that require modifications in dental care.

The kidneys have several important functions for quality of life. The kidneys regulate fluid volume, filter waste and toxins, maintain acid–base balance of plasma; synthesize and release hormones (erythropoietin, 1,25-dihydroxycholecalciferol, and renin). The kidneys are responsible for drug metabolism, and serve as the target organ for parathormone and aldosterone. Under normal physiologic conditions, 25% of the circulating blood perfuses the kidney each minute. The blood is filtered through a complex series of tubules and glomerular capillaries within the *nephron*, the functional unit of the kidney (Fig. 12.1). Ultrafiltrate, the precursor of urine, is produced in nephrons at a rate of about 125 mL/min/1.73 m².

Kidney disease can be caused by acute or chronic conditions. Acute conditions are often associated with bacterial infections, obstruction in the urinary tract, or damage to the renal parenchyma. Chronic kidney disease (CKD) is defined as the presence of kidney damage or decreased function, present for 3 months or longer. CKD results from direct damage to nephrons or from progressive, chronic bilateral deterioration of nephrons. In CKD, the kidney damage is rarely repaired; thus, progressive disease (i.e., uremia and kidney failure) can lead to death. The rate of destruction and severity of disease depend on the underlying causative disorders and contributing factors, with diabetes and hypertension recognized as the primary etiologies.

DEFINITION

The National Kidney Foundation defines a five-stage classification system for CKD (Table 12.1) based on the glomerular filtration rate (GFR). *Stage 1* is characterized by normal or only slightly increased GFR associated with some degree of kidney damage. This stage (>90 mL/min) usually is asymptomatic, with a slight (10%–20%) decline in renal function. *Stage 2* is marked by a mildly decreased GFR (60–89 mL/min) and persistent proteinuria. *Stage 3* is evidenced as a moderately decreased GFR (30–59 mL/min), with loss of 50% or more of normal renal function. Upon arriving at Stage 3, persons are at higher risk for progressive CKD. *Stage 4* is defined by a severely decreased GFR (15–29 mL/min). *Stage 5*, also known as *end-stage renal disease (ESRD)* or *renal failure*, is associated with a GFR <15 mL/min, wherein 75% or more of the approximately two million nephrons have lost function. Patients in Stage 5 require dialysis or transplant for survival.

As kidney disease progresses (Stages 2–5), nitrogen products accumulate in the blood, and fewer excretory, endocrine, and metabolic functions are performed by the kidneys, with eventual loss of the ability to maintain normal homeostasis. The resultant clinical syndrome—caused by renal failure, retention of excretory products, and interference with endocrine and metabolic functions—is called *uremia*.

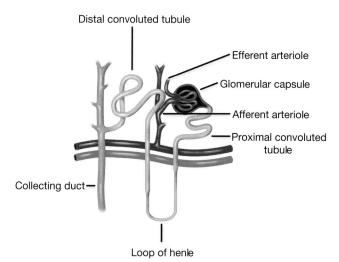

FIG. 12.1 The nephron. (Courtesy of Matt Hazzard, University of Kentucky.)

| TABLE 12.1 | Classification of Stages of Chronic Kidney Disease (CKD) and Associated Comorbid Conditions |

CKD Stage	Description	GFR (mL/min/1.73 m²)	Frequency of Comorbid Conditions
1	Chronic kidney damage; normal or ↑ GFR	≥90	Anemia: 4% HTN: 40% DM: 9%
2	Mild ↓ GFR	60–89	Anemia: 4% HTN: 40% DM: 13%
3	Moderate ↓ GFR	30–59	Anemia: 7%
3a		45–59	HTN: 55%
3b		30–44	DM: 20% HPT: >50% 5-yr mortality rate: 24%
4	Severe ↓ GFR	15–29	Anemia 29% HTN 77% DM 30% HPT >50% 5-yr mortality rate: 46%
5	Kidney failure— ESRD	<15 (or dialysis)	Anemia 69% HTN 75% DM 40% HPT >50% 5-yr mortality rate: >50%

DM, diabetes mellitus; *ESRD*, end-stage renal disease; *GFR*, glomerular filtration rate; *HPT*, hyperparathyroidism; *HTN*, hypertension.
Data from Mitch WE. Chronic kidney disease. In Goldman L, Ausiello D, eds. *Goldman-Cecil medicine*, 25th ed. Philadelphia, PA: Saunders; 2016:833–41.

EPIDEMIOLOGY

More than 35 million people (an estimated 15% of the adult population) in the United States have some form of kidney disease. The early stages of CKD (Stages 1–3) tend to be asymptomatic and constitute 96.5% of the disease. However, more than 661,000 people have ESRD, and each year more than 100,000 new cases of kidney failure are diagnosed.

CKD often develops between the ages of 45 and 64 years, although about 10% of patients are under the age of 18 years. CKD is observed most frequently in patients older than 65 years of age and in those who have diabetes and hypertension. CKD occurs more commonly in men and those with health disparities including Hispanics, African, Native, and Asian Americans. The higher prevalence of CKD in persons suffering from health disparities is often associated with differences in historical events, socioeconomic status, environmental influences, and personal behaviors.

CKD has established associations with cardiovascular disease, diabetes, and aging. Laboratory findings consistent with Stage 3 or higher CKD are present in 14% of persons with hypertension without diabetes, 20% of persons with diabetes, and 25% of persons older than 70 years of age. Approximately 50,000 Americans die annually as a result of kidney failure, mostly caused by cardiovascular system–related disease. The average dental practice that treats 2000 adults is likely to include 220 patients with physiologic evidence of CKD.

ETIOLOGY

ESRD is caused by conditions that destroy nephrons. The four most common causes of ESRD are diabetes mellitus (44%), hypertension (28%), chronic glomerulonephritis (16%), and polycystic kidney disease (4.5%). Other common causes, in decreasing order, are tubular interstitial nephritis, systemic lupus erythematosus, neoplasm, obstructive nephropathies, and acquired immunodeficiency syndrome nephropathy. Hereditary and environmental factors such as amyloidosis, congenital disease, hyperlipidemia, immunoglobulin A nephropathy, and silica and smoke exposure also contribute to the disease. Age older than 60 years is the highest risk factor for CKD.

PATHOPHYSIOLOGY AND COMPLICATIONS

The kidneys filter about 180 L/day through the function of approximately two million nephrons. Deterioration and destruction of functioning nephrons are the underlying pathologic processes of renal failure. The nephron includes the glomerulus, tubules, and vasculature. Various diseases affect different segments of the nephron at first, but the entire nephron eventually is affected. For example, whereas hypertension affects the vasculature first, glomerulonephritis affects the glomeruli first.

Importantly, nephrons that are lost are not replaced. However, because of compensatory hypertrophy of the remaining nephrons, normal renal function is maintained for a time. During this period of relative renal insufficiency, homeostasis is preserved. The patient remains asymptomatic and demonstrates minimal laboratory abnormalities such as a diminished GFR. Normal function is maintained until greater than 50% of nephrons are destroyed. Subsequently, compensatory mechanisms are overwhelmed, and the signs and symptoms of uremia appear. In terms of morphology, the end-stage kidney is markedly reduced in size, scarred, and nodular (Fig. 12.2).

A patient in early renal failure may remain asymptomatic, but physiologic changes invariably develop as the disease progresses. Such changes result from the loss of nephrons. Renal tubular malfunction causes the sodium pump to lose its effectiveness, and sodium excretion occurs. Along with sodium, excessive amounts of dilute urine are excreted, which accounts for the polyuria that is commonly encountered.

Patients with advanced renal disease develop *uremia,* which is uniformly fatal if not treated. Failing kidneys are unable to concentrate and filter the intake of sodium, which contributes to the drop in urine output,

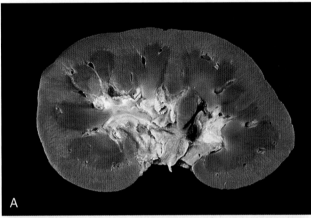

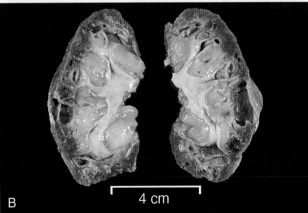

FIG. 12.2 Gross renal anatomy. (**A**) A normal kidney. (**B**) Atrophic kidneys from a patient with chronic glomerulonephritis. (From Klatt EC. *Robbins and Cotran Atlas of Pathology,* 2nd ed. Philadelphia, PA: Saunders; 2010.)

development of fluid overload, hypertension, insulin resistance, risk for severe electrolyte disturbances (sodium depletion and hyperkalemia—higher-than-normal levels of potassium), and cardiac disease. These cardiovascular system—related events cause approximately half of the deaths occurring annually among patients with ESRD.

The buildup of nonprotein nitrogen compounds in the blood, mainly urea, as a consequence of loss of glomerular filtration function, is called *azotemia.* The level of azotemia is measured as blood urea nitrogen (BUN). Acids also accumulate because of tubular impairment. The buildup of waste products serves as a substrate for the development of metabolic acidosis, and the resulting ammonia retention. In the later stages of renal failure, acidosis causes nausea, anorexia, and fatigue. Patients may hyperventilate to compensate for the metabolic acidosis. With acidosis superimposed on ESRD, adaptive mechanisms already are taxed beyond normal levels, and any increase in demand can lead to serious consequences. For example, sepsis or a febrile illness can result in profound acidosis and may be fatal.

Patients with ESRD demonstrate several hematologic abnormalities, including anemia, leukocyte and platelet dysfunction, and coagulopathy. Anemia, caused by iron deficiency, decreased erythropoietin production by the kidney, inhibition of red blood cell (RBC) production, hemolysis, bleeding episodes, and shortened RBC survival, is one of the most common manifestations of ESRD. Most of these effects result from unidentified toxic substances in uremic plasma and from other factors. Host defense is compromised by nutritional deficiencies, leukocyte dysfunction, depressed cellular immunity, and hypogammaglobulinemia. This diminished capacity leads to diminished granulocyte chemotaxis, phagocytosis, and bactericidal activity, making affected persons more susceptible to infection.

Hemorrhagic diatheses, characterized by tendency toward abnormal bleeding and bruising, are common in patients with ESRD and are attributed primarily to abnormal platelet aggregation and adhesiveness, decreased platelet factor 3, impaired prothrombin consumption, and loss of clotting factors with proteinuria. Defective platelet production also may play a role. Platelet factor 3 enhances the conversion of prothrombin to thrombin by activated factor X.

The cardiovascular system is affected by hyperlipidemia, athero- and arteriosclerosis, and arterial hypertension—the latter caused by sodium chloride retention, fluid overload, and inappropriately high renin levels. Congestive heart failure and hypertrophy of the left ventricle, which may compromise coronary artery blood flow, are relatively common developments. These complications, along with electrolyte disturbances, put patients with ESRD at increased risk for sudden death from myocardial infarction.

A variety of mineral bone disorders are seen in ESRD; these are collectively referred to as *renal osteodystrophy.*

Decreased kidney function results in decreased 1-α-hydroxylation of vitamin D, which leads to reduced intestinal absorption of calcium (thereby contributing to hypocalcemia). With advanced CKD and the loss of nephrons, renal phosphate excretion drops, and the bone attempts to buffer the acid buildup by releasing calcium and phosphates. This leads to demineralization, weak bones, and calcium–phosphate complexes in blood. The resulting low levels of serum ionized calcium stimulate the parathyroid glands to secrete parathyroid hormone (PTH), which results in *secondary hyperparathyroidism.* PTH has three main functions:

- Inhibiting the tubular reabsorption of phosphorus
- Stimulating renal production of the vitamin D necessary for calcium metabolism
- Enhancing vitamin D absorption within the intestine

High levels of PTH are sustained, however, because in ESRD the failing kidney does not synthesize 1,25-dihydroxycholecalciferol, the active metabolite of vitamin D; thus, calcium absorption in the gut is inhibited. PTH activates tumor necrosis factor and interleukin-1, which mediate bone remodeling, calcium mobilization from bones, and increased excretion of phosphorus, potentially leading to formation of renal and metastatic calcifications. Levels of fibroblast growth factor 23 (FGF-23), a key regulator of phosphorus and vitamin D metabolism, also increase and result in inhibition of osteoblast maturation and matrix mineralization. The progression of osseous changes is as follows: *osteomalacia* (increased unmineralized *osteoid* bone matrix) followed by *osteitis fibrosa* (bone resorption with lytic lesions and marrow fibrosis) (Fig. 12.3) and, finally, *osteosclerosis* of variable degree (enhanced bone density) (Fig. 12.4). With renal osteodystrophy in children, bone growth is impaired, along with a tendency for spontaneous fractures with slow healing, myopathy, aseptic necrosis of the hip, and extraosseous calcifications.

CLINICAL PRESENTATION

CKD is usually asymptomatic in its early stages. In contrast, the effects of renal failure are often widespread, vary with severity, and can involve multiple systems (e.g., >40% of patients with ESRD also have diabetes, and >25% have concurrent hypertension; Fig. 12.5).

Signs and Symptoms

Patients with CKD may show few clinical signs or symptoms until the condition progresses to Stage 3. At this stage and beyond, patients may complain of a general ill feeling, fatigue, weakness, headaches, nausea, loss of appetite, and weight loss. With further progression, anemia; leg cramps; insomnia; dark urine; and an increased need to urinate, especially at night (nocturia), often develop. The anemia produces pallor of the skin and mucous membranes and contributes to the symptoms of lethargy and dizziness.

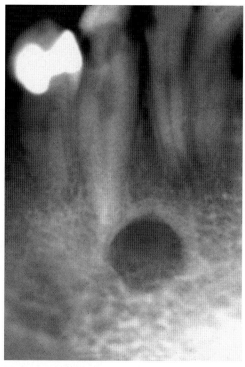

FIG. 12.3 Lytic lesion in the anterior mandible of a patient with hyperparathyroidism. (Courtesy of L.R. Bean, Lexington, KY.)

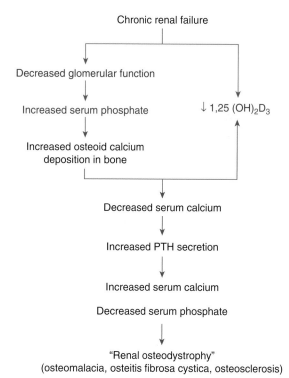

FIG. 12.4 Summary of changes that result in renal osteodystrophy. *PTH,* Parathyroid hormone.

Patients with renal failure are more likely to experience bone pain (e.g., pain in the lower back, hips, knees) and develop GI signs and symptoms such as anorexia, nausea, and vomiting, generalized gastroenteritis, and

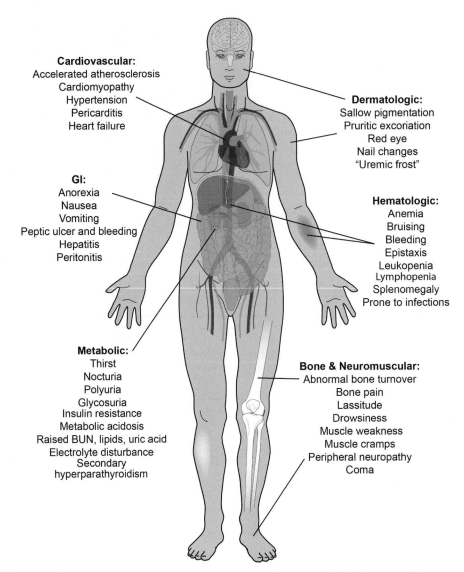

Cardiovascular:
Accelerated atherosclerosis
Cardiomyopathy
Hypertension
Pericarditis
Heart failure

GI:
Anorexia
Nausea
Vomiting
Peptic ulcer and bleeding
Hepatitis
Peritonitis

Metabolic:
Thirst
Nocturia
Polyuria
Glycosuria
Insulin resistance
Metabolic acidosis
Raised BUN, lipids, uric acid
Electrolyte disturbance
Secondary
hyperparathyroidism

Dermatologic:
Sallow pigmentation
Pruritic excoriation
Red eye
Nail changes
"Uremic frost"

Hematologic:
Anemia
Bruising
Bleeding
Epistaxis
Leukopenia
Lymphopenia
Splenomegaly
Prone to infections

Bone & Neuromuscular:
Abnormal bone turnover
Bone pain
Lassitude
Drowsiness
Muscle weakness
Muscle cramps
Peripheral neuropathy
Coma

FIG. 12.5 Clinical features of chronic renal failure. (Courtesy Matt Hazzard, University of Kentucky.)

peptic ulcer disease. Uremic syndrome commonly causes malnutrition and diarrhea. Patients can demonstrate cognitive impairment or depression or even psychotic symptoms in later stages. They also may exhibit signs of peripheral neuropathy and muscular hyperactivity (twitching, restless legs). Convulsions and cognitive impairment may be late manifestations that directly correlate with the degree of azotemia. Additional findings may include stomatitis manifested by oral ulceration and candidiasis (Fig. 12.6), parotitis, or smell and taste disturbances. A urine-like odor to the breath may be detected.

Because of bleeding diatheses that accompany ESRD, hemorrhagic episodes are common, particularly occult GI bleeding. In patients who receive dialysis, however, benefits include improved control of uremia and less severe bleeding. Skin manifestations associated with bleeding diatheses include ecchymoses, petechiae, purpura, and gingival or mucous membrane bleeding (e.g., epistaxis).

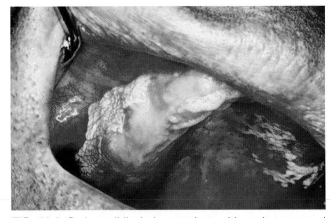

FIG. 12.6 Oral candidiasis in a patient with end-stage renal disease.

In addition, hyperpigmentation of the skin occurs with ESRD, which is characterized by a brownish-yellow appearance caused by the retention of carotene-like pigments normally excreted by the kidney. These pigments may cause profound pruritus. An occasional finding is a whitish coating on the skin of the trunk and arms produced by residual urea crystals left when perspiration evaporates ("uremic frost").

Cardiovascular manifestations of ESRD include hypertension, congestive heart failure (shortness of breath, orthopnea, dyspnea on exertion, peripheral edema), and pericarditis.

LABORATORY AND DIAGNOSTIC FINDINGS

The diagnosis of kidney disease is based on history; physical findings; laboratory evaluation; and, in select disorders, imaging and biopsy. Evaluation includes measures of blood pressure, GFR, urinalysis, serum BUN, serum creatinine, creatinine clearance (CrCl), and electrolytes.

The most basic test of kidney function is urinalysis, which is the physical, chemical, and microscopic examination of urine. Urinalysis typically looks for proteinuria, hematuria, cellular casts, specific gravity, pH, and a range of chemicals (see Fig. 12.7).

The GFR is the best measure of overall kidney function, and the most significant protein in the urine is albumin (albuminuria). Together these two measures are used to determine the severity and prognosis of CKD. Fig. 12.8 and Table 12.2 illustrate additional laboratory test results that help to measure kidney function.

Serum creatinine level is a measure of muscle breakdown and filtration capacity of the nephron. The creatinine concentration is proportional to the glomerular filtration and can be measured in serum as well as urine. The CrCl compares the creatinine concentrations in blood and urine (in a 24-h urine collection) and, like the GFR, can be determined using a variety of online calculators. BUN is a commonly used indicator of kidney function; however, it is not as specific as CrCl or serum creatinine level because BUN is also influenced by liver function and

TEST	RESULT	REFERENCE RANGE	UNITS	FLAG
PHYSICAL EXAMINATION				
Color	Yellow	Yellow		
Appearance	**Cloudy**	**Clear**		**Abnormal**
Specific gravity	1.020	1.005-1.030		
CHEMICAL EXAMINATION				
Glucose	Negative	Negative		
Bilirubin	Negative	Negative		
Ketone	Negative	Negative		
Blood	Negative	Negative		
pH	6.5	5-7.5		
Protein	Trace	Negative/Trace		
Urobilinogen	0.6	0.2-1.0	mg/dL	
Nitrite	**Positive**	**Negative**		**Abnormal**
Leukocytes	**2+**	**Negative**		**Abnormal**
MICROSCOPIC EXAMINATION				
WBC	**8-10**	**0-5**	**/HPF**	**Abnormal**
RBC	0-2	0-3	/HPF	
Epithelial Cells	0-8	0-10	/HPF	
Casts	None seen	None	/LPF	
Mucus Threads	Present	Not Established		
Bacteria	**Moderate**	**None Seen/ Few**	**/HPF**	**Abnormal**

FIG. 12.7 Typical urinalysis report. (From Health Testing Centers. 2022. HealthTeastingCenters.com. All rights reserved.)

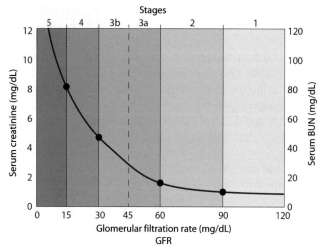

FIG. 12.8 Relationship of renal function to serum enzymes and glomerular filtration rate (GFR). Of note, patients often remain asymptomatic as renal failure develops until the GFR drops below 20 mL/min, albuminuria exceeds 300 mg/g, the creatinine clearance drops below 20 mL/min, and the blood urea nitrogen (BUN) is above 20 mg/dL. In fact, uremic syndrome is rare before the BUN concentration exceeds 60 mg/dL. (Courtesy of Matt Hazzard, University of Kentucky.)

conditions that affect blood flow. Other tests used to assess and monitor kidney disease include the concentrations of serum electrolytes involved in acid–base regulation and calcium and phosphorus metabolism (see Table 12.2), complete blood count, PTH levels, bone density measures, and urine immunoelectrophoresis.

MEDICAL MANAGEMENT

Conservative Care

Clinical practice guidelines for the management of CKD have been addressed by national and international organizations. The goals of treatment are to slow the progress of disease and to preserve the patient's quality of life. A conservative approach, which may be adequate for prolonged periods, is recommended for Stage 1 and Stage 2 CKD. Conservative care involves decreasing the retention of nitrogenous waste products and controlling hypertension, fluids, and electrolyte imbalances. These improvements are accomplished by dietary modifications, including instituting a low-protein diet and limiting fluid, sodium, and potassium intake. Comorbid conditions such as diabetes, hypertension, congestive heart failure, and hyperparathyroidism are corrected or controlled during the earliest stage possible. Anemia, malnutrition, and mineral bone disease (e.g., hyperparathyroidism) typically are managed beginning in Stage 3. By Stage 4, care by a nephrologist is recommended, and preparations for renal replacement therapy begin. In Stage 5, or when uremic features appear or intractable fluid overload occurs, dialysis is started. Renoprotective strategies for slowing progression of CKD and addressing comorbid conditions are summarized in Table 12.3.

Dialysis

Dialysis is a medical procedure that artificially filters blood. Dialysis becomes necessary when the number of nephrons diminishes to the point that azotemia is

TABLE 12.2   Laboratory Values for the Assessment of Renal Function and Failure

Laboratory Test	Reference Value	Indicator* of Renal Insufficiency (Stages II–IV)	Indicator of Renal Failure (Stage V)
Urine			
Albuminuria	<30 mg/g	30–300 mg/g	>300 mg/g
Creatinine clearance (CrCl)	85–125 mL/min (women) 97–140 mL/min[34]	50–90 mL/min	Moderate: 10–50 mL/min; severe: <10 mL/min
Glomerular filtration rate (GFR)[†]	100–150 mL/min	15–89 mL/min	Moderate: <15 mL/min; severe: <10 mL/min
Serum			
Blood urea nitrogen (BUN)	8–18 mg/dL (3–6.5 mmol/L)	20–30 mg/dL	Moderate: 30–50 mg/dL; severe: >50 mg/dL
Creatinine	0.6–1.20 mg/dL	2–3 mg/dL	Moderate: 3–6 mg/dL; severe: >6 mg/dL

*Secondary indicators of renal function. Normal reference values: calcium, 8.2–11.2 mg/dL; chloride, 95–103 mmol/L; inorganic phosphorus, 2.7–4.5 mg/dL; potassium, 3.8–5 mmol/L; sodium, 136–142 mmol/L; total carbon dioxide for venous blood, 22–26 mmol/L; and uric acid, 2.4–7.0 mg/dL.

[†]GFR is often calculated using the Cockcroft–Gault equation, the Modification of Diet in Renal Disease (MDRD) Study equation, or the Chronic Kidney Disease Epidemiology Collaboration (CKD-EPI) equation. https://www-uptodate-com.ezproxy.uky.edu/contents/calculator-glomerular-filtration-rate-estimate-by-abbreviated-mdrd-study-equation-in-adults?search=Kidney%20disease%20drug%20adjustment&topicRef=114914&source=see_link.

Adapted from National Kidney Foundation. K/DOQI clinical practice guidelines for chronic kidney disease: evaluation, classification, and stratification. *Am J Kidney Dis.* 2002;39:S1–S266 and Evaluation and management of chronic kidney disease: synopsis of the kidney disease: improving global outcomes 2012 clinical practice guideline. *Ann Intern Med.* 2013;158:825–30.

TABLE 12.3 Renoprotective Strategies for Slowing Progression* of Chronic Kidney Disease and Addressing Comorbid Conditions

Parameter	Goal	Intervention
Lifestyle modifications	Smoking cessation, achieving ideal body weight, exercising for 30 min 5× week	Counseling, exercise program, medical appointments every 3—6 months
Lipid lowering	LDL <100 mg/dL	Dietary counseling, statins
Blood pressure control (mm Hg)	<130/80 mm Hg for proteinuria with excretion <1 g protein/day; <125/75 mm Hg for proteinuria with excretion >1 g/day	ACE inhibitors, ARBs, sodium, restriction, diuretics, beta-blockers
Dietary protein and potassium restriction	<2 g/day and 40—70 mEq/day, respectively	Dietary counseling
Reduction in proteinuria	<0.5 g/day	ACE inhibitors, ARBs
Glycemic control	HgbA$_{1c}$ <7%	Dietary counseling, oral hypoglycemic agents, insulin
Anemia management	Hemoglobin 10—12 g/dL; serum ferritin concentration <100 ng/mL	Oral iron preparations, or injections of ferumoxytol IV (Feraheme), or recombinant human erythropoietin (epoetin alfa [Procrit, Epogen] or darbepoetin alfa [Aranesp]), or HIF stabilizers
Control of PTH levels to prevent secondary hyperparathyroidism	PTH: Stage 3, 35—70 pg/mL; Stage 4, 70—110 pg/mL; Stage 5, 150—300 pg/mL	Low-phosphate diet + use of nonaluminum phosphate binders (e.g., calcium carbonate) + vitamin D analogue

*One-third of Stage 4 CKD patients will progress to ESRD within 3 years.
ACE, angiotensin-converting enzyme; *ARB,* angiotensin receptor blocker; *HgbA$_{1c}$,* hemoglobin A1c; *HIF,* hypoxia-inducible factor; *IV,* intravenous; *LDL,* low-density lipoprotein; *PTH,* parathyroid hormone.
Adapted from Carey WD. *Cleveland Clinic: Current Clinical Medicine,* 2nd ed. St. Louis, MO: Saunders; 2010 and Abboud H, Henrich WL. Clinical practice. Stage IV chronic kidney disease. *N Engl J Med.* 2010;362:56—65; Macdougall IC. Intravenous iron use in the care of patients with kidney disease. Clin J Amer Soc Nephrol. 2019;14(10):1528—1530.

unpreventable or uncontrollable. The initiation of dialysis is an individual patient decision that becomes important when the GFR drops below 30 mL/min/1.73 m². About 468,000 people receive dialysis in the United States, at a cost of more than $28 billion a year. The procedure can be accomplished by peritoneal dialysis or hemodialysis.

Peritoneal dialysis is performed on about 36,000 Americans. It may be provided as continuous ambulatory peritoneal dialysis (CAPD) or automated peritoneal dialysis (APD). With both modalities, a hypertonic solution is instilled into the peritoneal cavity through a permanent peritoneal catheter. After a time, the solution and dissolved solutes (e.g., urea) are drawn out.

CAPD is the more commonly used procedure. Dialysis performed using this method (Fig. 12.9) requires shorter exchange periods of 30—45 min four to five times per day. Exchanges are performed manually, with instillation of 1.5—3 L of dialysate into the peritoneal cavity. The catheter is sealed, and every 3—6 h, the dialysate is allowed to drain into a bag strapped to the patient, and new dialysate is instilled by gravity. APD, in contrast, uses a machine to perform three to five dialysate exchanges at night while the patient sleeps (for 8—10 h). During the day, excretory fluids accumulate in the patient's abdomen until dialysis is repeated that evening.

The advantages of peritoneal dialysis are its relatively low initial cost, ease of performance, reduced likelihood of infectious disease transmission, and absence of requirement for anticoagulation. Disadvantages include the need for frequent sessions, risk of peritonitis (≈1 case per patient every 1.5 years), frequent association with abdominal hernia, and significantly lower effectiveness than that for hemodialysis. Its principal use is in patients in acute renal failure or those who require only occasional dialysis.

In the United States, most dialysis patients (88%) receive hemodialysis. Hemodialysis is the method of choice when azotemia occurs and dialysis is needed on a long-term basis. Treatments are performed every 2 or 3 days, generally in a dialysis center depending on need. Usually 3—4 h is required for each session (Fig. 12.10).

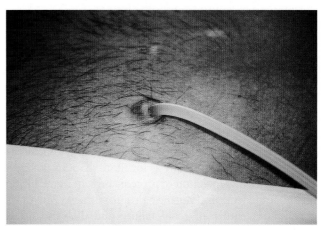

FIG. 12.9 Chronic ambulatory peritoneal dialysis catheter site in the abdominal wall. (From Lewis SM, Dirksen SR, Heitkemper MM, et al. *Medical Surgical Nursing,* 8th ed, St. Louis, MO, 2011. Courtesy of Mary Jo Holechek, Baltimore, MD.)

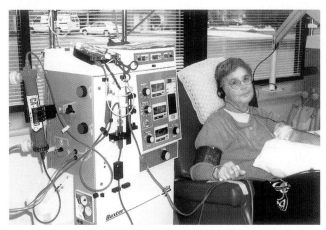

FIG. 12.10 Patient undergoing hemodialysis. (From Ignatavicius D, Workman ML. *Medical-Surgical Nursing: Patient-Centered Collaborative Care*, 6th ed. St. Louis, MO: Saunders; 2010.)

Hemodialysis consumes an enormous amount of the patient's time and is extremely confining. However, between dialysis sessions, patients lead relatively normal lives. Home hemodialysis offers an alternative to dialysis in a clinic setting and is used by about 3% of patients (see www.kidney.org/atoz/content/homehemo for more information).

More than 80% of the people who receive hemodialysis in the United States do so through a permanent and surgically created arteriovenous graft or fistula, usually placed in the forearm. Access is achieved by cannulation of the fistula with a large-gauge needle (Fig. 12.11). Approximately 18% of patients receive dialysis through a temporary or permanent central catheter while the permanent access site is healing or when all other access options have been exhausted. Patients are "plugged in" to the hemodialysis machine at the fistula or graft site, and blood is passed through the machine, filtered, and returned to the patient. Heparin usually is administered during the procedure to prevent clotting.

Although hemodialysis is a lifesaving technique, dialysis provides only about 15% of normal renal function, and complications develop as a result of the procedure. Serum calcium concentrations require close regulation that is achieved using calcium supplements, active forms of vitamin D (i.e., calcitriol, alfacalcidol, paricalcitol, or doxercalciferol), or dialysate that contains calcium. Improper blood levels contribute to muscle tetany and oversecretion of PTH. Dialysis-related amyloidosis is common in persons on dialysis for more than 5 years as a consequence of deposition of proteins present in the blood on joints and tendons, causing pain and stiffness. Anemia is a common feature of renal failure and dialysis and is treated with erythropoiesis-stimulating drugs (Table 12.3). The risk of hepatitis B, hepatitis C, and human immunodeficiency virus (HIV) infections is increased because dialyzers usually are disinfected—not sterilized—between uses, and patients usually have multiple blood exposures.

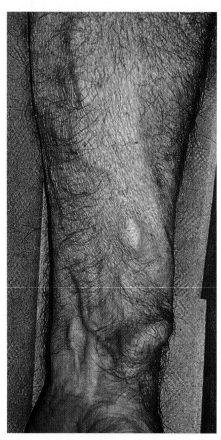

FIG. 12.11 Site of a surgically created arteriovenous fistula, with subsequent dilation and hypertrophy of the veins. (From Kumar P, Clark ML. *Kumar and Clark's Clinical Medicine*, 7th ed. Edinburgh: Saunders; 2009.)

National surveys report that among patients maintained on hemodialysis, the prevalence of hepatitis B surface antigen positivity (carriers of hepatitis B) ranges near 1.0%; of hepatitis C seropositive status, 5%–10%; and of HIV seropositivity, 1.5%. Although all three viruses constitute a reservoir of potential infection, only hepatitis B virus and hepatitis C virus have been reported to be transmitted nosocomially in dialysis centers in the United States.

Infection of the arteriovenous fistula is a possibility and can result in septicemia, septic emboli, infective endarteritis, and infective endocarditis. *Staphylococcus aureus* is the most common cause of vascular access infection and related bacteremia in these patients. The risk of fistula infection from surgical procedures (e.g., urogenital, oral surgical, dental) is considered to be low. A related concern is risk for infection and antibiotic-resistant infection. Of note, rates of tuberculosis and vancomycin- and methicillin-resistant infections are higher among patients maintained on long-term hemodialysis than in the general public.

As with all patients with ESRD, drugs that are metabolized primarily by the kidney or that are nephrotoxic must be avoided in patients receiving dialysis.

Another problem associated with dialysis is abnormal bleeding. Patients with ESRD have bleeding tendencies secondary to altered platelet aggregation and decreased platelet factor 3. Hemodialysis is associated with the additional problem of platelet destruction by mechanical trauma of the procedure. Aluminum contamination of the dialysate water may interfere with heme synthesis, contributing to the development of anemia and osteomalacia. Also, the process of hemodialysis may activate prostaglandin I_2 (prostacyclin), which can reduce platelet aggregation.

The 5-year survival rate of dialysis patients is 42%. An expected 7.1 years of remaining life occurs on average when dialysis is begun between age 50 and 54 years. An alternative to long-term dialysis is renal transplantation (see Chapter 21). There are approximately 193,000 people who have a functioning transplanted kidney and another 100,000 on the waiting list for a kidney transplant. Transplantation provides an average of 17.2 years of expected life remaining but also is associated with a significant number of issues.

DENTAL MANAGEMENT

Patient Under Conservative Care

Medical Considerations

Identification. The National Kidney Foundation's guidelines recommend that high-risk groups (i.e., patients with diabetes and hypertension) be screened for CKD. Thus, medical referrals should be made for screening when diabetes or hypertension are present and when other known risk factors are present (e.g., patients who are obese, smoke, have cardiovascular disease, or have family members with ESRD). Likewise, any patient who has signs and symptoms of kidney disease (e.g., hematuria, repeated urinary tract infections or edema) but has not been assessed should be referred to a physician for diagnosis and treatment. This simple step in coordinating care can improve the patient's awareness of his or her health and minimize patient morbidity and mortality associated with CKD.

Risk Assessment. Risk assessment begins with knowing the patient's GFR, the stage of CKD, and the extent of albuminuria. With CKD graded Stage 1–3, problems generally do not arise in the provision of outpatient dental care if the patient's disease is well controlled and conservative medical care is being provided. With CKD of Stage 4 or higher, consultation with the patient's physician is suggested before dental care is provided. If the patient is in advanced stages of renal failure or has another comorbid condition (e.g., diabetes mellitus, hypertension, systemic lupus erythematosus) or if severe albuminuria or electrolyte imbalance is present, dental care may best be provided after physician consultation in a hospital-like setting. Deferral of treatment may be required until the status of the patient has been ascertained and the CKD is adequately controlled (Box 12.1).

Recommendations. In developing recommendations for dental patients who have kidney disease, the dentist must consider the type and degree of kidney dysfunction, the medical care being provided, and the dental procedure planned.

Antibiotics. Patients who have CKD (Stages 1–3) and are not receiving dialysis generally have few issues with infection, so they generally do not require additional antibiotic considerations. However, when invasive procedures are planned for a patient with CKD in Stage 4 or 5, the dentist should consult with the physician to assess the need for antibiotics. Alterations in drug dosage may be needed, depending on the amount of renal function retained. If an orofacial infection occurs, aggressive management with the use of culture and sensitivity testing and appropriate antibiotics is generally necessary.

Bleeding. Because of the potential for bleeding problems, if an invasive procedure is planned, the patient should undergo pretreatment screening for bleeding disorders, and a platelet count should be obtained. The hematocrit level and hemoglobin count also should be obtained for assessment of anemia. Any abnormal values should be discussed with the physician. Few problems are encountered with nonhemorrhagic dental procedures when the hematocrit level is above 25%. If bleeding is anticipated, hematocrit levels can be raised with the use of erythropoiesis-stimulating agents under the guidance of the physician. A less desirable option is RBC transfusion, which carries the risks of sensitization and bloodborne infection.

When surgical procedures are undertaken, meticulous attention to good surgical technique is necessary to decrease the risks of excessive bleeding and infection. Local hemostatic agents (topical thrombin, microfibrillar collagen, absorbable gelatin sponge, suture) should be available and used during dental surgical procedures performed on patients with uremia. Desmopressin should be avoided. Conjugated estrogens are helpful when a longer duration of action is required; however, 1 week of therapy usually is needed to guarantee efficacy. High-purity plasma-derived products such as cryoprecipitate (a plasma derivative rich in factor VIII, fibrinogen, and fibronectin) may be used in refractory cases in consultation with the patient's hematologist. Platelet transfusions are used infrequently because of the associated risk of immunogenic sensitization.

Blood Pressure. When dental treatment is provided on an outpatient basis, blood pressure should be closely monitored before and during the procedure. Patients should be informed that good control of blood pressure will benefit both kidney and overall health.

Capacity to Tolerate Care. In patients whose kidney function is deteriorating (GFR <50 mL/min), elective dental care should be delayed until consultation is obtained and the patient is medically stable. Patients who take large doses of corticosteroids (e.g., ≥10 mg/day of prednisone or equivalent), as may be prescribed for medical management of ESRD, can develop adrenal insufficiency. To avoid an adrenal crisis in patients on such regimens, the dental clinician should ensure that the usual corticosteroid dose is taken before surgical procedures and monitor the patient closely during the postsurgical phase of care (see Chapter 15).

Drug Considerations. A major concern in the treatment of patients with ESRD is the potential for toxic effects on the kidneys and other adverse effects associated with drugs prescribed by the health care provider. Accordingly, dentists should know which drugs to use, which to avoid, and the correct drug dosage for the patient situation (Table 12.4). Some drugs are excreted primarily by the kidneys, and certain agents are inherently nephrotoxic. As a general rule, drugs excreted by the kidneys are eliminated twofold less efficiently when the GFR drops to 50 mL/min and thus may reach toxic levels at lower GFR. In such circumstances, the drug dosage needs to be reduced, and the timing of administration must be prolonged. Nephrotoxic drugs such as acyclovir, aminoglycosides, aspirin, nonsteroidal antiinflammatory drugs (NSAIDs), and tetracycline should generally be avoided in patients with renal impairment. NSAIDs inhibit prostaglandin synthesis, resulting in vasoconstriction and reduced renal perfusion. Acetaminophen also is nephrotoxic and may cause renal tubular necrosis at high doses, but it is probably safer than aspirin in these patients when used for a short time frame because acetaminophen is metabolized in the liver. An alternative analgesic is tramadol. Tetracyclines, except for doxycycline, worsen renal impairment by inhibiting protein synthesis and have been associated with kidney deterioration in the dental setting.

Drug frequency and dosage adjustments are required during advanced CKD for reasons besides nephrotoxicity and renal metabolism. For example, (1) a low serum albumin value reduces the number of binding sites for circulating drugs, thereby enhancing drug effects; (2) uremia can modify hepatic metabolism of drugs (increasing or decreasing clearance); (3) antacids can affect acid–base or electrolyte balance, further complicating uremic effects on electrolyte balance; (4) larger initial doses may be required in the presence of substantial edema or ascites, whereas smaller initial doses may be required if dehydration or severe debilitation is present; and (5) aspirin and other NSAIDs potentiate uremic platelet defects, so these antiplatelet agents may need to be avoided if invasive procedures are performed (see Table 12.4).

Nitrous oxide and diazepam are antianxiety agents that require little modification for use in patients with ESRD. However, the hematocrit or hemoglobin concentration should be measured before intravenous sedation, and the oxygen saturation measured before and during sedation to ensure adequate oxygenation. Drugs that depress the central nervous system (barbiturates,

narcotics) are best avoided in the presence of uremia because the blood–brain barrier may not be intact, so excessive sedation may result. Opioid use, if needed, requires dosage adjustment for CKD patients, and meperidine should be avoided in patients with CKD because its metabolite can accumulate, leading to seizures. When the hemoglobin concentration is below 10 g/100 mL, general anesthesia is not recommended for patients with ESRD.

Oral Complications and Manifestations. Box 12.2 lists some common oral manifestations of chronic renal failure. A red-orange discoloration of the cheeks and mucosa is associated with pruritus, and deposition of carotene-like pigments appears when renal filtration is decreased. Salivary flow may be diminished, resulting in xerostomia and parotid infections. Candidiasis is more frequent when salivary flow is diminished. Patients frequently complain of an altered or metallic taste, and saliva is altered in composition, has a higher pH, and may have a characteristic ammonia-like odor, which results from a high urea content. Poor oral hygiene, halitosis, gingivitis, periodontal disease, and tooth loss are more common in patients with Stage 3 or higher CKD.

Uremic stomatitis is a rare condition generally associated with acute renal failure (i.e., when BUN levels are >55 mg/dL). Early changes typically include red, burning mucosa covered with gray exudates and later by frank ulceration. Adherent white patches called *uremic frost* caused by urea crystal deposition are more common on the skin but may be seen on the oral mucosa and can resemble hairy leukoplakia. Bleeding tendencies are evident as petechiae and ecchymoses on the labial and buccal mucosa, soft palate, and margins of the tongue and as gingival bleeding (Fig. 12.12).

Tooth-specific changes may be seen. Enamel hypoplasia and hypocalcification are evident when ESRD begins at an early age. In the developing dentition, red-brown discoloration and a slight delay in eruption have been reported. Tooth erosion from persistent vomiting may be seen. Pulp narrowing or obliteration has been documented. Caries, however, is not a feature because salivary urea inhibits the metabolic end products of bacterial plaque and increases the buffering capacity of saliva, thus preventing a drop in pH sufficient to attain cariogenic levels.

Specific osseous changes of the jaws accompany chronic renal failure. The classical osseous changes described is the triad of loss of lamina dura, demineralized bone (resulting in a "ground-glass" appearance), and localized and expansile radiolucent jaw lesions (central giant cell granulomas, also called brown tumors), the latter from secondary hyperparathyroidism. Other osseous findings include widened trabeculations, loss of cortication, calcified extraction sites (so-called "socket sclerosis"), and metastatic calcifications within soft tissue and the skull. Vascular calcifications of the carotid arteries are common.

TABLE 12.4 Drug Adjustments in Chronic Renal Disease

Drug and Usual Dose	Dosage Adjustment for Renal Failure[a]		Removed by Dialysis
	GFR (ML/MIN)		
	10–50	**<10**	
Analgesics			
Acetaminophen 650 mg q4h	No adjustment needed	q8h	HD: Yes PD: No
Aspirin 650 mg q6h	50%	Avoid	Yes[b]
Celecoxib (Celebrex) 100–200 mg q12h	Avoid if GFR <30 mL/min	Avoid	No
Codeine 30–60 mg q4–6h	75%	Avoid	No
Ibuprofen (Motrin) 400–800 mg q8h	No adjustment needed	Avoid	No
Meperidined (Demerol) 50 mg q4h	75%	50%	No
Tramadol *(Ultram) 50–100 mg q6h*	q6–12h	50% q12h	No[a]
Anesthetics			
Articaine, lidocaine, mepivacaine, prilocaine	No adjustment needed	No	ND
Adjunctive analgesic			
Gabapentin (Neurontin) 200–600 mg q8h	200–600 mg q12–24h	<100 mg once daily	Yes[b]
Antimicrobials			
Acyclovir–*(Zovirax) 200–800 mg q4h*	q8h	q12h	Yes[b]
Amoxicillin *500 mg q8h*	q8–12h	q12–24h	Yes[a]
Azithromycin (Zithromax) 250–500 mg q24h	No adjustment needed	Avoid	ND
Cephalexin *(Keflex) 250–500 mg q6h*	q6–8h	q12–24h	Yes[b]
Clarithromycin 250 mg q12h	50%–100% q12h	50% q12h	ND
Clindamycin (Cleocin) 150–300 mg q6h	No adjustment needed	No	ND
Doxycycline (Vibramycin) 100 mg q12h	No adjustment needed	No	ND
Erythromycin 250–500 mg q6h	No adjustment needed	No	ND
Fluconazole *(Diflucan) 100–200 mg q24h*	50%	25%	Yes[b]
Metronidazole (Flagyl) 250–500 mg q8–12h	No adjustment needed	Yes[a]	ND
Tetracycline[c] *(Sumycin, Aureomycin) 250–500 mg q6–12h*	Avoid	Avoid	No
Benzodiazepine			
Diazepam (Valium),[d] 2–5 mg q12h, triazolam (Halcion) 0.125 mg at bedtime	No adjustment needed	No	ND
Corticosteroid			
Dexamethasone, hydrocortisone, prednisone 5–10 mg/day	No adjustment needed	No	ND
Sedative Hypnotic			
Chloral hydrate 250–500 mg/day	Contraindicated	Yes	ND

[a]25% means 25% of usual dosage.
[b]Supplement Dose After Hemodialysis.
[c]Acyclovir, tetracyclines, and aminoglycosides are nephrotoxic and should be avoided in patients with chronic kidney disease (CKD). Cevimeline (Evoxac), ceftriaxone, clindamycin, nafcillin, penicillin G, penicillin VK, and pilocarpine (Salagen) do not need dosage adjustment during CKD. Nonsteroidal antiinflammatory drugs can aggravate sodium retention and edema; full-dose aspirin can aggravate coagulopathy.
[d]Use with great caution. Active metabolites can accumulate in renal failure; reduce dose if drug will be given longer than a few days.
Italicized drugs are metabolized by the kidney.
GFR, glomerular filtration rate; *HD*, hemodialysis; *ND*, no data, *PD*, peritoneal dialysis; *q*, every.
Modified from Aronoff GR, Bennett WM, Berns JS, et al. *Drug Prescribing in Renal Failure: Dosing Guidelines for Adults and Children*, 5th ed. Philadelphia, PA: American College of Physicians; 2007 and Golightly LK, Teitelbaum I, Kiser TH, Levin DA et al., eds. *Renal Pharmacology*, New York, NY: Springer; 2013.

Patients with CKD who take calcium channel blocker (a hypotensive medication) may exhibit gingival enlargement. This condition also is seen in renal transplant recipients who take cyclosporine. The clinical presentation is similar to that caused by phenytoin (Dilantin).

BOX 12.1	Checklist for Dental Management of Patients With End-Stage Renal Disease

UNDER CONSERVATIVE CARE*

Preoperative Risk Assessment
- Review medical history, determine whether renal disease exists, and discuss relevant issues with the patient.
- Identify all medications and drugs being taken or supposed to be taken by the patient.
- Examine the patient for signs and symptoms of disease and obtain vital signs.
- Review recent laboratory test results or images required to assess risk.
- Confirm patient has a primary care provider and has taken medication(s) today.
- Obtain a medical consultation (i.e., refer to physician) if the patient is poorly controlled or if signs and symptoms point to an undiagnosed condition.
- If BP and vital signs are well controlled, routine dental procedures can be performed without special precautions.

A	
Analgesics	Dosage adjustment likely when GFR is <50 mL/min. Avoid long-term use of NSAIDs in CKD. Avoid narcotics in CKD because these drugs can cause prolonged sedation and respiratory depression.
Antibiotics	Dosage adjustments likely when GFR is <50 mL/min. Aggressively manage orofacial infections with culture and sensitivity testing and antibiotics. Consider hospitalization for severe infection or major procedures. A loading dose may be required when infection and CKD are concurrent.
Anesthetics (local)	Dosage adjustment generally is not required.
Antianxiety	Dosage adjustment for single-dose benzodiazepines is not necessary.

B	
Bleeding	Screen for bleeding disorder before invasive procedures. Pay meticulous attention to good surgical technique. Excessive bleeding may occur in the patient with untreated or poorly controlled CKD. Use topical hemostatic agents.
Blood pressure	Monitor BP closely because hypertension is common in CKD. Refer patient for physician evaluation if BP is elevated.

C	
Chair position	If patient is on antihypertensive medication, assist her or him to regain equilibrium in upright position before exiting dental chair.

D	
Devices	No issues.
Drugs (interactions, allergies, or supplementation)	Adjust dosage of drugs metabolized by the kidney when GFR is <50 mL/min, per Table 12.4. Avoid nephrotoxic drugs (aminoglycosides, acetaminophen in high doses, acyclovir, aspirin, other NSAIDs, tetracycline).

E	
Emergencies	Minimize risk for emergencies by avoiding invasive procedures and long appointments if disease is unstable (poorly controlled) or advanced (CKD Stage 3 or higher).

Receiving Hemodialysis

Preoperative risk assessment
- Same as for conservative care recommendations.
- Also determine liver function status and assess for presence of opportunistic infection in these patients because of increased risk for development of carrier state with hepatitis B and C viruses and human immunodeficiency virus.

Operative Concerns: Same as for conservative care recommendations, plus the following:

A	
Antibiotics	Consider antimicrobial prophylaxis if abscess is present (based on guidelines; see Box 12.3).

D	
Day of appointment	Avoid dental care on day of hemodialysis (especially within first 6 h afterward); best to treat on day after.
Devices	Avoid arm with AV shunt for blood pressure measurements. Avoid arm with AV shunt for delivery of IV medications (see Box 12.3).
Drugs (interactions, allergies, or supplementation)	Adjust drug dosages based on Table 12.4. Consider corticosteroid supplementation if indicated (see Table 15.2).

F	
Follow-up	• Patients who have had CKD should be contacted to ensure that the postoperative course proceeds without complications. • Ensure patient is receiving regular follow-up evaluation by physician.

*Strength of Recommendation Taxonomy (SORT) Grade: C (see Preface for further explanation).
AV, arteriovenous; *BP*, blood pressure; *CKD*, chronic kidney disease; *GFR*, glomerular filtration rate; *NSAID*, nonsteroidal antiinflammatory drug.

Treatment Planning Modifications. Persons with CKD often exhibit evidence of poor oral hygiene, low salivary flow, and unmet dental needs. In these patients, the goal of restoring dental health must address these factors while balancing their medical needs. Oral hygiene instruction and frequent periodic recall appointments are important for the maintenance of long-term oral health. Meticulous oral hygiene, frequent professional

---

BOX 12.2   **Oral Manifestations of Chronic Kidney Failure**

- Pallor; pigmentation, and petechiae (also ecchymosis) of oral mucosa
- Dry mouth (xerostomia), altered taste (dysgeusia), halitosis
- Infections: candidiasis, periodontitis, parotid infections
- Enamel defects of developing dentition (hypoplasia and hypocalcification)
- Osteodystrophy (radiolucent jaw lesions)
- Uremic stomatitis[a]

[a]Noted in severe end-stage renal disease.
Data from Proctor R, Kumar N, Stein A, et al. Oral and dental aspects of chronic renal failure. *J Dent Res.* 2005;84:199−208 and Patil S, Khaandelwal S, Doni B, et al. Oral manifestations in chronic renal failure patients attending two hospitals in North Karnataka, India. *Oral Health Dent Manag.* 2012;11:100−106.

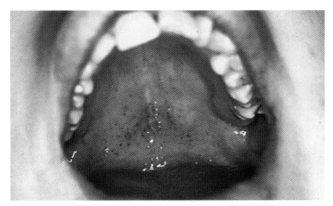

FIG. 12.12 Palatal petechiae in a patient with end-stage renal disease.

prophylaxis, and antiplaque measures (chlorhexidine or triclosan rinses) also help to reduce the effects of drug-induced gingival enlargement in transplant recipients taking cyclosporine. When an acceptable level of oral hygiene has been established, no contraindication exists to routine dental care, provided that proper attention is paid to the systemic health of the patient.

Patients Receiving Dialysis

Medical Considerations

Risk Assessment. In assessing risk for dental patients with kidney disease who receive dialysis, the dentist must consider the type dialysis, degree of kidney dysfunction, comorbidities (anemia, bone involvement, altered immune function and hemostasis), oral health status, and the dental procedure planned. For example, peritoneal dialysis presents no additional problems with respect to dental management. However, this is not the case with patients who are receiving hemodialysis (see Box 12.1). The arteriovenous fistula surgically created for the dialysis procedure in these patients is susceptible to infection (endarteritis) and may become a source of bacteremia, resulting in infective endocarditis. Infective endocarditis has been associated with hemodialysis even in the absence of preexisting cardiac defects. Although the risk

factors for infective endocarditis in this setting have not been fully established, altered host defenses, altered cardiac output and mechanical stresses, and bacterial seeding and growth on the shunt are recognized as important.

Infective endocarditis occurs in 2%−9% of patients receiving hemodialysis. This rate is significantly higher than that reported in persons with rheumatic heart disease. Most such infections are secondary to spread of staphylococcal infections that develop at the site of the graft, fistula, or catheter. Approximately 10%−17% of cases are caused by organisms that can arise from the oropharynx (*Streptococcus viridans, Lactobacillus* spp.). The following devices are considered to place the patient at increased risk for bacterial seeding over that associated with primary arteriovenous fistulas: dual-lumen cuffed venous catheters and polytetrafluoroethylene grafts, newly placed grafts, and long-term catheters.

Recommendations

Antibiotics. On the basis of an apparently low risk associated with oral bacteria, the current American Heart Association's guidelines do not include a recommendation for prophylactic antibiotics before invasive dental procedures are performed on patients with intravascular access devices to prevent endarteritis or infective endocarditis except if an abscess is being incised and drained (Box 12.3). This position is supported by systematic reviews of the literature.

Risk of Infection. Patients who are dependent on long-term dialysis, especially those with diabetes, are prone to infection. In addition, rates of tuberculosis and vancomycin- and methicillin-resistant infections are higher among such patients than in the general public. Thus, efforts should be directed at identifying signs of orofacial infections and eliminating oral sources of infection. Selection of antibiotics for hemodialysis patients with oral infections should be prudent and based on appropriate criteria (see Table 12.4).

BOX 12.3   **Antibiotic Prophylaxis Recommendations for Use With Existing Nonvalvular Cardiovascular Devices**

- Antibiotic prophylaxis is *NOT* routinely recommended after device placement for patients who undergo dental, respiratory, gastrointestinal, or genitourinary procedures.
- Antibiotic prophylaxis is recommended for patients with these devices if they undergo incision and drainage of infection at other sites (e.g., abscess) or replacement of an infected device.
- Antibiotic prophylaxis is recommended for patients with residual leak after device placement for attempted closure of the leak associated with patent ductus arteriosus, atrial septal defect, or ventricular septal defect.

Adapted from Baddour LM, Bettmann MA, Bolger AF, et al. AHA: Nonvalvular cardiovascular device-related infections. *Circulation.* 2003;108:2015−2031.

Patients who undergo hemodialysis can benefit from periodic testing for hepatitis viruses and HIV. The dentist should be aware that a negative test result in the past is not predictive of their current status. Patients may have acquired the disease since they were last tested, or they may be carriers of other infectious viruses (e.g., Epstein—Barr virus, cytomegalovirus) that can cause hepatic injury (see Chapter 10) or immune deficiency. Accordingly, the use of standard infection control procedures is warranted for dental procedures performed in all patients.

Patients who are carriers of hepatitis viruses may have altered hepatic function and may be at risk for developing liver cancer. Liver function should be assessed before hemorrhagic procedures are performed (see Chapter 10). Also proper follow-up with the patient's physician is advised as their physician can provide preventive measures (i.e., vaccinations) or needed treatment (i.e., antiviral agents).

Bleeding. Hemodialysis tends to aggravate bleeding tendencies through physical destruction of platelets and the associated use of heparin. Therefore, determination of the status of hemostasis is important before oral surgery is performed. Screening tests, such as activated partial thromboplastin time (aPTT) and platelet count, should be ordered. Higher risk occurs in patients who have elevated values on these laboratory tests and a history of GI bleeding (see Chapter 24). Although increased risk for bleeding is anticipated in these patients, several management modifications can be used to reduce the chance of serious bleeding:

- Providing dental treatment at the optimum time, usually on the day after hemodialysis, because on the day of dialysis, patients typically are fatigued and may have a tendency to bleed. The activity of heparin lasts for 3—6 h after infusion, and delay of treatment is prudent until that medication is eliminated from the bloodstream.
- Obtaining primary closure and, as needed, using pressure and local hemostatic agents (e.g., absorbable gelatin sponge, thrombin, oxidized cellulose, absorbable collagen, chitosan dressing, and cyanoacrylate). Tranexamic acid can be used (see Chapter 24), but the dosage should be adjusted in consultation with the physician.
- Performing major surgical procedures on the day after the end of the week of hemodialysis treatment to provide additional time for clot retention before dialysis is resumed. For example, for a patient on a Monday, Wednesday, Friday weekly hemodialysis regimen, surgery performed on Saturday allows an additional day for clot stabilization before hemodialysis is resumed on Monday of the following week.
- Contacting the nephrologist, as indicated, to request that the heparin dose be reduced or eliminated during the first hemodialysis session after the surgical procedure. Of note, hemodialysis can be performed without heparin when hemostasis and clot retention are especially critical.
- Administering protamine sulfate (usually by a physician) if dental care is necessary the day of hemodialysis. This agent will block the anticoagulant effects of heparin.

Blood Pressure. The clinician should be aware of other cardiovascular considerations in patients undergoing hemodialysis. For example, the arm that contains the arteriovenous shunt should be protected from application of the blood pressure cuff, blood drawing, and the introduction of intravenous medications. An inflated blood pressure cuff or tourniquet may potentially collapse the shunt, rendering it useless. Likewise, venipuncture of the shunt should be avoided to prevent the complication of phlebitis that can occur from administration of intravenous medications and thrombus development that may jeopardize the shunt.

Capacity to Tolerate Care. Comorbid conditions such as cardiovascular disease and diabetes are common in patients receiving dialysis. Moreover, approximately 40% of patients on dialysis have congestive heart failure, and 39% of them die of cardiovascular complications each year. These patients often take several medications to control hypertension, diabetes, congestive heart failure, or hypercoagulability (i.e., anticoagulation). Dental care must be provided only when the patient is medically stable, and treatment should be planned with an understanding of the required medications and the appropriate dental precautionary measures (see Chapters 3, 4, 6, and 24). In addition, patients receiving dialysis are at increased risk of bone fracture, so appropriate precautions should be implemented.

Drug Considerations. Dentists should be aware that hemodialysis removes some drugs from the circulating blood; this may shorten the duration of effect of prescribed medications. The chance that a given drug will be dialyzed is governed by four factors: (1) molecular weight and size, (2) degree of protein binding, (3) volume of drug distribution, and (4) endogenous drug clearance. For example, larger molecule (>500 Da) drugs are poorly dialyzed. Drugs removed during hemodialysis are those with low capacity for binding to plasma proteins. However, uremia may greatly alter the normal degree of protein binding. A drug such as phenytoin that normally is highly protein bound exhibits lower plasma protein binding during uremia and is available to a greater extent for dialysis removal. Drugs with high lipid affinity exhibit high tissue binding and are not available for dialysis removal. Also, efficient liver clearance of a drug greatly reduces the effect of dialysis treatment.

In general, dosing of drugs should be tailored to occur after dialysis to ensure active drug levels are reached until the next dosing, and dosage amounts and intervals should be adjusted in accordance with current evidence (see Table 12.4) and advice from the patient's physician.

Oral Complications and Manifestations. Hemodialysis reverses many of the severe oral pathologic changes associated with ESRD. However, uremic odor, dry mouth, taste change, and tongue and mucosal pain are signs and symptoms that persist in many of these patients. Petechiae, ecchymoses, higher plaque and calculus indices, and lower levels of salivary secretion are more common among patients undergoing hemodialysis than healthy patients. Secondary hyperparathyroidism along with the associated osseous changes in the jaws has been reported in more than 30% of patients receiving hemodialysis; high levels of PTH are associated with increased mortality.

Patient With Renal Transplant

Approximately 193,000 ESRD patients have a functioning transplanted kidney. Patients who have a transplanted kidney may require special management precautions, including the need for corticosteroids or antibiotic prophylaxis and the need for management of oral infection and gingival overgrowth caused by cyclosporine therapy (see Chapter 21).

BIBLIOGRAPHY

1. Aronoff GR, Bennett WM, Berns JS, et al. *Drug Prescribing in Renal Failure*. Philadelphia, PA: American College of Physicians; 2007.
2. Baddour LM, Bettmann MA, Bolger AF, et al. Nonvalvular cardiovascular device-related infections. *Circulation*. 2003;108(16):2015−2031.
3. Bargman JM, Skorecki K. Chronic kidney disease. In: Fauci AS, Braunwald E, Kasper DL, et al., eds. *Harrison's Principles of Internal Medicine*. New York, NY: McGraw Hill; 2008:1761−1771.
4. Carey WD, ed. *Cleveland Clinic: Current Clinical Medicine*. 2nd ed. St. Louis, MO: Saunders; 2010.
5. Centers for Disease Control, Prevention. Invasive methicillin-resistant *Staphylococcus aureus* infections among dialysis patients−United States, 2005. *MMWR Morb Mortal Wkly Rep*. 2007;56(9):197−199.
6. Chambrone L, Foz AM, Guglielmetti MR, et al. Periodontitis and chronic kidney disease: a systematic review of the association of diseases and the effect of periodontal treatment on estimated glomerular filtration rate. *J Clin Periodontol*. 2013;40(5):443−456.
7. Christensen L, Evans H, Cundick D, et al. Necrotizing fasciltis case presentation and literature review. *N Y State Dent J*. 2015;81(4):24−28.
8. Davidovich E, Davidovits M, Eidelman E, et al. Pathophysiology, therapy, and oral implications of renal failure in children and adolescents: an update. *Pediatr Dent*. 2005;27(2):98−106.
9. De Rossi SS, Glick M. Dental considerations for the patient with renal disease receiving hemodialysis. *J Am Dent Assoc*. 1996;127(2):211−219.
10. Finelli L, Miller JT, Tokars JI, et al. National surveillance of dialysis-associated diseases in the United States, 2002. *Semin Dial*. 2005;18(1):52−61.
11. Foundation NK Global Facts: About Kidney Disease. https://www.kidney.org/kidneydisease/global-facts-about-kidney-disease. Accessed June 18, 2021.
12. Gabardi S, Abramson S. Drug dosing in chronic kidney disease. *Med Clin*. 2005;89(3):649−687.
13. Galbusera M, Remuzzi G, Boccardo P. Treatment of bleeding in dialysis patients. *Semin Dial*. 2009;22(3):279−286.
14. Gavalda C, Bagan J, Scully C, et al. Renal hemodialysis patients: oral, salivary, dental and periodontal findings in 105 adult cases. *Oral Dis*. 1999;5(4):299−302.
15. Grams ME, Chow EK, Segev DL, et al. Lifetime incidence of CKD stages 3−5 in the United States. *Am J Kidney Dis*. 2013;62(2):245−252.
16. Han K, Park J-B. Tooth loss and risk of end-stage renal disease: a nationwide cohort study. *J Periodontol*. 2021;92(3):371−377.
17. Inker LA, Astor BC, Fox CH, et al. KDOQI US commentary on the 2012 KDIGO clinical practice guideline for the evaluation and management of CKD. *Am J Kidney Dis*. 2014;63(5):713−735.
18. Jadoul M, Bieber BA, Martin P, et al. Prevalence, incidence, and risk factors for hepatitis C virus infection in hemodialysis patients. *Kidney Int*. 2019;95(4):939−947.
19. Kho HS, Lee SW, Chung SC, et al. Oral manifestations and salivary flow rate, pH, and buffer capacity in patients with end-stage renal disease undergoing hemodialysis. *Oral Surg Oral Med Oral Pathol Oral Radiol Endod*. 1999;88(3):316−319.
20. Kidney Disease Statistics for the United States. https://www.niddk.nih.gov/health-information/health-statistics/kidney-disease#:∼:text=The%20overall%20prevalence%20of%20CKD,661%2C000%20Americans%20have%20kidney%20failure. Accessed March 6, 2021.
21. Kshirsagar AV, Moss KL, Elter JR, et al. Periodontal disease is associated with renal insufficiency in the Atherosclerosis Risk in Communities (ARIC) study. *Am J Kidney Dis*. 2005;45(4):650−657.
22. Landry DW, Bazari H. Approach to the patient with renal disease. In: Goldman L, ed. *Goldman-Cecil Medicine*. Philadelphia, PA: Saunders/Elsevier; 2016:728−736.
23. Lee JY, Antoniazzi MC, Perozini C, et al. Prevalence of carotid artery calcification in patients with chronic renal disease identified by panoramic radiography. *Oral Surg Oral Med Oral Pathol Oral Radiol*. 2014;118(5):612−618.
24. Levey AS, Coresh J, Balk E, et al. National Kidney Foundation practice guidelines for chronic kidney disease: evaluation, classification, and stratification. *Ann Intern Med*. 2003;139(2):137−147.
25. Lockhart PB, Gibson J, Pond SH, et al. Dental management considerations for the patient with an acquired coagulopathy. Part 1: coagulopathies from systemic disease. *Br Dent J*. 2003;195(8):439−445.
26. Lockhart PB, Loven B, Brennan MT, et al. The evidence base for the efficacy of antibiotic prophylaxis in dental practice. *J Am Dent Assoc*. 2007;138(4):458−474; quiz 534-5, 437.
27. Marik PE, Varon J. Requirement of perioperative stress doses of corticosteroids: a systematic review of the literature. *Arch Surg*. 2008;143(12):1222−1226.

28. Matzke GR, Aronoff GR, Atkinson Jr AJ, et al. Drug dosing consideration in patients with acute and chronic kidney disease-a clinical update from Kidney Disease: Improving Global Outcomes (KDIGO). *Kidney Int.* 2011;80(11):1122−1137.

29. Miller CS, McGarity GJ. Tetracycline-induced renal failure after dental treatment. *J Am Dent Assoc.* 2009;140(1): 56−60.

30. National Institute of Diabetes and Digestive and Kidney Diseases. Kidney Disease Statistics for the United States. U.S. Department of Health and Human Services. https://www.niddk.nih.gov/health-information/health-statistics/kidney-disease. Accessed June 18, 2021.

31. National Kidney and Urologic Diseases Information Clearinghouse (NKUDIC). *Treatment Methods for Kidney Failure: Peritoneal Dialysis*; 2010. Bethesda, MD https://www.niddk.nih.gov/health-information/kidney-disease/kidney-failure/peritoneal-dialysis. Accessed June 19, 2021.

32. National Kidney Foundation. K/DOQI Clinical practice guidelines for bone metabolism and disease in chronic kidney disease. *Am J Kidney Dis.* 2003;42(4 suppl 3):S1−S201.

33. National Kidney Foundation. K/DOQI Clinical practice guidelines for chronic kidney disease: evaluation, classification, and stratification. *Am J Kidney Dis.* 2002;39: S1−S266.

34. National Kidney Foundation. KDOQI clinical practice guideline for diabetes and CKD: 2012 update. *Am J Kidney Dis.* 2012;60(5):850−886.

35. Oliver R, Roberts GJ, Hooper L, et al. Antibiotics for the prophylaxis of bacterial endocarditis in dentistry. *Cochrane Database Syst Rev.* 2008;4:CD003813.

36. Proctor R, Kumar N, Stein A, et al. Oral and dental aspects of chronic renal failure. *J Dent Res.* 2005;84(3):199−208.

37. Pun PH, Smarz TR, Honeycutt EF, et al. Chronic kidney disease is associated with increased risk of sudden cardiac death among patients with coronary artery disease. *Kidney Int.* 2009;76(6):652−658.

38. Pharmacotherapy R. *Dosage Adjustment of Medications Eliminated by the Kidneys*. New York, NY: Springer; 2013.

39. Robinson DL, Fowler VG, Sexton DJ, et al. Bacterial endocarditis in hemodialysis patients. *Am J Kidney Dis.* 1997;30(4):521−524.

40. Saran R, Li Y, Robinson B, et al. US renal data system 2015 annual data report: Epidemiology of kidney disease in the United States. *Am J Kidney Dis.* 2016;67(3 suppl 1):A7−A8.

41. Slinin Y, Greer N, Ishani A, et al. Timing of dialysis initiation, duration and frequency of hemodialysis sessions, and membrane flux: a systematic review for a KDOQI clinical practice guideline. *Am J Kidney Dis.* 2015;66(5):823−836.

42. Stevens PE, Levin A, Kidney Disease: Improving Global Outcomes Chronic Kidney Disease Guideline Development Work Group M. Evaluation and management of chronic kidney disease: synopsis of the kidney disease: improving global outcomes 2012 clinical practice guideline. *Ann Intern Med.* 2013;158(11):825−830.

43. Tentori F, Wang M, Bieber BA, et al. Recent changes in therapeutic approaches and association with outcomes among patients with secondary hyperparathyroidism on chronic hemodialysis: the DOPPS study. *Clin J Am Soc Nephrol.* 2015;10(1):98−109.

44. Termine N, Panzarella V, Ciavarella D, et al. Antibiotic prophylaxis in dentistry and oral surgery: use and misuse. *Int Dent J.* 2009;59(5):263−270.

45. Thomas R, Kanso A, Sedor JR. Chronic kidney disease and its complications. *Prim Care.* 2008;35(2):329−344, vii.

46. Tokars JI, Miller ER, Alter MJ, et al. National surveillance of dialysis-associated diseases in the United States, 1997. *Semin Dial.* 2000;13(2):75−85.

47. Tokoff-Rubin N. Treatment of irreversible renal failure. In: Goldman L, Ausiello D, eds. *Cecil Medicine*. 23rd ed. Philadelphia, PA: Saunders Elsevier; 2008:936−947.

48. Tomas I, Marinho JS, Limeres J, et al. Changes in salivary composition in patients with renal failure. *Arch Oral Biol.* 2008;53(6):528−532.

49. Wakasugi M, Kawamura K, Yamamoto S, et al. High mortality rate of infectious diseases in dialysis patients: a comparison with the general population in Japan. *Ther Apher Dial.* 2012;16(3):226−231.

Sexually Transmitted Diseases

Sexually transmitted diseases (STDs) are a major global health problem. The worldwide burden is difficult to estimate across the more than 30 infectious diseases known to be transmitted through sexual contact (Box 13.1). However, the World Health Organization reports there are almost 1 million new cases each day. In 2018, there were estimated to be almost 68 million prevalent STD infections and 26 million incident (new) infections in the United States. These statistics are based on eight STDs, the three notifiable bacterial STDs (chlamydia, gonorrhea, and syphilis), plus trichomoniasis, human papillomavirus (HPV), herpes simplex virus (HSV), hepatitis B virus (HBV), and human immunodeficiency virus (HIV) infections. Of note, more than 50% of new infections occur in younger adults (aged 15–24 years). The cost to the US health care system is estimated to be greater than $15 billion. In a dental practice of 2000 patients, approximately 400 patients would be found to have an existing STD.

The morbidity and mortality of STDs vary from minor inconvenience to severe health consequences and death. The diagnosis of an STD also can have significant psychosocial effects. STDs have important implications for the dental team, and prompt recognition, diagnosis, and management of STDs are of paramount importance. Dental health professionals may intercept patients who have STDs while eliciting their history or by recognizing oral manifestations of STDs during the head and neck examination. However, it is important to remember that

patients may not always divulge that they have an STD, or they may have asymptomatic disease and be unaware that they have an active infection. STDs can be transmitted by contact with blood, saliva, and oral lesions (if present) or, in the case of some viral STDs, via asymptomatic viral shedding. As such, the dental team should assume that all patients are potentially infectious and must adhere to standard infection control precautions (see Appendix B). A single STD is accompanied by additional STDs in about 10% of cases, and STDs increase the risk for HIV infection. Prevention is critical, and dental health professionals can provide patient education to minimize transmission, particularly concerning oral contact.

Most dentists do not routinely obtain a sexual history on all patients but should be familiar with how to obtain a sexual history and do so as the need arise (Box 13.2). An understanding about the epidemiology, etiopathogenesis (the cause and development of a disease or abnormal condition), clinical course and manifestations, diagnosis, and medical management of STDs can provide a strong basis for the identification of the oral manifestations and dental considerations of patients with STDs. Discussion in this chapter is limited to gonorrhea, syphilis, selected human herpesviruses and HPV infections, because these entities are of special interest or importance to dental practice and serve to illustrate basic principles. Readers are referred to Chapters 10 and 18 for information about hepatitis B virus infection and HIV/AIDS.

BOX 13.1	Classification of Sexually Transmitted Diseases

Bacterial

Bacterial vaginosis	*Atopobium vaginae, Bacteroides* spp., *Fusobacterium* spp., *Gardnerella vaginalis, Mobiluncus* spp., *Mycoplasma hominis, Peptostreptococcus* spp., *Porphyromonas* spp., *Prevotella* spp., *Ureaplasma urealyticum*
Chancroid	*Haemophilus ducreyi*
Chlamydia	*Chlamydia trachomatis*
Giardiasis	*Giardia lamblia*
Gonorrhea	*Neisseria gonorrhoeae*
Granuloma inguinale (donovanosis)	*Klebsiella granulomatis*
Nongonococcal, nonchlamydial urethritis in men	*Mycoplasma genitalium* *Ureaplasma urealyticum*
Salmonellosis	*Salmonella* spp.
Shigellosis	*Shigella* spp.
Streptococcal infection	*Streptococcus* group B spp.
Syphilis	*Treponema pallidum*
Trichomoniasis	*Trichomoniasis vaginalis*

Ectoparasites

Pubic lice (crabs)	*Pthirus pubis*
Scabies	*Sarcoptes scabiei*

Fungal

Vulvovaginal candidiasis	*Candida* spp., *Torulopsis* spp.

Protozoal

Amebiasis	*Entamoeba histolytica*
Enterobiasis	*Enterobius vermicularis*

Viral

Condyloma acuminatum (anogenital and oral warts)	Human papillomavirus infection (HPV-6, HPV-11)
Cytomegalovirus infection	Cytomegalovirus (CMV)
Genital herpes	Herpes simplex viruses (HSV-1, HSV-2)
HIV infection/acquired immunodeficiency syndrome (AIDS)	Human immunodeficiency virus (HIV)
Hepatitis B	Hepatitis B virus (HBV)
Hepatitis C	Hepatitis C virus (HCV)
Molluscum contagiosum	Poxvirus
Zika virus infection	Zika virus

BOX 13.2	Taking a Sexual History

Partners
- Are you currently sexually active? (Are you having sex?)
  - If no, have you ever been sexually active?
- In recent months, how many sex partners have you had?
- In the past 12 months, how many sex partners have you had?
- Are your sex partners men, women, or both?

Practices
- I am going to be more explicit here about the kind of sex you've had over the past 12 months to better understand if you are at risk for sexually transmitted diseases (STDs).
- What kind of sexual contact do you have or have you had? Genital (penis in the vagina)? Anal (penis in the anus)? Oral (mouth on penis, vagina, or anus)?

Past History of STDs
- Have you ever been diagnosed with an STD? When? How were you treated?
- Have you had any recurring symptoms or diagnoses?
- Have you ever been tested for HIV or other STDs?
- Has your current partner or any former partners ever been diagnosed or treated for an STD? Were you tested for the same STD(s)?
- If yes, when were you tested? What was the diagnosis? How was it treated?

Protection From STDs
- Do you and your partner(s) use any protection against STDs?
- If so, what kind of protection do you use?
- How often do you use and have you used protection?

Adapted from the U.S. Department of Health and Human Services, Centers for Disease Control and Prevention, Atlanta, GA, 2014: *Guide to taking a sexual history.* https://www.cdc.gov/std/treatment/sexualhistory.pdf.

Gonorrhea primarily infects the urethra, cervix, rectum, and oropharynx, although it also can infect other sites such as the conjunctiva.

EPIDEMIOLOGY

Of the three nationally reported notifiable STDs (chlamydia, gonorrhea, and syphilis), gonorrhea is the second most common behind chlamydia with 538,405 new cases reported in the United States to the CDC in 2018. This represents a sustained increasing trend since 2014. Marginally more new cases were reported in men than women; more than 50% of cases are in 15- to 24-year-old individuals. Historical socioeconomic disparities contribute to the incidence among non-Hispanic blacks being more than 10 times the rates among whites.

ETIOLOGY

N. gonorrhoeae, an aerobic gram-negative β-proteobacteria, typically exists as diplococci with a marked tropism

GONORRHEA

Gonorrhea is caused by *Neisseria gonorrhoeae.* Humans are the only natural hosts for this disease, and gonorrhea is transmitted almost exclusively via sexual contact, whether genital–genital, oral–genital, or rectal–genital.

for human mucosae. It replicates easily in warm, moist areas and displays differential invasiveness based on the type of host epithelium with which it interacts. Columnar epithelium (as found in the mucosal lining of the urethra and cervix) and transitional epithelium (as in the pharynx and rectum) are highly susceptible to infection, but stratified squamous epithelium (skin and mucosal lining of the oral cavity) is generally resistant to infection. Fig. 13.1 depicts the areas of relative epithelial susceptibility to *N. gonorrhoeae* infection in the oral cavity and oropharynx. *N. gonorrhoeae* demonstrates a propensity for antibiotic resistance, which has become a major global issue.

CLINICAL PRESENTATION

Infection in men usually begins in the anterior urethra after sexual exposure and a 2–5 day incubation period. Typically, the acute infection is symptomatic and leads to urethritis, a purulent urethral discharge, and dysuria. Asymptomatic infection occurs in a minority of men. The infection may remain localized or may extend posteriorly to involve the epididymis, prostate, seminal vesicles, or bladder. Epididymitis can lead to infertility.

In contrast to men, infection in the majority of women is asymptomatic, which is problematic because patients may not seek medical care for their problem, creating a reservoir of infection. The incubation takes 5–10 days. Most symptomatic infections lead to a cervicitis with resultant purulent drainage and dyspareunia and less commonly urethritis. Bartholin glands and Skene ducts may also be affected. An ascending infection may involve the endometrium, fallopian tubes, ovaries, and pelvic peritoneum, and gonorrhea is a common cause of pelvic inflammatory disease (PID). PID can be symptomatic (backache and abdominal pain may be present) and may contribute to tubal scarring, leading to infertility or ectopic pregnancy. Perinatal transmission accounts for a small percentage of cases of gonorrhea in the United States, causing gonococcal conjunctivitis and arthritis of the newborn, which if untreated can cause blindness or joint infection.

In both genders, anorectal gonorrhea may occur after anal–genital intercourse. It typically has a milder course than a genital infection, and may include purulent discharge and pain. Oropharyngeal infection is detected most commonly following fellatio and while typically asymptomatic it may manifest as a mild sore throat associated with diffuse, nonspecific erythema with tiny pustules (Fig. 13.2), and can involve the palatine tonsils (which become enlarged with or without a yellowish exudate and may be associated with cervical lymphadenopathy). The likelihood of transmission of pharyngeal gonorrhea to the genitalia is less common than that of genital–pharynx or genital–genital transmission. Disseminated gonorrhea rarely occurs (1%–2% of cases) and may result in migratory arthritis, skin and mucous membrane lesions, endocarditis, meningitis, PID, and pericarditis.

LABORATORY AND DIAGNOSTIC FINDINGS

In symptomatic patients with a purulent discharge, Gram stain demonstrating gram-negative diplococci within neutrophils is the best point-of-care diagnostic for *N. gonorrhoeae* infection (Fig. 13.3). In an asymptomatic patient or a patient without purulent discharge (as may be the case in endocervical, rectal, or oropharyngeal infections), Gram staining has poor accuracy and is not indicated.

Culture and nucleic acid amplification testing (NAAT) are both widely available for gonorrhea testing. The CDC recommends NAAT as the first-line diagnostic for *N. gonorrhoeae*, for both symptomatic and asymptomatic genital tract and also for extragenital site infections. Given the strong likelihood for co-infection with *C. trachomatis*, these platforms are typically bundled to test for both organisms. Culture for *N. gonorrhoeae* is indicated in patients who have received a CDC-

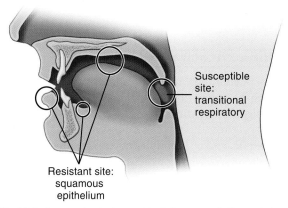

FIG. 13.1 Areas of relative epithelial susceptibility to infection by *Neisseria gonorrhoeae* within the oral cavity or oropharynx.

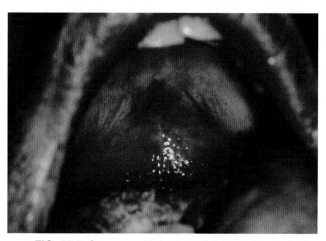

FIG. 13.2 Gonococcal infection of the oropharynx.

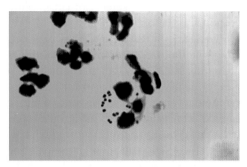

FIG. 13.3 Smear demonstrating gram-negative diplococci within neutrophils. (From http://www.public-domain-image. com/free-images/science/microscopy-images/gonorrhea-neisseria-gonorrhoeae/histopathology-in-an-acute-case-of-gonococcal-urethritis-using-gram-stain-technique/attachment/histopathology-in-an-acute-case-of-gonococcal-urethritis-using-gram-stain-technique.)

recommended antimicrobial regimen and yet have a persistent NAAT-positive result. Culture can be coupled with antimicrobial sensitivity testing, which is important given the propensity of *N. gonorrhoeae* for antimicrobial resistance.

MEDICAL MANAGEMENT

The CDC recommends a single dose of ceftriaxone 500 mg intramuscularly (IM) for the treatment of uncomplicated gonococcal infection of the cervix, urethra, pharynx, or rectum in adults (regimens for other sites, children, or during pregnancy are different). For persons weighing ≥150 kg (300 lbs), a single 1 g IM dose of ceftriaxone should be administered. Alternative regimens, when ceftriaxone is unavailable, include gentamycin 240 mg IM plus 2 g azithromycin orally, or cefixime 800 mg orally. If chlamydial infection has not been excluded, doxycycline 100 mg orally twice a day for 7 days is recommended. All sexual partners should be tested and treated, and patients who have been treated yet who have persistent signs or symptoms should undergo culture and antibiotic sensitivity testing.

DENTAL CONSIDERATIONS AND ORAL MANIFESTATIONS

A patient with a known recent gonorrhea infection who has been administered appropriate antibiotic therapy poses little threat of disease transmission to the dental team. Patients in this category can receive dental care within days of beginning antibiotic treatment. Patients with an active pharyngitis and other oral signs or symptoms suggestive of an active infection of unclear etiology should be promptly referred to a physician for further evaluation. Reports of gonorrhea involving the oral cavity (i.e., sites other than the oropharynx) are rare.

SYPHILIS

Syphilis is an STD caused by *Treponema pallidum*. As with gonorrhea, humans are the only known natural hosts for syphilis. Broadly, there are a number of distinct stages. Late-stage manifestations are diverse and have led to the historical designation of syphilis as the "great imitator" disease. Congenital syphilis is also possible. Syphilis remains an important infection in contemporary medicine because of the morbidity it can cause.

EPIDEMIOLOGY

The number of syphilis cases continue to rise, with 115,000 new cases (all stages and including congenital syphilis), and 35,000 new primary and secondary syphilis cases, reported in the United States to the CDC in 2018. More than 10 men are infected for every woman, with the highest incidence in black men, although the greatest increases have been reported in men who have sex with men (MSM), which is concerning because of the increased risk for the transmission of HIV infection.

In 2018, the rate of congenital syphilis was 33.1 per 100,000 live births, almost triple the incidence since 2014.

ETIOLOGY

Treponema pallidum is a slender, fragile microaerophilic spirochete. It is transmitted predominantly sexually, by genital–genital, oral–genital, or rectal–genital contact with contaminated sores. However, transmission also may occur through kissing or as a bloodborne infection and may be transmitted to fetuses, leading to congenital syphilis. *T. pallidum* is easily killed by heating, drying, disinfecting, and using soap and water; as such, transmission by fomites is unlikely. It is believed that *T. pallidum* does not invade completely intact skin; however, it can invade intact mucosal epithelium and gain entry via minute abrasions or hair follicles. Within a few hours after invasion, spread to the lymphatics and the bloodstream occurs, resulting in early widespread dissemination of the disease.

CLINICAL PRESENTATION

The case definitions of syphilis are classically divided according to stages of disease; each stage has its own unique signs and symptoms. These stages are primary, secondary, early nonprimary/nonsecondary, unknown duration/late, and congenital. Patients are most infectious during the first 2 years of the disease. It is important to note that many infected persons do not develop symptoms for years, yet they remain at risk for late complications if not treated.

Primary Syphilis

This stage is characterized by the chancre, a solitary (although multiple chancres are possible) round, often painless, somewhat firm lesion that develops at the site of contact with the infectious spirochete. The chancre usually occurs within 2–3 weeks (range, 10–90 days) after exposure (Figs. 13.4 and 13.5), and patients are infectious before it appears. The lesion begins as a small papule and enlarges to form a surface erosion or ulceration that commonly is covered by a yellowish hemorrhagic crust that is teeming with *T. pallidum.* Enlarged, painless, and firm regional lymphadenopathy is typically present. The chancre usually subsides in 3–6 weeks without treatment, leaving variable scarring in the form of a healed papule. More than 80% of chancres occur on the genitalia. The most common extragenital site is the oral cavity or oropharynx (others include the fingers, nipples, perineum, anus, and rectum). If adequate treatment is not provided, the infection progresses to secondary syphilis.

Secondary Syphilis

The manifestations of secondary syphilis typically appear 6–8 weeks after initial exposure and are associated with the hematogenous spread and associated systemic immunologic response to *T. pallidum.* The chancre may or may not have completely resolved by this time. There is a wide spectrum of systemic signs and symptoms, including fever, malaise, headache, arthralgias, generalized lymphadenopathy, and patchy hair loss and a generalized eruption of the skin and mucous membranes, including the oral cavity (see Oral Manifestations

section). In some cases, secondary syphilis can be asymptomatic. The skin rash is maculopapular (Fig. 13.6A) with well-demarcated and reddish-brown areas involving the trunk and with a predilection for the palms and soles; they are typically not itchy. Warty lesions, known as condyloma lata, may involve the genitalia, the oral cavity, or both. Lues maligna is a rare and severe manifestation of secondary syphilis in immunocompromised patients, such as those with HIV infection. The lesions of skin and mucous membranes are highly infectious. Without treatment, the signs and symptoms of secondary syphilis ultimately resolve; however, infection progresses.

Early Nonprimary Nonsecondary

These are patients with evidence of having acquired the disease within the preceding year, yet are asymptomatic, do not show clinical evidence of disease, but remain seroreactive (i.e., early latent infection).

Unknown Duration or Late

This case definition includes three seroreactive groups: those with no documented prior history of syphilis within the preceding year and are asymptomatic (i.e., later latent infection); those with a previous history of syphilis (but not acquired within the preceding year) who demonstrate increasing/sustained nontreponemal test titers but are asymptomatic (i.e., also a latent infection); and those with clinical signs and symptoms associated with neurologic, ocular, otic, or late stage disease (previously referred to as tertiary syphilis). It is important to note that neurosyphilis, ocular syphilis, or otosyphilis can occur during primary, secondary, or late-stage infection.

Late stage occurs in 10%–40% of untreated persons, generally many years after disease onset. It is the destructive stage of the disease, although patients are

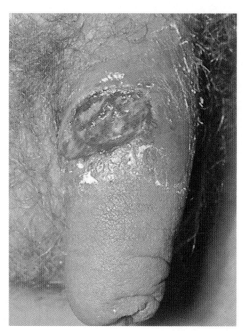

FIG. 13.4 Primary syphilis: chancre of the penis. (From Habif TP, Campbell JI Jr, Chapman MS et al. *Skin Disease: Diagnosis and Treatment.* 2nd ed. St. Louis, MO: Mosby; 2005.)

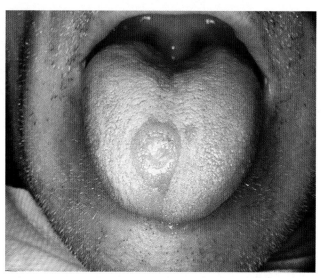

FIG. 13.5 Chancre on the tongue seen in primary syphilis. (From Ibsen DAC, Phelan JA. *Oral Pathology for the Hygienist.* 4th ed. St. Louis, MO: Saunders; 2003.)

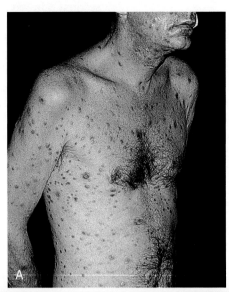

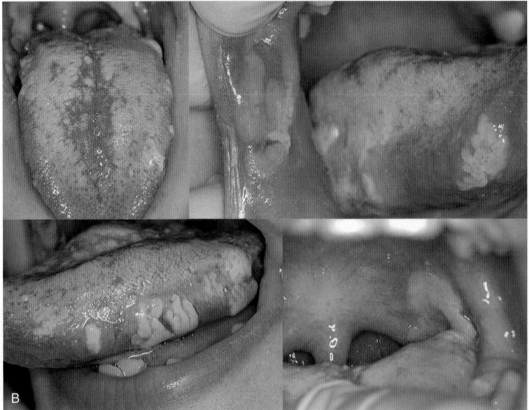

FIG. 13.6 Lesions of secondary syphilis. (**A**) Profuse papular rash. (**B**) Multiple oral lesions, including mucous patches, and nonwipeable white plaques. ((**A**) From Habif TP, Campbell JI Jr, Chapman MS et al. *Skin Disease: Diagnosis and Treatment.* 2nd ed. St. Louis,MO: Mosby; 2005. (**B**) From Dr. Stefania Leuci, Federico II University of Naples, Italy.)

considered noninfectious. Any organ of the body may become involved. Late neurosyphilis can result in a meningitis-like syndrome, Argyll Robertson pupils (which react to accommodation but not to light), altered tendon reflexes, general paresis, tabes dorsalis (degeneration of dorsal columns of the spinal cord and sensory nerve trunks), difficulty in coordinating muscle movements, or mental deterioration. Cardiovascular syphilis is the end product of an obliterative endarteritis and can manifest as an aneurysm of the ascending aorta. The *gumma*, which is the classic localized lesion of late-stage syphilis, may involve the skin, mucous membranes (including the oral cavity), bone, or within any organ. It is believed to be the end result of a hypersensitivity reaction and is basically a noninfectious inflammatory granulomatous lesion with a central zone of necrosis.

Congenital Syphilis

Syphilis may occur congenitally if the mother is infected while pregnant (i.e., secondary to treponemal bacteremia), and transplacental infection can occur as early as 9–10 weeks in utero. Approximately 25% of these pregnancies result in stillbirth, and 12% result in neonatal death. The majority of newborns (>80%) are asymptomatic. Congenital syphilis persists worldwide because a substantial number of women do not receive antenatal syphilis testing. Early signs, manifesting at birth or up to 2 years after birth, may include hepatomegaly and associated liver dysfunction, hematologic abnormalities, mucocutaneous findings (i.e., maculopapular rash, a rhinitis secondary to nasal inflammation, perioral and perineal condylomata lata), and bone changes (osteochondritis and periostitis causing pseudoparalysis) and, less commonly, neurologic manifestations. Late signs are rare, and there is a classic triad of congenital syphilis known as Hutchinson's triad that includes interstitial keratitis of the cornea, eighth nerve deafness, and dental abnormalities (see Oral Manifestations). In addition, rhinitis can lead to a saddle nose caused by cartilage destruction, rhagades, neurologic sequelae (including mental retardation), and bony abnormalities such as frontal bossing.

Laboratory and Diagnostic Findings

T. pallidum has never been cultured successfully on any type of medium and is difficult to stain for microscopic examination. Historically, the definitive diagnosis of syphilis has been made from microscopic examination of fresh lesion exudates during the primary and early secondary stages using positive dark-field microscopic examination. With the advent of serologic tests, the traditional diagnosis of syphilis is based on clinical findings in conjunction with a two-step testing algorithm using a nontreponemal "screening" test followed by a confirmatory specific treponemal test.

Nontreponemal Testing

The nontreponemal tests include the Venereal Disease Research Laboratory (VDRL) slide test and the rapid plasma reagin (RPR) test. These tests, both equally valid but noncomparable, detect an antibody-like substance called *reagin*, which is a surrogate for the immunologic response to a syphilis infection. They are less specific but can better assess current disease activity. The initial test is qualitative, and if positive, a quantitative step is performed that generates "titers," values reported as serologic dilutions (e.g., 1:2, 1:4, 1:8). They are consistently positive and yield the highest titers between 3 and 8 weeks after the appearance of the primary chancre. A fourfold change in titers (e.g., 1:4 to 1:16 (worsening infection) or 1:32 to 1:8 (improving infection)) is the

threshold signifying a clinically meaningful change in serial test results. In primary syphilis, nontreponemal test results usually revert to negative within 12 months after successful treatment. In secondary syphilis, up to 24 months may be required for the patient to become seronegative. Occasionally, a patient will remain seropositive for the rest of his or her life, or will test positive because of other infections or conditions (false positive). With late-stage syphilis, many patients remain seropositive for life.

Treponemal Testing. These include the fluorescent treponemal antibody absorption test (FTA-ABS), *T. pallidum* particle agglutination assay (TPPA), *T. pallidum* hemagglutination assay (TPHA), and various immunoassays (i.e., enzyme immunoassays [EIAs], chemiluminescent immunoassays [CIAs], and microbead immunoassays [MIAs]). These are highly specific, but a positive test result cannot differentiate between current and past infection because antibodies remain positive in most patients.

Treponemal testing is typically performed to confirm a positive screening RPR or VDRL nontreponemal test. However, some high-volume laboratories can screen first with treponemal tests ("reverse" algorithm) which can better capture those with a past history of infection and early stage disease. A treponemal EIA or CIA test is performed first and if reactive is followed by a qualitative nontreponemal test. If this second test result is negative, a different treponemal test is performed.

MEDICAL MANAGEMENT

Testing for concomitant HIV infection and the diagnosis and management of infection in the patient's sexual partners are recommended. Parenteral injection of long-acting benzathine penicillin G, 2.4 million IU IM in a single dose remains the recommended and predictable treatment for primary, secondary, or early latent syphilis in adults; 50,000 IU/kg of penicillin G should be used for children or infants. As with gonorrhea, infectiousness is reversed rapidly, probably within a matter of hours after injection. A more intensive regimen is indicated for those with unknown duration or late syphilis: injections of benzathine penicillin G, 2.4 million IU IM once a week for 3 weeks (i.e., total of 7.2 million IU). Neurosyphilis or ocular syphilis is managed more effectively with either 18–24 million IU of aqueous crystalline penicillin G delivered intravenously (IV) or 2.4 million IU procaine penicillin G given IM daily plus probenecid 500 mg four times a day, with both regimens given over a 10- to 14-day period. Neonates with possible congenital syphilis should be assessed by means of clinical, radiographic, and laboratory tests of blood and cerebrospinal fluid for VDRL. If results prove presence of the disease or suggest that syphilis is highly probable, then the infant should be treated with IV penicillin G for at least 10 days. The first-line drug for patients allergic to penicillin (except for pregnant patients) is oral doxycycline (100 mg orally twice a day for 2 weeks) or tetracycline 500 mg four times a day for 2 weeks. Desensitization to penicillin is recommended for pregnant patients allergic to penicillin. Patients with primary or secondary syphilis who are otherwise immunocompetent should be retested at 6 and 12 months to monitor for seroconversion. HIV-infected patients and those with "unknown duration or late syphilis" require more intensive or longer surveillance, respectively. The Jarisch–Herxheimer reaction is an acute febrile reaction that is frequently accompanied by chills, myalgias, and headache that occur within 24 h after initiation of antibiotic therapy for syphilis. It occurs most often (i.e., in 50% patients) after treatment for early syphilis.

DENTAL CONSIDERATIONS AND ORAL MANIFESTATIONS

Lesions of untreated primary and secondary syphilis are infectious, as are the patient's blood and saliva. Even after treatment has begun, its absolute effectiveness cannot be determined except through conversion of the positive serologic test to negative; however, early reversal of infectiousness is to be expected after antibiotic treatment has been initiated. The time required for this conversion varies from a few months to longer than 1 year. Therefore, patients who are currently under treatment or who remain seropositive for syphilis after receiving treatment should be viewed as potentially infectious. Still, any necessary dental care may be provided with adherence to standard precautions unless oral lesions are present. Dental treatment can commence after oral lesions have been successfully treated.

Oral syphilitic chancres and mucous patches are usually painless unless they become secondarily infected. Both lesions are highly infectious. Oral chancres (see Fig. 13.5) are typically solitary lesions that may involve the lips, tongue, oropharynx, or other oral sites and may be associated with lymphadenopathy. They begin as a round papule that erodes into a painless ulcer with a smooth surface. Size can vary from a few millimeters to more than 2 cm. Sometimes chancres may demonstrate induration. The oral manifestations of secondary syphilis (present in >30% of patients) (Fig. 13.6B) are highly variable and include single or multiple lesions such as mucous patches, maculopapular lesions (i.e., the likely counterpart to the skin rash), erosions, ulcerations including a peculiar "snail-track" variety, white plaques resembling leukoplakia, and papulonodular lesions. The intraoral mucous patch is often asymptomatic and appears as a slightly raised grayish plaque and may involve multiple oral sites. The oral gumma of late-stage syphilis is rare. It typically presents as a solitary lesion that most commonly involves the tongue or palate, which may be exophytic, indurated, and with surface ulceration. Palatal gummas may erode bone and perforate into the nasal cavity or maxillary sinus, creating an oronasal or oral-antral fistula. An atrophic or interstitial glossitis also has been reported in late stage syphilis. Oral manifestations of congenital syphilis include peg-shaped permanent central incisors with notching of the incisal edge (Hutchinson's incisors) (Fig. 13.7), defective molars with multiple supernumerary cusps (mulberry molars), a high narrow palate, and perioral rhagades (skin fissures).

The manifestations of syphilis can mimic malignant neoplasms; however, the evidence for syphilis as a causative agent for cancer has not been substantiated.

GENITAL HERPES SIMPLEX VIRUS INFECTIONS

Genital herpes is an incurable painful infection involving the anogenital region that is caused by one of two closely related types of HSV type 1 and type 2. The disease consists of acute and recurrent phases and is associated with high rates of subclinical infection and asymptomatic viral shedding.

EPIDEMIOLOGY

Genital herpes is an important STD in the United States and the world. Seroprevalence for genital HSV infection is challenging to assess. The serologic presence of antibodies (i.e., IgG to the glycoproteins G1 and G2) is indicative of past infection. HSV-2 antibodies correlate to sexual or genital transmission, but it is difficult to differentiate between oral versus genital HSV-1 infection. In 2018, approximately 18 million Americans have prevalent HSV-2 infection, with more than 750,000 new infections. Yet these estimates do not include HSV-1 genital infections which are rising and estimated to comprise as many as half of all new genital infections. HSV-2 seroprevalence is approximately twice as high for women (22%) as men (11%) and almost three times as high for non-Hispanic blacks (56%) as whites (21%). HSV-2 infection is associated with three times the risk for acquiring HIV infection.

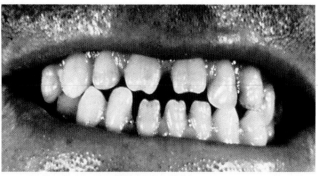

FIG. 13.7 Congenital syphilis: Hutchinson's teeth.

ETIOLOGY

Herpes simplex virus belongs to a family of eight human herpesviruses that includes cytomegalovirus (CMV), Epstein–Barr virus (EBV), varicella-zoster virus, human herpesvirus type 6 (HHV-6), human herpesvirus type 7 (HHV-7), and Kaposi sarcoma–associated herpesvirus (HHV-8). HSV-1 is the causative agent of most herpetic infections that occur above the waist, especially involving the oral mucosa (i.e., primary herpetic gingivostomatitis, recurrent herpes labialis, and recurrent intraoral herpes), nasal mucosa, eyes, brain, and skin. The majority of primary HSV-1 infections are subclinical; thus are never known to the infected person. Transmission to others occurs usually by transfer of infected saliva through close contact (i.e., touching, kissing, and via oral–oral or oral–anogenital sexual contact). Autoinoculation to the face, fingers, eyes, and genitalia also may occur. HSV-2 is transmitted predominantly by sexual contact, primarily through contact with an asymptomatic viral shedder, although it may also be transmitted nonsexually. HSV also may be transmitted to a newborn from an infected mother (neonatal herpes).

The pathogenesis of HSV-1 and HSV-2 infections is similar, and the lesions of skin and mucous membranes have a similar appearance. During the initial exposure, epithelial and epidermal and other permissive cells are "invaded" and viral replication occurs. Characteristic cellular changes include ballooning degeneration, intranuclear inclusion bodies, and the formation of multinucleated giant cells. With cellular destruction comes inflammation and increasing edema, which result in formation of papules that progress to fluid-filled vesicles. These vesicles rupture, leaving an ulcerated surface that if exposed to the air will crust over.

During the primary infection, progeny enter the ends of local peripheral neurons and migrate up the axon to the regional ganglia (HSV-1 primarily in the trigeminal and HSV-2 primarily in the sacral ganglia, respectively), where they reside as a latent infection. The virus reactivates after exposure to trauma, sunlight, menses, intercourse, or immune suppression. The reactivated progeny migrate down the axon and can produce a recurrent infection with lesions similar to the primary infection, albeit typically less severe in nature and more localized.

CLINICAL PRESENTATION

The clinical manifestations of genital herpes are divided into primary and recurrent infections.

Primary Infection

The clinical course of the primary HSV infection is variable, but lymphadenopathy and viremia are prominent features. In otherwise immunocompetent individuals, the infection is contained by the host's immune system and runs its course within 10–20 days. However, spread to other epidermal sites (e.g., herpetic whitlow [infection of the fingers], keratoconjunctivitis [eyes]) and in neonates during childbirth has been documented. In rare cases, infants and immunosuppressed persons can develop systemic and widespread infection that may result in significant morbidity and death.

Newly acquired genital infections may be symptomatic in approximately two-thirds of HSV-1 and 40% of HSV-2 infections; with a greater percentage of asymptomatic infections occurring in men. After a 2–10 day incubation period, the lesions of primary genital herpes may appear. In women, both internal and external genitalia may be involved, as well as the perineal region and the skin of the thighs and buttocks. In men, the external genitalia and the skin of the inguinal area may be involved. Lesions in moist areas tend to ulcerate early and depending on their location, may cause pain and dysuria. Lesions on exposed dry areas tend to remain pustular or vesicular and then crust over. Painful regional lymphadenopathy accompanies infection along with headache, malaise, myalgia, and symptoms of fever. These subside in approximately 2 weeks, and healing occurs in 3–5 weeks.

Recurrent Infection

Outbreaks of recurrent genital herpes typically occur two to six times per year and are generally less severe than the primary infection. Of the two serotypes, HSV-2 is more efficient in reactivating from the sacral ganglia (i.e., genital recurrences in those infected by HSV-2 are about four times as likely as those sacrally infected with HSV-1). Also, immune suppression increases the risk for more frequent and severe recurrences. A prodrome of localized itching, tingling, paresthesia, pain, and burning may be noted and is variably followed by a vesicular eruption (Fig. 13.8). Healing occurs in 10–14 days. Constitutional symptoms are generally absent.

HSV-1 and HSV-2 lesions are highly infectious and therefore can be transmitted to other individuals or to other sites on the patient. The infectious period coincides with the early stages before crusting. Therefore, one should assume that all herpetic lesions (i.e., papular, vesicular, pustular, and ulcerative) before completion of crusting are infectious. Between recurrences, infected persons intermittently shed the virus from the anogenital region (i.e., asymptomatic shedding), which can also lead to transmission.

LABORATORY AND DIAGNOSTIC FINDINGS

Culture, NAAT, and direct immunofluorescence (DIF) are widely available tests to evaluate active genital lesions to confirm viral types. Cytopathologic testing is typically not recommended, although staining for HSV infection may be helpful. Viral culture is slow (≈ 5 days), expensive, and technique sensitive (i.e., the specimen must be placed in viral transport medium and refrigerated). Real-

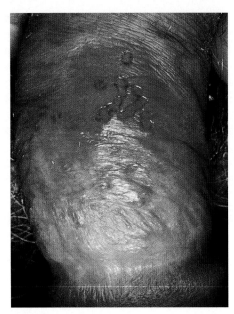

FIG. 13.8 Recurrent herpes simplex virus infection of the foreskin. (From Habif TP, Campbell JI Jr, Chapman MS et al. *Skin Disease: Diagnosis and Treatment.* 2nd ed. St. Louis, MO: Mosby; 2005.)

time PCR assays are highly accurate, rapid, and less technique sensitive; can provide quantitative results; and, importantly, can be used to assess asymptomatic viral shedding. DIF is a rapid test that requires rich fresh samples. Samples should be taken ideally within 24 h of the initial clinical manifestations and taken from the base of vesicular lesions.

Serology to detect HSV-1 or HSV-2 IgG is reliable to show past infection. HSV IgM serology is not reliable for a recent or early infection. Seroconversion can take several weeks to months in some cases, so repeat testing may be warranted if a patient tests seronegative at baseline.

MEDICAL MANAGEMENT

Evidence-based management strategies for genital herpes are related either to the treatment of patients diagnosed with an acute outbreak (either the primary or recurrent infections) or to prevent recurrent infections. All patients and their partners should receive counseling regarding the natural history of genital herpes, sexual and perinatal transmission, and ways to reduce transmission.

In those presenting with the first clinical episode of genital herpes, treatment includes oral antiviral therapy with acyclovir, famciclovir, or valacyclovir. All three are nucleoside analogue drugs that act as DNA chain terminators during virus replication in infected cells. Topical acyclovir therapy is substantially less effective than systemic drug administration, and its use is not recommended for genital herpes. Use of systemic antiviral drugs can shorten the duration, frequency, and

symptoms of outbreaks, and can reduce the frequency of asymptomatic shedding and the risk of transmission. However, antiviral agents do not eliminate the virus from the latent state, nor do they affect subsequent risk, frequency, or severity of recurrence after drug use is discontinued. However, antiviral drugs are effective when given suppressively (i.e., to prevent reactivation of a latent infection) or abortively (i.e., at least 1 day within the appearance of symptoms). Daily suppressive antiviral therapy can be implemented for patients with frequent recurrences (e.g., more than five recurrences per year). Safety and efficacy have been documented among patients given daily therapy with acyclovir for as long as 20 years and valacyclovir, a precursor of acyclovir, have repeatedly been demonstrated to have a similar safety profile. Suppressive therapy has not been associated with emergence of clinically significant acyclovir resistance among immunocompetent patients. Because the frequency of recurrence tends to diminish over time in many patients, current recommendations include discussing periodically the possibility of discontinuing suppressive therapy to reassess the need for continued therapy.

Acyclovir, famciclovir, and valacyclovir have been assigned pregnancy category C, B, and B, respectively, by the FDA. Accordingly, famciclovir and valacyclovir are considered relatively safe to administer to pregnant women.

Current treatment recommendations by the CDC (Box 13.3) are directed toward primary, recurrent, and suppressive genital herpes therapy. These protocols also may be used for oral infections. IV antiviral agents (acyclovir, cidofovir, and foscarnet) are reserved for severe or complicated infections and may be required for immune-suppressed patients.

Despite extensive research, there is currently no effective vaccine for HSV infection.

DENTAL CONSIDERATIONS AND ORAL MANIFESTATIONS

Genital herpes may rarely be transmitted from genital sites to the oral cavity (Fig. 13.9).

Herpes simplex virus–induced lesions involving the oral and perioral tissues, irrespective of cause or viral subtype, are infectious during the papular, vesicular, and ulcerative stages, and elective dental treatment should be delayed until the herpetic lesion has completely healed. Dental manipulation during these infectious stages poses risks of (1) inoculation to a new site on the patient, (2) infection to the dental health professional, and (3) aerosol or droplet inoculation of the conjunctivae of the patient or of dental personnel. After the lesion has crusted, the patient is considered noninfectious. Antiviral agents may be required to prevent dental treatment associated recurrence. Management of oral HSV infections is covered in Appendix C.

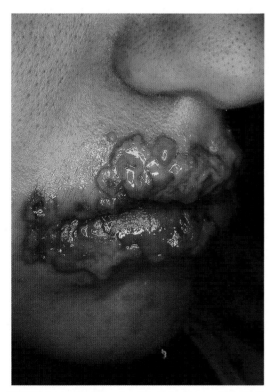

FIG. 13.9 Primary herpes simplex type 2 occurring in the oral cavity documented by laboratory testing. (From Sapp JP, Eversole LS, Wysocki GP. *Contemporary Oral and Maxillofacial Pathology.* 2nd ed. St. Louis, MO: Mosby; 2004.)

A problem of particular concern to dental health professionals is herpetic infection of the fingers or nail beds contracted by dermal contact with a herpetic lesion of the lip or oral cavity of a patient. The infection is called a herpetic whitlow or a herpetic paronychia (Fig. 13.10). It is serious, debilitating, and recurrent. Also, asymptomatic HSV shedding at oral or nonoral sites can trigger erythema multiforme, a mucocutaneous eruption characterized by "target" lesions and ulcers that result from an immune response to the virus and may be recurrent.

INFECTIOUS MONONUCLEOSIS

Although not classically defined as an STD, infectious mononucleosis is discussed in this chapter because transmission occurs through intimate personal contact. In more than 90% of cases, IM is caused by a primary EBV infection (the remaining approximately 10% of cases caused by other organisms, including CMV, HHV-6, HIV, adenovirus, and toxoplasmosis). Children, adolescents, and young adults are most commonly affected, and transmission of the virus occurs primarily by way of the oropharyngeal route during close personal contact (i.e., intimate kissing). Infectious mononucleosis produces a clinical triad of fever, sore throat, and lymphadenopathy, and is associated with lymphocytosis.

EPIDEMIOLOGY

More than 90% of adults worldwide have been infected with EBV. EBV seroprevalence increases during childhood, with socioeconomic factors contributing to the highest rates in non-Hispanic blacks aged 15–19 years ($\approx$78%). No gender predilection has been noted. Having numerous sexual partners increases the risk for acquisition of EBV. Only about 25% of teenagers who are infected with EBV develop infectious mononucleosis.

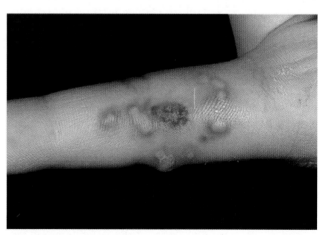

FIG. 13.10 Herpetic whitlow. (From Habif TP, Campbell JI Jr, Chapman MS et al. *Skin Disease: Diagnosis and Treatment.* 2nd ed. St. Louis, MO: Mosby; 2005.)

ETIOLOGY

Epstein—Barr virus is a B-lymphotropic herpesvirus that is transmitted primarily after exposure to oropharyngeal secretions, predominantly by kissing. Infrequently, it is transmitted through shared infected drinks, eating utensils, or infected blood products. The incubation time is approximately 6 weeks. A prodromal period of 3—5 days precedes the clinical phase, which typically lasts 7—20 days. During the prodromal phase, the virus infects oropharyngeal epithelial cells and spreads to B lymphocytes in the tonsillar crypts. Infected B lymphocytes circulate through the reticuloendothelial system, triggering a marked CD8+ T-lymphocytic response. The combination of reactive lymphocytes, the cytokines they produce, and the B cell—produced (heterophile) antibodies directed against EBV antigens contributes to the clinical manifestation of the acute infection. After the acute infection, the virus remains latent in B lymphocytes for the life of the host. About 40% of asymptomatic herpesvirus-seropositive adults carry EBV in their saliva on any given day.

CLINICAL PRESENTATION

Infectious mononucleosis usually is asymptomatic when found in children; however, when young adults are affected, about 75% are symptomatic. A meta-analysis of clinical features reported the most common presentations include lymphadenopathy (predominantly cervical), sore throat, malaise, and fatigue. Less common manifestations include palatal petechial hemorrhage; posterior cervical, axillary, or inguinal lymphadenopathy; pharyngeal or tonsillar exudate; and cutaneous rash. Other signs and symptoms include fever, headache, decreased appetite, nausea and vomiting, myalgias (body aches), arthralgias, splenomegaly, hepatomegaly, and jaundice. Symptoms typically dissipate within 3 weeks of onset.

Complications are rare (<1%) but can include splenic rupture (particularly in patients who play sports during the infection), airway obstruction caused by pharyngitis, meningoencephalitis, hemolytic anemia, and thrombocytopenia. Infectious mononucleosis and EBV infection are unlikely to be the underlying trigger for chronic fatigue syndrome, but EBV and a history of infectious mononucleosis are strong risk factors for the development of multiple sclerosis and other autoimmune diseases, EBV-associated lymphomas, and nasopharyngeal carcinoma.

LABORATORY AND DIAGNOSTIC FINDINGS

The diagnosis of infectious mononucleosis cannot be made by clinical examination alone, and laboratory testing is necessary for confirmation. A white blood cell count demonstrating lymphocytosis (>50%) with blood smears revealing more than 10% atypical "reactive" lymphocytes is highly predictive (Fig. 13.11). The heterophile antibody rapid latex agglutination test (Monospot test) has been largely replaced by EBV-specific antibody testing as the gold-standard for the diagnosis of IE. In immunocompetent patients, antibodies to the viral capsid antigen (VCA IgM and VCA IgG) and EBV nuclear antigen (EBNA-1 IgG) can help differentiate between a primary and past infection (a positive VCA IgM result is commensurate with the primary infection; positive results for VCA IgG and EBNA-1 IgG show a history of past infection). Antibody profiles are often equivocal in immunocompromised patients and PCR testing may be more useful for detecting primary infection, or for monitoring EBV-DNA copy numbers in the blood which correlates to severity and progression of the infection.

MEDICAL MANAGEMENT

Infectious mononucleosis is largely the result of the immune response to EBV, and there are no pharmacotherapies indicated for the disease. As such, treatment is tailored to symptoms and consists of bedrest, fluids, acetaminophen or nonsteroidal antiinflammatory agents for pain control, and gargling and irrigation with saline solution or lidocaine to relieve sore throat symptoms. There is poor evidence that antiviral drugs such as acyclovir are effective against acute infectious mononucleosis and they are not recommended. Systemic corticosteroids are not recommended unless there is evidence of airway obstruction. Vigorous activity is to be avoided to reduce the risk of splenic rupture. About 20% of patients with symptomatic infectious mononucleosis have concurrent β-hemolytic streptococcal pharyngotonsillitis and should be treated with penicillin VK if they are not allergic to penicillin. Most patients feel better and return to normal activities within 1 month.

Despite active research, there are currently no vaccines to prevent infectious mononucleosis.

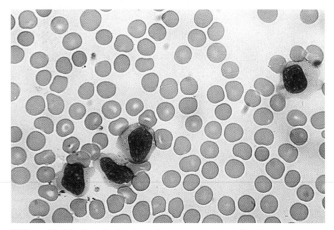

FIG. 13.11 Atypical lymphocytes in infectious mononucleosis. (From Kumar V, Abbas A, Fausto N. *Robbins & Cotran's Pathologic Basis of Disease.* 7th ed. Philadelphia, PA: Saunders; 2005.)

DENTAL CONSIDERATIONS AND ORAL MANIFESTATIONS

Patients (particularly adolescents) presenting with palatal petechiae, enlarged tonsils, pharyngitis with tonsillar exudate, and with cervical lymphadenopathy should raise suspicion of infectious mononucleosis, and these patients should be referred to a physician for evaluation and treatment. Routine dental treatment should be delayed for about 4 weeks until the patient has recovered. Patients with a history of infectious mononucleosis may be at risk for developing EBV-associated Hodgkin and non-Hodgkin lymphomas. These lymphomas may manifest as persistent cervical lymphadenopathy or oral cavity lesions.

HUMAN PAPILLOMAVIRUS INFECTIONS

Human papillomaviruses are small, double-stranded, non-enveloped DNA viruses that infect and replicate in mucosal and cutaneous sites. More than 120 genotypes of HPV have been identified, and more than 40 types are known to be sexually transmitted and to affect the anogenital epithelium. Each HPV subtype exhibits preferential anatomic sites of infection and a propensity for altering epithelial growth and replication. The spectrum of disease that is induced is dependent on the type of HPV infection, location, and immune response. Subtypes of HPV have been classified as "high-risk" or "low-risk" types. Low-risk HPVs (>90%, of subtypes are HPV-6 and -11) cause benign lesions (involving the anogenital area and other non-genital skin and mucosal sites), and high-risk HPV types (predominantly HPV-16 and -18) are strongly associated with intraepithelial lesions and carcinoma of the cervix, vagina, and anus. HPV-16 is also strongly associated with oropharynx cancer (base of tongue and palatine tonsils). Box 13.4 lists HPV-associated lesions and conditions.

EPIDEMIOLOGY

Globally, HPV-related infections are the most common STDs. In the United States, an estimated 80 million people have prevalent HPV infection, and more than 14 million new infections occur annually. More than 90% of these infections resolve over time, and the remainder become symptomatic, manifesting as either benign lesions (i.e., anogenital warts or oral lesions) or as premalignant or malignant disease (i.e., in those harboring high-risk genotypes infections). At least 50% of sexually active adults will acquire an HPV-related infection during their lifetime. Anogenital warts are common in both sexes, and the highest rates of infection occur between the ages of 19 and 26 years. By age 50 years, more than 80% of women will have acquired genital HPV infection. Socioeconomic factors contribute to infections being more common among African American women than white women. The lifetime number of sexual partners is the most important risk factor for the development of HPV-related infections.

BOX 13.4   **Papillomavirus Genotypes**
Non-Genital Benign Involving the Skin
Common warts (verrucae vulgaris) 1, 2, 4, 7
Flat plane warts 3, 10
Plantar warts 1, 2, 4, 63
Non-Genital Benign Involving Mucosae
Oral papillomata 6, 11
Focal epithelial hyperplasia (Heck's disease) 13, 32
Recurrent laryngeal papillomatosis 6, 11
Oral condylomata 6, 11
Florid oral papillomatosis (HIV-infected patients) 6, 7, 11, 16, 32
Genital Benign Lesions
Anogenital warts (condyloma acuminatum) 6, 11
Malignant and Potentially Malignant Disorders
Anal dysplasia and squamous cell carcinoma 16, 18
Cervical intraepithelial neoplasia and squamous cell carcinoma 16, 18, 31, 33, 35, 39, 45, 52, 58
Penile squamous cell carcinoma 16, 18
Oropharyngeal squamous cell carcinoma 16, 18
Vulvar squamous cell carcinoma 16, 18

There is a higher prevalence of HPV-related infections in HIV+ patients.

Based on data from 2013 to 2017, there are approximately 45,000 HPV-associated cancers diagnosed annually in the United States.

ETIOLOGY

Human papillomavirus can be transmitted by direct contact during sexual contact (i.e., penetrative: vaginal or anal, or nonpenetrative: oral–genital, genital–genital, or manual–genital). Fetal infection is rare but can lead to respiratory papillomatosis. HPV enters the epithelium or epidermis through microtears and infects the basal cell layer. When the virus is intracellular, it increases the turnover of infected cells. Nononcogenic subtypes, such as HPV-6 and -11 have a strong tendency to induce epithelial hyperplasia, leading to wart-like lesions known as condylomata. Some infections remain episomally in a latent state. Anogenital or oral lesions (condyloma acuminatum) usually appear after an incubation period of 3 weeks–8 months. There are at least 13 different oncogenic genotypes, of which HPV-16 and -18 are the most commonly detected in human cancers. All oncogenic genotypes have a propensity to induce malignancy, although it typically takes years to decades for malignant transformation to occur.

CLINICAL PRESENTATION

Anogenital warts (condylomata) are predominantly external, although they may be found intraanally, intravaginally, or involving the cervix and urethral meatus. Externally, they have a variable clinical appearance, ranging from small multiple confluent sessile papules (<1 mm) to grossly exophytic papillary or warty cauliflower-like lesions measuring up to several centimeters in diameter. In men, these growths may be found on the penis, scrotum, pubic region, and anal and rectal areas. In women, genital warts are commonly found on moist areas on the labia minora and vaginal opening (Fig. 13.12A). The borders are raised and rounded. The color varies from pink to dusky gray. Most condylomata are asymptomatic; however, patients may report itching, irritation, pain, or bleeding as a result of manipulation or trauma.

LABORATORY AND DIAGNOSTIC FINDINGS

Human papillomavirus does not grow in cell culture, and serologic tests are not routinely performed. Therefore, if the clinical diagnosis of condyloma acuminatum is uncertain, lesions should be biopsied and examined microscopically. The microscopic appearance consists of a sessile base, with raised epithelial borders, a thick spinous layer (acanthosis), hyperkeratosis, and often with the presence of koilocytes. If needed, the identification of HPV genotype is typically achieved with the use of commercial DNA and RNA in situ hybridization kits to detect HPV. Some kits can screen for low- versus high-risk HPV genotypes, and others can identify specific genotypes (Fig. 13.12D). Alternative diagnostics include PCR and immunohistochemistry using anti-HPV antibodies.

MEDICAL MANAGEMENT

As with all STDs, treatment should include the patient's sexual partner(s) to avoid reinfection and protective activities (i.e., abstinence, use of condoms) to reduce transmission. Without treatment, lesions may enlarge and spread, although spontaneous regression can occur.

Anogenital Warts

There is a strong evidence base for the management of genital warts that supports the use of a number of regimens that lead to clearance of warts, reduce recurrence, and prevent further transmission. These include surgical and ablative techniques or the administration of antiproliferative or immunomodulatory agents. Ablative techniques include scalpel excision; electrosurgery; laser removal (i.e., vaporization with a CO_2 laser); cryotherapy; photodynamic therapy; and chemical destruction with local application of trichloroacetic acid, bichloracetic acid, or potassium hydroxide. Nondestructive topical agents include podophyllotoxin, podophyllin, imiquimod, sinecatechins (e.g., Polyphenon E), cidofovir, and 5-fluorouracil. Other agents include systemic retinoids and interferon, which may be used topically,

intralesionally, or systemically. The CDC-recommended treatments are provided in Box 13.5.

Cancer

Management of patients diagnosed with HPV-associated cancers is site specific and may involve single or multimodality treatments including surgery, radiation therapy, chemotherapy, or targeted therapy.

HPV-Vaccine

A major advance occurred in 2006 with the introduction of the HPV vaccine, the most recent of which is a 9-valent HPV vaccine (Gardasil 9) that covers nononcogenic genotypes (6, 11) to prevent benign HPV-infection and anogenital warts, and seven oncogenic genotypes (16, 18, 31, 33, 45, 52, and 58) to prevent HPV-associated cancers. In 2020, the FDA expanded the indication for the HPV-vaccine to include the prevention of HPV-positive oropharynx cancer. The 2019 indications for the HPV-vaccine are included in Box 13.6.

ORAL MANIFESTATIONS AND DENTAL CONSIDERATIONS

Oral condylomata acuminatum commonly occurs as solitary or multiple lesions on the ventral tongue, gingivae, labial mucosae, and palate (Fig. 13.12B). Oral warts in HIV-infected patients, predominantly in the MSM population, may present as solitary lesions or as clusters of multiple lesions that may be florid in their presentation and that can be unesthetic (Fig. 13.12C). A number of different HPV genotypes may be detected in these lesions, some of which are high risk. Such lesions range in color (pink to white), surface topography (flat surfaced to papillary), and size (small 1–2 mm and confluent to large [>1 cm in diameter] and grossly exophytic).

Not all oral benign HPV-lesions are transmitted sexually, and when detected during a routine examination, dental health professionals should elicit a careful history to assess the likely mode of transmission. The identification of possible HPV-lesions resembling condylomata in children raises the suspicion of sexual abuse, particularly when autoinoculation by hand-to-genital contact, nonsexual contact, or maternal–fetal transmission has been ruled out. Failure to report signs of an STD to state health officials is a legal offense in some states.

Benign HPV lesions typically present little risk for transmission to the oral health care team. Solitary lesions may be surgically excised and submitted for histopathology. Management of florid oral lesions is challenging, and there is no evidence-based treatment. Lesions can be surgically excised or removed by electrocautery or laser. Clearance of warts with the use of topical, intralesional, or systemic agents such as podophyllin, imiquimod, cimetidine, interferon, or cidofovir

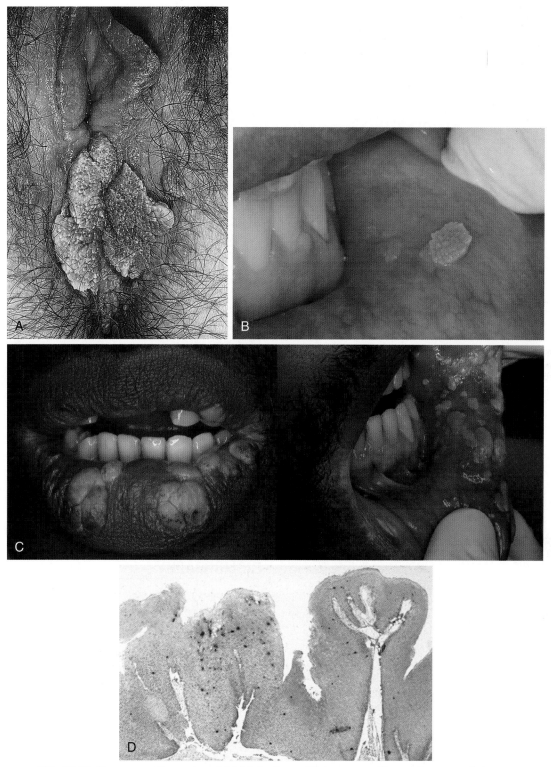

FIG. 13.12 Human papillomavirus (HPV) infections. (**A**) Large, cauliflower-like wart of the vagina. (**B**) Flat-topped papillary oral condylomata of the labial mucosa. (**C**) Multiple oral warts in an HIV-infected man who has sex with other men. (**D**) In situ hybridization showing HPV DNA as indicated by dark purple stains in the epithelium of a condyloma acuminatum. ((**A**) From Habif TP, Campbell JI Jr, Chapman MS et al. *Skin Disease: Diagnosis and Treatment.* 2nd ed. St. Louis, MO: Mosby; 2005.)

BOX 13.5 **Regimens Recommended by the Centers for Disease Control and Prevention for the Treatment of Anogenital Warts**

External Anogenital Warts (i.e., Penis, Groin, Scrotum, Vulva, Perineum, External Anus, and Perianus[a])

Patient Applied
Imiquimod 3.75% or 5% cream[b], or
Podofilox 0.5% solution or gel, or
Sinecatechins 15% ointment[b]

Provider Administered
Cryotherapy with liquid nitrogen or cryoprobe, or
Surgical removal:
- Tangential scissor excision, tangential shave excision, curettage or laser or
- Electrosurgery or
- TCA or BCA 80%–90% solution

Urethral Meatus Warts
Cryotherapy with liquid nitrogen, or
Surgical removal

Vaginal Warts
Cryotherapy with liquid nitrogen, or

Surgical removal, or
TCA or BCA 80%–90% solution
Note: The use of a cryoprobe in the vagina is not recommended because of the risk for vaginal perforation and fistula formation

Cervical Warts
Cryotherapy with liquid nitrogen, or
Surgical removal, or
TCA or BCA 80%–90% solution
Note: Management of cervical warts should include consultation with a specialist. For women who have exophytic cervical warts, a biopsy evaluation to exclude high-grade SIL must be performed before treatment is initiated.

Intraanal Warts
Cryotherapy with liquid nitrogen, or
Surgical removal, or
TCA or BCA 80%–90% solution
Note: Management of intraanal warts should include consultation with a specialist.

[a]Many persons with external anal warts also have intraanal warts. Thus, persons with external anal warts might benefit from an inspection of the anal canal by digital examination, standard anoscopy, or high-resolution anoscopy.
[b]Might weaken condoms and vaginal diaphragms.
BCA, Bichloroacetic acid; *SIL*, squamous intraepithelial lesion; *TCA*, trichloroacetic acid.

BOX 13.6 **HPV-Vaccine Recommendations[a]**

HPV vaccination is routinely recommended at age 11 or 12 y; vaccination can be given starting at age 9 y.

ACS Qualifying Statement: Routine HPV vaccination between ages 9–12 y is expected to achieve higher on-time vaccination rates, resulting in increased numbers of cancers prevented. Health care providers are encouraged to start offering the HPV vaccine at age 9 or 10 y.

Vaccination is recommended for all persons through age 26 y who are not adequately vaccinated.

ACS Qualifying Statement: Providers should inform individuals aged 22–26 y who have not been previously vaccinated or who have not completed the series that vaccination at older ages is less effective in lowering cancer risk.

Catch-up HPV vaccination is not recommended for all adults aged >26 y. Instead, shared clinical decision-making regarding HPV vaccination is recommended for some adults aged 27–45 y who are not adequately vaccinated.

The ACS does not endorse the recommendation for shared clinical decision-making for adults aged 27–45 y because of the low effectiveness and low cancer prevention potential of vaccination in this age group, the burden of decision-making on patients and clinicians, and the lack of sufficient guidance on selection of individuals who might benefit.

[a]American Cancer Society adaptation of the 2019 Advisory Committee on Immunization Practices HPV Vaccination Recommendations with qualifying statements in *italics*.

has been reported, although adverse effects are possible. Strict infection control procedures and high-speed evacuation should be used during laser therapy to avoid cross-contamination of surfaces and inhalation of the virion-laden plume.

BIBLIOGRAPHY

1. Abusalah MAH, Gan SH, Al-Hatamleh MAI, et al. Recent advances in diagnostic approaches for Epstein–Barr virus. *Pathogens.* 2020;9(226):2–17.
2. Bradley H, Markowitz LE, Gibson T, et al. Seroprevalence of herpes simplex virus types 1 and 2–United States, 1999–2010. *J Infect Dis.* 2014;209:325–333.
3. Compilato D, Amato S, Campisi G. Resurgence of syphilis: a diagnosis based on unusual oral mucosa lesions. *Oral Surg Oral Med Oral Pathol Oral Radiol Endod.* 2009;108:e45–e49.
4. Corey L, Wald A, Patel R, et al. Once-daily valacyclovir to reduce the risk of transmission of genital herpes. *N Engl J Med.* 2004;350:11–20.
5. Czerninski R, Pikovski A, Meir K, et al. Oral syphilis lesions–a diagnostic approach and histologic characteristics of secondary stage. *Quintessence Int.* 2011;42:883–889.
6. De Paor M, O'Brien K, Fahey T, Smith SM. Antiviral agents for infectious mononucleosis (glandular fever). *Cochrane Database Syst Rev.* 2016;12:CD011487.

7. Engelberg R, Carrell D, Krantz E, et al. Natural history of genital herpes simplex virus type 1 infection. *Sex Transm Dis*. 2003;30:174−177.

8. Kreisel KM, Spicknall IH, Gargano JW, Lewis FM, et al. Sexually transmitted Iinfections among US women and men: prevalence and incidence estimates, 2018. *Sex Transm Dis*. 2021;48:208−214.

9. Lennon P, Crotty M, Fenton JE. Infectious mononucleosis. *BMJ*. 2015;350:h1825.

10. Leuci S, Martina S, Adamo D, et al. Oral syphilis: a retrospective analysis of 12 cases and a review of the literature. *Oral Dis*. 2013;19:738−746.

11. Little JW. Gonorrhea: update. *Oral Surg Oral Med Oral Pathol Oral Radiol Endod*. 2006;101:137−143.

12. Little JW. Syphilis: an update. *Oral Surg Oral Med Oral Pathol Oral Radiol Endod*. 2005;100:3−9.

13. Meites E, Szilagyi PG, Chesson HW, et al. Human papillomavirus vaccination for adults: updated recommendations of the advisory committee on immunization practices. *MMWR Morb Mortal Wkly Rep*. 2019;68:698−702.

14. Miller CS, Cunningham LL, Lindroth JE, et al. The efficacy of valacyclovir in preventing recurrent herpes simplex virus infections associated with dental procedures. *J Am Dent Assoc*. 2004;135:1311−1318.

15. Miller CS, Avdiushko SA, Kryscio RJ, et al. Effect of prophylactic valacyclovir on the presence of human herpesvirus DNA in saliva of healthy individuals after dental treatment. *J Clin Microbiol*. 2005;43:2173−2180.

16. Nissanka-Jayasuriya EH, Odell EW, Phillips C. Dental stigmata of congenital syphilis: a historic review with present day relevance. *Head Neck Pathol*. 2016;10:327−331.

17. Rautava J, Syrjanen S. Human papillomavirus infections in the oral mucosa. *J Am Dent Assoc*. 2011;142:905−914.

18. Saslow D, Andrews KS, Manassaram-Baptiste D, Smith RA, et al. Human papillomavirus vaccination 2020 guideline update: American Cancer society guideline adaptation. *CA A Cancer J Clin*. 2020;70:274−280.

19. St Cyr S, Barbee L, Workowski KA, et al. Update to CDC's treatment guidelines for gonococcal infection, 2020. *Morb Mortal Wkly Rep*. 2020;69(50):1911−1916.

20. Tyring SK, Baker D, Snowden W. Valacyclovir for herpes simplex virus unfection: long-term safety and sustained efficacy after 20 years' experience with acyclovir. *J Infect Dis*. 2002;186(Suppl 1):S40−S46.

21. Unemo M, Del Rio C, Shafer WM. Antimicrobial resistance expressed by *Neisseria gonorrhoeae*: a major global public health problem in the 21st century. *Microbiol Spectr*. 2016;4(3):213−237.

22. Viens LJ, Henley SJ, Watson M, et al. Human papillomavirus-associated cancers − United States, 2008−2012. *MMWR Morb Mortal Wkly Rep*. 2016;65:661−666.

23. Workowski KA, Bachmann LH, Chan PA, et al. Sexually transmitted diseases treatment guidelines, 2021. *MMWR Recomm Rep (Morb Mortal Wkly Rep)*. 2021;70:1−187.

14

Diabetes Mellitus

KEY POINTS

- Diabetes mellitus is important because dentists regularly encounter patients with diabetes and will detect patients who are not yet diagnosed or poorly controlled.
- Diabetes negatively impacts oral health, and good oral health may positively impact diabetic control.
- Patients with diabetes undergoing dental treatment may be at risk for complications such as hypoglycemia, unconsciousness, dental infection, and drug interactions/side effects.
- Diabetics with a fasting blood glucose >300 mg/dL (16.6 mmol/L) should be referred to their physician or a hospital.

- Diabetics with no significant comorbidities and a preoperative fasting blood glucose between 80 and 200 mg/dL (4.4–11.2 mmol/L) can safely undergo dental and surgical procedures. Diabetics with comorbidities and/or fasting blood glucose outside these ranges require careful consideration before performing treatment.
- Diabetics are at risk for developing periodontal diseases, dental caries, odontogenic infections, xerostomia, and fungal infections.

Diabetes mellitus is a group of chronic metabolic diseases characterized by high blood glucose levels (hyperglycemia) and classified by the American Diabetes Association (ADA) into four general types (Box 14.1). Diabetes may affect persons of all ages, and persistent uncontrolled metabolic and hemodynamic changes can lead to both acute and chronic complications, and collectively these complications have an enormous impact on quality of life and mortality, not to mention health care costs. Careful determination of the level of disease severity/glycemic control, as well as the presence of diabetic complications is critical, and working in concert with the managing physician can help to develop a dental management plan that will be effective and safe for the patient.

EPIDEMIOLOGY

More than 400 million persons (>5%) have diabetes mellitus worldwide. In the United States there has been a sustained increasing trend. The year 2020 statistics report 34 million Americans have diabetes, representing more than 10% of the population. Twenty percent of diabetics are undiagnosed, and 88 million have prediabetes. Historical, political, and economic factors impacting health disparities have contributed to a disproportionately higher prevalence of diabetes in American Indians/Alaska Natives (15.9%), people of Hispanic origin (12.5%),

non-Hispanic Blacks (11.7%). Also, those with poor education (13.3% in those with less than high-school education) are more commonly affected. Diabetes mellitus accounts for about 85,000 deaths per year and is the seventh most common cause of death in the United States. Diabetics have higher rates of disability, a poorer quality of life, and lower life expectancy compared to those without diabetes.

Type 2 disease comprises >90% of diabetes mellitus. The incidence of type 2 diabetes increases with age and is primarily an adult disease. In contrast, type 1 diabetes is four times more prevalent than type 2 diabetes in persons younger than 20 years of age. The major reason for the increase in diabetes is the obesity epidemic, especially in relation to type 2 diabetes. In 2017, the annual health care costs for diabetes was $327 billion.

ETIOLOGY

Type 1 diabetes is the result of pancreatic β-cell destruction and is characterized by insulin deficiency. *Type 2 diabetes* is characterized by insulin resistance and relative insulin deficiency. The broad category of *other specific types* (Box 14.1) comprises numerous conditions (i.e., monogenic diabetes syndromes, diseases of the exocrine pancreas, and drug or chemical induced diabetes). *Gestational diabetes* is abnormal glucose tolerance

---

BOX 14.1 Classification of Diabetes

- **Type 1**: due to autoimmune β-cell destruction, usually leading to absolute insulin deficiency, including latent autoimmune diabetes of adulthood.
- **Type 2**: due to a progressive loss of adequate β-cell insulin secretion frequently on the background of insulin resistance.
- **Other specific types**: monogenic diabetes syndromes such as neonatal diabetes and maturity-onset diabetes of the young, diseases of the exocrine pancreas (such as cystic fibrosis and pancreatitis), and drug- or chemical-induced diabetes (such as with glucocorticoid use), in the treatment of HIV/AIDS, or after organ transplantation.
- **Gestational Diabetes**: diagnosed in the second or third trimester of pregnancy that was not clearly overt diabetes prior to gestation.

Data from American Diabetes Association. Standards of care—2021. *Diabetes Care.* 2021;44(suppl. 1):S15–S33.

---

that is detected during pregnancy. In addition, persons who have abnormal blood glucose levels that are not high enough to be classified as diabetes are assigned a diagnosis of *prediabetes*. Fig. 14.1 illustrates the disorders of glycemia by types of diabetes.

Type 1 diabetes is thought to be the result of autoimmunity to one or more different pancreatic islet antigens, likely triggered by environmental factors in the context of genetic susceptibility, and leads to pancreatic β-cell loss and ultimate diabetes and its progression over time Fig. 14.2. Genetics contributes to approximately half of those with type 1 diabetes, with candidate genes linked to the HLA region on chromosome 6, and, to a lesser extent, other non-HLA gene polymorphisms such as the insulin gene. Environmental triggers are less well established and may include exposure in utero or during early childhood to infections, diet, or toxins.

Type 2 diabetes is prominently linked to lifestyle and environmental factors in the context of genetic predisposition. An energy dense diet and a sedentary lifestyle predict an increase in body mass index (i.e., obesity), which is the strongest etiological predictor. Gene-wide association studies have identified a number of "susceptibility variants," and these are beginning to explain the complex interplay affecting insulin secretion by β-cells, target tissue insulin sensitivity, appetite regulation, and adipose storage. Table 14.1 compares the features of Type 1 and 2 diabetes.

PATHOPHYSIOLOGY AND COMPLICATIONS

Glucose is rapidly taken up by the pancreatic β-cells and serves as the most important stimulus for insulin secretion. Insulin remains in circulation for only several minutes (half-life, 4–8 min) and mediates glucose uptake and storage into target tissues (i.e., muscle, liver, kidney, and fat cells). Lack of insulin or a disruption in the action of insulin (i.e., insulin resistance) in diabetes leads to a constellation of downstream consequences (Fig. 14.3).

Persistently elevated blood glucose levels put persons at risk for diabetes. Approximately 10% of people with prediabetes develop overt diabetes each year. In an average dental practice of 2000 patients, approximately 200 patients will be diabetic and 500 will be prediabetic (90% of the diabetics will by type 2, and approximately 5% will be undiagnosed). Ten percent of diabetics will experience severe complications (requiring emergency medical intervention or hospitalization): almost 8% major cardiovascular events (i.e., myocardial infarction or stroke), 1% severe hypoglycemia, and 1% hyperglycemia (i.e., diabetic ketoacidosis (DKA) or hyperosmolar hyperglycemic syndrome).

In type 1 diabetes, the autoimmune-related inability of the pancreas to produce insulin results in hyperglycemia.

	Control of hyperglycemia		
	Insulin not required for control	Insulin required for control	Insulin required for survival
Diabetes types			
Type 1		+	+
Type 2	+[1]	+/–[1]	
Gestational	+[2]	+/–[2]	
Other specific types	+		

[1] In type 2 diabetics, glycemic control is typically achieved by medications other than insulin and modifications in lifestyle. In certain cases, insulin may be required.
[2] In gestational diabetes, glycemic control is typically achieved by diet control, although in some cases, insulin is required.

FIG. 14.1 Types of diabetes and requirements for insulin.

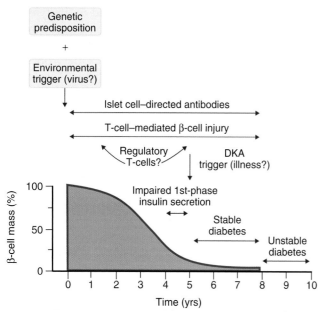

FIG. 14.2 Summary of the sequence of events that leads to pancreatic beta cell loss and ultimately to the clinical evolution of type 1 diabetes. *DKA,* Diabetic ketoacidosis.

The excess glucose is excreted by the kidneys into the urine (glycosuria) causing osmotic diuresis, dehydration, and electrolyte imbalance. Meanwhile, the target tissues become starved of glucose and enter a catabolic state leading to glycogenolysis, gluconeogenesis, proteolysis, and lipolysis with the release of ketone bodies. Ketosis precipitates metabolic acidosis and ultimately DKA, which can lead to coma and death in severe cases if it is not identified and treated promptly. In type 2 diabetes, adiposity-based chronic disease (ABCD, the current medical diagnostic terminology for overweight/obesity) causes the target tissues to become progressively resistant to insulin, and eventually the pancreas is unable to produce sufficient insulin to compensate. Type 2 diabetics typically undergo less severe lipolysis and ketosis, and, if left untreated, have a higher propensity for developing hyperglycemic hyperosmolar syndrome (HHS).

Irrespective of the type of diabetes, chronic hyperglycemia can have a profound effect on the vascular system, causing both macrovascular and microvascular disease and underlies the significant morbidity and mortality associated with diabetes. The mechanisms by which hyperglycemia may lead to macro and microvascular complications include increased accumulation of polyols through the aldose reductase pathway, advanced glycation end products, and increased production of vascular endothelial cell growth factor. Vessel changes include thickening of the intima, endothelial proliferation, and lipid deposition.

Macrovascular Complications

Macrovascular disease is similar to atherosclerosis and therefore associated with coronary, cerebral, and peripheral artery disease, the end-stages of which can result in complications such as myocardial infarction, stroke, renal failure, and gangrene. Diabetics are at a two- to fourfold greater risk for MI and stroke than persons without the disease, and the most common cause of death in patients with type 2 diabetes is myocardial infarction. Macrovascular disease (atherosclerosis) occurs earlier, is more widespread, and is more severe in diabetics. Hyperglycemia plays a role in the evolution of atherosclerotic plaques. Persons with uncontrolled diabetes have increased levels of low-density lipoprotein (LDL) cholesterol and reduced levels of high-density lipoprotein (HDL) cholesterol.

Microvascular Complications

Microvascular disease is specific to diabetes and leads to nephropathy, neuropathy, and retinopathy. In addition, there are a number of nonvascular complications such as

TABLE 14.1	Features of Type 1 and Type 2 Diabetes	
Feature	Type 1	Type 2
% of Persons with diabetes	5–10	90–95
Age at onset (yr)	15	40 and older
Body build	Normal or thin	Obese
Severity	Extreme	Mild
Need for insulin	Almost all	25%–30%
Ketoacidosis	More common	Less common
Long-term complications	Very common	Less common
Rate of clinical onset	Rapid	Slow
Stability	Unstable	Stable
Genetic locus	Chromosome 6	Chromosomes 2, 7, 12, 13, and 7
HLA and abnormal autoimmune reactions	Present	Not present
Insulin receptor defects	Less common	Very common

HLA, Human leukocyte antigen.

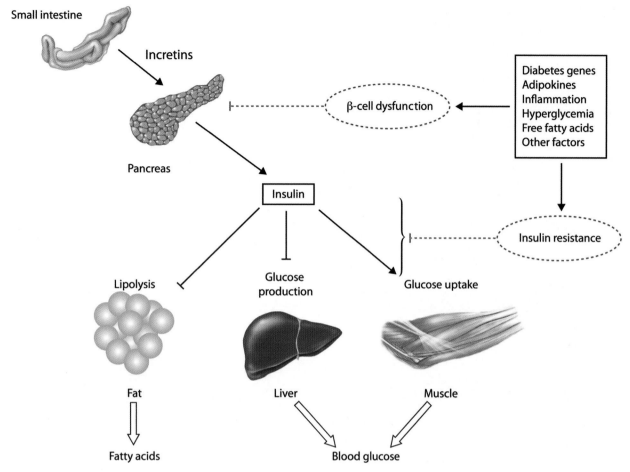

FIG. 14.3 Pathophysiology of hyperglycemia and target tissues. (Courtesy of Mary Lous Cahal, University of Kentucky.)

BOX 14.2 Complications of Diabetes Mellitus

- **Metabolic disturbances:** diabetic ketoacidosis (type 1) and hyperosmolar nonketotic coma (type 2 diabetes).
- **Cardiovascular:** accelerated atherosclerosis (coronary heart disease); high blood pressure; risk for stroke and myocardial infarction.
- **Eyes:** retinopathy, cataracts; blindness.
- **Kidney:** diabetic nephropathy; renal failure.
- **Extremities:** ulceration and gangrene of feet; non—accident-related leg and foot amputations.
- **Diabetic neuropathy:** dysphagia, gastric distention, diarrhea, impotence, muscle weakness or cramps, numbness, tingling, deep burning pain.
- **Early death:** diabetes is the seventh leading cause of death in the United States, most commonly caused by cardiovascular disease.

Data from Centers for Disease Control and Prevention. *National Diabetes Fact Sheet: National Estimates and General Information on Diabetes and Prediabetes in the United States, 2011.* Atlanta, GA, 2011, U.S. Department of Health and Human Services, Centers for Disease Control and Prevention.

---

increased risk for infections, dermatologic issues, hearing loss, and cognitive issues (Box 14.2). Retinopathy occurs in all forms of diabetes. It consists of nonproliferative changes (microaneurysms, retinal hemorrhages, retinal edema, and retinal exudates) and proliferative changes (neovascularization, glial proliferation, and vitreoretinal traction) and is the leading cause of blindness in the United States. Proliferative retinopathy is most common among patients with type 1 diabetes. Cataracts occur at an earlier age and with greater frequency in those with type 1 diabetes.

Individuals with diabetes are at high risk for end-stage renal disease (ESRD). Diabetic nephropathy, caused by microangiopathy of the capillaries of the glomerulus, leads to ESRD in 30%—40% of patients with type 1 diabetes (Fig. 14.4) and in 5% of patients with type 2 diabetes. Renal failure is the leading cause of death in patients with type 1 diabetes.

In the extremities, diabetic neuropathy may lead to progressive sensory and motor neuropathy with a range of signs and symptoms including tingling sensations, numbness, a deep burning pain, muscle cramps, or even muscle

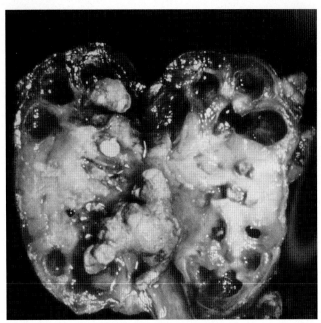

FIG. 14.4 Diabetic Nephropathy: cross section of a kidney. (Courtesy of Richard Estensen, MD, Minneapolis, Minnesota.)

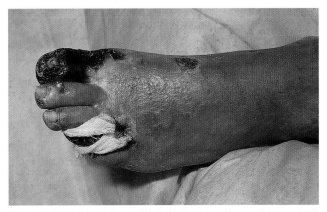

FIG. 14.5 Diabetic gangrene of the feet. (From Swartz MH. *Textbook of Physical Diagnosis: History and Examination.* 6th ed. Philadelphia, PA: Saunders; 2010.)

weakness. In addition, tendon reflexes, two-point discrimination, and position sense may be lost. Patients with peripheral neuropathy are prone to injury, ulceration, and poor wound healing. In the context of macrovascular disease, this can lead to progressive degeneration of a weight-bearing joint (Charcot joint) and gangrene (Fig. 14.5). The relative risk that patients with diabetes will require amputation of an extremity because of diabetic complications is more than 40 times that of normal persons. Diabetic neuropathy also may involve the autonomic nervous system. Esophageal dysfunction may cause dysphagia, stomach involvement may involve a loss of motility with gastric distention, and involvement of the small intestine may result in nocturnal diabetic diarrhea. Sexual impotence and bladder dysfunction also may occur.

Diabetes may be associated with other dermatologic complications such as decubitus ulcerations, skin rashes,

BOX 14.3   **Early Clinical Manifestations of Diabetes**

Type 1
- **Presenting "cardinal" symptoms:** polyuria (often at night), polydipsia, polyphagia, weight loss (without trying), blurry vision, numbness or tingling of hands or feet, very dry skin, sores that heal slowly, fatigue
- **Other signs and symptoms:** recurrence of bed wetting, repeated skin infections, marked irritability, headache, drowsiness, malaise, dry mouth, signs of periodontitis

Type 2
- **Frequent signs and symptoms**[a]**:** slight weight loss or gain, gastrointestinal upset, nausea, urination at night, vulvar pruritus, blurred vision, decreased vision, paresthesias, dry flushed skin, loss of sensation, impotence, postural hypotension, edentulism, signs of periodontitis

[a]The cardinal symptoms seen in type diabetes are far less common in type 2 diabetes.

and deposits of fat in the skin (xanthoma diabeticorum). Other organ system involvement such as cognitive issues and hearing loss also may be linked to diabetes.

CLINICAL PRESENTATION

The signs and symptoms of diabetes are variable and depend on the type of diabetes, disease severity, and associated complications (Box 14.3). In patients with type 1 diabetes, the onset of symptoms is sudden and acute, often developing over days or weeks. Typically, the diagnosis is made in non-obese children or adults younger than 40 years of age; however, it may occur at any age. Patients also may present with DKA, which if severe is accompanied by fruity breath, vomiting, abdominal pain, nausea, tachypnea, paralysis, and ultimately loss of consciousness.

Type 2 diabetes generally occurs after age 40 and more often affects obese individuals. The onset of symptoms in type 2 diabetes usually is insidious, and the manifestations and symptoms are less overt than in type 1 diabetes.

Other signs and symptoms are related to the chronic complications of diabetes.

Laboratory and Diagnostic Findings

The ADA recommends screening for diabetes in adults who are overweight or obese (BMI ≥25, or ≥23 in Asian Americans) or who have one or more of the following risk factors:

(1) first-degree relative with diabetes; (2) high-risk race/ethnicity (e.g., African American, Latino, Native American, Asian American, Pacific Islander); (3) history of cardiovascular disease; (4) hypertension (≥140/90 mmHg or on therapy for hypertension); (5) HDL cholesterol level <35 mg/dL (0.90 mmol/L) and/or a triglyceride level >250 mg/dL (2.82 mmol/L); (6) women with polycystic ovary syndrome; (7) physical inactivity;

TABLE 14.2	**Diagnostic Criteria for Diabetes Mellitus and Prediabetes**
Diabetes Mellitus	**Prediabetes[b]**
1. FGP ≥126 mg/dL (7.0 mmol/L). Fasting is defined as no caloric intake for at least 8 h.[a] or 2. 2-h Plasma Glucose ≥200 mg/dL (11.1 mmol/L) during OGTT. The test should be performed as described by WHO, using a glucose load containing the equivalent of 75 g anhydrous glucose dissolved in water.[a] or 3. A1C ≥6.5% (48 mmol/mol). The test should be performed in a laboratory using a method that is NGSP certified and standardized to the DCCT assay.[a] or 4. In a patient with classic symptoms of hyperglycemia or hyperglycemic crisis, a random plasma glucose ≥200 mg/dL (11.1 mmol/L).	1. FPG 100 mg/dL (5.6 mmol/L) —125 mg/dL (6.9 mmol/L) (IFG) or 2. 2-h PG during 75-g OGTT 140 mg/dL (7.8 mmol/L) to 199 mg/dL (11.0 mmol/L) (IGT) or 3. A1C 5.7% —6.4% (39 —47 mmol/mol)

[a]In the absence of unequivocal hyperglycemia, diagnosis requires two abnormal test results from the same sample or in two separate test samples.

[b]For all three prediabetes tests, risk is continuous, extending below the lower limit of the range and becoming disproportionately greater at the higher end of the range.

DCCT, Diabetes Control and Complications Trial; FPG, fasting plasma glucose; OGTT, oral glucose tolerance test; 2-h PG, 2-h plasma glucose; WHO, World Health Organization; 2-h PG, 2-h plasma glucose; IFG, impaired fasting glucose; IGT, impaired glucose tolerance.

Data from Classification and diagnosis of diabetes: standards of medical care in diabetes 2021. Diabetes Care. 2021;44(Suppl. 1):S15—S33.

and (8) other clinical conditions associated with insulin resistance.

Diabetes is diagnosed by four methods as defined by the ADA criteria (see Table 14.2). The primary diagnostic criteria for prediabetes include *impaired fasting glucose* (IFG) with FPG levels of 100 mg/dL (5.6 mmol/L) to 125 mg/dL (6.9 mmol/L), or *impaired glucose tolerance* (prediabetes) (IGT) with plasma glucose levels of 140 mg/dL (7.8 mmol/L) to 199 mg/dL (11.0 mmol/L) at 2 h in the OGTT, or A1C 5.7%—6.4% (39—47 mmol/mol).

Measurements of glucose are critical to the diagnosis and management of diabetes. Of note, levels of blood glucose are influenced by the source of blood (venous vs. capillary), the age of the patient, the nature of the diet, the physical activity level of the patient, and the measuring method used. Abnormalities in diet (e.g., diet poor in carbohydrate for several days) can lead to misdiagnoses. To minimize this possibility, the diet should contain at least 250—300 g of carbohydrate on each of the 3 days before testing. Patients should not participate in excessive physical activity immediately prior to testing because exercise tends to lower blood glucose levels.

The OGTT reflects how quickly glucose is cleared from the blood, taking into consideration the rate of absorption, uptake by tissues, and excretion in urine. A liquid 75 g glucose load in a 7-fl oz bottle is ingested, and venous blood samples are drawn from the arm just before (i.e., fasting plasma glucose) and 2 h after. The most characteristic alterations seen in diabetes are an increased fasting blood glucose (≥126 mg/dL (7.0 mmol/L)) and an increased 2 h value (≥200 mg/dL (11.1 mmol/L)) demonstrating a delayed return to normal.

The extent of glycosylation of hemoglobin A (a nonenzymatic addition of glucose) that results in formation of HbA_{1c} (i.e., glycated hemoglobin) in red blood cells is used to detect and assess the long-term level (and control) of hyperglycemia in patients with diabetes, and chronically elevated levels are the primary predictor for diabetic complications. The laboratory test to determine HbA_{1c} is known as the A1C assay. This assay measures the amount of sugar attached to hemoglobin; levels increase in the presence of hyperglycemia. The A1C reflects glucose levels in the blood over the preceding 3 months, which is the approximate life span of a red blood cell. In health, patients should have A1C levels less than 6%. In well-controlled diabetes, the level should stay below targets set by the patient's physician without the occurrence of clinically significant hypoglycemia. In newly diagnosed patients, glycemic targets are typically set for <7%; however, higher or lower targets may be set following considerations of risk for adverse effects from antidiabetic medications (i.e., hypoglycemia), duration of disease, life expectancy, important comorbidities, established vascular complications, patient motivation/self-care, and resources/patient support system (Table 14.3). It is standard practice to measure A1C levels at least twice a year in patients whose treatment goals are being met (and who have stable glycemic control) and quarterly in patients whose treatment has changed or whose goals are not being met. A1C levels may not gauge patients with significant glycemic variability, and therefore self-monitored blood glucose (SMBG) or continuous blood glucose (CMG) monitoring may be important.

MEDICAL MANAGEMENT

Diabetes mellitus is not a curable disease (aside from pancreas transplantation); however, strict glycemic control established through regular monitoring reduces complications. Hence, the guidelines published by the ADA, the American College of Endocrinology, and American College of Physicians rely not only on glycemic control but on other important targets such as improvements in lifestyle, modified nutrient intake and weight reduction (as appropriate), blood pressure control, and a favorable lipid profile.

The care of an individual with either type 1 or type 2 diabetes requires a multidisciplinary team. Central to the

TABLE 14.3   Glycemic Targets

Parameter	Target
A1C	<7%*.#
Preprandial plasma glucose	80—130 mg/dL(4.4—7.2 mmol/L)*
Peak postprandial plasma glucose	<180 mg/dL (10.0 mmol/L)*

*More or less stringent glycemic goals may be appropriate for individual patients. Goals should be individualized based on duration of diabetes, age/life expectancy, comorbid conditions, known CVD or advanced microvascular complications, hypoglycemia unawareness, and individual patient considerations.

#CGM may be used to assess glycemic target.

Adapted from Ludwig S: Practical diabetes care for healthcare professionals, 2nd ed. St. Louis, Elsevier, 2021.

BOX 14.4   Key Elements of a Comprehensive Management Plan for Patients With Diabetes Mellitus

Lifestyle Changes
- Healthy diet
- Aerobic exercise
- Weight control
- Smoking cessation
- Stress reduction

Control of Modifiable Metabolic Factors
- Glucose (lifestyle, antihyperglycemia agents, insulin, transplantation)
- Obesity (lifestyle, antiobesity agents, bariatric surgery)
- Lipids (lifestyle, antihyperlipidemia agents)
- Blood pressure (lifestyle, antihypertensives)

Preventive Care
- Regular medical screening examinations
- Regular screening for albuminuria
- Regular ophthalmologic examinations
- Regular podiatric examinations (and self-examinations)
- Regular dental check-ups
- Vaccinations

success of this team are the patient's participation, input, and enthusiasm, all of which are essential for optimal diabetes management. Members of the health care team include the primary care provider or the endocrinologist or diabetologist, a nutritionist, and a psychologist. In addition, when the complications of diabetes arise, subspecialists (including neurologists, nephrologists, vascular surgeons, cardiologists, ophthalmologists, and podiatrists) with experience in diabetes-related complications are essential.

For most patients, a comprehensive treatment plan (see Box 14.4) is devised that includes lifestyle modifications: healthy food choices and physical activity recommendations, along with long-term antihyperglycemic pharmacotherapy, medications to treat obesity, hypertension and hyperlipidemia, along with regular disease monitoring and adjustments. Bariatric surgery may be indicated for severe obesity. If the disease worsens, pancreas and kidney transplantation, or transplantation of pancreatic islet cells into the recipient's liver are options (see Chapter 21).

Because the complications of diabetes are related to glycemic control, normoglycemia is the desired but often elusive goal for most patients. Attempts to consistently normalize or near-normalize the plasma glucose for long periods of time is commensurate with improved outcomes (intensive treatment) (Fig. 14.6) but is challenging for patients. For some patients, striving for consistent normalization can lead to hypoglycemia and associated complications. Therefore, the target for glycemic control (as reflected by the A1C) must be individualized, and the goals of therapy should be developed in consultation with the patient after considering medical, social, and lifestyle issues. The ADA calls this a *patient-centered approach*, which suggests an individualized glycemic goal. For instance, the A1C goal in a young adult with type 1 diabetes may be 6.5%. A higher A1C goal (8.0% or 8.5%) may be appropriate for very young or old patients or individuals with limited life spans or who have comorbidities.

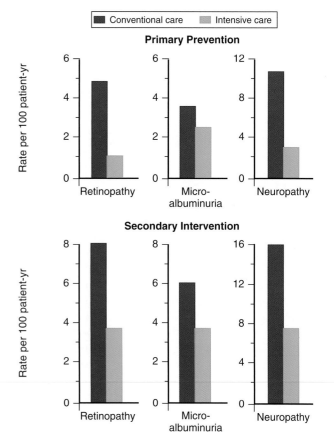

FIG. 14.6 Summary of the results of the diabetes control and complications trial (DCCT).

Type 1 Diabetes Mellitus

Because individuals with type 1 diabetes partially or completely lack endogenous insulin production, administration of insulin (basal insulin) is essential for preventing a catabolic state hallmarked by glycogen breakdown, gluconeogenesis, lipolysis, and ketogenesis. Insulin replacement also must be tailored to the patient's carbohydrate needs (prandial insulin). The treatment goal is therefore to design and implement customized insulin regimens that mimic both basal and prandial insulin secretion. The types of insulin selected for treatment are based on the speed of onset, peak effect, and duration of action.

Intensive diabetes management has the goal of achieving near-normal blood glucose. This approach requires continuing patient education, comprehensive recording of plasma glucose measurements (i.e., by repeated self-monitoring of blood glucose by use of finger-sticks and glucometer (SMBG), or continuous glucose monitoring (CGM)), tight carbohydrate counting by the patient, and a variable insulin regimen that matches glucose intake and insulin dose.

Insulin Preparations. Current insulin preparations are generated by recombinant DNA technology and consist of the amino acid sequence of human insulin or variations thereof to modulate activity (Table 14.4). Insulins can be classified as rapid, short, intermediate, or long acting. Rapid-acting insulin formulations include insulin lispro, an insulin analogue in which the 28th and 29th amino acids (lysine and proline) on the insulin B chain have been reversed by recombinant DNA technology.

Insulin aspart and insulin glulisine are genetically modified insulin analogues with properties similar to lispro. All three of the insulin analogues have full biologic activity but less tendency for self-aggregation, resulting in more rapid absorption and onset of action, and a shorter duration of action. Inhaled human insulin has recently been approved for use and is the most rapid acting. Rapidly acting insulins are associated with a decreased number of hypoglycemic episodes and they are therefore preferred over regular insulin for prandial coverage. Longer acting insulins include neutral protamine Hagedorn (NPH) insulin, insulin detemir (which has a fatty acid side chain that prolongs its action by slowing absorption and catabolism), insulin glargine (which is a biosynthetic human insulin), and insulin degludec. Basal insulin requirements are provided by intermediate or long-acting insulin formulations. These are usually prescribed with short-acting insulin in an attempt to mimic physiologic insulin release with meals.

Other than inhaled insulin, all insulin formulations are for subcutaneous injection, administered by needle, by insulin "pens" (which reduce the risk for intramuscular injection which leads to erratic effects), or for use in an insulin pump. There are multiple approaches to insulin therapy, all with the aim to adhere to glycemic targets, reduce the propensity for wide swings in glycemic control (i.e., hyperglycemia triggering ketoacidosis, and hypoglycemia), and ultimately reduce chronic complications. The two most common options are multiple daily injections (MDIs) of both prandial and

TABLE 14.4 Insulin Preparations Classified by Pharmacodynamic Profile*

	Onset	Peak	Duration
RAPID ACTING			
Inhaled human insulin	4—5 minutes	30—60 minutes	2—4 hours
Aspart	10—15 minutes	60—90 minutes	2—4 hours
Glulisine			
Lispro			
SHORT ACTING			
Regular human insulin	30—60 minutes	2—4 hours	6—8 hours
INTERMEDIATE ACTING			
NPH	1—3 hours	4—8 hours	12—16 hours
LONG ACTING			
Detemir	60 mins	No peak	12—24 hours
Glargine (U—100)	2—4 hours	No peak	20—24 hours
Glargine (U—300)	6 hours	No peak	24 hours
Degludec	30—90 minutes	No peak	>24 hours

*The time course of each insulin varies significantly between persons and in the same person on different days; therefore, the profiles listed should be used as guidelines only.
NPH, Neutral protamine Hagedorn.
Adapted from Ludwig S: Practical diabetes care for healthcare professionals, 2nd ed. St. Louis, Elsevier, 2021.

basal insulin, or the continuous subcutaneous infusion of insulin (CSII).

Irrespective of the insulin regimen, patients must be educated about how to appropriately dose their insulin. Although the insulin profiles are depicted as "smooth," symmetric curves, there is considerable patient-to-patient variation in the peak and duration. In general, individuals with type 1 diabetes require 0.5–1 U/kg per day of insulin divided into multiple doses, with about 50% of the insulin given as basal insulin. Longer-acting insulin is typically given at night and is dosed to regulate nighttime fasting glucose levels. Shorter-acting insulin (inhaled, rapid or short-acting) should be injected before, or just after a meal, or as dictated by the pharmacokinetics of the insulin preparation and glucose monitoring.

Continuous subcutaneous insulin infusion (CSII) devices pump rapid-acting insulin through a catheter inserted into the subcutaneous tissue of the patient's abdomen (Fig. 14.7) and can accurately deliver small doses of insulin (microliters per hour). They offer several advantages: (1) multiple basal infusion rates can be programmed to accommodate nocturnal versus daytime basal insulin requirement, (2) basal infusion rates can be altered during periods of exercise, (3) different waveforms of insulin infusion with meal-related bolus allow better matching of insulin depending on meal composition, and (4) programmed algorithms consider prior insulin administration and blood glucose values in calculating the insulin dose. Insulin infusion pumps present unique challenges, such as infection at the infusion site, unexplained hyperglycemia because the infusion set becomes obstructed, or DKA if the pump becomes disconnected. Essential to the safe use of infusion devices is thorough patient education about pump function and frequent glucose monitoring.

The regimens that most closely emulate endogenous insulin release entail intensive insulin regimens: more frequent plasma glucose measurements coupled with multiple daily insulin injections or use of an insulin pump. Self-monitoring of blood glucose (SMBG) is typically performed preprandially (meals and snacks), at bedtime, occasionally postprandially, before exercise, when low blood glucose is suspected, after treating low blood glucose until normoglycemic, and before critical tasks such as driving. Continuous glucose monitoring (CGM) systems can now measure blood glucose as often as every minute, sending real-time data to smart devices. Such intensive regimens have been demonstrated to reduce the risk for long-term complications and seem poised to become the standard of care for type 1 diabetes.

Sodium-glucose co-transporter-2 (SGLT2) inhibitors and α-glucosidase inhibitors may also be prescribed to type 1 diabetics and will be covered in the next section.

Type 2 Diabetes Mellitus

The goals of glycemia-controlling therapy for type 2 diabetes are similar to those in type 1 diabetes. Whereas glycemic control tends to dominate the management of type 1 diabetes, the care of individuals with type 2 diabetes must also include attention to the treatment of conditions associated with type 2 diabetes (e.g., obesity, hypertension, dyslipidemia, cardiovascular disease) and detection and management of diabetes-related complications. Reduction in cardiovascular risk is of paramount importance because this is the leading cause of death in these individuals.

Type 2 diabetes management should begin with lifestyle modifications, including diet, weight loss, and reduction of risk factors for cardiovascular disease. An exercise regimen to increase insulin sensitivity and promote weight loss also should be instituted. Pharmacologic approaches to the management of type 2 diabetes include oral glucose-lowering agents, insulin, and other agents that improve glucose control (Table 14.5). Monotherapy with oral glucose-lowering agents is the recommended initial pharmacologic choice, although combination therapy and/or insulin may be indicated at baseline for patients with more severe disease at diagnosis. The goal is an effective therapy that improves glycemic control, reduces "glucose toxicity" to beta cells, and improves endogenous insulin secretion. However, type 2 diabetes is a progressive disorder and ultimately requires multiple therapeutic agents, including insulin.

Antihyperglycemic Agents. Advances in the therapy of diabetes include the development of multiple antihyperglycemic agents that each target different pathophysiologic processes. Based on their mechanisms of action, these agents are subdivided into agents that

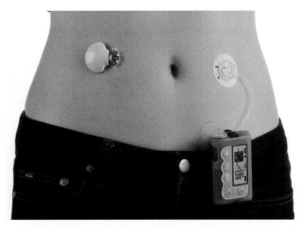

FIG. 14.7 MiniMed paradigm REAL-time revel system. The insulin pump is small and can be worn under clothing or on a belt. It delivers insulin through a tube or cannula (infusion set) that is inserted into the subcutaneous (SC) tissue. The pump can be disconnected for bathing, swimming, or changing clothes. A small sensor for glucose is inserted into the SC tissue using an automatic insertion device. Sensor data are sent to a transmitter that is attached to the skin with a waterproof adhesive patch. The transmitter sends data to the insulin pump using wireless technology. The sensor and tube (new tubing) from the pump must be relocated every 3 days to minimize the risk of infection obstruction of the tube. (Courtesy of Medtronics, Diabetes, Minneapolis, MN.)

TABLE 14.5 Noninsulin Antihyperglycemic Agents

Class Drug	Mechanism of Action (Target Tissue)	Warnings and Principal Adverse Effects	Drug Interaction(s)
Biguanides *Administer with meals.*			
Metformin	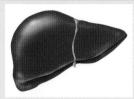 Reduced hepatic glucose production 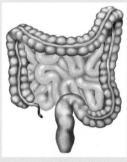 Reduced intestinal absorption of glucose. All target tissues: Increased insulin sensitivity (all target tissues).	GI disturbances (diarrhea, abdominal pain, nausea/vomiting, flatulence, metallic taste). Lactic acidosis (FDA warning). Vit B_{12} deficiency. Contraindicated in patients with renal impairment (eGFR<30 ml/min/1.73 m^2).	Avoid alcohol. Cationic drugs such as cimetidine, furosemide, and nifedipine are eliminated by the kidney and may lead to increased metformin levels.
Sulfonylureas (2nd generation) *Administer 30 min before meals.*			
Glipizide Glyburide Glimepiride	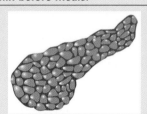 Enhanced insulin secretion. 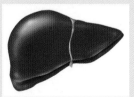 Reduced hepatic glucose release. 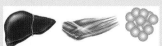 Increased insulin sensitivity.	Hypoglycemia. Weight gain. Possible increased cardiovascular risk. Contraindicated in patients with sulfa allergy. Caution using in patients with renal or hepatic impairment or with G6PD deficiency.	Avoid/limit sulfonureas and alcohol. The hypoglycemic effect of sulfonylureas may be enhanced by drugs that decrease hepatic metabolism, renal excretion, or lead to displacement from protein binding sites (i.e., aspirin/NSAIDs).

Continued

TABLE 14.5   Noninsulin Antihyperglycemic Agents—cont'd

Class Drug	Mechanism of Action (Target Tissue)	Warnings and Principal Adverse Effects	Drug Interaction(s)
Sodium glucose co-transporter 2 inhibitors (SLGT2 inhibitors)			
Dapagliflozin Empagliflozin Canagliflozin	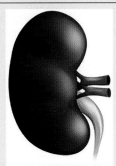 Reduced reabsorption and increased excretion of glucose.	Contraindicated in patients with impaired renal function. Genital fungal infections. Hypotension (with risk for syncope/falls). Increased risk for DKA Necrotizing fasciitis.	—
Glucagon-like peptide 1 (GLP-1) receptor agonists			
Administered by subcutaneous injection 15 min before meals. Exenatide Liraglutide Semaglutide Dulaglutide Lixisenatide Albiglutide	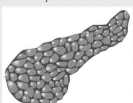 Enhance insulin secretion. Suppress prandial glucagon secretion. 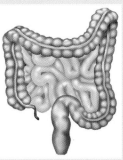 Delay gastric emptying.	GI adverse effects (nausea, vomiting, diarrhea). Injection site reactions. Thyroid C-cell tumors/thyroid medullary cancer (FDA warning). Contraindication in patients with MEN 2 or family history of MEN 2. End-stage renal disease (exenatide only).	GLP-1 receptor agonists may alter the pharmacokinetics of drugs that require rapid GI absorption, such as oral contraceptives and antibiotics (and reduce blood levels).
α-Glucosidase inhibitors (AGI) ***Administer just before meals.***			
Acarbose Miglitol	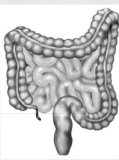 Delay carbohydrate digestion.	GI disturbances (abdominal pain, nausea, diarrhea, bloating) and contraindicated in patients with GI diseases. Elevated liver function tests (contraindicated in patients with hepatic diseases).	May lead to hypoglycemia in combination with other antihyperglycemic agents.

Dipeptidyl peptidase-4 inhibitors (DPP4i)

Administer once daily regardless of meals.

Linagliptin
Saxagliptin
Sitagliptin
Alogliptin

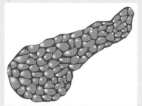

Inhibits enzymatic breakdown of GLP-1 and GIP; increases insulin secretion. Decreases glucagon secretion.

Runny nose (nasopharyngitis).
Increased risk for congestive heart failure (saxagliptin and alogliptin).

—

Thiazolidinediones (TZD)

Administer with meals.

Pioglitazone
Rosiglitazone

Improves target cell insulin sensitivity.

Weight gain flatulence.
May cause or exacerbate edema (including macular edema) and congestive heart failure. Contraindicated in patients with grade III/IV congestive heart failure (FDA warning).
May decrease hematocrit/hemoglobin.
Increase rate of fractures in women.
Possible risk for bladder cancer.
Safety in pregnancy is not established.

—

Glinides (GLN)
Administer 15 min before meals.

Repaglinide

Nateglinide

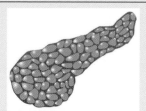

Glucose dependent enhanced insulin secretion.

Weight gain. Hypoglycemia (less than sulfonylureas).
Headache.

Avoid/limit alcohol with glinides.
Increased risk of hypoglycemia with other antidiabetic agents.
Strong interaction with CYP2C8 inhibitors such as gemfibrozil (will increase dose of glinides).
The hypoglycemic effect of sulfonylureas may be enhanced by drugs that lead to displacement from protein binding sites.

Colesevelam
Administer with meals.

Colesevelam

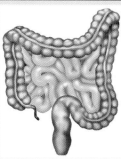

Binds to bile acids and leads to increased production of GLP-1 and inhibition of hepatic glyogenolysis.

GI disturbances (constipation).
Headache.
Contraindicated in patients with a history of bowel obstruction.

Avoid in patients taking mycophenolate.

Continued

TABLE 14.5   Noninsulin Antihyperglycemic Agents—cont'd

Class Drug	Mechanism of Action (Target Tissue)	Warnings and Principal Adverse Effects	Drug Interaction(s)
Bromocriptine *Administer with meals.*			
Bromocriptine	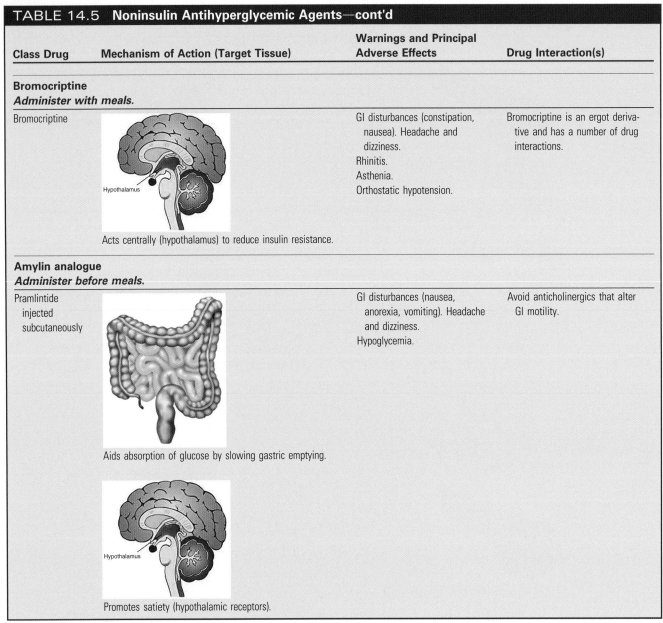 Acts centrally (hypothalamus) to reduce insulin resistance.	GI disturbances (constipation, nausea). Headache and dizziness. Rhinitis. Asthenia. Orthostatic hypotension.	Bromocriptine is an ergot derivative and has a number of drug interactions.
Amylin analogue *Administer before meals.*			
Pramlintide injected subcutaneously	Aids absorption of glucose by slowing gastric emptying. Promotes satiety (hypothalamic receptors).	GI disturbances (nausea, anorexia, vomiting). Headache and dizziness. Hypoglycemia.	Avoid anticholinergics that alter GI motility.

GI, Gastrointestinal; *GIP,* gastric inhibitory polypeptide; *GLP-1,* glucagon-like peptide 1.

increase insulin secretion, reduce glucose production, increase insulin sensitivity, enhance glucagon-like peptide 1 (GLP-1) action, or promote urinary excretion of glucose. Below is a listing of the most commonly prescribed antihyperglycemic agents, which are largely indicated for type 2 diabetes. Table 14.5 includes mechanism of action, warnings, adverse effects, and drug interactions.

Metformin. Metformin, a biguanide, reduces fasting plasma glucose and insulin levels, improves the lipid profile, and promotes modest weight loss. Because of its relatively slow onset of action and gastrointestinal (GI) symptoms with higher doses, the initial dose is low and escalated every 2–3 weeks based on glycemic targets. An extended-release form is available and may have fewer GI

side effects. Metformin is the recommended first-line monotherapy for type 2 diabetes, although it can be used in combination with other oral agents or with insulin.

Sodium-Glucose Co-Transporter 2 Inhibitors. Sodium-glucose co-transporter 2 (SGLT2) inhibitors lower the blood glucose and A1C by selectively inhibiting this cotransporter, which is expressed almost exclusively in the proximal convoluted tubule in the kidney. This inhibits glucose reabsorption, lowers the renal threshold for glucose, and leads to increased urinary glucose excretion. Because of the renal site of action, these agents have poor efficacy in patients with a low eGFR <45 mL/min/1.73 m^2. The glucose-lowering effect is insulin independent and not related to changes in insulin sensitivity or secretion. Most importantly, these agents reduce blood pressure, promote weight loss, and have a clinically significant benefit on cardiovascular and renal complications. These benefits have led to their recommendation as a second-line monotherapy (after metformin), or for use in dual or triple combination therapies, particularly in patients with cardiovascular comorbidities.

Glucagon-Like Peptide 1 Receptor Agonists. Glucagon-like peptide receptor agonists (GLP-1 RA) act like endogenously produced "incretins" to increase glucose-stimulated insulin secretion, suppress glucagon, and slow gastric emptying. GLP-1 RAs do not cause hypoglycemia because of the glucose-dependent nature of incretin-stimulated insulin secretion (unless they are used in combination with other agents that can cause hypoglycemia (e.g., sulfonylureas)). GLP-1 RAs have been shown to significantly reduce cardiovascular complications in type 2 diabetes. An important attribute of these agents is that they promote modest weight loss and appetite suppression. Treatment with these agents should start at a low dose to minimize initial side effects (nausea being the limiting one). GLP-1 RAs are available in twice-daily, daily, and weekly injectable formulations, can be used as second-line monotherapy if glycemic targets are not reached with metformin, or as part of dual or triple therapy with metformin (or other agents).

Second-Generation Sulfonylureas. Sulfonylureas have been used to treat diabetes since the 1950s. They are insulin secretagogues that stimulate insulin secretion by interacting with the ATP-sensitive potassium channel on the beta cell. These drugs are most effective in individuals with type 2 diabetes of relatively recent onset (<5 years) who have residual endogenous insulin production. Second-generations sulfonylureas reduce both fasting and postprandial glucose and should be initiated at low doses and increased at 1- to 2-week intervals based on glycemic targets. In general, sulfonylureas increase insulin acutely and thus should be taken shortly before a meal; with chronic therapy, though, the insulin release is more sustained. Glimepiride and glipizide can be given in a single daily dose and are preferred over glyburide. Sulfonylureas have the potential to cause hypoglycemia, especially in older individuals. Hypoglycemia is usually related to delayed meals, increased physical activity, alcohol intake, or renal insufficiency.

Glinides (Meglitinides). These agents are not sulfonylureas but also interact with the ATP-sensitive potassium channel in pancreatic β-cells. Because of their short half-lives, these agents are given with each meal or immediately before to reduce meal-related glucose excursions. Lesser degrees of hypoglycemia and weight gain are associated with the glinides than with sulfonylureas.

Dipeptidyl Peptidase 4 (DPP4) Inhibitors. DPP4 inhibitors block the enzyme responsible for the breakdown of incretins, and have been shown to provide good glycemic control as monotherapy or combined with metformin.

Thiazolidinediones. Thiazolidinediones (TZDs) reduce insulin resistance by binding to the PPAR-γ nuclear receptor, which is found at highest levels in adipocytes but is expressed at lower levels in many other tissues. They regulate a large number of genes, promote adipocyte differentiation, reduce hepatic fat accumulation, and promote fatty acid storage. TZDs promote a redistribution of fat from central to peripheral locations. Circulating insulin levels decrease with use of the thiazolidinediones, indicating a reduction in insulin resistance. Pioglitazone, but not rosiglitazone, has been demonstrated to exert cardiovascular benefits.

α-Glucosidase Inhibitors. α-Glucosidase inhibitors, such as acarbose and miglitol, reduce postprandial hyperglycemia by delaying glucose absorption by inhibiting the enzyme that cleaves oligosaccharides into simple sugars in the intestinal lumen. Therapy should be initiated at a low dose with the evening meal and increased to a maximal dose over weeks to months.

Other Agents. Pramlintide, colesevelam, and bromocriptine are prescribed less frequently (see Table 14.5).

Combination Therapy. Dual- or triple-drug therapy is typically indicated either when monotherapy fails to lead to glycemic targets or for patients who are diagnosed with more advanced stage disease and have a higher entry A1C (Fig. 14.8). In those with no residual β-cell function, insulin may be combined with other agents. A number of drug combinations have been formulated into single pills or injections.

Hypoglycemia

All diabetics are at risk for hypoglycemia, although those who are treated with insulin are at the highest risk and must closely adhere to their diets. If they fail to eat in accordance with their diabetes management plan (consumption of adequate calories at proper intervals) but continue to take their regular insulin injections, they may experience a hypoglycemic reaction caused by an excess of insulin (insulin shock). A hypoglycemic reaction also may be caused by an overdose of insulin or an oral hypoglycemic agent, particularly sulfonylureas. Reaction or shock caused by excess insulin usually occurs in three well-defined stages, each more severe and dangerous than the one preceding it (Box 14.5). Insulin shock can be corrected by giving the conscious patient sweetened fruit juice or anything with sugar in it (e.g., cake icing).

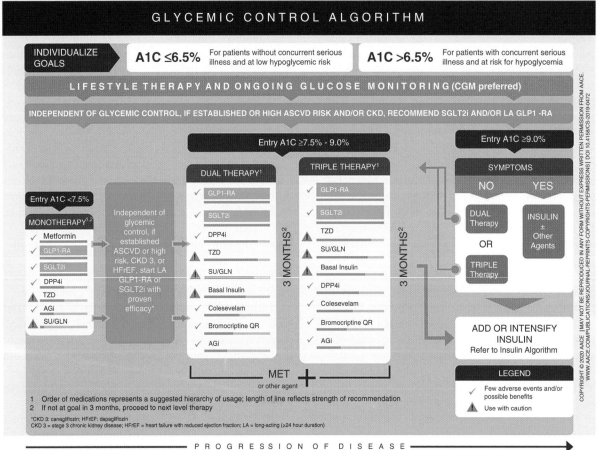

FIG. 14. 8 Management of type 2 diabetes based on A1C levels. (From Garber AJ, Handelsman Y, Grunberger G, et al. Consensus statement by the american association of clinical endocrinologists and American college of endocrinology on the comprehensive type 2 diabetes management algorithm — 2020 executive summary. Endocr Pract. 2020;26(1):107—139.)

Patients in the severe stage (unconsciousness) are best treated with an intravenous glucose solution; glucagon or epinephrine may be used for transient relief.

DENTAL MANAGEMENT

The dental office is a potential venue for diabetes screening, both by identifying the presenting signs and symptoms, and/or by performing chairside capillary blood glucose with a glucose monitor. Patients suspected to have undiagnosed diabetes should be promptly referred to a physician for diagnosis and treatment.

For those patients with an established diagnosis of diabetes, a careful history should be taken, including the type of diabetes, presence of complications, medical comorbidities (i.e., cardiovascular disease), and the medical treatment they are receiving (Box 14.6). Patients who are being treated with insulin should be asked about their daily insulin regimen, whether self-administered or using continuous subcutaneous insulin infusion. They should

indicate how often they self-monitor blood glucose levels, along with details about the glucose monitoring system and trends in recent values. The frequency of visits to the physician for diabetes follow-up should be recorded along with results of the last A1C and the trend over time. The frequency of insulin shock or other antihyperglycemic hypoglycemic reactions should be noted.

Vital signs also may indicate the level of disease control and precautions in the dental management of patients with diabetes. Patients with abnormal pulse rate and rhythm or elevated blood pressure should be approached with a measure of caution. Given the comorbidities associated with diabetes, poor functional capacity (i.e., <4 metabolic equivalent levels [METs]) (see Chapter 1), and increased risk of cardiovascular events during and after dental treatment, vital signs should be assessed in this population.

Consultation with the patient's physician at baseline is advised in order to establish the level of control. Patients who have not seen their physician recently (within the previous 6 months), who have had frequent episodes of

BOX 14.5	**Signs and Symptoms of Hypoglycemia**

Mild Stage
- Hunger
- Weakness
- Tachycardia
- Pallor
- Sweating
- Paresthesias

Moderate Stage
- Incoherence
- Uncooperativeness
- Belligerence
- Lack of judgment
- Poor orientation

Severe Stage
- Unconsciousness
- Tonic or clonic movements
- Hypotension
- Hypothermia
- Rapid, thready pulse

BOX 14.6	**Clinical Detection of Patients With Diabetes**

Patient With Known Diabetes
1. Detection by history
   a. Are you diabetic?
   b. What medications are you taking?
   c. Are you being treated by a physician?
2. Establishment of severity of disease and degree of "control"
   a. When were you first diagnosed as diabetic?
   b. What was your last blood glucose level, and when was it taken?
   c. What is the usual fasting level of blood glucose for you?
   d. How are you being treated for your diabetes?
   e. How often do you have insulin reactions or hypoglycemia?
   f. How much insulin do you take with each injection, and how often do you receive injections?
   g. How often do you test your blood glucose?
   h. When did you last visit your physician?
   i. Do you have any symptoms of diabetes at the present time?

Patient With Undiagnosed Diabetes
1. History of signs or symptoms of diabetes or its complications
2. High risk for developing diabetes:
   a. Presence of diabetes in a parent
   b. Giving birth to one or more large babies (>9 lb)
   c. History of spontaneous abortions or stillbirths
   d. Obesity
   e. Age older than 40 years
2. If diabetes is suspected, perform in-office fasting/casual blood glucose and/or refer for diabetes screening.

insulin shock/hypoglycemia, or who report signs and symptoms of diabetes indicating unstable disease should be referred to their physicians for reevaluation, or their physicians should be consulted to establish their current status.

Most patients with well-controlled diabetes without serious comorbidities such as renal disease, hypertension, or coronary artery disease require no special attention when receiving routine dental treatment. Those who are treated with insulin or who are under poor medical control of their diabetes or comorbidities may require additional consideration.

The decision to prescribe antibiotic prophylaxis before dental treatment would not be typical; i.e., there is little evidence supporting the need for antibiotic prophylaxis. Thus, this decision should be made on a case-by-case basis and in consultation with the patient's physician, when needed. Antibiotics in a postoperative setting should be reserved for poorly controlled diabetics with comorbidities (Box 14.7). For most patients with diabetes, routine use of local anesthetic with 1:100,000 epinephrine is well tolerated. In diabetic patients with hypertension, history of recent MI, or cardiac arrhythmia, caution may be indicated with use of epinephrine and guidelines for these patients are similar to those for patients with cardiovascular conditions (see Box 14.8). Careful and continuous monitoring of the patient's physical status are mandatory.

There is a paucity of well-designed research studies to compare the risk for complications in diabetics versus nondiabetic patients, or the relative risk stratified by glycemic control. There is a small risk for complications associated with restorative, dental cleaning/scaling and root-planing, and surgical procedures performed on diabetics in the dental office (low level evidence) and likely related to glycemic control during treatment and postoperatively, and those related to comorbidities (i.e., cardiovascular disease). Fasting blood glucose levels are a better predictor of glycemic control preoperatively. There are no published glycemic control threshold guidelines for oral surgical treatment of patients with diabetes that are based on high level evidence (i.e., randomized controlled trials). There is an increased risk for complications with increasing hyperglycemia to suggest that dental treatment (including surgery) should ideally be performed when the fasting blood glucose is adequately controlled, conservatively within the range of 80–200 mg/dL (4.4–11.2 mmol/L). Most patients can usually provide their blood glucose values preoperatively, although in some cases the dentist may need to perform chairside testing or send a patient for pre-operative testing. We strongly recommend dentists keep a glucometer on hand for this purpose. Patients with a fasting blood glucose below 70 mg/dL (4 mmol/L) and above 200 mg/dL (11.2 mmol/L) are at a higher risk for hypoglycemia and postoperative complications, respectively. Diabetics with fasting blood glucose outside these

BOX 14.7 | Checklist for Dental Management of Patient With Diabetes[a]

PREOPERATIVE RISK ASSESSMENT

R: Recognize risks

- Review medical history, determine whether diabetes exists, and discuss relevant issues with the patient.
- Identify all medications being taken or supposed to be taken by the patient.
- Examine the patient for signs and symptoms of disease and obtain vital signs.
- Obtain and review or obtain recent laboratory test results or images required to assess risk.
- Obtain a medical consultation if the patient has a poorly controlled or undiagnosed diabetes or if the patient's health status is uncertain.
- If diabetes is adequately controlled,[b] all routine dental procedures can be performed without special precautions. Morning appointments are preferable.

A

Antibiotics	Prophylactic antibiotics generally are not required, and may be given in the postoperative setting. Antibiotics may be considered for patients with very difficult to control diabetes for whom an invasive procedure is performed but whose oral health is poor and the fasting plasma glucose exceeds 200 mg/dL. Consider culture and sensitivity in poorly controlled diabetic patients with odontogenic infections.
Anesthesia	No issues if diabetes is well controlled. For diabetic patients with cardiovascular comorbidities, management should be customized accordingly. Caution to avoid high amounts of epinephrine.
Anxiety	Anxiety may impact glycemic control and trigger hypoglycemia.
Allergy	No issues.

B

Bleeding	For surgical procedures, see **Notes on Surgery** below.
Breathing	No issues.
Blood pressure	Monitor blood pressure.

C

Chair position	No issues.
Cardiovascular	Confirm cardiovascular status is stable.

D

Devices	A continuous monitoring device or insulin pump may be worn by the patient. Ensure these are attached and working properly. Antibiotic prophylaxis is not required.
Drugs	Patient advised to take usual insulin dosage and normal meals on day of dental appointment. Confirmed with patient medications taken that morning.

Drug interactions	Noninsulin antihyperglycemic drugs can interact with other medications. Perform multidrug check before prescribing medications. See Table 14.5.

E

Equipment	Use office glucometer to ensure adequate glucose control (pre-peri- or postoperatively).
Emergencies and urgencies	Advise patient to inform dentist or staff if symptoms of insulin reaction/hypoglycemia occur during dental visit. Have glucose source (orange juice, soda, cake icing) available if needed.

F

Follow-up	Postoperative analgesia:

- Aspirin and NSAIDs are highly bound to plasma proteins and may displace sulfonylureas/glinides and increase risk for hypoglycemia.
- Tramadol may cause severe hypoglycemia, particularly in diabetics taking bromocriptine. Other opioids may cause hyperglycemia and their sedating effects may reduce compliance of diet and diabetic drug regimens. Opioids should be avoided in diabetics, but if used, close glycemic monitoring is recommended.
- Acetaminophen may be safely prescribed to diabetics unless there are other contraindications.

Infections should be followed closely, particularly poorly healing infections which may require a change in the antibiotic regimen initially prescribed. Ensure patient is receiving routine and periodic follow-up evaluation by physician. Monitor for disease progression by update of diabetes history, and review of systems, check laboratory or chairside glycemic values, and re-examination for poor periodontal health, salivary gland hypofunction, and candidiasis.

Notes on Surgery

If extensive surgery is needed:

- Consult with patient's physician concerning dietary needs during postoperative period.
- If diabetes is not adequately controlled (i.e., fasting blood glucose <80 mg/dL or >200 mg/dL and comorbidities [post-MI, renal disease, CHF, symptomatic angina, old age, cardiac dysrhythmias, cerebrovascular accident] are present and blood pressure >180/110 mm Hg or functional capacity <4):
- Provide appropriate emergency care only.
- Request referral for medical evaluation, management, and risk factor modification.
- If patient is symptomatic (i.e., signs and symptoms of hypoglycemia or DKA/HHS), seek IMMEDIATE referral.
- If patient is asymptomatic, request routine referral.

[a]Unless otherwise specified, the Strength of Recommendation Taxonomy (SORT) for each dental management recommendation is Grade C (see Preface for further explanation).
[b]Adequately controlled: fasting blood glucose between 80 and 200 mg/dL and no complications (i.e., after myocardial infarction [MI], renal disease, congestive heart failure [CHF], symptomatic angina, old age, cardiac dysrhythmia, cerebrovascular accident), blood pressure <180/110 mm Hg, and functional capacity >4 metabolic equivalents (METs).
Note: special precautions may be needed for patients with complications of diabetes, renal disease, or heart disease.
NSAID, Nonsteroidal antiinflammatory drug.

BOX 14.8   Dental Management of Patients With Diabetes and Acute Odontogenic Infections

1. Non–insulin-controlled patients may require additional insulin; consultation with physician is indicated.
2. Insulin-controlled patients usually require increased dosage of insulin; consultation with physician is indicated.
3. Patient with poorly controlled diabetes or receiving high insulin dosage should have culture(s) taken from the infected area for antibiotic sensitivity testing.
   a. Culture is sent for testing.
   b. Antibiotic therapy is initiated.
   c. In cases of poor clinical responses to the first antibiotic, a more effective antibiotic is selected according to sensitivity test results.
4. Infection should be treated with the use of
   a. Incision and drainage
   b. Pulpotomy, pulpectomy, extractions
   c. Antibiotics
   d. Warm intraoral salt-water rinses

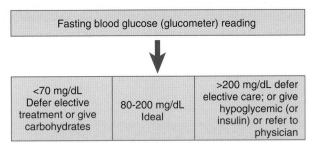

FIG. 14.9 Decision-making diagram for the dental treatment of patients with diabetes according to blood glucose (glucometer) reading. *Oral hypoglycemic agent/insulin prescribed by physician.

"normal" ranges, and those with comorbidities require careful consideration before performing treatment. In patients with preoperative blood glucose below 70 mg/dL (4 mmol/L), elective treatment should be deferred unless the patient consumes a carbohydrate (see below), restoring the levels to >80 mg/dL (4.4 mmol/L). All elective treatment should ideally be deferred in patients with fasting blood glucose levels >200 mg/dL or referred to a specialist/hospital setting (Fig. 14.9), although most procedures (other than extensive surgery) in these patients can be safely provided in a dental office with careful monitoring intraoperatively and postoperatively (see Box 14.8).

Patients prone to developing hypoglycemia are typically type 1 diabetics who have either not eaten preoperatively or have taken too much insulin. Patients should be told to take their usual insulin dosage and to eat normal meals before the appointment, which usually is best scheduled in the morning. When such a patient arrives, the dentist should confirm that the patient has taken insulin and has eaten breakfast, and ask them about their blood glucose levels. In addition, patients should be instructed to tell the dentist whether at any time during the appointment they are experiencing symptoms of hypoglycemia. A source of sugar such as orange juice, cake icing, or non-diet soft drink must be available in the dental office to be given to the patient if symptoms develop (see Box 14.6 and Appendix A).

The risk for postoperative issues such as infection or fluctuations in glycemic control in patients with diabetes is, in theory, directly related to preoperative fasting blood glucose levels (or A1C levels), the oral microbial burden, and the type of procedure. Diabetes aside, surgical procedures can exert a metabolic stress on patients, resulting in hyperglycemia. Therefore, any patient with diabetes who is going to undergo extensive periodontal or oral surgery procedures other than single simple extractions may be at an increased risk for complications; thus requiring carefully planned treatment, with input from the patient's physician to mitigate risk.

Individualized dietary instructions must take into account the patient's ability to masticate and swallow during the postsurgical healing. It is important that the total caloric content and the protein–carbohydrate–fat ratio of the diet do not deviate from normal so that glycemic control is maintained. One suggestion is to have the patient use a blender to prepare his or her usual diet so that it can be ingested with minimum discomfort; alternatively, special food supplements in a liquid form may be used. The physician also may alter the patient's insulin regimen, typically increasing the dose to offset the surgical stress (in the case of extensive surgery), and according to their ability to eat properly (see Box 14.6).

A protocol for intravenous sedation often involves fasting before the appointment (i.e., nothing by mouth after midnight), using only half the usual insulin dose, and then supplementing with intravenous glucose during the procedure. The physician may also recommend holding anti-hyperglycemic agents in some patients who must fast before the surgery. Patients with well-controlled diabetes may be given general anesthesia if available or necessary; however, coordination with the patient's physician is advised. Management with local anesthetics is preferable and is associated with lower risk, especially in outpatient office settings.

Diabetic patients presenting with an acute oral infection (postoperative or otherwise) may create the potential for a significant management problem (Box 14.8), particularly in patients with type 1 diabetes who take high doses of insulin. Infections may be associated with loss of glycemic control and may require hospitalization for adequate management. It is important to recognize infections promptly, manage them aggressively, and the best practice is to communicate with the patient's physician. The dentist should treat infections by incision and drainage, extraction, pulpotomy, warm rinses, and

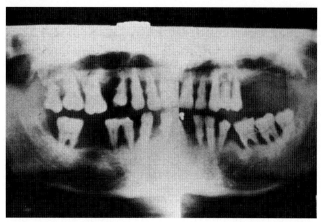

FIG. 14.10 Panoramic radiograph of a young adult with severe, progressive periodontitis. After positive screening for diabetes, the patient was referred to a physician, and the diagnosis of diabetes mellitus was established. The patient required insulin treatment.

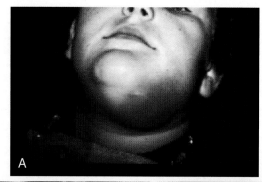

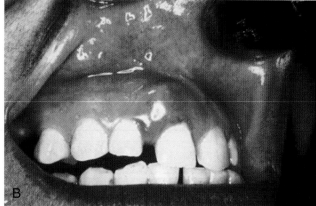

FIG. 14.11 A) Patient with cellulitis resulting from a mandibular tooth abscess. (**B**) Periodontal abscess in a patient with multiple abscesses. After evaluation by a physician, the diagnosis of diabetes was established.

antibiotics. Antibiotic sensitivity testing may be indicated for patients with diabetes that are difficult to control or for those who require high insulin dosage for control. For these patients, routine antibiotic therapy can be initiated. Then, if the clinical response is poor, a more effective antibiotic can be selected based on the results of antibiotic sensitivity testing.

Oral Complications and Manifestations

The reported oral complications of diabetes mellitus include hyposalivation, xerostomia; bacterial, viral, and fungal infections (including candidiasis); poor wound healing; increased incidence and severity of caries; periodontal and peri-implant diseases; odontogenic infections; and burning mouth symptoms (Figs. 14-10-14.13). The association between diabetes and each of these complications is variable and most likely attributed to poor glycemic control and associated dehydration; altered response to infection; microvascular changes; and, possibly, increased glucose concentrations in saliva.

The effects of hyperglycemia leads to excessive urination (polyuria), which deplete the extracellular fluids and reduce the secretion of saliva, resulting in dry mouth and reduced salivary levels of calcium, phosphate, and fluoride. Saliva glucose levels are elevated in persons with uncontrolled diabetes. There is an increased incidence and risk for progression of periodontal disease (Fig. 14.10) in patients with both type 1 and type 2 diabetes and the severity correlates to the degree of glycemic control. Diabetics have a sustained low-grade systemic inflammation, and this likely impacts periodontal tissue physiology. Furthermore, hyperglycemia likely drives the formation of advanced glycation end products, which leads to elevated levels of proinflammatory cytokines in periodontal tissues, and contributes to systemic inflammation. The precise mechanisms leading to tissue destruction have not been

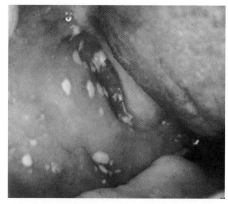

FIG. 14.12 Oral candidiasis in a patient with diabetes. The multiple small white lesions on the buccal mucosa were easily scraped off. Cytologic study and cultures confirmed the clinical impression of infection by *Candida albicans*.

elucidated. In type 2 diabetes, nonsurgical periodontal treatment with oral hygiene instruction improves periodontal indices and glycemic control (a clinically meaningful A1C reduction of approximately 0.5% at 3 months) and to a lesser extent is associated with reductions in markers of systemic inflammation (e.g., C-reactive protein levels). Stability of these findings after >6 months remain unclear.

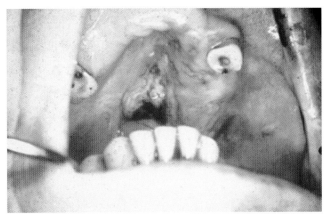

FIG. 14.13 Tan-dark brown lesion involving the palate in a patient with diabetes. Cultures established the diagnosis of mucormycosis, a serious fungal infection that may occur in patients with systemic diseases such as diabetes or cancer. Treatment usually includes control of diabetes, surgical excisions of the lesion, and administration of antibiotics and potent antifungals.

Poorly controlled diabetics are more likely to develop both coronal and root surface caries, and when encountering a patient with new or worsening caries, oral health care providers should consider undiagnosed or worsening glycemic control as a risk factor.

Oral fungal infections, including candidiasis (which is relatively common and often recurrent) and mucormycosis (which is rare) (Figs. 14.13 and 14.14), may be observed in the patient with uncontrolled diabetes. Treatment recommendations for these infections are found in Appendix C. Other oral mucosal lesions such as traumatic ulcers and lichenoid lesions also have been reported more commonly in patients with diabetes.

Diabetic neuropathy may lead to oral symptoms of dysesthesias and tingling, numbness, burning, and pain. Taste disturbances also may occur in diabetics.

BIBLIOGRAPHY

1. American Diabetes Association. Standards of medical care in diabetes-2021. Abridged for primary care providers. *Clin Diabetes.* 2020;39. Online Ahead of Print.
2. American Diabetes Association. Classification and diagnosis of diabetes: standards of medical care in diabetes-2021. *Diabetes Care.* 2021;44(suppl. 1):S15–S33.
3. American Diabetes Association. Comprehensive medical evaluation and assessment of comorbidities: standards of medical care in diabetes-2021. *Diabetes Care.* 2021;44(suppl. 1):S40–S52.
4. American Diabetes Association. Glycemic targets: standards of medical care in diabetes-2021. *Diabetes Care.* 2021;44(suppl. 1):S73–S84.
5. Aronovich S, Skope LW, Kelly JPW, Kyriakides TC. The relationship of glycemic control to the outcomes of dental extractions. *J Oral Maxillofac Surg.* 2010;68:2955–2961.
6. Baeza M, Morales A, Ciosterna C, et al. Effect of periodontal treatment in patients with periodontitis and diabetes: systematic review and meta-analysis. *J Appl Oral Sci.* 2020;28:e20190248.
7. Barasch A, Safford MM, Litaker MS, Gilbert GH. Risk factors for oral postoperative infection in patients with diabetes. *Spec Care Dent.* 2008;28(4):159–166.
8. Borgnakke WS, Chapple ILC. The multi-center randomized controlled trial (RCT) published by the Journal of the American Medical Association (JAMA) on the effect of periodontal therapy on glycated hemoglobin (HbA1c) has fundamental problems. *J Evid Base Dent Pract.* 2014;14(3):127–132.
9. Centers for Disease Control and Prevention. *National Diabetes Statistics Report, 2020.* Atlanta, GA: Centers for Disease Control and Prevention, US Department of Health and Human Services; 2020.
10. Chamberlain JJ, Kalyani RR, Leal S, et al. Treatment of type 1 diabetes: synopsis of the 2017 American diabetes association standards of medical care in diabetes. *Ann Intern Med.* 2017;167:493–498.
11. Chamberlain JJ, Johnson EL, Leal S, Rhinehart AS, Shubrook JH, Peterson L. Cardiovascular disease and risk management: review of the American diabetes association standards of medical care in diabetes 2018. *Ann Intern Med.* 2018;168:640–650.
12. Chamberlain JJ, Doyle-Delgado K, Peterson L, Skolnik N. Diabetes technology: review of the 2019 American diabetes association standards of medical care in diabetes. *Ann Intern Med.* 2019;171:415–420.
13. Chrcanovic BR, Albrektsson T, Wennerberg A. Diabetes and oral implant failure: a systematic review. *J Dent Res.* 2014;93(9):859–867.
14. Doyle-Delgado K, Chamberlain JJ, Shubrook JH, Skolnik N, Trujillo J. Pharmacologic approaches to glycemic treatment of type 2 diabetes: synopsis of the 2020 American diabetes association's standards of medical care in diabetes clinical guideline. *Ann Intern Med.* 2020;173:813–821.
15. Faggion Jr CM, Cullinan MP, Atieh M. An overview of systematic reviews on the effectiveness of periodontal treatment to improve glycaemic control. *J Periodontal Res.* 2016;51:716–725.
16. Fernandes KS, Glick M, de Souza MS, Kokron CM, Gallottini M. Association between immunologic parameters, glycemic control, and post-extraction complications in patients with type 2 diabetes. *J Am Dent Assoc.* 2015;146(8):592–599.
17. Garber AJ, Handelsman Y, Grunberger G, et al. Consensus statement by the American association of clinical endocrinologists and American college of endocrinology on the comprehensive type 2 diabetes management algorithm – 2020 executive summary. *Endocr Pract.* 2020;26(1):107–139.
18. Kidambi S, Patel SB. Diabetes mellitus. Considerations for dentistry. *J Am Dent Assoc.* 2008;139(10 suppl):8S–18S.
19. Laditka SB, Ladtika JN. Active life expectancy of Americans with diabetes: risks of heart disease, obesity, and inactivity. *Diabetes Res Clin Pract.* 2015;107:37–45.
20. McGowan K, Phillips T, Gielis E, et al. Developing a prototype for integrated dental and diabetes care: understanding needs and priorities. *Aust Dent J.* 2021;66:41–48.

21. Nascimento GG, Leite FRM, Vestergaard P, Scheutz F, Lopez R. Does diabetes increase the risk of periodontitis? A systematic review and meta-regression analysis of longitudinal prospective studies. *Acta Diabetol*. 2018;55: 653−667.

22. Philips KH, Zhang S Moss K, Ciarrocca K, Beck JD. Periodontal disease, undiagnosed diabetes, and body mass index. Implications for diabetes screening by dentists. *J Am Dent Assoc*. 2021;152(1):25−35.

23. Redondo MJ, STeck AK, Publiese A. Genetics of type 1 diabetes. *Pediatr Diabetes*. 2018;19(3):346−353.

24. Rewers M, Ludvigsson J. Environmental risk factors for type 1 diabetes. *Lancet*. 2016;387:2340−2348.

15

Adrenal Insufficiency

KEY POINTS

- Dentists should identify patients with adrenal dysfunction and ensure they are being evaluated on a consistent basis by their medical health care provider and are medically stable.
- Excess glucocorticoids in the body is associated with weight gain, a broad and round face ("moon facies"), a "buffalo hump" on the upper back, hypertension, and acne.
- Insufficient adrenal function is associated with weakness, fatigue, abdominal pain, and hyperpigmentation of the skin and oral mucosa.
- Clinicians should be aware that patients who chronically take glucocorticoids often have comorbidities (e.g., diabetes mellitus, heart failure, osteoporosis and

bone fractures, impaired healing, insomnia, peptic ulceration, cataract formation, and possibly psychological/mood disorders).
- Adrenal crisis is a rare but potentially life-threatening event in a patient who has adrenal insufficiency. It occurs more often under challenges of increased stress, pain, infection, illness, comorbidity, and surgery.
- Monitoring of blood pressure throughout an invasive dental procedure is a critical component for recognizing and preventing the development of an adrenal crisis in a patient with adrenal insufficiency.

The adrenal glands are small (6–8 g) endocrine glands located bilaterally at the superior pole of each kidney. Each gland contains an outer cortex and an inner medulla. The adrenal medulla functions as a sympathetic ganglion and secretes catecholamines, primarily epinephrine. The adrenal cortex secretes several steroid hormones with multiple actions (Fig. 15.1).

The adrenal cortex makes up about 90% of the gland and consists of three zones. The outer zone is the *zona glomerulosa*. The middle zone is the *zona fasciculata*, and the innermost zone is the *zona reticularis*. The cortex manufactures three classes of adrenal steroids: glucocorticoids, mineralocorticoids, and androgens. All are derived from cholesterol and share a common molecular nucleus. The predominant hormone of the zona glomerulosa is aldosterone, a mineralocorticoid that responds to hormones made by the kidneys (i.e., renin and angiotensin). Aldosterone regulates physiologic levels of sodium and potassium; these two electrolytes are important for control of intravascular volume and blood pressure. The zona fasciculata secretes glucocorticoids, and the zona reticularis secretes androgens, or sex hormones.

Cortisol, the primary glucocorticoid, has several important physiologic actions on digestion, metabolism, cardiovascular function, the immune system, and for maintaining homeostasis during periods of physical or emotional stress. Cortisol acts as an insulin antagonist (Fig. 15.2), increasing blood levels and peripheral use of glucose by activating key enzymes involved in hepatic gluconeogenesis and inhibiting glucose uptake in

peripheral tissues (i.e., skeletal muscles). In adipose tissue, cortisol activates lipolysis, resulting in the release of free fatty acids into circulation. Cortisol increases blood pressure by potentiating the vasoconstrictor action of catecholamines and angiotensin II on the kidney and vasculature. Its antiinflammatory action is modulated by its inhibitory action on (1) lysosome release, (2) prostaglandin production, (3) eicosanoid and cytokine release, (4) endothelial cell expression of intracellular and extracellular adhesion molecules (ICAMs and ECAMs, respectively) that attract neutrophils, and (5) leukocyte function. Cortisol also activates osteoclasts and inhibits osteoblasts.

Regulation of cortisol secretion occurs through activity of the hypothalamic–pituitary–adrenal (HPA) axis (Fig. 15.3). Central nervous system afferents mediating circadian rhythm and responses to stress stimulate the hypothalamus to release corticotropin-releasing hormone (CRH), which stimulates the production and secretion of adrenocorticotropic hormone (ACTH) by the anterior pituitary. Corticotropin (ACTH) then stimulates the adrenal cortex to produce and secrete cortisol. Plasma cortisol levels are increased within a few minutes after stimulation. Circulating levels of cortisol inhibit the production of CRH and ACTH, thus completing a negative feedback loop.

Cortisol secretion is pulsatile and normally follows a circadian pattern. Peak levels of plasma cortisol occur around the time of waking in the morning and are lowest in the evening and night (Fig. 15.4). This pattern is

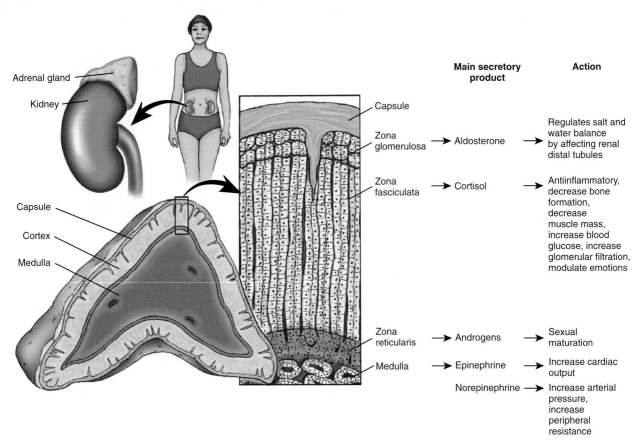

FIG. 15.1 Structure of the adrenal gland, representative zones, and their main secretory products and physiologic actions. (Adapted from Thibodeau GA, Patton KT. *Anatomy and Physiology.* 7th ed. St. Louis: Mosby; 2010.)

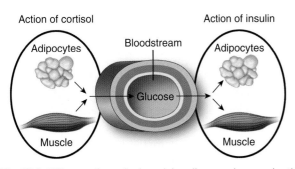

FIG. 15.2 Effects of cortisol and insulin on glucose in the bloodstream.

reversed in a person who habitually works the night shift and sleeps during the day. The normal secretion rate of cortisol over a 24-h period is approximately 20 mg. During periods of stress, the HPA axis is stimulated, resulting in increased secretion of cortisol. Anticipation of surgery or an athletic event usually is accompanied by only minimal increases in cortisol secretion. However, surgery itself is one of the most potent activators of the HPA axis. Also, various stressors such as trauma, illness, burns, fever, hypoglycemia, and emotional upset (e.g., anxiety) can trigger this effect. The most pronounced response is noted in the immediate postoperative period after surgery. However, this can be reduced by morphine-like analgesics, benzodiazepines, or local anesthesia, suggesting that the pain response mechanism increases the requirement for cortisol.

Synthetic glucocorticoids (cortisol-like drugs) used in the treatment of autoimmune and inflammatory diseases (e.g., rheumatoid arthritis, systemic lupus erythematosus, asthma, hepatitis, inflammatory bowel disease, dermatoses, mucositis) can affect adrenal function. Glucocorticoids are used on a long-term basis in patients during immunosuppressive therapy for organ transplantation and joint replacement. In dentistry, corticosteroids may be used during the perioperative period for the reduction of pain, edema, and trismus after oral surgical and endodontic procedures. Many synthetic glucocorticoids are available, and they differ in potency relative to cortisol and in their duration of action (Table 15.1).

MINERALOCORTICOIDS

Aldosterone is the primary mineralocorticoid secreted by the adrenal cortex. It is essential to sodium and potassium balance and to the maintenance of extracellular fluid (i.e., intravascular volume) and blood pressure. Its actions occur primarily on the distal tubule and the collecting

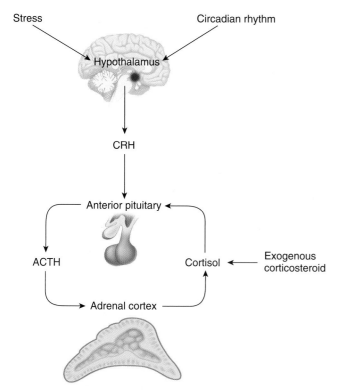

FIG. 15.3 Hypothalamic–pituitary–adrenal axis and the regulation of cortisol secretion. *ACTH*, adrenocorticotropic hormone; *CRH*, corticotropin-releasing hormone.

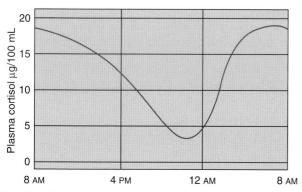

FIG. 15.4 Normal pattern of cortisol secretion over a 24-h period.

duct of the kidney, where it promotes sodium and water retention and potassium excretion. Aldosterone secretion is predominantly regulated by the renin–angiotensin system and extracellular potassium levels and less so by plasma sodium levels. Aldosterone secretion is stimulated by a fall in renal blood pressure, which results from decreased intravascular volume or a sodium imbalance. The drop in volume or pressure causes renin release from the kidney, which activates angiotensinogen to form angiotensin I and II. Angiotensin II, in turn, stimulates secretion of aldosterone from the adrenal cortex. When blood pressure rises, renin–angiotensin release diminishes, serving as a negative feedback loop that inhibits additional production of aldosterone (Fig. 15.5).

ADRENAL ANDROGENS

Dehydroepiandrosterone (DHEA) is the principal androgen secreted by the adrenal cortex. The effects of adrenal androgens are the same as those of testicular androgens (i.e., masculinization and the promotion of protein anabolism and growth). The activity of the adrenal androgens, however, is only about 20% that of the testicular androgens and is of relatively minor physiologic importance. Estrogen precursors are secreted from the zona reticularis of the adrenal cortex.

DEFINITION

Disorders of the adrenal glands can result in overproduction (hyperadrenalism) or underproduction (hypoadrenalism or adrenal insufficiency) of adrenal products.

Hyperadrenalism is characterized by excessive secretion of adrenal cortisol, mineralocorticoids, androgens, or estrogen in isolation or combination. The most common type of overproduction is due to glucocorticoid excess. When this is caused by pathophysiologic processes, the condition is known as *Cushing* disease. The term *Cushing syndrome* is a generalized state caused by excessive cortisol in the body, regardless of the cause.

Adrenal insufficiency (AI) is divided into three categories: primary, secondary, and tertiary. Primary adrenocortical insufficiency, also known as *Addison disease*, occurs when the adrenal cortex is destroyed or the gland is removed. Secondary AI is the consequence of pituitary disease, a lack of responsiveness of the adrenal glands to ACTH (corticotrophin) or caused by critical illness. Tertiary AI results from processes that impair function of the hypothalamus and secretion of corticotropin-releasing hormone, most commonly caused by chronic use of corticosteroids. Because abnormal adrenal function can be life-threatening, these conditions are of significant concern in clinical practice.

EPIDEMIOLOGY

Adrenal insufficiency occurs in 100–140 per 1 million persons of all ages, with about five new cases per million diagnosed each year. The diagnosis peaks in the fourth decade of life. Secondary AI is about two times more common than primary AI, and diagnosis peaks in the sixth decade. Both conditions are more common in women, and both conditions are associated with premature death. Approximately 2% of adults in the United States use corticosteroids on a chronic basis and thus are at risk for tertiary AI. A dental practice serving 2000 adults can expect to encounter 50 patients who use corticosteroids or who have potential adrenal abnormalities.

TABLE 15.1 Glucocorticoids and Their Relative Potency

Compound	Antiinflammatory Potency	Mineralocorticoid Potency	Equivalent Dose[a] (mg)
Short Acting (<12 h)			
Cortisol	1	2	20
Hydrocortisone	0.8	2	20
Intermediate Acting (12–36 h)			
Prednisone	4	1	5
Prednisolone	4	1	5
Triamcinolone	5	0	4
Methylprednisolone	5	0.5	4
Fludrocortisone	15	200	1.4
Long Acting (>36 h)			
Betamethasone	25	0	0.75
Dexamethasone	25	0	0.75
Inhaled			
Beclometasone dipropionate[b]	8 puffs 4 times a day equals 14 mg oral prednisone once a day	—	—

[a]Approximate.
[b]Fluticasone propionate is roughly twice as potent as beclometasone dipropionate and budesonide.
Data from Barnes N. Relative safety and efficacy of inhaled corticosteroids. *J Allergy Clin Immunol*. 1998;101:S460–S64; Schimmer BP, Parker KL. In: Brunton LL, Lazo JS, Parker KL, et al., eds. *Goodman and Gilman's the Pharmacological Basis of Therapeutics*. 11th ed. New York: McGraw-Hill; 2006; and Kroenberg HM, et al. *Williams Textbook of Endocrinology*. 11th ed. Philadelphia: Saunders; 2008.

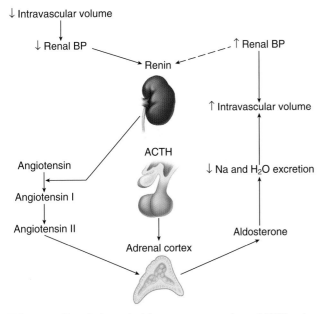

FIG. 15.5 Regulation of aldosterone secretion. *ACTH*, adrenocorticotropic hormone; *BP*, blood pressure.

ETIOLOGY

Primary adrenocortical insufficiency is caused by progressive destruction of the adrenal cortex, primarily because of autoimmune disease in adults and less frequently from chronic infectious disease (tuberculosis, human immunodeficiency virus [HIV] infection, cytomegalovirus infection, and fungal infection) or malignancy. The condition also may result from hemorrhage (e.g., heparin or low-molecular-weight heparin use), sepsis, adrenalectomy, genetic mutations (e.g., adrenoleukodystrophy, familial glucocorticoid deficiency), or drugs (e.g., that increase cortisol metabolism, inhibit gene transcription, or alter tissue resistance to glucocorticoids).

Secondary adrenocortical insufficiency is caused by structural lesions of the pituitary gland (e.g., tumor), removal of the pituitary gland, cranial irradiation of the pituitary gland, head trauma, and lack of responsiveness of the adrenal glands to ACTH (corticotrophin) or due to critical illness (e.g., sepsis, liver cirrhosis).

Tertiary AI results from defective hypothalamus function or, more commonly, as a result of chronic administration of exogenous corticosteroids. Prolonged corticosteroid use suppresses the hypothalamic–pituitary axis, which in turn inhibits ACTH production and adrenocortical production of cortisol (see Fig. 15.3). Less common causes include administration of specific drugs (Table 15.2) or a critical illness (burns, trauma, systemic infection).

PATHOPHYSIOLOGY AND COMPLICATIONS

Primary AI (Addison disease) is caused by the lack of the major hormones of the adrenal cortex: cortisol and aldosterone and to a lesser degree the androgens. Lack of

TABLE 15.2	Drugs that Interfere With Glucocorticoid Production and Increase Glucocorticoid Need
Drug Class	**Generic Drug Examples**
Antidepressant	Imipramine
Antifungal	Ketoconazole, fluconazole
Antipsychotic	Chlorpromazine
Antisteroid	Aminoglutethimide
Antiseizure	Phenytoin, topiramate
Antituberculosis	Rifampin
Barbiturate	Phenobarbital
Benzodiazepine	Midazolam
Diagnostic	Metyrapone
General anesthetic	Etomidate
Iron reducer (thalassemic drug)	Desferrioxamine

cortisol results in impaired metabolism of glucose, fat, and protein, as well as hypotension, increased ACTH secretion, impaired fluid excretion, excessive pigmentation, and an inability to tolerate stress. The relationship between corticosteroids and response to stress involves the maintenance of vascular reactivity to vasoactive agents and the maintenance of normal blood pressure and cardiac output. Aldosterone deficiency results in an inability to conserve sodium and eliminate potassium and hydrogen ions, leading to hypovolemia, hyperkalemia, and acidosis.

Secondary and tertiary AI are associated with low levels of cortisol. Unlike primary AI, aldosterone is not impaired with secondary or tertiary AI. This is because aldosterone secretion is ACTH independent.

Cushing syndrome refers to a condition caused by excessive cortisol in the body. When Cushing syndrome is caused by a pathophysiologic process (e.g., tumor of the pituitary gland or tumor of the adrenal gland), it is called Cushing disease. In Cushing disease, the endocrine tumor stimulates excessive circulating levels of glucocorticoids. Both Cushing disease and syndrome produce similar clinical features that result from high levels of cortisol that alters protein, carbohydrate, and fat metabolism, the effects of altered insulin and vasculature homeostasis. The most common cause of elevated cortisol levels in Cushing syndrome is the medical administration of corticosteroids (e.g., prednisone).

Corticosteroids can be administered by a variety of routes, and most medical regimens attempt to limit the dose so elevated cortisol levels, and thus adrenal suppression, do not occur. Corticosteroids that are topically applied or repeatedly locally injected or inhaled rarely induce adrenal suppression by absorption through the skin, subjacent tissues, or pulmonary alveoli. Although the amount of topical steroid required to treat small, noninflamed areas probably does not cause significant suppression, prolonged treatment of large inflamed areas may be a cause for concern, especially if occlusive

dressings are used with highly potent steroids. Similarly, the use of inhaled corticosteroids rarely causes adrenal suppression unless they are given in frequent and high doses. Doses above 400–500 µg/day in children or 800–1000 µg/day[,] of beclomethasone dipropionate equivalent in adults (depending on body mass) generally are considered to represent the cutoff point, indicating that adrenal suppression is probable.

In patients treated with corticosteroids, after administration ceases, the HPA axis begins to regain its responsiveness, and normal ACTH and cortisol secretion eventually resume. The time required to regain normal adrenal responsiveness is thought to range from days to months. However, studies from a large review demonstrated a return of HPA function to stress stimulation within 14 days even when supraphysiologic doses were given for 1 month or longer.

Adrenal Crisis

Adrenal crisis is a life-threatening emergency that occurs more often in those who have primary AI and are older or frail. The rate of occurrence is about 5–6 events per 100 patient-years. Adrenal crises are triggered by emotional and physical stress (e.g., infection, fever, sepsis, during or after surgery) when the body is unable to meet the increased demand for cortisol. The clinical signs of the impending crisis can be nonspecific, but evolve to manifest as hypotensive collapse, abdominal pain, myalgia, and fever.

CLINICAL PRESENTATION

Signs and Symptoms

Hypoadrenalism. Deficiencies of adrenocortical hormones produce signs and symptoms that are often nonspecific, leading to delays in diagnosis. Clinical evidence of adrenal deficiency generally appears only after 90% of the adrenal cortices have been destroyed.

Primary AI (Addison disease) produces signs and symptoms associated with a deficiency of all adrenocortical hormones (aldosterone, cortisol, androgens). The most common complaints are weakness, fatigue, abdominal pain, and hyperpigmentation of the skin (i.e., skin areas subjected to pressure: elbows, knuckles, palmar creases) and mucous membranes (Fig. 15.6). Hypotension, anorexia, salt craving, myalgia, hypoglycemia, and weight loss are additional commonly associated features. If a patient with Addison disease is challenged by emotional or physical stress (e.g., illness, infection, surgery), an *adrenal crisis* may be precipitated. This medical emergency evolves over a few hours and manifests as severe exacerbation of the patient's condition, including features described in Box 15.1. If not treated rapidly, the patient may develop hypothermia, severe hypotension, hypoglycemia, confusion, and circulatory collapse that can result in death.

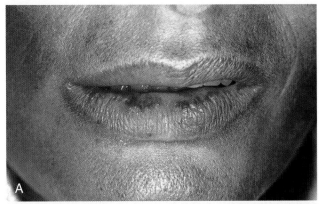

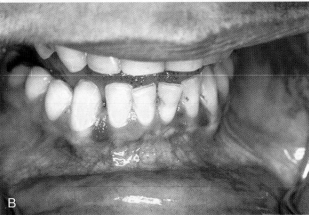

FIG. 15.6 Patient with Addison disease. Note bronzing of the skin with pigmentation of the lip (**A**) and the oral mucosa (**B**).

BOX 15.1 Features of an Adrenal Crisis

- Physical appearance: sunken eyes, profuse sweating, cyanosis
- Symptoms: headache, dyspnea, weakness
- Vitals: fever, hypotension, weak pulse
- Gastrointestinal: nausea, vomiting, dehydration,
- Musculoskeletal: myalgias, arthralgia,
- Blood laboratory: hyponatremia and eosinophilia

Secondary and tertiary AI may cause a partial insufficiency that is limited to glucocorticoids. The condition usually does not produce hyperpigmentation or any symptoms unless the patient is significantly stressed and does not have adequate circulating cortisol during times surrounding stress. In this event, an adrenal crisis is possible. However, an adrenal crisis in a patient with secondary or tertiary adrenal suppression is rare and tends not to be as severe as that seen with primary AI because aldosterone secretion is normal. Thus, hypotension, dehydration, and shock are seldom encountered.

Hyperadrenalism. Adrenal hyperfunction can produce four syndromes that are dependent on the adrenal product that is in excess—androgen, estrogen, mineralocorticoid, and cortisol. Androgen-related disorders are rare and primarily affect the reproductive organs.

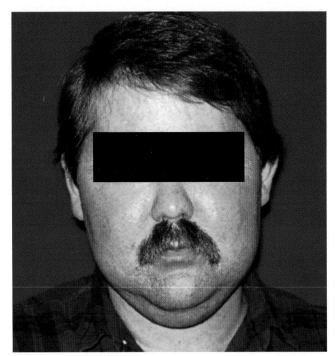

FIG. 15.7 "Moon-shaped face," a clinical manifestation of Cushing disease.

Mineralocorticoid excess (primary aldosteronism) is associated with hypertension, hypokalemia, and dependent edema (see Chapter 3). The most common form of hyperadrenalism is caused by glucocorticoid excess (endogenous or exogenous), and it leads to a syndrome known as Cushing syndrome. This syndrome classically produces weight gain, a broad and round face ("moon facies") (Fig. 15.7), a "buffalo hump" on the upper back, abdominal striae, hypertension, hirsutism, and acne. Other findings may include glucose intolerance (e.g., diabetes mellitus), heart failure, osteoporosis and bone fractures, impaired healing, and psychiatric disorders (mental depression, mania, anxiety disorders, cognitive dysfunction, and psychosis). Long-term steroid use also may increase risks for insomnia, peptic ulceration, cataract formation, glaucoma, growth suppression, and delayed wound healing.

LABORATORY AND DIAGNOSTIC FINDINGS

The presence of AI is determined by the presence of clinical features together with confirmation that cortisol secretion is inappropriately low. Low concentrations of serum or salivary cortisol in the early morning are strongly suggestive of AI. This relates to the fact that in the morning the adrenal gland is undergoing maximal secretion of cortisol (range, 10–20 μg/dL) compared with late afternoon when values are lower (3–10 μg/dL) owing to circadian rhythm. Clinicians also should be aware that cortisol levels vary in response to diet, stress, and sleep pattern.

Pairing the basal cortisol tests with plasma corticotropin concentration or with a provocative stimulation test of the HPA axis aids in the diagnosis. Levels of plasma corticotropin are high with primary AI and low with secondary AI.

The most common and reliable provocation test is the standard-dose corticotropin test. It is carried out by injecting 250 μg of exogenous corticotropin intravenously (IV) or intramuscularly (IM), and blood is collected 30 and 60 min after injection to determine stimulated cortisol levels. A positive response (i.e., an increase in plasma cortisol level after corticotropin administration) is indicative of adrenal reserve and function. A subnormal test response (60-min cortisol level <18 ng/mL) is suggestive of AI but has limited correlation with the patient's clinical ability to respond to stress.

The insulin tolerance test is used to assess the entire HPA axis when secondary AI is suspected. This test, however, is unpleasant for the patient because the insulin bolus induces severe hypoglycemia, and constant medical supervision is required during the 2-h test period.

Patients with AI may also experience low aldosterone concentration, hyponatremia, hyperkalemia, hypoglycemia, and high renin levels. Imaging of the adrenal gland and pituitary gland is recommended if malignancy, infiltrative disease, or hemorrhage is suspected.

MEDICAL MANAGEMENT

Primary Adrenal Insufficiency

The primary medical needs of patients with Addison disease are (1) management of the adrenal disease (e.g., elimination of the infectious agent or malignant disease) and (2) lifelong hormone replacement therapy. Glucocorticoid replacement is accomplished at levels that correspond to normal physiologic output of the adrenal cortex, usually about 20–25 mg/day of hydrocortisone or cortisone acetate, with a range of 12.5–50 mg/day. Standard practice is that half to two-thirds of the dose be given in the morning and one-third in the later afternoon in an attempt to reflect the normal diurnal cycle. Mineralocorticoid replacement is accomplished by single administration of 9α-fludrocortisone (0.05–0.2 mg) each morning. Patients also are encouraged to ingest adequate sodium and to monitor their blood pressure closely. Although patients with Addison disease can lead essentially normal lives with appropriate treatment, the need for supplemental glucocorticoids during periods of illness, trauma, or stress continues indefinitely. Target dose levels during periods of stress are 25–75 mg of hydrocortisone the day of minor to moderate surgery and 100–150 mg on the day of major surgery and the day after (Table 15.3). These target doses are based on the cortisol responses elicited by surgery, as explained below.

Surgery causes increased plasma corticosteroid levels during and after operations. Plasma cortisol levels peak at 2- to 10-fold above baseline between 4 and 10 h after the operation. The level of response is based on the magnitude of the surgery and whether general anesthesia is used. Postoperative pain is also contributory to elevated cortisol requirements. Kehlet and others estimate that adults secrete 75–200 mg a day in response to major surgery and 50 mg a day during minor procedures. Cortisol levels usually return to baseline within 24–48 h of surgery. Urine levels of cortisol metabolites, however, have been shown to remain increased for 3–6 days after the surgery.

Secondary Adrenal Insufficiency

Secondary AI results from destructive pituitary disorders. Treatment involves glucocorticoid replacement, albeit at a slightly lower dose than for primary disease. Hydrocortisone dosages of 10–20 mg are generally sufficient,

	TABLE 15.3 Recommendations for Steroid Supplementation During Surgery[a]	
	TARGET DOSE	
Procedure	**Primary Adrenal Insufficiency[b]**	**Secondary Adrenal Insufficiency[c]**
Routine dentistry	None	None
Minor surgery	25 mg of hydrocortisone equivalent, preoperatively on the day of surgery	Daily therapeutic dose
Moderate surgical stress	50–75 mg on day of surgery and up to 1 day after	Daily therapeutic dose
	Return to preoperative glucocorticoid dose on postoperative day 2	
Major surgical stress	100–150 mg per day of hydrocortisone equivalent given for 2–3 days	Daily therapeutic dose
	After preoperative dose, 50 mg of hydrocortisone IV every 8 h after the initial dose for the first 48–72 h after surgery	

[a]Guidelines based on patient's adrenal insufficiency status; however, requirements could increase if the patient's health is poor; if concurrent fear or anxiety, infection that is poorly managed, fever, or cirrhosis is present; and if major surgery or general anesthesia is being performed. Frequent monitoring of blood pressure during the first 8 h postoperatively is recommended.

[b]Data from Salem M, Tainsh Jr RE, Bromberg J, et al. Perioperative glucocorticoid coverage. A reassessment 42 years after emergence of a problem. *Ann Surg.* 1994;219:416–425.

[c]Data from Marik PE, Varon J. Requirement of perioperative stress doses of corticosteroids: a systematic review of the literature. *Arch Surg.* 2008;143:1222–1226. Supplemental doses can be provided if signs or symptoms of adrenal insufficiency (e.g., hypotension, abdominal pain, fatigue) appear.

IV, intravenous.

with stress-dose hydrocortisone coverage provided as needed. Mineralocorticoid replacement is not required.

Tertiary Adrenal Insufficiency

Tertiary AI is a condition involving interference with CRH secretion and occurs most often when corticosteroids are administered on a chronic basis. Here, the challenge for health care providers is to try and balance the beneficial effects of steroids with their unwanted adverse effects. Steroids are prescribed in the management of nonendocrine, inflammatory, and autoimmune disorders for their antiinflammatory and immunosuppressive properties. Selection is based on potency, route of administration, duration of action, and anticipated adverse effects. The goal is to achieve resolution of disease symptoms while minimizing adverse effects.

Depending on the condition, dosages prescribed generally are targeted to be the same as or less than the daily replacement dose of the preparation used. For example, hydrocortisone usually is dispensed at about 20 mg/day, prednisone or prednisolone at 5 mg/day, and dexamethasone at 0.3–0.5 mg/day (see Table 15.1). Such regimens given as a morning dose are less suppressive. Higher and divided daily doses are more suppressive and usually take at least 3 weeks to result in clinical manifestation of glucocorticoid deficiency. A method for minimizing the adverse effects of long-term systemic steroid therapy is the *alternate-day regimen*. This method consists of giving steroids in the morning every other day instead of daily but at a higher dose to maintain an elevated serum level. The alternate-day regimen allows the adrenal gland to function normally during the off day and thus does not tend to cause adrenal axis suppression. A *tapered dosage* schedule often is implemented for the discontinuation of steroid usage, but this approach may not be necessary in many cases.

The need for additional (i.e., supplemental) corticosteroids for patients taking daily or alternate-day steroids to prevent adrenal crisis during and after surgery has been a concern ever since Fraser and colleagues reported in 1952 that a patient who had taken cortisone for 8 months experienced refractory hypotension at the end of a routine surgical procedure and died 3 h later. A similar case was reported a year later. The general consensus for several decades was that "at-risk" patients who take corticosteroids should be provided supplemental steroids during periods of stress, trauma, or illness. More recent evidence, however, has led to revised recommendations (see Table 15.3).

The new recommendations, based on evidence-based reviews, suggest that only patients with primary AI receive supplemental doses of steroid, and those with secondary AI who take daily corticosteroids, regardless of the type of surgery, should receive only their usual daily dose of corticosteroid before the surgery. The rationale for these recommendations is that the vast majority of patients who take daily equivalent or lower doses of steroid (e.g., mean dose of 5–10 mg/day of prednisone) on a long-term basis for conditions such as renal transplantation or rheumatoid arthritis maintain adrenal function and do not experience adverse outcomes after minor or even major surgical procedures. In addition, patients who took 5–50 mg/day of prednisone for several years who had their glucocorticoid medications discontinued within 1 week before surgery have withstood general surgical procedures without the development of adrenal crisis. Clinicians should recognize that major surgery generally is performed in hospital-like environments, where close monitoring of blood pressure and fluid balance helps to ensure minimal adverse events during the surgical and postsurgical period. Thus, the recommendations listed in Table 15.3 include good operative and postoperative monitoring.

Inasmuch as the recommendations in Table 15.3 serve as guidelines, clinicians should be aware that the need for corticosteroid supplementation also can be influenced by factors that may complicate the postsurgical course and exacerbate AI. These factors include the overall physical status of the patient, including level of pain, liver dysfunction, febrile illness, sepsis, fluid loss, nausea and vomiting, and drugs taken. Clinicians are advised to monitor the patient for these conditions and to select medications carefully. Drugs that can lower plasma cortisol levels include general anesthetics, midazolam, barbiturates, aminoglutethimide (an adrenolytic), etomidate (an anesthetic agent), ketoconazole, and inducers of hepatic cytochrome P-450 oxygenases (e.g., phenytoin, barbiturates, rifampin) that accelerate degradation of cortisol (see Table 15.2). Also of note, the action of oral anticoagulants can be potentiated (resulting in increased risk of bleeding) by IV administration of high-dose methylprednisolone, which could lead to adrenal hemorrhage.

Adrenal Crisis

Adrenal crisis requires timely diagnosis and immediate treatment, including IV injection of a glucocorticoid—usually a 100-mg hydrocortisone bolus—and fluid and electrolyte replacement to reverse the hypotension, cortisol deficiency, and electrolyte abnormalities. IM injection results in slow absorption and is not preferred for emergency treatment. After the initial bolus, 50 mg of hydrocortisone is administered by IV slowly every 6–8 h for 24 h for a typical total dose of 100–200 mg per 24 h along with fluid replacement, vasopressors, continuous infusion of saline, and correction of hypoglycemia, if needed. Resolution of the precipitating event or condition also is required.

DENTAL MANAGEMENT

Identification. Any patient whose condition remains undiagnosed but who has signs and symptoms of adrenal disease should be referred to a physician for diagnosis and treatment. Laboratory testing and diagnostic imaging are helpful in identifying those who may have AI.

Risk Assessment. Risk assessment for primary or secondary AI should be determined by performing a thorough medical history, physical examination, and, if needed, laboratory tests and medical consultation. The dentist should be aware that a past or present history of tuberculosis, histoplasmosis, or HIV infection increases the risk for primary adrenal disease (insufficiency) because opportunistic infectious agents may attack the adrenal glands. In addition, adrenal crisis is more likely in patients with AI who have the following comorbidities: malignancy, major traumatic injury, severe pain, infection or sepsis, liver cirrhosis, administration of medications that alter cortisol metabolism or production, recent emergency or hospitalization visits, or need for stress-related corticoid dose self-adjustments. In general, patients with tertiary AI are at low risk for adrenal crisis unless they receive an invasive procedure and have one of the above-mentioned comorbidities in combination with recently discontinued high-dose corticosteroid treatment, simply do not take their glucocorticoid before a stressful surgical procedure, or present with low blood pressure before an invasive procedure. If the dentist is uncertain of the functional reserve of the patient, laboratory testing and medical consultation are advised before the performance of an invasive or prolonged (>1 h) procedure.

Recommendations. In developing recommendations for dental patients with adrenal disease, the dentist must consider the type and degree of adrenal dysfunction and the dental procedure planned.

Hyperadrenalism. Patients with hyperadrenalism or who take corticosteroids for prolonged periods have an increased likelihood of having hypertension, diabetes, delayed wound healing, osteoporosis, and peptic ulcer disease. To minimize the risk of an adverse outcome, blood pressure should be taken at baseline and monitored during dental appointments. Blood glucose levels should be determined, and invasive procedures should be performed during periods of good glucose control. Follow-up appointments should be arranged to assess proper wound healing. Because osteoporosis has a relationship with periodontal bone loss, implant placement, and bone fracture, periodic measures of periodontal bone loss are indicated. Also, measures should be instituted that promote bone mineralization, and extensive neck manipulation should be avoided if osteoporosis is severe. Because long-term steroid users are at risk of peptic ulceration, postoperative analgesics for these patients should not include aspirin or other nonsteroidal antiinflammatory drugs.

Adrenal Insufficiency

Antibiotics: Risk of Infection. No issues.

Bleeding. Generally, this is not an issue. An exception is the patient who take heparin or another anticoagulant, which places them at increased risk for adrenal hemorrhage, postsurgical bleeding, and hypotension.

Blood Pressure. Monitoring of blood pressure throughout invasive dental procedures of patients who have AI is critical for recognition of a developing adrenal crisis. During surgery, blood pressure should be evaluated at 5-min intervals and before the patient leaves the office. A systolic blood pressure below 100 mm Hg or a diastolic pressure at or below 60 mm Hg represents hypotension, which dictates that the clinician take corrective action. This includes proper patient positioning (i.e., head lower than feet), fluid replacement, administration of vasopressors, and evaluation for signs of adrenal dysfunction versus hypoglycemia. If adrenal crisis is determined to be occurring, a steroid bolus is required.

Capacity to Tolerate Care. Patients who have AI are potentially at risk for an adrenal crisis. The risk is highest in those with primary AI, especially those who are undiagnosed or untreated. In one study, 8% of patients with Addison disease needed hospital treatment annually for an adrenal crisis. In contrast, patients who have secondary or tertiary AI are at much lower risk. In fact, evidence indicates that the vast majority of patients with secondary or tertiary AI may undergo routine dental treatment without the need for supplemental glucocorticoids. Patients at risk for adrenal crisis are those who have a concomitant infection/illness/fever, comorbidity (e.g., pulmonary cardiac, malignant disease), or sustained trauma, or who are undergoing stressful surgical procedures or general anesthesia and have no, or extremely low, adrenal function because of primary or severe secondary AI. It is recommended to delay treatment for these patients and any patient who is undiagnosed or untreated until the patient has been medically stabilized.

Dentists should be aware that three factors influence the recommendation for supplemental corticosteroids: (1) type of AI, (2) medical status and stability, and (3) level and type of stress. Currently, only patients with primary AI are recommended to receive corticosteroid supplementation, and this recommendation applies only when surgery or general anesthesia is being performed or in the management of a dental or systemic infection (see Table 15.3). Patients with well-controlled secondary AI and those who take daily or alternate-day corticosteroids generally have enough exogenous and endogenous cortisol to handle routine dental procedures and surgery if their usual steroid dose (or parenteral dose equivalent) is taken the morning of the procedure. Thus, the recommendation is for patients to take their usual daily dose of steroid within 2 h of the surgical procedure and that the surgeon, anesthetist, and nurses be advised of possible complications associated with the patient's adrenal state. Routine dental procedures do not stimulate cortisol production at levels comparable with those that occur during and after surgery and do not require supplementation, even in patients with controlled primary AI.

Patients undergoing surgery should be closely monitored for blood and fluid loss and for hypotension during the postoperative period. If hypotension appears during monitoring, IV fluids are to be given and additional doses of corticosteroid considered if fluid replacement fails to rectify the blood pressure. Patients are returned to their usual glucocorticoid dosage as soon as their vital signs are stabilized.

Additional measures recommended to minimize the risk of adrenal crisis associated with surgical stress are shown in Box 15.2. Surgery should be scheduled in the morning when cortisol levels are highest. Proper stress reduction should be provided because fear and anxiety increase cortisol demand. Nitrous oxide—oxygen inhalation and benzodiazepine sedation are helpful in minimizing stress and reducing cortisol demand. In contrast, reversal of and recovery from general anesthesia and extubation, in addition to the trauma of the surgery, are major determinants of secretion, are major determinants

---

BOX 15.2   Checklist for Dental Management of Patients With Possible Adrenal Insufficiency[a]

PREOPERATIVE RISK ASSESSMENT
- Evaluate and determine whether primary, secondary, or tertiary adrenal sufficiency exists.
- Obtain medical consultation if condition is poorly controlled (e.g., acute infection), if clinical signs and symptoms point to an undiagnosed problem, or if diagnosis is uncertain.

A

Analgesics	Provide good postoperative pain control to avoid adrenal crisis.
Antibiotics	No issues.
Anesthesia	Provide adequate operative and postoperative anesthesia; routine use of epinephrine (1 : 100,000) is appropriate. Consider using long-acting local anesthetics (e.g., bupivacaine) at the end of the procedure to provide longer postoperative pain control. General anesthesia increases glucocorticoid demand and could render an adrenal-insufficient patient susceptible to adrenal crisis; therefore, use cautiously.
Anxiety	Anxiety and stress increase the risk of adrenal crisis if adrenal insufficiency is present. Use anxiety and stress reduction techniques as needed.

B

Bleeding	Minimize blood loss.
Blood pressure	Continuously monitor blood pressure throughout stressful and invasive procedures. Postoperative monitoring for at least 8 h is recommended for procedures involving moderate or major surgery. If blood pressure drops below 100/60 mm Hg, consider fluid replacement, vasopressive measures, and supplemental steroid administration, as needed.

C

Capacity to tolerate care[b]	Provide adequate supplemental corticosteroids according to Table 15.3.
Chair position	Hypotension (e.g., from severe adrenal insufficiency) may dictate a supine position. Otherwise, normal chair position can be used.

D

Devices	No issues.
Drugs	Provide steroid supplementation for primary adrenal insufficiency during surgical procedures or infection (see Table 15.2). Provide usual morning corticosteroid dose for patients who have secondary adrenal insufficiency and are undergoing surgical procedures. Avoid phenobarbital use because it increases the metabolism of cortisol and reduces blood levels of cortisol. Also, discontinue use of phenytoin, rifampicin, troglitazone (inducers of cortisol metabolism), ketoconazole, fluconazole, etomidate, metyrapone, and aminoglutethimide (inhibitors of corticosteroid production) at least 24 h before surgery, with the consent of the patient's physician.

E

Equipment Emergencies	Have an emergency medical kit readily available. Acute adrenal crisis is a medical emergency. Call 911. Apply cool wet or ice packs, assess and monitor vital signs, start IV saline solution, inject 100 IV of hydrocortisone followed by 100—200 mg of hydrocortisone in 5% glucose by continuous IV infusion, and transport patient to emergency medical facility.

F

Follow-up	Adrenal-insufficient patients should be monitored for good fluid balance and adequate blood pressure during the first 24 h postsurgery. Communicate with the patient at the end of the appointment and within 4 h postoperatively to determine whether features of weak pulse, hypotension, dyspnea, myalgias, arthralgia, ileus, and fever are present. Signs and symptoms of adrenal crisis dictate transport to a hospital for emergency care.

[b]Surgical procedures lasting longer than 1 h are more stressful than shorter procedures and are considered major surgery. Major surgery should be performed with the consideration for the need of steroid supplementation based on the overall health status of the patient. In addition, inadequate pain and anxiety control in the perioperative period increase the risk of adrenal crisis. Performance of major surgical procedures in a hospital environment is recommended to afford adequate patient monitoring during the postoperative phase.
[a]Strength of recommendation taxonomy (SORT) Grade: C (see Preface for further explanation).
IV, intravenous.

of secretion of ACTH, cortisol, and epinephrine. Thus, general anesthesia increases glucocorticoid demand for these patients. Barbiturates also should be used cautiously because these drugs enhance the metabolism of cortisol and reduce blood levels of cortisol. In addition, inhibitors of corticosteroid production (see Table 15.2) should be discontinued at least 24 h before surgery, with the consent of the patient's physician.

Surgeries that last longer than 1 h are more stressful than shorter surgeries and should be considered major surgical procedures that can require the need for steroid supplementation. Blood and fluid volume loss exacerbate hypotension, thereby increasing the risk for development of AI-like symptoms. Thus, methods that reduce blood loss are important in this setting. Clinicians should also realize that a fasting state can contribute to hypoglycemia, which can mimic features of an adrenal crisis but does not require glucocorticoids for resolution.

Drug Considerations and Interactions. Inadequate pain control during the postoperative period increases the risk of adrenal crisis. Clinicians should provide good postoperative pain control by means of long-acting local anesthetics (e.g., bupivacaine) given at the end of the procedure. Inasmuch as significant increases in cortisol levels generally are not seen before or during the operation but are increased in the postoperative period (i.e., 1–5 h after the procedure commensurate with the pain response) and the rise in cortisol levels is blunted by the use of analgesics and midazolam, good pain control with local anesthesia and analgesics is recommended for these patients.

Emergency Action. Immediate treatment during an adrenal crisis requires proper patient positioning (i.e., head lower than feet), fluid replacement, administration of vasopressors, administration of 100 mg of hydrocortisone or 4 mg of dexamethasone IV, and immediate transportation to a medical facility.

Oral Manifestations

Diffuse or focal brown macular pigmentation of the oral mucous membranes is a common finding in primary AI (see Fig. 15.6). Pigmentation of sun-exposed skin in areas of friction generally occurs after the appearance of oral pigmentation and is accompanied by lethargy. Patients with secondary or tertiary AI may be prone to delayed healing and may have increased susceptibility to infection but do not develop hyperpigmentation.

BIBLIOGRAPHY

1. Annetta M, Maviglia R, Proietti R, et al. Use of corticosteroids in critically ill septic patients: a review of mechanisms of adrenal insufficiency in sepsis and treatment. *Curr Drug Targets*. 2009;10(9):887–894.
2. Arlt W, Allolio B. Adrenal insufficiency. *Lancet*. 2003;361(9372):1881–1893.
3. Banks P. The adreno-cortical response to oral surgery. *Br J Oral Surg*. 1970;8(1):32–44.
4. Bergthorsdottir R, Leonsson-Zachrisson M, Oden A, et al. Premature mortality in patients with Addison's disease: a population-based study. *J Clin Endocrinol Metab*. 2006;91(12):4849–4853.
5. Bromberg JS, Baliga P, Cofer JB, et al. Stress steroids are not required for patients receiving a renal allograft and undergoing operation. *J Am Coll Surg*. 1995;180(5):532–536.
6. Broutsas MG, Seldin R. Adrenal crisis after tooth extractions in an adrenalectomized patient: report of case. *J Oral Surg*. 1972;30(4):301–302.
7. Cawson RA, James J. Adrenal crisis in a dental patient having systemic corticosteroids. *Br J Oral Surg*. 1973;10(3):305–309.
8. Charmandari E, Nicolaides NC, Chrousos GP. Adrenal insufficiency. *Lancet*. 2014;383(9935):2152–2167.
9. Chernow B, Alexander HR, Smallridge RC, et al. Hormonal responses to graded surgical stress. *Arch Intern Med*. 1987;147(7):1273–1278.
10. Collins S, Caron MG, Lefkowitz RJ. Beta-adrenergic receptors in hamster smooth muscle cells are transcriptionally regulated by glucocorticoids. *J Biol Chem*. 1988;263(19):9067–9070.
11. Cooper MS, Stewart PM. Corticosteroid insufficiency in acutely ill patients. *N Engl J Med*. 2003;348(8):727–734.
12. Coskey RJ. Adverse effects of corticosteroids: I. Topical and intralesional. *Clin Dermatol*. 1986;4(1):155–160.
13. Erichsen MM, Lovas K, Skinningsrud B, et al. Clinical, immunological, and genetic features of autoimmune primary adrenal insufficiency: observations from a Norwegian registry. *J Clin Endocrinol Metab*. 2009;94(12):4882–4890.
14. Costedoat-Chalumeau N, Amoura Z, Aymard G, et al. Potentiation of vitamin K antagonists by high-dose intravenous methylprednisolone. *Ann Intern Med*. 2000;132(8):631–635.
15. Dorin RI, Qualls CR, Crapo LM. Diagnosis of adrenal insufficiency. *Ann Intern Med*. 2003;139(3):194–204.
16. Falorni A, Minarelli V, Morelli S. Therapy of adrenal insufficiency: an update. *Endocrine*. 2013;43(3):514–528.
17. Findling JW, Raff H. Screening and diagnosis of Cushing's syndrome. *Endocrinol Metab Clin N Am*. 2005;34(2):385–402 (ix–x).
18. Fraser CG, Preuss FS, Bigford WD. Adrenal atrophy and irreversible shock associated with cortisone therapy. *J Am Med Assoc*. 1952;149(17):1542–1543.
19. Friedman RJ, Schiff CF, Bromberg JS. Use of supplemental steroids in patients having orthopaedic operations. *J Bone Joint Surg Am*. 1995;77(12):1801–1806.
20. George JM, Reier CE, Lanese RR, et al. Morphine anesthesia blocks cortisol and growth hormone response to surgical stress in humans. *J Clin Endocrinol Metab*. 1974;38(5):736–741.
21. Gersema L, Baker K. Use of corticosteroids in oral surgery. *J Oral Maxillofac Surg*. 1992;50(3):270–277.
22. Glick M. Glucocorticosteroid replacement therapy: a literature review and suggested replacement therapy. *Oral Surg Oral Med Oral Pathol*. 1989;67(5):614–620.
23. Grinspoon SK, Biller BM. Clinical review 62: laboratory assessment of adrenal insufficiency. *J Clin Endocrinol Metab*. 1994;79(4):923–931.

24. Hahner S, Loeffler M, Bleicken B, et al. Epidemiology of adrenal crisis in chronic adrenal insufficiency: the need for new prevention strategies. *Eur J Endocrinol.* 2010;162(3):597–602.

25. Hameed R, Zacharin MR. Cushing syndrome, adrenal suppression and local corticosteroid use. *J Paediatr Child Health.* 2006;42(6):392–394.

26. Hannig KE, Poulsen PL, Tonnesen EK, et al. Recommendations for supplementary intravenous glucocorticosteroids in patients on long-term steroid therapy—a systematic review. *Ugeskr Laeger.* 2012;174(50):3155–3159.

27. Hempenstall PD, Campbell JP, Bajurnow AT, et al. Cardiovascular, biochemical, and hormonal responses to intravenous sedation with local analgesia versus general anesthesia in patients undergoing oral surgery. *J Oral Maxillofac Surg.* 1986;44(6):441–446.

28. Jasani MK, Freeman PA, Boyle JA, et al. Cardiovascular and plasma cortisol responses to surgery in corticosteroid-treated R. A. patients. *Acta Rheumatol Scand.* 1968;14(1):65–70.

29. Jerjes W, Jerjes WK, Swinson B, et al. Midazolam in the reduction of surgical stress: a randomized clinical trial. *Oral Surg Oral Med Oral Pathol Oral Radiol Endod.* 2005;100(5):564–570.

30. Jung C, Inder WJ. Management of adrenal insufficiency during the stress of medical illness and surgery. *Med J Aust.* 2008;188(7):409–413.

31. Kaufman E, Heling I, Rotstein I, et al. Intraligamentary injection of slow-release methylprednisolone for the prevention of pain after endodontic treatment. *Oral Surg Oral Med Oral Pathol.* 1994;77(6):651–654.

32. Kehlet H. *Clinical Course and Hypothalamic-Pituitary-Adrenocortical Function in Glucocorticoid-Treated Surgical Patients.* Copenhagen: FADL's Forlag; 1976.

33. Kehlet H, Binder C. Adrenocortical function and clinical course during and after surgery in unsupplemented glucocorticoid-treated patients. *Br J Anaesth.* 1973;45(10):1043–1048.

34. Khalaf MW, Khader R, Cobetto G, et al. Risk of adrenal crisis in dental patients: results of a systematic search of the literature. *J Am Dent Assoc.* 2013;144(2):152–160.

35. Kelly HW, Nelson HS. Potential adverse effects of the inhaled corticosteroids. *J Allergy Clin Immunol.* 2003;112(3):469–478. quiz 79.

36. Lehtinen AM, Hovorka J, Widholm O. Modification of aspects of the endocrine response to tracheal intubation by lignocaine, halothane and thiopentone. *Br J Anaesth.* 1984;56(3):239–246.

37. Lewis L, Robinson RF, Yee J, et al. Fatal adrenal cortical insufficiency precipitated by surgery during prolonged continuous cortisone treatment. *Ann Intern Med.* 1953;39(1):116–126.

38. Lovas K, Husebye ES. High prevalence and increasing incidence of Addison's disease in western Norway. *Clin Endocrinol (Oxf).* 2002;56(6):787–791.

39. Lovas K, Husebye ES. Replacement therapy for Addison's disease: recent developments. *Expert Opin Investig Drugs.* 2008;17(4):497–509.

40. Mandanas S, Boudina M, Chrisoulidou A, et al. Acute adrenal insufficiency following arthroplasty: a case report and review of the literature. *BMC Res Notes.* 2013;6:370.

41. Marik PE, Pastores SM, Annane D, et al. Recommendations for the diagnosis and management of corticosteroid insufficiency in critically ill adult patients: consensus statements from an international task force by the American College of Critical Care Medicine. *Crit Care Med.* 2008;36(6):1937–1949.

42. Marik PE, Varon J. Requirement of perioperative stress doses of corticosteroids: a systematic review of the literature. *Arch Surg.* 2008;143(12):1222–1226.

43. Milenkovic A, Markovic D, Zdravkovic D, et al. Adrenal crisis provoked by dental infection: case report and review of the literature. *Oral Surg Oral Med Oral Pathol Oral Radiol Endod.* 2010;110(3):325–329.

44. Miller CS, Dembo JB, Falace DA, et al. Salivary cortisol response to dental treatment of varying stress. *Oral Surg Oral Med Oral Pathol Oral Radiol Endod.* 1995;79(4):436–441.

45. Miller CS, Little JW, Falace DA. Supplemental corticosteroids for dental patients with adrenal insufficiency: reconsideration of the problem. *J Am Dent Assoc.* 2001;132(11):1570–1579. quiz 96-7.

46. Molimard M, Girodet PO, Pollet C, et al. Inhaled corticosteroids and adrenal insufficiency: prevalence and clinical presentation. *Drug Saf.* 2008;31(9):769–774.

47. Napenas JJ, Kujan O, Arduino PG, et al. World Workship on Oral Medicine VI: controversies regarding dental management of medically complex patients: assessment of current recommendations. *Oral Surg Oral Med Oral Pathol Oral Radiol.* 2015;120(2):207–226.

48. Nieman LK, Chanco Turner ML. Addison's disease. *Clin Dermatol.* 2006;24(4):276–280.

49. Oyama T, Takiguchi M, Aoki N, et al. Adrenocortical function related to thiopental-nitrous oxide-oxygen anesthesia and surgery in man. *Anesth Analg.* 1971;50(5):727–731.

50. Patel L, Clayton PE, Addison GM, et al. Adrenal function following topical steroid treatment in children with atopic dermatitis. *Br J Dermatol.* 1995;132(6):950–955.

51. Parnell AG. Adrenal crisis and the dental surgeon. *Br Dent J.* 1964;116:294–298.

52. Plemons JM, Rees TD, Zachariah NY. Absorption of a topical steroid and evaluation of adrenal suppression in patients with erosive lichen planus. *Oral Surg Oral Med Oral Pathol.* 1990;69(6):688–693.

53. Plumpton FS, Besser GM, Cole PV. Corticosteroid treatment and surgery. 2. The management of steroid cover. *Anaesthesia.* 1969;24(1):12–18.

54. Puar TH, Stikkelbroeck NM, Smans LC, et al. Adrenal crisis: still a deadly event in the 21(st) century. *Am J Med.* 2016;129(3):339 e1–339 e9.

55. Raff H, Norton AJ, Flemma RJ, et al. Inhibition of the adrenocorticotropin response to surgery in humans: interaction between dexamethasone and fentanyl. *J Clin Endocrinol Metab.* 1987;65(2):295–298.

56. Reuter NG, Westgate PM, Ingram M, et al. Death related to dental treatment: a systematic review. *Oral Surg Oral Med Oral Pathol Oral Radiol.* 2017;123(2):194–204.

57. Reisch N, Arlt W. Fine tuning for quality of life: 21st century approach to treatment of Addison's disease. *Endocrinol Metab Clin N Am.* 2009;38(2):407–418 (ix–x).

58. Salem M, Tainsh Jr RE, Bromberg J, et al. Perioperative glucocorticoid coverage. A reassessment 42 years after emergence of a problem. *Ann Surg.* 1994;219(4):416–425.

59. Scheitler LE, Tucker WM, Christian DC. Adrenal insufficiency: report of case. *Spec Care Dent.* 1984;4(1):22–24.

60. Shannon IL, Isbell GM, Prigmore JR, et al. Stress in dental patients. II. The serum free 17-hydroxycorticosteroid response in routinely appointed patients undergoing simple exodontia. *Oral Surg Oral Med Oral Pathol.* 1962;15:1142–1146.

61. Shapiro R, Carroll PB, Tzakis AG, et al. Adrenal reserve in renal transplant recipients with cyclosporine, azathioprine, and prednisone immunosuppression. *Transplantation.* 1990;49(5):1011–1013.

62. Siker ES, Lipschitz E, Klein R. The effect of preanesthetic medications on the blood level of 17-hydroxycorticosteroids. *Ann Surg.* 1956;143(1):88–91.

63. Smans LCCJ, Van der Valk ES, Hermus Ad RMM, Zelissen PMJ. Incidence of adrenal crisis in patients with adrenal insufficiency. *Clin Endocrinol (Oxf).* January 2016;84(1):17–22.

64. Stewart PM, Newell-Price JDC. The adrenal cortex. In: Melmed S, Polonsky KS, Larsen R, et al., eds. *Williams Textbook of Endocrinology.* Philadelphia: Elsevier; 2016.

65. Thomasson B. Studies on the content of 17-hydroxycorticosteroids and its diurnal rhythm in the plasma of surgical patients. *Scand J Clin Lab Invest.* 1959;11(suppl 42):1–180.

66. Tomlinson JW, Holden N, Hills RK, et al. Association between premature mortality and hypopituitarism. West Midlands Prospective Hypopituitary Study Group. *Lancet.* 2001;357(9254):425–431.

67. Udelsman R, Holbrook NJ. Endocrine and molecular responses to surgical stress. *Curr Probl Surg.* 1994;31(8):653–720.

68. Udelsman R, Norton JA, Jelenich SE, et al. Responses of the hypothalamic-pituitary-adrenal and renin-angiotensin axes and the sympathetic system during controlled surgical and anesthetic stress. *J Clin Endocrinol Metab.* 1987;64(5):986–994.

69. Wallace I, Cunningham S, Lindsay J. The diagnosis and investigation of adrenal insufficiency in adults. *Ann Clin Biochem.* 2009;46(Pt 5):351–367.

70. White K, Arlt W. Adrenal crisis in treated Addison's disease: a predictable but under-managed event. *Eur J Endocrinol.* 2010;162(1):115–120.

71. Willis AC, Vince FP. The prevalence of Addison's disease in Coventry, UK. *Postgrad Med J.* 1997;73(859):286–288.

72. Yong SL, Coulthard P, Wrzosek A. Supplemental perioperative steroids for surgical patients with adrenal insufficiency. *Cochrane Database Syst Rev.* 2012;12:CD005367.

73. Ziccardi VB, Abubaker AO, Sotereanos GC, et al. Precipitation of an Addisonian crisis during dental surgery: recognition and management. *Compendium.* 1992;13(6):518, 20, 22–24.

16

Thyroid Diseases

KEY MESSAGES

1. Dentists can screen for thyroid disease and thyroid cancer through medical history and clinical examination.
2. Epinephrine should be minimized or even avoided in patients with poorly controlled hyperthyroidism, especially in those with existing cardiac disease.
3. Although exceedingly rare to encounter thyroid disease-related medical emergencies in the dental setting, myxedema coma in patients with poorly controlled hypothyroidism, and thyrotoxic storm in patients with poorly controlled hyperthyroidism, can both potentially be triggered by untreated odontogenic infection as well as surgical procedures.
4. Patients who have received radioactive iodine therapy (^{131}I) as treatment for thyroid cancer are at risk for developing chronic sialadenitis and may experience clinically significant salivary gland hypofunction and an increased risk of dental caries.

The thyroid gland plays a critical role in regulating a wide range of physiologic activities including growth and development, digestion and metabolism, cardiac function, and bone homeostasis; under normal healthy conditions, the gland is carefully regulated and maintains a "euthyroid" state with normal activity and function (Fig. 16.1). The four main categories of thyroid disease include hypothyroidism, hyperthyroidism (thyrotoxicosis), thyroiditis, and neoplasia/cancer (Table 16.1). While most patients with a history of thyroid disease can safely receive dental treatment without special precautions, dentists must be aware of certain risk assessment considerations including potentially high-risk medical emergencies. Further, dentists can screen for thyroid disease when obtaining a medical history and during clinical examination.

EPIDEMIOLOGY

Thyroid disease affects women at a higher frequency than men. While iodine deficiency is the most common cause of goiter (enlargement of the thyroid gland, Fig. 16.2) and hypothyroidism worldwide, this is relatively rare in the United States and developed world. Spontaneous hypothyroidism (most frequently due to Hashimoto thyroiditis) affects 1%–2% of the population and is more common in women and older individuals. Graves disease is the most common cause of hyperthyroidism in the United States, affecting 2% of women and 0.2% of men, primarily from the second to fifth decades.

Thyroiditis encompasses a group of conditions characterized by inflammation of the thyroid gland that, in many cases (e.g., Hashimoto thyroiditis), leads to eventual chronic hypothyroidism (Table 16.2). Subacute painless thyroiditis occurs in patients with underlying autoimmune thyroid disease and is reported in up to 5% of women 3–6 months after pregnancy (*postpartum thyroiditis*).

The American Cancer Society estimates that in the United States in 2020 there were 52,890 new cases of thyroid cancer (12,720 in men and 40,170 in women) and 2180 deaths from thyroid cancer (1040 men and 1140 women). Papillary thyroid carcinoma accounts for 85% of thyroid cancers. While the 5-year survival rate for thyroid cancer is 97%, poorly differentiated (e.g., medullary thyroid carcinoma) and anaplastic thyroid cancers, albeit rare, are associated with far poorer outcomes.

In an average dental practice of 2000 patients, an estimated 20–150 patients will have some form of thyroid disease.

ETIOLOGY

The most common cause of hypothyroidism is Hashimoto thyroiditis, an autoimmune disorder, with less frequent causes including developmental, pituitary disorders, pregnancy, and iodine deficiency. The most common cause of hyperthyroidism is Graves disease, also an autoimmune disorder, with other causes including toxic nodular goiter, acute thyroiditis, neoplasia, and iatrogenic due to overmedication with synthetic thyroid hormone in hypothyroid individuals. Three autoantibodies are most often involved in autoimmune thyroid disease: TSH receptor antibodies (TSHRAb, blocking and activating), thyroid peroxidase antibodies (TPoAb), and thyroglobulin antibodies (TgAb). For example, in Graves disease, thyroid-stimulating immunoglobulins bind to and activate thyrotrophic receptors, causing the gland to grow and stimulating increased T4 and T3 synthesis. This disorder is much more common in women

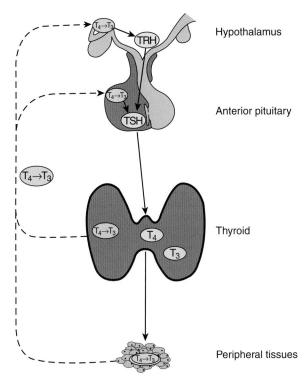

FIG. 16.1 The hypothalamic–pituitary–thyroid axis. *Solid lines* correspond to stimulatory effects, and *dotted lines* depict inhibitory effects. Conversion of thyroxine (T₄) to triiodothyronine (T₃) in the pituitary and the hypothalamus is mediated by 5′-deiodinase type II. This event also is important throughout the central nervous system, thyroid, and muscle. 5′-Deiodinase type I (propylthiouracil sensitive) plays a major role in liver, kidney, and thyroid function. *TRH,* thyrotropin-releasing hormone; *TSH,* thyroid-stimulating hormone. (Redrawn from DeGroot LJ, Jameson JL. *Endocrinology.* 5th ed., vol. 2. Philadelphia: Saunders; 2006.)

(with a male-to-female ratio of 10:1) and may manifest during puberty or pregnancy or at menopause.

Patients with hyperthyroidism who are untreated or incompletely treated may develop thyrotoxic crisis, a rare but serious complication of abrupt onset that may occur at any age. Most patients who develop thyrotoxic crisis have a goiter, wide pulse pressure, ophthalmic signs, and a long-standing history of thyrotoxicosis. Precipitating factors include infection, trauma, surgical emergencies, and operations.

Thyroid cancer is the most common of the endocrine cancers and with very few identified risk factors. Disease variants are characterized histologically (differentiated, medullary, and anaplastic) and by various mutations in the MAPK and PI3K-AKT pathways including the BRAF, RAS, RET, and ALK genes. While overall survival outcomes are excellent, there is significant variability based on specific diagnosis (Table 16.2). Multiple endocrine neoplasia type 2 (MEN2) syndrome is associated with risk of medullary thyroid carcinoma, pheochromocytoma, and parathyroid hyperplasia or adenoma. In addition, primary lymphomas may occur in the thyroid gland, and other cancers may metastasize to the thyroid.

PATHOPHYSIOLOGY AND COMPLICATIONS

The thyroid gland is a small, butterfly-shaped endocrine gland located in the base of the neck that secretes three hormones: thyroxine (T4), triiodothyronine (T3), and calcitonin. T3 and T4 collectively are termed "thyroid hormone," which influences the growth and maturation of tissues, cell respiration, and total energy expenditure (Fig. 16.1). Calcitonin is involved, along with parathyroid hormone and vitamin D, in regulating serum calcium and phosphorus levels and skeletal remodeling. Under normal conditions, thyrotropin-releasing hormone (TRH) is released by the hypothalamus in response to external stimuli (e.g., stress, illness, metabolic demand, low levels of T3 and, to a lesser extent, T4). TRH stimulates the pituitary to release thyroid-stimulating hormone (TSH), which causes the thyroid gland to secrete T4 and T3. In the blood, T4 and T3 are almost entirely bound to plasma proteins, with the most important being thyroid hormone–binding serum protein (TBG), which binds about 70% of T4 and 75%–80% of T3.

Thyroiditis is defined as inflammation of the thyroid gland, which may occur due to multiple causes. Five types of thyroiditis have been identified: Hashimoto, subacute painful, subacute painless, acute suppurative, and Riedel (Table 16.3). In some cases (e.g., subacute painful thyroiditis), inflammation may be associated only with transient hyper/hypoactivity before returning to normal function, while in others (e.g., Hashimoto thyroiditis leading to hypothyroidism) the inflammation results in progressive and permanent dysfunction.

Untreated hypothyroidism can lead to goiter development, cardiac disease, peripheral neuropathy, depression, and myxedema (a condition of severe hypothyroidism), as well as infertility and risk of birth defects in women (Fig. 16.3). Complications in patients with hypothyroidism include an exaggerated response to central nervous system (CNS) depressants (sedatives and narcotic analgesics) and myxedematous coma, a rare life-threatening condition in long-standing undiagnosed hypothyroidism precipitated by CNS depressants, infection, severe stress, or surgical procedures.

Hyperthyroidism is characterized by thyrotoxicosis, an excess of T4 and T3 in the bloodstream, leading to a hypermetabolic state. Increased metabolic activity caused by excessive hormone secretion increases circulatory demand which can result in palpitations, supraventricular cardiac dysrhythmias, and congestive heart failure. Ophthalmopathy associated with Graves disease can lead to vision loss. Thyrotoxic crisis or storm, which can be precipitated by infection or surgical procedures, is rare and can be life-threatening requiring emergency intervention.

TABLE 16.1   Thyroid Disorders

Thyroid Condition	Causes
Hyperthyroidism	**Primary thyroid hyperfunction** • Graves disease • Toxic multinodular goiter • Toxic adenoma **Secondary thyroid hyperfunction** • Pituitary adenoma—TSH secretion • Inappropriate TSH secretion (pituitary) • Trophoblastic hCG secretion **Without thyroid hyperfunction** • Hormonal leakage—subacute thyroiditis • Bovine thyroid in ground beef • Metastatic thyroid cancer • Iatrogenic (overdosage of thyroid hormone) • Thyroid hormone use (factitia)

Hypothyroidism (cretinism, myxedema)	**Primary atrophic hypothyroidism**
	• Insufficient amount of functioning thyroid tissue
	  • Destruction of tissue by autoimmune process: Hashimoto thyroiditis, Graves disease (end stage)
	  • Destruction of tissue by iatrogenic procedures: ^{131}I therapy, surgical thyroidectomy, external radiation to thyroid gland
	  • Destruction of tissue by infiltrative process: amyloidosis, lymphoma, scleroderma
	• Defects of thyroid hormone biosynthesis
	  • Congenital enzyme defects
	  • Congenital mutations in TSH receptor
	  • Iodine deficiency of excess
	  • Drug-induced: thionamides, lithium, others
	• Agenesis or dysplasia
	Secondary hypothyroidism
	• Pituitary
	  • Panhypopituitarism (neoplasm, irradiation, surgery)
	  • Isolated TSH deficiency
	• Hypothalamic
	  • Congenital
	  • Infection
	  • Infiltration (sarcoidosis, granulomas)
	Transient hypothyroidism
	• Silent and subacute thyroiditis
	• Thyroxine withdrawal
	Generalized resistance to thyroid hormone

Thyroiditis	Acute suppurative Subacute painful Subacute painless Hashimoto Chronic fibrosing (Riedel)
Thyroid neoplasms	Adenomas Carcinomas Others

hCG, Human chorionic gonadotropin; *TSH,* thyroid-stimulating hormone.

Thyroid cancers are heterogeneous with variable pathology, biological characteristics, therapeutic approaches, and survival outcomes. While tumors may secrete excess thyroid hormone and lead to a state of hyperthyroidism, and aggressive cancers may metastasize and lead to complications in distant sites and organs (including rarely the oral cavity; Fig. 16.4), most medical complications associated with thyroid cancers arise secondary to treatment of the cancer. Of the various treatment modalities used in the management of thyroid cancers (e.g., surgery, chemotherapy, targeted therapy, radiation therapy), the only treatment-related complication unique to thyroid cancer is risk of salivary gland sialadenitis and hypofunction following treatment with radioactive iodine (^{131}I), due to uptake in the salivary glands. This complication may present with generalized

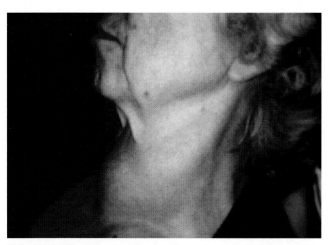

FIG. 16.2 Diffuse enlargement of the thyroid gland caused by Graves disease (goiter).

TABLE 16.2 Classification of Thyroid Cancer

Type (Histologic)	Frequency (%)	5-Year Survival Rate (%)
Differentiated—papillary	75–80	Near 100
Differentiated—follicular	8–10	98
Differentiated—Hürthle cell	1	70
Anaplastic	1–5	7
Medullary	5–8	90
Lymphoma	1–5	Determined by lymphoma diagnosis/stage
Metastases to the thyroid	<1	Determined by primary

discomfort with or without swelling of the salivary glands along with typical signs and symptoms of radiation-induced salivary gland dysfunction and xerostomia.

CLINICAL PRESENTATION

Hypothyroidism. Typical signs and symptoms of hypothyroidism include fatigue, weight gain, poor memory, poor ability to concentrate, dry and rough skin, and dry, brittle, and coarse hair (Fig. 16.5, Table 16.4). Hashimoto thyroiditis typically presents as an asymptomatic diffuse goiter, and most patients are already found to be hypothyroid upon diagnosis (Fig. 16.6).

Neonatal hypothyroidism (cretinism) is characterized by dwarfism, intellectual disability, and characteristic facial features including a broad flat nose, wide-set eyes, thick lips, a large protruding tongue, delayed eruption of teeth and malocclusions; all of which can be prevented by early detection and management (Fig. 16.7).

Hyperthyroidism (Thyrotoxicosis) and Thyrotoxic Storm. The most common signs and symptoms of uncontrolled hyperthyroidism include nervousness, fatigue, rapid heartbeat or palpitations, heat intolerance, and

weight loss (Table 16.4). With increasing age, weight loss and decreased appetite become more common, and irritability and heat intolerance are less common. Atrial fibrillation is rare in patients younger than 50 years of age but occurs in approximately 20% of older patients. The skin may be warm and moist and the complexion rosy with easy blushing. Hair may become fine and friable and nails may soften.

Graves ophthalmopathy affects approximately 50% of patients and is characterized by edema and inflammation of the extraocular muscles, as well as an increase in orbital connective tissue and fat, leading to characteristic features of "exophthalmos" or bulging eyes (Fig. 16.8).

Thyrotoxic storm is characterized by fever, profuse sweating, marked tachycardia and cardiac arrhythmias, pulmonary edema, and congestive heart failure which can lead to severe hypotension, coma, and death.

Thyroid Cancer. Thyroid cancers may present variably: as a solitary lump in the region of the gland; a dominant nodule(s) in multinodular goiter; a hard, painless mass with possible fixation to adjacent structures; sometimes associated with enlarged cervical lymph nodes; and symptoms of hoarseness, stridor, and dysphagia may be present (Fig. 16.4).

Laboratory and Diagnostic Findings

Several tests are available that measure thyroid function (Table 16.5). Serum T_4 and T_3 concentrations can be measured, with elevated levels usually indicating hyperthyroidism, and lower levels usually indicating hypothyroidism. Measurement of basal serum TSH concentration is also useful in the diagnosis of hyperthyroidism (low TSH) and hypothyroidism (high TSH).

T_4, T_3, TBG, and TSH tests are used to screen for hyperthyroidism. Radioassay techniques are used to detect various pathogenic antibodies (i.e., TSHRAb, TSHR-blocking Ab, TPoAb, and TgAb). A thyroid scan (using ^{123}I or ^{99}Tc) may be used to localize thyroid nodules and to locate functional ectopic thyroid tissue (Fig. 16.9).

Thyroid nodules are typically evaluated by ultrasonography (US) and fine-needle aspiration biopsy (Fig. 16.10). US may be used to detect thyroid lesions/nodules as small as 1–2 mm in size and can distinguish solid from cystic lesions. US, CT, MRI, and PET imaging are used in the diagnosis and monitoring of thyroid cancers.

MEDICAL MANAGEMENT

Hypothyroidism and Myxedema Coma. Patients with hypothyroidism are treated with synthetic preparations that contain sodium levothyroxine (LT_4) or sodium liothyronine (LT_3) to restore a euthyroid state (Table 16.4). Patients with untreated hypothyroidism are sensitive to the actions of narcotics, barbiturates, and tranquilizers due to generalized CNS depression, so these drugs must

TABLE 16.3 Thyroiditis

Type	Cause	Clinical Findings	Thyroid Function	Treatment
Hashimoto thyroiditis	Autoimmune related	Goiter—moderate in size, rubbery, firm	Euthyroid early Few cases with transient hyperfunction Hypothyroidism develops in most cases	Thyroid hormone In rare cases of compression of vital tissues, surgery is indicated
Subacute painful thyroiditis	Possible viral infection	Enlarged, firm, tender, gland with pain that may radiate to ear, jaw, or occipital region	Hyperthyroidism with return to euthyroid state	Aspirin Prednisone Propranolol for symptoms of thyrotoxicosis
Acute suppurative thyroiditis	Bacterial infection	Pain and tenderness in gland; fever, malaise; skin over the gland warm and red	Euthyroid	Incision and drainage, appropriate antibiotics
Chronic fibrosing thyroiditis (Riedel)	Unknown	Enlarged gland that is stony hard and fixed to surrounding tissues	Usually remain euthyroid but in some cases hypothyroidism may occur	Usually none; if vital structures are compressed, surgery is indicated; thyroid hormone
Subacute painless thyroiditis (postpartum thyroiditis)	Not established but related to autoimmune thyroid disease	Enlarged gland that is firm and nontender; may occur in women 5–6 months after pregnancy	Hyperthyroidism for 5–6 months; then return to euthyroid state	Propranolol for symptoms of thyrotoxicosis

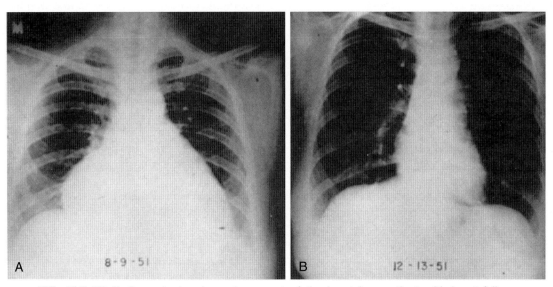

FIG. 16.3 (A) Radiograph showing enlargement of the heart in a patient with heart failure caused by myxedema. **(B)** After treatment with thyroid hormone, the radiograph shows a return to normal heart size. (From Melmed S, et al. *Williams Textbook of Endocrinology*. 12th ed. Philadelphia: Saunders; 2011.)

be used with caution. Myxedematous coma is treated by parenteral levothyroxine (T_4) and corticosteroids, and the patient is covered to conserve heat.

Hyperthyroidism and Thyrotoxic Crisis

Treatment of patients with thyrotoxicosis may involve antithyroid agents that block hormone synthesis, iodides, ^{131}I, or subtotal thyroidectomy (Table 16.4). The antithyroid agents most often used in the United States are propylthiouracil and methimazole, both of which inhibit thyroid peroxidase and thus the synthesis of thyroid hormone. Propylthiouracil also blocks extrathyroidal deiodination of T_4 to T_3. Treatment duration is typically 1–2 years. Administration of ^{131}I is the preferred initial treatment for patients with Graves disease in North America and is associated with risk of developing hypothyroidism. Subtotal thyroidectomy is preferred by some patients with a large goiter and is indicated in those with a coexistent thyroid nodule whose nature is unclear. Beta blockers (e.g., propranolol) are used for management of adrenergic effects (e.g., tremor, tachycardia) of hyperthyroidism.

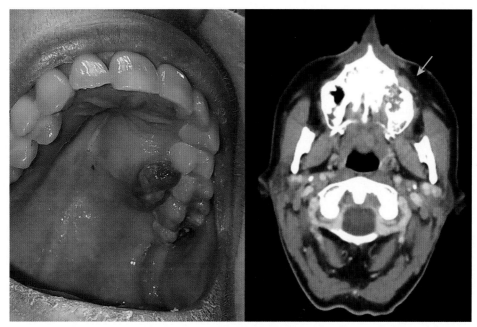

FIG. 16.4 A 56-year-old with metastatic anaplastic thyroid cancer, with metastasis to the left upper alveolar ridge and protrusion into the oral cavity. (Courtesy of Jochen Lorch, MD, Dana-Farber Cancer Institute, Boston, MA.)

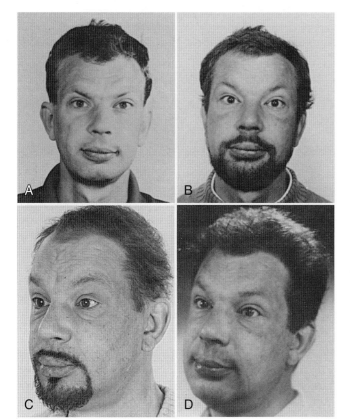

FIG. 16.5 Appearance of a 47-year-old man 12 years (A), 5 years (B), and 3 years (C) before hypothyroidism secondary to atrophic myxedema (D) was diagnosed. Note the typical myxedema face characterized by puffy nonpitting swelling of the skin and coarse facial features. (Editor(s): from Jameson JL, et al. *Endocrinology: Adult and Pediatric.* 7th ed. Philadelphia: Saunders; 2016. Reproduced with permission of the patient.)

Emergency management of thyrotoxic crisis consists of administration of large doses of antithyroid medication (propylthiouracil), potassium iodide, propranolol, corticosteroids, IV glucose, vitamin B complex, wet packs, fans, and ice packs. Cardiopulmonary resuscitation may be indicated.

Thyroid Cancer. Treatment of thyroid cancer depends on the specific diagnosis, stage, clinical features, and patient factors such as comorbidities and life expectancy. Treatment modalities include surgery, radioiodine ablation (^{131}I), external beam radiation therapy, chemotherapy, targeted therapy, and immunotherapy (Fig. 16.11).

DENTAL MANAGEMENT

Risk Assessment

A new patient and periodically updated medical history should include any history of and treatment for thyroid disease, and any related medical complications. The thyroid gland should be inspected and palpated as part of the routine head and neck examination performed by the dentist (see Chapter 1). Although difficult to detect, the normal thyroid gland can be palpated in many patients and has a somewhat rubbery consistency. If a thyroid abnormality is detected (e.g., nodule/mass, diffuse enlargement), the patient should be referred to their primary care physician for evaluation.

Patients with a history of thyroid disease who have received prior successful corrective therapy or who are on

TABLE 16.4   Clinical Features and Management of Thyroid Disorders

Condition	Signs and Symptoms	Laboratory Tests	Treatment
Hyperthyroidism	*Skeletal*—osteoporosis *Cardiovascular*—palpitations, tachycardia, arrhythmias, hypertension, cardiomegaly, congestive heart failure, angina, myocardial infarction *GI*—weight loss, increased appetite, pernicious anemia *CNS*—anxiety, restlessness, sleep disturbances, emotional lability, impaired concentration, weakness, tremors (hands, fingers, tongue) *Skin*—erythema, thin fine hair, areas of alopecia, soft nails *Eyes*—retraction of upper eyelid, exophthalmos, corneal ulceration, ocular muscle weakness *Other*—increased risk for diabetes, decreased serum cholesterol level, increased risk for thrombocytopenia, sweating	T_4—elevated T_3—elevated TSH—none or very low TBG—elevated Normal range: T_4—5–12 µg/dL or 64–154 nmol/L T_3—80–190 ng/dL or 1.2–2.9 nmol/L TSH—0.5–4.5 mIU/L TBG—1–25 ng/mL	Antithyroid agents: pro-pylthiouracil, carbima-zole, methimazole RAI Subtotal thyroidectomy Propranolol for adrenergic component in thyrotoxi-cosis (sweating, tremor, and tachycardia)
Hypothyroidism	*Musculoskeletal*—arthritis, muscle cramps *Cardiovascular*—shortness of breath, hypotension, slow pulse *GI*—constipation, nausea or vomiting, weight gain *CNS*—mental and physical slowness, sleepiness, headache *General*—dry, thick skin and dry hair; fatigue; edema (puffy hand, face, eyes), cold intolerance; hoarseness; weight gain	T_4—decreased T_3—decreased TSH—elevated TBG—decreased	Levothyroxine (synthetic T_4) or Liothyronine (syn-thetic T_3)
Thyroiditis	*Hashimoto*—rubbery firm goiter, hypothyroidism develops later	Later in disease: T_4, T_3, and TBG are decreased; TSH becomes elevated	Thyroid hormone; surgery in rare cases (compres-sion of vital tissues)
	Subacute painful—enlarged, firm, tender gland, pain that may radiate to ear or jaw	Hyperthyroid returning to euthyroid status	Aspirin, prednisone, pro-pranolol for symptoms of thyrotoxicosis
	Acute suppurative—pain, tenderness in gland, fever, malaise	Euthyroid	Incision and drainage, appropriate antibiotics
	Riedel/Chronic fibrosing—hard, fixed, enlarged gland	Usually remains euthyroid; hypothyroid status can occur	Usually none; surgery if vi-tal tissues compressed, thyroid hormone
	Subacute painless—firm, nontender, enlarged gland	Hyperthyroid for 5–6 months, returning to euthyroid status	Propranolol for symptoms of thyrotoxicosis

CNS, central nervous system; *GI*, gastrointestinal; *RAI*, radioactive iodine; T_3, triiodothyronine; T_4, tetraiodothyronine (thyroxine); *TBG*, thyroid-binding globulin; *TSH*, thyroid-stimulating hormone.

therapy and euthyroid do not require any special pre-cautions or measures. Patients with a history of poorly controlled disease should be evaluated for signs and symptoms and referred to their physician if indicated. Medical consultation with the patient's physician to evaluate risk is essential in those with a known history of serious medical complications such as thyrotoxic storm, myxedematous coma, or advanced cardiac complications (e.g., congestive heart failure). Medical complications and emergencies that may potentially be encountered during or associated with provision of dental treatment of patients with undiagnosed or poorly controlled thyroid disease are summarized in Box 16.1.

Prevention and Management Recommendations (Box 16.2)

Antibiotics and Risk of Infection. Acute and chronic odontogenic infections should be actively treated to avoid risk of infection-related complications in patients with poorly controlled disease. Infection and surgical procedures can precipitate a myxedematous coma and a thyrotoxic storm in patients with poorly controlled hypothyroidism and hyperthyroidism, respectively.

Bleeding. There is little to no risk of bleeding abnor-malities in patients with thyroid disease except in hy-perthyroid patients concurrently taking warfarin and propylthiouracil.

Capacity to Tolerate Care. When a patient with thyroid disease is under good medical management, dental treatment can proceed without alteration. While the following situations are both exceedingly rare, poorly controlled hypothyroid patients are at risk for myxedema coma, and poorly controlled hyperthyroid patients are at risk for

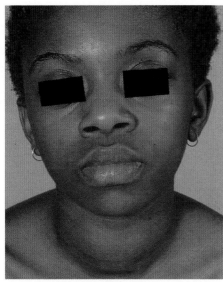

FIG. 16.6 Hashimoto disease is the most common cause of goitrous hypothyroidism. The initial lesion consists of a diffuse goiter, and the patient may be euthyroid. Later the patient becomes hypothyroid, and very late in the disease, the gland atrophies. (From Forbes CD, Jackson WF. *Color Atlas and Text of Clinical Medicine*. 3rd ed. Edinburgh: Mosby; 2003.)

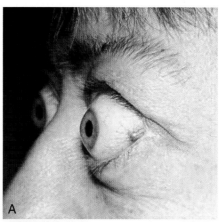

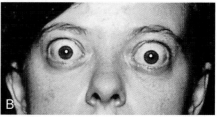

FIG. 16.8 Exophthalmos of Graves disease. (**A**) Eyelid retraction is a common eye sign in Graves disease. It is recognized when the sclera is visible between the lower margin of the upper eyelid and the cornea. (**B**) Proptosis in Graves disease results from enlargement of muscles and fat within the orbit as a result of mucopolysaccharide infiltration. ((**A**) From Goldman L, Ausiello D. *Cecil Textbook of Medicine*. 23rd ed. Philadelphia: Saunders; 2008. (**B**) From Seidel H. *Mosby's Guide to Physical Examination*. 4th ed. St. Louis: Mosby; 1999.)

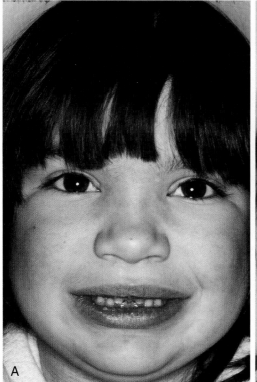

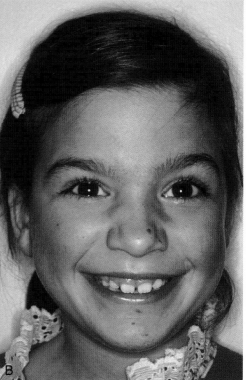

FIG. 16.7 (**A**) A 9-year-old girl with severe hypothyroidism. (**B**) The same patient 1 year after treatment with thyroid hormone replacement. Note the return to normal facial appearance. (From Neville B, Damm D, Alley C, et al. *Oral and Maxillofacial Pathology*. 3rd ed. St. Louis: Saunders; 2009.)

TABLE 16.5 Laboratory Tests

Test	Normal Range	Interpretation
Radioactive iodine uptake (RIU)	5%–30%	Elevated: hyperthyroidism Decreased: hypothyroidism
Thyroid-stimulating hormone (TSH)	0.5–4.5 mIU/L	Elevated: hypothyroidism Suppressed: hyperthyroidism
Total serum T$_4$ (TT$_4$)	5–12 μg/dL 64–154 nmol/L	High: hyperthyroidism Low: hypothyroidism
Free T$_4$ (FT$_4$)	1.0–3.0 ng/dL 13–39 pmol/L	Increased: hyperthyroidism Decreased: hypothyroidism
Total serum T$_3$ (TT$_3$)	1.2–2.9 nmol/L 80–190 ng/dL	High: hyperthyroidism Low: hypothyroidism
Free T$_3$ (FT$_3$)	0.25–0.65 ng/dL 3.8–10 nmol/L	Increased: hyperthyroidism Decreased: hypothyroidism

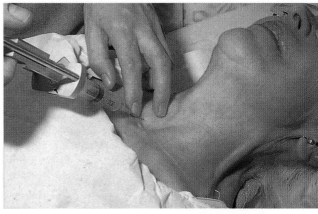

FIG. 16.10 Fine-needle aspiration biopsy of a thyroid nodule is the investigation of choice in a patient with a solitary nodule. (From Forbes CD, Jackson WF. *Color Atlas and Text of Clinical Medicine*. 3rd ed. Edinburgh: Mosby; 2003.)

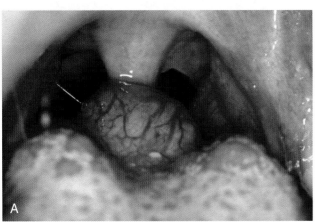

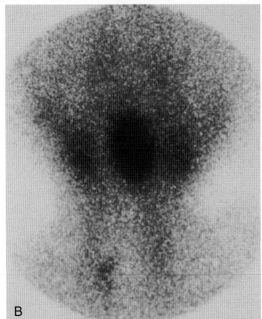

FIG. 16.9 (A) Lingual thyroid nodule in a 4-year-old girl. **(B)** Thyroid scan of the nodule. (From Neville BW, et al. *Oral and Maxillofacial Pathology*. 3rd ed. St. Louis: Saunders; 2009.)

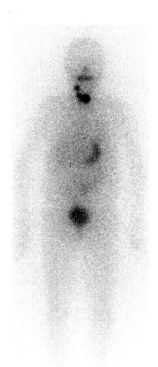

FIG. 16.11 A 31-year-old female with papillary thyroid carcinoma who underwent near-total thyroidectomy and then was recommended for ^{131}I treatment. She was administered 30mCi ^{131}I, and the attached whole-body scan was performed 4 days thereafter. Images demonstrate uptake in the neck, but separately iodine avidity in the right lateral neck consistent with local metastatic lymph node disease. Physiologic excretion of the isotope is seen in the bowel and bladder, as well as uptake in the cranial sinuses. (Courtesy of Erik Alexander, MD, Brigham and Women's Hospital, Boston, MA.)

thyrotoxic storm. Dental surgical procedures could potentially trigger such emergency situations. If a patient's disease status is unclear, or they appear unstable, medical consultation is indicated, and dental treatment should be postponed unless emergency care is required.

BOX 16.1 Medical Complications Potentially Encountered in Patients With Undiagnosed or Poorly Controlled Thyroid Disease

Hyperthyroidism

Adverse interaction with epinephrine

Life-threatening cardiac arrhythmias

Congestive heart failure

Complications of underlying cardiovascular pathologic conditions

Thyrotoxic crisis can be precipitated by:
- Infection
- Surgical procedures

Hypothyroidism

Exaggerated response to CNS depressants (sedatives, opioid analgesics)

Myxedematous coma can be precipitated by:
- CNS depressants
- Infection
- Surgical procedures

CNS, central nervous system.

Drug Considerations. Use of CNS depressants, sedatives, and narcotic analgesics may result in an exaggerated response in patients with uncontrolled hypothyroidism and should be used with caution. Use of epinephrine or other vasopressors should be avoided in untreated or inadequately managed thyrotoxic patients. In such patients with poorly controlled disease, dental treatment should be limited to emergency care and coordinated closely with the patient's physician.

Antithyroid medications (propylthiouracil and methimazole) can rarely cause agranulocytosis thereby increasing risk of infection.

Emergencies. Albeit exceedingly unlikely in the dental care setting, in case of a medical emergency of myxedema coma or thyrotoxic storm, the dentist must recognize the clinical signs and symptoms, stop treatment and ensure that the patient is safe and secure, and seek immediate medical assistance as these can be life-threatening situations. Basic measures including monitoring of vital signs should be initiated while awaiting emergency medical assistance.

BOX 16.2 | Checklist for Dental Management of Patients With Thyroid Disease[a]

PREOPERATIVE RISK ASSESSMENT (SEE BOX 16.1)	
• Evaluate and determine whether a hyper-, hypo-, or euthyroid condition exists	
• Obtain medical consultation if poorly controlled or undiagnosed problem or if uncertain	

A	
Antibiotics	Treat acute infection aggressively in patients with untreated or poorly controlled disease
Anesthesia	Avoid using epinephrine in local anesthetics in patients with untreated or poorly controlled hyperthyroidism
Anxiety	Patients with untreated or poorly controlled hyperthyroidism may appear very anxious
	Avoid CNS depressants such as narcotics, barbiturates, and sedatives in patients with untreated or poorly controlled hypothyroidism

B	
Bleeding	
Blood pressure and vital sign monitoring	Blood pressure be elevated in patients with untreated or poorly controlled hyperthyroidism.
	Patients with untreated or poorly controlled hyperthyroidism may be subject to cardiac arrhythmias.

C	
Chair position	

D	
Devices	
Drugs	Antithyroid medications (propylthiouracil and methimazole) can rarely cause agranulocytosis thereby increasing risk of infection.
	Hyperthyroid patients concurrently taking warfarin and propylthiouracil may be at increased risk for bleeding.
	Avoid CNS depressants such as narcotics, barbiturates, and sedatives in patients with untreated or poorly controlled hypothyroidism.

E	
Emergencies and urgent care	Thyrotoxic crisis: Seek medical aid; vital signs must be monitored and CPR initiated if necessary; apply wet packs or ice packs; inject 100–300 mg of hydrocortisone, IV glucose solution; administer propylthiouracil; and transport patient to emergency medical facilities.
	Myxedema coma: Seek medical aid; vital signs must be monitored and CPR initiated if necessary. Cover patient to conserve body heat; inject 100–300 mg of hydrocortisone, thyroxine (1.8 µg/kg daily with a 500 µg loading dose), IV saline, and glucose; transport to medical emergency facility.

F	
Follow-up care	Routine unless patient develops complications; no specific precautions.

[a]Strength of recommendation taxonomy (SORT) Grade: C (see Preface for further explanation).

ORAL MANIFESTATIONS

Hypothyroidism

Infants and children with hypothyroidism may present with thick lips, enlarged tongue, and delayed eruption of teeth with resulting malocclusion (Fig. 16.7). Adults with acquired hypothyroidism can display an enlarged tongue and diminished salivary flow. Hashimoto thyroiditis can be accompanied by salivary gland dysfunction, resulting in dry mouth. Studies suggest an association between thyroid disease (i.e., hypothyroidism or its pharmacologic treatment) and oral lichen planus but the relationship remains uncertain.

Hyperthyroidism

In children, the teeth and jaws develop rapidly, and premature loss of deciduous teeth with early eruption of permanent teeth is common. Patients with thyrotoxicosis are infrequently found to have a lingual "thyroid" consisting of thyroid tissue posterior to the foramen cecum (Fig. 16.9). If a lingual thyroid is suspected, the patient should be referred for further evaluation (e.g., radioactive iodine scan) rather than biopsy.

Thyroid Cancer

Patients who have been treated with ^{131}I are at risk for developing chronic salivary gland dysfunction and sialadenitis and an increased rate of dental caries (see Chapter 26). Patients suffering from chronic painful sialadenitis may benefit from sialadenoscopy with intraductal lavage.

BIBLIOGRAPHY

1. Allweiss P, Braunstein GD, Katz A, Waxman A. Sialadenitis following I-131 therapy for thyroid carcinoma: concise communication. *J Nucl Med.* July 1984;25(7): 755–758.
2. Fagin JA, Wells Jr SA. Biologic and clinical perspectives on thyroid cancer. *N Engl J Med.* 2016;375:1054–1067.
3. Ferri FF, ed. *Ferri's Clinical Advisor.* Philadelphia, PA: Elsevier (Saunders); 2020.
4. Franklin N, Tessler FN, Middleton WD, Grant EG. Thyroid imaging reporting and data system (TI-RADS): a user's guide. *Radiol Clin N Am.* 2018;287:29–36.
5. Garber JR, Cobin RH, Gharib H, et al. American Association of Clinical Endocrinologists and American Thyroid Association taskforce on hypothyroidism in adults. Clinical practice guidelines for hypothyroidism in adults: cosponsored by the American Association of Clinical Endocrinologists and the American Thyroid Association. *Thyroid.* December 2012;22(12):1200–1235. https://doi.org/10.1089/thy.2012.0205. Epub 2012 Nov 6. Erratum in: Thyroid. 2013 Feb;23(2):251. Erratum in: Thyroid. 2013 Jan;23(1):129.
6. Goldman L, Schafer AI, eds. *Goldman-Cecil Medicine.* 26th ed. Philadelphia, PA: Elsevier (Saunders); 2019.
7. Grewal RK, Larson SM, Pentlow CE, et al. Salivary gland side effects commonly develop several weeks after initial radioactive iodine ablation. *J Nucl Med.* 2009;50(10): 1605–1610.
8. Huber MA, Terézhalmy GT. Risk stratification and dental management of the patient with thyroid dysfunction. *Quintessence Int.* February 2008;39(2):139–150.
9. Jonklaas J, Bianco AC, Bauer AJ, et al. American Thyroid Association Task Force on Thyroid Hormone Replacement. Guidelines for the treatment of hypothyroidism: prepared by the American thyroid association task force on thyroid hormone replacement. *Thyroid.* December 2014;24(12):1670–1751. https://doi.org/10.1089/thy. 2014.0028. PMID: 25266247; PMCID: PMC4267409.
10. Lee SL. Complications of radioactive iodine treatment of thyroid carcinoma. *J Natl Compr Cancer Netw.* 2010;8(11):1277–1287.
11. Lele SJ, Hamiter M, Fourrier TL, Nathan CA. Sialendoscopy with intraductal steroid irrigation in patients with sialadenitis without sialoliths. *Ear Nose Throat J.* June 2019;98(5):291–294.
12. Li Q, Lin X, Shao Y, Xiang F, Samir AE. Imaging and screening of thyroid cancer. *Radiol Clin North Am.* 2017;55:1261–1271.
13. Little JW. Thyroid disorders: part I, hyperthyroidism. *Oral Surg Oral Med Oral Pathol Oral Radiol Endod.* 2006;101(3):276–284.
14. Little JW. Thyroid disorders: part II, hypothyroidism and thyroiditis. *Oral Surg Oral Med Oral Pathol Oral Radiol Endod.* 2006;102(2):148–153.
15. Little JW. Thyroid disorders: part III, thyroid neoplasms. *Oral Surg Oral Med Oral Pathol Oral Radiol Endod.* 2006;102(3):275–280.
16. National Cancer Institute. *SEER: Surveillance, Epidemiology and End Results. Cancer Stat Facts: Thyroid Cancer;* 2022. https://seer.cancer.gov/statfacts/html/thyro.html.
17. Neville BW, Damm DD, Allen CM, Chi AC. *Oral and Maxillofacial Pathology.* 4th ed. St. Louis, MO: Elsevier; 2016.
18. Pinto A, Glick M. Management of patients with thyroid disease: oral health considerations. *J Am Dent Assoc.* 2002;133(7):849–858.
19. Robledo-Sierra J, Mattsson U, Jontell M. Use of systemic medication in patients with oral lichen planus—a possible association with hypothyroidism. *Oral Dis.* April 2013; 19(3):313–319.
20. Ross DS, Burch HB, Cooper DS, et al. 2016 American Thyroid Association guidelines for diagnosis and management of hyperthyroidism and other causes of thyrotoxicosis. *Thyroid.* October 2016;26(10):1343–1421. https://doi.org/10.1089/thy.2016.0229. Erratum in: Thyroid. 2017 Nov;27(11):1462. PMID: 27521067.
21. Siponen M, Huuskonen L, Laara E, et al. Association of oral lichen planus with thyroid disease in a Finnish population: a retrospective case-control study. *Oral Surg Oral Med Oral Pathol Oral Radiol Endod.* 2010;110(3):319–324.
22. Vanderpump MPJ. The epidemiology of thyroid disease. *Br Med Bull.* 2011;99:39–51.

Women's Health Issues

PREGNANCY

A pregnant patient poses a unique set of management considerations for the dentist. Dental care must be rendered to the mother without adversely affecting the developing fetus, and although routine dental care of pregnant patients is generally safe, the delivery of dental care involves some potentially harmful elements, including the use of ionizing radiation and drug administration. Thus, practitioners must balance the beneficial aspects of dentistry while minimizing or avoiding exposure of the patient (and the developing fetus) to potentially harmful procedures.

Additional considerations arise during the postpartum period if the mother elects to breastfeed her infant. Although most drugs are only minimally transmitted from maternal serum to breast milk, and the infant's exposure is not significant, the dentist should avoid using any drug that is known to be harmful to infants.

Approximately 3.7 million babies were born in 2019 in the United States. The average age of women having their first child is approximately 26 years old. A typical dental practice serving 2000 patients will have approximately 15 patients in various stages of pregnancy.

PATHOPHYSIOLOGY AND COMPLICATIONS

Endocrine changes are the most significant basic alterations that occur with pregnancy. They result from the increased production of maternal and placental hormones and from modified activity of target end organs.

Fatigue is a common physiologic finding during the first trimester that may have a psychological impact. A tendency toward syncope and postural hypotension may be present. During the second trimester, patients typically have a sense of well-being and relatively few symptoms. During the third trimester, increasing fatigue and discomfort and mild depression may be reported. Several cardiovascular changes occur as well. Blood volume increases by 40%–50%, and cardiac output increases by 30%–50%, but red blood cell (RBC) volume increases by only about 15%–20%, resulting in a fall in the maternal hematocrit. Despite the increase in cardiac output, blood pressure falls (usually to ≤100/70 mm Hg) during the second trimester, and a modest increase is noted in the last month of pregnancy. This increase in blood volume is associated with high-flow, low-resistance circulation; tachycardia; and heart murmurs, and it may unmask glomerulopathies, peripartum cardiomyopathy, arterial aneurysms, or arteriovenous malformations. A benign systolic ejection murmur occurs in more than 90% of pregnant women, and disappears shortly after delivery. A murmur of this type is considered physiologic or functional.

During late pregnancy, a phenomenon known as *supine hypotensive syndrome* may occur that manifests as an abrupt fall in blood pressure, bradycardia, sweating, nausea, weakness, and dyspnea when the patient is in a supine position. Symptoms are caused by impaired venous return to the heart that results from compression of the inferior vena cava by the gravid uterus. This leads to decreased blood pressure, reduced cardiac output, and impairment or loss of consciousness. The remedy for the problem is to roll the patient over onto her left side, which lifts the uterus off the vena cava. Blood pressure should rapidly return to normal.

Blood changes in pregnancy include anemia and a decreased hematocrit value. Anemia occurs because blood volume increases more rapidly than RBC mass. As a result, a fall in hemoglobin and a marked need for additional folate and iron occur. The majority of pregnant women have insufficient iron stores, a problem that is exaggerated by significant blood loss. However, there is disagreement over whether or not to routinely provide iron supplementation. Although changes in platelets are usually clinically insignificant, most studies show a mild decrease in platelets during pregnancy. Several blood-clotting factors, especially fibrinogen and factors VII, VIII, IX, and X, are increased. As a result of the increase in many of the coagulation factors, combined with venous stasis, pregnancy is associated with a hypercoagulable state. The overall risk of thromboembolism in pregnancy is estimated to be 1 in 1500 and accounts for 25% of maternal deaths in the United States.

Several white blood cell (WBC) and immunologic changes occur. The WBC count increases progressively throughout pregnancy primarily because of an increase in neutrophils and is nearly doubled by term. The reason for the increase is unclear, but it may be due to elevated estrogen and cortisol levels. This increase of neutrophils may complicate the interpretation of the complete blood count during infection. Also, during pregnancy, the immune system shifts from helper T-cell 1 (Th1) dominance to Th2 dominance. This can lead to immune suppression. Clinically, the decrease in cellular immunity leads to increased susceptibility to infections with pathogens. During the postpartum period, rebound and heightened inflammatory activity occur.

Changes in respiratory function during pregnancy include elevation of the diaphragm, which decreases the volume of the lungs in the resting state, thereby reducing total lung capacity by 5% and the functional residual capacity, the volume of air in the lungs at the end of quiet exhalation, by 20%. These ventilatory changes produce an increased rate of respiration (tachypnea) and dyspnea that is worsened by the supine position. Thus, it is not surprising that sleep during pregnancy is impaired, especially during the third trimester.

Pregnancy predisposes the expectant mother to an increased appetite and often a craving for unusual foods. As a result, the diet may be unbalanced, high in sugars, or nonnutritious. This can adversely affect the mother's dentition and contribute to significant weight gain. Taste alterations and an increased gag response are also common. Nausea and vomiting, or "morning sickness," complicate up to 70% of pregnancies. Typical onset is between 4 and 8 weeks' gestation, with improvement before 16 weeks; however, 10%−25% of women still experience symptoms at 20−22 weeks' gestation, and some women experience this throughout the pregnancy. The cause is not well understood.

The general pattern of fetal development should be understood when dental management plans are being formulated. Normal pregnancy lasts approximately 40 weeks. During the first trimester, organs and systems are formed (organogenesis). Thus, fetuses are most susceptible to malformation during this period. After the first trimester, the majority of formation is complete, and the remainder of fetal development is devoted primarily to growth and maturation. Thus, the chances of malformation are markedly diminished after the first trimester. A notable exception to this is the fetal dentition, which is susceptible to malformation from toxins or radiation and to tooth discoloration caused by administration of certain tetracyclines.

Common complications during pregnancy include infection, inflammatory response, glucose abnormalities, and hypertension. Each complication increases the risks for preterm delivery, perinatal mortality, and congenital anomalies. Insulin resistance is a contributing factor to the development of gestational diabetes mellitus (GDM), which occurs in 2%−6% of pregnant women. GDM increases the risks for infection and large birth weight babies. Hypertension can lead to end-organ damage or preeclampsia, a clinical condition of pregnancy that manifests as hypertension, proteinuria, edema, and blurred vision. During preeclampsia, which is a pregnancy complication characterized by high blood pressure and signs of damage to another organ system, most often the liver and kidneys usually begins after 20 weeks of pregnancy in women whose blood pressure had been previously normal. Symptoms include unusual weight gain, edema, and hypertension. Risk factors include kidney disease and vitamin D deficiency.

Preeclampsia may progress to eclampsia, a very serious, life-threatening condition with increasing blood pressure, and seizures or coma may develop. Symptoms that signal an increasing risk of eclampsia include upper right abdominal pain, severe headache, and vision and mental status changes. The cause of eclampsia is unknown but appears to involve sympathetic overactivity associated with insulin resistance, the renin−angiotensin system, lipid peroxidation, and inflammatory mediators. Complications of pregnancy that are unresponsive to diet modification and palliative care ultimately require drugs or hospitalization for adequate control.

Miscarriage or spontaneous abortion is the natural termination of pregnancy before the 20th week of gestation, and occurs in approximately 15% of all pregnancies. The most common causes of spontaneous abortion are morphologic or chromosomal abnormalities that prevent successful implantation. Febrile illness and sepsis also can precipitate a miscarriage.

Because of immature liver and enzyme systems, fetuses have a limited ability to metabolize drugs. Pharmacologic challenge of fetuses is to be avoided when possible.

During the postpartum period, the mother may suffer from lack of sleep and postpartum depression. Also during the postpartum period, risks are increased for the development of autoimmune disease, particularly rheumatoid arthritis, multiple sclerosis, thyroiditis, and oral vesiculobullous conditions.

DENTAL MANAGEMENT

Management recommendations during pregnancy should be viewed as general guidelines, not immutable rules. The dentist should assess the general health of the patient through a thorough medical history. Inquiries should be made regarding the patient's current physician;

BOX 17.1	Checklist for Dental Management of Pregnant Patients[1]

P: PREOPERATIVE RISK ASSESSMENT (SEE BOX 1.1)

- Determine patient's stage of pregnancy, prenatal medical care, previous outcomes,
- Determine comorbid conditions (e.g., hypertension, diabetes)

A

Antibiotics	If antibiotics are required, consult with the physician. Use those with FDA classification A or B unless otherwise approved by the physician.
Analgesics	If analgesics are required, consult with the physician. Acetaminophen is the drug of choice. If other analgesics are required, use with approval of physician.
Anesthesia	The usual local anesthetics with vasoconstrictors are safe to use, provided care is taken not to exceed the recommended dose.
Anxiety	Avoid the use of most anxiolytics. Short-term use of nitrous oxide can be used, if needed, provided 50% oxygen is used.

B

Bleeding	No issues.
Breathing	Patient may have difficulty breathing in the supine position.

Blood pressure	Watch for supine hypotension if patient is in the supine position, most likely in late third trimester. Roll patient on left side if hypotension occurs.

C

Chair position	Patient may not be able to tolerate a supine chair position in the third trimester.
Cardiovascular	Elevated BP could be a sign of preeclampsia; refer to physician for follow-up care.

D

Drugs	Avoid all drugs, if possible. If drugs are needed, use FDA category A or B if possible.

E

Equipment	Take only necessary radiographs; use a lead apron and thyroid collar.
Emergencies	Anticipate the possibility of supine hypotension if in the third trimester.

F

Follow-up	Postoperative communication to determine any complications. Advise continuing pernatal medical visits. Patient should have teeth cleaned during pregnancy and be advised of importance of health and baby's oral health and not to put the baby to bed with a bottle.

[1]Strength of Recommendation Taxonomy (SORT) Grade: C (see Preface for further explanation).
BP, Blood pressure; *FDA*, Food and Drug Administration.

medications taken; use of tobacco, alcohol, or illicit drugs; history of GDM; miscarriage; hypertension; and morning sickness. If the need arises, the patient's obstetrician should be consulted, particularly with the use of certain medications (Box 17.1).

As with all patients, measuring vital signs is important for identifying undiagnosed abnormalities and the need for corrective action. At a minimum, blood pressure and pulse should be measured. Systolic pressure at or above 140 mm Hg and diastolic pressure at or above 90 mm Hg are signs of hypertension (see Chapter 3). Also, there is concern if a patient's systolic blood pressure increases 30 mm Hg or more or diastolic blood pressure increases 15 mm Hg or more compared with prepregnancy values because this can be a sign of preeclampsia. Confirmed hypertensive values dictate that the patient should be referred to a physician to ensure that preeclampsia and other cardiovascular disorders are properly diagnosed and managed.

PREVENTIVE PROGRAM

An important objective in planning dental treatment for a pregnant patient is to establish a healthy oral environment and an optimum level of oral hygiene. This essentially consists of a plaque control program that minimizes the exaggerated inflammatory response of gingival tissues that commonly accompany the hormonal changes of pregnancy when local irritants are present.

Personal oral hygiene and preventive plaque control measures should be encouraged and emphasized throughout pregnancy, including the first trimester, to benefit the pregnant mother and the developing baby. Coronal scaling and polishing or root curettage may be performed whenever necessary. Chlorhexidine 0.12% mouth rinse may be used safely during pregnancy, if needed.

The benefits of prenatal fluoride are controversial, and in 2001, the CDC indicated that there was a lack of evidence to support a recommendation for the use of prenatal fluoride.

Dental Treatment Timing

The American Dental Association acknowledges that preventive, diagnostic, and restorative dental treatment to promote health and eliminate disease is safe throughout pregnancy and is effective in improving and maintaining the oral health of the mother and her child. However, during the first trimester, the pregnant patient may experience symptoms that make dental treatment

TABLE 17.1	Treatment Timing During Pregnancy	
First Trimester	Second Trimester	Third Trimester
Plaque control	Plaque control	Plaque control
Oral hygiene instruction	Oral hygiene instruction	Oral hygiene instruction
Scaling, polishing, curettage	Scaling, polishing, curettage	Scaling, polishing, curettage
Avoid elective treatment; urgent care only	Routine dental care	Routine dental care

unpleasant (Table 17.1). Febrile illness and sepsis can precipitate a miscarriage; therefore, prompt treatment of odontogenic infection and periodontitis is advised. The second trimester is the safest period during which routine dental care can be provided. Emphasis should be placed on controlling active disease and eliminating potential problems that could occur later in pregnancy or during the immediate postpartum period, because providing dental care during these periods is often difficult. Extensive reconstruction or significant surgical procedures are best postponed until after delivery.

The early part of the third trimester is a safe and generally stable time to provide routine dental care. However, after the middle of the third trimester, elective dental care is best postponed. This is because of the increasing feeling of discomfort that many expectant mothers may experience. Prolonged time in the dental chair should be avoided to prevent the complication of supine hypotension. If supine hypotension develops, rolling the patient onto her left side affords return of circulation to the heart. Scheduling short appointments, allowing the patient to assume a semireclined position, and encouraging frequent changes of position can help minimize problems.

Dental Radiographs

Dental radiography is one of the more controversial areas in the management of pregnant patients. Pregnant patients who require radiographs often have anxiety about the adverse effects of X-rays to their developing fetus. In some instances, their obstetrician or primary care physician may reinforce these fears. In almost all cases involving dental radiography, these fears are unfounded. The safety of dental radiography has been well established, provided adequate safety measures are maintained and especially with the use of digital radiography, which markedly reduces radiation exposure.

Ionizing radiation should be avoided, if possible, during pregnancy, especially during the first trimester, because developing fetuses are particularly susceptible to radiation damage. However, if dental treatment becomes necessary, radiographs may be required to accurately diagnose and treat the patient. The American Academy of Pediatrics (AAP) and the American College of Obstetricians and Gynecologists have published guidelines stating: "Diagnostic radiologic procedures should not be performed during pregnancy unless the information to be obtained from them is necessary for the care of the patient and cannot be obtained by other means." Therefore, the dentist should understand the risks of ionizing radiation and know how to proceed as safely as possible in the event that radiographs are needed.

The teratogenicity of ionizing radiation is dose dependent. Increased risk of adverse outcomes has not been detected among animals with continuous low-dose exposure less than 5 rad (5 cGy) throughout pregnancy. The NCRP concluded that exposures less than 5 rads (5 cGy) were not associated with increased risk of malformations. Available animal and human data support the conclusion that an increase in gross congenital anomalies or intrauterine growth retardation does not occur as a result of exposures during pregnancy totaling less than 5 cGy (5 rad). Table 17.2 provides a comparison of ionizing radiation exposures expressed in cGy, demonstrating that exposures from typical dental radiographs are less than natural daily background radiation. It should be noted, however, that maternal thyroid exposure to diagnostic radiation in excess of 0.4 cGy has been associated with a slight decrease in birth weight. This finding reinforces the importance of using a thyroid collar on pregnant patients.

Teratogenicity also is dependent on the gestational age of the fetus at the time of exposure. During the organogenesis period (from the end of the second to the eighth week postconception), fetuses are extremely sensitive to the teratogenic effect of ionizing radiation, particularly the central nervous system (CNS) between the 8th and 15th weeks of pregnancy. From the 16th to the 25th week, there is a reduction in the radiosensitivity of the CNS and in many of the other organs. After the 25th week, the CNS becomes relatively radioresistant, and major fetal malformations and functional anomalies are highly improbable.

When risks of dental radiography are assessed during pregnancy, the following evidence should be kept in mind and can be used to explain the risk to a patient.

1. The maximum risk attributable to 1 cGy (which is more than 1000 full-mouth series with E-speed film and rectangular collimation or 10%−20% of the threshold dose) of in utero radiation exposure is estimated to be approximately 0.1%. This is a quantity thousands of times less than the normal anticipated risks of spontaneous abortion, malformation, or genetic disease.
2. The gonadal or fetal dose of two periapical dental films (when a lead apron is used) is 700 times less than 1 day of average exposure to natural background radiation in the United States.

TABLE 17.2 Effective Dose from Radiographic Examinations and Equivalent Background Exposure

Examination	Effective Dose (μSv)	Equivalent Background Exposure (days)
Intraoral[a]		
Rectangular Collimation		
Posterior bitewings: PSP or F-speed film	5	0.6
Full-mouth: PSP or F-speed film	35	4
Full-mouth: CCD sensor (estimated)	17	2
Round Collimation		
Full-mouth: D-speed film	388	46
Full-mouth: PSP or F-speed film	171	20
Full-mouth: CCD sensor (estimated)	85	10
Extraoral		
Panoramic[a–c]	9–24	1–3
Cephalometric[a,b,d]	2–6	0.3–0.7
Cone-beam CT[e,f]		
Large field of view	68–1073	8–126
Medium field of view	45–860	5–101
Small field of view	19–652	2–77
Multislice CT		
Head: Conventional protocol[f,g,h,i]	860–1500	101–177
Head: Low-dose protocol[f,h]	180–534	21–63
Abdomen[g]	5300	624
Chest[g]	5800	682
Plain Films[j]		
Skull	70	8
Chest	20	2
Barium enema	7200	847

[a]Data from Ludlow JB, Davies-Ludlow LE, White SC. Patient risk related to common dental radiographic examinations: the impact of 2007 international commission on radiological protection recommendations regarding dose calculation. *J Am Dent Assoc* 2008;139:1237–1243.

[b]Data from Lecomber AR, Yoneyama Y, Lovelock DJ et al. Comparison of patient dose from imaging protocols for dental implant planning using conventional radiography and computed tomography. *Dentomaxillofac Radiol* 2001;30:255–259.

[c]Data from Ludlow JB, Davies-Ludlow LE, Brooks SL. Dosimetry of two extraoral direct digital imaging devices: NewTom cone beam CT and Orthophos Plus DS panoramic unit. *Dentomaxillofac Radiol* 2003;32:229–234.

[d]Data from Gijbels F, Sanderink G, Wyatt J, et al. Radiation doses of indirect and direct digital cephalometric radiography. *Br Dent J* 2004;197:149–152.

[e]Data from Pauwels R, Beinsberger J, Collaert B et al. Effective dose range for dental cone beam computed tomography scanners. *Eur J Radiol* 2012;81:267–271.

[f]Data from Ludlow JB, Ivanovic M. Comparative dosimetry of dental CBCT devices and 64-slice CT for oral and maxillofacial radiology. *Oral Surg Oral Med Oral Pathol Oral Radiol Endod* 2008;106:106–114.

[g]Data from Shrimpton PC, Hillier MC, Lewis MA et al. National survey of doses from CT in the UK: 2003. *Br J Radiol* 2006;79:968–980.

[h]Data from Loubele M, Jacobs R, Maes F et al. Radiation dose versus image quality for low-dose CT protocols of the head for maxillofacial surgery and oral implant planning. *Radiat Prot Dosimetry* 2005;117:211–216.

[i]Data from Loubele M, Bogaerts R, Van Dijck E et al. Comparison between effective radiation dose of CBCT and MSCT scanners for dentomaxillofacial applications. *Eur J Radiol* 2009;71:461–468.

[j]Data from European Commission: *Referral guidelines for imaging*, Radiation Protection 2007;118. http://www.sergas.es/Docs/Profesional/BoaPraticaClinica/RP118.pdf.

CCD, Charge-coupled device; *CT*, computed tomography; *PSP*, photostimulable phosphor.

Adapted from White SC, Pharoah MJ. *Oral Radiol.* 7th ed., St. Louis: Elsevier; 2014.

3. The risk of a first-generation fetal defect from a dental radiographic examination is estimated to be 9 in 1 billion.

4. The gonadal dose to women after full-mouth radiography using a lead apron is less than 0.01 μSv, which is at least 1000-fold below the threshold shown to cause congenital damage to newborns.

Together these data indicate that with use of a lead apron, rectangular collimation, and E-speed film or faster techniques, one or two intraoral films are truly of minute significance in terms of radiation effects on a developing fetus.

REDUCTION OF RADIATION DOSE TO PREGNANT PATIENTS

During pregnancy, radiographs should be used selectively and only when necessary and appropriate to aid in diagnosis and treatment. Several methods can be employed to reduce radiation dose to follow the principles of ALARA (as low as reasonably achievable).

Selection criteria for dental imaging: Not every dental patient requires radiographic examinations. A clinical examination should precede any radiographic order. There should not be a routine imaging protocol for a new dental patient. After a clinical examination, the ordering doctor should evaluate the risk of radiation against the diagnostic benefits. The benefit to the patient must outweigh the risk.

Image receptor: For intraoral imaging, digital sensors or E/F speed should be used to decrease the radiation dose by at least 50% compared to D speed films. Recent reports indicate that in the United States, about 63% of film-based radiography is still conducted with D speed films. Digital sensors, either PSP or CCD/CMOS, are increasingly being adopted and are replacing film-based imaging.

X-ray tube energy: The X-ray tubes for intraoral imaging should have 60 to 80 kVp. Machines operating at a lower potential deposits substantial amount of X-ray photons on skin, leading to unnecessary exposure. Machines operating at higher than 80 kVp unnecessarily expose the opposite side of the arch. Most intraoral machines currently sold for intraoral imaging do not operate below 60 kVp or higher than 70 kVp.

Collimation: The X-ray beam should be collimated to the shape of the receptor or the area of interest. For intraoral radiography, the beam should be rectangular, either by a collimator attached to the positioning indicating device or receptor holding device. The effective dose from a rectangular collimation is four to five times less than round collimation. For extra-oral imaging, e.g., cephalometric radiography, the beam should be collimated to the area of interest. Similarly, for cone beam computed tomography (CBCT) examinations, the field of view should be as small as possible. Collimating the X-ray beam not only reduces the radiation dose but also improves the image quality by reducing scatter radiation.

Exposure time: Compared to film-based radiography, digital sensors require a shorter exposure time, therefore reducing radiation dose. Exposure time can be particularly adjusted in case of CBCT examination. A shorter scan time not only reduces radiation dose but also helps in case of patient movement. A pulsed radiation can reduce the radiation dose compared to a continuous exposure.

Lead apron: Lead aprons were advocated when X-ray beams were not adequately collimated or the X-ray tubes were not properly filtered. Newer intraoral or panoramic machines deliver a small dose to the gonadal area or to the fetus. The dose to the gonads is primarily from internal scatter. Use of a lead apron does not provide protection against internal scatter. NCRP currently do not advocate the use of a lead apron. The UK Guidance/National Radiation Protection Board, the European Commission on Radiation Protection, and the Australian Radiation Protection and Nuclear Safety Agency do not recommend the use of a lead apron for intraoral radiography. The Australian Radiation Protection and Nuclear Safety Agency recommends the use of lead apron in case of maxillary occlusal radiography. With the advent of CBCT, maxillary occlusal projection is rarely used. Several states also do not require a lead apron for intraoral or panoramic radiography. The practitioner should review the local regulations before abandoning the use of a lead apron. A patient may request a lead apron out of concern of harmful effects of radiation. There is, however, no contraindication of using a lead apron. A lead apron still has beneficial role if a round collimation is used.

Thyroid shielding: Dental radiography can expose the thyroid gland, a radiosensitive organ. Whenever a thyroid shield does not interfere with an imaging technique, it should be used in addition to the lead apron. For panoramic and CBCT examinations, a thyroid shield may interfere with image production.

REDUCTION OF RADIATION DOSE TO PREGNANT OPERATORS

Radiation dose to the fetus of a patient from dental radiography is minimal. In case of a pregnant X-ray operator, the radiation dose to the fetus may become high if proper procedures are not followed. The maximum permissible radiation dose for whole-body exposure of the pregnant dental care worker is 0.005 Gy or 5 mSv per year. This is equivalent to the maximum permissible radiation dose of the nonoccupationally exposed public and 10-fold less than the level of occupationally exposed nonpregnant workers (50 mSv). The National Council on Radiation Protection and Measurements reports that production of congenital defects is negligible from fetal exposures of 50 mSv. To further ensure safety, a pregnant operator should wear a film badge; stand more than 2 m (6 feet) from the tube head; and position herself at between 90 and 130 degrees of the beam, preferably behind a protective wall (Fig. 17.1). When these guidelines are followed, no contraindication to pregnant women operating an X-ray machine occurs. However, dentists should familiarize themselves with federal (Code of Federal Regulations, Code 10, Part 20, Section 20.201) and state regulations that would supersede these guidelines.

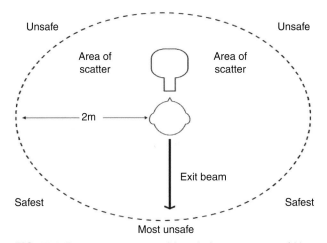

FIG 17.1 Proper operator position during exposure of X-rays.

Restraining a patient: If a patient needs restraining or a sensor needs to be held by hand, such action should be done by patient's family or caregiver. The person providing the help should be protected with lead apron and lead gloves. The operator, whether pregnant or not, should not be holding the receptor for the patient.

Handheld X-ray equipment: Handheld X-ray machines pose a challenge due to the design of the lead shield mounted on the unit, weight of the unit, and potential of incorrect use. The units approved by Food and Drug Administration (FDA) have been shown to be safe to the operator. For an FDA-approved handheld equipment, the operator does not have to wear a protective garment.

Drug Administration

Another important area in the treatment of pregnant dental patients is drug administration. The principal concern is that a drug may cross the placenta and be toxic or teratogenic to the fetus.

Ideally, drug administration should be avoided during pregnancy, especially during the first trimester. However, adhering to this rule is sometimes difficult. Moreover, 75% of pregnant women in the United States are taking some type of medication. Fortunately, most of the commonly used drugs in dental practice can be given during pregnancy with relative safety, although a few exceptions are notable. Table 17.3 presents a suggested approach to drug usage for pregnant patients.

Before prescribing or administering a drug to a pregnant patient, the dentist should be familiar with the US FDA categorization of prescription drugs for pregnancy based on their potential risk of fetal injury. The five pregnancy risk classification categories, although not without limitations, are meant to aid clinicians and patients in making decisions about drug therapy (see below or https://chemm.nlm.nih.gov/pregnancycategories.htm). Counseling should be provided to ensure that women who are pregnant clearly understand the nature and magnitude of the risk associated with a drug.

Category A: Adequate and well-controlled studies have failed to demonstrate a risk to the fetus in the first trimester of pregnancy (and there is no evidence of risk in later trimesters).

Category B: Animal reproduction studies have failed to demonstrate a risk to the fetus and there are no adequate and well-controlled studies in pregnant women.

Category C: Animal reproduction studies have shown an adverse effect on the fetus and there are no adequate and well-controlled studies in humans, but potential benefits may warrant use of the drug in pregnant women despite potential risks.

Category D: There is positive evidence of human fetal risk based on adverse reaction data from investigational or marketing experience or studies in humans, but potential benefits may warrant use of the drug in pregnant women despite potential risks.

Category X: Studies in animals or humans have demonstrated fetal abnormalities and/or there is positive evidence of human fetal risk based on adverse reaction data from investigational or marketing experience, and the risks involved in use of the drug in pregnant women clearly outweigh potential benefits.

TABLE 17.3 Key Medication Considerations During Pregnancy and Breastfeeding

Agent	FDA PR[a] Category	Safe During Pregnancy?	Safe During Breastfeeding?
Analgesics and antiinflammatories[b]			
Acetaminophen	B	Yes	Yes
Aspirin	C/D	Avoid	Avoid
Codeine	C	Use with caution	Yes
Glucocorticoids (dexamethasone, prednisone)	C	Avoid[c]	Yes
Hydrocodone	C	Use with caution	Use with caution
Ibuprofen[d]	C/D	Avoid use in third trimester	Yes
Oxycodone	B	Use with caution	Use with caution
Antibiotics[e,f]			
Amoxicillin	B	Yes	Yes
Azithromycin	B	Yes	Yes

Continued

TABLE 17.3   Key Medication Considerations During Pregnancy and Breastfeeding—cont'd

Agent	FDA PR[a] Category	Safe During Pregnancy?	Safe During Breastfeeding?
Cephalexin	B	Yes	Yes
Chlorhexidine (topical)	B	Yes	Yes
Clarithromycin	C	Use with caution	Use with caution
Clindamycin	B	Yes	Yes
Clotrimazole (topical)	B	Yes	Yes
Doxycycline	D	Avoid	Avoid
Erythromycin	B	Yes	Use with caution
Fluconazole	C/D	Yes (single-dose regimens)	Yes
Metronidazole	B	Yes	Avoid; may give breast milk an unpleasant taste
Nystatin	C	Yes	Yes
Penicillin	B	Yes	Yes
Terconazole (topical)	B	Yes	Yes
Tetracycline	D	Avoid	Avoid
Local anesthetics			
Articaine	C	Use with caution	Use with caution
Bupivacaine	C	Use with caution	Yes
Lidocaine (with or without epinephrine)	B	Yes	Yes
Mepivacaine (with or without levonordefrin)	C	Use with caution	Yes
Prilocaine	B	Yes	Yes
Benzocaine (topical)	C	Use with caution	Use with caution
Dyclonine (topical)	C	Yes	Yes
Lidocaine (topical)	B	Yes	Yes
Tetracaine (topical)	C	Use with caution	Use with caution
Sedatives			
Benzodiazepines	D/X	Avoid	Avoid
Zaleplon	C	Use with caution	Use with caution
Zolpidem	C	Use with caution	Yes
Emergency medications			
Albuterol	C	Steroid and β_2-agonist inhalers are safe	Yes
Diphenhydramine	B	Yes	Avoid
Epinephrine	C	Use with caution	Yes
Flumazenil	C	Use with caution	Use with caution
Naloxone	C	Use with caution	Use with caution
Nitroglycerin	C	Use with caution	Use with caution

[a]FDA PR: US Food and Drug Administration Pregnancy Risk. See Table 17.1 for FDA PR category definitions.

[b]In the case of combination products (such as oxycodone with acetaminophen), the safety with respect to either pregnancy or breastfeeding is dependent on the highest-risk moiety. In the example of oxycodone with acetaminophen, the combination of these two drugs should be used with caution, because the oxycodone moiety carries a higher risk than the acetaminophen moiety.

[c]Oral steroids should not be withheld from patients with acute severe asthma.

[d]Ibuprofen is representative of all nonsteroidal antiinflammatory drugs. In breastfeeding patients, avoid cyclooxygenase selective inhibitors such as celecoxib, as few data regarding their safe use in this population are available, and avoid doses of aspirin higher than 100 mg because of risk of platelet dysfunction and Reye syndrome.

[e]Antibiotic use during pregnancy: The patient should receive the full adult dose and for the usual length of treatment. Serious infections should be treated aggressively. Penicillins and cephalosporins are considered safe. Use higher-dose regimens (such as cephalexin 500 mg three times per day rather than 250 mg three times per day), as they are cleared from the system more quickly because of the increase in glomerular filtration rate in pregnancy.

[f]Antibiotic use during breastfeeding: These agents may cause altered bowel flora and, thus, diarrhea in the baby. If the infant develops a fever, the clinician should take into account maternal antibiotic treatment.

Drugs in categories A or B are preferable for prescribing during pregnancy. However, many commonly prescribed drugs used in dentistry fall into category C, and thus the safety of their use is often uncertain. Drugs in category C present the greatest difficulty for the dentist and the physician in terms of therapeutic and medicolegal decisions, and therefore, consultation with the physician may be needed. Drugs in categories D or X should be avoided.

Physicians may advise against the use of some of the approved drugs (i.e., analgesics) or conversely may suggest the use of an uncertain or questionable drug (i.e., antibiotics). The FDA categories are general guidelines and may be incomplete, and therefore require clinical judgment.

Local Anesthetics. Common local anesthetics (lidocaine, prilocaine) administered with epinephrine are generally considered safe for use during pregnancy. Articaine, bupivacaine, and mepivacaine are typically safe, although some caution should be exercised. Although both the local anesthetic and the vasoconstrictor cross the placenta, subtoxic threshold doses have not been shown to cause fetal abnormalities. Because of adverse effects associated with high levels of local anesthetics, it is important not to exceed the manufacturer's recommended maximum dose.

Most topical anesthetics, including topical lidocaine, are acceptable when small amounts are used.

Analgesics. The analgesic of choice during pregnancy is acetaminophen. Aspirin and nonsteroidal antiinflammatory drugs convey risks for constriction of the ductus arteriosus, as well as for postpartum hemorrhage and delayed labor (see Table 17.3). The risk of these adverse events increases when agents are administered during the third trimester. Therefore, it is best to avoid these analgesics (especially in the third trimester) or use them with caution. Most opioids, including codeine, are associated with multiple congenital defects and should be avoided.

Antibiotics. Penicillins (including amoxicillin), erythromycin (except in estolate form), cephalosporins, metronidazole, and clindamycin are generally considered to be safe for expectant mothers and developing fetuses. The use of tetracyclines generally is contraindicated during pregnancy. Tetracyclines bind to hydroxyapatite, causing brown discoloration of teeth, hypoplastic enamel, inhibition of bone growth, and other skeletal abnormalities. Clarithromycin should be avoided or used with caution.

Antibiotics and Oral Contraceptives. The concern for potential interactions between antibiotics and oral contraceptives requires mention in this chapter. This concern arises from the ability of select antibiotics such as rifampin, an antituberculosis drug, to reduce plasma levels of circulating oral contraceptives. It has been speculated that this interaction also may be seen with other antibiotics; however, studies to date regarding other antibiotics have been less convincing. To address this concern, the American Dental Association Council on Scientific Affairs issued the following recommendations when prescribing antibiotics to a female patient who takes oral contraceptives: "The dentist should (1) advise the patient of the potential risk of the antibiotic's reducing the effectiveness of the oral contraceptive, (2) recommend that the patient discuss with her physician the use of an additional nonhormonal means of contraception, [and] (3) advise the patient to maintain compliance with oral contraceptives when concurrently using antibiotics."

Anxiolytics. Few anxiolytics are considered safe to use during pregnancy. Therefore, most of them should be avoided. Benzodiazepines, zaleplon, and zolpidem should be avoided. However, a single, short-term exposure to nitrous oxide–oxygen (N_2O-O_2) for less than 30 minutes is considered safe. Nitrous oxide may cause inactivation of methionine synthetase and vitamin B_{12}, resulting in altered DNA metabolism that can lead to cellular abnormalities in animals and birth defects. Accordingly, the following guidelines are recommended if N_2O-O_2 is used during pregnancy:

- Use of N_2O-O_2 inhalation should be minimized to 30 minutes.
- At least 50% oxygen should be delivered to ensure adequate oxygenation at all times.
- Appropriate oxygenation should be provided to avoid diffusion hypoxia at the termination of administration.
- Repeated and prolonged exposures to nitrous oxide are to be prevented.
- The second and third trimester are safer periods for treatment because organogenesis occurs during the first trimester.

An additional consideration involves female dentists or dental auxiliaries who are pregnant. These individuals should not be exposed to persistent trace levels of nitrous oxide in the operatory. The use of appropriate scavenging equipment is required and can help alleviate this problem. Female dental health care workers who are chronically exposed to nitrous oxide for more than 3 hours per week, when scavenging equipment is not used, have decreased fertility and increased rates of spontaneous abortion. Implementation of National Institute for Occupational Safety and Health recommendations can reduce occupational exposure to nitrous oxide (Box 17.2).

Breastfeeding/Nursing. A potential problem arises when a nursing mother requires the administration of a drug in the course of dental treatment. The concern is that the administered drug may enter the breast milk and be transferred to the nursing infant, in whom exposure may result in adverse effects.

Data on which to draw definitive conclusions about drug dosages and effects via breast milk are limited. However, retrospective clinical studies and empiric

BOX 17.2 Control of Nitrous Oxide in the Dental Office During Pregnancy

1. Inspect nitrous oxide equipment and replace defective tubing and parts.
2. Check pressure connections for leaks; fix leaks.
3. Ensure that mask fits well and is secure. Check that the reservoir bag is not over- or underinflated.
4. Provide operatory ventilation of 10 or more room air exchanges per hour.
5. Use a scavenging system and appropriate mask sizes. Vacuum should provide up to 45 L/min.
6. Connect and turn on the vacuum pump of the scavenging system before providing nitrous oxide.
7. Regularly conduct air sampling. Maintain low exposure limits (e.g., 25 ppm[1]) when pregnant dental health care workers are involved.

[1]This limit is a National Institute for Occupational Safety and Health recommendation. In contrast, Yagiela65 suggests a time-weighted average lower limit of 100 ppm for an 8-hour workday.
Modified from McGlothlin JD, Crouch KG, Mickelsen RL. *Control of nitrous oxide in dental operatories.* Cincinnati, OH, 1994, U.S. Department of Health and Human Services, Public Health Service, Centers for Disease Control and Prevention, National Institute for Occupational Safety and Health, Division of Physical Sciences and Engineering, Engineering Control Technology Branch. DHHS publication no. (NIOSH) 94–129. ETTB report no. 166–04.

observations, coupled with known pharmacologic pathways, allow recommendations to be made. The AAP concludes that "most drugs likely to be prescribed to the nursing mother should have no effect on milk supply or on infant well-being." A significant fact is that the amount of drug excreted in the breast milk usually is not more than about 1%–2% of the maternal dose. Therefore, most drugs are of little pharmacologic significance to infants.

Agreement exists that a few drugs, or categories of drugs, are definitely contraindicated for nursing mothers. These include lithium, anticancer drugs, radioactive pharmaceuticals, and phenindione. Table 17.3 contains recommendations adapted from the AAP regarding the administration of commonly used dental drugs during breastfeeding. As with drug use during pregnancy, individual physicians may wish to modify these recommendations, which should be viewed only as general guidelines for treatment.

In addition to careful drug selection, nursing mothers may take the drug just after breastfeeding and avoid nursing for 4 hours or longer if possible. This should result in reduced drug concentrations in the breast milk.

TREATMENT PLANNING MODIFICATIONS

No technical modifications are required for pregnant patients. However, full-mouth radiographs, reconstruction, crown and bridge procedures, and significant

surgery are best delayed until after pregnancy. A prominent gag reflex also may dictate a delay in certain dental procedures. Many patients have a concern about mercury exposure from amalgam restorations. In 2009, the FDA concluded that "although data are limited, existing data do not suggest that fetuses are at risk for adverse health effects due to maternal exposure to mercury vapors from dental amalgam." The FDA does note, however, that "maternal exposures are likely to increase temporarily when new dental amalgams are inserted or existing dental amalgams are removed." The FDA furthermore concluded that "existing data support a finding that infants are not at risk for adverse health effects from the breast milk of women exposed to mercury vapors from dental amalgams." Practitioners should be aware, however, that several European countries and Canada have national recommendations advising dentists to limit or avoid the placement and replacement of amalgam restorations during pregnancy.

ORAL COMPLICATIONS AND MANIFESTATIONS

The most common oral complication of pregnancy is pregnancy gingivitis (Fig. 17.2). This condition results from an exaggerated inflammatory response to local irritants and less than meticulous oral hygiene during periods of increased secretion of estrogen and progesterone and altered fibrinolysis. Pregnancy gingivitis begins at the marginal and interdental gingiva, usually in the second month of pregnancy. Progression of this condition leads to fiery red and edematous interproximal papillae that are tender to palpation. In approximately 1% of gravid women, the hyperplastic response may exacerbate in a localized area, resulting in a pyogenic granuloma or "pregnancy tumor" (Fig. 17.3). The most common location for a pyogenic granuloma is the labial aspect of the interdental papilla. The lesion is generally

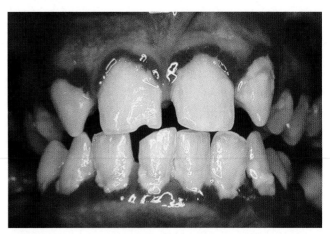

FIG 17.2 Generalized gingivitis ("pregnancy gingivitis") in a woman in the sixth month of pregnancy.

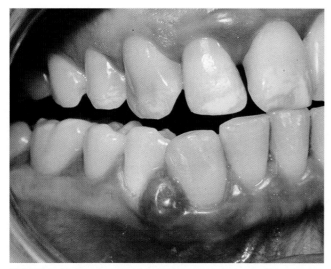

FIG 17.3 Pyogenic granuloma ("pregnancy tumor") occurring during pregnancy.

asymptomatic; however, tooth brushing may traumatize the lesion and cause bleeding. Hyperplastic gingival changes become apparent around the second month and continue until after parturition, at which time the gingival tissues usually regress and return to normal, provided proper oral hygiene measures are implemented and any calculus present is removed. Surgical or laser excision is occasionally required if symptoms, bleeding, or interference with mastication dictates. Pregnancy does not cause periodontal disease but may modify and worsen what is already present. Febrile illness and sepsis also can precipitate a miscarriage; therefore, prompt treatment of odontogenic infection and periodontitis is advised.

Pregnant women often have a hypersensitive gag reflex. This, in combination with morning sickness, may contribute to episodes of regurgitation and lead to halitosis and enamel erosion. The dentist should advise the patient to rinse after regurgitation with a solution that neutralizes the acid (e.g., baking soda, water).

OSTEOPOROSIS

Osteoporosis is defined as a skeletal disorder that compromises bone strength due to inhibited calcium intake and mineral loss, predisposing a person to an increased risk of bone fracture. According to World Health Organization criteria, osteoporosis occurs when the bone mineral density (BMD) is measured to be 2.5 standard deviations (SDs) less than the average value for young healthy women (a T-score of <2.5 SD). Osteoporosis can be characterized as either primary or secondary. Primary osteoporosis occurs in both genders at all ages but typically follows menopause in women and occurs later in life in men. Secondary osteoporosis is the result of medications (glucocorticoids), other conditions (hypogonadism), or diseases (celiac disease, cystic fibrosis).

EPIDEMIOLOGY

The National Osteoporosis Foundation estimates that more than 10 million people older than 50 years of age have osteoporosis, and another 34 million are at risk for the disease. Bone fractures among older adults reduce mobility and potentially increase the need for long-term care. Hip fractures are particularly problematic; one in three older adults who lived independently before a hip fracture remained in a nursing home for at least 1 year after his or her injury.

PATHOPHYSIOLOGY AND COMPLICATIONS

Osteoporosis is caused by an uncoupling of bone resorption from bone formation such that the activities of osteoclasts far outweigh those of the osteoblasts. Peak bone mass is achieved in early adulthood and, after this point, both women and men lose bone with increasing age. However, this process is accelerated in postmenopausal women whereby the loss of estrogen is associated with an increase in osteoclast activity. Decades of research indicate that estrogen plays a dominant multifactorial role in maintaining cortical bone formation by supporting osteoblasts and preventing bone resorption by suppressing osteoclast formation and stimulating osteoclast apoptosis.

Fig. 17.4 illustrates normal bone remodeling through a balanced regulation of osteoblastic and osteoclastic activity. Osteoporosis occurs when this balance shifts to increased osteoclastic activity. The integrity of the skeleton is also intricately linked to appetite and energy balance, and the underlying mechanism by which bone mass is regulated by the brain is through a leptin-mediated brain-derived serotonin pathway. In addition, glucocorticoid-induced osteoporosis is one of the most common and serious adverse effects associated with glucocorticoid use, which significantly increase risk of fractures with long-term use.

LABORATORY AND DIAGNOSTIC TESTING

Conventional radiography is used for the diagnosis of osteoporosis, but approximately 75% of cases are not diagnosed until late in the disease process because imaging is not a routine part of primary medical care. A new method for point-of-care osteoporosis screening and diagnostics has emerged that is effective for early diagnosis of osteoporosis. Axial dual-energy X-ray absorptiometry is an ultrasound method for osteoporosis diagnostics at primary health care facilities. This method provides an estimate of BMD (i.e., density index). Areal BMD measurements at the femoral neck (BMD_{neck}) and total hip (BMD_{total}) are used for women older than 50 years of age. Osteoporosis is diagnosed in individuals with a bone density of 2.5 SDs below the adult mean (i.e., T-score of −2.5 or less) in the total hip or femoral neck.

Serum biomarkers may be helpful in the diagnosis of osteoporosis. Table 17.4 outlines some of the diagnostic

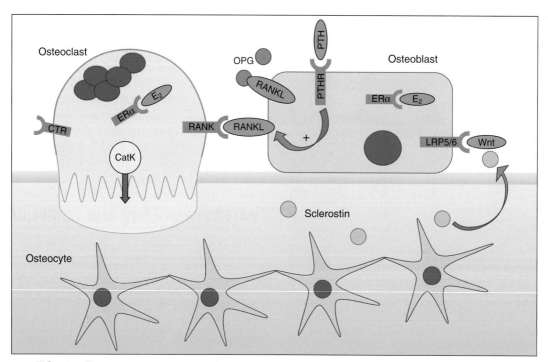

FIG 17.4 The cells responsible for bone remodeling, highlighting key signaling pathways that are targets for therapies recommended for the prevention of osteoporotic fracture. Osteocytes are embedded within mineralized bone and, in response to mechanical loading or micro-damage, provide signals to osteoclasts to resorb. Osteoclast differentiation and function are dependent on the RANKL—RANK (receptor activator of nuclear factor-κB ligand—receptor activator of nuclear factor-κB) signaling pathway, which is negatively regulated by osteoprotegerin (OPG) in vivo. Circulating parathyroid hormone (PTH) is a physiologic regulator of plasma calcium and binds to parathyroid hormone receptor (PTHR) on osteoblasts indirectly stimulating osteoclast activity via upregulation of RANKL and downregulation of OPG expression. Calcitonin binds to the calcitonin receptor (CTR) expressed on mature osteoclasts to reversibly inhibit osteoclast function, although the exact physiologic relevance for calcitonin is not fully understood. Estrogen (E2) has a positive effect on bone through effects on osteoblasts and osteoclasts via estrogen receptor (ERα). Cathepsin K (CatK) is secreted by resorbing osteoclasts across the convoluted ruffled border membrane and is required to degrade collagen. Osteoclast activity releases factors from the bone, which attract osteoblasts to the site of resorption. Osteoblast differentiation and function are controlled by the Wnt signaling pathway via the lipoprotein-related protein 5/6 (LRP5/6) and Frizzled coreceptors, which is regulated by endogenous inhibitors such as sclerostin, expressed by osteocytes and upregulated in response to unloading.

TABLE 17.4	Serum Biomarkers for Osteoporosis
Osteoblastic Activity Markers	**Osteoclastic Activity Markers**
Total or bone-specific alkaline phosphatase	Tartrate-resistant acid phosphatase (TRAP)
Osteocalcin	C-terminal telopeptide of collagen type I (ICTP)
N- or C-terminal propeptide of protocollagen type I	β-CrossLaps (β-CTX)
	N-terminal telopeptide of collagen type I (NTX)

Adapted from Torres E, Mezquita P, DeLa Higuera M, Fernandez D, Munoz M. Actualizacion sobre la determinacion de marcadores de remodelado oseo. *Endocrinol Nutr* 2003;50(6):237–243.

serum markers. Serum alkaline phosphate levels are indicators of osteoblastic activity. Tartrate-resistant acid phosphatase (TRAP), C-terminal telopeptide of collagen type I (CTP), and beta-crosslaps (beta-CTX) are indicators of increased osteoclastic activity.

MEDICAL MANAGEMENT

Box 17.3 provides general indications for the treatment of osteoporosis. The primary drugs used to treat osteoporosis are the bisphosphonates, which act by suppressing osteoclast activity and increasing BMD (Fig. 17.5). Both oral and intravenous (IV) bisphosphonates are used to treat osteoporosis and osteopenia (decrease of calcification and bone density). Table 17.5 lists some of the IV

BOX 17.3   A Summary of the National Institute for Clinical Excellence (NICE) Guidelines[1] for the Therapeutic Management of Primary and Secondary Osteoporotic Fractures in Postmenopausal Women

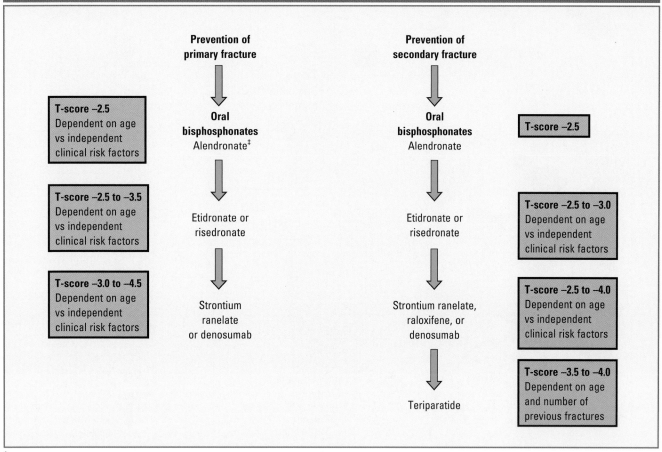

[1]Available at https://pathways.nice.org.uk/pathways/osteoporosis.
‡Alendronate is the treatment of choice in each case, but for those intolerant or contraindicated for alendronate, a hierarchy of treatment choices is recommended, and patients are assigned to each treatment based on T-score, the magnitude of which depends on age and the number of independent clinical risk factors.

and orally administered bisphosphonate agents and their associated effects.

Secondary osteoporosis is defined as osteoporosis that develops as a consequence of an unrelated underlying cause such as drug treatment (e.g., chronic corticosteroid use), hypogonadism, malnutrition, or eating disorders such as anorexia nervosa, excessive exercise, and neoplastic disorders. Because these comorbid conditions increase the risk of fractures among patients with osteoporosis, these patients may require more aggressive treatment with bisphosphonate drugs (i.e., teriparatide, risedronate, and etidronate or denosumab, romosozumab) to decrease their risk of vertebral fracture. Appropriate recommendations for calcium and vitamin D supplements as well as low impact exercise to increase bone density also should be implemented.

ORAL HEALTH IMPLICATIONS OF OSTEOPOROSIS

Studies have shown that mandibular and maxillary bone densities, as well as alveolar BMD and height, are modestly correlated with other skeletal sites. However, it does not appear that low BMD in the jaw results in other adverse periodontal changes such as gingival bleeding, greater probing depth, and gingival recession.

Smoking tobacco, radiation therapy, and diabetes have been shown to be associated with the progression of osteoporosis and subsequent risk factors for dental implant failure. Dentists should be aware of the implications and possible risks when patients are medicated with bisphosphonate agents (as well as other drugs) that might place them at risk for osteonecrosis of the jaw (ONJ).

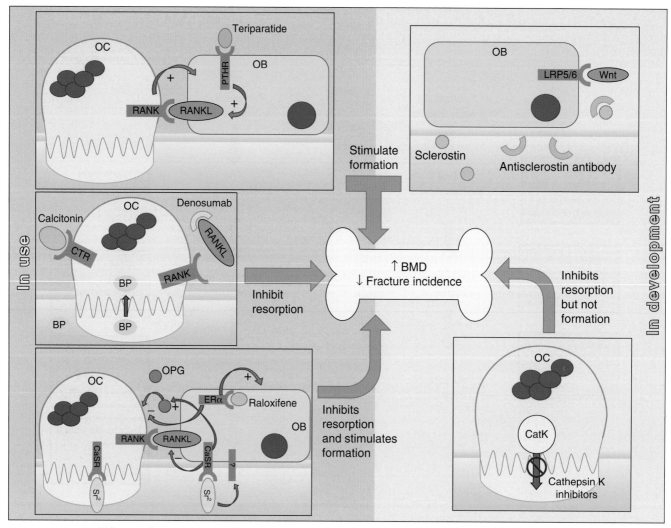

FIG 17.5 Sites of action of different classes of drugs that are either in clinical use (*left*) or in development (*right*). *Drugs that inhibit resorption*: Bisphosphonate (BPs) are internalized and inactivate resorbing osteoclasts, and calcitonin binds to a cell-surface receptor to inhibit osteoclast (OC) function. Denosumab prevents receptor activator of nuclear factor-κB ligand (RANKL) interacting with receptor activator of nuclear factor-κB (RANK), therefore potentially inhibiting both the differentiation of OCs and the function of mature OCs. *Drugs that stimulate formation*: Teriparatide, an analogue of parathyroid hormone (PTH), binds to the parathyroid hormone receptor (PTHR) on osteoblasts (OBs), and after a transient increase in OC activity, a coupled increase in OB activity is observed. Antisclerostin antibodies prevent sclerostin binding to the lipoprotein-related protein 5/6 (LRP5/6) coreceptor, thereby allowing Wnt ligands to activate the canonical signaling pathway in OBs. *Drugs that uncouple bone formation from resorption*: Raloxifene interacts with intracellular estrogen receptor (ERα) in OBs and, via upregulation of osteoprotegerin (OPG) and downregulation of RANKL, inhibits OCs. Raloxifene also has positive effects on OB proliferation. Strontium ranelate (Sr2) substitutes for Ca2 in the bone and interacts with the calcium-sensing receptor (CaSR) on OBs, upregulating OPG expression and downregulating RANKL expression to indirectly inhibit OCs while acting directly on the CaSR on OCs themselves to induce apoptosis. The anabolic effect of strontium ranelate on OBs is also mediated via the CaSR as well as potentially other, unidentified receptors. Cathepsin K inhibitors uncouple resorption from formation because the cross-talk between inactive OCs and OBs is maintained. *BMD*, Bone mineral density; *CatK*, cathepsin K; *CTR*, calcitonin receptor.

TABLE 17.5 Examples of Bisphosphonate Agents With Relative Potency

Bisphosphonate Agent		Potency	Route
Didronel	Etidronate	1	PO
Bonefos Clasteon (Canada)	Clodronate	10×	PO or IV
Skelid	Tiludronate	10×	PO
Aredia[a]	Pamidronate	100×	IV
	Neridronate[a]	100×	PO
	Olpadronate[a]	1000×	IV
Fosamax[a]	Alendronate	1000×	Oral
Boniva[a]	Ibandronate	5000×	PO or IV
Actonel[a]	Risidronate	5000×	PO
Reclast[a]	Zoledronate	10,000×	IV once per year
Zometa[a]			IV q3–4 week

[a]These agents have been shown to be associated with osteonecrosis.
IV, Intravenous; *PO*, oral; *q*, every.

OSTEONECROSIS

Bisphosphonates are synthetic analogues of inorganic pyrophosphate that have a high affinity for calcium. Bisphosphonates also are potent inhibitors of osteoclastic activity. All bisphosphonate compounds accumulate over extended periods of time in mineralized bone matrix. Depending on the duration of the treatment and the specific bisphosphonate prescribed, the drug may remain in the body for years.

Patients treated with bisphosphonates (as well as other antiresorptive agents) are at risk of developing ONJ (see Fig. 17.6). Several medications have been associated with the onset of ONJ; therefore, the current description of this condition is termed medication-related osteonecrosis of the jaw (MRONJ). Other drugs that have been associated with MRONJ include the RANK (receptor activator of nuclear factor-κB) ligand inhibitor denosumab, some antiangiogenic agents (i.e., ranibizumab and bevacizumab), and some monoclonal antibodies (i.e., rituximab, adalimumab, infliximab, and romosozumab).

ONJ can occur with the oral administration of bisphosphonates but is rare (<0.01%). In contrast, ONJ is a more common complication of injected bisphosphonates (2%–4%). The exact mechanism that leads to the induction of ONJ is unknown. However, risk factors include previous use of IV bisphosphonates (i.e., etidronate [Didronel], pamidronate [Aredia], zoledronic acid [Zometa]), diabetes mellitus, overall cancer (breast, prostate, multiple myeloma) stage and tumor burden, overall systemic and immune health, immunosuppressive drug use, any periodontal or other oral infection, and history of radiation to the jaws. Of note, posterior sites are at higher risk than anterior sites, and the mandible is more often affected than the maxilla.

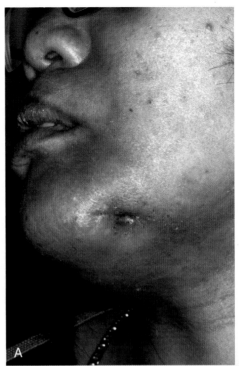

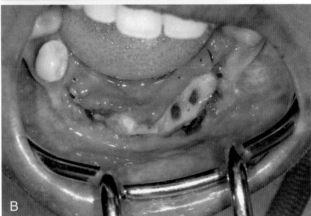

FIG 17.6 (A), Extraoral and **(B)**, Intraoral views of medication-associated osteonecrosis of the mandible in a patient with metastatic breast cancer. (Courtesy of Dr. Denis Lynch, Milwaukee, WI.)

Patients treated with IV bisphosphonates have a higher risk of developing MRONJ. This risk increases when the duration of therapy exceeds 2 years.

Bone remodeling is a physiologic function that occurs in normal bone. During remodeling, the drug is taken up by osteoclasts and internalized in the cell cytoplasm, where it inhibits osteoclastic function and induces apoptotic cell death. It also inhibits osteoblast-mediated osteoclastic resorption and has antiangiogenic properties (see Fig. 17.4). As a result, bone turnover becomes profoundly suppressed, and over time, the bone shows little physiologic remodeling. The bone becomes brittle and unable to repair physiologic microfractures that occur in the human skeleton with daily activity (e.g., common masticatory forces). In the oral cavity, the

TABLE 17.6   Staging and Treatment Strategies

Staging of Medication-Related Osteonecrosis of the Jaw[a]	Treatment Strategies[b]
At risk: No apparent necrotic bone in patients who have been treated with oral or intravenous bisphosphonates	No treatment indicated Patient education
Stage 0: No clinical evidence of necrotic bone but nonspecific clinical findings, radiographic changes, and symptoms	Systemic management, including use of pain medication and antibiotics
Stage 1: Exposed and necrotic bone or fistulas that probe to bone in patients who are asymptomatic and have no evidence of infection	Antibacterial mouth rinse Clinical follow-up on a quarterly basis Patient education and review of indications for continued bisphosphonate therapy
Stage 2: Exposed and necrotic bone or fistulas that probe to bone associated with infection as evidenced by pain and erythema in the region of exposed bone with or without purulent drainage	Symptomatic treatment with oral antibiotics Oral antibacterial mouth rinse Pain control Debridement to relieve soft tissue irritation and infection control
Stage 3: Exposed and necrotic bone or a fistula that probes to bone in patients with pain, infection, and one or more of the following: exposed and necrotic bone extending beyond the region of alveolar bone (i.e., inferior border and ramus in mandible, maxillary sinus, and zygoma in maxilla) resulting in pathologic fracture, extraoral fistula, oral antral or oral nasal communication, or osteolysis extending to inferior border of the mandible or sinus floor	Antibacterial mouth rinse Antibiotic therapy and pain control Surgical debridement or resection for longer-term palliation of infection and pain

[a]Exposed or probable bone in the maxillofacial region without resolution for longer than 8 weeks in patients treated with an antiresorptive or an antiangiogenic agent who have not received radiation therapy to the jaws.

[b]Regardless of disease stage, mobile segments of bony sequestrum should be removed without exposing uninvolved bone. Extraction of symptomatic teeth within exposed necrotic bone should be considered because it is unlikely that extraction will exacerbate the established necrotic process.

Adapted from Ruggiero SL, Dodson TB, Fantasia J et al. American Association of Oral and Maxillofacial Surgeons: American Association of Oral and Maxillofacial Surgeons position paper on medication-related osteonecrosis of the jaw—2014 update. *J Oral Maxillofac Surg* 2014;72(10):1938–1956.

maxilla and mandible are subjected to constant stress from masticatory forces.

Physiologic microdamage and microfractures occur daily in the oral cavity. Although the exact cause of MRONJ is not known, it is theorized that in a patient taking a bisphosphonate, the resulting microdamage is not repaired, setting the stage for oral osteonecrosis to occur. Therefore, MRONJ results from a complex interplay of bone metabolism, local trauma, increased demand for bone repair, infection, and hypovascularity.

In the early stages of oral MRONJ, radiographic manifestations may not be seen, but in some cases, thickening of the lamina dura and a density in the medullary bone are seen. Patients usually are asymptomatic but may develop pain because the necrotic bone becomes infected secondarily after it is exposed to the oral environment. The osteonecrosis often is progressive, potentially leading to extensive areas of bony exposure and dehiscence. When tissues are acutely infected, patients may complain of severe pain or lack of sensory sensation (paresthesia). Either symptom may be an indication of inflammation, necrosis, and peripheral nerve compression (see Fig. 17.6).

In patients in whom MRONJ develops spontaneously, the most common initial complaint is the sudden presence of intraoral discomfort and the presence of roughness that may progress to traumatize the oral soft tissues surrounding the area of necrotic bone. Therefore, the diagnosis of MRONJ is based on the medical and dental history or each patient, as well as the observation of clinical signs and symptoms of this pathologic process. According to the most recent recommendations from the American Academy of Oral Medicine (see Chapter 26) and American Association of Oral and Maxillofacial Surgeons AAOMS, the working definition of MRONJ is based on the following criteria:

1. Current or previous treatment with a bisphosphonate (or other drug known to be associated with a higher risk of ONJ).
2. Exposed bone in the maxillofacial region that has persisted for more than 8 weeks.
3. No history of radiation therapy to the jaws.

The AAOMS staging (four stages) for MRONJ is summarized in Table 17.6.

TREATMENT STRATEGIES

Treatment strategies seek resolution and healing of ONJ. However, to date, effective strategies have been elusive. In fact, many cases have poor outcomes despite therapy, progressing to extensive dehiscence and exposure of bone. Recommended strategies included local surgical debridement, bone curettage, local irrigation with antibiotics, and hyperbaric oxygen therapy. Unfortunately,

---

> **BOX 17.4 Dental Treatment Recommendations for Patients Treated With Bisphosphonates**
>
> - Treat active oral infections.
> - Eliminate sites at high risk for infection. Remove nonrestorable teeth and teeth with substantial periodontal bone loss. Encourage routine dental care, oral examinations, and cleanings. Minimize periodontal inflammation, restorative treatment of caries, and endodontic therapy when indicated.
> - Seek alternatives to surgical oral procedures with appropriate local and systemic antibiotics.
> - Conduct extractions and other surgery using as little bone manipulation as possible, appropriate local and systemic antibiotics, and close follow-up to monitor healing.
> - Consider additional imaging studies such as computed tomography scans.
> - Remove necrotic bone as necessary with minimal trauma to adjacent tissue.
> - Prescribe oral rinses, such as chlorhexidine gluconate 0.12%.
> - Prescribe systemic antibiotics and analgesics if needed.
> - Fabricate a soft acrylic stent to cover areas of exposed bone, protect adjacent soft tissues, and improve comfort.
> - Suggest cessation of bisphosphonate therapy until osteonecrosis heals or the underlying diseases progresses (discussion with patient's medical providers).

Adapted from Kelsey JL. Musculoskeletal conditions. In: Lamster IB, Northridge ME, eds. *Improving oral health for the elderly*, New York, 2008, Springer, with permission.

their limited success rate compromises the nutritional and oral management of affected patients. Prevention of this condition is of paramount importance for these patients so that they can receive the proper therapies required for the best possible outcome of their disease. The most current recommendations for the dental management of patients with MRONJ are summarized in Box 17.4. The recommendations to dental professionals for managing patients on bisphosphonates therapy are also presented in Box 17.4.

BIBLIOGRAPHY

1. Montella K. Common medical problems in pregnancy. In: Goldman L, Schafer AI, eds. *Cecil Textbook of Medicine*. 25th ed. Elsevier; 2015:1555–1565. ISBN 978-1-4377-1604-7 (Chapter 247).

2. NCHS Dataset. http://www.cdc.gov/nchs/data_access/vitalstatsonline.htmftp://ftp.cdc.gov/pub/Health_Statistics/NCHS/Dataset_Documentation/DVS/natality/UserGuide2014.pdf and http://www.businessinsider.com/average-age-of-mother-having-first-child-going-up-2015-6. [Accessed January 16, 2017].

3. FDA. http://www.fda.gov/Drugs/DevelopmentApprovalProcess/DevelopmentResources/Labeling/ucm093307.htm. Pregnancy drug labeling. [Accessed January 16, 2017].

4. Donaldson M, Goodchild JH. Pregnancy, beast-feeding and drugs used in dentistry. *J Am Dent Assoc*. 2012;143(8):858–864. http://jada.ada.org.

5. Michalowicz BS, Hodges JS, DiAngelis AJ, et al. OPT Study. Treatment of periodontal disease and the risk of preterm birth. *N Engl J Med*. 2006;355(18):1885–1894.

6. White SC, Pharoah MJ. *Oral radiology. Principles and interpretation*. 6th ed. St. Louis: Mosby Elsevier; 2009.

7. FDA. Drug administration during pregnancy and breast feeding in dental patients. http://www.fda.gov/Drugs/DevelopmentApprovalProcess/DevelopmentResources/Labeling/ucm093307.htm.

8. Patrick SW, Dudley J, Martin PR, et al. Prescription opioid epidemic and infant outcomes. *Pediatrics*. 2015;135(5):842–850.

9. Rayburn WF, Amanze AC. Prescribing medications safely during pregnancy. *Med Clin North Am*. 2008;92(5):1227–1237 (xii).

10. Publication no. 1750-992399. *Osteoporosis: pathophysiology and treatment*. WHO; 2016. www.who.int/chp/topics/Osteoporosis.pdf.

11. Rosen C. Osteoporosis. In: Goldman L, Schafer AI, eds. *Cecil textbook of medicine*. 25th ed. Elsevier; 2015:1577–1587. ISBN 978-1-4377-1604-7 (Chapter 251) www.dentistryiq.com/articles/2013/11/what-does-osteoporosis-have-to-do-with-oral-health.html [Accessed March 2, 2017].

12. Migliorati CA, Casiglia J, Epstein J, et al. Managing the care of patients with bisphosphonate-associated osteonecrosis: an American Academy of Oral Medicine position paper. *J Am Dent Assoc*. 2005;136:1658–1668.

13. Ruggiero SL, Dodson TB, Fantasia J, et al. American Association of Oral and Maxillofacial Surgeons position paper on medication-related osteonecrosis of the jaw—2014 update. *J Oral Maxillofac Surg*. 2014;72:1938–1956.

14. Medication-Related Osteonecrosis of Jaws (MRONJ) Prevention and Diagnosis: Italian Consensus Update 2020. *Int J Environ Res Public Health*. 2020;17(16):5998. https://www.ncbi.nlm.nih.gov/pmc/articles/PMC7460511/. [Accessed April 20, 2021].

18

AIDS, HIV Infection, and Related Conditions

KEY POINTS

- Patients who have human immunodeficiency virus (HIV) infection or acquired immunodeficiency syndrome (AIDS) may be undiagnosed, and screening can be performed in a dental setting.
- Patients who have HIV/AIDS are at increased risk for oral opportunistic infections, cardiovascular disease, and cancer.
- Patients who have HIV/AIDS may be at risk for complications from dental treatment such as infection, bleeding, drug interactions, and side effects.
- Risk assessment of patients who have HIV involves knowledge of their complete blood count, HIV load, and CD4 lymphocyte count.
- Patients with HIV/AIDS are more likely to have a history of tobacco, alcohol, and substance use disorders.

Since June 5, 1981, when the Centers for Disease Control and Prevention (CDC) reported five cases of Pneumocystis pneumonia in young men who have sex with men (MSM) in Los Angeles, and subsequently led to the identification of human immunodeficiency virus (HIV) as the underlying cause for this opportunistic infection, more than 75 million persons have been infected with HIV, and more than 32 million have died of HIV-related illness worldwide. Acquired immunodeficiency syndrome (AIDS) is the most advanced stage of HIV infection. HIV is a bloodborne infectious disease that is transmitted predominantly through intimate sexual contact and by parenteral means. HIV has been rarely transmitted from patients to health care workers, and patients with HIV infection or AIDS may be medically compromised and may need special dental management considerations. An average dental practice of 2000 patients will encounter at least two patients infected with HIV per year.

EPIDEMIOLOGY

An estimated 1.7 million people across the globe were newly infected with HIV in 2019, which is a >20% decline since 2010. Of the approximately 38 million patients living with HIV in 2019, more than 50% are women, and the majority live in low- to middle-income regions (with almost 70% living in Africa, largely Sub-Saharan Africa). Of these, 36.2 million infections are in adults, and 1.8 million infections are in children (aged 0–14). The United Nations Program for HIV/AIDS (UNAIDS) set a 2020 goal for "90–90–90" (i.e., 90% of HIV-infected patients will know their status, 90% of

those who know their status will be on antiretroviral therapy (ART), and 90% of patients on ART will be virally suppressed). This remains a challenging goal and as of 2019, these targets only were at "81–67–59."

Disparities in HIV incidence in the United States are impacted by social, economic, and historical factors, as well as differences in environment, personal behavior, and habits. Approximately 38,000 incident HIV infections occurred in the United States in 2018 (11.5/ 10,000), a 7% reduction compared to 2014. The highest incidence was in the southern United States (15.6/ 100,000), 79% of infections in the United States occurred in males, 19% in females, and 2% in transgender adults and adolescents. Other epidemiological trends are shown in Figs. 18.1, 18.2 and 18.3. From 2014 through 2018, 66% of all HIV infections occurred as a result of male-to-male sexual contact, followed by heterosexual transmission (24%), injected drug use (<10%), and a small number of other modes of transmission (e.g., perinatal).

Since the introduction of protease inhibitors in 1996 and the advent of ART, the epidemic of HIV/AIDS in the United States has slowed and stabilized. In 2018, there were 15,280 deaths (5.7/100,000). With improved survival there are more people living with HIV infection (>1 million in the United States) and therefore more people who may seek dental treatment.

ETIOLOGY

HIV is a nontransforming retrovirus of the lentivirus family. There are two HIV subtypes, HIV-1 and HIV-2 (each with multiple strains). HIV-1 was first identified

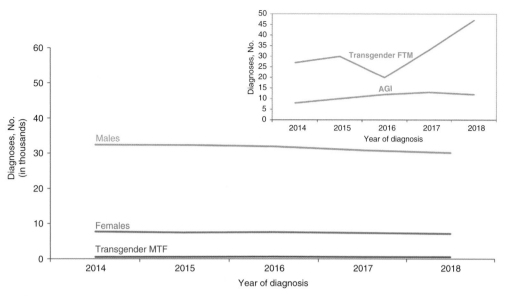

FIG. 18.1 Diagnoses of HIV infection among adults and adolescents, by gender, 2014–2018—United States. There was an overall decrease in males and females and an increase in transgender (female to male) and adolescents.

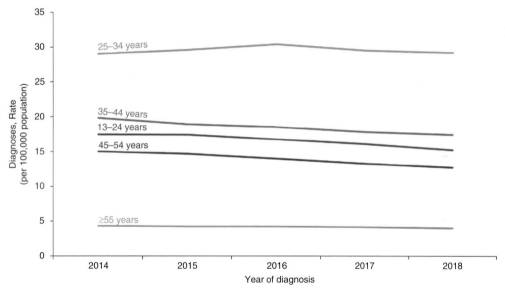

FIG. 18.2 Rates of diagnoses of HIV infection among adults and adolescents by age at diagnosis, 2014–2018 (United States). HIV-infection rates decreased in all age strata, except the 15–19 and 25–34 age groups where the rates have remained stable since 2014. The highest incidence is in the 25–34 age group.

in 1983 by Francoise Barre-Sinoussi in the laboratory of Luc Montaignier of the Pasteur Institute and it was initially named *lymphadenopathy-associated virus*. Within 1 year of this discovery, a team led by Robert Gallo from the National Institutes of Health (NIH) isolated a retrovirus identified as the human T-lymphotropic virus III (HTLV-III) and labeled it as the etiologic agent for AIDS. In 1984, Jay Levy's team in San Francisco also isolated a retrovirus, AIDS-related virus, and designated it as the causative agent for AIDS. All three viruses were similar retroviruses, but minor differences were observed in their amino acid sequences. Variation in disease patterns is attributed to the sequence differences among HIV strains, and variation in genomic sequences explains in

part the difficulty in engineering a vaccine. In 1986, the World Health Organization (WHO) recommended the name human immunodeficiency virus.

HIV is an enveloped RNA retrovirus about 100 nM in diameter (Fig. 18.4). Glycoproteins (gp41 and gp120) stud the surface of the envelope and serve as binding domains to human cells. Internal to the envelope is a protein capsid (p24) that surrounds essential viral enzymes (protease, integrase, reverse transcriptase) and an inner core containing RNA. The cells most commonly infected are those with CD4+ receptors, including T helper lymphocytes (CD4+ cells) and macrophages. Additional coreceptors that allow HIV to infect human cells include CCR5, CXCR4 (fusin), and CCR2.

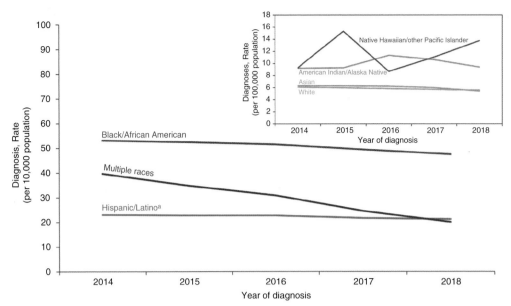

FIG. 18.3 Rates of diagnoses of HIV infection among adults and adolescents, by race/ethnicity, 2014–2018 (United States). Whites and Asians experience the lowest incidence and Blacks/African Americans experience the highest incidence. Native Hawaiians/other Pacific Islanders and Native Indians/Alaskan Natives were the only two race groups with increasing rates of infection.

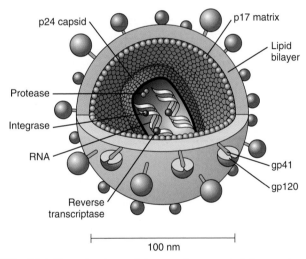

FIG. 18.4 The structure of human immunodeficiency virus, showing the p24 capsid protein surrounding two strands of viral RNA. (From Copstead LC, Banasik JL: *Pathophysiology*, ed 4, St. Louis, 2010, Saunders.)

HIV infection occurs in steps: *entry, reverse transcription* of RNA to DNA, export of the viral DNA from the cytoplasm to the nucleus and *integration* into the host chromosome, *transcription, translation,* and cleavage of the polyproteins produced, *assembly* of virions, and budding of virions. The process is largely regulated by the proteins tat, rev, and nef, which are necessary for viral replication. Virulence has been mapped to the carboxyl-terminal half of the gp120, which has been referred to as the V_3 loop.

Pathophysiology and Complications

Transmission of HIV is by exchange of infected bodily fluids from sexual contact, and through blood and blood products. The most common method of sexual transmission in the United States is anal intercourse in men who have sex with men (MSM), followed by heterosexual transmission (male to female or female to male) through sexual contact (i.e., penetrative intercourse or oral sex with HIV+ partners). Transmission from injected drug use (i.e., sharing contaminated needles) is the third largest group affected in the United States. Blood, semen, breast milk, and vaginal secretions are the main fluids associated with transmission of the virus. Transmission through saliva has not been documented. Vertical transmission, from mother to infant, can occur during pregnancy, at birth, or during breastfeeding. Casual contact has not been demonstrated as a means of transmission. Inflammation and breaks in the skin or mucosa (e.g., due to the coexistence of other inflammatory sexually transmitted diseases) and high concentrations of HIV in bodily fluids increase the risk of transmission. The risk of transmission from a blood transfusion is estimated to be less than one in a million because of current blood screening measures. Occupational exposure is a source of transmission, and transmission from health care provider to patient has occurred.

After HIV has gained access to the bloodstream, the virus selectively seeks out T lymphocytes (specifically CD4+ T helper lymphocytes) (Fig. 18.5). The virus binds to the CD4+ lymphocyte cell surface specifically through the highly glycosylated outer surface envelope (gp120) proteins. Upon infection, reverse transcriptase catalyzes the synthesis of a haploid, double-stranded DNA provirus, which integrates into the chromosomal DNA of the host cell. After integration, the provirus genetic material may remain latent in an unexpressed form until events occur to activate it. Activation leads to DNA

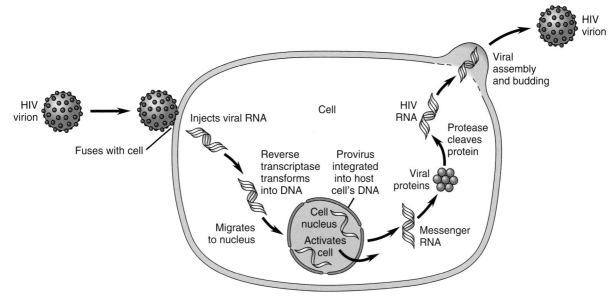

FIG. 18.5 Life cycle of the human immunodeficiency virus. (From Copstead LC, Banasik JL: *Pathophysiology*, ed 4, St. Louis, 2010, Saunders.)

transcription and the production of new virions. Viral infection causes progressive reduction in the total number of T helper cells and a marked reversal in the ratio of CD4+ to CD8+ lymphocytes (the normal ratio of is approximately 2:1). This marked and progressive reduction in T helper lymphocytes, to a great degree, explains the lack of an effective immune response seen in patients with HIV-infection, it is the basis for the staging of HIV-infection, and explains the increase in opportunistic illness (i.e., infections and malignancies).

The case definition and staging of HIV-infection is provided in Table 18.1. Upon laboratory confirmation of HIV-1 or HIV-2 infection, the disease is classified into stages 1, 2, or 3 based upon the degree in reduction of

TABLE 18.1	Features of HIV Infection and Disease Progression and Centers for Disease Control and Prevention Case Definition for HIV-Infection in Patients >6 years old[a] (2014)		
Status/Case Definition	**Signs/Symptoms**	**Laboratory Findings**	**Comments**
Stage 0: A sequence of discordant test results indicative of early HIV infection in which a negative or indeterminate result was within 180 days of a positive result.	No signs or symptoms.	Only p24 antigen and HIV. RNA/DNA are detected and these remain positive throughout all stages.	Patient is unaware of his or her HIV infection. Can transmit the infection by blood or sexual activity.
Stage 1: Acute seroconversion syndrome	Symptoms occur within about 1–3 weeks after infection in ≈70% of infected patients: Fever, weakness, diarrhea, nausea, vomiting, myalgia, headache, weight loss, pharyngitis, skin rashes (roseolalike or urticarial), lymphadenopathy; symptoms clear in about 1–2 weeks.	HIV antibody becomes detectable at the end of the seroconversion syndrome. CD4+ lymphocytes begin to decline but remain ≥500 cells/mm^3 or CD4+ lymphocyte percentage of total lymphocytes of ≥26%. After acute symptoms, CD4+ counts tend to return toward normal levels.	The severity of the acute syndrome varies among infected persons. The period for seroconversion of 30% of patients without acute symptoms varies and can be 1–6 months or longer.
Stage 2: Latent period (asymptomatic stage) Stage 2	Median time from initial infection to onset of clinical symptoms: 8–10 years ≈50%–70% of patients develop PGL.	A slow but usually steady increase in viral load. Usually, a steady decline in CD4+ lymphocytes but no AIDS-defining conditions and CD4+ T lymphocyte count of 200–499 cells/mm^3 or CD4+ T lymphocyte percentage of total lymphocytes of 14%–28%.	Viral replication is ongoing and progressive. A steady decline in CD4+ cell counts occurs, except in the fewer than 1% who are nonprogressors (also have low viral load).

Continued

TABLE 18.1   Features of HIV Infection and Disease Progression and Centers for Disease Control and Prevention Case Definition for HIV-Infection in Patients >6 years old[a] (2014)—cont'd

Status/Case Definition	Signs/Symptoms	Laboratory Findings	Comments
Stage 2: Early symptomatic stage	Without treatment, lasts for 1–3 years; any of the following: PGL, fungal infections, vaginal yeast and trichomonal infections, oral hairy leukoplakia, herpes zoster, herpes simplex, HIV retinopathy. Constitutional symptoms: Fever, night sweats, fatigue, diarrhea, weight loss, weakness.	Signs and symptoms increase as CD4+ cell count declines and approaches 200/mm^3; Viral load continues to increase.	The spectrum of disease changes as CD4+ cell count declines.
Stage 3: AIDS	Opportunistic infection(s): *Pneumocystis jiroveci* pneumonia, cryptococcosis, tuberculosis, toxoplasmosis, histoplasmosis, others. Malignancies: Kaposi sarcoma, Burkitt lymphoma, nonHodgkin lymphoma, primary CNS lymphoma, invasive cervical cancer, carcinoma of rectum, slim (wasting) disease (Box 18.2).	High viral load; CD4+ T lymphocyte count is < 200 cells/mm^3 or CD4+ T lymphocyte percentage of total lymphocytes is <14% or documentation of a stage-3 defining opportunistic illness. Other cytopenias are possible.	Death usually occurs because of wasting, opportunistic infection, or malignancies.

AIDS, Acquired immunodeficiency syndrome; *CNS,* central nervous system; *HIV,* human immunodeficiency virus; *PGL,* persistent generalized lymphadenopathy.
[a]Threshold CD4 counts differ for newborns and children <6 years old.

CD4+ counts and presence of stage-3 or AIDS defining opportunistic illness. This definition also provides criteria for stage 0 and "unknown" staging and includes minor updates in stage-3 defining opportunistic illnesses (Box 18.1). Of note, because of the provision of antiretroviral drug regimens, not all patients progress to stage 3 disease. HIV-2 occurs less commonly throughout the world and most cases of HIV-2 infection have occurred in West Africa. Most persons infected with HIV-2 are long-term nonprogressors because viral loads generally are low, and immunosuppression is typically not as severe compared to HIV-1.

Table 18.1 presents the clinical stages of HIV infection through to frank AIDS (stage 3). In stage 1 more than 50% of persons exposed to HIV develop a seroconversion sickness associated with an acute and brief viremia within 2–6 weeks of exposure, and develop antibodies (anti-gag, anti-gp120, anti-p24) between weeks 6 and 12. Some patients may take 6 months or longer to achieve seroconversion. During stage 1 (i.e., early phase of HIV infection), the virus disseminates throughout lymphoid tissue, incubates, replicates, and alters many physiologic processes, resulting in hyperimmune activation, persistent inflammation, and impaired gut function and flora.

As time progresses, the patient enters stage 2 infection, which is characterized by a steady-state viremia and several thousand copies of HIV detected in the blood (Fig. 18.6). Although the infection is clinically latent, there is a progressive decline in immune function evident by the progressive depletion of CD4+ lymphocytes.

In untreated persons the CD4+ count continues to decline while HIV proliferates. As the CD4+ count drops and approaches 200 cells/mm^3, persons can exhibit weight loss, diarrhea, and night sweats (Fig. 18.6) and

BOX 18.1   Stage-3 Defining Opportunistic Illness

- Bacterial infections, multiple or recurrent[a]
- Candidiasis of bronchi, trachea, or lungs
- Candidiasis of esophagus
- Cervical cancer, invasive[b]
- Coccidioidomycosis, disseminated or extrapulmonary
- Cryptococcosis, extrapulmonary
- Cryptosporidiosis, chronic intestinal (>1 month in duration)
- Cytomegalovirus disease (other than liver, spleen, or nodes), onset at age >1 month
- Cytomegalovirus retinitis (with loss of vision)
- Encephalopathy, HIV related
- Herpes simplex: chronic ulcers (>1 month's duration) or bronchitis, pneumonitis, or esophagitis (onset at age >1 month)
- Histoplasmosis, disseminated or extrapulmonary
- Isosporiasis, chronic intestinal (>1 month's duration)
- Kaposi sarcoma
- Lymphoma, Burkitt (or equivalent term)
- Lymphoma, immunoblastic (or equivalent term)
- Lymphoma, primary, of brain
- *Mycobacterium avium* complex or *Mycobacterium kansasii* infection, disseminated or extrapulmonary
- *Mycobacterium tuberculosis* infection of any site, pulmonary,[b] disseminated, or extrapulmonary
- Mycobacterium infection, other species or unidentified species, disseminated or extrapulmonary
- *Pneumocystis jiroveci* pneumonia
- Pneumonia, recurrent[b]
- Progressive multifocal leukoencephalopathy
- *Salmonella* septicemia, recurrent
- Toxoplasmosis of brain, onset at age >1 month
- Wasting syndrome attributed to HIV

[a]Only among children age <6.
[b]Only among those ≥6 years of age.

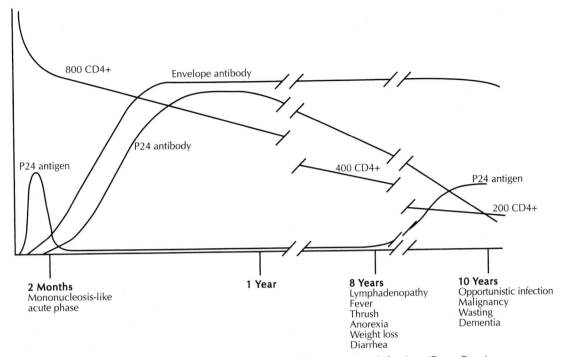

FIG. 18.6 The natural history of human immunodeficiency virus infection. (From Brookmeyer R, Gail MH: *AIDS epidemiology: a quantitative approach*, New York, 1994, Oxford University Press.)

eventually the person enters into the most severe stage 3 disease where they become susceptible to opportunistic illnesses (Box 18.1).

HIV can lead to bone marrow suppression and HIV+ patients are at a higher risk for developing cytopenias such as anemia, neutropenia, and thrombocytopenia, although the risk in well-controlled patients is rare. Longstanding HIV infection also leads to immune activation and dysregulated lipid metabolism, resulting in hyperlipidemia, hypertension, cardiovascular events, diabetes, premature aging, and noninfectious disease related cancers. HIV+ patients have higher rates of tobacco, alcohol, and substance use disorders, further magnifying the risk for these comorbidities.

Evidence suggests that persons most susceptible to developing AIDS are those with repeated exposure to the virus and who also have an immune system that has been challenged by repeated exposure to various antigens. The median time from primary infection to the development of AIDS in untreated patients is about 10–15 years, and notably, there are gender-based differences in HIV-pathogenesis with progression to AIDS being faster in women than men. Given the advances in the treatment of HIV-infection, the potential for long-term survival with HIV infection is now a reality.

CLINICAL PRESENTATION

Signs and Symptoms

The acute viremia during stage 1 infection can range from being asymptomatic to causing lymphadenopathy, fever,

pharyngitis, and a skin rash. Following resolution of these acute signs and symptoms patients are HIV antibody positive but may remain asymptomatic and show no other laboratory abnormalities for months. Stage 2 is characterized by "clinical latency" and eventually progressive immunosuppression and symptomatic disease. Patients will demonstrate various laboratory changes (i.e., decreasing CD4 counts, a ratio of T helper to T suppressor of <1, and increasing viral load) in addition to clinical signs or symptoms, such as enlarged lymph nodes, night sweats, weight loss, fever, malaise, diarrhea, and oral opportunistic infections such as oral candidiasis. This risk for opportunistic diseases predominates as the CD4+ T count approximates and then declines below 200 cells/mm^3; the latter finding defining entry into Stage 3. Neurologic disease is common and may be related not only to opportunistic infections but also to the effects of primary HIV infection of macrophages, neurons, and microglial cells in the CNS. Signs and symptoms may include confusion and short-term memory deficits. Some patients develop severe depression, paranoia, suicidal tendencies, and dementia. Persons in stage 3/AIDS can demonstrate a variety of opportunistic diseases' each with different manifestations.

Laboratory and Diagnostic Findings

There are three types of testing used for HIV-infections and these include nucleic acid tests (NAT), combined antigen/antibody tests (Ag/Ab), and antibody tests (Ab). Each test type is employed in different situations (i.e., initial screening, following initial diagnosis, and for

---

BOX 18.2 Screening Indications for HIV-infection

Clinical Indications
- Whenever STD[a] screening is done on a patient who is not known to have HIV
- Pregnancy at both the first prenatal visit and during the third trimester
- Tuberculosis (TB) (both TB infection and suspected TB)
- Suspected Acute HIV—persistent flulike symptoms starting 1–4 weeks following a potential HIV exposure

Routine Screening
- Every 3–5 years for all sexually active individuals
- Every year if the patient or their partner:
  - is sexually active and has had condomless anal or vaginal sex with a new partner since the patient's most recent HIV test
  - has had *any* new STD[a] within the last 12 months
- Every 3–6 months if the patient or their partner:
  - is a man who is gay, bisexual, or has sex with men
  - injects nonprescription drugs/hormones/cosmetic fillers
  - exchanges sex for money/drugs/housing
  - has a sex partner living with HIV whose viral load is greater than 200 copies/mL[3] or not known

[a]*STD*: sexually transmitted disease.

---

disease monitoring). There are a number of different indications for HIV screening (Box 18.2) and while most screening occurs almost exclusively in medical clinics, dental clinics have been successfully utilized. If blood can be drawn, a serum or plasma HIV 1/2 Ag/Ab combination screening test "with reflex" is indicated. This tests for HIV-1 and 2 antibodies and HIV-1 p24 antigen (i.e., the presence of acute HIV-infection). Reflex tells the lab to proceed with additional testing on the same specimen if indicated. Following initial diagnosis, several additional tests are typically performed, including HIV quantitative viral load testing, CD4 count, HIV-1 genotyping and HLA-B*5701 testing and CCR5 coreceptor tropism assay (required for purposes of selection of certain antiretroviral agents), along with other baseline tests important for medical management (i.e., complete blood count, routine metabolic panel, testing for sexually transmitted infections, and hepatitis). HIV-1 RNA NAT and CD4 counts are the preferred monitoring tests to assess disease progression or response to treatment.

MEDICAL MANAGEMENT

Medical management of the HIV-infected patient has four main treatment goals: (1) to reduce HIV-associated morbidity and prolong the duration and quality of survival, (2) to restore and preserve immunologic function, (3) to maximally and durably suppress plasma HIV viral load, and (4) to prevent HIV transmission. Physicians managing these patients should be experts in

infectious disease and in the use of antiretroviral drugs. Antiretroviral therapy (ART) should be used in a manner to achieve viral suppression and immune reconstitution while simultaneously preventing emergence of resistance and limiting drug toxicity. Long-term goals are to delay disease progression, prolong life, and improve quality of life. Treatment is often categorized into three major areas: (1) ART, (2) prophylaxis for opportunistic infections, and (3) treatment of HIV-related complications. Monitoring response to therapy and disease control is critical to long-term survival.

ART

Enormous progress has been made in the treatment of HIV to the point that the life expectancy of patients who are controlled on stable ART regimens is approaching that of the general population. ART involves the use antiretroviral drugs in combination to target multiple pathways in viral pathogenesis.

ART increases survival, reduces systemic complications, and improves the quality of life in patients infected with HIV. The initial goal of ART is to inhibit HIV replication such that the HIV-RNA viral load is <200 copies/mL at 3–6 months; the standard of care is to initiate ART as soon as possible, ideally at the time of HIV diagnosis. There are seven classes of antiretrovirals (ARV), and more than 30 of these drugs have been FDA approved, mostly used in combination (Table 18.2). These classes include nucleoside/nucleotide reverse transcriptase inhibitors (NRTIs), nonnucleoside reverse transcriptase inhibitors (NNRTIs), protease inhibitors (PIs), integrase strand transfer inhibitors (INSTIs), a fusion inhibitor, a CCR5 antagonist, and a CD4 T lymphocyte (CD4) postattachment inhibitor. In addition, two drugs, ritonavir (RTV) and cobicistat (COBI), are used as pharmacokinetic enhancers (or boosters) to improve the pharmacokinetic profiles of PIs and the INSTI elvitegravir (EVG).

Evidence-based regimens in treatment-naïve HIV-infected patients typically include integrase strand transfer inhibitors in combination with various other drugs (Box 18.3) and their selection is based on a number of considerations including pretreatment viral load and CD4 count, HIV genotypic drug resistance, predicted adherence factors, timing relative to baseline diagnosis, drug interaction and potential adverse effect profile, individual preferences, and availability/cost.

Patients who are on ART must be closely monitored for drug effectiveness, development of antiviral resistance, drug toxicity, and drug interactions. Important toxicities include hyperlactemia, mitochondrial dysfunction, peripheral neuropathy, hepatotoxicity, and lipodystrophy. Adherence also is a major challenge for patients in view of recognized drug toxicities, costs, and inconvenience. When cocktails of ARVs began to be used, some patients were expected to take two dozen or more pills a day. The formulation of combination agents

TABLE 18.2 Antiretroviral Drugs Used to Treat HIV Infection.

Drug	Adverse Effects	Drug Interactions	Coformulations
Integrase Strand Transfer Inhibitors (INSTIs)	Nausea, diarrhea, headache, insomnia, weight gain, depression/suicidality rare among those with preexisting psychiatric conditions. Increases creatinine (without affecting glomerular filtration). Pregnancy testing advised before considering INSTIs (may be contraindicated).	Reduction in absorption when given concomitantly with polyvalent cations (i.e., Fe, Mg, Ca, Al, Zn).	
Bictigravir (BIC)		P-gp, CYP3A4 (minor) and UGT1A1 substrate; inhibitor of drug transporters OCT2 and MATE1. Cyclosporine may increase BIC levels.	**BIC**/TAF/FTC
Dolutegravir (DTG)		P-gp, CYP3A4 (minor) and UGT1A1 substrate; inhibitor of drug transporter OCT2 and MATE2.	**DTG**/3TC **DTG**/ABC/3TC
Elvitegravir (EVG)		P-gp, CYP3A4 and UGT1A1 substrate, CYP2C9 inhibitor Due to boosting with cobicistat: Benzodiazepines (alprazolam, clonazepam, diazepam), calcineurin inhibitors (cyclosporine, tacrolimus), and systemic/injected corticosteroids levels may increase. Opioid levels may increase or decrease (complex metabolism). Carbamazepine and oxcarbazepine may decrease EVG levels.	**EVG**/c/TAF/FTC **EVG**/c/TDF/FTC
Raltegravir (RAL)	Myositis, rhabdomyolysis and elevated creatine kinase levels possible. Rare skin/systemic hypersensitivity reactions.	UGT1A1 substrate	**RAL**
Cabotegravir (CAB)		UGT1A1 substrate	**CAB**/RPV
NNRTIs		Carbamazepine and oxcarbazepine will lead to decreased NNRTI levels.	
Doravirine (DOR)		CYP3A4, 3A5 substrate	**DOR**/TDF/3TC
Efavirenz (EFV)	Neuropsychiatric effects such as abnormal dreams, dizziness, headache, depression (largely short-term only). Delayed neurotoxicity, dyslipidemia, QTc interval prolongation.	CYP2B6 (primary), 3A4 (major) substrate, CYP3A4 (weak) inhibitor, CYP3A4 (moderate), 2B6 (moderate), 2C19 (weak) inducer Benzodiazepines (alprazolam, clonazepam, and diazepam), calcineurin inhibitors (cyclosporine, tacrolimus) and corticosteroids levels may decrease. Morphine and hydromorphone levels may increase, oxycodone and tramadol levels may decrease, meperidine use may lead to seizures. Bupropion levels may decrease (i.e., if prescribed by a dentist for smoking cessation).	**EFV**/TDF/FTC
Etravirine (ETR)	Skin rash, dyslipidemia, increased glucose	CYP3A4, 2C9, 2C19 substrate (strong), CYP2C9, 2C19 inhibitor (weak), CYP3A4 inducer (moderate), P-gP inducer Benzodiazepines (alprazolam, clonazepam, and diazepam), calcineurin inhibitors (cyclosporine, tacrolimus) and corticosteroid levels may decrease.	**ETR**
Rilpivirine (RPV)	Depressive symptoms. QTc interval prolongation.	Contraindicated with PPIs and caution with H2-blockers. CYP3A4 substrate. GI absorption is pH dependent. RPV levels may be decrease with systemic dexamethasone.	**RPV**/TAF/FTC **RPV**/TDF/FTC CAB/**RPV**
NRTIs Tenofovir alafenamide (TAF)	Reduction in bone density. Possible weight gain.	P-gp, BCRP, OATP substrate	BIC/**TAF**/FTC DRV/c/**TAF**/FTC EVG/c/**TAF**/FTC RPV/**TAF**/FTC **TAF**/FTC

Continued

TABLE 18.2   Antiretroviral Drugs Used to Treat HIV Infection.—cont'd

Drug	Adverse Effects	Drug Interactions	Coformulations
Tenofovir disoproxil fumarate (TDF)	New onset or worsening renal impairment (renal function/urinalysis monitoring and avoid if CrCl<60 mL/min). Avoid in patients with osteoporosis.	P-gp, OATP, MRP substrate	DOR/**TDF**/3TC EFV/**TDF**/FTC EVG/c/**TDF**/FTC RPV/**TDF**/FTC **TDF**/3TC **TDF**/FTC
Abacavir (ABC)	Hypersensitivity reaction (contraindicated in HLA-B*5701+ patients). Possible risk for myocardial infarction (use with caution in patients with cardiovascular risk).	UGT1A1 substrate, alcohol dehydrogenase substrate	**ABC**/3TC DTG/**ABC**/3TC
Emtricitabine (FTC)	Possible exacerbation of hepatitis B infection after discontinuing. Dizziness, nausea, headache, abnormal dreams.	MATE1 substrate	BIC/TAF/**FTC** DRV/c/TAF/**FTC** EFV/TDF/**FTC** EVG/c/TAF/**FTC** EVG/c/TDF/**FTC** RPV/TAF/**FTC** RPV/TDF/**FTC** TAF/**FTC** TDF/**FTC**
Lamivudine (3TC)	Possible exacerbation of hepatitis B infection after discontinuing. Dizziness, fatigue nausea, diarrhea, headache, abnormal dreams, skin rash.	Substrate of MATE1/2; OCT2. Sorbitol-containing drugs can cause decrease in 3TC levels.	ABC/**3TC** DOR/TDF/**3TC** DTG/**3TC** DTG/ABC/**3TC** EFV/TDF/**3TC** TDF/**3TC**
PIs Atazanavir (ATV)	Diarrhea Reversible indirect hyperbilirubinemia without elevated transaminases (with possible jaundice). Cholelithiasis, nephrolithiasis (with possible nephrotoxicity) and caution in those with compromised kidney function.	GI absorption is pH dependent. Reduction in absorption when given with acid lowering agents (PPIs/H2 blockers). CYP3A4 inhibitor. Due to boosting with cobicistat or ritonavir: Benzodiazepines (alprazolam, clonazepam, and diazepam), calcineurin inhibitors (tacrolimus) and systemic/injected corticosteroids levels may increase. Tricyclic antidepressants (given for neuropathic pain) in combination with boosted PIs may prolong QT interval. Due to boosting with cobicistat or ritonavir, opioid levels may increase or decrease (complex metabolism). Carbamazepine and oxcarbazepine may decrease ATV levels.	**ATV**/c **ATV**/r
Darunavir (DRV)	Skin rash, increase in serum transaminases, hyperlipidemia, higher cardiovascular risk.	Due to boosting with cobicistat or ritonavir: Benzodiazepines (alprazolam, clonazepam, and diazepam), calcineurin inhibitors (tacrolimus) and systemic/injected corticosteroids levels may increase. Tricyclic antidepressants (given for neuropathic pain) in combination with boosted PIs may prolong QT interval. Due to boosting with cobicistat or ritonavir, opioid levels may increase or decrease (complex metabolism). Carbamazepine and oxcarbazepine may decrease DRV levels.	**DRV**/c **DRV**/c/TAF/FTC **DRV**/r
Ritonavir (r) Used as a booster agent.	Skin rash, flushing, abdominal pain, diarrhea, dysgeusia, dizziness, fatigue, backpain, cough.	Due to boosting with cobicistat or ritonavir: Benzodiazepines (alprazolam, clonazepam, and diazepam), calcineurin inhibitors (tacrolimus) and systemic/injected corticosteroids levels may increase.	DRV/**r** ATV/**r**

Continued

		Tricyclic antidepressants (given for neuropathic pain) in combination with boosted PIs may prolong QT interval. Due to boosting with ritonavir, opioid levels may increase or decrease (complex metabolism). Carbamazepine and oxcarbazepine may decrease ritonavir levels.	
Others **Booster agent** Cobicistat (c)	Hyperbilirubinemia	CYP3A4 and 2D6 substrate and inhibitor. P-gP, BCRP, OATP, OCT, MATE1 inhibitor. Due to boosting with cobicistat: Benzodiazepines (alprazolam, clonazepam, and diazepam), calcineurin inhibitors (tacrolimus) and systemic/injected corticosteroids levels may increase. Tricyclic antidepressants (given for neuropathic pain) in combination with boosted PIs may prolong QT interval. Due to boosting with cobicistat or ritonavir, opioid levels may increase or decrease (complex metabolism). Carbamazepine and oxcarbazepine may decrease cobicistat levels.	ATV/**c** DRV/**c** DRV/**c**/TAF/FTC EVG/**c**/TAF/FTC EVG/**c**/TDF/FTC
CCR5 inhibitor Maraviroc (MVC)	Skin rash, vomiting, cough, fever	P-gp substrate, CYP3A4 substrate	**MVC**
Fusion inhibitor Enfuvirtide (T-20)	Diarrhea, nausea, fatigue, insomnia, injection site reaction.	None	**T-20**
Post-attachment inhibitor Ibalizumab (IBA)	Diarrhea, dizziness.	None	**IBA**

P-gp, efflux transporter P-glycoprotein in the intestines;
CYP3A4: the most common enzyme in the cytochrome p450 system responsible for hepatic drug metabolism. Other less common cytochrome p450 enzymes are designated with a different suffix (i.e., 2C19, 2D6, etc.). Those ARVs which are substrates for CYP3A4 (or other enzymes) will be affected by concomitant use of medications that either induce or inhibit this enzyme (i.e., reduce or increase ARV blood levels, respectively). Some drugs can act as an enzyme substrate, inhibitor, and inducer;

UGT1A1, uridine diphosphate glucuronosyltransferase (UGT) 1A1 hepatic enzyme;
OCT2, organic cation transporter 2;
MATE1, multidrug and toxin extrusion;
OATP, organic anion transporting polypeptide;
BCRP, breast cancer resistance protein;
MRP, multidrug resistance protein;
Note: Drug interactions of concern in dentistry are covered in Appendix C.

into single pills has markedly improved compliance, and the recent FDA approval of long-acting injectable combination ARVs (cabotegravir (CAB) and rilpivirine (RPV)) to replace standard ART in patients on stable oral ART offers further promise in the optimal delivery of ART over the long term.

Following the initiation of ART, a patient's viral load and CD4 counts will be monitored every 3–4 months. If, after 2 years, the viral load is persistently suppressed, the viral load can be measured every 6 months and the CD4 count can be measured every 12 months (if the CD4 is 300–500 cells/mm^3) or optionally if CD4 is >500 cells/mm^3. In addition, a complete blood count (CBC) with differential is recommended when the CD4 count is evaluated, basic chemistry and liver function testing every 6 months, and lipids/glucose testing annually. Virologic failure in ART-experienced patients requires careful reevaluation by the patient's physician.

Approximately 10% of patients, particularly those with very low CD4+ T-cell counts, experience an exacerbation of opportunistic infections (e.g., tuberculosis, herpes zoster, or cryptococcal meningitis) during immune reconstitution, a few weeks after initiation of ART. This is known as *immune reconstitution inflammatory syndrome* (IRIS). The pathogenesis of IRIS is unclear and the opportunistic infections may be preexisting ("paradoxical" IRIS) or new ("unmasking" IRIS).

HIV-infected patients have a high prevalence of substance use disorders, which predict poor adherence to ART.

PrEP

Preexposure prophylaxis is indicated for HIV-negative persons who may have sexual contact with a HIV-positive person or injection drug user, to help prevent the transmission of HIV. Two ARV regimens have been

BOX 18.3   ART Regimens for ARV-Naïve Patients[a]

Recommended Initial Antiretroviral Regimens for Most People with HIV
- INSTI + 2 NRTIs
  - BIC/TAF/FTC
  - DTG/ABC/3TC (if HLA-B*5701 negative)
  - DTG + (TAF or TDF) + (FTC or 3TC)
  - RAL + (TAF or TDF) + FTC or 3TC)
- INSTI + 1 NRTI
  - DTG/3TC (except if HIV RNA >500,000 copies/mL, HBV coinfection, or if results of genotypic resistance is pending)

Alternative Recommended Initial Antiretroviral Regimens
- INSTI+ 2 NRTIs
  - EVG/c/(TAF or TDF)/FTC
- Boosted PI + 2 NRTIs
  - (DRV/c or DRV/r) + (TAF or TDF) + (FTC or 3TC)
  - (ATV/c or ATV/r) + (TAF or TDF) + (FTC or 3TC)
  - (DRV/c or DRV/r) + ABC/3TC (if HLA-B*5701 negative)
- NNRTI + 2 NRTIs
  - DOR/TDF/3TC or DOR + TAF/FTC
  - EVF + (TAF or TDF) + (FTC or 3TC)
  - RPV/(TAF or TDF)/FTC (if HIV RNA<100,000 copies/mL and CD4 count >200 cells/mm^3)
- Regimens when ABC, TAF or TDF cannot be used
  - DTG/3TC (except if HIV RNA >500,000 copies/mL, HBV coinfection, or if results of genotypic resistance is pending)
  - DRV/r + RAL (if HIV RNA <100,000 copies/mL and CD4 count >200 cells/mm^3)
  - DRV/r + 3TC

3TC, lamivudine; *ABC*, abacavir; *ATV*, atazanavir; *BIC*, bictegravir; */c*, boosted with cobicistat; *DOR*, doravirine; *DRV*, darunavir; *DTG*, dolutegravir; *EVF*, efavirenz; *EVG*, elvitigravir; *FTC*, emtricitabine; *INSTI*, integrase strand transfer inhibitor; *NNRTI*, nonnucleoside reverse transcriptase inhibitor; *NRTI*, nucleoside reverse transcriptase inhibitor; *PI*, protease inhibitor; */r*, boosted with ritonavir; *RAL*, raltegravir; *TAF*, tenofovir alafenamide; *TDF*, tenofovir disoproxil fumarate.

[a]A pregnancy test should be performed before prescribing dolutegravir and other INSTIs and alternative regimens should be considered.

approved for daily prophylactic use: emtricitabine/tenofovir disoproxil fumarate or emtricitabine/tenofovir alafenamide. These medications are prescribed in conjunction with other preventive activities (e.g., condom use). PrEP is taken daily for extended periods of sexual activity, and is not to be taken on an "as needed basis."

U = U

The concept of "Undetectable = Untransmissible" is based on data that patients with durable undetectable HIV-infection do not pose a risk for transmission to others. It allows serodiscordant couples to engage sexually without protection. These patients require annual physician contact.

Prophylaxis Versus Opportunistic Infections

Prophylaxis regimens are recommended for HIV+ patients with low CD4+ lymphocyte counts to prevent new infectious diseases or to suppress a developing opportunistic infection. These regimens exist for the prevention of *Pneumocystis jiroveci* pneumonia and toxoplasmosis. Also, select vaccines (e.g., vs. Hepatitis B, human papillomavirus, influenza) are recommended for HIV-infected adults. At present, there is no effective vaccine to prevent HIV infection, although large research efforts have and continue to be made in this area.

DENTAL MANAGEMENT

Health history, head and neck examination, intraoral soft tissue examination, and complete periodontal and dental examinations should be performed on all new patients. History and clinical findings may suggest that the patient has HIV infection. It is important to note that patients who know they are seropositive or who have engaged in high-risk behaviors may not divulge their history honestly because of the stigma associated with the disease and concern for privacy. Accordingly, the patient history should be obtained whenever possible with this understanding; verbal communication in a quiet, private location; and the sharing of knowledge and facts in an atmosphere of honesty and openness.

Clinicians who, on the basis of history (i.e., sexual history, injecting drug use, and others) or clinical findings, encounter patients at high risk for HIV infection should emphasize the importance of testing and prompt referral to a medical facility for confidential testing and medical care. While dentists can undertake point-of-care saliva diagnostic testing (e.g., OraQuick Advance; OraSure Technologies, Bethlehem, PA) they must maintain tests as per manufacturer standards, be able to provide appropriate pre and posttest counseling, and have an established referral pathway for patients who test positive.

Federal law dictates that a patient with HIV infection who needs dental treatment may not be refused care simply because the dental provider does not want to treat HIV+ patients. Patients with known HIV infection should be treated in a manner identical to that for any other patient—that is, with standard infection control precautions. When considering the treatment of patients infected with HIV, the dentist should determine if he or she has the need of another's skills, knowledge, equipment, or expertise, and if so, consultation or referral may be indicated. Decisions regarding the type of dental treatment provided or referrals made or suggested should be made on the same basis as they are made with other patients. The dentist should also determine, after consultation with the patient's physician, if appropriate, if the patient's health status would be significantly compromised by the provision of dental treatment.

Infected dentists should inform their patients of their HIV serostatus and should receive consent, otherwise the dentist should refrain from performing invasive procedures.

Treatment Planning Considerations

The major considerations in dental treatment of the patient who has HIV infection involve determining the level of immunosuppression related to HIV-infection and appreciating other medical comorbidities that are prevalent in this population (e.g., cardiovascular disease, viral hepatitis, substance use disorder, and others). Disease control and immunosuppression may be gauged by current viral load, CD4+ lymphocyte count and CBC, and these values must be interpreted in the context of whether or not the patient is on ART. The dentist should be knowledgeable about the current or past history and status of opportunistic infections and their treatment. Patients who are HIV+ with undetectable viral loads secondary to durable viral suppression may safely receive all indicated dental treatment without specific HIV-related modifications. Patients with CD4+ cell counts <200 cells/mm^3 are profoundly immunosuppressed and at increased risk for opportunistic infections as well as other cytopenias. Any oral lesions found should be diagnosed and then managed by appropriate local and/or systemic treatment or referred for diagnosis and treatment.

In planning invasive dental procedures, attention must be paid to the prevention of perioperative and postoperative complications, such as excessive bleeding or infection. HIV patients are at potential risk for anemia, neutropenia, and/or thrombocytopenia, particularly those who are not on ART or with a low CD4 count <200 cells/mm^3. Consultation with the patient's physician and preoperative blood work (i.e., CBC with differential) should be considered for those with poorly controlled HIV infection (i.e., not on ART and with a trend of decreasing CD4 counts/increasing viral load) or with a history of anemia, neutropenia, or thrombocytopenia. Elective dental treatment should be postponed until the cytopenia stabilizes. Antibiotic prophylaxis is recommended if there is severe neutropenia (i.e., absolute neutrophil count <500 cells/mm^3). Patients with severe thrombocytopenia (i.e., platelet count <50,000) may require platelet transfusion before surgical procedures, including scaling and curettage. Surgical procedures are contraindicated in patients with severe anemia (i.e., hemoglobin <11 g/dL).

Some ARVs are substrates for cytochrome P450 (CYP$_{450}$) and other metabolic pathway systems, and their drug levels may be affected by CYP$_{450}$ inducers or inhibitors (Table 18.2). Dentists who prescribe medications to HIV-infected patients must consider risks for ARV drug interactions. Furthermore, consideration about potential drug interactions with alcohol and illicit substance use (e.g., stimulants such as methamphetamines or cocaine, or "depressants" such as opioids or benzodiazepines) is prudent (see Chapter 29).

People living with HIV experience a higher burden of dental issues. It is important to restore missing teeth and provide optimal mastication and esthetics. Following clinical and radiographic examination, diagnosis, risk factor assessment, and prompt treatment of existing active dental issues (dental caries/periapical infections, or periodontal diseases) is warranted. Risk factors for caries include poor diet, suboptimal oral hygiene, and may include xerostomia (due to polypharmacy, substance use disorders, or to HIV-related salivary gland hypofunction).

BOX 18.4 PostExposure ARV Prophylaxis Regimen Following Occupational Exposure

Preferred HIV PEP Regimen
Raltegravir (RAL) 400 mg PO Twice Daily
PLUS
Tenofovir DF (TDF) 300 mg/emtricitabine (FTC) 200 mg PO Once Daily

Alternative Regimens
(May combine one drug or drug pair from the left column with one pair of nucleoside/nucleotide reverse transcriptase inhibitors from the right column[a])

Raltegravir (RAL)	Tenofovir DF (TDF) + emtricitabine (FTC)
Darunavir (DRV) + ritonavir (RTV)	Tenofovir DF (TDF) + lamivudine (3TC)
Etravirine (ETR)	Zidovudine (ZDV; AZT) + lamivudine (3TC)
Rilpivirine (RPV)	Zidovudine (ZDV; AZT) + emtricitabine (FTC)
Atazanavir (ATV) + ritonavir (RTV)	
Lopinavir/ritonavir (LPV/RTV)	

[a]Prescribers unfamiliar with these agents/regimens should consult physicians familiar with the agents and their toxicities, and this includes consideration of PEP in pregnant health care workers.

BOX 18.5	Checklist for Dental Management Considerations of Patients With HIV Infection or AIDS[a]

PREOPERATIVE RISK ASSESSMENT

- Review medical history, determine whether HIV infection exists, and discuss relevant issues with the patient.
- Identify all medications and drugs being taken or supposed to be taken by the patient.
- Examine the patient for signs and symptoms of disease and obtain vital signs.
- Review recent laboratory test results or images required to assess risk.
- Confirm patient has a primary care provider.
- Obtain a medical consultation (i.e., refer to physician) if the patient is poorly controlled or is undiagnosed or if uncertain.
- If laboratory tests indicate patient is well controlled, routine dental procedures can be performed without special precautions.

A

Analgesics and drugs for neuropathic pain	The risk for renal impairment of NSAIDs is potentially higher in patients taking TDF (tenofovir disoproxil fumarate). This does not contraindicate use of NSAIDs, but judicious use is warranted. Aspirin and other NSAID use can worsen bleeding in a patient who has thrombocytopenia. Check drug or potential substance use interactions before prescribing. Opioid metabolism (including tramadol) may be affected by co-administration with boosted ARVs (i.e., those containing ritonavir or cobicistat) or EFV resulting in either increased or, in some cases, decreased opioid levels. Meperidine is contraindicated in patients taking EFV because of seizure risk. TCAs (tricyclic antidepressants) may interact with PIs to increase risk for arrhythmias. Monitor for cardiac AEs. Carbamazepine or oxcarbazepine may reduce ARVs levels (NNRTIs, boosted PIs, and RAL) and should be avoided. Lamotrigine levels will be reduced by ARVs boosted with ritonavir. Clonazepam, alprazolam, and diazepam levels will be increased by boosted ARVs (i.e., those drugs containing ritonavir or cobicistat).
Antibiotics	Prophylactic use not required unless severe neutropenia (<500 cells/mm³) is present. Manage odontogenic infections with usual antibiotic regimens. There are no significant ART interactions with antibiotics typically prescribed by dentists.
Anesthesia	No issues.
Anxiety	This patient population has a higher risk of dental phobia.
Allergy	No issues.

B

Bleeding	Excessive bleeding may occur in patients with untreated or poorly controlled disease as a result of thrombocytopenia. Order CBC. Platelet counts <50,000 may require transfusion.
Breathing	Ensure that patient does not have a pulmonary infection. Delay treatment until pulmonary infections are resolved.
Blood pressure	No issues.

C

Chair position	No issues.
Cardiovascular	HIV-infected patients are at a higher risk for cardiovascular disease. Confirm cardiovascular status. Some ARVs, such as PIs, can increase risk for arrhythmias by extending QT prolongation.

D

Devices	No issues.
Drugs	There are possible drug interactions and drug toxicities associated with ART and clinicians are advised to check drug reference resources before prescribing medications. In addition to those interactions described above: Benzodiazepeine levels (diazepam and alprazolam) may be increased with boosted ARVs and reduced by EFV and ETR. Systemic and injected corticosteroid levels (i.e., prednisolone, prednisone, dexamethasone, and triamcinolone (injected)) are increased by boosted ARVs (i.e., those containing ritonavir or cobicistat). Short-term use (<2 weeks) is usually not associated with an interaction, but co-administration for longer periods is not recommended unless benefit outweighs risk. There is little data on chronic oral topical corticosteroids. EFV/ETR and RVP may reduce systemic dexamethasone levels (i.e., >a single dose). EFV may reduce bupropion levels (i.e., bupropion given for smoking cessation). Systemic cyclosporine may increase BIC levels; everolimus, sirolimus, cyclosporine, or tacrolimus levels may be increased by boosted ARVs, or reduced by EFV and ETV. There is no data on chronic use of topical tacrolimus or pimecrolimus.

E

Equipment	No issues.
Emergencies/urgencies	No issues.

F

Follow-up	Routine and periodic follow-up evaluation is advised for HIV-infected patients. Request recent bloodwork and inspect for oral lesions to monitor for disease progression or ART failure. Patients in stage 2 or 3 may require more frequent follow-up and additional bloodwork investigations.

[a]Strength of Recommendation Taxonomy (SORT) Grade: C (see Preface for further explanation).

ART, antiretroviral therapy; *ARV,* antiretroviral; *BIC,* bictegravir; *COBI,* cobistat; *EFV,* efavirenz; *ETR,* etravirine; *FTR,* fostemsavir; *NSAID,* nonsteroidal antiinflammatory drug; *RPV,* rilpirivine; *RTV,* ritonavir.

HIV-infected patients are also at higher risk for gingival and periodontal diseases. Necrotizing ulcerative periodontitis (NUP), necrotizing ulcerative gingivitis (NUG), and linear gingival erythema are encountered less frequently with the advent of ART. However, chronic periodontitis remains an important issue. Dentists should monitor patients for progression, which may indicate significant immunosuppression.

Customized preventive plans for home-care include oral hygiene instruction, fluoride regimens (for those with high-caries risk), and antibacterial rinses (e.g., chlorhexidine) for those unable to maintain adequate biofilm

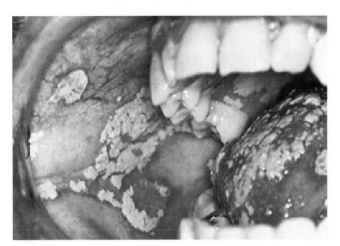

FIG. 18.7 Note the white lesions on the oral mucosa. The diagnosis of pseudomembranous candidiasis was established. (Courtesy of Eric Haus, Chicago, IL.)

control. In stable HIV-infected patients there is no evidence to contraindicate restorative care, endodontics, scaling/root-planing, or invasive surgical procedures including implant placement. Patients with a history of periodontal disease or other oral diseases who do not respond to conventional treatment should be referred to a specialist. It is important to provide evidence-based tobacco cessation and refer patients with alcohol and substance use disorders to experts. Regular recall appointments allow for reevaluation of oral disease and maintenance of oral health.

Occupational Exposure to HIV

The risk of HIV transmission from infected patients to health care workers is very low, 0.3% following a percutaneous injury (i.e., a needlestick). In comparison, the risk of infection from a needlestick is 3% for hepatitis C and is 30% for hepatitis B. Factors increasing the risk of transmission include the presence of blood on the sharp instrument or needle, use of a hollow-bore needle, a deep injury, and a patient with a high viral load. These statistics underly the importance of implementing administrative and engineering controls to minimize accidental exposure. An occupational exposure is an emergency and the rate of transmission of HIV can be reduced by postexposure prophylaxis (PEP). PEP is offered to all exposed health care workers, irrespective of degree of risk of transmission (i.e., even if the source patient has an undetectable viral load). The CDC recommends PEP as soon as possible after exposure to HIV-infected blood (i.e., ideally within 2 h, but not longer

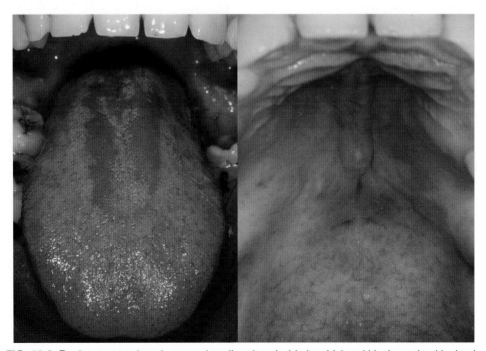

FIG. 18.8 Erythematous dorsal tongue (median rhomboid glossitis) and kissing palatal lesion in an HIV-infected patient. Smears taken from the lesion showed hyphae and spores consistent with *Candida*. The lesion healed after a 2-week course of antifungal medications. (Courtesy of Ross Kerr, New York, NY.)

than 72 h) with a recommended regimen (Box 18.4). Institutional or dental office protocols should be in place to help manage an exposure, including counseling, PEP initiation, HIV testing, and follow-up. In the United States there is a PEP hotline 888-448-4911 or website http://www.nccc.ucsf.edu/about_nccc/pepline/. PEP should be continued for 4 weeks, during which time the exposed health care worker should be provided expert consultation and follow-up monitoring for compliance, adverse events, and possible seroconversion. Tests for seroconversion should be performed at 3, 6, and 12 months.

Risk of Transmission From Health Care Personnel

The risk of transmission in the dental setting is minimized by adherence to standard infection control precautions (see Appendix B).

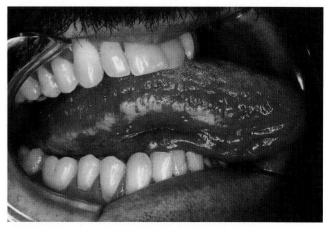

FIG. 18.11 Diffuse white lesion involving the tongue. Biopsy supported the diagnosis of hairy leukoplakia. (From Silverman S Jr: *Color atlas of oral manifestations of AIDS*, ed 2, St. Louis, 1996, Mosby.)

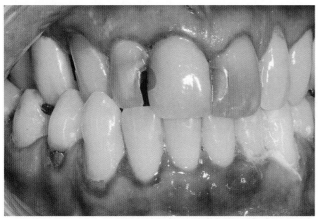

FIG. 18.9 Band of linear gingival erythema involving the free gingival margin of a human immunodeficiency virus–infected patient. (From Neville B, Damm D, Allen C: *Oral and maxillofacial pathology*, ed 3, St. Louis, 2009, Saunders.)

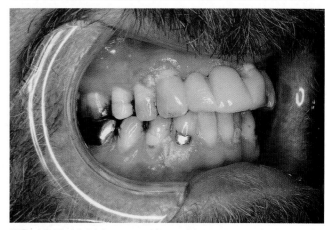

FIG. 18.12 Multiple areas of condylomata acuminata on the gingivae of an HIV-infected patient. (From Silverman S Jr: *Color atlas of oral manifestations of AIDS*, ed 2, St. Louis, 1996, Mosby.)

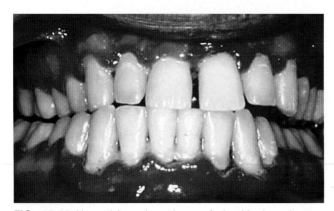

FIG. 18.10 Necrotizing ulcerative periodontitis in a human immunodeficiency virus–infected patient. The diagnosis was established after the patient was referred for medical evaluation. (Courtesy of Sol Silverman, San Francisco, CA.)

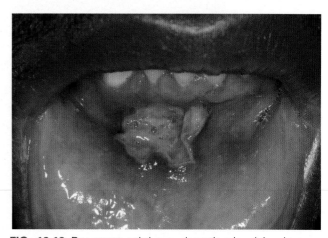

FIG. 18.13 Recurrent aphthous ulceration involving in a patient suspected and confirmed to be HIV-infected (baseline CD4 count was <100 cells/mm^3). (Courtesy of Ross Kerr, New York, NY.)

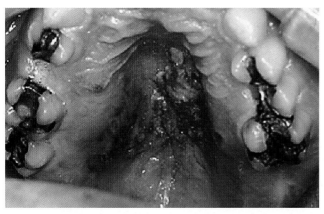

FIG. 18.14 Palatal lesion in a patient with AIDS (macular form). Biopsy revealed Kaposi sarcoma. (Courtesy of Sol Silverman, San Francisco, CA.)

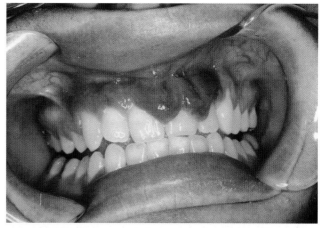

FIG. 18.15 Kaposi sarcoma of the gingiva (nodular form). (From Silverman S Jr: *Color atlas of oral manifestations of AIDS*, ed 2, St. Louis, 1996, Mosby.)

TABLE 18.3 Head, Neck, and Oral Lesions and Conditions Associated With HIV Infection and AIDS

Oral Condition	Features	Treatment
Persistent generalized lymphadenopathy	An early sign of HIV infection found in about 70% of infected patients during the latent stage of infection. Must be present >3 months and in two or more extra-inguinal locations. Anterior and posterior cervical, submandibular, occipital, and axillary nodes are most frequently involved.	Usually not treated directly; may need imaging or fine need aspiration to rule out other etiologies including infectious conditions (e.g., tuberculosis or nontuberculous mycobacterial, viral or fungal infections), immune reconstitution inflammatory syndrome (IRIS), or malignant neoplasms (e.g., lymphoma)
Oral candidiasis: Pseudomembranous Erythematous Hyperplastic Angular cheilitis	Most common intraoral manifestation of HIV infection. First found during the early symptomatic stage of infection. ≈90% of patients with AIDS will develop oral candidiasis at some time during their disease course. IRIS-related oral candidiasis is common. May affect any mucosal site.	All regimens 7—14 days First line: fluconazole tablets 100 mg PO od for 7—14 days[a] Alternatives: Topical miconazole 50 mg buccal tablet od OR clotrimazole 10 mg troche 5×/day OR nystatin suspension 100,000 U/mL 4—6 mL or pastilles 500,000 U 4×/day OR gentian violet (0.00165%) applied bid Itraconazole and posaconazole are effective but have more drug—drug interactions than fluconazole. Refractory disease (i.e., fluconazole resistance): Posaconazole suspension 400 mg bid × 28 days. Alternatives include itraconazole, and if azoles fail, then IV amphotericin B can be administered. Prophylaxis for recurrent disease is recommended if recurrences are frequent or severe.
HIV-associated gingival or periodontal diseases		
Linear gingival erythema (LGE)	LGE associated with candidiasis and does not respond to standard plaque control. May precede NUG. Involves the free marginal gingivae.	LGE usually responds to superficial debridement, improved oral hygiene, and chlorhexidine rinses. Persistent cases usually respond to local measures plus systemic antifungal medications.
Necrotizing ulcerative gingivitis (NUG)	NUG relates to ulceration and necrosis of one or more interdental papillae with no loss of periodontal attachment. Radiographs are needed to differentiate between NUG and NUP.	Therapy for NUG, NUP, and NS involves debridement (removal of necrotic tissue and 0.12% chlorhexidine or 10% povidone—iodine irrigation), and home care with chlorhexidine or povidone-iodine rinses, metronidazole 250 mg 3×/day for 7—14 days (for more severe or refractory cases, and concomitant antifungal regimen to prevent candidiasis), follow-up care, and long-term maintenance.
Necrotizing ulcerative periodontitis (NUP)	NUP consists of gingival ulceration and necrosis with attachment loss and does not respond to conventional periodontal therapy.	
Necrotizing stomatitis (NS)	May be seen as an extension of NUP or may involve oral mucosal sites separate from the gingiva.	
Herpes simplex virus (HSV) infection	Seroprevalence of HSV is higher in the HIV population. Oral HSV infections in HIV-infected patients are typically similar to those in HIV negative patients.	Patients with herpes labialis may be treated episodically (for 5—10 days) with acyclovir 400 mg PO tid, valacyclovir 1 g PO bid or famciclovir 500 mg PO bid. OR suppressively (if

Continued

TABLE 18.3	Head, Neck, and Oral Lesions and Conditions Associated With HIV Infection and AIDS—cont'd	
Oral Condition	**Features**	**Treatment**
Varicella-zoster virus (VZV) infection	Atypical HSV infections may be seen in profoundly immunosuppressed patients and may affect keratinized and nonkeratinized oral sites. Disseminated infections are very rare. PCR or viral culture of active lesions may facilitate diagnosis if atypical. Secondary VZV infection is 3 times more common in HIV-infected patients and head and neck manifestations can cause significant morbidity. May affect any of the three divisions of the trigeminal nerve.	frequent and severe recurrences) with acyclovir 400 mg PO bid, valacyclovir 500 mg PO bid or famciclovir 500 mg PO bid (reevaluated annually). Acyclovir resistance should be suspected for refractory disease, and phenotypic testing of viral isolates performed. IV foscarnet may be indicated. Vaccination to prevent primary infection may be recommended for patients aged ≥8 who are seronegative for VZV (live attenuated varicella vaccine, except in severely immunocompromised patients), and to prevent reactivation in those aged ≥50 who are seropositive (recombinant zoster vaccine). Secondary disease (Shingles): Similar regimen for 7–10 days. IV acyclovir may be needed for severe disease in patients with immunosuppression.
Oral hairy leukoplakia (OHL)	Corrugated white lesion(s) most often found on the lateral border of the tongue, bilaterally. OHL on rare occasions has been found on the buccal mucosa, soft palate, and pharynx. It is associated with EBV infection. In an untreated patient with HIV symptomatic infection, the finding of OHL is predictive for disease progression. Despite the name, this condition has no malignant potential.	HIV therapy with ART can result in significant regression.
Human papillomavirus (HPV)	Lesions may be solitary or multifocal (florid HPV infection), and presentations may range from pink to white, and exhibit smooth to papillary surface. Common nononcogenic HPV genotypes are typically found in oral lesions (i.e., HPV-6 and 11, but some uncommon variants such as HPV-7 and HPV-32 may be found). May involve keratinized or nonkeratinized mucosal sites.	Treatment of choice for solitary lesions is surgical removal. Treatment of multifocal lesions may include laser ablation and electrosurgery (care must be taken because the plume may contain infectious HPV). Other low evidence treatment modalities include topical podophyllin, interferon, and cryosurgery.
Aphthous stomatitis (major, minor, herpetiform)	Severity is correlated with degree of immunosuppression. Biopsy (or other testing) may be indicated to rule out infectious etiology or malignant neoplasm for lesions that do not respond to conventional treatment. May involve keratinized or nonkeratinized mucosal sites.	Treatment of major lesions that persist involves potent topical, intralesional or systemic corticosteroids. Thalidomide treatment has yielded good response although adverse effects are possible (i.e., peripheral neuropathy, or increasing viral load).
HIV-associated salivary gland disease	Can occur any time during HIV infection and includes xerostomia/salivary gland hypofunction (SGH) and/or salivary gland enlargement. SGH is multifactorial. The parotid glands are most commonly involved, and typically there is bilateral nontender enlargement due to cystic lymphoid hyperplasia (CLH), or diffuse lymphocytosis syndrome (DILS). DILS is associated with a predominant CD8+ lymphocyte infiltrate and patients are at increased risk for nonHodgkin lymphoma.	Associated xerostomia can be managed with sialogogues and saliva substitutes. ART will typically lead to resolution of CLH/DILS.
Hyperpigmentation	Oral pigmentation has been reported to occur in HIV-infected patients and is multifactorial (i.e., intrinsic to HIV-pathogenesis, medication related, postinflammatory, or related to adrenal gland dysfunction). May involve keratinized or nonkeratinized mucosal sites.	Usually no treatment is indicated. Solitary and evolving lesions may indicate biopsy to rule out mucosal melanoma.
Kaposi sarcoma (KS)	HHV-8 is involved in KS development. ~50% of patients with KS have oral lesions, and the oral cavity is the initial site of involvement in 20%–25% of cases. The most common sites are the hard palate,	Often regresses with ART. Treatment may include radiation and local/or systemic chemotherapy. Focal symptomatic lesions can be excised or injected with vinblastine or a sclerosing agent (sodium tetradecyl sulfate). Other options

Continued

	gingiva, and tongue. KS that occurs in an HIV-infected patient is diagnostic of AIDS.	include cryotherapy, laser ablation, and electrosurgery (care must be taken to protect operating personnel from plume when using laser/electrosurgery).
Lymphoma	Approximately 5% of HIV-infected patients develop lymphomas (all sites). Most head and neck lymphomas in HIV+ patients are high grade nonHodgkin (NHL) lymphomas (plasmablastic or diffuse large B-cell lymphomas) and are typically related to EBV. Extranodal locations are common, particularly the maxilla. NHL that occurs in an HIV-infected patient is diagnostic of AIDS.	Treatment usually involves a combination of chemotherapy and radiation and is used for local control of disease. The prognosis is very poor, with death occurring within months of the diagnosis. ART has reduced the prevalence of opportunistic infections and KS in HIV-infected patients but has not affected the prevalence of lymphoma.
Oral potentially malignant disorders (i.e., leukoplakia/erythroplakia) and squamous cell carcinoma (SCC) of the oral cavity and oropharynx.	Can be found in the oral cavity, pharynx, and larynx in HIV-infected persons. Similar risk factors apply as for the general population, but the cancer occurs at a younger age. HIV-infected patients are at higher risk for HPV associated oral and oropharynx SCCs. May involve any mucosal sites.	Treatment of oral cavity and oropharynx SCC is the same as for non–HIV-infected patients: Surgery, radiation, chemotherapy, or combination therapy.

AIDS, Acquired immunodeficiency syndrome; *ART*, antiretroviral therapy; *CLH*, cystic lymphoid hyperplasia; *DILS*, diffuse lymphocytosis syndrome; *EBV*, Epstein–Barr virus; *HHV-8*, human herpes virus type; *HIV*, human immunodeficiency virus; *IV*, intravenous; *KS*, Kaposi sarcoma; *HPV*, human papillomavirus; *PO*, oral; *tid*, three times a day. *SGH*, salivary gland hypofunction.
aContraindicated during pregnancy.

Oral Complications and Manifestations

The detection of oral "lesions" or conditions, in HIV+ individuals, may correlate with the degree of immunosuppression. An oral lesion can be one of the presenting signs of HIV infection or be indicative of treatment failure and disease progression (Box 18.5). Clinicians should be cognizant of the oral/head and neck manifestations of HIV infection and should perform head and neck and intraoral soft tissue examinations on all patients. Upon detection, appropriate steps must be taken to establish the diagnosis for oral lesions, including tissue biopsy if indicated. Head and neck lymphadenopathy may be an early finding in patients infected with HIV and often remains persistent (i.e., persistent generalized lymphadenopathy). Lymphadenopathy may also indicate a malignant neoplasm, and consideration for referral for medical evaluation, diagnosis, and treatment is prudent.

The overall prevalence of oral manifestations has significantly decreased since the advent of effective ART in the mid-1990s. The most common oral manifestation is candidiasis (pseudomembranous, erythematous, or hyperplastic) (Figs. 18.7 and 18.8). Other oral conditions that may occur in association with HIV infection are gingival and periodontal diseases (i.e., linear gingival erythema) (Fig. 18.9), NUG, NUP (Fig. 18.10)), herpes virus infections (i.e., herpes simplex virus (HSV), varicella-zoster virus (VZV), cytomegalovirus (CMV), and Epstein Barr virus (EBV) (i.e., hairy leukoplakia Fig. 18.11), oral human papillomavirus infections (HPV) (Fig. 18.12), bacterial infections (e.g., tuberculosis and syphilis), deep fungal infections (e.g., cryptococcus, histoplasmosis), recurrent aphthous ulcerations (Fig. 18.13), hyperpigmentation, salivary gland disease, facial palsy, trigeminal neuropathy, and malignant neoplasms (i.e.,

Kaposi sarcoma (Figs. 18.14 and 18.15), non-Hodgkin lymphoma, plasmablastic lymphoma, diffuse large B-cell lymphoma, and oral squamous cell carcinoma). Features and management of the oral manifestations of HIV infection are covered in Table 18.3.

BIBLIOGRAPHY

1. Aberg JA, Gallant JE, Ghanem KG, et al. Primary care Guidelines for the management of persons infected with HIV: 2013 update by the HIV medicine association of the infectious diseases Society of America. *Clin Infect Dis*. 2014;58(1):e1–e34.
2. Akdag D, Knudsen AD, Thudium RF, et al. Increased risk of anemia, neutropenia, and thrombocytopenia in people with human immunodeficiency virus and well-controlled viral replication. *J Infect Dis*. 2019;220:1834–1842.
3. Baccaglini B, Atkinson JC, Patton LL, et al. Management of oral lesions in HIV-positive patients. *Oral Surg Oral Med Oral Pathol Oral Radiol Endod*. 2007;103(suppl 1): S50.e1–S50.e23.
4. Barré-Sinoussi F, Chermann JC, Rey F, et al. Isolation of a T-lymphotropic retrovirus from a patient at risk for acquired immune deficiency syndrome (AIDS). *Science*. 1983;220:868–871.
5. Beachler DC, D'Souza G. Oral HPV infection and head and neck cancers in HIV-infected individuals. *Curr Opin Oncol*. September 2013;25(5):503–510.
6. Campo J, Cano J, del Romero J, et al. Oral complication risks after invasive and non-invasive dental procedures in HIV-positive patients. *Oral Dis*. 2007;13:110–116.
7. Centers for Disease Control and Prevention. HIV, https://www.cdc.gov/hiv/default.html.
8. Centers for Disease Control and Prevention. *HIV Surveillance Report*. Vol 31. 2018. Updated) http://www.cdc.gov/hiv/library/reports/hiv-surveillance.html. Published May 2020. Accessed March 2021.

9. Centers for Disease Control and Prevention. US Public Health Service: Preexposure Prophylaxis for the Prevention of HIV Infection in the United States—2017 Update: Clinical Providers' Supplement. Published March 2018 https://www.cdc.gov/hiv/pdf/risk/prep-cdc-hiv-prep-provider-supplement-2017.pdf.

10. Centers for Disease Control and Prevention. Updated U.S. Public Health Service Guidelines for the Management of Occupational Exposures to HIV and Recommendations for Postexposure Prophylaxis. Update https://stacks.cdc.gov/view/cdc/20711 CDC Stacks. Accessed May 23, 2018.

11. Challacombe SJ. Global inequalities in HIV infection. *Oral Dis.* 2020;26(suppl. 1):16—21.

12. Chung R, ILeung S-YJ, Abel SN, et al. HIV screening in the dental setting in New York State. *PLoS One.* 2020:1—16. https://doi.org/10.1371/journal.pone.0231638.

13. Dale Sannisha K, Traeger L, O'Cleirigh C, et al. High prevalence of metabolic syndrome and cardiovascular disease risk among people with HIV on stable ART. *AIDS Patient Care STDS.* 2016;30(5):215—220. https://doi.org/10.1089/apc.2015.0340.

14. de Oliveira MA, Pallos D, Mecca F, et al. Dental implants in patients seropositive for HIV. A 12-year follow-up study. *J Am Dent Assoc.* 2020;151(11):863—869.

15. Eshleman SH, Khaki L, Laeyendecker O, et al. Detection of individuals with acute HIV-1 infection using the ARCHITECT HIV Ag/Ab Combo assay. *J Acquir Immune Defic Syndr.* 2009;52:121—124.

16. Fact Sheet. UNAIDS World AIDS Day Dec 2020. https://www.unaids.org/sites/default/files/media_asset/UNAIDS_FactSheet_en.pdf.

17. Feller L, Chandran R, Kramer B, et al. Melanocyte biology and function with reference to oral melanin hyperpigmentation in HIV-seropositive subjects. *AIDS Res Hum Retroviruses.* 2014;30(9):837—843.

18. Gallo RC, Salahuddin SZ, Popovic M, et al. Frequent detection and isolation of cytopathic retroviruses (HTLV-III) from patients with AIDS and at risk for AIDS. *Science.* 1984;224:500—503.

19. Gbabe OF, Okwundu CI, Dedicoat M, Freeman EE. Treatment of severe or progressive Kaposi's sarcoma in HIV-infected adults. *Cochrane Database Syst Rev.* 2014;(9):CD003256.

20. Glushko T, He L, McNamee W, Babu AS, Simpson SA. HIV Lymphadenopathy: differential diagnosis and important imaging features. *Am J Roentgenol.* 2021;216:526—533.

21. Greenspan D, Canchola AJ, MacPhail LA, et al. Effect of highly active antiretroviral therapy on frequency of oral warts. *Lancet.* 2001;357(9266):1411—1412.

22. Greenspan JS, Greenspan D, Webster-Cyriaque J. Hairy leukoplakia; lessons learned: 30-plus years. *Oral Dis.* 2016;22(suppl 1):120—127 (1).

23. Hillis DM. AIDS. Origins of HIV. *Science.* 2000;288:1757—1759.

24. Hodgson TA, Greenspan D, Greenspan JS. Oral lesions of HIV disease and HAART in industrialized countries. *Adv Dent Res.* 2006;19:57—62.

25. Levy JA, Hoffman AD, Kramer SM, et al. Isolation of lymphocytopathic retroviruses from San Francisco patients with AIDS. *Science.* 1984;225:840—842.

26. Maddi A. *Management of Periodontal Disease.* New York State: Department of Health AIDS Institute Clinical Guideline; March 2020. https://www.hivguidelines.org/hiv-care/hiv-related-periodontal-disease/. Accessed December 1, 2021.

27. McGowan JP, Fine SM, Merrick ST, et al. *ART Drug-Drug Interactions.* New York State: Department of Health AIDS Institute Clinical Guideline; February 2021. https://www.hivguidelines.org/antiretroviral-therapy/ddis/. Accessed December 7, 2021.

28. Meer S. Human immunodeficiency virus and salivary gland pathology: an update. *Oral Surg Oral Med Oral Pathol Oral Radiol.* 2019;128(1):52—59.

29. Moswin AH, Epstein JB. Essential medical issues related to HIV in dentistry. *J Can Dent Assoc.* 2007;73:945—948.

30. Müller M, Wandel S, Colebunders R, et al. IeDEA Southern and Central Africa: immune reconstitution inflammatory syndrome in patients starting antiretroviral therapy for HIV infection: a systematic review and meta-analysis. *Lancet Infect Dis.* 2010;10:251—261.

31. Muyanja D, Muzoora C, Muyingo A, et al. High prevalence of metabolic syndrome and cardiovascular disease risk among people with HIV on stable ART in Southwestern Uganda. *AIDS Patient Care STDS.* 2016;30(1):4—10. https://doi.org/10.1089/apc.2015.0213.

32. Nwaiwu CA, Egro FM, Smith S, Harper JD, Spiess AM. Seroconversion rate among health care workers exposed to HIV- contaminated body fluids: the University of Pittsburgh 13-year experience. *Am J Infect Control.* 2017;45:896—900.

33. Panel for Antiretroviral Guidelines for Adults and Adolescent. Guidelines for the Use of Antiretroviral Agents in Adults and Adolescents with HIV. Department of Health and Human Services. Available at: http://www.aidsinfo.nih.gov/ContentFiles/Adultand AdolescentGL.pdf. Accessed March 15, 2021.

34. Patton LL. Current strategies for prevention of oral manifestations of human immunodeficiency virus. *Oral Surg Oral Med Oral Pathol Oral Radiol.* 2016;121:29—38.

35. Patton LL, Shugars DC. Immunologic and viral markers of HIV-1 disease progression: implications for dentistry. *J Am Dent Assoc.* 1999;130:1313—1322.

36. Patton LL. Oral lesions associated with human immunodeficiency virus disease dent. *Clin North Am.* 2013;57:673—698.

37. Revised Surveillance Case Definition for HIV Infection — United States, 2014. *MMWR Recomm Rep.* 2014;63(3). https://www.cdc.gov/mmwr/pdf/rr/rr6303.pdf.

38. Robbins MR. Recent recommendations for management of human immunodeficiency virus—positive patients. *Dent Clin North Am.* 2017;61:365—387.

39. Shiboski CH, Patton LL, Webster-Cyriaque JY, et al. The Oral HIV/AIDS Research Alliance: updated case definitions of oral disease endpoints. *J Oral Pathol Med.* 2009;38:481—488.

40. Treatment. Early ART reduces transmission, non-AIDS related health issues. *AIDS Pol Law.* 2015;30(10):1—4.

Allergy

EPIDEMIOLOGY

Allergy is an abnormal or hypersensitive response of the immune system to a substance introduced into the body. It is estimated that more than 25% of Americans demonstrate an allergy to some substance, including approximately 10%−20% who have allergic rhino-conjunctivitis, approximately 7% who have a diagnosed food allergy, approximately 7% who have asthma, approximately 4% who are allergic to insect stings, and between 5% and 10% who are allergic to one or more drugs. Allergic reactions account for up to 10% of all adverse drug reactions. Over 12 million medical office visits per year are due to allergic reactions.

Drugs are the most common cause of urticarial reactions in adults, whereas in children the most common causes are food and infection. Urticaria occurs in 15%−20% of young adults. In approximately 70% of patients with chronic urticaria, an etiologic agent cannot be identified.

Anaphylaxis in dental practice is estimated to occur in 0.004−0.015 cases per dentist per year. Antibiotics account for most drug allergies, with penicillin being one of the more common instigators. About 10% of people who take penicillin develop an allergic reaction, and 0.04%−0.2% of them experience anaphylaxis. Death occurs in about 1%−10% of those persons who experience an anaphylactic reaction, and usually death occurs within 15 min after administration of the drug. Most often, the allergic reaction starts immediately after drug administration. About 70% of affected patients report that they have taken penicillin previously without incident. The most common causes of anaphylactic death are penicillin, bee stings, and wasp stings. People with a history of atopy are more susceptible to anaphylactic death than are patients with no history of allergy. Significant causes of anaphylaxis in clinical practice are listed in Box 19.1.

ETIOLOGY

Allergic reactions classically involve contact with foreign substances, called *allergens* or *antigens*, that trigger hypersensitivity reactions, which involve elements of the innate, humoral, and cellular immune system and the release of chemical mediators (Fig. 19.1). The primary underlying factor is aberrant regulatory activity of T lymphocytes. The CD4+ T helper (T_h) cells, specifically the T_h2 lymphocytes, produce cytokines (interleukins-4, -13, and -5) that stimulate B-lymphocyte synthesis of IgE antibody, which attracts and activates eosinophils. Binding of IgE to mast cells and basophils leads to degranulation and release of additional vasoactive substances.

PATHOPHYSIOLOGY AND COMPLICATIONS

Several drugs used in dentistry and medicine can cause allergic reactions. For example, parabens (used as preservatives in local anesthetics) have caused anaphylactoid reactions. Sulfites (sodium metabisulfite or acetone sodium bisulfite) used in local anesthetic solutions to prevent oxidation of the vasoconstrictors can cause serious allergic reactions. Persons most susceptible to allergic reactions caused by sulfites (i.e., 25 million persons in the United States) are those diagnosed with asthma. Iodinated organic compounds used in radiographic contrast media results in laryngeal edema, seizure, or unconsciousness in about 3% of diagnostic procedures and between one and five deaths per million procedures.

Humoral Immune System

B lymphocytes recognize specific foreign chemical configurations via receptors on their cell membranes. For the antigen to be recognized by specific B lymphocytes, it must first be processed by T lymphocytes and macrophages. Each clone (family) of B lymphocytes recognizes its own specific chemical structure. Once recognition has occurred, B lymphocytes differentiate and multiply, forming plasma cells and memory B lymphocytes. Memory B lymphocytes remain inactive until contact is made with the same type of antigen, transforming the memory cell into a plasma cell that produces immunoglobulins (antibodies) specific for the antigen involved. Box 19.2 lists the five classes of immunoglobulins and their functions. Note that immunoglobulin E is the key antibody involved in the pathogenesis of type I hypersensitivity reactions. Normal functions of the humoral immune system are shown in Box 19.3.

Type I, II, and III hypersensitivity reactions involve elements of the humoral immune system.

Type I Hypersensitivity. Type I hypersensitivity involves contact with common exposures such as dust, mites, pollens, animal danders, food (e.g., shellfish, nuts, eggs, milk), drugs (e.g., antibiotics: sulfa drugs, penicillins, cephalosporins), or insect bites (e.g., bee stings). This is an IgE-mediated reaction that leads to the release of chemical mediators from mast cells and basophils in various target tissues, which leads to release of histamine, leukotrienes, and interleukins. These mediators cause

vascular dilation and endothelial leakage and can induce smooth muscle contraction. In addition, these molecules attract CD4+ T lymphocytes, eosinophils, and basophils, which can extend the reaction time and alter healing. Usually type I reactions occur soon after second contact with an antigen; however, many people have repeated contacts with a specific drug or material before developing an allergic reaction (Fig. 19.2). Type I hypersensitivity include atopy (clinically appears as hay fever, asthma, urticaria, or angioedema), and anaphylaxis.

Atopy is a hypersensitivity state that is influenced by hereditary factors. Hay fever, asthma, urticaria, and angioedema are examples of atopic reactions. Lesions most commonly associated with atopic reactions include *urticaria*, a superficial lesion of the skin, and *angioedema*, which is edema that occurs in the deeper layers (i.e., dermis or subcutaneous tissues) and often involves diffuse enlargement of the lips, infraorbital tissues, larynx, or tongue. In true allergic reactions, these lesions result from the effects of antigens and their antibodies on mast cells in various locations in the body. As is typical for type I hypersensitivity, the antigen—antibody complex causes the release of mediators (histamine) from mast cells. These mediators then produce increased permeability of adjacent vascular structures, resulting in leakage of intravascular fluid into surrounding tissue spaces—this is seen clinically as urticaria, angioedema, and secretions associated with hay fever.

There are several types of angioedema and three types of interest to dentistry: allergic, acquired, and hereditary angioedema. *Acquired angioedema* is allergic (histamine) based. For the *allergic type* see the previous Type I hypersensitivity. *Drug-induced angioedema* is also form of acquired angioedema which results from impaired bradykinin degradation after administration of certain drugs, such as angiotensin-converting enzyme inhibitors. *Hereditary angioedema* is a rare genetic disorder caused by a deficiency or dysfunction of complement C1 esterase inhibitor, which can be triggered by stress, trauma (e.g., extractions, oral surgery), or infections. These triggers lead to activation of the complement cascade and Hageman factor (factor XII) and overproduction of bradykinin. The hereditary form can produce variable manifestations, including recurrent and sudden episodes of angioedema with swelling of the skin or mucosa of the extremities, oropharynx, or abdominal structures, the latter resulting in severe abdominal pain.

Anaphylaxis is an acute reaction involving the smooth muscle of the bronchi in which antigen—IgE antibody complexes form on the surface of mast cells, resulting in sudden histamine release from these cells. The release of histamine, as well as other vasoactive mediators, leads to smooth muscle contraction and increased vascular permeability. The potential end result is acute respiratory compromise, cardiovascular collapse, and death.

Type II Hypersensitivity. Type II (cytotoxic) hypersensitivity are IgG- or IgM-mediated reactions that result in

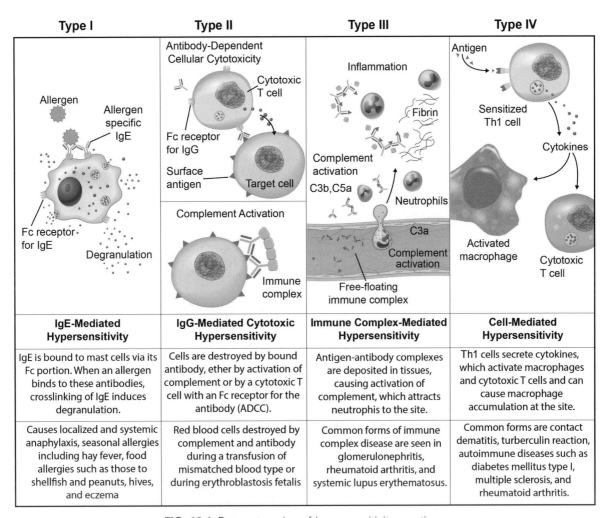

Type I	Type II	Type III	Type IV
IgE-Mediated Hypersensitivity	**IgG-Mediated Cytotoxic Hypersensitivity**	**Immune Complex-Mediated Hypersensitivity**	**Cell-Mediated Hypersensitivity**
IgE is bound to mast cells via its Fc portion. When an allergen binds to these antibodies, crosslinking of IgE induces degranulation.	Cells are destroyed by bound antibody, ether by activation of complement or by a cytotoxic T cell with an Fc receptor for the antibody (ADCC).	Antigen-antibody complexes are deposited in tissues, causing activation of complement, which attracts neutrophis to the site.	Th1 cells secrete cytokines, which activate macrophages and cytotoxic T cells and can cause macrophage accumulation at the site.
Causes localized and systemic anaphylaxis, seasonal allergies including hay fever, food allergies such as those to shellfish and peanuts, hives, and eczema	Red blood cells destroyed by complement and antibody during a transfusion of mismatched blood type or during erythroblastosis fetalis	Common forms of immune complex disease are seen in glomerulonephritis, rheumatoid arthritis, and systemic lupus erythematosus.	Common forms are contact dematitis, turberculin reaction, autoimmune diseases such as diabetes mellitus type I, multiple sclerosis, and rheumatoid arthritis.

FIG. 19.1 Four categories of hypersensitivity reactions.

destruction of the targeted cells by complement and antibodies. The classic example of type II hypersensitivity is transfusion reaction caused by mismatched blood.

Type III Hypersensitivity. Type III hypersensitivity, or *immune complex—mediated hypersensitivity*, occurs when there is excess antigen in the bloodstream. These antigens are bound with antibody, forming immune complexes of different size within blood vessels. The antigen—antibody complexes migrate under the basement membrane of small blood vessels, which sets off the complement cascade, particularly involving C3b and C5aa. Macrophages remove the large complexes, but the small complexes are ineffectively removed and accumulate in small blood vessels (capillaries and glomeruli) and in joints. This leads to an inflammatory response with key features of vasculitis, swelling, and pain. Clinical examples include serum sickness, vasculitis, and streptococcal glomerulonephritis.

Cellular Immune System

In the cellular or delayed immune system, T lymphocytes play the central role. The primary function of this system is to recognize and eradicate antigens that are fixed in tissues or within cells. This system is involved in protection against viruses, tuberculosis, and leprosy. Antibodies are not operative in the cell-mediated immune system; however, effector T lymphocytes produce various cytokines that serve as active agents of this system. For example, T_h1 lymphocytes can produce cytokines (IL-4, -5, -13) that stimulate B lymphocytes to produce IgE antibody.

Type IV Hypersensitivity. Type IV *delayed* hypersensitivity reactions involve the cellular immune system and cytokine release; they are not antibody mediated. Common conditions associated with type IV hypersensitivity are contact dermatitis, transplant rejection, and graft-versus-host disease. The sequential events involved in type IV hypersensitivity include dendritic cells and Langerhans cells that ingest a foreign antigen and present it to undifferentiated T lymphocytes. This response is mediated by sensitized CD4+ T lymphocytes, which release cytokines (IL-2 and interferon gamma). The lymphokines promote a T_h1 reaction mediated by macrophages that begins in hours and peaks in 2—3 days, hence the term *delayed hypersensitivity*.

BOX 19.2 Functions of Immunoglobulins

- Immunoglobulin (Ig) G
  - Most abundant immunoglobulin
  - Small size allows diffusion into tissue spaces
  - Can cross the placenta
  - Opsonizing antibody—facilitates phagocytosis of microorganisms by neutrophils
  - Four subclasses: IgG1, IgG2, IgG3, IgG4 (IgG can bind to mast cells)
- IgA
  - Two types
  - Secretory (dimer, secretory components)—found in saliva, tears, and nasal mucus; secretory component protects from proteolysis
  - Serum (monomer)
  - Does not cross the placenta
  - Last immunoglobulin to appear in childhood
- IgM
  - Large molecule
  - Confined to intravascular space
  - First immunoglobulin produced
  - Activates complement
  - Good agglutinating antibody
- IgE
  - Very low concentration in serum (0.004%)
  - Increased in parasitic and atopic diseases
  - Binds to mast cells and basophils
  - Key antibody in pathogenesis of type I hypersensitivity reactions
- IgD
  - Low concentration in serum
  - Minor importance

BOX 19.3 Functions of the Humoral Immune System

1. First encounter with antigen (primary response)
   a. Latent period
      - Antigen is processed
      - B lymphocyte clone is selected
      - Differentiation and proliferation
      - Plasma cells produce specific immunoglobulins.
   b. Specific immunoglobulin (Ig)M level increases first in serum followed by IgG.
   c. IgM levels later fall to zero.
   d. IgG levels fall; however, some stay the same.
2. Second encounter with antigen (secondary response)
   a. Latent period is shorter
      - Antigen is processed
      - Memory cells are selected; become plasma cells
      - Plasma cells produce specific immunoglobulins.
   b. IgM levels increase first.
   c. IgG levels increase to 50 times the level found in the primary response.
   d. IgM levels fall later.
   e. IgG levels fall later, but a significant serum level is usually maintained.

Some of the more common antigens that cause contact dermatitis include metal jewelry, perfumes, rubber products, chemicals such as formaldehyde, and drugs such as topical anesthetics. Contact allergy occurs when a substance of low molecular weight that is not antigenic by itself comes in contact with a tissue component (primarily a protein) and forms an antigenic complex. This small molecule is called a *hapten* (or one-half of an antigen), and the resulting complex causes sensitization of T lymphocytes.

Poison ivy is an example of a contact allergy wherein the reaction is delayed (with response occurring 48–72 h after contact is made with the allergen). Infectious-type allergic reactions are exemplified by the tuberculin skin test, in which a person who has previously been exposed to *Mycobacterium tuberculosis* develops a delayed response, usually within 48–72 h after a second exposure to components of the bacteria. This response is characterized by induration, erythema, swelling, and sometimes ulceration at the site of injection.

Graft rejection occurs when organs or tissues from one body are transplanted into another body. Cellular rejection of transplanted tissue occurs unless the donor and

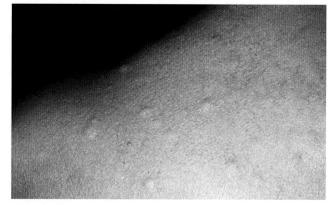

FIG. 19.2 This generalized urticarial reaction occurred after injection of penicillin for treatment of an acute oral infection. The patient had previously taken penicillin a number of times without any problem.

recipient are appropriately HLA matched or the host immune response has been suppressed by immunomodulatory medications. Graft-versus-host reaction is an unusual phenomenon that occurs in bone marrow transplant recipients whose cellular immune system, which has been effectively replaced by the donor cells, recognizes host tissues as foreign and mounts an inflammatory response that has been rendered deficient by whole-body irradiation. Lymphocytes transferred to the host attempt to destroy host tissues.

Other examples of Type IV hypersensitivity include diabetes type 1 in which pancreatic beta cells are attacked, the lymphocytic attack of oligodendrocyte proteins causing the demyelinated disease multiple sclerosis, and the lymphocytic infiltrate that occurs with Hashimoto thyroiditis.

Nonallergic Reactions or Pseudoallergy

Other agents may cause mast cells to release their mediators without inciting a true allergic reaction; this occurs in cases of chronic urticaria caused by certain drugs (e.g., meperidine), temperature changes, emotional states, and in some reactions to drugs. Most so-called anaphylactic reactions to local anesthetics do not involve an antigen–antibody reaction but result from damage to the mast cells caused by other mechanisms. These reactions are referred to as anaphylactoid or *anaphylaxis-like* reactions, and from a clinical standpoint, the approach to management of these patients are similar.

Nonallergic cases of urticaria, angioedema, and anaphylactoid reactions are caused by the nonspecific release of vasoactive amines from mast cells or by the activation of other forms of nonspecific immunologic effectors involving the complement system and Hageman factor–dependent pathway. One example is hereditary angioedema, in which tissue swelling is triggered by stress, trauma, or infections because of an underlying absence or dysfunction of C1 inhibitor, a protein that regulates the complement cascade pathway and the production of bradykinin.

LABORATORY AND DIAGNOSTIC FINDINGS

Patients with IgE-mediated allergy can have elevated levels of total IgE, allergen-specific IgE, and eosinophils in their serum or nasal passages and test positive to a specific allergen after skin testing (patch or skin-prick testing) performed by an allergist. Tryptase blood tests are helpful in diagnosing anaphylaxis. Patients who have hereditary angioedema typically have low C4 levels and low levels of C1 inhibitor or low functional activity of C1 inhibitor and mutations in the C1-inhibitor/*SERPING1* gene as determined by genetic testing.

MEDICAL MANAGEMENT

Patients with atopy may be given serial, increasing doses of the antigen by injection over several weeks to gradually desensitize them so that they are no longer allergic to the antigen. Patients with asthma (see Chapter 7), immune complex injury, or cytotoxic immune reactions may be treated with systemic steroids, and those with hay fever or urticaria are treated with antihistamines. Newer antihistamines are highly effective and produce fewer adverse effects (e.g., drowsiness) than older antihistamines (Table 19.1).

A variety of treatments, including topical steroids, have been used for patients with contact dermatitis. From a dental standpoint, a patient who is being treated for

TABLE 19.1 Examples of Second- and Third-Generation Antihistamines

Drug	Trade Name(s)	OTC[a]
Acrivastine	Semprex, Benadryl Allergy Relief capsules	No
Cetirizine	Zyrtec	Yes
Desloratadine	Neoclarityn	No
Fexofenadine	Telfast 120, Telfast 180, Allegra	No
Levocetirizine	Xyzal	No
Loratadine	Claritin, Clarityn, Clarityne, Boots antihistamine tablets	Yes
Mizolastine	Mizollen, Mistamine (superseded by fexofenadine)	No
Rupatadine	Rupafin, Rupax, Ralif	No

[a]Some of these medicines can be purchased without a doctor's prescription in the United States.
OTC, over the counter.

allergies has an increased chance of being allergic to another substance. In addition, if the person is taking steroids, the body's reaction to stress may be impaired (see Chapter 15).

DENTAL MANAGEMENT

Identification and Risk Assessment

Dentists should identify patients with allergies from their medical history. Efforts should be directed toward determining the type, extent, length of the reaction, and what was done to treat it. One of the most common concerns is a patient who reports allergy to a local anesthetic, antibiotic, or analgesic. In this case, the history must be expanded, with specific efforts made to determine exactly what the offending substance was and exactly how the patient reacted. If the adverse reaction was of an allergic nature, one or more of the classic signs or symptoms of allergy should have been present (Box 19.4). If these signs or symptoms were not reported, the patient probably did not experience a true allergic reaction. Common examples of reactions mislabeled as "allergy" are syncope after injection of a local anesthetic, and nausea or vomiting after ingestion of an opioid (e.g., codeine). An adverse drug reaction may be mistaken for allergy and efforts should be made to determine the actual condition. Types of adverse drug reactions are listed in Box 19.5.

Anesthetics

A common "nonallergic" reaction to local anesthetics involves an anxious patient who, because of concern about receiving a "shot," experiences a psychogenic reaction that includes hyperventilation, tachycardia, sweating, pallor, and syncope. True allergic reactions to the local anesthetics (amides) used in dentistry are rare.

BOX 19.4   Signs and Symptoms Suggestive of an Allergic Reaction

- Urticaria
- Swelling
- Skin rash
- Chest tightness
- Dyspnea, shortness of breath
- Rhinorrhea
- Conjunctivitis

BOX 19.5   Adverse Drug Reactions

Predictable
- Dose related
- No immunologic basis
- Account for about 80% of all adverse reactions to drugs
- Direct toxicity
- Overdose
- Drug interaction
- Adverse effects of drugs

Unpredictable
- Not dose related
- Unrelated to expected pharmacologic effects
- Allergy
- Pseudoallergy (anaphylactoid reactions)
- Idiosyncrasy
- Intolerance
- Paradoxical reactions (cause histamine release but not IgE-mediated)
- Underlying genetic defect often present

Data from Lichtenstein LM, Busse WW, Geha R, eds. *Current Therapy in Allergy, Immunology, and Rheumatology.* 6th ed. St. Louis: Mosby; 2004.

BOX 19.6   Adverse Reactions to Local Anesthetics

- Allergic reaction
- Anxiety (syncope)
- CNS stimulation → CNS depression → Toxicity (talkativeness, excitement, euphoria; slurred speech, dizziness, depression, convulsions)
- Vasoconstrictor effects (heart palpitations)

CNS, central nervous system.

Data from Malamed SF. Allergy and toxic reactions to local anesthetics. *Dent Today.* 22:114–116, 118–121, 2003.

Local anesthetics containing a vasoconstrictor can cause an epinephrine reaction (tachycardia, sweating, paleness), which usually results from inadvertent intravenous injection (Box 19.6). Excessive amounts of an anesthetic (e.g., multiple carpules) also can cause a toxic reaction. Signs and symptoms associated with toxic reactions to a local anesthetic are characterized by talkativeness, slurred speech, dizziness, disorientation, euphoria, and nausea followed by muscle twitching or convulsions, mental and respiratory depression, unconsciousness, coma, and cardiovascular collapse.

If the patient reports having experienced a toxic or vasoconstrictor reaction, the dentist should explain the likely cause of the previous reaction and should avoid injecting the local anesthetic solution intravenously by aspirating before injection and limiting the amount of solution. If the patient's history supports a fainting episode and not a toxic or allergic reaction, the dentist's primary task is to reduce the patient's anxiety before and during the dental visit.

If the history supports a true allergic reaction to a local anesthetic, the dentist should try to identify the type of local anesthetic that was used. After this has been ascertained, a new anesthetic with a different basic chemical structure can be used. The two main groups of local anesthetics in dentistry consist of the following:

1. *Para*-aminobenzoic acid (PABA) esters (procaine [Novocain] and tetracaine [Pontocaine])
2. Amides (articaine [Septocaine], bupivacaine [Marcaine], lidocaine [Xylocaine], mepivacaine [Carbocaine], and prilocaine [Citanest])

The benzoic acid ester anesthetics may cross-react with each other, but amide anesthetics usually do not cross-react. Cross-reaction does not occur between ester and amide local anesthetics.

Procaine is the local anesthetic associated with the highest incidence of allergic reactions. Currently, it is available only in multidose vials. Its antigenic component appears to be PABA, one of the metabolic breakdown products of procaine. Lidocaine or another amide local anesthetic should be used for patients with a history of allergy to procaine.

Patients who have been allergic to local anesthetics but who cannot identify the specific agent to which they reacted present more of a diagnostic problem. The nature of the reaction must be established (Box 19.7), by referral to an allergist to determine the nature and extent of the actual allergy. If indeed it is consistent with an allergic reaction, the next step should be to attempt to identify the actual anesthetic used. When the patient is unable to provide this information, the dentist can attempt to contact the previous dentist involved. If this fails, two additional options are available:

- An antihistamine (e.g., diphenhydramine [Benadryl]) can be used as the local anesthetic.
- The patient may be referred to an allergist for provocative dose testing (PDT).

BOX 19.7	Checklist for Dental Management of Patients With a Drug Allergy[a]

PREOPERATIVE RISK ASSESSMENT
- Review medical history, determine whether drug allergy exists.
- Determine the type and severity or previous allergic reaction(s).
- Obtain a medical consultation (i.e., refer to physician) if undiagnosed of if uncertain.

A

Anesthesia	Establish history of reaction after use of local anesthetic.
Anxiety	Distinguish that the reaction is not a vasovagal or syncopal reaction associated with anxiety.
Allergy	Determine the type of anesthetic used that triggered the allergy. A patient experiencing a true allergic reaction will demonstrate one or more of the following: soft tissue swelling, skin rash, rhinitis, or difficulty breathing. If the reaction is consistent with allergic reaction, the following should be done: Select anesthetic from a different chemical group: (1) Para-aminobenzoic acid (procaine) (2) Amide (lidocaine, mepivacaine, articaine) Aspirate, inject 1 drop of alternate anesthetic, and wait 5 min; if no reaction occurs, inject after the rest of the anesthetic needed is aspirated (be prepared to deal with an allergic reaction if one occurs).

B

Bleeding	No issues.
Breathing	Breathing difficulties can be avoided by avoiding the allergen (e.g., local anesthetic) until after allergy testing is completed; thereafter use a drug (e.g., local anesthetic) to which patient is not allergic.
Blood pressure	Monitor blood pressure during severe allergic reaction.

C

Chair position	During allergic reaction with a conscious patient, place in comfortable position. With unconscious patient, place in supine position.

D

Drugs	In cases of allergic reaction to several local anesthetic agents or when a previously used anesthetic cannot be identified, consider using diphenhydramine. Have injectable epinephrine (1:1000) and diphenhydramine available.

E

Equipment	Emergency kit should be up to date and readily available.
Emergencies or urgencies	For severe allergic reaction (e.g., anaphylaxis), inject 0.3–0.5 mL of 1:1000 epinephrine through an IM (into the tongue) or SC route; supplement with IV diphenhydramine 50–100 mg if needed. Support respiration, if indicated, by mouth-to-mouth breathing or bag and mask.

F

Follow-up	If history includes allergy to multiple substances, or if type of local anesthetic used previously cannot be identified, refer the patient to an allergist for PDT. Follow up with physician regarding results of tests.

[a]Strength of recommendation taxonomy (SORT) Grade: C (see Preface for further explanation).
IM, intramuscular; *IV*, intravenous; *PDT*, provocative dose testing; *SC*, subcutaneous.

The use of diphenhydramine often is the more practical option. A 1% solution of diphenhydramine that contains 1:100,000 epinephrine can be easily compounded by a pharmacist. This solution induces anesthesia for approximately 30 min and can be used for infiltration or block injection. When it is used for a mandibular block, 1–4 mL of solution is needed. Some patients have reported a burning sensation, swelling, or erythema after a mandibular block with 1% diphenhydramine, but these effects were not serious and cleared within 1 or 2 days. No more than 50 mg of diphenhydramine should be given during a single appointment. Diphenhydramine also can be used in patients who report a previous allergic reaction to either an ester or amide local anesthetic.

The dentist may elect to refer the patient to an allergist for evaluation and testing, which usually includes both skin testing and PDT. Skin testing alone for allergy to local anesthetics is of little benefit because false-positive results are common; therefore, the allergist also should perform PDT.

The allergist, based on the patient's history, selects a local anesthetic for testing that is least likely to cause an allergic reaction; this usually is an anesthetic from the amide group because they generally do not cross-react with each other. At 15-min intervals, 0.1 mL of test solution is injected subcutaneously, with concentrations increasing from 1:10,000 to 1:1000 to 1:100 to 1:10, followed by undiluted solution; next, 0.5 mL of undiluted test solution is tried; and finally, 1 mL of undiluted solution is given. During PDT, the allergist should be prepared to deal with any adverse reaction that might occur and should report to the dentist on the drug selected, the final dose given, and the presence or absence of any adverse reaction. After testing, a local anesthetic that does not cause a reaction can be used safely, with the risk of an allergic reaction being no greater than in the general population.

When administering an alternative anesthetic to a patient with a history of a true local anesthetic allergy, the dentist should follow these steps:

1. Inject slowly, aspirating first to make sure that a vessel is not being injected.
2. Place 1 drop of the solution into the tissues.
3. Withdraw the needle and wait 5 min to observe for any potential reaction (e.g., urticaria, rhinitis, edema, etc.). If an allergic reaction does not occur, the anesthetic can be delivered at the recommended dose for the procedure. Be sure to aspirate before giving the second injection.

Antibiotics: Penicillin

Penicillin is used frequently throughout the world and is a common cause of drug allergy. In the United States, up to 10% of the population is allergic to penicillin and penicillin-related drugs. About 1–5 in 10,000 patients treated with penicillin develop an anaphylactic reaction, which is fatal in about 1 in 100,000 of penicillin-treated patients, accounting for some 400 to 800 deaths per year. The possibility of sensitizing a patient to penicillin varies with different routes of administration, as follows: Oral administration results in sensitization of only about 0.1% of patients, and intramuscular injection in about 1%–2%. Thus, the oral route is preferable for administration whenever possible. Parenteral administration of penicillin evokes a more serious reaction than that typically associated with oral administration. Antibodies produced against penicillin cross-react with the semisynthetic penicillins (i.e., Ampicillin, Penicillinase, Cloxacillin, Methicillin, et al.) and may cause severe reactions in patients who are allergic to penicillin. Nevertheless, the synthetic penicillins seem to cause fewer new sensitizations in patients who are not allergic to penicillin at the time of administration.

Skin testing for allergy to penicillin is more reliable than is skin testing for allergy to a local anesthetic; however, some risk is involved, and the vast majority (~90%) are negative when skin tested. Thus to be cost-effective, the test should be conducted only on patients with a history of penicillin reaction who need penicillin for a serious infection. Penicillin reactivity declines with time; hence, a patient may have reacted to the drug years ago but is now no longer sensitive by testing (i.e., negative skin test result). Most anaphylactic reactions to penicillin occur in patients who have been treated in the past with penicillin but reported no adverse reactions.

In dentistry, a patient who self-reports allergy to penicillin should be carefully interviewed to determine the plausibility of the allergy. If the information provided is convincing, then the patient is generally best treated with an alternative antibiotic. For example, patients with a history of penicillin allergy should be given an alternate antibiotic for the treatment of oral infection or a cephalosporin, azithromycin, or clarithromycin for prophylaxis against infective endocarditis.

Although cephalosporins are often used as alternatives to penicillins, cephalosporins cross-react in 5%–10% of penicillin-sensitive patients (Box 19.8). The risk is

---

BOX 19.8   Use of Cephalosporins in Patients With a History of Penicillin Hypersensitivity

Cephaloyl, a major metabolite of cephalosporins, can cross-react with major determinant of penicillin (penicilloyl polylysine).

Risk of adverse reaction to cephalosporin is controversial.

- Greatest with first- or second-generation drugs:
  - Cephaloridine (16.5%), cephalothin (5%), cephalexin (5.4%)
- Anaphylaxis
  - Positive history of penicillin reaction, 0.1%
  - Negative history of penicillin reaction, 0.4%
- Urticaria
  - Positive history of penicillin reaction, 1.3%
  - Negative history of penicillin reaction, 0.4%

Patient with history of penicillin reaction: first skin test for penicillin sensitivity

- Negative—Use penicillin or a cephalosporin.
- Positive
  - Avoid penicillin.
  - Skin test is specific for cephalosporin; use cephalosporin if result is negative.

Data from Lichtenstein LM, Busse WW, Geha RS. *Current Therapy in Allergy, Immunology and Rheumatology.* 6th ed. London: Mosby; 2004.

---

greatest with first- and second-generation drugs. Cephalosporins are metabolized to their major determinant, cephaloyl, which may cross-react with the major determinant of penicillin. Cephalosporins usually can be used in patients with a history of distant past, nonserious reaction to penicillin. However, skin testing is recommended for these patients. If the patient's penicillin skin test result is negative, then penicillin or a cephalosporin may be used. If the penicillin skin test result is positive, a skin test for the specific cephalosporin selected should be performed (Box 19.9).

Analgesics

Allergic reactions to aspirin can be serious and deaths have been reported. Aspirin provokes a severe reaction in some patients with asthma. They may react in the same way to other nonsteroidal antiinflammatory drugs (NSAIDs) that inhibit cyclooxygenase, which is the key enzyme involved in the generation of prostaglandin from arachidonic acid. The typical reaction consists of acute bronchospasm, rhinorrhea, and urticaria. Most patients with asthma who react to NSAIDs also have nasal polyps and nasal eosinophilia. The mechanism for this reaction involves abnormal (increased) leukotriene E4 levels as a result of synthesis by the eosinophils. NSAIDs should not be given to these patients, and the dentist should be aware of the many combination analgesic preparations that include aspirin or other salicylates. These agents must not be given to the patient who may develop an adverse reaction associated with aspirin or other

---

BOX 19.9   Procedures for Prevention of a Penicillin Reaction

1. Have emergency kit available.
2. Take medical history on all patients, including the following:
   a. Previous contact with penicillin
   b. Reactions to penicillin
   c. Allergic reactions to other agents
3. Do not use penicillin in patient with a history of reactions to drugs.
4. Inform patient.
5. Do not use penicillin in topical preparations; instead use oral formulations when indicated.
6. Do not use penicillinase-resistant penicillins unless infection is caused by penicillinase-producing staphylococci.
7. Use disposable syringes for injection of penicillin.
8. Have patient wait in office for 30 min after first dose of penicillin is given.
9. Inform patient about signs and symptoms of allergic reaction to penicillin and, if these occur, to seek immediate medical assistance.

---

salicylates. Also, NSAIDs should not be given to certain patients with an ulcer or hemorrhagic disease, pregnant or nursing mothers, and patients with advanced renal disease.

Dental Materials and Products

Type I, III, and IV hypersensitivity reactions have been reported to result from various dental materials and products. Topical anesthetic agents have been reported to cause type I reactions consisting of urticarial swelling. Mouth rinses and toothpastes containing phenolic compounds, antiseptics, astringents, or flavoring agents have been known to cause type I, III, and IV hypersensitivity reactions involving the oral mucosa or lips, characterized by erythema, swelling, and itching. Hand soaps used by dental care workers also have been reported as a cause of type IV reactions. Some dental agents that can lead to type IV hypersensitivity of the oral mucosa (contact stomatitis) include dental amalgam, acrylic, composite resin, nickel, palladium, chromium, cobalt, eugenol, rubber products, talcum powder, mouthwashes, and toothpastes.

Latex Rubber Products. A number of reports have demonstrated that certain health care workers and patients are at risk for hypersensitivity reactions to latex or agents used in the production of rubber gloves or related materials (e.g., rubber dam, blood pressure cuff, catheters). Up to 6% of the general public and up to 18% of health care providers are hypersensitive to latex. Although most cases in health providers are type IV reactions, caused by agents used in the production of rubber products, serious type I hypersensitivity reactions

may occur in physicians, dentists, other health care workers, and patients as the result of contact with latex products such as gloves, rubber dams, or catheters.

Dentists should be aware that latex allergy can manifest as anaphylaxis when the patient or the dentist has been sensitized to latex. Studies have shown that latex-allergic persons have IgE antibodies for specific latex proteins. Latex skin tests are a satisfactory means of identifying individuals who may be sensitized to latex. Nitrile gloves and latex-free rubber dam should be considered for use to minimize these adverse reactions to latex proteins.

Hereditary Angioedema

Hereditary angioedema is a condition that can be provoked by infection, stress, trauma, or dental surgery. It is best managed by implementation of preventive measures but could possibly progress to severe angioedema. Attenuated androgens, such as danazol and stanozolol, are used prophylactically to increase hepatic production of C1 inhibitor and help decrease the number and severity of attacks. Recombinant C1 inhibitor concentrate (Cinryze or Berinert), while expensive, may be indicated in more severe cases. Use of such preventive agents is important because hereditary angioedema does not respond well to epinephrine or antihistamines. Fresh frozen plasma or antifibrinolytic agents may be used as well.

Treatment Planning Modifications

Dentists should obtain a history of any allergic reactions when obtaining a patient's medical history. If a patient has a history of allergy to drugs or materials that may be used in dentistry, a clear entry should be made in the dental record, and any further contact with or use of the antigen(s) should be avoided in that patient. Most allergic patients can receive any indicated dental treatment as long as the antigen is avoided and precautions are taken for patients receiving steroids or who are predisposed to angioedema. Drugs that can abort an allergic reaction should be readily available in all dental offices.

ORAL COMPLICATIONS AND MANIFESTATIONS

Hypersensitivity

Type I Hypersensitivity. Oral lesions can be produced by type I hypersensitivity reactions. Atopic reactions to various foods, drugs, or anesthetic agents may occur within or around the oral cavity and usually are characterized by urticarial swelling or angioedema (Fig. 19.3). The reaction generally is rapid, with soft tissue swelling developing within a short time after coming into contact with the antigen. The painless swelling, produced by transudate from the surrounding vessels, may cause

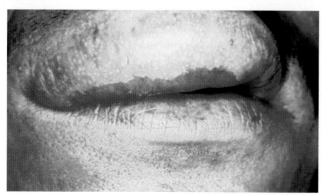

FIG. 19.3 Angioedema of the upper lip that occurred soon after injection of a local anesthetic.

itching and burning. The lesion can last for 1–3 days if untreated but will resolve spontaneously. Oral antihistamines should be given; oral diphenhydramine, 25–50 mg every 4–6 h, as needed. Treatment is provided for 1–3 days. Further contact with the antigen must be avoided (Box 19.10).

Type III Hypersensitivity. Foods, drugs, or agents that are placed within the oral cavity can cause white, erythematous, or ulcerative lesions representative of type III hypersensitivity or immune complex reactions. These lesions develop usually within a 24-h period, after contact is made with the offending antigen. Some cases of aphthous stomatitis (Fig. 19.4) may be caused by type III hypersensitivity, but most are related to immune dysfunction that has not been fully characterized. Fig. 19.5 shows an allergic dermatitis that occurred after orthodontic brackets and archwires (containing nickel) were placed. Hypersensitivity reactions to orthodontic appliances are rare and seldom occur unless the patient has nickel hypersensitivity and a history of previous cutaneous or skin piercing.

Erythema multiforme represents an immune complex reaction that appears as polymorphous eruption of macules, erosions, and characteristic "target" lesions that are symmetrically distributed on the skin or mucosa. Common sites in the mouth are the lips, buccal mucosa, and tongue (Fig. 19.6). In about half of affected patients, a predisposing factor such as a drug allergy or a herpes simplex infection is involved in the onset of their disease. Sulfa antibiotics are frequently associated with the onset of erythema multiforme. Sulfonyl urea hypoglycemic agents (e.g., tolbutamide, tolazamide, glyburide, glipizide) used to treat diabetes also have been associated with the onset of erythema multiforme. Many patients with erythema multiforme can be treated with symptomatic therapy, including a bland mouth rinse, syrup of diphenhydramine, and topical or systemic corticosteroids (see Appendix C for treatment regimens). If a drug appears to be associated with onset of the disease, the drug should be withdrawn and any further contact with it should be avoided.

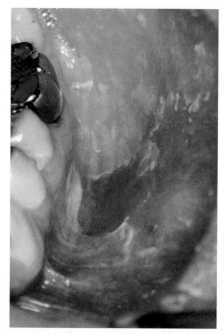

FIG. 19.4 Stomatitis in a patient who was found to be allergic to the toothpaste he was using. (From Neville BW, Damm DD, Allen CM, et al. *Oral and Maxillofacial Pathology.* 3rd ed. St. Louis: Saunders; 2009.)

Type IV Hypersensitivity. Contact stomatitis is a delayed allergic reaction that often is associated with the cellular immune response. Because of the delayed nature of the reaction after contact is made with the allergen, the dentist must inquire about contacts with materials that may have occurred days before the lesions appeared. The antigen may be found in dental materials, toothpaste, mouth rinses, lipsticks, cosmetics, and so forth. In many cases, no further treatment is necessary after the source of

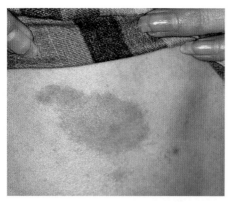

FIG. 19.5 Allergic rash on the abdomen of a patient in whom orthodontic brackets and archwires were just placed. The patient was tested and was found to be allergic to the nickel in the wires.

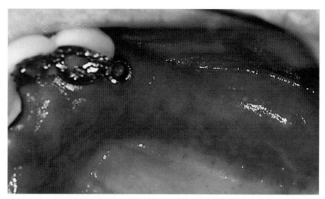

FIG. 19.7 Allergic reaction to removable partial denture framework. Note the erythematous demarcation.

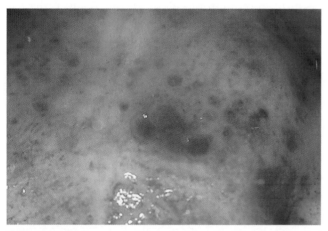

FIG. 19.6 Erythema multiforme that developed after oral administration of a drug used to treat an oral infection. Ulceration of the palatal mucosa.

the antigen has been identified and removed from further contact with the patient; however, if the tissue reaction is severe or persistent, topical corticosteroids should be used (see Appendix C for treatment regimens).

Various dental materials have been reported as the cause of allergic reactions in patients. Impression materials containing an aromatic sulfonate catalyst have been reported to cause a delayed allergic reaction in postmenopausal women. The reactive lesion consists of tissue ulceration and necrosis that becomes progressively worse with each exposure.

Some investigators have reported that oral lesions may be found in close association with amalgam restorations. These (mucosal) lesions appear as whitish, reddish, ulcerative, or "lichenoid" and appear to be a hypersensitivity reaction to components of the amalgam restoration. When these restorations are removed, the lesions are most often clear. Reports have suggested that some of the oral lesions resulted from toxic injury to the mucosa, and the majority are a result of type IV hypersensitivity reaction to heavy metals in amalgam.

Several studies performed to date have not correlated symptoms such as depression, fatigue, and headache with the effects of mercury in amalgam restorations. The practice of avoiding the use of amalgam restorations in patients with these nonspecific symptoms has, at present, no scientific basis. However, removal of any amalgam restorations in contact with oral mucosa that shows lesions consistent with a toxic or hypersensitivity reaction to mercury is rational.

On rare occasions, dental composite materials have been reported to cause allergic reactions. The acrylic monomer used in denture construction has caused an allergic reaction; however, the vast majority of tissue changes under dentures result from trauma and secondary infection with bacteria or fungi. Gold, nickel, and mercury have been reported to cause allergic reactions that result in tissue erythema and ulceration (Fig. 19.7).

The dentist may wish to test agents that are thought to be possible antigens that cause oral lesions. Oral epimucous testing for contact stomatitis consists of placing the suspected antigen in contact with the oral mucosa and observing for any reaction over a period of several days (e.g., erythema, sloughing, ulceration) that might indicate an allergy to the test material. In most cases, a reaction is not expected to develop for at least 48–72 h. Various techniques have been used to conduct epimucous testing for suspected allergens. One of these involves placing the suspected allergen in a rubber suction cup, placing the cup on the buccal mucosa, and observing at intervals for erythema or ulceration under the cup. Another technique is to place a sample of the suspected antigen in a depression on the palatal aspect of an overlay denture. The denture is inserted and holds the allergen in contact with the palatal mucosa.

Another technique consists of incorporating the allergen into Orabase, applying the Orabase to the mucobuccal fold, and periodically observing for a reaction. Alternately, the antigen can be incorporated into an oral adhesive spray. Skin testing and oral epimucous testing for potential antigens are not foolproof by any means; in certain patients, they yield unreliable tissue responses. The response in some cases may be caused by trauma; in other cases, in which a tissue reaction does not occur, the patient may still be allergic to the substance.

Basic management of contact stomatitis requires removal of common sources of antigens known to cause hypersensitivity reactions and assessment for lesion healing. After the offending agent or antigen has been identified, the patient should be told to avoid any future contact with the antigen. Again, if the lesions persist, topical steroids can be applied (see Appendix C).

Lichenoid Drug Eruptions

Some patients with skin or oral lesions identical to those of lichen planus will be found to be taking certain drugs that cause lichenoid reactions. If the offending drug is withdrawn, the lesions clear within several days (in most patients) or within a few weeks. The agents most commonly associated with the onset of lichenoid lesions are levamisole (Levantine) and quinidine drugs. Other agents associated with such lesions are thiazides, gold, mercury, methyldopa, phenothiazines, quinidine, and certain antibiotics. A biopsy, if performed, will show a microscopic picture similar to that seen in lichen planus, with the additional finding of eosinophils in the subepithelial infiltrate.

Management of Severe Type I Hypersensitivity Reactions

Even when the dentist has taken appropriate precautions, an allergic reaction may occur. Most of these reactions are mild and of a nonemergency nature; however, some may be severe and life threatening (anaphylactic). The dentist must be ready to deal with either type. In handling the anaphylactic reaction, the dentist should remember that it has an allergic origin. In other words, the reaction occurs soon (within minutes) after the injection, ingestion, or application of a topical anesthetic, medication, drug, local anesthetic, or dental product. The dentist must immediately take the following actions (see Appendix A):

- Place the patient in a head-down or supine position.
- Make certain that the airway is open.
- Administer oxygen.

- Be prepared to send for help and support respiration and circulation. The rate and depth of respiration should be noted, as should the patient's other vital signs. Most reactions in dental patients consist of simple fainting, which can be well managed by the preceding actions. In addition, the dentist may administer aromatic spirits of ammonia through inhalation, which encourages breathing through reflex stimulation.
- If these initial steps have not solved the emergency problem and the cause is highly likely to be allergic, an edematous-type or anaphylactic reaction should be considered.

Angioedema

If an immediate type I hypersensitivity reaction results in edema of the tongue, pharyngeal tissues, or larynx, the dentist must take additional emergency steps to prevent death from respiratory failure. At this point, if the patient has not responded to the initial procedures and is in acute respiratory distress, the dentist should do the following:

- Activate emergency medical service (EMS; call 911).
- Inject 0.3–0.5 mL of 1:1000 epinephrine by an intramuscular (into the tongue) or subcutaneous route.
- Supplement with intravenous diphenhydramine 50–100 mg if needed.
- Support respiration, if indicated, by mouth-to-mouth breathing or bag and mask; the dentist should make sure the chest rises and falls when either of these methods is used.
- Check the carotid or femoral pulse; if a pulse cannot be detected, closed chest cardiac massage per current guidelines should be initiated.
- Confirm EMS is on their way and transport to medical facility if needed.

Anaphylaxis

Anaphylaxis is a potentially life-threatening emergency that usually occurs rapidly (i.e., within minutes) but may take longer. The signs and symptoms associated with anaphylactic reactions are shown in Fig. 19.8. In contrast with a severe edematous reaction, in which respiratory distress occurs first, both respiratory and circulatory components of depression occur early in the anaphylactic reaction. Anaphylaxis often is fatal unless vigorous, immediate action is taken. Because it occurs often within minutes after contact with the antigen, the dentist should take the sequential steps delineated in Box 19.11.

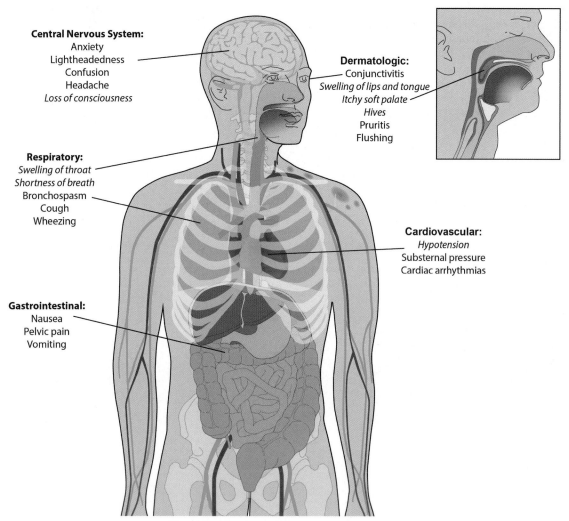

Central Nervous System:
Anxiety
Lightheadedness
Confusion
Headache
Loss of consciousness

Dermatologic:
Conjunctivitis
Swelling of lips and tongue
Itchy soft palate
Hives
Pruritis
Flushing

Respiratory:
Swelling of throat
Shortness of breath
Bronchospasm
Cough
Wheezing

Cardiovascular:
Hypotension
Substernal pressure
Cardiac arrhythmias

Gastrointestinal:
Nausea
Pelvic pain
Vomiting

FIG. 19.8 Signs and symptoms of anaphylaxis.

BOX 19.11 Anaphylaxis Management

1. Call 911 to activate EMS.
2. Place patient in the supine position.
3. Check for and establish an open airway.
4. Administer oxygen.
5. Check pulse, blood pressure, and respiration.
    a. If any of the vital signs are depressed or absent, inject 0.3 −0.5 mL 1:1000 epinephrine IM into the thigh or tongue.
    b. Provide CPR if needed. Support respiration by mouth-to-mouth breathing.
    c. Repeat IM injection of 0.5 mL 1:1000 epinephrine as needed every 5 min to control symptoms and blood pressure until emergency medical response arrives.

CPR, cardiopulmonary resuscitation; *EMSs*, emergency medical services; *IM*, intramuscular.

BIBLIOGRAPHY

1. https://www.aaaai.org/about-aaaai/newsroom/allergy-statistics.
2. Boyce JA, Austen KF. Allergies, anaphylaxis and systemic mastocytosis. Copyright ©. In: Jameson, Fauci, Kasper, et al., eds. *Harrison's*^TM *Principles of Internal Medicine.* 20th ed. Vol. 1.
3. Malamed SF. Managing medical emergencies. *J Am Dent Assoc.* 1993;124(8):40−53.
4. Albin S, Agarwal S. Prevalence and characteristics of reported penicillin allergy in an urban outpatient adult population. *Allergy Asthma Proc.* 2014;35(6):489−494.
5. Adkinson NF, Bochner BS, Burks WA, et al. *Middleton's Allergy: Principles and Practice.* 8th ed. St. Louis: Mosby/Elsevier; 2014.
6. Gell PGH, Coombs RRA, Lachman PJ. *Aspects of Immunology.* 3rd ed. Oxford, United Kingdom: Blackwell Scientific; 1975.
7. Bernstein JA, Lang DM, Khan DA, et al. The diagnosis and management of acute and chronic urticaria: 2014 update. *J Allergy Clin Immunol.* 2014;133(5):1270−1277.
8. Neugut AI, Ghatak AT, Miller RL. Anaphylaxis in the United States. An investigation into its epidemiology. *Arch Intern Med.* 2001;161(1):15−21. https://doi.org/10.1001/archinte.161.1.15.
9. Malamed SF. Allergy and toxic reactions to local anesthetics. *Dent Today.* 2003;22(4):114−116, 18-21.

10. Becker DE. Drug allergies and implications for dental practice. *Anesth Prog.* 2013;60(4):188–197.

11. Yagiela JA, Dowd FJ, Johnson B, et al. *Pharmacology and Therapeutics for Dentistry.* 6th ed. St. Louis, MO: Mosby/ Elsevier; 2011.

12. Cullinan P, Brown R, Field A, et al. Latex allergy. A position paper of the British Society of Allergy and Clinical Immunology. *Clin Exp Allergy.* 2003;33(11):1484–1499.

13. Stoopler ET, Sollecito TP. Oral mucosal diseases: evaluation and management. *Med Clin N Am.* 2014;98(6):1323–1352.

14. Syed M, Chopra R, Sachdev V. Allergic reactions to dental materials-a systematic review. *J Clin Diagn Res.* 2015;9(10):ZE04–ZE09.

15. Yuan A, Woo SB. Adverse drug events in the oral cavity. *Oral Surg Oral Med Oral Pathol Oral Radiol.* 2015;119(1):35–47.

Rheumatologic Disorders

Arthritis is a nonspecific term meaning "inflammation of the joints" that manifests as joint dysfunction. The term *arthritis* is often used interchangeably with *rheumatism* or *rheumatoid arthritis* (RA) to denote aches, pains, and stiffness in the joints and muscles, but these terms are neither synonymous nor inclusive. Rheumatologic disorders are also referred to as systemic autoimmune disorders or systemic autoimmune rheumatic diseases or musculoskeletal or connective tissue diseases. Rheumatologic disorders include RA, osteoarthritis (OA), psoriatic arthritis (PsA), systemic lupus erythematosus (SLE), juvenile rheumatoid arthritis (JRA), progressive systemic sclerosis or scleroderma (SD), Sjögren syndrome (SS), gout, ankylosing spondylitis, Lyme disease, giant cell arteritis (GCA or temporal arteritis), and fibromyalgia syndrome (FMS).

In this chapter, RA, OA, SLE, and SS are presented in more detail, and PsA, Lyme disease, GCA, and FMS are discussed to a lesser degree.

Rheumatologic disorders have significant personal and economic impact. According to the Arthritis Foundation, more than 40 million Americans have various forms of arthritis, and more than 8 million of them are considered "disabled." In terms of its overall economic impact, arthritis costs the American economy more than $20 billion annually and accounts for nearly 30 million lost workdays per year.

CATEGORIES OF RHEUMATOLOGIC DISORDERS

Rheumatologic disorders can be classified into nine categories, defined predominantly by the affected tissues, such as joint, synovium, cartilage, or connective tissues (Table 20.1).

ANATOMY OF THE JOINT

Structures commonly involved in rheumatologic disorders include the joint, joint cavity, synovial fluid, and periarticular structures. The lining membrane, known as the *synovium*, consists of a thin layer of macrophages (type A cells) and fibroblasts (type B cells) with a sublining of rich, vascular, loose connective tissue. Hyaline cartilage overlies the bony endplates and provides a cushion to joint motion. The cartilage has high water content and obtains its nutrition solely from the synovial fluid. The synovial fluid is comprised of ultrafiltrate of plasma and specialized molecules (e.g., hyaluronic acid) derived primarily from the synovium. The joint capsule and ligaments provide support for the joint and its movement. Periarticular anatomy is equally important and includes the tendons, bursae, and muscles associated with the joint.

OVERVIEW OF THE TYPES

Synovial inflammatory disorders, such as RA, begin in the synovium and damage secondarily the cartilage, joint capsule, and bone. Inflammation at entheses, the insertion sites of tendons or ligaments on bone, is characteristic of the spondyloarthropathies, such as ankylosing spondylitis. Crystal deposition disorders, such as gout or pseudogout, may also cause articular inflammation. Infections involve primarily the joint cavity (septic arthritis) or bone (osteomyelitis). OA is a degenerative disease caused by natural wearing down of cartilage that leads to cartilage loss, subchondral new bone formation, and marginal bony overgrowth. Osteonecrosis of bone may be associated with secondary cartilage damage after collapse of the bony endplate. Inflammatory diseases of the muscle usually manifest with painless proximal

TABLE 20.1 Classification of Musculoskeletal Diseases

Category	Prototype(s)	Useful Test(s)	Treatment(s)[a]
Synovitis	Rheumatoid arthritis	Rheumatoid factor, ESR	DMARDs and biologic agents
	Autoimmune diseases	ANA test	Prednisone and immunosuppressive drugs
Enthesopathy	Ankylosing spondylitis and spondyloarthropathies	Sacroiliac radiographs	NSAIDs, MTX, and biologic agents
Crystal-induced synovitis	Gout	Joint fluid crystal examination	NSAIDs
	CPPD (pseudogout)	Radiographic chondrocalcinosis	NSAIDs
Joint space disease	Septic arthritis	Joint fluid culture	Antibiotics
Cartilage degeneration	Osteoarthritis	Radiographs of affected area	NSAIDs, analgesics, and physical therapy
Osteoarticular disease	Osteonecrosis	Radiographs, magnetic resonance imaging	Core decompression or prosthetic joint replacement
Inflammatory myopathy	Polymyositis Dermatomyositis Inclusion body myositis	Muscle enzymes, electromyography, muscle biopsy	Corticosteroids and immunosuppressive drugs
Local and regional conditions	Tendonitis or bursitis	Aspirate bursa if infection is suspected	Local injections
General conditions	Polymyalgia rheumatica	Elevated ESR	Corticosteroids
	Fibromyalgia	Normal ESR	Aerobic exercise, stretches, and sleep medications

[a]Biologic agents include antitumor necrosis factor) drugs and others.
ANA, antinuclear antibody; *CPPD,* calcium pyrophosphate crystal deposition disease; *DMARDs,* disease-modifying antirheumatic drugs; *ESR,* erythrocyte sedimentation rate; *MTX,* methotrexate; *NSAIDs,* nonsteroidal antiinflammatory drugs.

weakness. Periarticular inflammation may involve tendons or bursae, and these structures are common causes of pain and stiffness. Fibromyalgia (FM; widespread muscle pain) is characterized by soft tissue pain with local tenderness in specific points but without abnormal blood studies.

RHEUMATOID ARTHRITIS

Rheumatoid arthritis is an autoimmune disease of unknown origin characterized by symmetric inflammation of joints, especially of the hands, feet, and knees. The severity of the disease varies widely from patient to patient and fluctuates over time. Onset usually occurs between ages 35 and 50 years. RA is more prevalent in women than in men by a 3:1 ratio.

EPIDEMIOLOGY AND ETIOLOGY

Prevalence estimates range from 1% to 2% of the US population are affected by RA. The cause of RA is unknown; however, evidence seems to implicate an interrelationship of infectious agents, genetics, and autoimmunity. One theory suggests that a viral agent alters the immune system in a genetically predisposed person, leading to destruction of synovial tissues. Although the disease can occur within families, suggesting a genetic component, specific associated genes have not been identified. Nevertheless, many people who

develop RA have a genetic predisposition that occurs in association with a tissue marker called HLA-DR4; however, not everyone with this tissue type develops the disease.

PATHOPHYSIOLOGY AND COMPLICATIONS

The fundamental abnormality of RA involves microvascular endothelial cell activation and injury. Primary changes occur within the synovium; the inner lining of the joint capsule (Fig. 20.1). Edema of the synovium occurs followed by thickening and folding. This excessive tissue, composed of proliferative and invasive granulation tissue, is referred to as *pannus.* Lymphocytes and plasma cells also infiltrate the joint capsule. Eventually, granulation tissue covers the articular surfaces and destroys the cartilage and subchondral bone through enzymatic activity (Fig. 20.2). This process, if untreated, extends to the capsule and ligaments, causing distention and rupture. New bone or fibrous tissue then is deposited, resulting in loss of mobility.

The sequence of pathologic events begins with a synovitis that stimulates immunoglobulin G (IgG) antibodies. These antibodies form antigenic aggregates in the joint space, leading to the production of rheumatoid factor (RF; autoantibodies). RF then complexes with IgG complement, a process that produces an inflammatory reaction that injures the joint space. The key drivers of RA include proinflammatory cytokines such as tumor

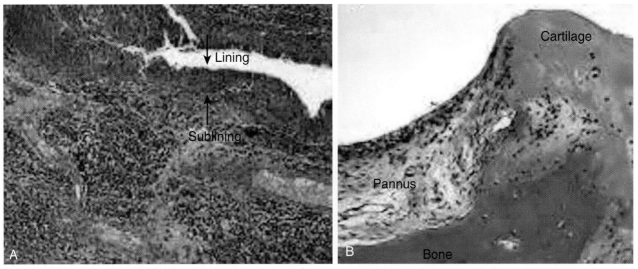

FIG. 20.1 Micrograph images of severe synovitis in rheumatoid arthritis.

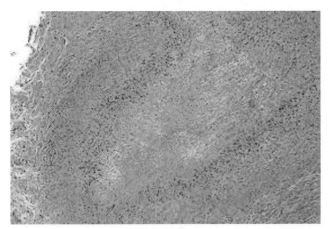

FIG. 20.2 A micrograph of a nodule resulting from severe synovitis in rheumatoid arthritis.

necrosis factor-α (TNFα), interleukin-1 (IL-1), and interleukin-6 (IL-6).

Subcutaneous nodules are found in 20% of patients with RA and commonly occur around the elbow and finger joints. These nodules are thought to arise from the same antigen–antibody complex found in the joint. Antigen-mediated vasculitis confined to small- and medium-sized vessels also may occur.

Rheumatoid arthritis is a pleomorphic disease with variable expression. The most progressive period of the disease occurs during the earlier years; thereafter, it slows. Onset is gradual in more than 50% of patients, and as many as 20% follow a limited course that abates within 2 years. Approximately 10% of patients with RA who do not receive adequate treatment experience relentless crippling that leads to nearly complete disability. The remaining patients have a polycyclic or progressive course. The long-term prognosis for individuals with abrupt onset is similar to that for those with gradual disease onset. The course and severity of RA are unpredictable, but the disorder is characterized by remissions and exacerbations. For most patients, however, the disease is a sustained, lifelong problem that can be managed to allow a normal or nearly normal life.

The life expectancy of persons with severe RA is shortened by 10–15 years. This increased mortality rate usually is attributed to infection, pulmonary and renal disease, and gastrointestinal bleeding.

Many complications may accompany RA, including keratoconjunctivitis sicca and SS, digital gangrene, temporomandibular joint (TMJ) involvement, pulmonary interstitial fibrosis, pericarditis, amyloidosis, anemia, thrombocytopenia, neutropenia, and splenomegaly (Felty syndrome).

CLINICAL PRESENTATION

The usual onset of RA is gradual and subtle (Table 20.2). RA is commonly preceded by a prodromal phase of general fatigue and weakness with joint and muscle aches. Characteristically, these symptoms come and go over varying periods. Then, painful joint swelling, especially of the hands and feet, occurs in several joints and progresses to other joints in a symmetric fashion (Fig. 20.3). Joint involvement persists and gradually progresses to immobility, contractures, subluxation, deviation, and other deformities. Features include pain in the affected joints aggravated by movement, generalized joint stiffness after inactivity, and morning stiffness that lasts longer than 1 h. The joints most commonly affected are fingers, wrists, feet, ankles, knees, and elbows. Multiple joint changes noted in the hands include a symmetric spindle-shaped swelling of the proximal interphalangeal (PIP) joints, with dorsal swelling and characteristic volar subluxation of the metacarpophalangeal (MCP) joint (Fig. 20.3). TMJ involvement occurs in up to 75% of RA patients. Because of the variable rate of progression and pain intensity, the median period between onset of symptoms of RA and its diagnosis is 36 weeks.

TABLE 20.2   Comparison of the Clinical Features of Rheumatoid Arthritis and Osteoarthritis

Rheumatoid Arthritis	Osteoarthritis
Multiple symmetric joint involvement	Usually one or two joints (or groups) involved
Significant joint inflammation	Joint pain usually without inflammation
Morning joint stiffness lasting longer than 1 h	Morning joint stiffness lasting less than 15 min
Symmetric, spindle-shaped swelling of PIP joints and volar subluxation of MCP joints and Bouchard's nodes of PIP joints	Heberden nodes of DIP joints
Systemic manifestations (fatigue, weakness, malaise)	No systemic involvement

DIP, distal interphalangeal; *MCP*, metacarpophalangeal; *PIP*, proximal interphalangeal.

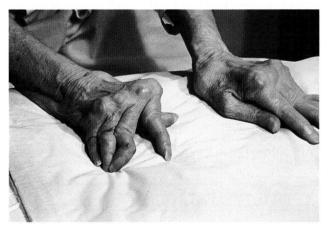

FIG. 20.3 Hands of a patient with advanced rheumatoid arthritis. (From Damjanov I. *Pathology for the Health Professions.* 4th ed. St. Louis: Saunders; 2012.)

Extraarticular manifestations include rheumatoid nodules, vasculitis, skin ulcers, SS, muscle atrophy, interstitial lung disease, pericarditis, cervical spine instability, entrapment neuropathies, and ischemic neuropathies.

LABORATORY AND DIAGNOSTIC FINDINGS

Laboratory tests are not pathognomonic or diagnostic of RA, although they are used in conjunction with clinical findings to confirm the diagnosis. Laboratory findings most commonly seen in RA include an increased erythrocyte sedimentation rate (ESR), elevated C-reactive protein (CRP), a positive RF (in 85% of affected patients), and a hypochromic microcytic anemia. In patients with Felty syndrome (RA with splenomegaly), a marked neutropenia may be present.

Autoantibodies to cyclic citrullinated proteins (CCPs) are highly specific for RA and are present in 70%–80% of patients with RA. These antibodies may appear before any sign or symptom of RA and therefore may prove beneficial as early screening markers for earlier diagnosis and intervention of RA.

The American College of Rheumatology (ACR) has established criteria for the diagnosis of RA (see Box 20.1), the classification of severity by radiography, functional classes, and definition of remission. Although the criteria were not designed for managing individual patients, they are useful as a frame of reference and for describing clinical phenomena.

By definition, the diagnosis of RA cannot be made until the disease has been present for at least several weeks. Many extraarticular features of RA, the characteristic symmetry of inflammation, and typical serologic findings may not be evident during the first few months after disease onset. Therefore, the diagnosis of RA usually is presumptive early in its course.

Although extraarticular manifestations may dominate in some patients, documentation of an inflammatory synovitis is essential for diagnosis. Inflammatory synovitis can be documented by demonstration of synovial fluid leukocytosis, defined as white blood cell (WBC) counts greater than 2000/μL, histologic evidence of synovitis, or radiographic evidence of characteristic joint erosions.

MEDICAL MANAGEMENT

Treatment of RA focuses on use of antiinflammatory drugs and disease-modifying antirheumatic drugs (DMARDs), which are helpful in controlling the disease and limiting joint damage. The treatment approach is mostly palliative because no cure exists yet for RA. The ultimate aims of management are to achieve disease remission and maintain or regain functional activity.

Clinical tools for monitoring the patient's well-being and the efficacy of therapy include self-assessment of the duration of morning stiffness and severity of fatigue, as well as functional, social, emotional, and pain status, as measured by a health assessment questionnaire. A patient-derived global assessment based on a visual analogue scale is a simple and effective means of recording patient well-being. The number of tender and swollen joints is a useful measure of disease activity, as is the presence of anemia, thrombocytosis, and elevated ESR or CRP. Serial radiographs of target joints, including the hands, are helpful in assessing disease progression.

Patients are best served by a multidisciplinary approach with early referral to a rheumatologist and other specially trained medical personnel, including nurses, counselors, and occupational and physical therapists who are skilled and knowledgeable about RA. Appropriate medical care of patients with RA encompasses attention to smoking cessation, immunizations, prompt treatment of infections, and management of

BOX 20.1   Criteria for the Diagnosis of Rheumatoid Arthritis

- Morning stiffness
- Arthritis of three or more joint areas
- Arthritis of hand joints
- Symmetric arthritis
- Rheumatoid nodules
- Serum rheumatoid factor
- Radiographic changes

Adapted from Arnett FC, Edworthy SM, Bloch DA, et al. The American Rheumatism Association 1987 revised criteria for the classification of rheumatoid arthritis. *Arthritis Rheum*. 1988;31:315–324.

comorbid conditions such as diabetes, hypertension, and osteoporosis. Practical treatment goals are to reduce joint inflammation and swelling, relieve pain and stiffness, and facilitate and encourage normal function. These goals are accomplished through a basic treatment program that consists of patient education, rest, exercise, physical therapy, and various drugs.

Drugs for the management of RA have been traditionally, but imperfectly, divided into two groups: those used primarily for the control of joint pain and swelling and those intended to limit joint damage and improve long-term outcome (Table 20.3). Symptoms of pain and swelling in RA are mediated, at least in part, by intense cytokine activity. NSAIDs inhibit proinflammatory prostaglandins and are effective treatments for pain, swelling, and stiffness, but they have no effect on the disease course or on risk of joint damage. On the other hand, antiinflammatory properties have been noted for several DMARDs, which are used principally to control the disease and to limit joint damage. DMARDs include methotrexate and biologic response modifiers with actions targeted against specific cytokines, such as TNF-α. Corticosteroids are powerful, nonspecific inhibitors of cytokines that are used episodically to reduce inflammation and delay joint erosion.

Many different drugs are used in the treatment of patients with RA. Some are used primarily to ease the symptoms of RA; others are used to slow or stop the course of the disease and to inhibit structural damage. Most of these drugs fall into one of the following categories.

NSAIDs

NSAIDs, including aspirin, constitute the cornerstone of treatment, as these drugs effectively reduce arthritis pain and inflammation. A common approach is to start a patient on three 5-grain tablets four times a day, then adjust the dosage based on patient response. The most common sign of aspirin toxicity is tinnitus. If this occurs, the dosage is decreased. In addition to aspirin, NSAIDs can be used (see Table 20.3). All NSAIDs, including aspirin, can cause a qualitative platelet defect that may result in prolonged bleeding, especially when given in high doses. Aspirin's effects are irreversible for the life of the platelet (10–12 days); thus, this effect continues until new platelets replace the old. The effect of the other NSAIDs on platelets is reversible and lasts only as long as the drug is present in the plasma (see Chapter 24). Celecoxib (Celebrex), a COX-2 inhibitor, is designed to be safer for the stomach. In addition to NSAIDs, a variety of other drugs can be used to treat patients with RA (Table 20.3).

Corticosteroids

Corticosteroids, including prednisone, prednisolone, and methylprednisolone, are potent and quick-acting antiinflammatory medications. These medications provide immediate control of inflammation while waiting for NSAIDs and DMARDs take effect. Because of the risk of side effects with corticosteroids, they are prescribed for as short a time as possible and in doses as low as possible.

DMARDS

Disease-modifying antirheumatic drugs modify the course of the disease through various mechanisms. The most commonly used DMARD for RA is methotrexate. Other frequently used DMARDs include hydroxychloroquine (Plaquenil), sulfasalazine (Azulfidine, Azulfidine EN-Tabs), leflunomide (Arava), and azathioprine (Imuran).

An individual diagnosed with RA is likely to be prescribed a DMARD fairly early in the course of the disease because studies have demonstrated that starting these drugs early can help prevent irreparable joint damage.

Biologic Agents

Biologic agents are highly targeted DMARDs that have revolutionized the management of RA (Table 20.4). Biologics have been shown to help slow progression of RA when all other treatments have failed to do so. Aggressive RA treatment is known to help prevent long-term disability from RA.

Each of the biologics targets a specific molecular mediator in the inflammation cascade. They are administered by injection or IV infusion. The mechanism of action for these agents are found in Table 20.4. At present, the TNF-α blockers etanercept (e.g., Enbrel, Immunex) and infliximab (Remicade) are known to be highly effective in the treatment of patients with early RA relative to the "gold standard" agent, methotrexate. Both have been shown to significantly reduce signs, symptoms, and progression of RA. However, both are costly and difficult to administer (etanercept—requiring an injectable route), and infliximab (requiring intravenous (IV) administration). The most common side effect seen with biologics is pain and rash at the injection site, occurring in fewer than 30% of patients. Allergic infusion reactions are possible with infliximab, hence

TABLE 20.3 Drugs Used in the Management of Rheumatologic Disorders

Drug(s) (Trade Name)	Dental and Oral Considerations
Salicylates	
Aspirin, Ascriptin, Bufferin, Anacin, Ecotrin, Empirin	Prolonged bleeding but not usually clinically significant
Nonsteroidal Antiinflammatory Drugs	
Ibuprofen (Motrin), fenoprofen (Nalfon), indomethacin (Indocin), naproxen (Naprosyn), meclofenamate (Meclomen), piroxicam (Feldene), sulindac (Sulindac), tolmetin (Tolectin), diclofenac (Voltaren), flurbiprofen (Ansaid), diflunisal (Dolobid), etodolac (Lodine), nabumetone (Relafen), oxaprozin, ketorolac	Prolonged bleeding but not usually clinically significant; oral ulceration, stomatitis
Cyclooxygenase-2 Inhibitors	
Celecoxib	None
Rofecoxib	
Tumor Necrosis Factor-α Inhibitors	
Etanercept	None
Adalimumab	
Infliximab	
Injectable Glucocorticoids	
Triamcinolone hexacetonide	Adrenal suppression, impaired healing
Triamcinolone acetonide	
Prednisolone tebutate	
Methylprednisolone acetate	
Dexamethasone acetate	
Hydrocortisone acetate	
Triamcinolone diacetate	
Betamethasone sodium phosphate and acetate	
Dexamethasone sodium phosphate	
Prednisolone sodium phosphate	
Systemic Glucocorticoids	
Hydrocortisone, cortisone, prednisone, prednisolone, dexamethasone, methylprednisolone	Adrenal suppression, impaired healing
Disease-Modifying Antirheumatic Drugs	
Antimalarial Agents	
Hydroxychloroquine, quinine, chloroquine	Non
Penicillamines	
Cuprimine, Depen	None
GOLD Compounds	
Gold sodium thiomalate (Auranofin), aurothioglucose (Myochrysine Ridaura, Solganal)	Increased infections, delayed healing, prolonged bleeding, oral ulcerations
Sulfasalazine	Increased infections, delayed healing, prolonged bleeding, intraoral pigmentation
Immunosuppressives	
Azathioprine, cyclophosphamide	Increased infections, delayed healing, prolonged bleeding
Methotrexate, cyclosporine, azathioprine chlorambucil	Increased infections, delayed healing, prolonged bleeding, stomatitis

patients are monitored during infusions. Symptoms of infusion reactions include flulike illness, fever, chills, nausea, and headache. Biologics also have been implicated in increased risk of infections. In one study, patients taking high-dose biologics were nearly 2.5 times more likely to have a serious infection than control participants. Thus, people taking biologics should seek immediate medical attention if they develop persistent fever or unexplained symptoms. Vaccinations that prevent infections should be considered before taking biologics. While taking biologic medications, people should not receive live vaccines.

TABLE 20.4 General Categories and Descriptions of Drugs to Treat Rheumatologic Disorders

There are many different drugs used in the treatment of rheumatologic disorders. Some are used primarily to ease the symptoms, and others are used to slow or stop the course of the disease and to inhibit structural damage. Most of these drugs fall into one of the following categories:

1. **Nonsteroidal antiinflammatory drugs (NSAIDs)** include more than a dozen different medications—some available over the counter, some available by prescription only—used to help ease arthritis pain and inflammation. NSAIDs include such drugs as ibuprofen (Advil, Motrin), ketoprofen (Actron, Orudis KT), and naproxen sodium (Aleve), among others. If you have had or are at risk of stomach ulcers, your doctor may prescribe celecoxib (Celebrex), a type of NSAID called a cyclooxygenase-2 inhibitor, which is designed to be safer for the stomach.

2. **Corticosteroids:** Corticosteroid medications, including prednisone, prednisolone, and methylprednisolone, are potent and quick-acting antiinflammatory medications. They may be used in patients with rheumatoid arthritis (RAs) to get potentially damaging inflammation under control while waiting for NSAIDs and DMARDs (below) to take effect. Because of the risk of side effects with these drugs, doctors prefer to use them for as short a time as possible and in doses as low as possible.

3. **Disease-modifying antirheumatic drugs (DMARDs):** DMARDs are drugs that work slowly to actually modify the course of the disease. In recent years, the most commonly used DMARD for rheumatoid arthritis is methotrexate. But there are about a dozen others that fall into this category. They include hydroxychloroquine (Plaquenil), sulfasalazine (Azulfidine, Azulfidine EN-Tabs), leflunomide (Arava), and azathioprine (Imuran). Patients diagnosed with RA today are likely to be prescribed a DMARD fairly early in the course of their disease because doctors have found that starting these drugs early on can help prevent irreparable joint damage that might occur if their use was delayed.

4. **Biologic agents:** The newest category of medications used for rheumatoid arthritis is a subset of DMARDs called biologic response modifiers, or biologics. There are currently several agents approved for RA: abatacept (Orencia), adalimumab (Humira), anakinra (Kineret), certolizumab pegol (Cimzia), etanercept (Enbrel), infliximab (Remicade), golimumab (Simponi), and rituximab (Rituxan), belimumuab (Benlysta), canakinumab (Ilaris), infliximab (Remicade), Ixekizumab (Taltz), Sarilumab (Kevzara). Each of the biologics blocks a specific step in the inflammation process. Cimzia, Enbrel, Humira, Remicade, and Simponi block a cytokine called tumor necrosis factor-α (TNF-α) and therefore often are called TNF inhibitors. Kineret blocks a cytokine called interleukin-1 (IL-1). Orencia blocks the activation of T cells. Rituxan blocks B cells. Actemra blocks a cytokine called interleukin-6 (IL-6). Because these agents target specific steps in the process, they do not wipe out the entire immune response as some other RA treatments do, and in many people, a biologic agent can slow, modify, or stop the disease even when other treatments have not helped much.

5. **Janus kinase (JAK) inhibitors:** Tofacitinib (Xeljanz) is being compared to biologics. However, it is part of a new subcategory of DMARDs known as JAK inhibitors that block Janus kinase, or JAK, pathways, which are involved in the body's immune response. Unlike biologics, it can be taken orally.

Janus-Associated Kinase Inhibitors

Tofacitinib (Xeljanz) is a Janus-associated kinase inhibitor that disrupts cytokine and growth factor signaling pathways, thereby effectively reducing inflammation.

Prosthetic Joints

A potential long-term complication of RA, OA, and other joint disorders is the destruction of particular joint structures to the degree that the joint must be replaced with synthetic materials. Patients who have recently received a prosthetic joint (particularly the knee) are at increased risk (up to nine times more likely) of having a thromboembolic event (including a possible myocardial infarction) within 1 month of the implant, and are more likely to have a pulmonary embolism for several years after their implant. Patients with prosthetic joints (most commonly, hip and knee replacement, followed by shoulder, elbow, wrist, and ankle) often are encountered in dental practice; when this occurs, a question concerning the need for antibiotic prophylaxis to prevent infection of the prosthesis can arise.

DENTAL MANAGEMENT

Depending on which joints are involved, patients may not be comfortable in a supine position in the dental chair. Consideration should be given to providing a more upright chair position, using neck, back, and leg supports, and scheduling short appointments (Box 20.2).

Dental appointments should be kept as short as possible, and the patient should be allowed to make frequent position changes as needed to accommodate joint pain and immobility (Box 20.2). The patient also may be more comfortable in a sitting or semisupine position, as opposed to a supine one. Physical supports, such as a pillow or a rolled towel, may be used to provide support for deformed limbs, joints, or the neck.

The most significant complications associated with RA are drug related (Table 20.3). Aspirin and other NSAIDs can interfere with platelet function and cause prolonged bleeding; however, this effect alone generally is not found to be of clinical significance unless another bleeding problem is present. A patient who is taking both aspirin and a corticosteroid may be at greater risk for bleeding (see Chapter 24).

Patients who are taking gold salts, penicillamine, sulfasalazine, or immunosuppressive agents are susceptible to bone marrow suppression, which can result in anemia, agranulocytosis, and thrombocytopenia. If a patient has not undergone recent laboratory testing, a complete blood cell count with a differential WBC count should be ordered. Abnormal results should be discussed with the patient's physician. Patients being treated with corticosteroid therapy are at risk for a number of adverse effects (see Table 20.3), including adrenal suppression (see Chapter 15).

Prosthetic Joint Infection

Rarely, patients who have had a joint replaced may acquire an infection of the artificial joint. It appears that wound contamination or skin infection (staphylococci) is the source of the vast majority of late prosthetic joint

BOX 20.2   Checklist for Dental Management of Patients With Patients With Rheumatologic Disorders[a]

PREOPERATIVE RISK ASSESSMENT
- Evaluation is directed at determining the nature, severity, control, and stability of disease
- Review relevant lab values (AST, ALT, bilirubin, aPTT, bleeding time, see Chapter 24)
- Determine comorbid conditions (HTN, renal disease, etc.)
- Medical consult may be necessary

POTENTIAL ISSUES AND FACTORS OF CONCERN DURING TREATMENT

A	
Analgesics	If patient is taking aspirin or another NSAID or acetaminophen, be aware of dosing and the possibility that pain may be refractory to some analgesics; dosing and analgesic choices may need to be modified in consultation with the physician.
Antibiotics	Antibiotic prophylaxis is generally not needed. If needed, follow ADA (2015) guidelines (see Boxes 20.3 and 20.4).
Anesthesia	No issues.
Allergy	Allergic reactions or lichenoid reactions are possible in patients taking many medications.

B	
Bleeding	Excessive bleeding may occur if surgery is performed on patients who take aspirin or other NSAIDs. Bleeding usually is not clinically significant and can be controlled with local hemostatic measures.
Blood pressure	No issues.

C	
Chair position	Ensure comfortable chair position. Consider shorter appointments, and use supports as needed (e.g., pillows, towels).

D	
Devices	Patients who have a prosthetic joint replacement should be managed according to ADA (2003) guidelines (see Boxes 20.3 and 20.4).
Drugs	Obtain blood cell count with differential if surgery is planned for patients taking gold salts, penicillamine, antimalarials, or immunosuppressives. If patient is taking corticosteroids, secondary adrenal suppression is possible (see Chapter 15).

E	
Equipment	No issues.
Emergencies	If surgery is performed, supplemental techniques may be necessary to control bleeding.

F	
Follow-up	Monitor dental and periodontal health; routine follow-up evaluation is appropriate.

[a]Strength of recommendation taxonomy (SORT) Grade: C (see Preface for further explanation).
ADA, American Dental Association; *NSAID*, nonsteroidal antiinflammatory drug.

infections (LPJIs). Only a few cases of LPJI have been remotely associated with bacteria (streptococci) found in the oral cavity. Most of these infections were more likely to result from physiologically occurring bacteremia or bacteremia caused by acute or chronic infection rather than from invasive dental procedures. Many orthopedic surgeons have persisted in requesting that these patients continue to receive antibiotic prophylaxis for all dental procedures despite the lack of evidence.

2015 Summary of American Dental Association and the American Academy of Orthopedic Surgeons

In an effort to resolve controversies in this area the American Dental Association (ADA) Council on Scientific Affairs published a clinical practice guideline based on a review of the literature that considered information about antibiotic resistance, adverse drug reactions, and costs associated with prescribing antibiotics for PJI prophylaxis. The results of the most recent task force (2015) are summarized in Table 20.5. The current recommendation is that *"in general, patients with prosthetic joints ARE NOT recommended to receive prophylactic antibiotics before dental treatment."* Consistent with this Berbari and colleagues have demonstrated that the clear majority of PJIs are caused by *Staphylococcus* species, gram-negative bacteria and anaerobic bacteria not associated with the oral cavity.

As with any recommendations, certain caveats and exceptions must be taken into account in making the decision to prescribe prophylactic antibiotics before dental treatment. Those factors may include other systemic comorbid conditions that may render the individual patient susceptible to infection, or prior or existing infection of the prosthetic joint. Box 20.3 lists some of the comorbid medical conditions that may increase the risk for PJI. Therefore, a careful, comprehensive review of the patient's medical conditions and status and possible consultation with the physician may be in order.

A further recommendation of the ADA was: *"In cases where antibiotic prophylaxis is deemed necessary by the orthopedic surgeon, it is appropriate for them to recommend the appropriate antibiotic and when reasonable, to write the prescription ...."*

TABLE 20.5 Management of Patients With Prosthetic Joints Undergoing Dental Procedures

Clinical Recommendation

In general, for patients with prosthetic joint implants, prophylactic antibiotics are *not* recommended before dental procedures to prevent prosthetic joint infection.

For patients with a history of complications associated with their joint replacement surgery who are undergoing dental procedures that include gingival manipulation or mucosal incision, prophylactic antibiotics should only be considered after consultation with the patient and orthopedic surgeon.[a] To assess a patient's medical status, a complete health history is always recommended when making final decisions regarding the need for antibiotic prophylaxis.

Clinical Reasoning for the Recommendation

- Most prosthetic joint infections are caused by *Staphylococcus aureus*, which is not an inhabitant of the oral cavity.
- There is evidence that dental procedures are not associated with prosthetic joint implant infections.
- There is evidence that antibiotics provided before oral care do not prevent prosthetic joint implant infections.
- There are potential harms of antibiotics, including risk for anaphylaxis, antibiotic resistance, and opportunistic infections such as *Clostridium difficile*.
- The benefits of antibiotic prophylaxis may not exceed the harms for most patients.
- The individual patient's circumstances and preferences should be considered when deciding whether to prescribe prophylactic antibiotics prior to dental procedures.

[a]In cases in which antibiotics are deemed necessary, it is most appropriate that the orthopedic surgeon recommend the appropriate antibiotic regimen and when reasonable write the prescription.

Adapted from Sollecito TP, Abt E, Lockhart PB, et al. The use of prophylactic antibiotics prior to dental procedures in patients with prosthetic joints: evidence-based clinical practice guideline for dental practitioners—a report of the American Dental Association Council on Scientific Affairs. *J Am Dent Assoc.* 2015;146(1):11–16.

These recommendations are intended to provide rational insight and guidance to the individual dental practitioner to exercise good clinical judgment and to make the best treatment decisions for the individual patient.

Box 20.4 provides the suggested antibiotic regimens when prophylaxis is indicated. Because of the risk of potential complications, it is best to defer elective dental treatment for at least 30 days after a total joint replacement.

Treatment Planning Modifications

Treatment planning modifications are dictated by the patient's physical disabilities. RA is a progressive disease that ultimately may lead to severe disability and crippling in some patients, which can make providing dental care difficult. Therefore, the dentist should be diligent in providing ongoing preventive care and should attempt to identify and treat or eliminate potential problems before the disease progresses.

Disabled patients may have significant difficulty cleaning their teeth. Cleaning aids such as floss holders, toothpicks, irrigating devices, and mechanical toothbrushes may be recommended. If replacement of missing teeth is desired, consideration should be given to procedures that minimize chair time needed for mouth preparation, the potential for TMJ involvement, and the abilities of the patient to clean a dental implant, fixed or removable oral prosthesis.

Oral Complications and Manifestations

The most significant complication of the oral and maxillofacial complex is TMJ involvement, which affects up to 75% of patients with RA. This may present as bilateral

---

BOX 20.3 Patients With Prosthetic Joints at Increased Risk for Joint Infection

Immunocompromised or Immunosuppressed Patients
- Inflammatory arthropathies: rheumatoid arthritis; systemic lupus erythematosus; disease, immunosuppression

Other Patients
- Insulin-dependent (type 1) diabetes
- First 2 years after joint replacement
- Previous prosthetic joint infections
- Malnourishment
- Hemophilia

BOX 20.4 Suggested Antibiotic Prophylaxis Regimens for Select Patient With Prosthetic Joints Who Are Consider to Be at Risk for Infection[a]

Patients Not Allergic to Penicillin: Cephalexin, Cefradine, or Amoxicillin
- 2 g orally 30 min to 1 h before the dental procedure

Patients Not Allergic to Penicillin and Unable to Take Oral Medications: Cefazolin or Ampicillin
- Cefazolin 1 g *or* ampicillin 2 g intramuscularly or intravenously 30 min to 1 h before the dental procedure

[a]In general, patients with prosthetic joints ARE NOT recommended to receive prophylactic antibiotics before dental treatment.

preauricular pain, tenderness, swelling, stiffness, and decreased mobility of the TMJ, or it may be asymptomatic. Periods of remission and exacerbation may occur, as with other joint involvement. Fibrosis or bony ankylosis can occur; therefore, treatment should be initiated promptly. Clinically, patients may present with tenderness over the lateral pole of the condyle, crepitus, and limited opening. Radiographic changes initially may show increased joint space caused by inflammation in the joint. Later, these inflammatory changes progress to erosive degenerative changes and changes in size and shape of the joint and can involve both the condyles and the fossa.

A potential dental complication is the development of an anterior open bite, caused by destruction of the condylar heads and loss of condylar height (Fig. 20.4). Although palliative treatment such as interocclusal splints, physical therapy, and medication may prove to be helpful, surgical intervention can become necessary to decrease pain, improve appearance, or restore function.

Meticulous oral hygiene combined with more frequent dental prophylaxis are important for reducing periodontal problems. An additional complication that may be seen in patients with RA is severe stomatitis that occurs after administration of drugs such as gold compounds, penicillamine, or immunosuppressive agents. Stomatitis may be an indication of drug toxicity and should be reported to the physician. Treatment for this problem should include consideration for changing the offending drug and palliative mouth rinses, diphenhydramine elixir, or a topical emollient such as Orabase (see Appendix C).

OSTEOARTHRITIS

OA or degenerative joint disease is the most common form of arthritis. Nearly all individuals older than 60 years of age develop some degree of OA, and approximately 17 million people in the United States have painful OA. It is the leading cause of disability within the elderly

population. Osteoarthritis usually affects often-used joints such as hips, knees, feet, spine, and hands. The TMJ also may be affected. Osteoarthritis and RA are two conditions that are very frequently confused, often because of the family of pathology to which they belong, i.e., rheumatologic disorders. However, they are indeed different and many of their symptoms are distinct. OA is deemed a mechanical condition characterized by the gradual wearing down of cartilage in the joints. Aging is the most common risk factor for OA. RA, on the other hand, is not caused by the normal wear and tear of bones. Instead, it is an inflammation that leads to the secretion of substances, gradually destroying the structure of the joint. It can be of infectious, genetic, or metabolic origin.

EPIDEMIOLOGY AND ETIOLOGY

It is estimated that 12% of the US population has OA. The prevalence of OA increases with age and women are affected twice as often as men. It is generally a disease of middle to older age, first appearing after 40 years of age. Although the exact cause of OA is not known, it is believed to result from normal wear and tear on joints over a long period. Other contributing factors may include preexisting structural joint abnormalities, intrinsic aging, metabolic factors, genetic predisposition, obesity leading to overloaded joints, and macro- or microtrauma.

PATHOPHYSIOLOGY AND COMPLICATIONS

The trigger of OA is often unknown, but begins with tissue damage from mechanical injury, transmission of inflammatory mediators from the synovium into the articular cartilage, or defects in cartilage metabolism. As a result, the articular cartilage becomes thicker, and water content and the synthesis of proteoglycans are increased. This reflects a repair effort by the chondrocytes

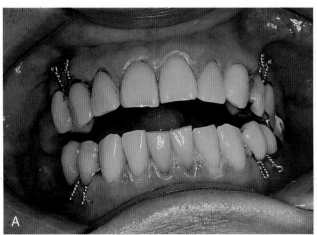
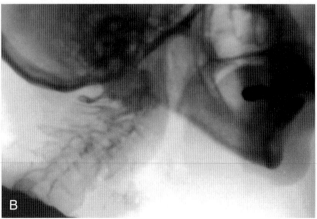

FIG. 20.4 (**A**) Anterior open bite resulting from progressive bilateral condylar resorption in a patient with advanced rheumatoid arthritis. (**B**) Lateral skull film shows a swan-neck deformity. (From Quinn PD. *Color Atlas of Temporomandibular Joint Surgery*. St. Louis: Mosby; 1998.)

that may last for several years. Ultimately, the joint surface thins and proteoglycan concentration decreases, leading to softening of the cartilage. Progressive splitting and abrasion of cartilage down to the subchondral bone occur. The exposed bone becomes polished and sclerotic, resembling ivory (eburnation). Some resurfacing with cartilage may occur if the disorder is arrested or stabilized. New bone forms at the margin of the articular cartilage in the non–weight-bearing part of the joint, creating osteophytes (or spurs), often covered by cartilage, that augment the degree of deformity.

The two most important complications associated with OA are pain and disability. Although RA is a more serious disease with more significant joint complications, OA has a 30-fold greater economic impact. One form of OA, called *primary generalized osteoarthritis,* is characterized by involvement of three or more joints or groups of joints. It occurs most often in women and affects the hands, knees, hips, and spine.

CLINICAL PRESENTATION

The primary symptom of OA is pain, typically localized to one or two joints (see Table 20.2). The pain is described as a dull ache accompanied by stiffness that is typically worse in the morning or after a period of inactivity. Usually the pain and stiffness last no longer than 15 min. Joint noises or grinding sounds (crepitus) may be detected with movement.

The most common sign of OA is appearance of painless bony growths on the medial and lateral aspects of the PIP joints, called Heberden nodes. When these enlargements occur on the distal interphalangeal joints, they are called Bouchard nodes (Fig. 20.5). On occasion, some pain may be associated with these nodes. Redness and swelling are uncommon.

Depending on which joint or group of joints is involved, patients may experience varying degrees of loss of range of motion and incapacitation. Hip and knee

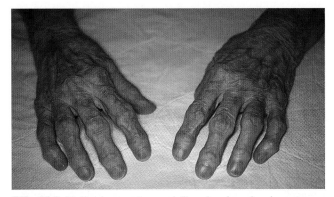

FIG. 20.5 Heberden nodes and Bouchard nodes in osteoarthritis. (From Swartz MH. *Textbook of Physical Diagnosis: History and Examination.* 6th ed. Philadelphia: Saunders; 2010.)

joints are particularly troublesome and are a common source of disability.

Radiographic signs of OA include narrowing of the joint space, articular surface irregularities and remodeling, and osteophytes or spurs. In addition, subchondral sclerosis (eburnation) and ankylosis may be seen. Symptoms often are not well correlated with radiographic signs.

LABORATORY AND DIAGNOSTIC FINDINGS

Laboratory findings in OA are essentially unremarkable. The ESR is usually normal, except for a mild elevation in primary generalized cases. Radiographic changes include narrowing of the joint space, increased density of subchondral bone, bony remodeling, and osteophytes (or spurs).

MEDICAL MANAGEMENT

Management targets the relief of pain and maintenance of joint flexibility and function. Patient education, physical therapy, exercise, weight reduction, and joint protection are all important aspects of management. Drug therapy often involves use of acetaminophen, which is recommended as a first-line drug, at doses of 1 g four times daily. Aspirin or NSAIDs also are commonly used when acetaminophen is not effective (see Table 20.3). Narcotic analgesics are generally used only for acute flares for short periods. Alternatively, duloxetine, a serotonin norepinephrine reuptake inhibitor, can be used to help reduce the pain caused by OA. Intraarticular steroid injections may be used intermittently for acute flares for short periods to reduce acute pain and inflammation. Surgery, including joint replacement, may be required to improve function or relieve pain.

DENTAL MANAGEMENT

Dental management and treatment planning modifications are essentially the same as for patients with RA (see Box 20.2).

Oral Complications and Manifestations

The TMJ may be affected by osteoarthritic changes (Fig. 20.6). This is characterized by insidious onset of unilateral preauricular aching and pain with stiffness after a period of inactivity that decreases with mild activity. Severe pain may be elicited on wide opening, and pain occurs with normal function and worsens during the day. Adjacent muscle splinting and spasm may occur. Crepitus is a common finding in the affected joint. In most cases, osteoarthritic pain in the TMJ resolves within 6–12 months of onset. Radiographic changes include decreased joint space, sclerosis, remodeling, and osteophytes (see Fig. 20.6). No correlation exists between TMJ symptoms and radiographic or histologic signs of OA.

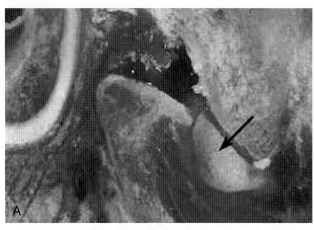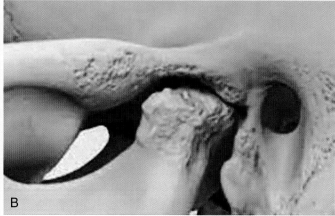

FIG. 20.6 (A) Surgical section of the temporomandibular joint demonstrating osteoarthritic changes especially of the condyle. **(B)** Postmortem dry skull section of the temporomandibular joint demonstrating osteoarthritic changes especially of the condyle.

Treatment of OA of the TMJ consists of acetaminophen, aspirin or NSAIDs, muscle relaxants, approaches to limit jaw function, physical therapy (heat, ice, ultrasound, controlled exercise), and occlusal splints to decrease joint loading. Conservative therapy is successful in controlling symptoms in most cases; however, if pain or dysfunction is severe and persistent, TMJ surgery may be necessary.

SYSTEMIC LUPUS ERYTHEMATOSUS

There are two types of lupus erythematosus (LE): *discoid* (*DLE*), which predominantly affects the skin, and a more generalized *systemic form* (*SLE*), which affects multiple organ systems. DLE is characterized by chronic, erythematous, scaly plaques on the face, scalp, or ears. Most patients with DLE have very few systemic manifestations, and the course tends to be benign. SLE involves the skin and other organ systems and is the more serious form. This section focuses on SLE.

Systemic lupus erythematosus is an autoimmune disease of unknown etiology. A strong familial aggregation exists, with a much higher frequency noted among first-degree relatives of patients. Studies of patients with SLE suggest that the disease is caused by genetically determined immune abnormalities that can be triggered by exogenous and endogenous factors. Among these triggering factors are infectious agents, stress, diet, toxins, drugs, and sunlight.

EPIDEMIOLOGY

Systemic lupus erythematosus is a prototypical autoimmune disease that predominantly affects women of childbearing age with a female-to-male ratio as high as 10:1. The disease is more common and more severe among African Americans and Hispanics compared with whites.

PATHOPHYSIOLOGY AND COMPLICATIONS

In SLE, antibody and immune complex deposition lead to inflammation and vasculopathy. Circulating autoantibodies form antigen–antibody complexes, which are deposited in a wide variety of tissues and organs, including the kidneys, skin, blood vessels, muscles and joints, heart, lungs, brain, gastrointestinal tract, lymphatics, and eyes.

Complications of SLE include infection, coronary artery disease, renal and pulmonary disease, and osteonecrosis. The leading causes of death in patients with SLE are infectious complications as well as lupus-related acute vascular neurologic events, renal failure, and cardiovascular or pulmonary involvement, with 10-year survival rates of ≥80%, respectively.

CLINICAL PRESENTATION

Because of the widespread systemic involvement of SLE, multiple manifestations are observed in many tissues and organs. The typical presentation is a woman with polyarthritis and a butterfly-shaped erythematous rash across the nose and cheeks (Fig. 20.7). The clinical presentation varies widely from mild to severe and depends largely on the extent and type of organ involvement.

Arthritis affects nearly three-quarters of patients. It affects the small joints and is migratory, with the pain typically out of proportion compared with clinical signs.

Serious renal abnormalities occur in fewer than one-third of patients with SLE. Renal failure, one of the most serious problems, is the best clinical indicator of a poor prognosis. Autoimmune hepatitis may occur with SLE and may result in liver damage (see Chapter 10).

Neuropsychiatric symptoms are common and include organic brain syndrome (a state of diffuse cerebral dysfunction associated with a disturbance in consciousness, cognition, mood, affect, and behavior in the absence of drugs, infection, or a metabolic cause), psychosis,

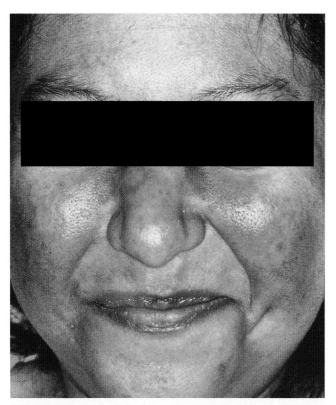

FIG. 20.7 Characteristic butterfly-shaped rash of systemic lupus erythematosus. (From Ignatavicius D, Workman ML. *Medical-Surgical Nursing: Patient-Centered Collaborative Care.* 6th ed. St. Louis: Saunders; 2010.)

seizures, stroke, movement disorders, and peripheral neuropathy. Thromboembolism associated with antiphospholipid antibody is an important cause of abnormalities in the central nervous system.

Pulmonary manifestations of SLE include pleuritis, infection, pulmonary edema, pneumonitis, and pulmonary hypertension. Cardiac involvement is common and consists of pericarditis, myocarditis, endocarditis, and coronary artery disease. Libman-Sacks endocarditis (nonbacterial verrucous endocarditis) is found at autopsy in 50% of patients with SLE.

LABORATORY AND DIAGNOSTIC FINDINGS

Laboratory tests are required to differentiate SLE from other connective tissue (CT) disorders. Routine testing includes antinuclear antibodies (ANA), anti-double-stranded (ds) DNA (anti-dsDNA), complete blood count, urinalysis, and chemistry profiling to rule out concurrent renal or liver disease involvement.

Antibody testing is useful in the diagnosis of SLE but is not 100% accurate and can result in false-positive results. The most relied-on test for defining SLE is the ANA; this test is positive in 95% of SLE patients; however, a positive result also occurs in patients with other CT diseases. Results of anti-DNA assays—double helix and single helix—are elevated in 65%–80% of patients with active untreated SLE.

Common hematologic abnormalities include hemolytic anemia, leukopenia, lymphopenia, and thrombocytopenia as well as a variety of clotting abnormalities. The most common clotting abnormality is the lupus anticoagulant, which is associated with elevated partial thromboplastin time (PTT) and the presence of antiphospholipid antibodies. Antiphospholipid antibodies are a group of immune proteins (antibodies) that the body mistakenly produces against itself in an autoimmune response to phospholipids. A positive test to antiphospholipids increase the risk of excessive blood clotting.

SLE-related nephritis is associated with urine proteinuria, hematuria, and white blood cell casts.

MEDICAL MANAGEMENT

Treatment for patients with SLE uses many of the medications used in the treatment other rheumatologic disorders (see Table 20.3) but with a greater degree of observation for renal, cardiac, and clotting abnormalities. Patients with SLE are advised to avoid sun exposure because this may trigger onset or exacerbation of the disease. Aspirin and NSAIDs are often used for mild disease, antimalarials for dermatologic disease, glucocorticoids for more severe symptoms, and cytotoxic agents for symptoms unresponsive to other therapies or as adjuncts in severe disease.

A specific set of quality indicators (QIs) to evaluate the monitoring of SLE patients in routine clinical practice have been integrated into the recently developed European League Against Rheumatism (EULAR) recommendations for monitoring SLE patients in routine clinical practice and observational studies. Eleven QIs have been developed including the general evaluation of drug toxicity, evaluation of comorbid conditions, eye evaluation, laboratory assessment, evaluation of the presence of chronic viral infections, documentation of vaccination, and antibody testing at baseline.

DENTAL MANAGEMENT

Because SLE is a varied disease with so many potential problems caused by the disease or its treatment, pretreatment consultation with the patient's physician is advised (Box 20.5). As in RA, drug considerations and adverse effects in SLE are of major importance. Table 20.3 lists the dental and oral considerations associated with the use of these drugs. In patients who are taking corticosteroids or cytotoxins who also have leukopenia, the use of prophylactic antibiotics for periodontal and oral surgical procedures may be considered. Patients who are taking corticosteroids also may develop significant adrenal suppression and could require supplementation, especially for surgical procedures or in cases of extreme anxiety (see Chapter 15).

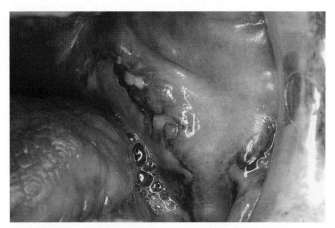

FIG. 20.8 Ulceration of the buccal mucosa in a patient with systemic lupus erythematosus. (From Neville BW, Damm D, Allen C, et al. *Oral and Maxillofacial Pathology*. 3rd ed. St. Louis: Saunders; 2009.)

erythematous with white spots or radiating peripheral lines; they also may occur as painful ulcerations (Fig. 20.8). Lesions frequently resemble lichen planus or leukoplakia. When they occur on the lip, a silvery, scaly margin, similar to that seen on the skin, may develop. Skin and lip lesions frequently are noted after exposure to the sun. Treatment of these lesions is symptomatic, and future sun exposure is to be avoided (see Appendix C).

SJÖGREN SYNDROME

Sjögren syndrome is an autoimmune disease that causes exocrinopathy and affects the salivary and lacrimal glands. SS can be categorized as primary SS and secondary SS. Primary SS manifests clinically with keratoconjunctivitis sicca and salivary gland dysfunction (xerostomia) in the absence of an associated connective tissue disorder. Secondary SS (SS-2) manifests with the same clinical features as primary SS in the presence of a diagnosed systemic connective tissue disease (e.g., RA, SLE, primary biliary cirrhosis, FM, mixed connective tissue disease, polymyositis, Raynaud syndrome).

EPIDEMIOLOGY AND ETIOLOGY

The prevalence of SS in the adult population is estimated to be 2.7%; thus it is the second most common rheumatoid disorder. More than 90% of patients with SS are female.

Sjögren syndrome typically manifests during the fourth or fifth decade of life, although isolated cases of SS have been reported in children. The precise cause of SS, as of many of the autoimmune rheumatic disorders, is unknown, although several contributing factors have been identified. One theory is that the disease results from complications of viral infection with Epstein—Barr virus (EBV). Exposure to, or reactivation of, EBV elicits expression of the human lymphocyte antigen (HLA)

Abnormal bleeding caused by thrombocytopenia is a potential problem in some patients with SLE. Therefore, a platelet count should be obtained. A platelet count lower than 50,000/mL may indicate inadequate platelet activity and potential bleeding problems.

Cardiac valvular abnormalities are found in 25%−50% of patients who have SLE and often are not clinically detectable. Because of these valve abnormalities the potential exists for bacterial endocarditis resulting from physiologic bacteremia. However, the current American Heart Association's guidelines for endocarditis prevention do not recommend antibiotic prophylaxis for patients with valvular disease associated with SLE when receiving invasive dental procedures. Patients with SLE-associated renal failure have the potential for altered drug metabolism, hematologic disorders, and infection (see Chapter 12).

Treatment Planning Considerations

Consideration should be given to physical disabilities related to arthritis and myalgia.

Oral Complications and Manifestations

Oral lesions of the lips and mucous membranes have been reported to occur in up to 5%−25% of patients with SLE. These lesions are rather nonspecific and may be complex; this is recognized by the T-cell (CD4+) lymphocytes and results in the release of cytokines (TNF, IL-2, interferon-γ [IFN-γ], and others). Current evidence has shown that both innate and adaptive genetic alteration are involved in SS. Chronic inflammation, infiltration of lymphocytes, and ultimate destruction of exocrine gland tissue follow.

PATHOPHYSIOLOGY AND COMPLICATIONS

Sjögren syndrome is a chronic, progressive autoimmune disorder that is characterized by exocrinopathy and generalized lymphoproliferation that primarily affect the salivary and lacrimal glands. Systemic manifestations of SS include involvement of the pancreas, biliary tract, and lungs.

Progression to lymphoma occurs in about 5% of SS patients. Lymphoma in these patients occurs independent of a history of other cancers or prior radiation therapy or chemotherapy, although the relative risk may be as high as 100 times greater when prior cancer therapy has occurred (see Chapter 23). Clinical findings associated with lymphoma (see Chapter 23) include chronic parotid enlargement, lymphadenopathy (enlarged cervical and axillary nodes), anemia, cryoglobulinemia, lymphopenia, cutaneous vasculitis, and peripheral neuropathy.

The most common type of lymphoma in patients with SS involves mucosa-associated lymphoid tissue (MALT); 70% of cases are low-grade, nonaggressive lymphomas, and 15% are the high-grade lymphoblastic type. IL-6 and TNF-α are associated with lesions that undergo transformation to lymphoma, as well as the presence of B-cell monoclonality in labial minor salivary gland tissue.

CLINICAL PRESENTATION

Sjögren syndrome is characterized by eye dryness, hyposalivation, and enlargement of the parotid glands. Secondary outcomes of persistent oral dryness are fissured tongue, dysgeusia (taste dysfunction), difficulty tolerating and swallowing certain foods, secondary infection, and an increased caries rate (Table 20.6). *Candida* infections, such as angular cheilitis, are very common in patients who have Sjögren syndrome.

LABORATORY AND DIAGNOSTIC FINDINGS

Precise diagnostic criteria for SS remain controversial, although specific laboratory tests are available for the major diagnostic categories of salivary and tear production, histopathologic changes, and serologic inflammatory markers (Box 20.6). Several published criteria (e.g., ACR) are available for the diagnosis of SS with values that are slightly different. Common characteristics and variations are summarized in Box 20.6.

Labial salivary gland histopathologic examination has been accepted almost universally as the prima facie

TABLE 20.6	Clinical Manifestations of Sjögren Syndrome[a]
Clinical Manifestation	Prevalence (% of Affected Patients)
Orcheilosis or angular cheilitis	75
Glossitis	60
Mucositis	30
Glossodynia	45
Dysgeusia	75
Dysphagia	45
Candidiasis	75
Dental caries	100
Periodontitis	60–100

[a]From 62 consecutive patients with Sjögren syndrome who presented to the University of Minnesota Xerostomia Clinic.
Data from Rhodus NL. Xerostomia and glossodynia in patients with autoimmune disorders. *Ear Nose Throat J.* 1989;68:791–794 and Rhodus NL, Colby S, Moller K, Bereuter J. Quantitative assessment of dysphagia in patients with primary and secondary Sjögren's syndrome. *Oral Surg Oral Med Oral Pathol Oral Radiol Endod.* 1995;79:305–310.

BOX 20.6 Diagnostic Criteria for Sjögren Syndrome

Subjects must meet four of six criteria; labial biopsy or serologic studies must be performed.

Ocular Symptoms (1:3)	Ocular Signs (1:2)
Daily dry eyes >3 months	+ Schirmer test (<5 mm/5 min)
Sand or gravel sensitivity	Rose Bengal score (>4 vBs)
Use of tear substitutes (>3 times daily)	
Oral symptoms (1:3)	Oral signs: salivary function (1:3)
Daily dry mouth >3 months	+ Scintigraphy
Swollen salivary glands	+ Sialography
Need fluids to swallow food	WUSF <1.5 mL/15 min (0.1 mL/min)
Labial SG histology	Autoantibodies (1:2)
Focus scope biopsy > ¼ mm >50 mononuclear cells per field	anti—SS-Ro anti—SS-La

SG, salivary gland; *vBs,* von Blisterberg score for eyes; *WUSF,* whole unstimulated saliva flow.

diagnostic indicator for definitive diagnosis of SS. The classic histopathologic feature of the minor salivary glands in SS is seen as lymphocytic infiltration that includes benign lymphosialadenopathy (focal lymphocytic sialadenitis or benign lymphoepithelial lesion in the major salivary glands). This benign lymphosialadenopathy may manifest as parotid hypertrophy, particularly in patients with primary SS. Small clusters of intralobular ducts enlarge to replace the acinar epithelial parenchyma.

The lesion comprises primarily CD4+ T-cell lymphocytes, along with polyclonal B cells and plasma cells that are acquired late. Among the lymphocytic foci, approximately 75% are T cells, and 5%–10% are B cells. As the inflammatory process progresses, fibrosis and atrophy of the salivary glands occur, and hyposalivation progresses.

Hypergammaglobulinemia is the most frequent laboratory finding (80%) among patients with SS. Hyperactivity of B lymphocytes results in increased RF antibodies, such as ANAs and antibodies against organ-specific antigens including salivary duct epithelia or thyroid tissue. The ANAs include SS-A (Ro), which is present in approximately 70% of patients with SS-1 and 15% –90% with SS-1 and SS-B (La) antibodies, which are present in approximately 50% of patients with SS-1 and 5%–30% with SS-2. These ANAs also may be found in other autoimmune disorders. Elevated ESR, mild anemia ($\approx$25%), and leukopenia ($\approx$10%) also are found in patients with SS.

Sialometry is useful as an initial screening tool for hyposalivation associated with SS and as an assessment for the level of severity of SS. To be valuable as a diagnostic technique, unstimulated and stimulated salivary flow should be assessed over a period of at least 5 min (often up to 15 min).

DENTAL MANAGEMENT

Dental management of patients with SS requires three levels of care that include (1) provision of moisture and lubrication by stimulation or simulation, (2) treatment of secondary mucosal conditions (such as mucositis or candidiasis), and (3) prevention of oral disease, provision of maintenance and general support (e.g., nutrition) (Table 20.7).

Patients with SS should be counseled to drink plenty of water (8–10 glasses per day) and to avoid diuretics such as caffeine, tobacco, and alcoholic beverages. Salivary substitutes, oral moisturizers, and artificial salivas may provide some xerostomia relief. Pilocarpine HCl (Salagen) and cevimeline HCl (Evoxac) are effective for the treatment of patients with SS with signs and symptoms of hyposalivation. Administration of pilocarpine or cevimeline effectively stimulates only the salivary acinar tissue, which remains functional. Therefore, patients with SS who have lost most of the salivary acinar tissue capable of fluid production benefit little from these drugs.

Oral Complications and Manifestations

Patients who have SS and hyposalivation are at significant increased risk of caries as well as enamel erosion. Of particular risk is the cervical–cementoenamel junction portion of the tooth. Recommendations for patients with SS with dry mouth are as follows: meticulous oral hygiene with minimally abrasive fluoridated dentifrices and irrigation devices is paramount; 3–4 month professional hygiene recall intervals; topical daily fluoride use

TABLE 20.7 Management of Salivary Dysfunction[a] (See Appendix C)

General Measures	Specific Agents or Measures[a,b]
Moisture and Lubrication (Continuous, as Needed)	
1. Drink (sip water, liquids)	1. Artificial saliva, or moisturizers (especially at night)
2. Use sugarless candy or gum	2. Pilocarpine hydrochloride, 5 mg three times daily)
3. Avoid ethanol	*or*
4. Avoid tobacco	3. Cevimeline hydrochloride (Evoxac, 30 mg three times daily)
5. Avoid coffee, tea, and other caffeinated beverages	4. Sodium carboxymethylcellulose, 0.5% solution
Soft Tissue Lesions and Soreness (Treatment and Maintenance)	
Magic mouthwash	1. Benadryl + Maalox + nystatin elixir
	2. (Carafate, optional)
	3. (Lidocaine 2%, optional, for acute lesions)
	4. Orabase-HCA (for acute lesions)
	5. Mycelex 60-mg troches (for candidiasis)
	6. Mycolog II ointment (inflamed lips and tongue)
Prevention of Caries and Periodontal Disease (Continuous)	
1. Meticulous perioral hygiene	1. Biotene toothpaste (neutral sodium fluoride, 1.0%, trays)
2. Avoid acids	2. Prevident, 5000 ppm[c]
3. Regular hygiene and prophylaxis recalls	3. Peridex (chlorhexidine gluconate) (optional)
4. Sodium bicarbonate rinses (optional)	4. Waterpik

[a]Specific treatments are dependent on the diagnosis. **(See Appendix C)**.
[b]Manufacturers: Oral Balance, Laclede Pharmaceuticals; Salagen, MGI Pharmaceuticals; Mouthkote, Parnell Pharmaceuticals; Optimoist, Colgate-Hoyt; Salivart, Gebauer; Biotene, Laclede Pharmaceuticals; Benadryl, Parke-Davis; Maalox, Novartis Pharmaceuticals; Carafate, Hoechst, Marion, Roussel Pharmaceuticals; Decadron, Merck & Co. Pharmaceuticals; Orabase, Colgate-Palmolive; Mycelex, ALZA Prevident, Colgate-Hoyte; Peridex, Procter & Gamble; Waterpik, Teledyne.
[c]Prevident neutral sodium fluoride, 1.0%, to be applied in trays 2 times daily.
‡Benadryl, 25 mg/10 mL + Maalox, 64 mL + nystatin, 100,000 IU/mL = 16 mL.
§Decadron elixir, 0.5%/5 mL. Dispense 100 mL; to be swished and expectorated, 5 mL three times daily.
Adapted from Rhodus NL: Diagnosis and treatment of Sjögren's syndrome, *Quintessence Int* 30:689–699, 1999.

(concentrated fluorides delivered as a direct brush-on treatment or with custom-made trays) as well as fluoride varnishes, gels, or rinses; chlorhexidine administration and calcium-phosphate–based remineralizing agents use as adjunctive therapy.

Patients with SS and xerostomia may report symptoms of glossodynia (burning tongue). The tongue often becomes depapillated and fissured appearance (Fig. 20.9). The dorsal epithelium often is atrophic or eroded, erythematous, and potentially secondarily infected. Pain and burning may be spontaneous or elicited with acidic or spicy foods, such as those containing ascorbic or acetic acid. The tongue is commonly infected with *Candida albicans* in patients with SS. Acute candidal infections must be treated with antifungals, and maintenance therapy is generally required to prevent recurrence of the fungal infection (see Table 20.5).

PSORIATIC ARTHRITIS

Psoriatic arthritis is an inflammatory arthritis associated with the chronic inflammatory skin condition psoriasis. Although most cases arise in patients with established cutaneous disease, some patients (particularly children) have arthritis that antedates the appearance of the skin lesions. Risk factors for the development of PsA are a family history of PsA, early age onset of psoriasis, and in some studies the severity psoriasis.

EPIDEMIOLOGY

Psoriatic arthritis is estimated to occur in 0.1%–1% of the US population, and develops in 5%–10% of patients with psoriasis. The age at onset can range from 30 to 55 years, with an equal predilection for women and men.

PATHOPHYSIOLOGY AND COMPLICATIONS

The genetic associations with PsA are complex. Psoriasis itself is associated with HLA-B13, HLA-B16, HLA-B17, and HLA-Cw6. By contrast, HLA-B39 and HLA-B27 have been associated with sacroiliitis and axial involvement. No etiologic agent has been proved in PsA, although some investigators have proposed that the disease process represents RA in response to cutaneous bacteria. PsA can be progressive with the potential for aggressive osteolysis, fibrous ankylosis, and heterotopic new bone formation.

CLINICAL PRESENTATION

Psoriatic arthritis has a variable manifestation and disease course, but several clinical patterns have been identified. The clinical subsets are not mutually exclusive, nor are they static over time. The most common form (30% –50% of patients) is an asymmetric oligoarthritis that may involve both large and small joints. In the second subset (10%–15% of patients), there is selective targeting of the distal interphalangeal joints. These changes are strongly associated with nail dystrophy, of which the features are onycholysis, subungual keratosis, pitting, and oil drop–like staining (Fig. 20.10). The third subset (15%–30% of patients) has a symmetric polyarthritis that mimics RA in many ways except for the absence of rheumatoid nodules and RF. The fourth clinical variant is psoriatic spondylitis (20% of patients) in which 50% of patients are HLA-B27 positive. The fifth subset, arthritis mutilans (5% of patients), is a destructive, erosive arthritis that affects large and small joints and can be associated with marked deformities and significant disability.

LABORATORY AND DIAGNOSTIC FINDINGS

Psoriatic arthritis is a diagnosis of exclusion. The RF antibody test is usually negative and so is the anti-CCP, which helps rule out RA. The histopathology of the synovitis of PsA is comparable to that of the other SpAs. Radiographic changes in PsA involve soft tissue swelling (particularly in the case of dactylitis), erosions, and periostitis. Axial involvement may lead to the appearance

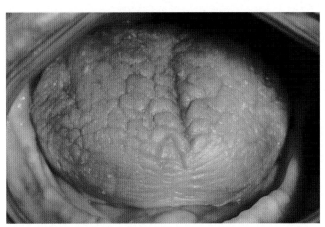

FIG. 20.9 Dry and fissured tongue in a patient with Sjögren syndrome. (From Neville BW, Damm D, Allen C, et al. *Oral and Maxillofacial Pathology.* 3rd ed. St. Louis: Saunders; 2009.)

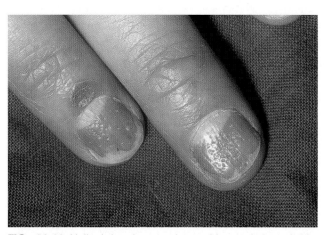

FIG. 20.10 Nail pitting in a patient with psoriatic arthritis. (From Goldman L, Ausiello D, eds. *Cecil Textbook of Medicine.* 23rd ed. Philadelphia: Saunders; 2008.)

of asymmetric sacroiliitis with syndesmophytes that are bulky, asymmetric, and nonmarginal. The classic "pencil-in-cup" deformity may be seen in patients with distal interphalangeal joint disease or arthritis mutilans. Acroosteolysis is noted in a minority of patients and reflects an aggressive erosive process.

MEDICAL MANAGEMENT

Treatment is directed at reducing joint inflammation and controlling skin lesions. Several DMARDs are available for use including methotrexate, TNF-α antagonists, etanercept (Enbrel), and biologic agents such as abatacept (Orencia). Abatacept is a modified antibody that selectively inhibits T-cell activation via competitive binding to CD80 or CD86, and decreases serum levels of cytokines and inflammatory proteins implicated in the pathogenesis of PsA.

DENTAL MANAGEMENT

Dental management and treatment planning modifications for PsA are similar to those for RA and are reviewed in Box 20.2.

GIANT CELL ARTERITIS

Giant cell arteritis (GCA) is a systemic vasculitis involving medium-sized and large arteries, most commonly the extracranial branches of the carotid artery and specifically the temporal artery ("temporal arteritis").

EPIDEMIOLOGY AND ETIOLOGY

This inflammatory disorder affects women more often than men (as do most autoimmune diseases), almost exclusively after 50 years of age, and the average age is 72 years. Histologically, GCA is characterized by a mononuclear cell infiltrate of T cells and macrophages that penetrates through the wall of arteries (Fig. 20.11). Approximately 50% of patients with GCA also have polymyalgia rheumatica. GCA is occlusive in nature because of the narrowing of vascular lumen, thus it has associations with cranial pain, blindness, transient ischemic attacks, and stroke.

CLINICAL PRESENTATION

Symptoms and signs of GCA include excessive sweating, fever, malaise, anorexia, headaches and scalp tenderness, muscle aches (including muscles of mastication), and jaw pain (Box 20.7).

LABORATORY AND DIAGNOSTIC FINDINGS

There are no specific laboratory tests for GCA. Typically, patients exhibit a high ESR and CRP, but these values are nonspecific. Angiography (particularly magnetic

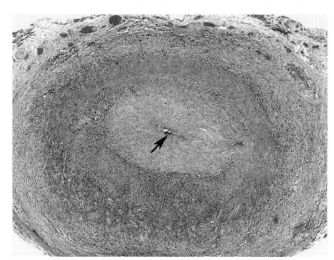

FIG. 20.11 Histology of giant cell arteritis (GCAs). A typical temporal artery affected by GCA shows characteristics such as panmural mononuclear inflammatory infiltrate, destruction of the internal and external elastic laminae, and concentric intimal hyperplasia. (From Albert DM, Robinson P, Nelson D, et al. *Albert & Jakobiec's Principles & Practice of Ophthalmology.* 3rd ed. Edinburgh: Saunders; 2008.)

BOX 20.7	Signs and Symptoms of Giant Cell Arteritis

Commonly Reported Signs and Symptoms
- Excessive sweating
- Fever
- General ill feeling
- Jaw pain (intermittent or when chewing)
- Loss of appetite
- Muscle aches
- Throbbing headache on one side of the head or the back of the head
- Scalp sensitivity; tenderness when touching the scalp
- Vision difficulties
- Blurred vision
- Double vision
- Reduced vision (blindness in one eye)
- Weakness, excessive tiredness
- Weight loss (>5% of total body weight)

Other, Less Common Signs and Symptoms
- Bleeding gums
- Face pain
- Hearing loss
- Joint stiffness
- Joint pain
- Mouth sores

resonance angiography) can be helpful in making the diagnosis. Temporal artery biopsy demonstrates features that include panmural mononuclear inflammatory infiltrate, destruction of the internal and external elastic laminae, and concentric intimal hyperplasia (Fig. 20.11).

MEDICAL MANAGEMENT

The universal treatment for GCA is glucocorticoid therapy. Prednisone (60 mg/day) is the usual initial therapy. After the immune response has subsided and symptoms diminish, prednisone may be reduced by 10% per week. However, therapy may need to be resumed when symptoms return. Adjunctive therapy with aspirin may also be helpful to reduce ischemic events in the obstructed vessels.

DENTAL MANAGEMENT

From a dental perspective, GCA is significant for several reasons. Major manifestations are temporal headaches and jaw claudication. Additionally, orofacial manifestations of GCA can lead to misdiagnosis of GCA as TM disorder. GCA should be included in the differential diagnosis for orofacial pain in older adults on the basis of knowledge of related signs and symptoms, including masticatory muscle pain, resistance to motion at the end of range (end-feel limitation), and temporal headache. Early diagnosis and treatment are essential to avoid severe complications.

LYME DISEASE

Lyme disease is a multisystem inflammatory disease caused by the tick-borne spirochete of the *Borrelia species*. *Borrelia burgdorferi* is the primary agent in the United States, however *B. mayonii*, *B. afzelli*, and *B. garinii* are responsible in Europe and Asia. The disease was first identified in the United States in 1975 during an outbreak around Lyme, Connecticut, of an inflammatory condition presumed to be JRA. The classical pattern of Lyme disease is a characteristic macular skin rash (erythema migrans) that appears within a month after the bite of the tick *of the Ixodes species* (i.e., *I scapularis*, *I. pacificus*, *I. ricinus*, *and I. persulcatus*). Several different manifestations, including neurologic, articular, and cardiac, may follow.

EPIDEMIOLOGY

Lyme disease has been reported in North America, Europe, and Asia. In the United States, more than 90% of all cases of Lyme disease have been reported in only eight states (New York, Connecticut, Pennsylvania, Massachusetts, Rhode Island, New Jersey, Wisconsin, and Minnesota). Differences in the organism and in the immunogenetics of the affected population may explain the differences in clinical presentation of Lyme disease. Only about 30% of patients can recall an associated tick bite.

PATHOPHYSIOLOGY AND COMPLICATIONS

B. burgdorferi enters the skin and within 3 to about 30 days migrates to the lymphatics where it can cause adenopathy or disseminate in the blood to organs or other skin sites. Vasculitis ensues which has been implicated in some cases of peripheral neuropathy, and can cause a vascular lesion resembling endarteritis obliterans in the meninges and synovium of affected patients.

The clinical manifestations of Lyme disease can be divided into three phases: early localized, early disseminated, and late disease. Patients with a diagnosis of Lyme disease may not be identified until later stages of the disease. Early localized disease includes erythema migrans and associated findings. Erythema migrans occurs in 50%–80% of infected patients within 1 month of the tick bite. Erythema migrans presents as a "target" or "bull's eye" lesion that typically appears in or near the axilla or belt line because ticks like warm, moist areas of the human body (Fig. 20.12). Most often, the lesion is asymptomatic, although it may itch, burn, or hurt. The lesion typically expands and enlarges over the course of a few days and can cause multiple lesions or a rash. Patients also may have an acute viremia-like syndrome with fever, malaise, nausea, myalgia, fatigue, headache, and arthralgias.

The next phase of clinical presentation is early disseminated disease, which may occur within a few days to a few months after the tick bite, possibly without preceding erythema migrans. The clinical manifestations of this phase are flu-like syndrome, lingering malaise and fatigue, cardiac involvement, and neurologic problems. In the absence of treatment, about 8% of patients infected with Lyme disease manifest cardiac problems including heart block, myopericarditis, and cardiomegaly. In most cases, the carditis begins to resolve, even without antibiotic therapy. Neurologic damage occurs in approximately 10% of untreated patients. Primary

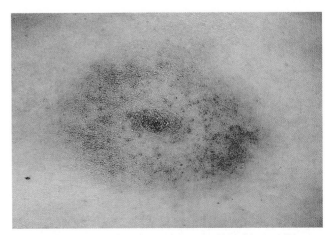

FIG. 20.12 Classic erythema migrans lesion of Lyme disease. (From Swartz M. *Textbook of Physical Diagnosis*. 6th ed. St. Louis: Saunders; 2010.)

manifestations include lymphocytic meningitis, cranial nerve palsy (especially of the facial nerve), and radiculoneuritis.

In the late disease stage, which may occur months to years after the infection and may not be preceded by the earlier manifestations, musculoskeletal problems are the primary manifestation. Intermittent, migratory episodes of polyarthritis that mimic the "juvenile arthritis" originally described in cases of Lyme disease occur in approximately 50% of patients. Chronic arthritis of the knee is common, along with erosion of bone and cartilage. Chronic inflammatory joint disease may last for 5–8 years.

Late neurologic manifestations of Lyme disease, called *tertiary neuroborreliosis,* consist of encephalopathy, neurocognitive dysfunction, and peripheral neuropathy. Symptoms may be subtle and may be reported as headache and fatigue in addition to cognitive, mood, and sleep disturbances. Neuropsychological testing may be useful in confirming the diagnosis.

LABORATORY AND DIAGNOSTIC FINDINGS

Although the diagnosis of Lyme disease is based on clinical findings, serologic testing (antibodies against the pathogen) is important and necessary. Current practice is to confirm enzyme-linked immunosorbent assay results with Western blot analysis. Many other conditions (e.g., EBV infections, SLE, infective endocarditis) may mimic Lyme disease; therefore, laboratory testing should be performed for a definitive diagnosis. Antibody responses may be undetectable in infections of less than 6 weeks' duration, and early antibiotic therapy based on symptoms may render the infected patient seronegative. Most patients with late disease manifestations are strongly seropositive.

MEDICAL MANAGEMENT

Antibiotic therapy is effective for the treatment of Lyme disease. Prompt antibiotic therapy when early symptoms are reported usually prevents progression to later stages of Lyme disease. Oral doses of 100 mg of doxycycline given twice daily for 3–4 weeks provide first-line treatment for early infection. Alternatively, amoxicillin (500 mg three times daily) or ceftriaxone may be given. In the late disseminated stages of Lyme disease and in pregnant women, IV antibiotics (e.g., ceftriaxone) are often used. Some patients with arthritis are refractory to antibiotic therapy. These patients may benefit from intraarticular corticosteroid injections or hydroxychloroquine. Adequate therapy for neurologic damage is elusive, and recovery may be very slow.

DENTAL MANAGEMENT

The major dental consideration in Lyme disease is the identification of unusual symptoms in the absence of a clear medical condition. Symptoms of fatigue, malaise, arthralgia, neuritis, or neuralgia, including facial palsy, may indicate the possibility of Lyme disease and the need for referral for proper medical diagnosis. Numerous reports have described facial nerve palsy that closely resembles Bell palsy caused by Lyme disease. The presentation of this facial palsy may be combined with other neurologic deficits or may stand alone. Involvement of the parotid glands (acute parotitis) has been reported. Along with facial nerve palsy, facial and dental neuralgia and TMJ symptoms have been reported to occur with Lyme disease.

FIBROMYALGIA

Fibromyalgia (FM) is a common cause of chronic pain in the United States. The diagnosis of FM is typically difficult and lengthy because there are so many other potential causes for the widespread pain, including head and neck pain, back and extremity pain, and others. Chronic (several years) diffuse (muscle) pain accompanied by fatigue, sleep disturbance, and neuropathies (or other neurologic symptoms) are all cardinal symptoms of FM.

EPIDEMIOLOGY AND ETIOLOGY

Fibromyalgia affects up to 4% of the population, primarily women, presenting with a spectrum of signs and symptoms (Box 20.8). Current evidence supports that FM is associated with stress and may be a centrally mediated pain disorder.

CLINICAL PRESENTATION

Patients with FM typically have diffuse aches and pain together with fatigue, muscle strain, and mental cloudiness. To meet the diagnostic criteria (Fig. 20.13), the patient must have chronic (present for >3 months) widespread pain in all four quadrants of the body, and 11

BOX 20.8 Symptoms of Fibromyalgia

- Body aches
- Chronic facial muscle pain or aching
- Fatigue
- Irritable bowel syndrome
- Memory difficulties and cognitive difficulties
- Multiple tender areas (muscle and joint pain) on the back of the neck, shoulders, sternum, lower back, hips, shins, elbows, knees
- Numbness and tingling
- Palpitations
- Reduced exercise tolerance
- Sleep disturbances
- Tension or migraine headache

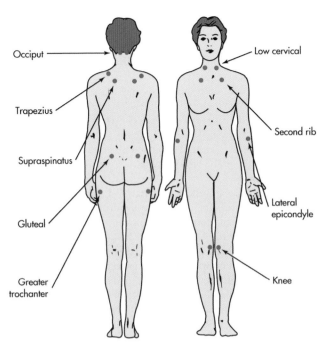

Occiput

Trapezius

Supraspinatus

Gluteal

Greater trochanter

Low cervical

Second rib

Lateral epicondyle

Knee

FIG. 20.13 The American College of Rheumatology defines fibromyalgia as consistent tender points in 11 of these 18 anatomic locations. (Redrawn from Freundlich B, Leventhal L. The fibromyalgia syndrome. In: Schumacher Jr HR, et al., eds. *Primer on the Rheumatic Diseases.* 11th ed. Atlanta: Arthritis Foundation; 1997. Reprinted with permission from The Arthritis Foundation, 1330 W. Peachtree St., Atlanta, GA 30309.)

of the 18 points must be painful on application of only 4 kg of pressure.

MEDICAL MANAGEMENT

Successful management of FM requires a thorough analysis of the patient's biopsychosocial issues, including fatigue, sleep, pain, psychological distress, diet, and stress factors. Patients are encouraged to get exercise, sound and sufficient sleep, apply heat to affected areas, and receive gentle massage along with stress management. Heterocyclic antidepressant agents (amitriptyline, trazadone, or nortriptyline) that target management of central sensitization and can improve sleep are generally beneficial. Highly selective serotonin reuptake inhibitors such as fluoxetine exhibit a modest pain benefit in patients with FM. Anticonvulsant medications such as gabapentin, topiramate, or pregabalin are effective and are recommended as adjuncts to exercise. Opioids are to be avoided.

DENTAL MANAGEMENT

The major discomfort with FM is muscle pain. Depending on which muscles are involved, patients may not be comfortable in a supine position in a dental chair. Therefore, just as with RA or OA, consideration should

be given to providing a more upright chair position; using neck, back, and leg supports; and scheduling short appointments (see Box 20.2).

Oral Complications and Manifestations

Patients affected with FM may experience TMD-like features, resulting in severe pain upon wide opening, and pain occurring even with normal function, which worsens throughout the day. Adjacent muscle splinting and spasm may occur. Crepitus is a common finding in the affected joint.

The regional pain found with myofascial pain syndrome (MFP) needs to be distinguished from the widespread muscular pain associated with FM. In both cases, the pain is often described as a "chronic dull aching pain" and is central to the diagnosis of both disorders. It should be further noted that when the muscle pain is primarily due to the FM, it may not respond as well as the jaw pain from MFP because FM is a systemic and not a local condition, and muscle pain is a typical presentation in FM.

BIBLIOGRAPHY

1. American College of Rheumatology clinical practice guidelines; 2016. http://www.rheumatology.org/Practice-Quality/Clinical-Support/Clinical-Practice-Guidelines. Accessed April 20, 2021.
2. American College of Rheumatology diagnostic classification of rheumatoid disorders. http://www.rheumatology.org/Diagnosticclassification. Accessed April 20, 2021.
3. Arthritis Foundation. Rheumatoid arthritis. http://www.arthritis.org. Accessed April 20, 2021.
4. Arthritis Foundation. Osteoarthritis; 2016. www.arthritis.org/osteoarthritis. Accessed April 20, 2021.
5. Berbari EF, Osmon DR, Carr A, et al. Dental procedures as risk factors for prosthetic hip or knee infection: a hospital-based prospective case-control study. *Clin Infect Dis.* 2010;50:8−19.
6. WebMD. Complications from biologic treatment of arthritis. www.webmd.com/rheumatology/news. Accessed April 20, 2021.
7. Emamian ES, Leon JM, Lessard CJ, et al. Peripheral blood gene expression profiling in Sjogren's syndrome. *Gene Immun.* 2009;10:285−296.
8. Felson D. Osteoarthritis. In: In Harrison's Principles of Internal Medicine, 20th ed.. Jameson, Fauci, Kasper, et al. Copyright © 2018. McGraw- Hill Publishers. Volume Vol. 1 eBook ISBN 978-1-259-64400-9; MHID 1-259-64400-6; Volume 2 eBook ISBN 978-1-259-64402-3; MHID 1-259-64402-2 [Chapter 326].
9. Langford CA, Gilliand BC. Fibromyalgia and chronic fatigue syndrome. In Harrison's Principles of Internal Medicine, 20th ed.. Jameson, Fauci, Kasper, et al. Copyright © 2018. McGraw- Hill Publishers. Volume Vol. 1 eBook ISBN 978-1-259-64400-9; MHID 1-259-64400-6; Volume 2 eBook ISBN 978-1-259-64402-3; MHID 1-259-64402-2 [Chapter 329].
10. Lessard CJ, Rasmussen A, Li H, et al. Identification of multiple genetic variants associated with Sjögren's syndrome

involved in both the innate and adaptive immune responses. *Nat Genet.* 2013. https://doi.org/10.1038/ng.2792.

11. Little J. Patients with prosthetic joints: are they at risk when undergoing dental procedures? *Spec Care Dent.* 1997;17:153−160.

12. Little JW, Jacobson JJ, Lockhart PB, et al. The dental treatment of patients with joint replacements. *J Am Dental Assoc.* 2010;141:667−671.

13. Lipsky P, Diamond K. Autoimmunity and autoimmune disorders. In: Harrison's Principles of Internal Medicine, 20th ed.. Jameson, Fauci, Kasper, et al. Copyright © 2018. McGraw- Hill Publishers. Volume Vol. 1 eBook ISBN 978-1-259-64400-9; MHID 1-259-64400-6; Volume 2 eBook ISBN 978-1-259-64402-3; MHID 1-259-64402-2. Chapter 312].

14. Lipsky P. Rheumatoid arthritis. In Harrison's Principles of Internal Medicine, 20th ed.. Jameson, Fauci, Kasper, et al. Copyright © 2018. McGraw- Hill Publishers. Volume Vol. 1 eBook ISBN 978-1-259-64400-9; MHID 1-259-64400-6; Volume 2 eBook ISBN 978-1-259-64402-3; MHID 1-259-64402-2. [Chapter 314].

15. Lockhart PB, Loven B, Brennan MT, et al. The evidence base for the efficacy of antibiotic prophylaxis in dental practice. *J Am Dent Assoc.* 2007;138:458−474. www.aaos.org/research/guidelines/PUDP/PUDP_guideline.pdf. Accessed April 20, 2021.

16. Nazmul-Hossien A, Morarasu GM, Schmidt S, et al. A current perspective on Sjogren's syndrome. *J Calif Dent Assoc.* 2011;39(9):631−637.

17. Rasmussen A, Ice JA, Li H, et al. Comparison of the American-European Consensus Group Sjögren's syndrome classification criteria to newly proposed American College of Rheumatology criteria in a large, carefully characterized sicca cohort. *Ann Rheum Dis.* 2013;10:1−8. https://doi.org/10.1136/annrheumdis-2014.

18. Rethman MP, Watters 3rd W, Abt E, et al, American Academy of Orthopaedic Surgeons; American Dental Association. The American Academy of Orthopaedic Surgeons and the American Dental Association clinical practice guideline on the prevention of orthopaedic implant infection in patients undergoing dental procedures. *J Bone Joint Surg Am.* 2013;95(8):745−747.

19. Rhodus NL, Johnson DK. The prevalence of oral manifestations of systemic lupus erythematosus. *Quintessence Int.* 1990;21:461−465.

20. Rhodus NL. Perspectives on Sjogren's syndrome. *J Missouri Dent Assn.* 2014;98(1):16−24.

21. Rhodus NL, Falace DA. Oral concerns in Lyme disease. *NW Dent.* 2002;81:17−18.

22. Rhodus NL, Fricton JF, Carlson P, et al. Oral symptoms in patients with Fibromyalgia. *J Rheumatol.* 2003;30:1841−1844.

23. Shiboski SC, Shiboski CH, Criswell L, et al. New classification criteria for Sjögren's syndrome: a data-driven expert-clinician consensus approach within the SICCA Cohort. *Arthritis Care Res.* 2012;64:475−487.

24. Sollecito T, Abt E, Lockhart P, et al. The use of prophylactic antibiotics prior to dental procedures in patients with prosthetic joints: evidence-based clinical practice guideline for dental practitioners—a report of the American Dental Association Council on Scientific Affairs. *J Am Dent Assoc.* 2015;146(1):1117. http://jada.ada.org. Accessed April 20, 2021.

25. Tai ST, Bergari A, Tande M. Microbiology of hip and knew periprosthetic joint infections. *Clin Microbiol Infect.* 2021;12. S1198-743X.

26. von Bültzingslöwen I, Sollecito T, Fox PC, et al. Salivary dysfunction associated with systemic diseases—systematic review and clinical management recommendations. *Oral Surg Oral Med Oral Pathol Oral Radiol Endod.* 2007;103(3s1):57−64.

27. WebMD. Rheumatoid arthritis drug guide. http://www.webmd.com/rheumatoid-arthritis/guide/rheumatoid-arthritis-medications. Accessed April 20, 2021.

28. WebMD. Biologics for rheumatoid arthritis treatment. http://www.webmd.com/rheumatoid-arthritis/guide/biologics. Accessed April 20, 2021.

29. Zero D, Brennan MT, Daniels T, et al. Clinical practice guidelines for oral management in Sjögren's disease: dental caries prevention. *J Am Dent Assoc.* 2015;8:15.

Organ Transplantation

KEY POINTS

- Patients who are awaiting organ transplantation may, depending on the organ and indication for transplantation, be medically unstable and at imminent risk for death.
- Dental clearance should be performed prior to organ transplantation to reduce risk of infection during the period of profound immunosuppression.
- Oral infections are common in organ transplant recipients who are receiving long-term immunosuppressive therapy; odontogenic infections may not appear with typical signs of swelling, erythema, and purulence; and nonodontogenic

infections (e.g., candidiasis, herpes simplex virus recrudescence) may present with atypical and more extensive features.
- Chronic graft-versus-host disease is a unique immune-mediated complication of allogeneic hematopoietic cell transplantation that frequently affects the oral cavity and is associated with significant morbidity.
- Organ transplant recipients, particularly those with chronic graft-versus-host disease after allogeneic hematopoietic cell transplantation, are at increased risk for head and neck squamous cell carcinoma.

Organ transplantation can effectively restore vital organ function in patients with a variety of medical conditions, including inherited and genetic disorders (e.g., bone marrow failure syndromes, sickle cell disease, congenital cardiac disease), end-organ damage caused by chronic disease (e.g., diabetes-associated chronic renal disease, cardiomyopathy, Crohn disease), and cancer (e.g., leukemia, multiple myeloma, hepatocellular carcinoma). Organ transplantation may be the only available option and essential for survival, or, may offer the potential for improved disease control and better quality of life. In addition to intensive immunosuppression at the time of transplantation, most patients remain on long-term immunosuppressive therapy to prevent and manage chronic rejection, in the case of solid organ transplantation, and chronic graft-versus-host disease, in the case of allogeneic hematopoietic cell transplantation. While all solid organ transplantations are allogeneic, from a donor, there is a procedure referred to as autologous hematopoietic cell transplantation. However, this is not actually a transplantation, but rather a stem cell rescue therapy, using the patient's own cells, after very high-dose myeloablative chemotherapy. The dentist must understand the basic principles of risk assessment and dental treatment planning before organ transplantation, as well as be able to provide safe and appropriate comprehensive oral health care management in the posttransplantation setting.

EPIDEMIOLOGY

The various clinical indications for organ transplantation are summarized in Box 21.1. It must be recognized that in

aggregate, most patients with these medical diagnoses will not be managed with organ transplantation for many different reasons. The frequency of and outcomes for solid organ transplantation in the United States are summarized in Table 21.1 (adults) and Table 21.2 (children). Allogeneic hematopoietic cell transplantation (alloHCT) was performed in approximately 10,000 patients in the United States in 2020; outcomes are highly variable based on underlying disease (e.g., malignant vs. nonmalignant disease) and risk factors.

ETIOLOGY

The remarkable successes in transplant medicine have been related to advances in the understanding of key clinical immunologic principles of donor–recipient matching, establishment and coordination of organ donor networks, optimization of immunosuppression regimens, and improvements in supportive care. Human leukocyte antigen (HLA) matching of donor and recipient reduces the risk of graft rejection (and in the case of alloHCT, graft-versus-host disease), a major complication of organ transplantation characterized by a host immune response to tissues expressing non–self-histocompatibility antigens.

Donors and recipients are matched using two different laboratory tests. First, HLA antigen expression is determined on donor and recipient leukocytes through serologic or more frequently DNA-typing assays. The second test is serologic cross-matching, which functionally measures recipient immune cell response to exposure to donor cell antigens, and, in the case of alloHCT, donor immune cell response to recipient cell antigens. This test exposes

BOX 21.1 Organ Transplantation Indications

Renal Transplantation
End-stage renal disease secondary to glomerulonephritis, pyelonephritis, diabetic nephropathy; congenital kidney disorders.

Heart Transplantation
Severe cardiomyopathy, severe coronary artery disease, congenital heart disease.

Liver Transplantation
Acute liver failure and end-stage liver disease related to extrahepatic biliary atresia, primary biliary cirrhosis, chronic HCV infection, advanced cirrhosis, sclerosing cholangitis, nonalcoholic steatohepatitis, alcoholic liver disease, fulminant hepatic failure, hepatobiliary cancers.

Pancreas and Islet Cell Transplantation
Pancreas transplantation restores normal blood glucose levels, effectively curing diabetes and limiting the progression of diabetes-related complications in high risk patients.

Lung Transplantation
Chronic obstructive pulmonary disease, α_1-antitrypsin deficiency, idiopathic pulmonary fibrosis, cystic fibrosis, idiopathic pulmonary arterial hypertension (IPAH). Patients may be considered for single lung or bilateral lung transplantation and less frequently combined heart–lung transplantation.

Intestinal Transplantation
Intestinal transplantation is a lifesaving procedure indicated for management of intestinal failure (IF) secondary to a range of pathologic conditions. With advances in medical management of IF, the number of intestinal transplants performed annually is decreasing.

Bone Marrow/Hematopoietic Cell Transplantation
Acute and chronic leukemia, myelodysplastic syndrome, lymphoma, multiple myeloma, aplastic anemia, severe immunodeficiency syndromes, inherited metabolic disorders, hemoglobinopathies.

Vascularized Composite Tissue Allotransplantation
Composite tissues that may be transplanted include skin, mucosa, muscle, and bone, among other structures, and may be used to replace lost or dysfunctional anatomic structures, with the potential to greatly improve the recipient's quality of life. Because the procedure requires long-term immunosuppression, this carries risks of opportunistic infection, organ failure, and cancer.

Transplanted composite tissues include upper and lower extremities, face, abdominal wall, larynx, and penis.

TABLE 21.1 Adult Survival Rates After Organ Transplantation[a]

Organ	Organs Transplanted in United States—Adults (2020)[a] (n)	1-Year Patient Survival Rate (Deceased/Living Donor)[b] (%)	3-Year Patient Survival Rate (Deceased/Living Donor)[b] (%)
Kidney	22,107	97.0/99.0	93.0/97.0
Pancreas (all)	939		
Pancreas alone		98.4	98.1
Pancreas after kidney		96.1	94.7
Pancreas–kidney (SPK)	822	97.7	95.4
Liver	8404	93.7/96.3	87.3/90.5
Heart	3197	91.7	86.0
Lung	2507	89.9	74.3
Heart–lung	54	83.9	71.8
Intestine	57	77.2	66.2

[a]Data from Organ Procurement and Transplantation Network. https://optn.transplant.hrsa.gov/data.
[b]Data from OPTN/SRTR 2019/20 Annual Data Report, Jan 2021 https://www.srtr.org/.

donor cells to recipient serum and evaluates for the detection of antibodies to red blood cell or HLA antigens, both of which correlate with acute graft rejection. The Organ Procurement and Transplant Network (OPTN) requires HLA-A, HLA-B, and HLA-DR antigen typing of the donor and recipient. The National Marrow Donor Program (NMDP), which coordinates unrelated donor matching for alloHCT in the United States, requires high-resolution DNA-based matching of HLA-A, HLA-B, HLA-C, and DRB1, with a four of four match, or if not possible, then a single mismatch at one of the four loci.

Most organ donations within the United States are coordinated through the OPTN (for solid organs) and NMDP (for alloHCT). The United Network for Organ Sharing (UNOS; https://www.unos.org) is a nonprofit organization that operates the OPTN under a long-term contract from the US Department of Health and Human Services. The Organ Center of the OPTN/UNOS

TABLE 21.2 Pediatric Survival Rates After Organ Transplantation[a]

Organ	Organs Transplanted in United States—Pediatric (2020)[a] (*n*)	1-Year Patient Survival Rate (Deceased/Living Donor)[b] (%)	3-Year Patient Survival Rate (Deceased/Living Donor)[b] (%)
Kidney	710	99.6/99.7	99.1/98.2
Pancreas (all)[c]	23		
Pancreas alone			
Pancreas after kidney			
Pancreas—kidney (SPK)	5		
Liver	502	95.8/95.5	92.9/95.6
Heart	431	92.47	89.44
Lung	32	89.18	64.71
Heart—lung	4		
Intestine	34	84.59	75.65

[a]Data from Organ Procurement and Transplantation Network. Data. https://optn.transplant.hrsa.gov/data.
[b]Data from OPTN/SRTR 2019/20 Annual Data Report, Jan 2021. https://www.srtr.org/.
[c]No pediatric survival is calculated for this organ.

supports the US transplant community 24 h a day, 365 days a year, through providing resource support about organ-sharing policies and processes, managing the computerized donor—recipient match results, coordinating donation of deceased donor organs, and arranging transportation for shared organs. Approximately 70% of patients requiring alloHCT do not have a matched related donor, necessitating coordination of matched unrelated graft donations through the NMDP.

PATHOPHYSIOLOGY AND COMPLICATIONS

Complications associated with organ transplantation include graft rejection, problems related to chronic immunosuppressive therapy, and special considerations specific to the transplanted organ (see Box 21.2 and Fig. 21.1).

Graft Rejection. Graft rejection can occur despite donor—recipient matching and the administration of immunosuppressive medications. *Hyperacute rejection* of solid organs occurs within 48 h of surgical anastomosis and is mediated by preformed antibodies and complement activation and requires immediate graft removal; this is generally avoidable through cross-matching. *Acute rejection*, mediated by T cells and antibodies, occurs within the first 90 days after transplantation and

---

BOX 21.2 Organ-Specific Posttransplant Complications

Kidney Transplantation
- Particularly susceptible to BK virus nephropathy
- Graft rejection monitored primarily by serum creatinine (rather than biopsy)
- If graft failure occurs, hemodialysis can be initiated

Heart Transplantation
- Allograft vasculopathy leads to coronary artery disease; symptoms of angina may not be noted due to surgery-related denervation; monitored by angiography
- All heart transplant recipients receive lifelong statin therapy (regardless of lipid levels)
- Surveillance for graft failure by endomyocardial biopsy
- Rejection may present with typical symptoms of heart failure

Liver Transplantation
- In addition to graft rejection, recurrent underlying disease for which transplant was indicated is a potentially serious complication and can lead to transplant failure

Lung Transplantation
- Lung function is monitored by spirometry with transbronchial lung biopsy performed as needed to rule out/confirm acute rejection
- Bronchiolitis obliterans is the characteristic feature of chronic rejection and is less readily determined by transbronchial biopsy and is therefore monitored based primarily on spirometric measures and changes over time
- Rejection may present with dyspnea, cough, and hypoxia

Bone Marrow/Hematopoietic Cell Transplantation
- Acute GVHD typically occurs within the first 100 days and is characterized by skin rash, elevated liver transaminases, and diarrhea
- Chronic GVHD typically occurs after day +100, affecting most frequently the skin, mouth, eyes, liver, and lungs, contributing to significant morbidity and mortality

Vascularized Composite Tissue Allotransplantation
- Graft rejection of transplanted skin and oral mucosa in face transplantation may present with GVHD-like features

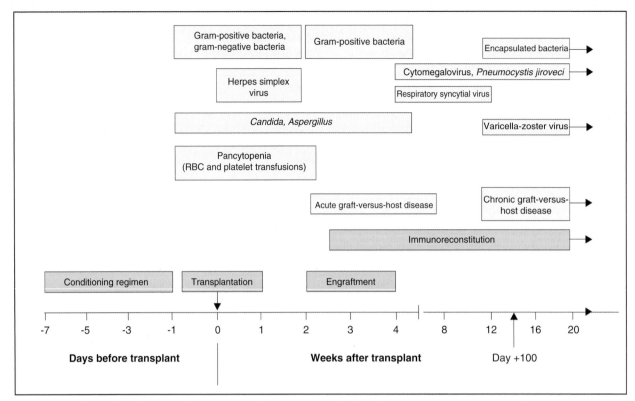

FIG. 21.1 Course of events and risks associated with allogeneic hematopoietic cell transplantation. (Leger CS, Nevill TJ. Hematopoietic stem cell transplantation: a primer for the primary care physician. *CMAJ.* 2004;170:1569–1577.)

generally responds to high-dose steroids and antilymphocyte therapies. *Chronic rejection* of solid organs is primarily antibody mediated and, despite treatment with immunosuppressive medications, is generally irreversible.

Although graft rejection is relatively uncommon in alloHCT, graft-versus-host disease (GVHD) is a serious and potentially life-threatening complication in which the transplanted immune cells attack the patient/host. Acute GVHD typically occurs before day +100 (after alloHCT) and tends to be self-limiting, affecting the skin, liver, and GI tract (but rarely the oral cavity), whereas chronic GVHD typically occurs after day +100 and is characterized by inflammation, fibrosis, and disability, often requiring years of active therapy, with the most frequent target organs including mouth, skin, eyes, liver, and lungs (Fig. 21.2).

Immunosuppression and Infection Risk. Immunosuppressive medications inhibit T- and B-cell activity as well as innate immunity effector cells and pathways, increasing infection risk. Signs and symptoms of infection may be subtle or even nonexistent due to immunosuppression. Patients with chronic rejection or chronic GVHD require more intense and longer-duration immunosuppression and are therefore at higher risk.

In the immediate early posttransplant period, patients are primarily at risk for nosocomial infections

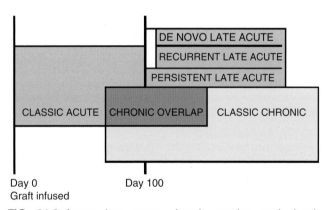

FIG. 21.2 Acute, late acute, chronic overlap, and classic chronic GVHD. The box sizes do not reflect prevalence. (Lee S. *Blood.* 2017; 129(1):30–37.)

(e.g., methicillin-resistant *Staphylococcus aureus* [MRSA]), opportunistic infections (e.g., oropharyngeal candidiasis, aspergillus), and donor-derived infections. *Viridans streptococci* is frequently isolated from blood cultures of patients undergoing alloHCT and has been associated with poor oral health. For the first 6 months posttransplantation, when patients tend to be most highly immunosuppressed, there is high risk of both opportunistic infections (e.g., BK virus, adenovirus) and reactivation of latent infections (e.g., CMV). Infections occurring more than 6 months after transplantation tend to be typical community-acquired infections (e.g., pneumonia) but may have more severe manifestations than in the general population.

In addition to infection risk, there are additional important noninfectious complications associated with frequently administered immunosuppressive medications (Table 21.3).

Cancer Risk. Organ transplant recipients are at increased risk for posttransplant lymphoproliferative disease (PTLD), a rare lymphoma-like condition that is Epstein–Barr virus-associated and typically develops in the early posttransplant period. Nonmelanoma skin cancers are related to the intensity and duration of immunosuppressive therapy as well as sun exposure. In addition to nonmelanoma skin cancers, recipients of alloHCT (and especially those who develop chronic GVHD) are at increased risk for oral squamous cell carcinoma as well as other solid cancers.

CLINICAL PRESENTATION

In the absence of treatment-related comorbidities (e.g., chronic rejection, GVHD, infections), transplant recipients generally have normal function and performance status, similar to the general population. With chronic rejection of solid organs, depending on the extent of organ function compromise, the clinical presentation may eventually resemble that of the pretransplant status. Signs and symptoms of GVHD vary widely, with diffuse erythematous maculopapular skin rash, diarrhea, and elevated liver transaminases most common in the acute setting and more variable skin rash and fibrosis, oral lichenoid inflammation and

TABLE 21.3 Immunosuppressive Medications Commonly Used in Transplant Medicine

Agent	Class	Mechanism of Action	Side Effects	Monitoring	Drug Interactions	Oral Complications
Prednisone	Corticosteroid	Blocks cytokine gene transcription, broadly immunosuppressant	Cushing syndrome, hyperlipidemia, diabetes, hypertension, myopathy, avascular necrosis, osteoporosis, glaucoma, cataracts	Triglycerides, fasting blood glucose, bone density, BP	Potentiates effects of concomitant therapy with other immunosuppressive medications	Increases risk of oral candidiasis, recrudescent HSV infection, poor healing
Cyclosporine	Calcineurin inhibitor	Inhibits IL-2 gene transcription, reduces T-cell activation	Hypertension, nephrotoxicity, tremors	BUN/Cr, LFTs, potassium, magnesium, lipid panel, serum drug levels	Fluconazole may increase cyclosporine levels	Gingival overgrowth
Tacrolimus	Calcineurin inhibitor	Inhibits IL-2 gene transcription, reduces T-cell activation	Hypertension, nephrotoxicity, tremors	Cr, potassium, fasting blood glucose, serum drug levels, BP	Fluconazole may increase tacrolimus levels	Pyogenic granuloma—like lesions
Azathioprine	Nucleoside inhibitor	Inhibits purine synthesis, impairs DNA synthesis, inhibits T- and B-cell proliferation	Leukopenia, myelosuppression, hepatotoxicity	CBC, Cr, LFTs; consider TPMT screening		
Mycophenolate mofetil	Nucleoside inhibitor	Inhibitor of inosine-5′-monophosphate dehydrogenase, impairs DNA synthesis, inhibits T- and B-cell proliferation	Hypertension, anemia, leukopenia, diarrhea	CBC, Cr		Oral ulcers rarely described
Sirolimus	mTOR inhibitor	Inhibits IL-2 sensitivity, reduces T-cell proliferation	Hyperlipidemia, diabetes	Lipid panel, serum drug levels	Fluconazole may increase sirolimus levels	Aphthous-like ulcers
Everolimus	mTOR inhibitor	Inhibits IL-2 sensitivity, reduces T-cell proliferation	Hyperlipidemia, diabetes	Lipid panel, fasting blood glucose, serum drug levels	Fluconazole may increase everolimus levels	Aphthous-like ulcers

BP, blood pressure; *BUN*, blood urea nitrogen; *CBC*, complete blood count; *Cr*, creatinine; *HSV*, herpes simplex virus; *IL-2*, interleukin-2; *LFT*, liver function test; *mTOR*, mammalian target of rapamycin; *TPMT*, thiopurine methyltransferase, enzyme deficiency associated with myelosuppression.

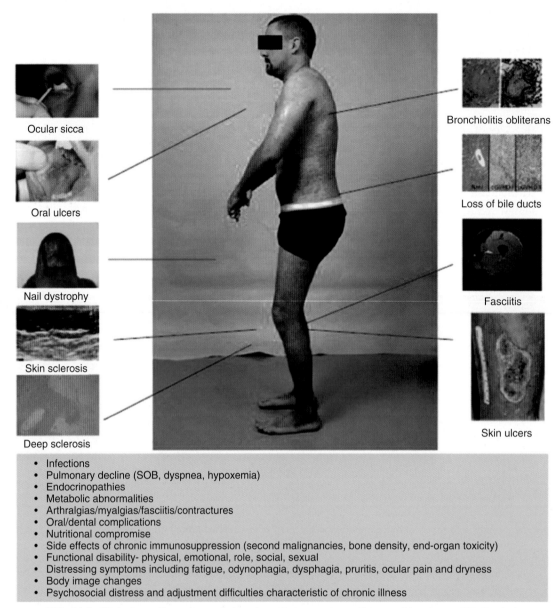

Ocular sicca

Oral ulcers

Nail dystrophy

Skin sclerosis

Deep sclerosis

Bronchiolitis obliterans

Loss of bile ducts

Fasciitis

Skin ulcers

- Infections
- Pulmonary decline (SOB, dyspnea, hypoxemia)
- Endocrinopathies
- Metabolic abnormalities
- Arthralgias/myalgias/fasciitis/contractures
- Oral/dental complications
- Nutritional compromise
- Side effects of chronic immunosuppression (second malignancies, bone density, end-organ toxicity)
- Functional disability- physical, emotional, role, social, sexual
- Distressing symptoms including fatigue, odynophagia, dysphagia, pruritis, ocular pain and dryness
- Body image changes
- Psychosocial distress and adjustment difficulties characteristic of chronic illness

FIG. 21.3 Clinical manifestations of chronic graft-versus-host disease. (Vogelsang GB, Pavletic SZ. *Chronic Graft Versus Host Disease: Interdisciplinary Management.* From Cambridge University Press; 2009. https://doi.org/10.1017/CBO9780511576751.)

salivary gland dysfunction, and eye dryness and discomfort most common in the chronic setting (Fig. 21.3, Table 21.4).

LABORATORY AND DIAGNOSTIC FINDINGS

Laboratory testing is critical for monitoring organ and immune function, levels and metabolism of medications, and infectious diseases. Testing protocols vary depending on the transplanted organ and institutional preferences. Blood pressure is monitored at every visit. A lipid panel and diabetes screening test should be ordered every 6–12 months, especially in patients on long-term calcineurin inhibitor (CNI) and corticosteroid therapies. Monitoring of serum creatinine is important in renal transplant recipients to screen for rejection, as well as in all patients on

CNIs (and other immunosuppressive agents) because of potential renal toxicity. Similarly, liver function testing is routinely performed in liver transplant recipients because rejection causes elevated transaminases, bilirubin, and alkaline phosphatase. The liver is also a frequent target of GVHD and is similarly monitored. Pulmonary function is evaluated by spirometry (referred to generally as pulmonary function tests) and indicated in lung transplant patients as well as alloHCT patients with chronic GVHD affecting the lungs. Pancreas transplant rejection may manifest with compromised endocrine function or an increase in amylase levels. Recipients of alloHCT are followed using many different tests that may include complete blood counts, flow cytometry, molecular testing, and PET scans.

TABLE 21.4 Signs and Symptoms of Chronic Graft-Versus-Host Disease

Organ or Site	Diagnostic (Sufficient to Establish the Diagnosis of Chronic GVHD)	Distinctive[a] (Seen in Chronic GVHD, but Insufficient Alone to Establish a Diagnosis)	Other Features or Unclassified Entities[b]	Common[c] (Seen With Both Acute and Chronic GVHD)
Skin	Poikiloderma Lichen planus—like features Sclerotic features Morphea-like features Lichen sclerosus—like features	Depigmentation Papulosquamous lesions	Sweat impairment Ichthyosis Keratosis Pilaris Hypopigmentation Hyperpigmentation	Erythema Maculopapular rash Pruritus
Nails		Dystrophy longitudinal ridging, splitting or brittle features Onycholysis Pterygium unguis Nail loss (usually symmetric, affects most nails)		
Scalp and body hair		New onset of scarring or nonscarring scalp Alopecia (after recovery from chemoradiotherapy) Loss of body hair Scaling	Thinning scalp hair, typically patchy, coarse or dull (not explained by endocrine or other causes) Premature gray hair	
Mouth	Lichen planus—like changes	Xerostomia Mucoceles Mucosal atrophy Ulcers Pseudomembranes		Gingivitis Mucositis Erythema Pain
Eyes		New onset dry, gritty, or painful eyes Cicatricial conjunctivitis KCS Confluent areas of punctate keratopathy	Photophobia Periorbital hyperpigmentation Blepharitis (erythema of the eyelids with edema)	
Genitalia	Lichen planus—like features Lichen sclerosus—like features	Erosions Fissures		
Females	Vaginal scarring or clitoral/labial agglutination	Ulcers		
Males	Phimosis or urethral/meatus scarring or stenosis			
GI tract	Esophageal web Strictures or stenosis in the upper to mid-third of the esophagus		Exocrine pancreatic insufficiency	Anorexia nausea vomiting diarrhea weight loss Failure to thrive (infants and children Total bilirubin, alkaline
Liver				Phosphatase > 2 × upper Limit of normal ALT > 2 × upper limit of normal
Lung	Bronchiolitis obliterans diagnosed with lung biopsy BOS[d]	Air trapping and bronchiectasis on chest CT	Cryptogenic organizing pneumonia Restrictive lung disease[e]	
Muscles, fascia, joints	Fasciitis Joint stiffness or contractures secondary to fasciitis or sclerosis	Myositis or polymyositis[f]	Edema Muscle cramps Arthralgia or arthritis	

Continued

TABLE 21.4 **Signs and Symptoms of Chronic Graft-Versus-Host Disease—cont'd**

Organ or Site	Diagnostic (Sufficient to Establish the Diagnosis of Chronic GVHD)	Distinctive[a] (Seen in Chronic GVHD, but Insufficient Alone to Establish a Diagnosis)	Other Features or Unclassified Entities[b]	Common[c] (Seen With Both Acute and Chronic GVHD)
Hematopoietic and immune			Thrombocytopenia Eosinophilia Lymphopenia Hypo- or hypergammaglobulinemia autoantibodies (AIHA, ITP) Raynaud's phenomenon	
Other			Pericardial or pleural effusions Ascites Peripheral neuropathy Nephrotic syndrome Myasthenia gravis Cardiac conduction abnormality or cardiomyopathy	

[a]In all cases, infection, drug effect, malignancy, or other causes must be excluded.
[b]Can be acknowledged as part of the chronic GVHD manifestations if diagnosis is confirmed.
[c]Common refers to shared features by both acute and chronic GVHD.
[d]BOS can be diagnostic for lung chronic GVHD only if distinctive sign or symptom present in another organ (see text).
[e]Pulmonary entities under investigation or unclassified.
[f]Diagnosis of chronic GVHD requires biopsy.
ALT, indicates alanine aminotransferase; *AIHA*, autoimmune hemolytic anemia; *ITP*, idiopathic thrombocytopenic purpura.
From Jagasia MH, Greinix HT, Arora M, et al. National institutes of health consensus development project on criteria for clinical trials in chronic graft-versus-host disease: I. The 2014 diagnosis and staging working group report. *Biol Blood Marrow Transplant.* March 2015;21(3):389–401.

Surveillance needle biopsy is routinely performed for most solid organs to screen for rejection. In the early transplant period biopsies may be obtained weekly or monthly, and then less frequently (e.g., annually) thereafter; protocols vary among centers. GVHD can often be diagnosed from clinical features alone, but biopsy (e.g., skin, oral mucosa, GI) may be helpful in supporting or ruling out the diagnosis. Cyclosporine, tacrolimus, and sirolimus are monitored by routine measurement of serum trough levels, with doses adjusted accordingly if needed. CMV reactivation is monitored by quantitative polymerase chain reaction, with a positive assay triggering initiation of preemptive therapy with ganciclovir, a reduction in the intensity of immunosuppression (if feasible), and intensified monitoring. Transplant patients with a history of invasive fungal infection may be monitored for evidence of recurrent infection by serum glucan and galactomannan antigen testing.

MEDICAL AND SURGICAL MANAGEMENT

Medical management of organ transplant patients is largely based on principles of immunosuppression for prevention and management of graft rejection (or GVHD), prevention and aggressive management of infections, and screening for and management of late complications. The specifics of transplant surgery and the surgical management of graft failure and other organ-specific complications are beyond the scope of this chapter.

Immunosuppressive therapy (Table 21.3) is initiated at the time of transplantation ("induction" in solid organ, "conditioning" and "GVHD prophylaxis" in alloHCT), and although regimens are generally similar, there is some degree of variability based on the transplanted organ, patient-specific factors, and institutional preferences. In solid organ transplantation, this typically consists of triple-drug therapy with a corticosteroid (prednisone, which is typically tapered over a period of weeks), a CNI (cyclosporine or tacrolimus), and a purine synthesis inhibitor (mycophenolate mofetil). Antilymphocyte therapy (e.g., ATG, or antithymocyte globulin) is sometimes included as part of the initial immunosuppressive therapy or used in the management of rejection episodes. Sirolimus is variably used in some protocols to spare the need for CNI therapy; for example, in renal transplantation to minimize CNI-associated nephrotoxicity. In most cases patients require lifelong immunosuppression to prevent graft rejection.

In alloHCT, GVHD prophylaxis regimens typically consist of a short course of methotrexate (for several days after graft infusion) combined with a CNI that, in the absence of GVHD, is tapered over a 3- to 6-month period. First-line therapy for rejection and GVHD is corticosteroids, with second-line therapies including rituximab, alemtuzumab, mycophenolate mofetil, extracorporeal photopheresis, and, in GVHD specifically, ibrutinib, and ruxolitinib. Relapse of underlying hematologic malignancy after alloHCT is managed with rapid tapering of immunosuppressive therapy and donor lymphocyte infusion, both of which are intended to stimulate a potent graft-versus-tumor effect but also frequently trigger GVHD.

Guidelines are available for long-term preventive and screening practices for organ transplant recipients. Many recommendations are organ and disease specific, as well as age specific in pediatric transplantation, but many are related to administration of immunosuppressive medications and generally universal to all organ transplant patients.

DENTAL MANAGEMENT

General Principles and Basic Oral Care

Because of the anticipated period of profound immunosuppression after transplantation, it is standard of care for all transplant candidates to undergo pretransplant dental screening and clearance to reduce the risk of infectious complications. In case of rejection, or GVHD, long-term immunosuppressive therapy may be required, prolonging the period of risk, and further reinforcing the importance of oral health care maintenance. All transplant patients should perform basic oral care to maintain good oral health, consisting at minimum of tooth brushing with a soft toothbrush and fluoride toothpaste at least twice a day and flossing daily. Patients with a history of gingivitis or periodontitis may benefit from daily chlorhexidine gluconate rinses, which is often included in oral care regimens at alloHCT centers. Removable prostheses should be cleaned and disinfected overnight (e.g., using a brush and a commercial disinfecting solution).

There are no universally agreed-upon indications for antibiotic prophylaxis before dental treatment in transplant patients due to immunosuppression alone. The American Heart Association (AHA) guidelines for prevention of infectious endocarditis recommend antibiotic prophylaxis in cardiac transplant recipients who develop cardiac valvulopathy. The American Academy of Pediatric Dentistry guidelines recommend considering prescribing prophylactic antibiotics according to the AHA guidelines for pediatric dental patients at risk for infection (e.g., $<2000\ mm^3$), including transplant recipients on immunosuppressive therapy.

Risk Assessment

Risk assessment requires an understanding of the indication for transplantation, the schedule and timeline of transplantation, organ function status, medications, pertinent laboratory results, and history of complications. Patients scheduled for organ transplantation may be at risk for bleeding because of antithrombotic therapy, anticoagulant therapy, advanced liver disease, or thrombocytopenia. Risk for infection in the pretransplant setting is generally low and not significantly different from the general population in most solid organ transplant candidates. However, in patients with hematologic malignancies scheduled for alloHCT, there may be high risk of infection requiring careful attention to the complete blood count and absolute neutrophil count.

Pretransplant Dental Screening and Clearance

The National Institute of Craniofacial Research, as well as the joint task force of the Multinational Association of Supportive Care in Cancer/International Society of Oral Oncology (MASCC/ISOO) and the European Society for Blood and Marrow Transplantation (EBMT), recommend that all patients receive a comprehensive dental and oral evaluation as early as possible before organ transplantation to identify and eliminate any potential odontogenic sources of infection (Table 21.5). The pretransplant dental screening includes a dental history, dental radiographs, soft tissue examination, charting of caries and defective restorations, vitality testing, periodontal evaluation, and assessment of third molars. All patients should receive a professional dental prophylaxis before transplantation. The amount of time available for completion of the pretransplant dental clearance can vary

TABLE 21.5	Dental Clearance Prior to Organ Transplantation	
Risk Factor	**Evaluation or Test**	**Treatment**
Soft tissue infection	Examination, culture, biopsy	Definitive antimicrobial therapy; prophylactic therapy during high-risk periods
Dental caries	Clinical examination, dental radiographs, vitality testing	Treat caries; provide endodontic therapy or extraction of abscessed and nonvital teeth and teeth with untreated periapical radiolucencies; extraction of nonrestorable teeth
Periodontal disease	Periodontal examination, dental radiographs	Scaling and root planing; extraction of mobile and hopeless teeth
Pericoronitis	History of recurrent pain or swelling associated with third molars, examination, dental radiographs	Extraction of associated third molar

Dental clearance reduces the risk of infection during the period of intense immunosuppression and may be required for a patient to become eligible to be listed for solid organ transplantation and for final payor approval for alloHCT.

depending on several factors, including the indication for transplantation and donor organ availability. This may require scheduling of multiple visits in a short span of time and prioritizing certain items (e.g., teeth with active infection) with the dental treatment plan. All necessary dental treatment and dental extractions should be completed at least 2 weeks before transplantation, when feasible, to allow for adequate healing prior to immunosuppression.

The AAPD has published guidelines for pediatric patients undergoing alloHCT, which can be generalized to all pediatric organ transplant patients and are similar to those described above. Orthodontic appliances and space maintainers can be left in place if nonirritating and if the patient is maintaining adequate oral hygiene.

Posttransplant Dental Care

The dental management of patients after transplantation can be divided into three phases: (1) immediate posttransplant period; (2) stable graft period (or, in alloHCT, absence of GVHD); and (3) chronic rejection period, or in alloHCT, the onset of significant chronic GVHD, requiring intensive and sustained immunosuppression (Table 21.6). Elective dental care is generally deferred during the immediate posttransplant period due to profound immunosuppression and risk for infection. However, in the case of actual dental infection during this period, emergency care can be provided, following

the same risk assessment principles as before transplantation. Infections should be managed aggressively and may require extended courses of antimicrobial therapy.

When the graft is stable with good function, and any acute rejection reaction (or acute GVHD) has been controlled, the patient is considered stable. During the stable period, patients should receive routine dental care without restrictions. The medical history should be updated, and blood counts and other relevant labs, if being monitored, should be reviewed.

During chronic rejection or chronic GVHD, transplant recipients are at significantly higher risk for infection because of more intensive and prolonged immunosuppressive therapy. In addition, in solid organ transplant recipients with chronic rejection, organ function may be compromised such that their status may resemble the pretransplant period, and with chronic GVHD, there can be considerable end organ fibrosis and damage, especially when the lungs are affected.

Oral Complications and Manifestations

Both infectious and noninfectious oral complications may be encountered in organ transplant patients (Table 21.7). Patient evaluation begins with a comprehensive medical history, review of current medications, and assessment of pertinent laboratory results (per above, generally readily available from the patient's medical team; especially if patient is at risk for neutropenia and/or thrombocytopenia). Physical evaluation includes careful extraoral and intraoral examinations. Soft tissue abnormalities should be described based on location, size, color, consistency, and symptoms. Additional tests may be indicated, including microbiologic cultures, imaging, and tissue biopsy. Management of oral complications depends on an accurate and timely diagnosis and careful coordination of care with the primary medical team (Box 21.3).

Oral Mucositis

Oral mucositis is a complication that is unique to alloHCT and related to both the intensive conditioning regimen as well as the course of methotrexate given for GVHD prophylaxis. Oral mucositis develops 7–10 days after initiation of conditioning and does not resolve until engraftment and resolution of the white blood cell count. The incidence and severity of mucositis are greatly lessened with "reduced-intensity" conditioning regimens, as well as GVHD prophylaxis regimens that do not include methotrexate. Clinical features are characterized by diffuse, nonspecific erythema and ulcerations of the nonkeratinized oral mucosa that compromise oral function and quality of life (Fig. 21.4). Management includes diet modifications (e.g., soft, bland foods), palliative rinses (e.g., viscous lidocaine, magic mouthwash, Appendix C), devices (various coating agents), and systemic analgesics.

TABLE 21.6 Dental Management of the Organ Transplant Recipient

Immediate Posttransplantation Period (≤6 Months)
Consultation with physician(s)
1. Defer routine dental treatment.
2. Continue oral hygiene procedures.
3. Provide emergency dental care as needed (eliminate infections).

Stable Graft Period
Consultation with physician(s)
1. Continue oral hygiene procedures.
2. Initiate active recall program with appointments every 3–6 months.
3. Monitor blood pressure in patients taking cyclosporine, tacrolimus, or prednisone; if blood pressure increases above established baseline, refer for medical evaluation.
4. Treat all new dental disease; no contraindications to routine dental care.
5. Examine for oral signs and symptoms of oral complications.
6. Alter drug selection or reduce dosage.
   a. Liver or kidney failure
   b. Limit drugs toxic to liver or kidney (i.e., acetaminophen, NSAIDs)
   c. Drug interactions

Chronic Rejection Period
Consultation with physician(s)
1. Follow recommendations for stable graft period.
2. Manage odontogenic infections aggressively.
3. Monitor medical status and medications; continually reassess risk.

NSAID, nonsteroidal antiinflammatory drug.

TABLE 21.7 Oral Complications in Organ Transplantation

	Oral Complication	Diagnosis	Management
Infectious	Oral candidiasis	History and examination findings, culture, cytology	• Antifungal therapy • Disinfection of oral prostheses
Noninfectious	HSV recrudescence	History and examination findings, culture, cytology	• Antiviral therapy
	Gingival overgrowth (cyclosporine associated)	History and examination findings	• Improve oral hygiene • Periodontal therapy • Gingivectomy
	Aphthous stomatitis (mTOR inhibitor —associated)	History and examination findings	• Topical steroid therapy • Intralesional steroid therapy • mTOR inhibitor dose reduction or discontinuation if severe
	Pyogenic granuloma (tacrolimus associated)	Examination and biopsy	• Surgical excision
	Orofacial granulomatosis	Examination and biopsy	• Topical steroid therapy if symptomatic
	Oral hairy leukoplakia	Examination and biopsy	• No specific therapy indicated
	Squamous cell carcinoma	Examination and biopsy	• Refer to oncology center
Unique to alloHCT	Oral mucositis	History and examination findings	• Palliative care, analgesics, bland soft diet
	Chronic GVHD	History of alloHCT, lichenoid white reticulations throughout oral mucosa and lips with variable erythema and ulceration, palatal superficial mucoceles common, salivary gland dysfunction	• Topical tacrolimus ointment for lips • Topical steroid therapy for mucosal disease (e.g., dexamethasone solution) • Xerostomia management with over-the-counter products and prescription sialogogue therapy, fluoride

alloHCT, allogeneic hematopoietic cell transplantation; *GVHD*, graft-versus-host disease; *mTOR*, mammalian target of rapamycin.

Medication-Related Oral Complications

Aside from infections (discussed later), several important potential oral complications are associated with immunosuppressive medications commonly used in organ transplantation. These are relatively uncommon and may not be dose related. An understanding of these conditions is essential for correct diagnosis and appropriate management.

Gingival Overgrowth

Cyclosporine-associated gingival overgrowth is characterized by fibro-inflammatory enlargement of the gingiva, which appears edematous, swollen, and "overgrown," often involving the interdental regions (Fig. 21.5). Poor oral hygiene increases the risk significantly. Management includes intensive periodontal care, improved oral hygiene, and if necessary surgical excision by gingivectomy. As tacrolimus is being used more often in place of cyclosporine, cases of gingival overgrowth are on the decline.

Pyogenic Granuloma

Tacrolimus has been associated with oral soft tissue pyogenic granuloma-like lesions (Fig. 21.6). These appear as exophytic ulcerated fibrous lobulated masses,

measuring up to 4 cm in diameter. Symptoms are variable and are typically associated with secondary trauma. The pathophysiologic mechanisms and relationship with tacrolimus therapy remain unclear. Management is surgical excision.

mTOR Inhibitor–Associated Stomatitis

mTOR inhibitor therapy with sirolimus and everolimus is associated with development of aphthous-like oral ulcers, referred to as *mTOR inhibitor–associated stomatitis* (mIAS; Fig. 21.7). Ulcers typically develop within the first few weeks of initiating therapy and tend to diminish with time despite continuation of therapy. Management with topical and intralesional steroid therapy is generally effective.

Orofacial Granulomatosis-Like Lesions

Atypical orofacial granulomatosis-like oral lesions have been described infrequently in pediatric solid organ transplant recipients who received tacrolimus. Features include multiple spherical nodules of the tongue, mucosal fissuring, and lip swelling (Fig. 21.8). Food allergy has been proposed as a contributing factor, but very little is known about this condition.

BOX 21.3	Checklist for Dental Management of Organ Transplant Recipients[a]

PREOPERATIVE RISK ASSESSMENT
- Review medical history, determine whether there are any infectious or organ-specific complications.
- Identify all medications being taken or supposed to be taken by the patient.
- Review recent laboratory test results to assess risk.
- Obtain a medical consultation (i.e., refer to physician) if the patient reports undiagnosed or previously unreported signs/symptoms.
- If organ function stable, routine dental procedures can be performed without special precautions.

A

Antibiotics	There is no consensus on the need for antibiotic prophylaxis in an organ transplant recipient who is receiving immunosuppressive therapy. The American Academy of Pediatric Dentists (AAPD) suggests consideration of antibiotic prophylaxis when ANC is between 1000 and 2000 cells/mm³; when ANC is <1000 the AAPD recommends antibiotic prophylaxis and consideration of an extended course of antibiotics.
Analgesics	Limit drugs toxic to the liver or kidney (i.e., acetaminophen, NSAIDs). In patients who are at risk for bleeding (e.g., liver transplant rejection, persistent thrombocytopenia after alloHCT), avoid aspirin and NSAIDs.
Anesthesia	N/A
Anxiety	N/A

B

Bleeding	Assess liver function in liver transplant recipients; consult with transplant physician in case of chronic rejection. Assess platelet count in alloHCT recipients (if has trended below normal).
Breathing	Lung transplant recipients with chronic rejection, as well as alloHCT recipients with pulmonary chronic GVHD, may be oxygen dependent and require supplemental oxygen during care.
Blood pressure	Blood pressure should be monitored at every visit due to organ (e.g., renal) and medication (e.g., tacrolimus) risks.

C

Capacity to tolerate care	Most organ transplant recipients can tolerate dental care. Modifications in appointment length, patient positioning, and treatment planning may be indicated in patients with significant disability.

D

Drugs	Fluconazole and other azole antifungals (including clotrimazole) can increase levels of tacrolimus and sirolimus, increasing risk of toxicity. Serum levels of tacrolimus and sirolimus are routinely monitored as standard of care practice. Use of these antifungal medications should be coordinated with the patient's medical team.
Devices	N/A

E

Equipment	N/A
Emergencies	N/A

F—Postoperative Care

Follow-up care	Consider postoperative antibiotics after invasive procedures (e.g., dental extractions) in patients who are receiving immunosuppressive therapy.

[a]Strength of recommendation taxonomy (SORT) Grade: C (see Preface for further explanation).
alloHCT, allogeneic hematopoietic cell transplantation; *NSAID*, nonsteroidal antiinflammatory drug.

Oral Hairy Leukoplakia

Oral hairy leukoplakia (OHL) is a painless, benign condition that appears as corrugated white plaques on the ventrolateral tongue that cannot be removed (Fig. 21.9). It is associated with Epstein–Barr virus (EBV) replication and encountered in patients with immunodeficiency, including human immunodeficiency virus (HIV) disease and organ transplant recipients. Biopsy is diagnostic and demonstrates characteristic changes of EBV infection. Lesions may resolve with antiviral therapy; however, OHL is asymptomatic and does not require treatment.

Oral Infections

Oral infection is common in organ transplant recipients. Aside from odontogenic infections (discussed under Dental Management), oral bacterial infections are exceedingly rare. The most frequently encountered oral infections in transplant recipients are candidiasis and recrudescent HSV, and although these rarely progress to systemic disease, both infections can cause significant morbidity and should be managed accordingly.

Candidiasis. In addition to medication-induced immunosuppression, other potential risk factors for development of oral candidiasis in organ transplant recipients include topical steroid use (e.g., treatment of oral GVHD, use of steroid inhalers), salivary gland hypofunction (related to medications and chronic GVHD), and use of an oral prosthesis. Infection typically appears with generalized white curd-like papules and plaques throughout the oral cavity (i.e., pseudomembranous candidiasis Fig. 21.10), although some cases are erythematous, presenting with

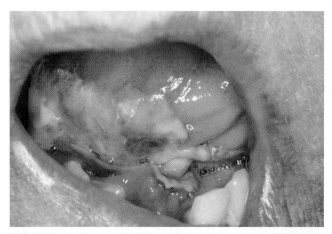

FIG. 21.4 Oral mucositis in a patient with acute myelogenous leukemia undergoing myeloablative allogeneic hematopoietic cell transplantation. (From Wingard JR, Gastineau DA, Leather HL, et al. *Hematopoietic Stem Cell Transplantation: A Handbook for Clinicians.* 2nd ed. American Association of Blood Banks; 2015.)

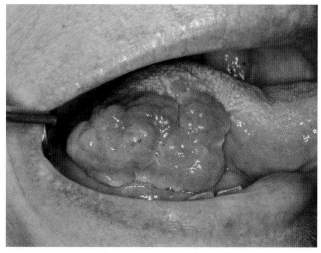

FIG. 21.6 Multilobulated pyogenic granuloma–like lesion in a hematopoietic cell transplant recipient treated with tacrolimus. (From Antin J, Yolin-Raley D. *Manual of Stem Cell and Bone Marrow Transplantation.* 2nd ed. Cambridge University Press; 2013.)

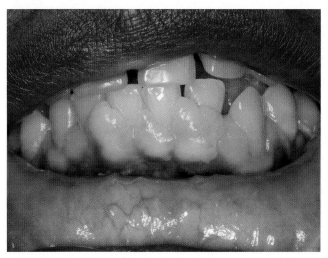

FIG. 21.5 Cyclosporine-associated gingival overgrowth in a renal transplant recipient.

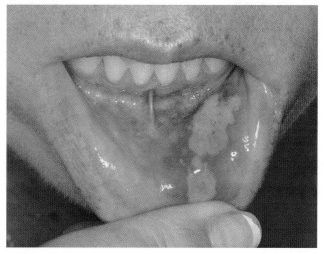

FIG. 21.7 Aphthous-like ulceration of the lower labial mucosa in a patient receiving mTOR inhibitor therapy. (From Sonis S, Treister N, Chawla S, et al. Preliminary characterization of oral lesions associated with inhibitors of mammalian target of rapamycin in cancer patients. *Cancer.* 2010;116:210–215.)

generalized or patchy redness (Fig. 21.11). Symptoms are more common with the erythematous form and can include burning, which may extend into the throat.

Candidiasis can often be diagnosed clinically; however, cytology is confirmatory. A positive fungal culture does not indicate infection per se, especially in the absence of obvious signs of infection. Topical antifungal therapy is generally effective but systemic therapy (e.g., fluconazole) may be indicated. Because cyclosporine, tacrolimus, and sirolimus are metabolized through the cytochrome p450 pathway, fluconazole, and to lesser extent topical clotrimazole, may lead to increased levels of these drugs and therefore requires attentive monitoring or dosage adjustment. Removable oral prostheses should be removed, cleaned, and disinfected nightly. Antifungal prophylaxis (e.g., fluconazole 100–200 mg 1–2/times weekly) is effective in cases of chronic recurrent infection (see Appendix A).

Herpes Simplex Virus Recrudescence. The risk of HSV recrudescence is so high that all seropositive organ transplant recipients receive acyclovir prophylaxis during periods of profound immunosuppression. Breakthrough infections despite acyclovir therapy are possible, and even after acyclovir is discontinued, patients continue to be immunosuppressed and at risk for recrudescence. Lesions appear as painful irregularly shaped shallow ulcerations that can affect both keratinized and nonkeratinized surfaces, with the lips and tongue most frequently affected (Fig. 21.12). Diagnosis can be confirmed by multiple assays (e.g., PCR, culture), but therapy should generally be initiated empirically in case of suspected infection. Management requires systemic antiviral therapy with

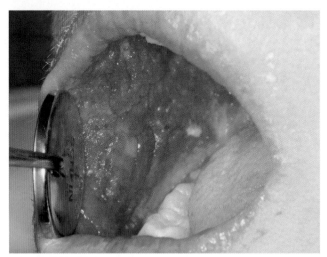

FIG. 21.8 Orofacial granulomatosis-like features in a child after allogeneic hematopoietic cell transplantation.

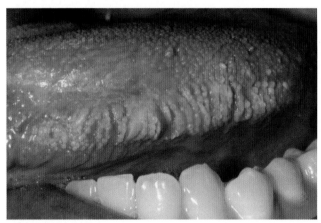

FIG. 21.9 Oral hairy leukoplakia. (From Neville B, Damm D, Allen C, et al. *Oral and Maxillofacial Pathology*. 3rd ed. St. Louis: Saunders; 2008.)

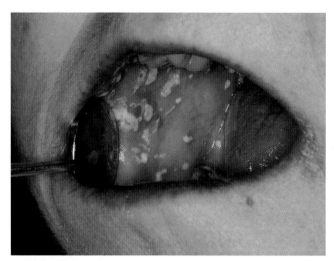

FIG. 21.10 Pseudomembranous candidiasis of the right buccal mucosa. Angular cheilitis is also evident.

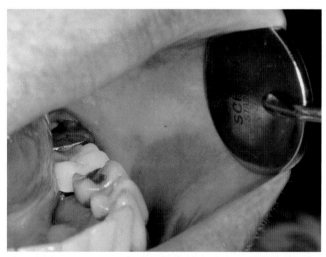

FIG. 21.11 Erythematous candidiasis of the left buccal mucosa.

acyclovir or valacyclovir, or rarely foscarnet in cases of acyclovir resistance, as well as symptom control with topical and systemic analgesics (see Appendix C).

Other Infrequent Infections. Invasive fungal infection (most frequently aspergillus) may present intraorally as an ulcerated mass, typically in the maxilla as an extension of sinopulmonary involvement. Management includes a combination of surgery and intensive antifungal therapy. CMV reactivation rarely causes painful nonspecific ulcerations that require biopsy and immunostaining for diagnosis. Management is ganciclovir.

Graft-Versus-Host Disease

Graft-versus-host disease is a major complication of alloHCT and the leading cause of non−relapse-related mortality. Although infrequently involved, oral features of acute GVHD are similar to those of erythema multiforme and are managed with systemic and topical steroids (Fig. 21.13). In contrast, the oral cavity is one of the most frequent targets of chronic GVHD with clinical features including lichenoid changes and associated mouth and lip discomfort and sensitivity (Fig. 21.14), salivary gland dysfunction with xerostomia and high risk for dental decay (Fig. 21.15), and less frequently fibrosis of oral and perioral tissues leading to limited mobility and function. Superficial mucoceles are a common feature characterized by superficial saliva-filled blisters that develop primarily on the palate caused by inflammation of minor salivary glands and do not generally require any specific therapy (Fig. 21.16).

Management of oral chronic GVHD is directed at controlling symptoms and reducing the risk of and screening for complications (see Table 21.4). Many patients, due to multisystem involvement, will require systemic treatment for month or even years; many of these will continue to require additional ancillary therapy for the oral cavity. Oral mucosal disease can be effectively treated with topical steroids and topical tacrolimus (see Appendix C). The lips can be safely and effectively

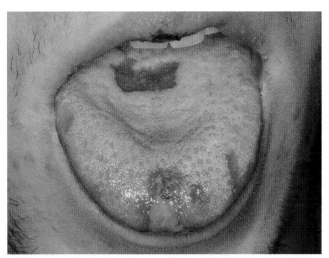

FIG. 21.12 Recrudescent herpes simplex virus infection affecting the anterior and posterior tongue dorsum in an organ transplant recipient.

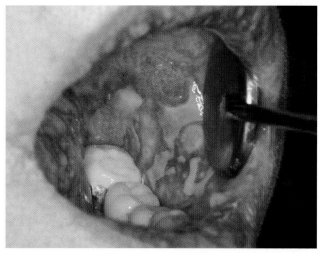

FIG. 21.14 Lichenoid changes associated with chronic graft-versus-host disease.

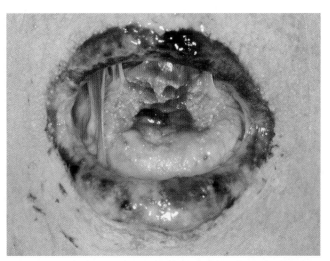

FIG. 21.13 Oral features of acute graft-versus-host disease with diffuse ulcerations of the lips and tongue. (From Kuten-Shorrer M, Woo SB, Treister NS. Oral graft-versus-host disease. *Dent Clin N Am.* 2014;58:351−368.)

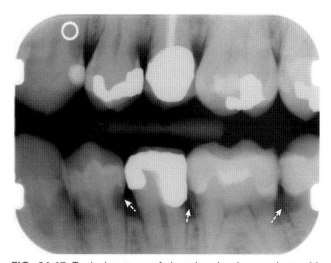

FIG. 21.15 Typical pattern of dental caries in a patient with salivary gland chronic graft-versus-host disease. (From Kuten-Shorrer M, Woo SB, Treister NS. Oral graft-versus-host disease. *Dent Clin N Am.* 2014;58:351−368.)

treated with topical tacrolimus ointment. Prescription topical fluoride should be prescribed for patients with significant salivary gland dysfunction, and all patients should see a dentist for a professional cleaning and examination with periodic radiographs at least twice per year. Patients with salivary gland hypofunction at high risk for dental caries may require more frequent bitewing radiographs.

Graft rejection episodes in recipients of composite tissue facial allografts may appear clinically similar to acute and chronic GVHD of the skin and oral mucosa.

Cancer

Organ transplant patients are at increased risk for developing cancer due to long-term immunosuppression

(Fig. 21.17). Patients with hematologic malignancies who undergo alloHCT remain at risk for relapse of primary disease (e.g., AML), typically within the first 1−2 years after transplantation. Extramedullary disease (e.g., granulocytic sarcoma or plasmacytoma), albeit rare, can appear in the oral cavity as a nonspecific mass or ulceration (Fig. 21.18). Posttransplant lymphoproliferative disease can similarly appear in the oral cavity as a mass or ulceration (Fig. 21.19). Risk of oral cavity and lip squamous cell carcinoma (SCC) is increased significantly in posttransplant patients, with patients with oral chronic GVHD after alloHCT being at particularly high risk. Oral SCC appears with the same clinical features as in the general population but may be challenging to detect in the context of active GVHD changes (Fig. 21.20). All transplant patients should receive annual oral cavity cancer screening.

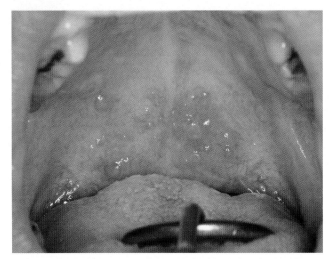

FIG. 21.16 Superficial mucoceles of the soft palate. (From Kuten-Shorrer M, Woo SB, Treister NS. Oral graft-versus-host disease. *Dent Clin N Am.* 2014;58:351–368.)

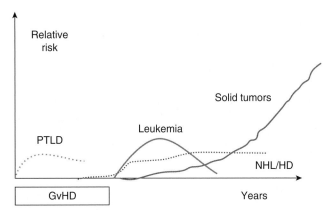

FIG. 21.17 Scheme of time course and relative risk of second malignancies after allogeneic hematopoietic cell transplantation. *HD*, Hodgkin disease; *NHL*, non-Hodgkin lymphoma; *PTLD*, posttransplant lymphoproliferative disease. (From Ades L, et al. *Blood Rev.* 2002;16:135–146.)

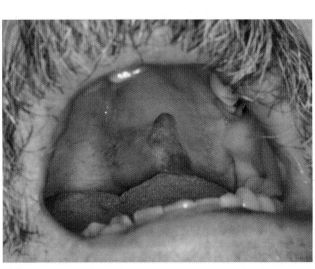

FIG. 21.18 Extramedullary relapse of acute myeloid leukemia presenting as a palatal ulceration in a patient after hematopoietic cell transplantation.

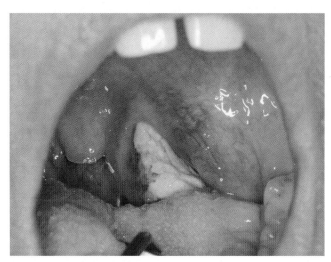

FIG. 21.19 Posttransplant lymphoproliferative disease presenting as a palatal ulceration in a patient after hematopoietic cell transplantation.

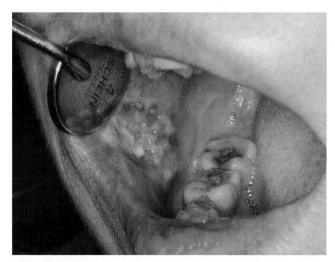

FIG. 21.20 Squamous cell carcinoma of the right buccal mucosa arising in the background of active oral chronic graft-versus-host disease in a patient after hematopoietic cell transplantation. (From Bruch JM, Treister NS. *Clinical Oral Medicine and Pathology.* New York: Humana Press; 2010.)

BIBLIOGRAPHY

1. American Academy of Pediatric Dentistry. Dental management of pediatric patients receiving immunosuppressive therapy and/or radiation therapy. In: *The Reference Manual of Pediatric Dentistry.* Chicago, IL: American Academy of Pediatric Dentistry; 2020:453–461.
2. American Academy of Pediatric Dentistry. Antibiotic prophylaxis for dental patients at risk for infection. In: *The Reference Manual of Pediatric Dentistry.* Chicago, IL: American Academy of Pediatric Dentistry; 2020:447–452.
3. Antin JH. Clinical practice. Long-term care after hematopoietic-cell transplantation in adults. *N Engl J Med.* 2002;347:36–42.
4. Bray RA, Hurley CK, Kamani NR, et al. National marrow donor program HLA matching guidelines for unrelated

adult donor hematopoietic cell transplants. *Biol Blood Marrow Transplant.* 2008;14:45–53.

5. Brown RS, Belton AM, Martin JM, et al. Evolution of quality at the Organ Center of the Organ Procurement and Transplantation Network/United Network for Organ Sharing. *Prog Transplant.* 2009;19:221–226.

6. Chinen J, Buckley RH. Transplantation immunology: solid organ and bone marrow. *J Allergy Clin Immunol.* 2010;125:S324–S335.

7. Colvin M, Smith JM, Skeans MA, et al. Heart. *Am J Transplant.* 2016;16(suppl 2):115–140.

8. Cutler C, Antin JH. Chronic graft-versus-host disease. *Curr Opin Oncol.* 2006;18:126–131.

9. Curtis RE, Rowlings PA, Deeg HJ, et al. Solid cancers after bone marrow transplantation. *N Engl J Med.* 1997;336:897–904.

10. Dierickx D, Tousseyn T, Gheysens O. How I treat posttransplant lymphoproliferative disorders. *Blood.* 2015;126:2274–2283.

11. D'Souza A, Fretham C, Lee SJ, et al. Current use of and trends in hematopoietic cell transplantation in the United States. *Biol Blood Marrow Transplant.* May 11, 2020;(20):S1083–S8791 30225-1. https://doi.org/10.1016/j.bbmt.2020.04.013. PMID 32438042.

12. Dubernard JM, Lengele B, Morelon E, et al. Outcomes 18 months after the first human partial face transplantation. *N Engl J Med.* 2007;357:2451–2460.

13. Elad S, Meyerowitz C, Shapira MY, et al. Oral post-transplantation lymphoproliferative disorder: an uncommon site for an uncommon disorder. *Oral Surg Oral Med Oral Pathol Oral Radiol Endod.* 2008;105:59–64.

14. Elad S, Raber-Durlacher JE, Brennan MT, et al. Basic oral care for hematology-oncology patients and hematopoietic stem cell transplantation recipients: a position paper from the joint task force of the Multinational Association of Supportive Care in Cancer/International Society of Oral Oncology (MASCC/ISOO) and the European Society for Blood and Marrow Transplantation (EBMT). *Support Care Cancer.* 2015;23:223–236.

15. Eng HS, Leffell MS. Histocompatibility testing after fifty years of transplantation. *J Immunol Methods.* 2011;369:1–21.

16. Engels EA, Pfeiffer RM, Fraumeni Jr JF, et al. Spectrum of cancer risk among US solid organ transplant recipients. *JAMA.* 2011;306:1891–1901.

17. Epstein JB, Raber-Durlacher JE, Wilkins A, et al. Advances in hematologic stem cell transplant: an update for oral health care providers. *Oral Surg Oral Med Oral Pathol Oral Radiol Endod.* 2009;107:301–312.

18. Fischer SA, Lu K, Practice ASTIDCo. Screening of donor and recipient in solid organ transplantation. *Am J Transplant.* 2013;13(suppl 4):9–21.

19. Fishman JA. Infection in solid-organ transplant recipients. *N Engl J Med.* 2007;357:2601–2614.

20. Flowers ME, Martin PJ. How we treat chronic graft-versus-host disease. *Blood.* 2015;125:606–615.

21. Green M. Introduction: infections in solid organ transplantation. *Am J Transplant.* 2013;13(suppl 4):3–8.

22. Guggenheimer J, Eghtesad B, Stock DJ. Dental management of the (solid) organ transplant patient. *Oral Surg Oral Med Oral Pathol Oral Radiol Endod.* 2003;95:383–389.

23. Hart A, Smith JM, Skeans MA, et al. Kidney. *Am J Transplant.* 2016;16(suppl 2):11–46.

24. Ion D, Stevenson K, Woo SB, et al. Characterization of oral involvement in acute graft-versus-host disease. *Biol Blood Marrow Transplant.* 2014;20:1717–1721.

25. Jagasia MH, Greinix HT, Arora M, et al. National institutes of health consensus development project on criteria for clinical trials in chronic graft-versus-host disease: I. The 2014 diagnosis and staging working group report. *Biol Blood Marrow Transplant.* 2015;21:389–401.e1.

26. Kandaswamy R, Skeans MA, Gustafson SK, et al. Pancreas. *Am J Transplant.* 2016;16(suppl 2):47–68.

27. Kim WR, Lake JR, Smith JM, et al. Liver. *Am J Transplant.* 2016;16(suppl 2):69–98.

28. Leger CS, Nevill TJ. Hematopoietic stem cell transplantation: a primer for the primary care physician. *CMAJ (Can Med Assoc J).* 2004;170:1569–1577.

29. Majhail NS, Rizzo JD, Lee SJ, et al. Recommended screening and preventive practices for long-term survivors after hematopoietic cell transplantation. *Biol Blood Marrow Transplant.* 2012;18:348–371.

30. Opelz G, Dohler B. Lymphomas after solid organ transplantation: a collaborative transplant study report. *Am J Transplant.* 2004;4:222–230.

31. Palmason S, Marty FM, Treister NS. How do we manage oral infections in allogeneic stem cell transplantation and other severely immunocompromised patients? *Oral Maxillofac Surg Clin.* 2011;23:579–599.

32. Pappas PG, Kauffman CA, Andes D, et al. Clinical practice guidelines for the management of candidiasis: 2009 update by the Infectious Diseases Society of America. *Clin Infect Dis.* 2009;48:503–535.

33. Sayegh MH, Carpenter CB. Transplantation 50 years later—progress, challenges, and promises. *N Engl J Med.* 2004;351:2761–2766.

34. Smith JM, Skeans MA, Horslen SP, et al. Intestine. *Am J Transplant.* 2016;16(suppl 2):99–114.

35. Stites E, Le Quintrec M, Thurman JM. The complement system and antibody-mediated transplant rejection. *J Immunol.* 2015;195:5525–5531.

36. Sonis S, Treister N, Chawla S, et al. Preliminary characterization of oral lesions associated with inhibitors of mammalian target of rapamycin in cancer patients. *Cancer.* 2010;116:210–215.

37. Storek J. Immunological reconstitution after hematopoietic cell transplantation - its relation to the contents of the graft. *Expert Opin Biol Ther.* 2008;8:583–597.

38. Swearingen B, Ravindra K, Xu H, et al. Science of composite tissue allotransplantation. *Transplantation.* 2008;86:627–635.

39. Treister N, Duncan C, Cutler C, et al. How we treat oral chronic graft-versus-host disease. *Blood.* 2012;120:3407–3418.

40. Valapour M, Skeans MA, Smith JM, et al. Lung. *Am J Transplant.* 2016;16(suppl 2):141–168.

41. Vivas AP, Bomfin LE, Costa Jr WI, et al. Oral granulomatosis-like lesions in liver-transplanted pediatric patients. *Oral Dis.* 2014;20:e97–e102.

42. Wall A, Bueno E, Pomahac B, et al. Intraoral features and considerations in face transplantation. *Oral Dis.* 2016;22:93–103.

43. Wijdicks EF, Varelas PN, Gronseth GS, et al. Evidence-based guideline update: determining brain death in adults: report of the Quality Standards Subcommittee of the American Academy of Neurology. *Neurology.* 2010;74:1911–1918.

44. Wong CJ, Pagalilauan G. Primary care of the solid organ transplant recipient. *Med Clin N Am.* 2015;99:1075–1103.

45. Woo SB, Matin K. Off-site dental evaluation program for prospective bone marrow transplant recipients. *J Am Dent Assoc.* 1997;128:189–193.

22

Disorders of Red Blood Cells

KEY POINTS

- The dentist serves an important role in detecting patients with previously undiagnosed anemia through history, clinical examination, and laboratory screening tests.
- Clinical recognition of anemia can significantly affect morbidity and mortality risks, as it is a systemic disease that requires medical management.

- Anemia is an independent risk factor for adverse cardiovascular outcomes (i.e., acute myocardial infarction and death) in a variety of patient populations (as defined by chronic kidney disease, acute coronary syndrome, or old age).
- Dental management may require modification in patients with poorly controlled disease.

Anemia, defined as a reduction in the oxygen-carrying capacity of the blood, is usually associated with a decreased number of circulating red blood cells (RBCs) or an abnormality in the hemoglobin (Hb) contained within the RBCs. Anemia is not a disease but rather a symptom complex that may result from one of three underlying causes: (1) decreased production of RBCs (iron deficiency, folate deficiency, pernicious anemia), (2) blood loss, or (3) increased rate of destruction of circulating RBCs (hypersplenism, autoimmune destruction) (Fig. 22.1).

Oxygen demand (hypoxia) serves as the stimulus for erythropoiesis (RBC production). The kidney serves as the primary sensor for determining the level of oxygenation. If the level is low, the kidney releases erythropoietin, a hormone that stimulates the bone marrow to release RBCs. The oxygen-carrying molecule of RBCs is Hb, and consists of two pairs of globin chains (i.e., α plus β, δ, or γ) that form a shell around four oxygen-binding heme groups. The normal RBC is about 33% Hb by volume or 13–17 g/dL (see Table 1.2).

TYPES OF ANEMIA (SEE TABLE 22.1)

Iron Deficiency Anemia

Iron deficiency anemia is a microcytic anemia (Fig. 22.2) caused by excessive blood loss, poor iron intake, poor iron absorption, or increased demand for iron.

Folate Deficiency Anemia and Pernicious Anemia

Vitamin B_{12} (cobalamin) and folic acid are required for RBC formation and growth within bone marrow. A deficiency in daily intake or absorption of these vitamins can result in anemia.

Hemolytic Anemia

Hemolytic anemias consist of sickle cell anemia, thalassemia, and glucose-6-phosphate dehydrogenase (G6PD) deficiency. These anemias are caused by diverse factors including immune attack, extrinsic factors (infection, splenomegaly, drugs, eclampsia), disorders of

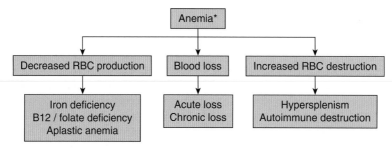

*Anemia may also be attributed to inflammation, neoplasia and / or chronic disease.

FIG. 22.1 Common causes of anemias.

TABLE 22.1 Overview of Anemias

Type	Pathophysiology	Major Signs/Symptoms	Treatment
Iron deficiency[a]	Excessive blood loss Poor iron intake/absorption Increased demand for iron	Pallor, fatigue, lethargy, palpitations, shortness of breath, impaired immunity	Eliminate source of internal bleeding (if present) Iron supplementation
(a) Folate deficiency (b) Pernicious	(a) Deficiency in intake or absorption of folic acid (b) Deficiency of intrinsic factor necessary for absorption of vitamin B_{12}	(a) and (b) Pallor, fatigue, lethargy, palpitations, shortness of breath	(a) Folic acid supplementation (b) Vitamin B_{12} supplementation
Sickle cell	Inherited structurally deficient vhemoglobin protein	Pallor, fatigue, lethargy, palpitations, shortness of breath, dactylitis, leg ulcers	Antibiotics Medications to stimulate production of hemoglobin proteins
Thalassemias	Inherited decrease in production of globin chains on hemoglobin molecule	Pallor, fatigue, lethargy, palpitations, shortness of breath, loss of appetite	Blood transfusions Hematopoietic stem cell transplant
Glucose 6-Phosphate dehydrogenase (G6PD)	Inherited deficit of G6PD enzyme	Pallor, fatigue, lethargy, palpitations, shortness of breath, acute intravascular hemolysis	Prescreening and avoidance of oxidative medication triggers
Aplastic	Complete bone marrow suppression and depletion of all hematopoietic cell lines	Pallor, fatigue, lethargy, palpitations, shortness of breath, petechiae, ecchymosis	Bone marrow transplant Immunosuppressants

[a]Most common type of anemia in the United States.

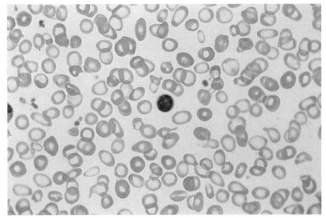

FIG. 22.2 Microcytic anemia associated with iron deficiency. Peripheral blood smear shows red blood cells that are small and have marked hypochromic central pallor.

the RBC membrane (spherocytosis), enzymopathies, and hemoglobinopathies.

Sickle Cell Anemia

The two most common types of sickle cell disorders are sickle cell trait and sickle cell (disease) anemia. Sickle cell trait is the heterozygous state in which the affected person carries one gene for sickle cell hemoglobin (HbS), the result of substitution of a single amino acid—valine for glutamic acid—at the sixth residue of the β-hemoglobin chain. In patients with sickle cell anemia, more than 80% of the Hb is HbS.

Thalassemias

Thalassemias, another type of hemoglobinopathy, are caused by deletions or mutations of the α- or β-globin gene that results in defective globin synthesis (reduced or absent synthesis of one or more globin chains). Mutations affecting one or two genes result in a trait status.

Glucose-6-Phosphate Dehydrogenase Deficiency

Glucose-6-phosphate dehydrogenase is an enzyme that enables the RBC to convert carbohydrates into energy via the hexose monophosphate shunt pathway. Blockade of this enzymatic pathway in persons with G6PD deficiency results in production of methemoglobin and denatured Hb, which leads to cell membrane alterations and hemolysis of the cell (hemolytic anemia).

Aplastic Anemia

Aplastic anemia occurs when the bone marrow is unable to produce adequate numbers of RBCs, white blood cells (WBCs), and platelets due to inability of the hematopoietic stem cells to proliferate, differentiate, or give rise to mature blood cells.

EPIDEMIOLOGY

It is estimated that anemia affects 1.62 billion people globally and 3.4 million Americans. Approximately 4% of men and 8% of women in the United States have anemia, defined as Hb values below 13.5 g/dL for men and below 12 g/dL for women. In the United States, iron deficiency anemia is the most common type. Folate deficiency anemia occurs in about 4 of 100,000 people. The sickle cell trait is carried by approximately 8%–10% of African Americans. In western Africa, 25%–30% of the population may be carriers. Approximately 50,000 African Americans (≈0.003%–0.15%), or 1 in 600, have sickle cell anemia. Worldwide, an estimated 1.7% of the population has α- or β-thalassemia trait and is estimated to occur in about 44 per 100,000 live births. Historically, α-thalassemia is more prevalent in persons of African and Southeast Asian descent, and β-thalassemia is most common in persons of Mediterranean, African, and Southeast Asian descent. The incidence of aplastic anemia in the United States is about 2 cases per 1 million persons per year, and in 4 cases per million in Asia.

Of the approximately 2000 patients treated in the average dental practice, about 12 men and 24 women will be anemic. In most of these patients, the condition may be undiagnosed.

ETIOLOGY

Anemia has numerous causes, including genetic disorders that produce aberrant RBCs that result in RBC destruction (hemolysis), nutritional disorders that limit the production of RBCs, immune-mediated disorders that result in attacks on RBCs, bleeding disorders that cause loss of RBCs, chronic diseases (e.g., rheumatoid arthritis), infections, and diseases of bone marrow (Table 22.2).

PATHOPHYSIOLOGY AND COMPLICATIONS

In general, anemia increases the risk for acute myocardial infarction, chronic kidney disease, acute coronary syndrome, and death. The type of anemia dictates the types of complications seen in these patients.

Iron Deficiency Anemia

Depletion of iron commonly occurs with blood loss caused by menstruation, pregnancy, or bleeding from the

gastrointestinal (GI) tract. During pregnancy, the expectant mother experiences an increased demand for additional iron and vitamins to support fetal growth, and unless sufficient amounts of these nutrients have been provided, she may become anemic. Anemia in men usually indicates the presence of an underlying medical problem (e.g., GI bleeding, malignancy). Poor intake is more common in children who live in developing countries, where cereals and formula fortified with iron are not readily available. Malabsorption of iron can result from gastrectomy or intestinal disease that reduces absorption of iron from the duodenum and the jejunum. Increased demand is associated with chronic inflammation (autoimmune disease).

Folate Deficiency and Pernicious Anemia

Vitamin B_{12} (cobalamin) and folic acid are needed for RBC formation and growth within bone marrow. Vitamin B_{12} is a cofactor in methionine-associated enzymatic reactions required of protein synthesis and thus in the maturation of RBCs. Folate is needed for enzymatic reactions required for the synthesis of purines and pyrimidines of deoxyribonucleic acid (DNA) and ribonucleic acid (RNA) and thus for the synthesis of proteins. Risk factors for folate deficiency include poor diet (frequently encountered in individuals with lower socioeconomic status, older adults, and people who do not eat fresh fruits or leafy vegetables), alcoholism, history of malabsorption disorders, and pregnancy (especially during the third trimester).

Pernicious anemia is caused by a deficiency of intrinsic factor, a substance secreted by the gastric parietal cells that is necessary for absorption of vitamin B_{12}. Most patients with pernicious anemia have chronic atrophic gastritis with decreased intrinsic factor and hydrochloric acid secretion. Antibodies against parietal cells and intrinsic factor also are present in the sera of most patients. This finding strongly suggests that the disease is of autoimmune origin. Long-standing pernicious anemia is associated with increased risk for development of gastric carcinoma. In addition, an association between pernicious anemia with myxedema, rheumatoid arthritis, and neuropsychiatric and neuromuscular abnormalities (caused by a defect in myelin synthesis) has been reported.

Sickle Cell Anemia

Sickle cell hemoglobin is the result of substitution of a single amino acid—valine for glutamic acid—at the sixth residue of the β chain. Sickle cell disorders are distinguished by the number of globin genes affected. Whereas sickle cell trait is the heterozygous state in which the affected person carries one gene for HbS, sickle cell anemia is the homozygous state. In patients with sickle cell anemia, more than 80% of the Hb is HbS. Distortion of the RBC into a sickled shape results from deoxygenation or decreased blood pH, causing partial crystallization of HbS, polymerization, and realignment of the defective Hb molecule (Fig. 22.3). Cellular rigidity and membrane damage occur, and irreversible sickling is the

TABLE 22.2   Types of Anemia

Classification by RBC Size and Shape	Cause
MICROCYTIC (MCV ≤80 FL[a])	
Iron deficiency anemia	Decreased production of RBCs
Thalassemias	Defective hemoglobin synthesis
Lead poisoning	Inhibition of hemoglobin synthesis
NORMOCYTIC (MCV 80–100 FL[a])	
Hemolytic anemia	Increased destruction of RBCs
• sickle cell anemia	
• G6PD deficiency	
Aplastic anemia	Decreased production of RBCs
Renal failure	Decreased production of RBCs
Anemia of chronic disease	Decreased production of RBCs
MACROCYTIC (MCV > 100 FL[a])	
Pernicious anemia	Decreased production of RBCs
Folate deficiency	Decreased production of RBCs
Hypothyroidism	Decreased production of RBCs

[a]Also expressed in μm^3 units.

fL, Femtoliter; *G6PD,* glucose-6-phosphate dehydrogenase; *MCV,* mean corpuscular volume; *RBC,* red blood cell.

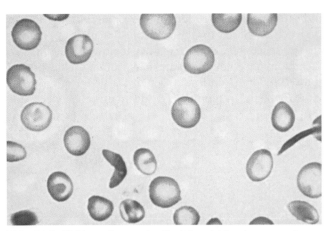

FIG. 22.3 Sickle cell anemia. Peripheral blood smear shows characteristic abnormal sickle-shaped red blood cells.

result. The net effects of these changes are erythrostasis, increased blood viscosity, reduced blood flow, hypoxia, increased adhesion of RBCs, vascular occlusion, and further sickling.

Complications of sickle cell anemia can occur at any age, but patients in the following age groups are more likely to manifest certain complications:

1. *Birth to 20 years of age:* painful events, stroke, acute chest syndrome (fever, chest pain, wheezing, cough, and hypoxia), acute anemia, and infection.
2. *From 20 to 40 years of age:* osteonecrosis of hip and shoulder joints, leg ulcers, priapism, liver disease, and gallstones.
3. *Older than 40 years of age:* pulmonary hypertension, nephropathy, proliferative retinopathy, and cardiac enlargement, heart murmurs, and sudden death from arrhythmias.
4. Sickle cell anemia has a high rate of mortality with, about 50% of patients at risk of death before the age of 30 years, if not adequately treated (see Medical Management section).

Thalassemias

Pathophysiology of α-thalassemia is characterized by insufficient synthesis of α-globin chains, resulting in excess β-like globin chains. Classification of α-thalassemia is based on the number of gene deletions. A single-gene deletion results in α-thalassemia silent carrier status. The two-gene deletion causes α-thalassemia trait (minor). The three-gene deletion results in significant production of HbH, which has four β-chains, resulting in α-thalassemia intermedia. The four-gene deletion, or α-thalassemia major, results in significant production of Hb Bart's, which has four γ-chains and typically results in fetal death.

β-Thalassemia is caused by mutations resulting in a single nucleotide substitution, small deletions or insertions within the β-globin gene or its immediate flanking sequence, or, in rare cases, gross deletions. These mutations result in reduced production of β-globin chains and HbA. The one gene defect is classified as β-thalassemia trait (minor). When the synthesis from both genes is severely reduced or absent, the person has β-thalassemia major, also known as Cooley anemia. Complications of thalassemias depend on severity of disease ranging from none in mild disease to hepatosplenomegaly, life-threatening infections, thrombosis, and heart failure in severe cases.

Aplastic Anemia

An abnormal T-cell response facilitated by genetic predisposition has been postulated as the pathogenic mechanism of aplastic anemia leading to the overproduction of bone marrow–inhibiting cytokines. Viral infections (e.g., cytomegalovirus, HIV), drugs (e.g., chloramphenicol, sulfonamides), and/or genetic mutations may trigger the disease process that leads to production of autoreactive T cells resulting in pancytopenias. Complications of aplastic anemia depend upon severity of disease with fatigue, easy bruising, and bleeding in mild cases to life-threatening hemorrhage, infection, arrhythmia, and heart failure in severe cases.

CLINICAL PRESENTATION

Signs and Symptoms

Symptoms of anemia occur in proportion to the rate of anemia development; rapidly developing anemia has more profound features than slowly developing disease. Since anemia develops slowly in most affected patients, few symptoms are typically experienced until the condition worsens. Table 22.3 provides an overview of the signs and symptoms of anemia. Clinical features of sickle cell anemia include leg ulcers and dactylitis (hand and foot warmth and tenderness) (Fig. 22.4). Premature graying of hair and yellowing of the skin (caused by jaundice) have been reported with pernicious anemia (Fig. 22.5). Patients with anemia also may describe a sore or painful tongue (glossitis), a smooth tongue, or redness of the tongue or cheilosis (Fig. 22.6).

LABORATORY AND DIAGNOSTIC FINDINGS

A patient with signs or symptoms suggestive of anemia should be referred to a physician for evaluation and subsequently undergo laboratory testing for a complete blood count with differential. The Hb level, hematocrit, and RBC indices (mean corpuscular volume [MCV], mean corpuscular hemoglobin [MCH], RBC distribution width [RDW], and mean corpuscular hemoglobin concentration [MCHC]) are tests used to screen for anemia. In addition, total WBC count and platelet count should be obtained to determine whether a generalized bone marrow defect has occurred and to evaluate for hypersegmented neutrophils (see Chapter 23).

Anemia is generally defined as Hb level less than 12 g/dL for women and less than 13.5 g/dL for men. In accordance with the size of RBCs, anemia is classified as microcytic (MCV <80 fL [or μm³]), macrocytic (MCV > 100 fL), or normocytic (MCV of 80–100 fL). Whereas a reticulocyte count (based on percentage of RBCs) of less than 0.5% indicates inadequate RBC production in the bone marrow, a value greater than 1.5%

indicates increased production in response to bleeding or destruction. Based on the absolute reticulocyte count in the presence of anemia, a value below 75,000/μL indicates hypoproliferative anemias, and a value greater than 100,000/μL indicates hemolysis or an appropriate erythropoietic response. To distinguish between the

TABLE 22.3	Signs and Symptoms of Anemia
Type of Anemia	**Signs/Symptoms**
General	Pallor, fatigue, lethargy, palpitations, shortness of breath, jaundice, splitting/spooning of fingernails, abdominal pain, bone pain, tinnitus, irritability, dizziness, tingling of fingers and toes, muscular weakness, hepatosplenomegaly, lymphadenopathy, melena, glossodynia, glossitis, cheilosis, loss of taste.
Iron deficiency	(+) Impaired immunity, diminished exercise tolerance, and work performance.
G6PD deficiency	(+) Acute intravascular hemolysis, dyspnea
Sickle cell	(+) Dactylitis (hand and foot warmth and tenderness), leg ulcers, organomegaly, cardiac failure, stroke, delays in growth and development.
Thalassemias	(+) Loss of appetite, poor growth, skeletal abnormalities.
Aplastic	(+) Weakness, headaches, dyspnea with exertion, petechiae, ecchymoses, epistaxis, metrorrhagia, infection, gingival bleeding.

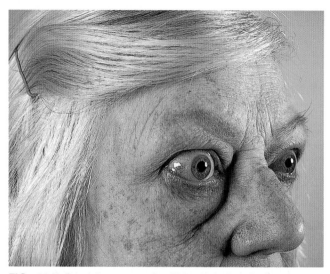

FIG. 22.5 Pernicious anemia. This 38-year-old woman has blue eyes and vitiligo and shows premature graying of the hair—three features that are more common in patients with pernicious anemia than in control subjects. (From Hoffbrand AV, Pettit JE: *Color atlas of clinical hematology,* ed 4, London, 2010, Mosby.)

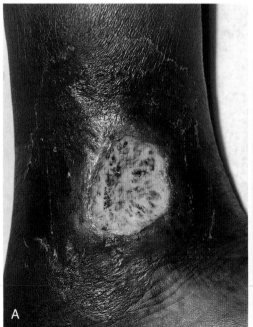

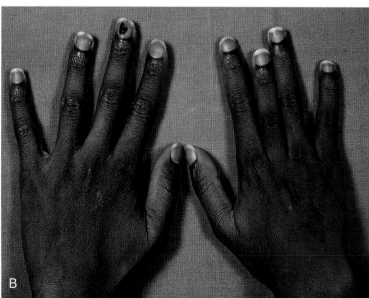

FIG. 22.4 Sickle cell anemia may cause various complications. **A**, Leg ulcer secondary to a vasoocclusive attack. **B**, Growth deformation of the middle finger from dactylitis of the growth plate. (From Hoffbrand AV, Pettit JE: *Color atlas of clinical hematology,* ed 4, London, 2010, Mosby.)

various types of anemias, key laboratory tests, as shown in Table 22.4, are performed.

Deficiencies in iron reveal a microcytic anemia, low serum ferritin, low serum iron, and high total iron-binding capacity (TIBC). Deficiencies of vitamin B_{12} and folic acid are associated with macrocytic anemia and the presence of hypersegmented polymorphonuclear leukocytes in the peripheral blood smear (Fig. 22.7). Measures of serum methylmalonic acid and homocysteine levels and serologic testing for parietal cell and intrinsic factor antibodies are used to further screen for the deficiency. Use of the serum cobalamin assay followed by the Schilling test helps to establish the diagnosis of pernicious anemia. For the Schilling test, the fasting patient receives a small oral dose of radioactive vitamin B_{12} and then a larger dose of nonradioactive vitamin B_{12} as a parenteral flush. At 24 h, the amount of radioactive cyanocobalamin in the urine is measured. About 7% of the radioactive vitamin B_{12} dose is excreted during the first 24 h; however, persons with pernicious anemia excrete less than 3%. The Schilling test is used occasionally; serologic testing for parietal cell and intrinsic factor antibodies is more commonly used to diagnose pernicious anemia.

Screening tests for Heinz bodies (Hb precipitates) (Fig. 22.8) or nicotinamide adenine dinucleotide phosphate (NADPH) may be used to detect G6PD deficiency. More sensitive tests use direct fluorescent measures of NADPH. Other tests used to detect this deficiency include the cyanide-ascorbate assay, the quantitative assay of G6PD, and G6PD-tetrazolium cytochemical test.

Newborn babies are screened for sickle cell status (disease or trait) as early as 24–48 hours after birth. All African American patients should be asked whether sickle cell disease is present in their family histories. If the

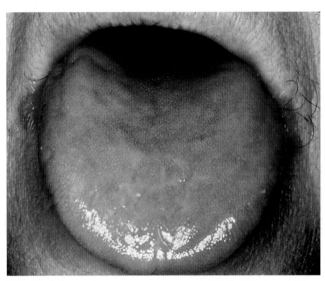

FIG. 22.6 Smooth red tongue and angular cheilitis in a patient found to have iron deficiency anemia.

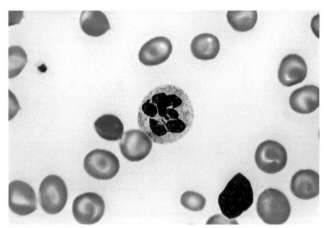

FIG. 22.7 Megaloblastic anemia. Peripheral blood smear shows a hypersegmented neutrophil with a six-lobed nucleus. (From Kumar V, Abbas A, Fausto N: *Robbins and Cotran pathologic basis of disease*, ed 8, Philadelphia, Saunders, 2010. Courtesy of Dr. Robert W. McKenna, Department of Pathology, University of Texas Southwestern Medical School, Dallas, TX.)

TABLE 22.4	Laboratory Assessments to Aid in the Diagnosis of Anemia[a]	
Type	**Etiology**	**Tests to Discriminate Types of Anemia**
Microcytic anemia	Iron deficiency	Serum iron, ferritin, TIBC, transferrin saturation, bone marrow aspirate; also, stool examination for occult blood
Macrocytic anemia	Folate deficiency	CBC, serum folate level
Macrocytic anemia	Pernicious anemia	CBC, serum vitamin B_{12} (cobalamin) assay levels, schilling test, serum antiparietal cell, and intrinsic factor antibodies
Normocytic anemia	G6PD	Staining peripheral blood smear with methyl or crystal violet, cyanide-ascorbate assay, qualitative (fluorescent spot) test and quantitative test for G6PD, reticulocyte count, indirect bilirubin levels
Normocytic anemia	Sickle cell anemia	Sickledex, high-performance liquid chromatography, hemoglobin electrophoresis, reticulocyte count, indirect bilirubin levels
Normocytic anemia	Aplastic anemia	Erythropoietin levels, bone marrow aspirate

[a]*MCH,* Mean corpuscular hemoglobin; *MCHC,* mean corpuscular hemoglobin concentration; *MCV,* mean corpuscular volume has been assessed, and values indicate that anemia is present. These tests are ordered after the initial complete blood count (CBC) and differential, including red blood cell indices.
G6PD, Glucose-6-phosphate dehydrogenase; *TIBC,* total iron-binding capacity.

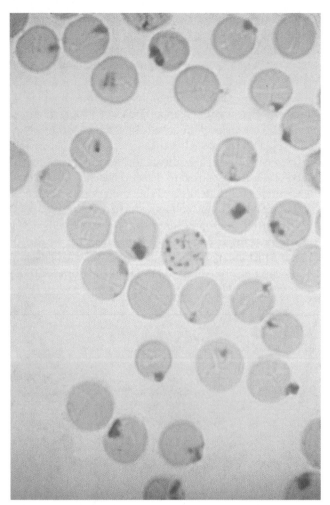

FIG. 22.8 Deficiency of glucose 6-phosphate dehydrogenase: Peripheral blood film shows Heinz bodies in red blood cells and a single reticulocyte. (Supravital new methylene blue stain.). (From Hoffbrand AV, Pettit JE: *Color atlas of clinical hematology,* ed 4, London, 2010, Mosby.)

patient or family members have not been screened, the dentist should consider referring these individuals to their physicians for appropriate screening. This can be done in the dental office with the Sickledex test (Streck, Inc., Omaha, NE), in a commercial clinical laboratory, or by a physician. The Sickledex test uses deoxygenating agents, which will cause defective RBCs to sickle in shape. Electrophoresis or high-performance liquid chromatography is performed as a confirmatory test.

If thalassemia is suspected on the basis of the physical examination, personal and family history, and red-cell indexes (low mean corpuscular volume, low mean corpuscular hemoglobin level, and normal red-cell distribution width), the diagnosis can be confirmed by means of hemoglobin electrophoresis or high-performance liquid chromatography. DNA analysis may be required to confirm the diagnosis and identify the specific disease genotypes.

The diagnosis of aplastic anemia is based on the presence of anemia (normochromic, normocytic),

thrombocytopenia (normal sized platelets), neutropenia, and the absence of abnormal cells in the leukocyte differential. The diagnosis is confirmed by findings on bone marrow biopsy and examination consisting of numerous bone spicules with empty fatty spaces and few hematopoietic cells. Lymphocytes, plasma cells, and mast cells are increased in numbers and represent more than 65% of the cells found in the samples.

MEDICAL MANAGEMENT

The goal of treatment is to eliminate the underlying cause. In microcytic anemia (iron deficiency), the physician should investigate a source of internal bleeding (peptic ulcer, GI malignancy) or menses; hence, management needs to be specific for the underlying cause. Iron deficiency associated with pregnancy often resolves after childbirth. In children, iron supplements (ferrous sulfate, 2–6 mg/kg/day) are recommended to arrest motor and cognitive impairment brought on by iron deficiency. In patients who have undergone a gastrectomy, iron supplements (ferrous sulfate, ferrous fumarate, or ferrous gluconate) are provided on a long-term basis. The preferred route of iron administration is oral. In cases in which blood loss is uncontrollable, iron cannot be absorbed, or iron is not tolerated, parenteral iron is given by either intravenous (IV) or intramuscular injection.

Folate deficiency is managed by administering folic acid supplements and by increasing the intake of green, leafy vegetables and citrus fruits. In the case of poor intestinal absorption, such as in patients with gastric bypass, replacement therapy with folic acid or supplemental iron may be lifelong. Cyanocobalamin injections are used to treat patients with pernicious anemia. Injections generally are given daily for the first week and then are tapered eventually to once a month, as needed.

Without medical management, 50% of persons with sickle cell anemia will die before the age of 30 years; however, because of advances in medical care, sickle cell anemia is now considered a chronic adult disease. Management of sickle cell anemia includes routine prophylactic penicillin for infants and the early use of antibiotics to prevent severe infection. Children should receive vaccination against *Streptococcus pneumoniae*, *Haemophilus influenzae*, hepatitis B, and influenza. Folic acid dietary supplements are given daily to most patients with sickle cell anemia because folic acid deficiency may play a role in the causes of crises. In addition, penicillin prophylaxis is used for at least the first 5 years of life. Therapeutic strategies include the use of hydroxyurea (with or without erythropoietin), which induces production of HbF and thus prevents formation of HbS polymers. Newer therapeutic agents, such as voxelotor, Crizanlinzumab, and L-Glutamine, are used as replacement or add-on therapies for management of sickle cell anemia. When a crisis occurs, high doses of folic acid, analgesics for pain, hydration, and blood transfusions are used. Hematopoietic stem cell transplantation can cure sickle cell anemia, however, patient eligibility depends on disease type, age, complications, and whether an appropriate donor is available. The source in a majority of cases is from sibling donors, which carries a 10% mortality rate and a 90% overall survival rate at a mean follow-up of 54 months. Patients older than 16 years of age are less likely to have successful grafts. Only about 1% of the patients with sickle cell anemia meet the criteria for stem cell transplantation.

Management of thalassemias is dependent on type and severity of the condition. Periodic and lifelong blood transfusions are required for patients with β-thalassemia major and may be clinically necessary for those with intermedia disease (α- and β-). Hematopoietic stem cell transplantation in childhood is the only curative therapy for β-thalassemia major with disease-free survival rates exceeding 90%.

After the diagnosis of aplastic anemia is established, family human leukocyte antigen (HLA) typing is recommended for patients 50 years of age or younger for possible stem cell transplantation from a histocompatible sibling. Transplantation is curative but is associated with an early mortality rate of 10% in children and young adults and more than 20% in older patients. HLA-matched related bone marrow transplantation is curative for 80%–90% of patients. In long-term survivors, the development of chronic graft-versus-host disease (GVHD) is common (see Chapter 21). GVHD occurs in about 20% of the patients younger than 20 years of age and in about 40% of those older than 40 years of age. Immunosuppression with antithymocyte globulin alone or with cyclosporine is the most common therapy for aplastic anemia. Other treatments include Eltrombopag, an oral thrombopoeitin receptor agonist previously used for treatment of chronic idiopathic thrombocytopenic purpura and immunosuppressive therapy.

DENTAL MANAGEMENT

Medical Considerations

Identification and Risk Assessment. The dentist should obtain a careful history to identify conditions associated with anemia. The assessment should include questions concerning dietary intake, malnutrition, alcohol or drug use, use of nonsteroidal antiinflammatory drugs, menstrual blood loss, pregnancies, hypothyroidism, jaundice, gallstones, splenectomy, bleeding disorders and abnormal Hb, and organ transplantation. Historical information concerning family members also is important for identifying hereditary risk for hemolytic anemias. In children, the history should identify patterns of growth. Women should be queried regarding the onset, nature, and regularity of the menstrual cycle. Women with a history of regular periods but with heavy flow may be anemic and should be referred for appropriate medical evaluation and treatment. Patients who report a change in the

pattern, onset, duration, or rate of menstrual flow should be encouraged to seek medical evaluation. Patients who stopped having periods prematurely should be referred for medical evaluation, as should those who have experienced bleeding between regular periods. In addition, in women who are pregnant or who recently experienced childbirth, the history should establish whether the patient had excessive bleeding during pregnancy and whether the patient has other children and when they were born because the closer together the pregnancies were, the greater is the risk for development of iron deficiency anemia. The mother may lose additional iron during delivery and breastfeeding.

The dentist may identify signs and symptoms of anemia in patients seeking dental treatment (Fig. 22.9). A patient with classic signs or symptoms of anemia should be referred to a physician and screened by appropriate laboratory tests (Table 22.4). Screening tests should include complete and differential blood counts, a smear for cell morphologic study, determination of Hb or hematocrit, a Sickledex test (for African American patients), and platelet count. If screening tests are ordered by the dentist and the results of one or more are abnormal, the patient should be referred for medical evaluation and treatment.

Patients with anemia may have an underlying disease such as peptic ulcer or carcinoma, for which early detection may be lifesaving. Patients with sickle cell anemia may be at increased risk of complications if the disease is not detected before dental treatment is started. Thus, it is important for the dentist to attempt to identify these patients through history and clinical examination before starting any treatment.

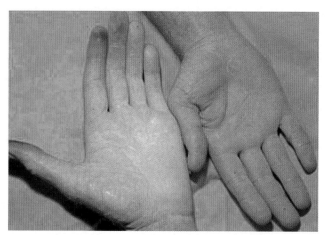

FIG. 22.9 Pallor of the hand in anemia is obvious in this patient, especially when compared with the physician's hand on the right. The patient's hemoglobin level was 7 g/dL. The patient's hand also shows that he was a heavy smoker. The cause of the anemia was chronic blood loss from carcinoma of the esophagus. (From Forbes CD, Jackson WF: *Color atlas and text of clinical medicine*, ed 3, Edinburgh, 2003, Mosby.)

Assessment of the severity of a patient's anemia is important for preventing complications. The dentist should ensure that the patient's underlying condition is stable before proceeding with routine dental treatment. In many cases, anemia is associated with chronic illness; thus, treatment may be provided in the presence of anemia.

Recommendations

To minimize the risk of medical complications, Hb levels should be above 11 g/dL, and the patient should be free from symptoms. Patients who are short of breath and in whom Hb levels are less than 11 g/dL, have an abnormal heart rate, or have an oxygen saturation less than 91% (as determined by pulse oximetry) are considered medically unstable, and routine treatment should be deferred until their health status improves.

Patients with G6PD deficiency exhibit an increased incidence of drug sensitivity with sulfonamides (sulfamethoxazole), aspirin, and chloramphenicol being the prime offenders. Penicillin, streptomycin, and isoniazid also have been linked to hemolysis in these patients. Dental infection may accelerate the rate of hemolysis in patients with this type of anemia. Thus, dental infections should be avoided, and if they occur, they must be managed effectively. The astute clinician will recognize that febrile illness and elevated bilirubin are features of this condition. The drugs listed previously should not be used in these patients.

African Americans with sickle cell anemia can receive routine dental care during noncrisis periods; however, long and complicated procedures should be avoided. Appropriate restorative and preventive dental care are important because oral infection can precipitate a crisis. If infection occurs, it must be treated expeditiously using local and systemic measures, such as incision and drainage, heat, therapeutic doses of appropriate antibiotics, pulpectomy, or extraction. If cellulitis develops, the patient's physician must be consulted and hospitalization considered. Adequate fluid intake is important for avoiding dehydration. Dental management considerations for patients with sickle cell anemia are summarized in Box 22.1. There are no contraindications for providing routine dental care for thalassemia patients under proper medical management. Dental management of patients who are immunosuppressed and/or after receiving a bone marrow transplant are referred to Chapter 21.

Anesthesia. For routine dental care, appointments should be short for patients with sickle cell anemia to minimize stress. The use of a local anesthetic is acceptable (avoid prilocaine and general anesthesia); however, inclusion of small amounts of epinephrine in the local anesthetic is controversial as it may impair circulation and cause vascular occlusion. The benefits of a vasoconstrictor probably outweigh the risk of local impairment of circulation. Thus, the use of a local anesthetic

with epinephrine 1:100,000 to attain hemostasis and profound anesthesia is warranted within the context of limiting the total dose of epinephrine (limit the dose to <3 carpules). Stronger concentrations of epinephrine must be avoided. If required, nitrous oxide–oxygen (N_2O–O_2) should be used for short periods, with at least 50% oxygen concentration provided.

Intravenous sedation must be used with extreme caution in patients who have a history of sickle cell anemia. Barbiturates and narcotics should be avoided because suppression of the respiratory center by these agents leads to hypoxia and acidosis, which may precipitate an acute crisis. Light sedation can be provided with midazolam (versed) or nalbuphine hydrochloride. Additional oxygen provided by nasal cannula and liberal use of IV fluids during sedation are advised. General anesthesia is not recommended when the Hb level falls below 10 g/dL. High doses of salicylates should be avoided because the "acid" effect can precipitate a crisis. Pain control may be attempted with use of acetaminophen and small doses of codeine.

Although the evidence is weak, prophylactic antibiotics are often recommended for sickle cell anemia when major surgical procedures are performed to prevent wound infection or osteomyelitis. Penicillin is the drug of choice in nonallergic patients; however, amoxicillin and doxycycline with metronidazole also are considered acceptable for prophylaxis. Intramuscular or IV antibiotics should be considered for use in patients with sickle cell anemia who have an acute dental infection. The dentist must establish the patient's status and if blood transfusion is indicated prior to surgery. Accordingly, consultation with the patient's physician is recommended before any surgical procedure to establish the severity of the anemia and how best to manage any complications. Dehydration must be avoided during surgery and the postoperative period.

Bleeding. Persons with aplastic anemia are susceptible to infection and bleeding, so clinical recognition of such patients before invasive dental procedures are performed is important. Patients with signs and symptoms of anemia, petechiae, ecchymoses, and gingival bleeding should be referred to a physician for evaluation, diagnosis, and treatment as indicated. Dental extractions in a patient with thrombocytopenia (platelets <50,000/mm^3) may be associated with excessive bleeding and the reader is referred to Chapter 24 for management considerations. In addition, the dental management of the patient treated by immunosuppression or bone marrow transplantation is covered in Chapter 21.

Capacity to Tolerate Care. Patients who are short of breath or have Hb levels below 11 g/dL, an abnormal heart rate, or oxygen saturation less than 91% are considered medically unstable, and routine treatment should be deferred until their health status improves. Delays in dental treatment also may be required for

| BOX 22.1 | Checklist for Dental Management of Patients With Red Blood Cell Disorders[a] |

PREOPERATIVE RISK ASSESSMENT

R: Recognize Risks
- Be **aware** of adverse events that may occur in the management of a patient who has a medical condition.

P: Patient Evaluation
- Review **medical history** and discuss relevant issues with the patient.
- Identify all **medications and drugs** being taken or supposed to be taken by the patient.
- **Examine** the patient for signs and symptoms of disease and obtain vital signs.
- Review or obtain recent **laboratory test** results or **images** required to assess risk.
- Obtain a **medical consultation** if the patient has a poorly controlled or undiagnosed problem or if the patient's health status is uncertain, and before surgical procedures are performed.

A	
Analgesics	Avoid strong narcotics and high doses of salicylates. Use acetaminophen with or without small doses of codeine.
Antibiotics	Antibiotic prophylaxis is generally recommended for major surgical procedures in patients with sickle cell anemia.
Anesthesia	Consider using local anesthetic without epinephrine for routine dental care. For surgical procedures, use 1:100,000 epinephrine in local anesthetic, limit the dose to <3 carpules. Avoid general anesthesia, particularly if the hemoglobin level is below 10 g/dL.
Anxiety	No issues.

B	
Bleeding	No issues with exception of aplastic anemia.
Blood pressure and vital sign monitoring	Obtain pretreatment vital signs.

C	
Capacity to tolerate care	Patients with active, symptomatic disease may defer elective dental treatment until condition(s) are stable.
Chair position	No issues.

D	
Devices	No issues.
Drugs	Avoid barbiturates and strong narcotics; sedation may be obtained with midazolam (versed). When using nitrous oxide, provide oxygen at greater than 50% with high flow rate and good ventilation.

E	
Equipment	Use pulse oximeter and maintain oxygen saturation above 95%.
Emergencies and urgent care	Treat acute infection with incision and drainage if indicated; local heat and high doses of appropriate antibiotics will help avoid a crisis. Dehydration should be avoided. If sickling crisis occurs, hospitalization is indicated.

Postoperative care F	
Follow-up care	Follow-up consultation with patient's physician is advised.

[a]Recommendations based on SORT taxonomy C.

patients who have anemia caused by severe underlying conditions.

Treatment Planning Modifications

Treatment planning modifications are directed primarily toward patients who have severe anemia or sickle cell anemia. Elective surgical procedures are best avoided in patients with sickle cell anemia. Since these patients may be at higher risk for bone complications, dental implant therapy should be considered judiciously and on a case-by-case basis. Routine dental care can be rendered for patients with sickle cell trait and for those in whom the disease is in a noncrisis state. Special emphasis should be placed on oral hygiene procedures to avoid development of dental caries, gingival inflammation, and infection, which can lead to osteomyelitis. Adequate oxygenation should be provided during nitrous oxide inhalation procedures. Pulse oximetry monitoring is prudent during invasive dental treatment of all patients with anemia.

ORAL MANIFESTATIONS

Oral findings in patients with anemia usually relate to the underlying cause of the anemia. The oral mucosa may appear pale. Patients with nutritional causes of anemia (e.g., vitamin B_{12} or iron deficiency) may show loss of papillae from the tongue and atrophic changes in the oral mucosa (see Fig. 22.6). Angular cheilitis and aphthae may be observed. Patients also may report a burning or sore tongue. Some patients with iron deficiency anemia develop Plummer–Vinson syndrome (Fig. 22.10), which is characterized by a sore mouth, dysphagia (resulting from muscular degeneration in the esophagus with esophageal stenosis or "webbing"), and an increased frequency of carcinoma of the oral cavity and pharynx. Patients with this syndrome should be monitored closely for any oral or pharyngeal tissue changes that might be early indicators of carcinoma.

Patients with hemolytic anemia (e.g., sickle cell anemia) may show pallor and oral evidence of jaundice

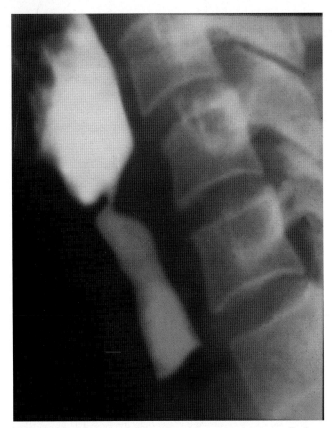

FIG. 22.10 Feature of Plummer–Vinson syndrome. Barium contrast radiograph demonstrates esophageal webbing. (From Bricker SL, Langlais RP, Miller CS: *Oral diagnosis, oral medicine, and treatment planning*, ed 2, Hamilton, Ontario, 2002, BC Decker. Courtesy of Dr. Thomas J. Vaughan.)

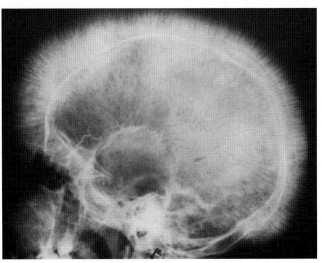

FIG. 22.12 Skull film in a patient with hemolytic anemia shows new bone formation on the outer table, producing perpendicular radiations or "hair on end" appearance. (From Kumar V, Abbas A, Fausto N: *Robbins and Cotran pathologic basis of disease*, ed 8, Philadelphia, 2010, Saunders. Courtesy of Dr. Jack Reynolds, Department of Radiology, University of Texas Southwestern Medical School, Dallas, TX.)

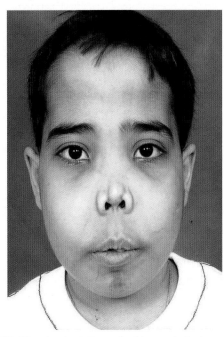

FIG. 22.13 Classic depiction of *chipmunk facies*, characterized by maxillary expansion, saddle nose, frontal bossing, and depressed cranial vault. (From Singh A, Varma S. β-Thalassaemia intermedia masquerading as β-thalassaemia major. BMJ Case Rep. 2014; 2014:bcr2014207637.)

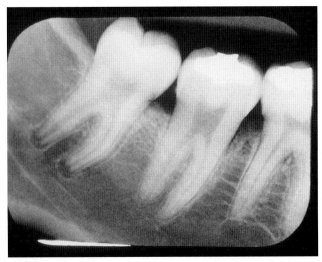

FIG. 22.11 Periapical radiograph of the mandible in a patient with sickle cell anemia. Note the prominent horizontal trabeculations and the dense lamina dura.

caused by hyperbilirubinemia caused by excessive erythrocyte destruction. The trabecular pattern of the bone on dental radiographs may be affected because of

hyperplasia of marrow elements in response to increased destruction of RBCs. Therefore, dental radiographs may show enlarged bone marrow (medullary) spaces associated with bone marrow hyperplasia, increased widening and decreased numbers of

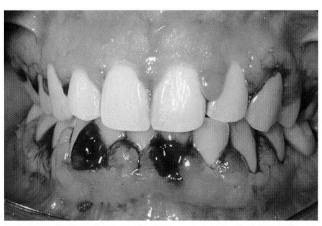

FIG. 22.14 Aplastic anemia. Diffuse gingival hyperplasia with sulcal hemorrhage. (From Neville BW, Damm DD, Allen CM et al., editors: *Oral and maxillofacial pathology*, ed 3, St. Louis, 2009, Saunders.)

trabeculations, and generalized osteoporosis (thinning of the inferior border of the mandible). Because of compensatory marrow expansion, the bone appears more radiolucent, with prominent lamellar striations. Specifically, the trabeculae between teeth may appear as horizontal rows or in a "stepladder" configuration (Fig. 22.11). This can also manifest as frontal bossing or "hair-on-end" appearance in the cortical regions of a skull film (Fig. 22.12). Vaso-occlusive events can promote asymptomatic pulpal necrosis, osteomyelitis, ischemic necrosis within the mandible, and peripheral neuropathy. Patients with sickle cell anemia often have delayed eruption of teeth and dental hypoplasia.

Orofacial findings associated with thalassemias mainly affect the craniofacial bones and occur more frequently in patients with β-thalassemia. These include Class II malocclusion, lateral displacement of orbits and development of *chipmunk facies*, which is characterized by maxillary expansion, saddle nose, frontal bossing, and depressed cranial vault (Fig. 22.13). Other reported potential findings include spiky-shaped and short roots, taurodontism, increased caries risk, and reduced levels of salivary phosphorus, IgA, and urea.

The oral findings associated with aplastic anemia include petechiae, ecchymoses, mucosal pallor, ulceration (infection), gingival bleeding, and/or swelling (Fig. 22.14). Another oral finding of aplastic anemia is necrotizing gingivostomatitis. For more information about oral complications of immunosuppression and bone marrow transplantation and their management associated with aplastic anemia, see Chapter 21.

BIBLIOGRAPHY

1. World Health Organization. Global anaemia prevalence and number of individuals affected. Available at: https://www.who.int/vmnis/anaemia/prevalence/summary/anaemia_data_status_t2/en/. Accessed June 7, 2021.
2. Abed H, Sharma SP, Balkhoyor A, et al. Special care dentistry for patients diagnosed with sickle cell disease: an update for dentists. *Gen Dent.* 2019;67:40–44.
3. Acharya S. Oral and dental considerations in management of sickle cell anemia. *Int J Clin Pediatr Dent.* 2015;8:141–144.
4. Antony AC. Megaloblastic anemias. In: Hoffman R, Benz Jr E, Shattil S, et al., eds. *Hematology: Basic Principles and Practice.* 5th ed. Philadelphia: Churchill Livingstone; 2009:491–524.
5. Avsever IH, Orhan K, Tuncer O, et al. Evaluation of mandibular bone structure in sickle cell anaemia patients. *Gulhane Med J.* 2015;57:11–15.
6. Green R, Mitra A Datta. Folate, cobalamin and megaloblastic anemias. In: Kaushansky K, Prchal J, Burns L, Lichtman M, Levi M, Linch D, eds. *Williams Hematology.* 10th. New York: McGraw-Hill; 2021:e1–e79.
7. Bizzaro N, Antico A. Diagnosis and classification of pernicious anemia. *Autoimmun Rev.* 2014;13:565–568.
8. Brittenham GM. Disorders of iron metabolism: iron deficiency and iron overload. In: Hoffman R, Benz Jr E, Shattil S, et al., eds. *Hematology: Basic Principles and Practice.* 5th ed. Philadelphia: Churchill Livingstone; 2009:453–468.
9. Bsoul SA. Sickle cell disease. *Quintessence Int.* 2003;34:76–77.
10. Castro-Malaspina H, O'Reilly RJ. Aplastic anemia and related disorders. In: Goldman L, Ausiello D, eds. *Cecil Medicine.* 23rd ed. Philadelphia: Saunders; 2008:1241–1247.
11. Cavusoglu E. Usefulness of anemia in men as an independent predictor of two-year cardiovascular outcome in patients presenting with acute coronary syndrome. *Am J Cardiol.* 2006;98:580–584.
12. Centers for Disease Control and Prevention. Recommendation to prevent and control iron deficiency in the United States. *MMWR Recomm Rep.* 1998;47:1–29.
13. Davies SC, Gilmore A. The role of hydroxyurea in the management of sickle cell disease. *Blood Rev.* 2003;17:99–109.
14. Chekroun M, Chérifi H, Fournier B, et al. Oral manifestations of sickle cell disease. *Br Dent J.* 2019;226:27–31.
15. DeRossi SS, Garfunkel A, Greenberg MS. Hematologic diseases. In: Lynch MA, ed. *Burket's Oral Medicine: Diagnosis and Treatment.* 10th ed. Hamilton, Ontario: BCDecker; 2003.
16. Derossi SS, Raghavendra S. *Anemia. Oral Surg Oral Med Oral Pathol Oral Radiol Endod.* 2003;95:131–141.
17. Desai B, Sollecito TP. Hematological disease. In: Patton LL, Glick M, eds. *The ADA Practical Guide to Patients with Medical Conditions.* 2nd ed. Hoboken: John Wiley and Sons, Inc.; 2015:153–182.
18. Elghetany MT, Banki K. Erythrocytic disorders. In: McPherson RA, Pincus MR, eds. *Henry's Clinical Diagnosis and Management by Laboratory Methods.* 21st ed. Philadelphia: Saunders; 2007.
19. Frith-Terhune AL. Iron deficiency anemia: higher prevalence in Mexican American than in non-Hispanic white females in the Third National Health and Nutrition Examination Survey, 1988-1994. *Am J Clin Nutr.* 2000;72:963–968.
20. Forbes CD, Jackson WF. *Color Atlas and Text of Clinical Medicine.* 3rd ed. St. Louis: Mosby; 2003.

21. Gallagher PG, Jarolim P. Red blood cell membrane disorders. In: Hoffman R, Benz Jr E, Shattil S, et al., eds. *Hematology: Basic Principles and Practice*. 5th ed. Philadelphia: Churchill Livingstone; 2009:623–643.

22. Giardia PJ, Forget BG. Thalassemia syndromes. In: Hoffman R, Benz Jr E, Shattil S, et al., eds. *Hematology: Basic Principles and Practice*. 5th ed. Philadelphia: Churchill Livingstone; 2009:535–564.

23. Ginder GD. Microcytic and hypochromic anemias. In: Goldman L, Ausiello D, eds. *Cecil Medicine*. 23rd ed. Philadelphia: Saunders; 2008:1187–1193.

24. Golan DE. Hemolytic anemias: red cell membrane and metabolic defects. In: Goldman L, Ausiello D, eds. *Cecil Medicine*. 23rd ed. Philadelphia: Saunders; 2008:1203–1211.

25. Gregg XT, Prchal JT. Red blood cell enzymopathies. In: Hoffman R, Benz Jr E, Shattil S, et al., eds. *Hematology: Basic Principles and Practice*. 5th ed. Philadelphia: Churchill Livingstone; 2009:611–622.

26. Helmi N, Bashir M, Shireen A, et al. Thalassemia review: features, dental considerations and management. *Electron Physician*. 2017;9:4003–4008.

27. Hsu LL, Fan-Hsu J. Evidence-based dental management in the new era of sickle cell disease: a scoping review. *J Am Dent Assoc*. 2020;151:668–677.e9.

28. Huber MA, Sankar V. Hematologic diseases. In: Glick M, ed. *Burket's Oral Medicine*. 12th ed. Shelton: PMPH; 2015:435–462.

29. Javed F, Correa FO, Nooh N, et al. Orofacial manifestations in patients with sickle cell disease. *Am J Med Sci*. 2013;3 45:234–237.

30. Johnson-Wimbley TD, Graham DY. Diagnosis and management of iron deficiency anemia in the 21st century. *Therap Adv Gastroenterol*. 2011;4:177–184.

31. Le CH. The prevalence of anemia and moderate-severe anemia in the US population (NHANES 2003-2012). *PLoS One*. 2016;11:e0166635.

32. Lockhart PB. *Dental Care of the Medically Complex Patient*. 5th ed. St. Louis: Wright Elsevier; 2004.

33. Marks PW, Gladere B. Approach to anemia in the adult and child. In: Hoffman R, Benz Jr E, Shattil S, et al., eds. *Hematology: Basic Principles and Practice*. 5th ed. Philadelphia: Churchill Livingstone; 2009:439–446.

34. McCord C, Johnson L. Oral manifestations of hematologic disease. *Atlas Oral Maxillofac Surg Clin North Am*. 2017;(2):149–162.

35. Miano M, Dufour C. The diagnosis and treatment of aplastic anemia: a review. *Int J Hematol*. 2015;101:527–535.

36. Micromedex. *Drug Information for the Health Care Professional*. Taunton, Mass: Thomson Micromedex; 2006.

37. Muncie Jr HL, Campbell J. Alpha and beta thalassemia. *Am Fam Physician*. 2009;80:339–344.

38. Neville BW, Damm DD, Allen CM, Chi AC. Hematologic disorders. In: Neville BW, Damm DD, Allen CM, Chi AC, eds. *Oral and Maxillofacial Pathology*. 4th ed. St. Louis: Elsevier; 2016:533–571.

39. Neville BW, Damm DD, Allen CM, Bouquot J. *Hematologic Disorders. Oral and Maxillofacial Pathology*. 3rd ed. St. Louis: WB Saunders; 2009:571–612.

40. Shafer WG, Hine MK, Levy BM. *A Textbook of Oral Pathology*. 4th ed. Philadelphia: WB Saunders; 1983.

41. Pecker LH, Lanzkron S. Sickle cell disease. *Ann Intern Med*. 2021;174:ITC1–ITC16.

42. Penninx BW. Anemia in old age is associated with increased mortality and hospitalization. *J Gerontol A Biol Sci Med Sci*. 2006;61(5):474–479.

43. Peslak SA, Olson T, Babushok DV. Diagnosis and treatment of aplastic anemia. *Curr Treat Options Oncol*. 2017;18:70.

44. Ruwende C, Hill A. Glucose-6 phosphate dehydrogenase deficiency and malaria. *J Mol Med*. 1998;76:581–588.

45. Sansevere JJ, Milles M. Management of the oral and maxillofacial surgery patient with sickle cell disease and related hemoglobinopathies. *J Oral Maxillofac Surg*. 1993;51:912–916.

46. Saunthararajah Y, Vichinsky EP. Sickle cell disease. Clinical features and management. In: Hoffman R, Benz Jr E, Shattil S, et al., eds. *Hematology: Basic Principles and Practice*. 5th ed. Philadelphia: Churchill Livingstone; 2009:577–602.

47. Silver BJ. Anemia. In: Carey WD, ed. *Current Clinical Medicine 2009*. Cleveland Clinic. Philadelphia: Saunders; 2009:615–620.

48. Singh A, Varma S. β-Thalassaemia intermedia masquerading as β-thalassaemia major. *BMJ Case Rep*. 2014;2014. bcr2014207637.

49. Smith HB, McDonald DK, Miller RI. Dental management of patients with sickle cell disorders. *J Am Dent Assoc*. 1987;114:85–87.

50. Stanley AC, Christian JM. Sickle cell disease and perioperative considerations: review and retrospective report. *J Oral Maxillofac Surg*. 2013;71:1027–1033.

51. Steinberg MH. Sickle cell disease and associated hemoglobinopathies. In: Goldman L, Ausiello D, eds. *Cecil Medicine*. 23rd ed. Philadelphia: Saunders; 2008:1217–1225.

52. Suresh L, Radfar L. Pregnancy and lactation. *Oral Surg Oral Med Oral Pathol Oral Radiol Endod*. 2004;97:672–682.

53. Swaak A. Anemia of chronic disease in patients with rheumatoid arthritis: aspects of prevalence, outcome, diagnosis, and the effect of treatment on disease activity. *J Rheumatol*. 2006;33:1467–1468.

54. Taher AT, Musallam KM, Cappellini MD. β-Thalassemias. *N Engl J Med*. 2021;384:727–743.

55. Tewari S, Tewari S, Sharma RK, Abrol P, Sen R, et al. Necrotizing stomatitis: a possible periodontal manifestation of deferiprone-induced agranulocytosis. *Oral Surg Oral Med Oral Pathol Oral Radiol Endod*. 2009;108(4):e13–e19.

56. Walker AM. Anemia as a predictor of cardiovascular events in patients with elevated serum creatinine. *J Am Soc Nephrol*. 2006;17:2293–2298.

57. Wilson A. Prevalence and outcomes of anemia in rheumatoid arthritis: a systematic review of the literature. *Am J Med*. 2004;(7A):50S–57S.

58. Young NS. Bone marrow failure syndromes including aplastic anemia and myelodysplasia. In: Loscalzo J, Fauci A, Kasper D, Hauser S, Longo D, Jameson J, eds. *Harrison's Principles of Internal Medicine*. 21st ed. New York: McGraw-Hill; 2022:e1–e22.

59. Young NS, Maciejewski JP. Aplastic anemia. In: Hoffman R, Benz Jr E, Shattil S, et al., eds. *Hematology: Basic Principles and Practice*. 5th ed. Philadelphia: Churchill Livingstone; 2009:359–384.

60. Zuckerman KS. Approach to the anemias. In: Goldman L, Ausiello D, eds. *Cecil Medicine*. 23rd ed. Philadelphia: Saunders; 2008:1179–1188.

23

Disorders of White Blood Cells

KEY POINTS

- Disorders of white blood cells (WBCs) in dental patients can substantially influence clinical decision-making and delivery of care.
- Defects in WBCs can manifest as delayed healing, infection, mucosal ulceration, nodal and extranodal enlargement, and in some cases, may be fatal.
- Dentists should be able to identify possible WBC abnormalities through history, clinical examination, and screening laboratory tests and provide prompt referral to a physician for further evaluation and management before invasive dental procedures are performed.
- Patients with life-threatening WBC disorders under medical care should not receive dental care until after consultation with the patient's medical provider(s).

WBCs constitute the primary defense against microbial infections and are critical for mounting an immune response. Three groups of WBCs are found in the peripheral circulation: granulocytes, lymphocytes, and monocytes. Of the granulocyte population, 90% is composed of neutrophils; the remainder consists of eosinophils and basophils. Circulating lymphocytes are of three types: T lymphocytes (thymus mediated), B lymphocytes (bursa derived), and natural killer (NK) cells. Lymphocytes are subdivided by the surface markers they exhibit and by the cytokines they produce.

The primary function of neutrophils is to defend the body against certain infectious agents (primarily bacteria) through phagocytosis and enzymatic destruction. Eosinophils and basophils are involved in inflammatory allergic reactions and mediate these reactions through release of their cytoplasmic granules. Eosinophils also combat infection by parasites. T lymphocytes (T cells) are involved with the delayed, or cellular, immune reaction. In contrast, B lymphocytes (B cells) play an important role in the immediate, or humoral, immune system involving the production of plasma cells and immunoglobulins (IgA, IgD, IgE, IgG, and IgM). Monocytes have diverse functions that include phagocytosis; intracellular killing (especially of mycobacteria, fungi, and protozoa); and mediating the immune and inflammatory response through the production of biologically active substances, such as cytokines and growth factors, that increase the activity of lymphocytes. In addition, monocytes serve as antigen-presenting cells and migrate into tissues. In tissue, these antigen-presenting cells are known as dendritic cells (in lymph nodes) or Langerhans cells (in skin and mucosa). Monocytes in tissue that phagocytose microbes are known as macrophages.

Most WBCs are produced primarily in the bone marrow (granulocytes and monocytes), and these cells form several "pools" in the marrow: (1) the mitotic pool, which consists of immature precursor cells; (2) a maturing pool, which consists of cells undergoing maturation; and (3) a storage pool of functional cells, which can be released as needed.

WBCs released from the bone marrow that circulate in the peripheral blood account for only 5% of the total WBC mass and form two pools of cells: (1) marginal and (2) circulating. Cells in the marginal pool adhere to vessel walls and are readily available. When infection threatens the body, the storage and marginal pools can be recruited to help fight the invading organisms.

Growth-promoting substances called colony-stimulating factors (CSFs) are responsible for the growth of committed granulocyte–monocyte stem cells. The major function of CSFs is to amplify leukopoiesis rather than recruit new stem cells into the granulocyte–monocyte differentiation pathway. Thus, through the local release of CSFs, the bone marrow can increase the production of granulocytes and monocytes. This process occurs in response to infection.

Lymphocytes localize primarily in three regions: lymph nodes, the spleen, and the mucosa-associated lymphoid tissue (MALT) lining the respiratory and gastrointestinal tracts. At these sites, microbial antigens are trapped and presented to B or T lymphocytes (cells). Antigens bind B cells through cell surface immunoglobulins, whereupon B cells are activated, proliferate, and produce large amounts of immunoglobulin to aid in opsonization. Antigens are presented to CD4+ (helper) T cells by major histocompatibility complex (MHC) class I molecules and to CD8+ T cells by MHC class II molecules. CD4+ T cells activate B cells and macrophages by producing cytokines and through direct contact. CD8+ T cells kill virus-infected cells. NK cells also kill virus-infected cells and tumor cells.

LEUKOCYTOSIS AND LEUKOPENIA

The number of circulating WBCs normally ranges from 4500 to 11,000/μL in adults. The differential WBC count is an estimation of the percentage of each cell type per microliter of blood. A normal differential count consists of 50%–70% neutrophils, 20%–40% lymphocytes, 2%–8% monocytes, 1%–4% eosinophils, and less than 1% basophils. The term *leukocytosis* is defined as an increase in the number of circulating WBCs (lymphocytes or granulocytes) to greater than 11,000/μL, and *leukopenia* as a reduction in the number of circulating WBCs (<4500/μL).

Exercise, pregnancy, and emotional stress can lead to increased numbers of WBCs in the peripheral circulation resulting in physiologic leukocytosis. Pathologic leukocytosis can be caused by infection, neoplasia, or necrosis. Pyogenic infections induce a type of leukocytosis that is characterized by an increased number of neutrophils. A "shift to the left" results from excessive numbers of immature neutrophils (bands or stab cells) released into the circulation in response to a bacterial infection. Tuberculosis, syphilis, and viral infections produce a type of leukocytosis that is characterized by increased numbers of lymphocytes. Protozoal infections often produce a type of leukocytosis that increases the numbers of monocytes. Allergies and parasitic infections caused by certain helminths increase the numbers of circulating eosinophils. Cellular necrosis increases the numbers of circulating neutrophils. Leukemia (cancer of the WBCs) is characterized by a substantial increase in the numbers of circulating immature leukocytes. Carcinoma of glandular tissues may cause an increase in the number of circulating neutrophils. Acute bleeding also can result in leukocytosis.

Leukopenia may occur in the early phases of leukemia and lymphoma as a result of bone marrow replacement through excessive proliferation of WBCs. Leukopenia also occurs during agranulocytosis (reduction of granulocytes) and pancytopenia (decreased WBCs and red blood cells [RBCs]) that result from toxic effects of drugs and chemicals. Leukopenia is a common complication of drugs and chemicals (e.g., cancer chemotherapy).

Cyclic Neutropenia

An important form of leukopenia involving the cyclic depression of circulating neutrophils is a disorder called cyclic neutropenia. It is associated with mutations at locus 19q13 of the neutrophil elastase gene (*ELANE*). The estimated frequency of cyclic neutropenia is about 1 in 1 million. In this condition, patients have a periodic decrease (at least a 40% drop) in the number of neutrophils (about every 21–28 days). During the period in which few circulating neutrophils are present, the patient is susceptible to infection and oral manifestations (see Oral Manifestations). Up to 10% of patients die from pneumonia, cellulitis, or peritonitis.

Patients with leukocytosis or leukopenia may have bone marrow abnormalities that can cause thrombocytopenia. Examination of the patient's bone marrow aspirate is important for making the final diagnosis. Infectious diseases that can cause leukocytosis and leukopenia are discussed in Chapters 7, 13, and 18.

Leukemia and Lymphoma

The remainder of this chapter focuses on leukemia and malignancies of lymphoid cells (lymphoma and multiple myeloma [MM]; Box 23.1). These conditions are associated with high morbidity and mortality if not properly identified and patients do not receive appropriate medical care. In addition, patients are usually immunosuppressed as a result of the disease itself or because of the treatment used to manage it. Hence, they are prone to develop serious infection and often bleed easily because of thrombocytopenia.

About every 3 min, a person in the United States is diagnosed with a blood cancer. Approximately 186,400 people in the United States are diagnosed with leukemia, lymphoma, or myeloma annually. New cases of leukemia, lymphoma, and myeloma account for 9.8% of the estimated 1,898,160 new cases diagnosed in the United States annually. An estimated 1,519,907 people in the United States are either living with or are in remission from leukemia, lymphoma, or myeloma. These diseases were expected to account for 9.5% of the deaths (608,570) from cancer annually. A dental practice that manages 2000 patients is predicted to have one to three patients who have or develop leukemia or a malignancy of lymphoid cells.

Leukemia

Leukemia is cancer of the WBCs that affects the bone marrow and circulating blood. It involves exponential proliferation of a clonal myeloid or lymphoid cell and occurs in both acute and chronic forms. Acute leukemia is a rapidly progressive disease that results from accumulation of immature, nonfunctional WBCs in the marrow and blood. Chronic leukemias have a slower onset, which allows production of larger numbers of more mature (terminally differentiated), functional cells. This section focuses on four types of leukemia: (1) acute myelogenous (myeloid) leukemia (AML), (2) acute lymphoblastic leukemia (ALL), (3) chronic myelogenous (myeloid) leukemia (CML), and (4) chronic lymphocytic leukemia (CLL).

The cause of leukemia remains unknown. Increased risk is associated with large doses of ionizing radiation, certain chemicals (benzene), and infection with specific viruses (e.g., Epstein–Barr virus [EBV], human lymphotropic virus [HTLV]-1). Cigarette smoking and exposure to electromagnetic fields also have been proposed to be causative.

Annually, 61,090 people are expected to be diagnosed with leukemia. There are an estimated 397,501 people living with or in remission from leukemia in the United States. The overall 5-year relative survival rate for leukemia has more than quadrupled since 1960. From 2010

BOX 23.1 World Health Organization of Hematologic Malignancies (Abridged Version).

MYELOID NEOPLASMS

Subtype	Putative cell of origin
Acute myeloid leukemia (AML)	Early myeloid progenitor
AML with recurrent genetic aberrations	
AML without recurrent genetic aberrations	
AML following cytotoxic therapy	
Myeloproliferative neoplasms	Hematopoietic stem cell or early myeloid progenitor
Chronic myeloid leukemia	
Polycythemia vera	
Essential thrombocytopenia	
Chronic eosinophilic leukemia	
Primary myelofibrosis	
Myelodysplastic syndromes	Early myeloid progenitor

LYMPHOID NEOPLASMS

Immature B-cell and T-cell tumors	Early B-cell progenitor
B-cell acute lymphoblastic leukemia/lymphoma	Early T-cell progenitor
T-cell acute lymphoblastic leukemia/lymphoma	
Mature B-cell tumors	Postgerminal center B cell
aChronic lymphocytic leukemia/small lymphocytic lymphoma	Naïve B cell
	Germinal center B cell
Mantle cell lymphoma	Germinal center B cell
aFollicular lymphoma	Germinal center or postgerminal center B cell
Burkitt lymphoma	
aDiffuse large B-cell lymphoma	
Plasma cell tumors and related entities	Postgerminal center B cell
Multiple myeloma	Mature B ell
Lymphoplasmacytic lymphoma	
Mature T-cell and natural killer cell tumors	Mature T-cell or natural killer cell
Hodgkin lymphoma	Germinal center or postgerminal center B cell

aMost common types of non-Hodgkin lymphoma (86 subtypes).
Adapted from Aster JC, Fleming M. Introduction to hematologic malignancies. In: Aster JC, Bunn HF, eds. *Pathophysiology of Blood Disorders*. 2nd edn. New York: McGraw Hill Education; 2017:1–12.

to 2016, the 5-year relative survival rates were (1) AML—29.8%, (2) ALL—72.1%, (3) CML—71.7%, and (4) CLL—88.6%. From 2013 to 2017, leukemia was the sixth most common cause of cancer deaths in men and the seventh most common in women in the United States. A comparison of acute and chronic leukemia is presented in Table 23.1.

ACUTE MYELOGENOUS (MYELOID) LEUKEMIA

AML is a neoplasm of myeloid (immature) WBCs, which demonstrate uncontrolled proliferation in the bone marrow and subsequently appear in the peripheral blood.

EPIDEMIOLOGY

AML occurs in about 20,240 persons in the United States annually and accounts for 33.0% of all leukemias. AML

TABLE 23.1 Comparison of Acute and Chronic Leukemias

Parameter	Acute	Chronic
Clinical onset	Sudden	Insidious
Course (untreated)	<6 months	2–6 years
Leukemic cells	Immature	Mature
Anemia	Mild to severe	Mild
Thrombocytopenia	Mild to severe	Mild
White blood cell count	Variable	Increased
Organomegaly	Mild	Prominent
Age	Adults and children	Adults

Data from Harming DM. *Clinical Hematology and Fundamentals of Hemostasis*. Philadelphia: FA Davis; 2009.

is the most common acute leukemia in adult patients. The incidence increases with age and rises rapidly after the age of 60 years, reaching 28 per 100,000 by age 80 years. The median age of persons at time of AML diagnosis is 68 years.

ETIOLOGY

AML arises de novo or secondarily as a consequence of myelodysplastic syndromes or other myeloproliferative neoplasms. These are a diverse group of clonal disorders of hematopoietic stem or progenitor cells resulting in abnormal cellular differentiation that places an individual at high risk for AML. Environmental factors such as tobacco smoke, benzene-containing products, chemotherapies for cancer, and radiation exposure are risk factors for AML. Genetic factors (e.g., familial mutations of *CEBPA, DDX41, RUNX1*) may cause cytogenetic abnormalities that affect transcriptional cascades of myeloid precursor cells leading to uncontrolled proliferation of these cells. The most frequently identified gene mutation in AML is FMS-like tyrosine kinase 3 (*FLT3*). Certain genetic disorders, including Trisomy 21, Klinefelter syndrome, Fanconi anemia, and von Recklinghausen disease, increase the risk for AML.

PATHOPHYSIOLOGY AND COMPLICATIONS

AML has a sudden onset and leads to death on average in 1–3 months if left untreated. It involves increased numbers of immature myeloid WBCs in the bone marrow space and peripheral circulation (Fig. 23.1). As a result, patients are susceptible to excessive bleeding, anemia, poor healing, and infection. Hemorrhage and infection, also frequent complications of chemotherapy, are the chief causes of death. The overall survival rate for AML patients is only 30%. The prognosis of AML in adults who are 60 years or older is poorer with only 25% −40% of these individuals expected to survive 3 years or more.

CLINICAL PRESENTATION

AML produces a leukemic infiltration of marrow and organs that causes cytopenia and diverse nonspecific signs and symptoms, including fatigue, easy bruising, and bone pain. Many patients complain of flu-like symptoms for 4–6 weeks before the diagnosis. Anemia and thrombocytopenia usually manifest as malaise, pallor, dyspnea on exertion, and bleeding and small hemorrhage (petechiae, ecchymoses) in the skin and mucous membranes (Fig. 23.2A). At least one-third of patients have recurrent infections (nonhealing wounds), oral ulcerations, and fever due to granulocytopenia. Enlargement of the tonsils, lymph nodes, spleen, and gingiva (Fig. 23.2B) occurs as a result of leukemic infiltration of these tissues. Infiltration of the CNS occurs in about 35% of the cases of AML with increased eosinophils. Most of these patients are asymptomatic, but some present with meningeal signs and symptoms associated with increased intracranial pressure. Skin lesions, consisting of

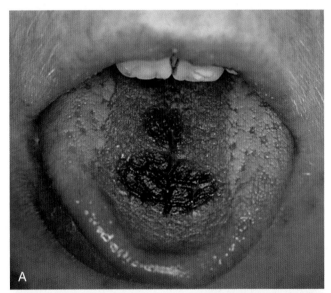

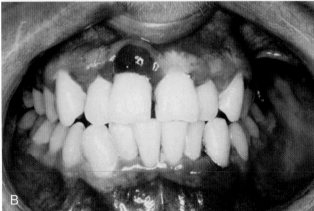

FIG. 23.2 **(A)** Acute myeloid leukemia presenting as bleeding and ecchymosis of the tongue in a 14-year-old patient. **(B)** Gingival leukemia infiltrate in a patient with acute myeloid leukemia.

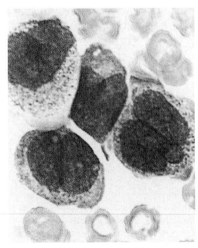

FIG. 23.1 Acute myeloid leukemia. Peripheral blood smear shows many myeloid cells with large nuclei and azurophilic granules. (From Hoffbrand AV, Pettit JE. *Color Atlas of Clinical Hematology.* 4th ed. London: Mosby; 2010. Courtesy of Prof. J.M. Chessells.)

collections of leukemic cells termed leukemia cutis, granulocytic sarcomas (also known as myeloid sarcomas, chloromas) may occur.

Laboratory and Diagnostic Findings

The diagnosis of leukemia is made through examination of peripheral blood and bone marrow stained with Wright-Giemsa. Cytochemical staining, immunophenotyping, and cytogenetic analyses are used to characterize the type and subtype, to allow for specific treatment approaches, and to detect residual disease after therapy is provided. Granulocytopenia and thrombocytopenia are common.

The diagnosis of AML is made when myeloblasts are found in the bone marrow or peripheral blood at a rate of at least 20%. In addition, immunophenotyping by flow cytometry is used to confirm the myeloid origin of malignant blast populations. Cytogenetic analysis allows for recognition of AML subgroups defined by the presence of specific recurrent genetic abnormalities, including balanced translocations, gene fusions, or single molecular mutations. AML is classified using the World Health Organization (WHO) classification system based on a combination of cytogenetic and molecular abnormalities, clinical features, and light microscope morphology (Table 23.2).

ACUTE LYMPHOBLASTIC LEUKEMIA

ALL (also known as acute lymphocytic leukemia or acute lymphoid leukemia) is the result of uncontrolled monoclonal proliferation of immature lymphoid cells in the bone marrow and peripheral blood. These neoplastic cells may also expand in the lymph nodes, liver, spleen, or CNS.

EPIDEMIOLOGY

Approximately 5690 cases of ALL occur in the United States annually. ALL occurs at an incidence of 1.7 in 100,000 and typically occurs in children. It accounts for 75% of leukemias in children and approximately 20% of all childhood cancers. Peak incidence occurs in children ages 1–4 years and is the most common cancer in children and adolescents <20 years. Boys are affected slightly more often than girls. About 20% of cases occur after age 55 years.

ETIOLOGY

Although environmental, infectious, and genetic factors are considered likely causes of the disease, definitive etiology for ALL has not been established. Congenital syndromes predisposing to ALL include Fanconi anemia and Bloom syndrome. The disease is 18- to 20-fold more common in patients with Down syndrome (Trisomy 21). Inherited gene variants

TABLE 23.2	World Health Organization Classification of Acute Myeloid Leukemia and Related Neoplasms

Acute Myeloid Leukemia (AML) With Recurrent Genetic Abnormalities

AML with t(8;21)(q22;q22); RUNX1-RUNX1T1
AML with inv(16)(p13.1q22) or t(16;16)(p13.1;q22); *CBFB-MYH11*

Acute Promyelocytic Leukemia With *PML-RARA*

AML with t(9;11)(p21.3;q23.3); *MLLT3-KMT2A*
AML with t(6;9)(p23;q34.1); *DEK-NUP214*
AML with inv(3)(q21.3q26.2) or t(3;3)(q21.3;q26.2); *GATA2, MECOM*
AML (megakaryoblastic) with t(1;22)(p13.3;q13.3); *RBM15-MKL1* provisional entity: AML with BCR-ABL1
AML with mutated *NPM1*
AML with biallelic mutations of *CEBPA* provisional entity: AML with mutated RUNX1

AML With Myelodysplasia-Related Changes

Therapy-related myeloid neoplasms

AML, Not Otherwise Specified (NOS)

AML with minimal differentiation AML without maturation
AML with maturation
Acute myelomonocytic leukemia
Acute monoblastic/monocytic leukemia pure erythroid leukemia
Acute megakaryoblastic leukemia acute basophilic leukemia
Acute panmyelosis with myelofibrosis

Myeloid Sarcoma
Myeloid Proliferations Related to Down Syndrome

Transient abnormal myelopoiesis (TAMs)
Myeloid leukemia associated with Down syndrome

Note: Marrow blast count of ≥20% is required, except for AML with the recurrent genetic abnormalities t(15;17), t(8;21), inv(16), or t(16;16).
Adapted from: Blum W, Bloomfield CD. Acute myeloid leukemia. In: Jameson J, et al., eds. *Harrison's Principles of Internal Medicine,* 20e. New York: McGraw Hill; 2018:1–21.

associated with ALL include *ARID5B*, *IKZF1*, *CEBPE*, *CDKN2A/2B*, and *PIP4K2A*. Cytogenetic studies display the Philadelphia chromosome [t(9;22)], *BCR-ABL1*, in 5% of children and 25% of adults with the condition. Patients with the Philadelphia chromosome have slightly lower complete remission rates and greatly reduced remission durations.

PATHOPHYSIOLOGY AND COMPLICATIONS

Similar to AML, ALL results in suppression of normal hematopoiesis, leaving patients susceptible to excessive bleeding, anemia, poor healing, and infection. Treatment of children results in remission rates that exceed 90% and cure rates above 70%. In adults, long-term survival from ALL occurs at rates of about 70%.

CLINICAL PRESENTATION

The clinical presentation of ALL can be acute or insidious. Presenting signs and symptoms relate to anemia, thrombocytopenia, fever, neutropenia, as well as bone and joint pain that can affect walking. Patients can present with infection or fever, hemorrhagic episodes, and enlargement of the liver, spleen, and lymph nodes. A higher propensity toward CNS disease occurs with ALL compared with AML; thus patients may present with cranial nerve deficiencies.

Laboratory and Diagnostic Findings

Diagnosis of ALL integrates the characteristics of cell morphology, immunophenotypes, genetics, and cytogenetics. Massive replacement of the bone marrow space with leukemic blast cells is observed in ALL (Fig. 23.3). A correspondingly high number of lymphoblasts are detected in the peripheral blood smear, and levels of hemoglobin, hematocrit, and platelets are depressed, reflecting replacement of marrow by lymphoblasts. Flow cytometry and immunophenotyping is the preferred method of lineage assignment and assessment of cell maturation. T-lineage lymphoblasts are positive for cytoplasmic or surface *CD3* and negative for myeloperoxidase and B-cell antigens. B-lineage lymphoblasts are often positive for B-cell markers, such as *CD19*, cytoplasmic *CD22*, and cytoplasmic *CD79a*; negative for *CD3* and myeloperoxidase. The WHO classifies ALL based on the immunophenotype of the leukemia cell and is the most commonly used classification system in medicine for this disorder (Table 23.3).

MEDICAL MANAGEMENT OF ACUTE LEUKEMIA

The ability to cure a patient of acute leukemia is related to inducing complete remission of the disease and prolonging survival. Complete remission (CR) is defined as a normal peripheral blood count (absolute neutrophil count $>1000/mm^3$ and platelet count $>100,000/mm^3$) and normocellular marrow with $<5\%$ blasts in the marrow and no signs or symptoms of the disease. In addition, no signs or symptoms are evident of CNS leukemia or other extramedullary infiltration.

Treatment of the newly diagnosed patient AML is usually divided into two phases, induction and consolidation (postremission). The purpose of the induction phase is to induce a state of CR by killing tumor cells with cytotoxic agents (chemotherapy). The consolidation (postremission) phase is designed to eradicate residual (typically undetectable) leukemic cells to prevent relapse and prolong survival. Therapies for both phases are chosen based on the patient's age, overall fitness, and cytogenetic/molecular risk. Common classes of drugs commonly used to treat acute leukemia are shown in Table 23.4.

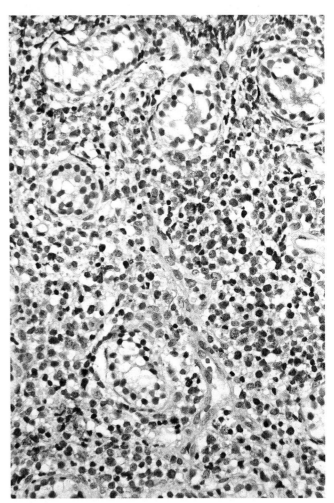

FIG. 23.3 Peripheral blood smear of acute lymphoblastic leukemia. (From Hoffbrand AV, Pettit JE. *Color Atlas of Clinical Hematology.* 4th ed. London: Mosby; 2010.)

TABLE 23.3	World Health Organization Classification of Acute Lymphoblastic Leukemia
Type of Lymphoblast	**WHO Subtype**
Precursor B cell	B lymphoblastic leukemia/lymphoma, not otherwise specified, NOS
Precursor B cell	B lymphoblastic leukemia/lymphoma with recurrent cytogenetic abnormalities [e.g., t(9;22)]
Precursor T cell	T lymphoblastic leukemia/lymphoma

Adapted from Canadian Cancer Society. https://cancer.ca/en/. Accessed November 29, 2021.

The most commonly used induction regimens for AML consist of combination chemotherapy with cytarabine and an anthracycline (e.g., daunorubicin, idarubicin). Cytarabine used at standard dose is administered

TABLE 23.4 Classes of Drugs Commonly Used to Treat Leukemia

Drug Class	Chemotherapeutic Agent(s)	Mechanism of Action
Alkylating agents	Cyclophosphamide	Produce alkyl radicals, causing cross-linking of DNA and inhibition of DNA synthesis in rapidly replicating tumor cells
Anthracyclines	Daunorubicin, idarubicin	Disrupt cellular functions, such as RNA synthesis, or inhibit mitosis
Antimetabolites	Antifolates: methotrexate	Disrupt enzymatic processes or nucleic acid synthesis
	Purine analogues: fludarabine, 6-mercaptopurine	
	Pyrimidine analogues: cytarabine	
Antineoplastics	Arsenic trioxide	Inorganic compound affecting intracellular signal transduction inducing apoptosis
	Venetoclax	Selective inhibitor of the B-cell lymphoma 2 (*BCL2*), leading to programmed cell death
Biologics	Rituximab	Monoclonal antibody to *CD*20
	Ofatumumab	Monoclonal antibody to *CD*20
	Obinutuzumab	Monoclonal antibody to *CD*20
	All-*trans* retinoic acid (ATRA; tretinoin)	Binds antigen target on malignant lymphocyte
		Induces differentiation and apoptosis of malignant promyelocytes in APML
Chimeric antigen receptor T-cell (CAR T-cell)	Tisagenlecleucel	Autologous T-cells modified to produce chimeric antigen receptors (CARs) that target tumor antigens (e.g., *CD19*)
Corticosteroids	Prednisone	Hormone that has antiinflammatory and antilymphocytic properties
Enzymes	Asparaginase	Inhibits synthesis of asparagines, which is required for protein synthesis in leukemic lymphoblasts
Mitotic inhibitors	Vincristine	Act as mitotic spindle inhibitors, causing metaphase arrest
Tyrosine kinase inhibitors	Imatinib	Inhibits signal transduction in cancer cells
	Ibrutinib	
	FLT3 inhibitors: Midostaurin Gilteritinib	Inhibits Fms related receptor tyrosine kinase 3 (*FLT3*) signal transduction in patients with identified mutation.

APML, Acute promyelocytic leukemia.
Adapted from: Blum W, Bloomfield CD. Acute myeloid leukemia. In: Jameson J, et al., eds. *Harrison's Principles of Internal Medicine, 20e.* New York: McGraw Hill; 2018:1–21. Hoelzer D. Acute lymphoid leukemia. In: Jameson J, et al., eds. *Harrison's Principles of Internal Medicine, 20e.* New York: McGraw Hill; 2018:1–13; Kantarjian H, Cortes J. Chronic myeloid leukemia. In: Jameson J, et al., eds. *Harrison's Principles of Internal Medicine, 20e.* New York: McGraw Hill; 2018:1–18; Hallek M, Shanafelt TD, Eichhorst B. Chronic lymphocytic leukemia. *Lancet.* 2018;391:1524–1537.

as a continuous intravenous infusion for 7 days with cytarabine, daunorubicin, or idarubicin administered on days 1, 2, and 3. With this regimen, 60%–80% of patients <65 years and 33%–60% of patients >65 years (among suitable candidates) with primary AML achieve CR. Venetoclax is a selective inhibitor of the B-cell lymphoma 2 (*BCL-2*) gene used in combination with standard induction therapy or targeted agents, such as *FLT-3* inhibitors (e.g., gilteritinib), which has led to improved clinical outcomes in AML.

Following induction therapy, consolidation with chemotherapy or allogeneic hematopoietic cell transplantation (HCT) is complex and based on age, risk, and practical considerations. While cytarabine at varying doses according to age appears to be effective, allogeneic HCT is the best relapse-prevention strategy currently available for AML. It is recommended in patients <75 years who do not have favorable-risk disease and who have a human leukocyte antigen (HLA)-matched donor (related or unrelated). The relapse risk reduction

associated with allogeneic HCT is partially offset by the increase in fatal treatment related-toxicities, such as graft-versus-host disease (GVHD). Additional information regarding allogeneic HCT and GVHD can be found in Chapters 21 and 26.

ALL treatment consists of induction, consolidation, and maintenance therapy. Induction therapy regimens include vincristine, corticosteroids, and asparaginase with the possible addition of anthracycline in high-risk patients. The majority of *BCR-ABL1*-negative ALL patients achieve CR after completion of induction therapy, whereas *BCR-ABL1*-positive ALL children benefit from receiving tyrosine kinase inhibitors [TKIs]; (e.g., imatinib or dasatinib). Consolidation therapy is started after CR is achieved, typically lasts 6–8 weeks, and includes various drug combinations, such as anthracyclines, alkylating agents, cytarabine, and methotrexate. Maintenance chemotherapy for children often consists of daily oral 6-mercaptopurine and weekly methotrexate with periodic vincristine, prednisone, and intrathecal therapy.

Allogeneic HCT may be considered for high-risk ALL patients, those with a poor initial response to therapy and adults with specific chromosomal abnormalities. Cellular immunotherapy with chimeric antigen receptor (CAR) T-cells directed against *CD19* represents the most recent advance in treating ALL and additional information regarding CAR T therapy is found in Chapter 26.

Another concern related to treatment of patients with acute leukemia is that leukemic cells can migrate to areas in the body where chemotherapeutic agents cannot reach them. These areas are called sanctuaries, and they require special treatment. The most important sanctuary in patients with ALL is the CNS. Thus, patients with ALL are treated with systemic chemotherapy plus high-dose methotrexate intravenously and cytarabine or intrathecal methotrexate and radiation to the cranium plus high-dose systemic chemotherapy. Another important sanctuary (in male patients) is the testes.

Oral Manifestations of Acute Leukemia

Patients with acute leukemia are prone to develop gingival enlargement, ulceration, and oral infection. Localized or generalized gingival enlargement is caused by inflammation and infiltration of atypical and immature WBCs (Fig. 23.2B). It occurs in up to 40% of those with acute leukemia and in about 10% of those with chronic leukemia. The gingiva is boggy and bleeds easily, and multiple tooth sites are typically affected. Generalized gingival enlargement is more common in AML and is particularly prevalent when oral hygiene is poor in patients who have AML. The combination of poor oral hygiene and gingival enlargement contributes to gingival bleeding and fetor oris. Gingival bleeding is exacerbated by the presence of thrombocytopenia. Plaque control measures, chlorhexidine, and chemotherapy promote resolution of the condition.

A localized mass of leukemic cells is specifically known as a granulocytic sarcoma (also known as myeloid sarcoma or chloroma*). These extramedullary tumors have been observed in the hard tissues (maxilla, palate) and soft tissues (gingiva, tongue, oral mucosa) of the maxillofacial complex.

CHRONIC MYELOGENOUS (MYELOID) LEUKEMIA

CML is a neoplasm of mature myeloid WBCs.

EPIDEMIOLOGY

CML has an incidence of 1.5 cases per 100,000 with a slight male predilection and 9110 cases in the United States annually. It accounts for 15%–20% of all leukemias and is less common than CLL in the United States. The median age of diagnosis is 55–65 years, and the incidence increases with age. CML causes 3% of childhood leukemias.

ETIOLOGY

The etiology of CML is unknown, but radiation exposure increases risk for the disease. The genetic defect consists of a balanced reciprocal translocation between the long arms of chromosomes 9 and 22, generating a hybrid oncogene, *BCR-ABL1*, and is evident in more than 90% of cases of CML. This oncogene is also present in ALL. This fusion gene directs for increased tyrosine kinase activity and myeloid proliferation.

PATHOPHYSIOLOGY AND COMPLICATIONS

CML progresses through a chronic (indolent) phase, an accelerated phase, followed by blast crisis. More than 90% of patients, when first diagnosed, are in the chronic phase of the disease. During the chronic phase of CML (average 3–5 years), leukemic cells are functional; thus, infection is not a major problem. In the accelerated phase, the number of immature blast cells rise, new chromosomal changes may occur and clinical signs / symptoms of disease emerge. After transformation to the blast stage, the leukemic cells are immature and nonfunctional. As a result, anemia, thrombocytopenia, and infection typically develop. About 25% of patients with CML per year exhibit progression to the blast phase of the disease 6–12 months after diagnosis. The blast phase is characterized by 30% or more leukemic blast cells in the peripheral blood or marrow. Patients treated in the chronic phase with TKIs (e.g., imatinib) obtain complete remission, and about 70% of the patients remain in remission after 5 years. Allogeneic transplantation is used as secondary treatment for those patients who progress through or are intolerant to multiple TKIs. Patients treated in the accelerated or blast phase of the disease have a much poorer prognosis, with cure rates of <15%.

CLINICAL PRESENTATION

In nearly 90% of patients, CML is diagnosed during the chronic phase. 50%–60% of patients are asymptomatic, and the diagnosis is based on their complete blood count (CBC). Common symptoms are fatigue, weakness, abdominal (upper left quadrant) pain, abdominal fullness, weight loss, night sweats caused by anemia, an enlarged and painful spleen (splenomegaly), and altered hematopoiesis. Hyperviscosity of the blood increases risk of stroke.

Laboratory and Diagnostic Findings

Patients are identified by marked elevation of their WBC count during routine examination (Fig. 23.4). WBC count usually is above 50,000/μL at the time of diagnosis, and basophilia and eosinophilia are present. Cytogenetic analysis reveals *BCR-ABL1* in more than 90% of cases.

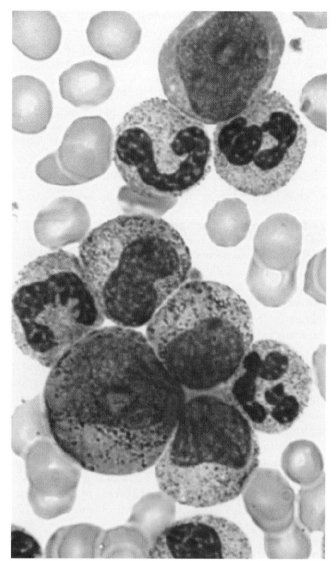

FIG. 23.4 Chronic myeloid leukemia. Peripheral blood smear shows myeloblasts, promyelocytes, and segmented neutrophils. (From Hoffbrand AV, Pettit JE. *Color Atlas of Clinical Hematology*. 3rd ed. London: Mosby; 2000.)

Serum chemistry reveals elevated levels of lactate dehydrogenase (LDH) and low levels of leukocyte alkaline phosphatase. The bone marrow is markedly hypercellular.

MEDICAL MANAGEMENT

Patients with CML were historically treated during the chronic phase with hydroxyurea or busulfan; this approach resulted in good symptom and blood count control along with significant toxicity. Imatinib, an inhibitor of tyrosine kinase, is widely used today as first-line treatment for CML. Second-generation TKIs, dasatinib, nilotinib, and bosutinib, have demonstrated faster responses, but no improvement in overall survival. Allogeneic HCT is associated with long-term survival

rates of 40%−60% when treatment is provided before the blastic phase. CML patients are monitored regularly by quantitative PCR measurement in the peripheral blood for *BCR-ABL1* transcripts.

Oral Manifestations

Chronic forms of leukemia are less likely to demonstrate oral manifestations compared with acute forms of leukemia. Generalized lymphadenopathy, pallor of the oral mucosa, and soft tissue infection may be present.

CHRONIC LYMPHOCYTIC LEUKEMIA

CLL (also referred to as small lymphocytic anemia) is a neoplasm of mature and typically *CD5+* B lymphocytes.

EPIDEMIOLOGY

CLL is the most common type of leukemia in adults >19 years. Approximately 21,250 cases of CLL occur in the United States annually. The incidence rate is 4−5 cases per 100,000 and the median age at diagnosis is 72 years. CLL is very uncommon before the age of 45 years and infrequent in patients younger than 65 years of age. The 5-year survival rate is 88.6%, with >95,000 patients living with CLL. It is more common in men than in women and in Jewish people from Russian or Eastern European ancestry. This disease is rare in Asia and in children throughout the world.

ETIOLOGY

The etiology of CLL is unknown, and risk factors are more related to familial inheritance than to exposure to harmful environmental agents. Neoplastic B cells have various genetic aberrations, most commonly gene deletions (e.g., on chromosome 11, 13, 14, or 17) that lead to loss of cell cycle control. The specific genetic defect dictates the course of the disease. Cytogenetic analysis shows the following abnormalities: 13q deletion (55%), trisomy 12 (10%−20%), 11q deletion (10%), and 17p deletion (5%−8%). Neoplastic B cells express *CD19*, *CD20*, and *CD23* and demonstrate a variety of genetic aberrations.

PATHOPHYSIOLOGY AND COMPLICATIONS

The pathophysiology of CLL relates directly to the slow lymphocytic infiltration of the bone marrow. This eventually results in marrow failure and anemia, hepatosplenomegaly, hypogammaglobulinemia, and risk for infection. Although the course of the disease is variable, median survival is 10 years.

CLL is staged using the Rai and Binet Systems in the United States and Europe, respectively (Table 23.5). Median life expectancy for patients with Low Risk (stage 0)/Stage A disease is 13 years; with Intermediate Risk

TABLE 23.5 Staging of Chronic Lymphocytic Leukemia (CLL)

Rai Staging System

Low risk (stage 0) lymphocytosis only

Intermediate risk (stage I/II) lymphocytosis with lymphadenopathy, with or without splenomegaly or hepatomegaly

High risk (stage III/IV) lymphocytosis with anemia or thrombocytopenia due to bone marrow involvement

Binet Staging System

A <3 areas of lymphadenopathy

B ≥3 areas of lymphadenopathy

C Hemoglobin ≤10 g/dL and/or platelets <100,000/μL

Adapted from Woyach JA, Byrd JC. Chronic lymphocytic leukemia. In: Jameson J, et al., eds. *Harrison's Principles of Internal Medicine, 20e.* New York: McGraw Hill; 2018:1–13.

(stage I/II)/Stage B, about 8 years; and with High Risk (stage III/IV)/Stage C, about 2 years.

CLINICAL PRESENTATION

Most patients with CLL are asymptomatic at presentation. When symptoms occur, fatigue, anorexia, and weight loss are the most common complaints. Patients have an enlarged spleen, lymphadenopathy (Fig. 23.5), and hypogammaglobulinemia that contribute to susceptibility to infection. Less frequently, patients with CLL develop autoantibodies against RBCs or platelets that produce hemolytic anemia or thrombocytopenia. Second malignancies occur because of immune defects associated with the disease. In about 15% of patients, CLL evolves

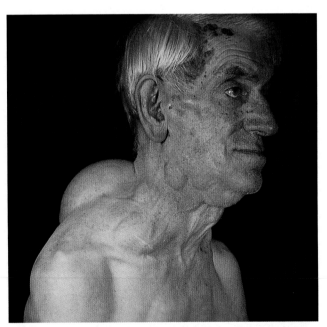

FIG. 23.5 Chronic lymphocytic leukemia in a 65-year-old man with bilateral cervical lymphadenopathy. (From Hoffbrand AV, Pettit JE. *Color Atlas of Clinical Hematology.* 3rd ed. London: Mosby; 2000.)

into a more aggressive malignancy with increasing lymphadenopathy, hepatosplenomegaly, fever, abdominal pain, weight loss, progressive anemia, and thrombocytopenia. Survival is typically less than 1 year.

Laboratory and Diagnostic Findings

CLL requires the presence of more than 5000 mature lymphocytes per microliter in the peripheral blood smear. Also evident in the smear are numerous small, round lymphocytes with scant cytoplasm. Immunotyping reveals the neoplastic cells to be B lymphocytes that are positive for *CD19, CD20,* and *CD23.*

MEDICAL MANAGEMENT

Treatment is not necessary for all patients with CLL and observation is usually indicated in individuals with early-stage asymptomatic CLL. Treatment is indicated in patients with advanced-stage, high tumor burden, disease-related anemia, or thrombocytopenia. Several regimens are considered for first-line CLL therapy, including FCR (fludarabine, cyclophosphamide, and anti-*CD20* rituximab) and ibrutinib (TKI) with or without rituximab. Other anti-*CD20* agents used in combination chemotherapy regimens to treat CLL include ofatumumab and obinutuzumab. Venetoclax is used for patients with relapsed or refractory CLL with 17p deletion and in combination with obinutuzumab for patients with previously untreated CLL. Stem cell transplantation is not frequently used in CLL due to significant morbidity and mortality in the typical age group affected by this disease. Radiation therapy is used to shrink problematic areas of lymphadenopathy.

Oral Manifestations

Generalized lymphadenopathy and pallor of the oral mucosa are features of CLL. Oral soft tissue infection, petechiae, and/or ecchymosis may become evident as the patient develops hypoglobulinemia.

LYMPHOMAS

Lymphoma is cancer of the lymphoid organs and tissues that often presents as discrete tissue masses. The WHO lymphoma classification system comprises more than 80 types of mature lymphoid neoplasms (B-cell, T-cell, and Hodgkin lymphomas), which are defined according to their morphology, immunophenotype, genetic lesions and molecular profiles, clinical features, and cellular derivation. The classification also recognizes both incipient and indolent lymphoid neoplasms with a low potential of progression. Three common lymphomas (Hodgkin lymphoma [HL], non-Hodgkin lymphoma [NHL], Burkitt lymphoma [BL], an aggressive subtype of NHL) and a plasma cell malignancy (MM) are considered here. These diseases are of importance in dental management because initial signs may occur in the mouth (e.g., Waldeyer ring)

TABLE 23.6 Comparison of Hodgkin and Non-Hodgkin Lymphomas

Parameter	Hodgkin Lymphoma [HL]	Non-Hodgkin Lymphoma [NHL]
Cellular derivation site	B cell	B cell > T cell or NK cell
Localized	Common	Uncommon
Waldeyer ring	Rarely involved	Commonly involved
Extranodal	Uncommon	Common
Abdominal (mesenteric nodes)	Uncommon	Common
Mediastinal	Common	Uncommon
Bone marrow	Uncommon	Common
"B" symptoms (fever, night sweats, weight loss)	Common	Uncommon
Curability	More favorable than NHL	Less favorable than HL

NK, natural killer.
Data from Armitage JO, Longo DL. Malignancies of lymphoid cells. In: Kasper DL, et al., eds. *Harrison's Principles of Internal Medicine.* 16th ed. New York: McGraw-Hill; 2005.

and in the head and neck region, and precautions must be taken before any dental treatment is provided.

Approximately 90,390 new cases of lymphoma occur in the United States (8830 cases of HL; 81,560 cases of NHL) annually. There are an estimated 825,651 people living with or in remission from lymphoma in the United States. The 5-year relative survival rate for people with HL has more than doubled, from 40% in whites from 1960 to 1963 (only data available) to 89.6% for all races from 2010 to 2016. HL is considered to be one of the most curable forms of cancer. Approximately 21,680 people are expected to die from lymphoma (960 from HL; 20,720 from NHL) annually. HL and NHL are compared in Table 23.6.

HODGKIN LYMPHOMA

HL is a neoplasm of B lymphocytes that was named for Thomas Hodgkin, the British pathologist who first described it. This neoplasm contains a characteristic tumor cell called the *Reed-Sternberg cell* that represents usually less than 1% of the cellular infiltrate in affected tissues. HL is subdivided into classical HL and the rare nodular lymphocyte predominant HL (NLPHL), which differ in histopathology, clinical characteristics, therapy and outcomes.

EPIDEMIOLOGY

HL is the most common lymphoma in adolescents and young adults. HL has a bimodal incidence pattern that appears around the age of 20–30 years and subsequently at the age of 50–70 years. Men are at slightly higher risk

for developing the disease (2.9 per 100,000 for males, 2.3 per 100,000 for females). In developing countries, HL is found primarily in children and adolescents, with the most common age range affected being 15–19 years. The incidence decreases with age, in contrast with industrialized countries, where it is uncommon in children. Patients with NLPHL are typically young males in the 2nd to 4th decades.

ETIOLOGY

The cause of HL is unknown, but EBV has been causally related in up to 40% of HL cases. Increased risk is associated with presence of the disease in first-degree relatives and with human immunodeficiency virus (HIV) —seropositive status.

PATHOPHYSIOLOGY AND COMPLICATIONS

Enlarging tumorous nodes may cause lung or vascular obstruction, and enlarging mediastinal nodes can cause cough, shortness of breath, or dysphagia. The disease spreads predictably over weeks to months, first to other lymphoid sites (other lymph nodes and spleen) and then hematogenously to extranodal sites, including the bone marrow, liver, and lung. Without treatment, death occurs as a result of complications from bone marrow failure or infection.

CLINICAL PRESENTATION

HL presents most commonly as a painless mass or a group of firm, nontender, enlarged lymph nodes, often affecting the mediastinal nodes or the neck nodes (in >50% of cases) (Fig. 23.6A). Enlarged lymph nodes in the underarm or groin are also common. Fever, weight loss, and night sweats occur in about one-third of patients. Pruritus and fatigue develop and may precede the appearance of enlarging lymph nodes. Palpation of the lymph nodes typically reveals a rubbery consistency. NLPHL typically involves nodes in cervical, axillary, inguinal, or mesenteric locations.

Laboratory and Diagnostic Findings

The diagnosis of lymphoma is made based on nodal biopsy or bone marrow aspirate. Microscopically, tumorous tissue typically shows large, multinucleated Reed-Sternberg reticulum (monoclonal B) cells (Fig. 23.6B). Immunophenotyping of Reed-Sternberg cells demonstrates *CD30* and *CD15*. The four histopathologic variants of classic HL are (1) nodular sclerosing, (2) mixed cellularity, (3) lymphocyte-depleted type, and (4) lymphocyte-predominant type. Together, nodular sclerosing and mixed cellularity types account for nearly 95% of cases. NLPHL is characterized by the presence of lymphocyte predominant cells with strong expression of the B-cell marker, *OCT2*, and the presence

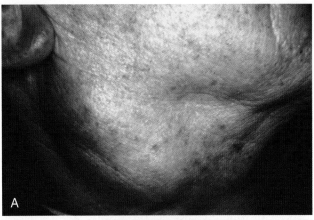

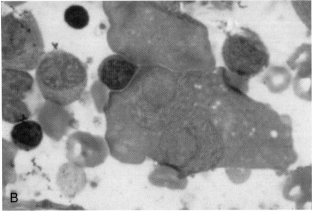

FIG. 23.6 Hodgkin lymphoma. (**A**) Cervical lymphadenopathy caused by tumor infiltrate. (**B**) Large Reed-Sternberg cells are seen in this bone marrow specimen.

of *PD-1*-positive T-follicular helper (TFH) cells surrounding the neoplastic cells.

MEDICAL MANAGEMENT

Effective management requires accurate staging of the disease. HL patients are staged using the Ann Arbor staging system with Cotswold modification. More recently, the Lugano classification incorporated use of fluorodeoxyglucose (FDG) PET-CT for staging (Fig. 23.7).

For early stage disease, the most common treatment is chemotherapy using the ABVD (adriamycin, bleomycin, vinblastine, and dacarbazine) regimen. This may be followed by involved field radiation therapy (IFRT). For advanced stage disease, additional chemotherapy regimens such as Stanford V (doxorubicin, vinblastine, mechlorethamine, etoposide, vincristine, bleomycin, and prednisone) and escalated-BEACOPP (bleomycin, etoposide, doxorubicin, cyclophosphamide, vincristine, procarbazine, and prednisone) may be considered. Patients with relapsed disease may benefit from additional very high-dose chemotherapy and may receive an autologous stem cell rescue. Brentuximab vedotin, an anti-*CD30* antibody linked to a microtubule toxin, is used for patients with advanced stage disease in whom salvage chemotherapy and autologous HCT fails. Immune checkpoint inhibitor therapy with nivolumab or pembrolizumab, monoclonal antibodies blocking *PD-1* pathway signaling, are used in combination with brentuximab vedotin, in patients who have relapsed or

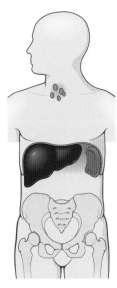

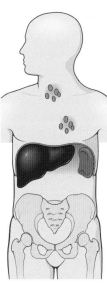

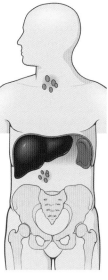

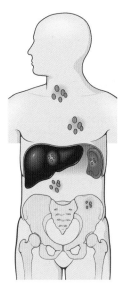

Stage I
Involvement of single lymph node or group of nodes

Stage II
Involvement of two or more sites on same side of diaphragm; often involves the mediastinum

Stage III
Disease on both sides of diaphragm; may include spleen

Stage IV
Widespread extralymphatic involvement (liver, bone marrow, lung, skin)

FIG. 23.7 Staging of Hodgkin lymphoma. (From Chabner D. *The Language of Medicine.* 12th ed. St. Louis: Elsevier; 2021.)

progressed after autologous HCT. Patients with early stage NLPHL are treated with definitive radiotherapy while advanced stage disease may be managed with chemotherapeutic regimens used for HL and NHL.

The current cure rate for HL is about 90%. Poorer survival rates are associated with mixed cellularity and lymphocyte-depleted types, male sex, presence of B symptoms (>10% of baseline weight loss, night sweats, and persistent fever), a large number of involved nodal sites, and bulky disease. The prognosis of early-stage NLPHL is excellent, with progression-free survival and overall survival rates exceeding 90% after treatment.

Long-term complications of chemotherapy and radiation therapy used to manage patients with HL can occur in the lungs, heart, thyroid, breasts, and gonads. Radiation pneumonitis occurs in <10% of irradiated patients with mediastinal lymphadenopathy. Myocarditis, myocardial necrosis, arrhythmias, myocardial infarction, and pericarditis occur in <4% of patients receiving chemotherapy and radiation treatment. Valvular heart disease and coronary artery disease have been reported as late complications of radiation therapy to the chest area. Secondary neoplasia is a complication of treatment of HL and includes acute leukemia, lung cancer, breast cancer, and thyroid cancer.

NON-HODGKIN LYMPHOMA

NHL comprises a large group of lymphoproliferative disorders derived from B-cell progenitors, T-cell progenitors, mature T cells, mature B cells, or natural killer cells. The WHO classification system is based on morphology, immunophenotype, genetic, molecular, and clinical features to distinguish the many types of NHL (Table 23.7).

EPIDEMIOLOGY

NHL is the seventh most common cancer in the United States; accounting for about 81,560 cases per year. The age-adjusted incidence rate of NHL rose by 74.1% from 1975 to 2017 and all races and age groups are affected. NHL results in about 22,000 deaths per year and is the eighth leading cause of death in the United States. The median age at the time of diagnosis is 67 years.

ETIOLOGY

The cause of NHL is unknown, but genetic factors, infectious agents, herbicides, radiation, and some forms of chemotherapy are recognized as causative agents. At the molecular level, malignant lymphocytes have chromosomal translocations or mutations in genes that regulate lymphocyte growth (*BCL6*) or survival (*BCL2*). Persistent inflammation from *H. pylori* infection of the stomach contributes to gastric MALT lymphomas. Oncogenic viruses such as EBV, Kaposi sarcoma herpesvirus

TABLE 23.7	WHO Classification of the Non-Hodgkin Lymphomas

The Indolent Lymphomas

B-cell Neoplasms

Small lymphocytic lymphoma/B-cell chronic lymphocytic leukemia
Lymphoplasmacytic lymphoma (±Waldenstrom's macroglobulinemia)
Plasma cell myeloma/plasmacytoma
Hairy cell leukemia
Follicular lymphoma (grade I and II)
Marginal zone B-cell lymphoma
Mantle cell lymphoma

T-cell Neoplasms

T-cell large granular lymphocyte leukemia
Mycosis fungoides
T-cell prolymphocytic leukemia

Natural Killer Cell Neoplasms

Natural killer cell large granular lymphocyte leukemia

The Aggressive Lymphomas

B-cell neoplasms
Follicular lymphoma (grade III)
Diffuse large B-cell lymphoma
Mantle cell lymphoma

T-cell Neoplasms

Peripheral T-cell lymphoma
Anaplastic large cell lymphoma, T/null cell

The Highly Aggressive Lymphomas

B-cell neoplasms
Burkitt's lymphoma
Precursor B lymphoblastic leukemia/lymphoma
T-cell neoplasms
Adult T-cell lymphoma/leukemia
Precursor T lymphoblastic leukemia/lymphoma

Source: Adapted from UpToDate, December 2021.

(KSHV), and retroviruses are associated with several types of NHL. Patients with autoimmune disease (Sjögren syndrome) or immunodeficiency states (acquired immunodeficiency syndrome [AIDS], after chemotherapy) are at increased risk for the disease.

Pathophysiology and Complications

The course of NHL varies from highly proliferative and rapidly fatal disorders (aggressive) to slowly progressing (indolent) malignancies that are tolerated for decades. Tumorous cells behave in similar fashion to that for the cell of origin: B cells congregate in follicular regions of lymph nodes, and T cells have a propensity for paracortical T-cell zones. These neoplasms cause tumorous enlargements and abnormalities of the immune system. Tumors often are widespread at the time of diagnosis and more variable in location (involving various organs such as liver and spleen) than in HL. Anemic and leukemic manifestations are common.

CLINICAL PRESENTATION

NHL may occur at any age and often is marked by enlarged lymph nodes, fever, and weight loss. In contrast with HL, which often begins with a single focus of tumor, NHL usually is multifocal when first detected. About 20%–40% of lymphomas develop outside of lymph nodes and are termed *extranodal lymphomas*. The most prominent sign of NHL is a painless lymph node(s) swelling of longer than 2 weeks' duration. Additional signs and symptoms include persistent fever of unknown cause, weight loss, malaise, sweating, tender lymphadenopathy, abdominal or chest pain, and, on occasion, extranodal tumors. *B symptoms,* defined as fever, drenching night sweats, and weight loss of more than 10%, as seen with HL, indicate a more aggressive clinical course.

Laboratory and Diagnostic Findings

The diagnosis of NHL is based on findings on excisional biopsy of the involved lymph node. Tumorous cells are classified first by lineage (B, T, or NK cell) and second by level of differentiation. Immunologic and molecular genetic assays are performed to facilitate diagnosis. Proper staging of disease requires CBC count, chemistry screen, chest radiographs, PET-CT scans, and bone marrow biopsy. The Lugano Classification system previously described may be used to stage NHL.

MEDICAL MANAGEMENT

Radiotherapy is used to treat all subtypes and stages of NHL as it is a radiosensitive tumor. This may be curative for patients with indolent lymphoma, and for those with aggressive disease, radiotherapy is used after or to consolidate chemotherapy, and for palliative treatment. Optimal radiation dosing for both indolent and aggressive lymphoma is unclear. Adults with NHL who were treated either with standard high-dose radiation (40–45 Gy in both indolent and aggressive NHL) or low-dose radiation (24 Gy in indolent NHL or 30 Gy in aggressive NHL) demonstrated similar efficacy. Chemotherapy regimens differ between indolent or aggressive lymphoma. Various prognostic and treatment indices are available for NHL, including the International Prognostic Index (IPI), which is utilized for all types of NHL, although originally developed for B-cell and T-cell lymphomas. Medical treatment of the two most common subtypes of NHL are briefly discussed.

Diffuse large B-cell lymphoma (DLBCL) is the most common histologic subtype of NHL diagnosed, representing approximately 33% of all cases. Combination chemotherapy offers potentially curative therapy for DLBCL, regardless of stage. Standard first-line chemotherapy consists of R-CHOP (cyclophosphamide, doxorubicin, vincristine, and prednisone) and rituximab. On average, 60%–65% of patients with DLBCL are cured

with this approach. Patients with relapsed or refractory disease may be cured with salvage chemotherapy followed by autologous HCT. Immune checkpoint inhibitor (e.g., polatuzumab vedotin-piiq) and CAR T-cell therapy may also be considered in these cases.

Follicular lymphoma (FL) is the second leading NHL diagnosis accounting for at least 30% of NHL in the United States. Observation may be indicated for asymptomatic individuals. Up to 15% of patients with FL have localized disease, which usually is treated with IRFT, with overall survival rates of 60%–70%. R-CHOP is first-line chemotherapy and autologous and allogeneic HCT may be curative in patients with relapsed disease. New treatment approaches for relapsed FL include idelalisib (*PI3K* inhibitor), ibrutinib, and *PD-1* inhibitors. Of clinical importance, patients with FL have a high rate of histologic transformation to DLBCL (approximately 3% per year).

Oral Manifestations

Patients with HL or NHL may develop cervical lymphadenopathy and extranodal or intraoral tumors (Fig. 23.8). Lymphoma in the oral cavity usually appears as extranodal disease. This situation is of particular concern in immunosuppressed patients and in those with Sjögren syndrome, who are at increased risk for the development of lymphoma. These patients should be

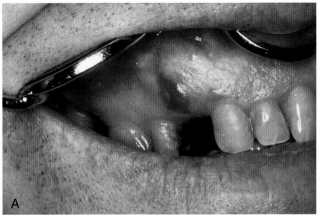

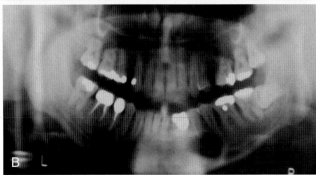

FIG. 23.8 Non-Hodgkin lymphoma manifesting as a gingival enlargement that also involved the underlying alveolar bone (**A**) and an osteolytic lesion of the mandible (**B**).

periodically monitored for the development of orofacial neoplasia.

Intraoral lymphoma commonly involves Waldeyer ring (soft palate and oropharynx), and less often the salivary glands and mandible. These lymphomas appear as rapidly expanding (or chronic), nonspecific swellings of the head and neck lymph nodes, palate, gingiva, buccal sulcus, or floor of the mouth. Enlargements may be painless or painful. The presence of these orofacial abnormalities requires prompt evaluation by biopsy using needle, incisional, or excisional techniques. Ulceration, paresthesia, and mobile teeth are also oral findings associated with lymphoma.

Patients with lymphoma who have received medical treatment for their disease sometimes report oral discomfort akin to burning, similar to those noted by patients with leukemia, which may be related to drug toxicity, hyposalivation, candidiasis, or anemia (see Appendix C for management regimens). Patients who have received more than 25 Gy of radiation to the head and neck region are susceptible to xerostomia and may benefit from salivary substitutes or pilocarpine. Radiation also can damage taste buds, cause trismus of the masticatory muscles, and stunt craniomandibular growth and development.

BURKITT LYMPHOMA

BL is an aggressive B-cell (non-Hodgkin) lymphoma that originally was described by Denis Burkitt.

EPIDEMIOLOGY

BL accounts for approximately 40% of childhood NHL in the United States; affecting children and young adults at a rate of 0.5 cases per 100,000. The disease is more common in men. The WHO classifies BL into three types: (1) endemic, (2) sporadic, and (3) immunodeficiency associated. BL that is found most often in Central Africa is known as endemic BL and affects children with a peak prevalence of about 6 years of age. More than 50% −70% of endemic cases present in the jaws (90% in 3-year-old patients and 25% in patients older than age 15 years). Sporadic BL is more common in Western societies with a median age of diagnosis of 45 years. Immunodeficiency-associated BL occurs in persons infected with HIV.

ETIOLOGY

BL is a mature B-cell lymphoma expressing pan B-cell surface markers CD10, 19, 20, 22, 79, and BCL6, but lacks BCL2. Translocations of the c-MYC gene on chromosome 8 is the hallmark of BL, occurring in approximately 95% of cases. The t(8;14)(q24;q32) is the most common translocation in BL, occurring in 70% −80% of cases. In addition to the characteristic

translocation of c-MYC, many gene mutations have been identified, including truncating mutations of ARID1A, amplification of MCL1 and truncating alterations of PTEN, NOTCH, and ATM. More than 90% of endemic tumors contain latent EBV. EBV is present in about 15% −20% of sporadic BL and in about 25% of HIV-associated tumors.

PATHOPHYSIOLOGY AND COMPLICATIONS

This malignancy is aggressive and grows very rapidly. Tumors can double in size every 3 days; thus, obstruction of the airway, alimentary canal, and vasculature is possible. The tumor also has a propensity for spread to the CNS.

CLINICAL PRESENTATION

Most cases arise at extranodal sites. The endemic form shows a predilection for tumors of the jaw and for involvement of select abdominal organs, particularly the kidneys, ovaries, and adrenal glands. Jaw involvement is more common in patients younger than 5 years of age than among those older than age 10 years (Fig. 23.9). Sporadic BL often presents as an abdominal mass that involves the lymph nodes of the intestine and peritoneum, with jaw lesions being less common. Tumors that enlarge as abdominal masses are accompanied by fluid accumulation, pain, and possibly vomiting. The bone marrow is infrequently involved.

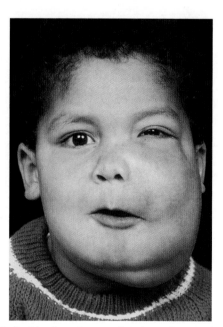

FIG. 23.9 Burkitt lymphoma showing characteristic facial swelling caused by extensive tumor involvement of the mandible and surrounding soft tissues. (From Hoffbrand AV, Pettit JE. *Color Atlas of Clinical Hematology.* 4th ed. London: Mosby; 2010. Courtesy of Prof. J.M. Chessells.)

Laboratory and Diagnostic Findings

The diagnosis is based on biopsy of the involved tissue, flow cytometry, chromosome analysis, and immunophenotyping. Biopsy of affected tissue demonstrates a histologic pattern of numerous small B lymphocytes interspersed with lightly stained histiocytes ("starry sky" pattern) (Fig. 23.10). Histologically, tumor cells are darkly stained and have small prominent nucleoli and a high mitotic index. Flow cytometry demonstrates IgM and the aforementioned B-cell surface markers. Radiographic evaluation of jaw lesions typically demonstrate osteolytic jaw lesions with ill-defined margins and tooth displacement (floating teeth) typically posterior to the molars.

MEDICAL MANAGEMENT

Staging of BL frequently occurs per the Lugano Classification system. Patients with a localized tumor that was completely excised may be on a short course (<2 months) of chemotherapy, utilizing multiagent regimens, such as

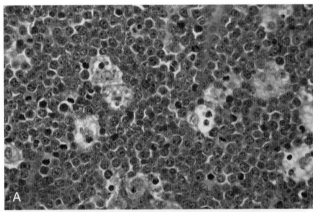
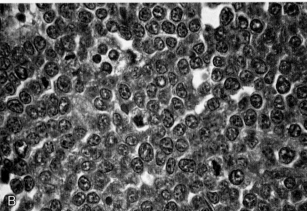

FIG. 23.10 Burkitt lymphoma. (**A**) At low power, numerous pale macrophages are evident, interspersed among the tumor cells, producing a "starry sky" appearance. (**B**) At high power, tumor cells are seen to have multiple small nucleoli and a high mitotic index. ((**A**) and (**B**) from Kumar V, Abbas A, Fausto N, eds. *Robbins & Cotran Pathologic Basis of Disease.* 7th ed. Philadelphia: Saunders; 2005. (**B**) courtesy of Dr. Jose Hernandez, Department of Pathology, University of Texas Southwestern Medical School, Dallas, TX.)

etoposide, prednisone, vincristine, cyclophosphamide, and doxorubicin (DA-EPOCH), in combination with rituximab. In cases where the tumor cannot be surgically removed and does not involve the CNS, chemotherapy may be used for 4 months with the same agents with the addition of cytarabine and methotrexate. Patients with CNS involvement receive 6 months of chemotherapy with similar agents. As BL responds well to high-dose chemotherapy, disease remission is achieved in more than 90% of patients. Those who live beyond 2 years often experience long-term remission. Relapsed and refractory BL is associated with very poor outcomes.

Oral Manifestations

Endemic BL often presents as a rapidly expanding tumorous mass in the posterior region of the maxilla or mandible with about 50%–70% of the cases demonstrating jaw lesions. Rapid growth displaces adjacent teeth, resulting in mobile and abnormally positioned teeth. Pain and paresthesia accompany the condition. Radiographically, the tumor produces an osteolytic lesion with poorly demarcated margins, erosion of the cortical plate, and soft tissue involvement.

MULTIPLE MYELOMA

MM is a lymphoproliferative disorder caused from overproduction of clonal malignant plasma cells that results in multiple tumorous masses scattered throughout the skeletal system. Malignant plasma cells secrete monoclonal immunoglobulins and various cytokines. Monoclonal gammopathy of undetermined significance (MGUS), consisting of increased numbers of plasma cells with no indicators of active disease, is considered part of the spectrum of monoclonal gammopathies. MGUS has a progression risk to MM of 1% annually. Another condition within the spectrum is smoldering multiple myeloma (SMM), considered to be an asymptomatic, intermediate stage of myeloma between MGUS and active MM. SMM is at a higher progression risk to MM of 10% per year.

EPIDEMIOLOGY

Approximately 34,920 new cases of myeloma (19,320 males and 15,600 females) are diagnosed in the United States annually. An estimated 138,415 people in the United States are living with or in remission from myeloma. The 3-year survival rate is 70% (for all races and ethnicities). Approximately 12,410 deaths are expected from myeloma. The lifetime risk for MM is 1 in 132 (0.76%). The median age at diagnosis of MM is 69 years and is seldom diagnosed in people younger than 40 years of age.

ETIOLOGY

Risk factors for MM include chronic exposure to low-dose ionizing radiation, occupational exposure (e.g., chemicals), genetic factors, and chronic antigenic stimulation. The initiating event driving development of malignancy is either the acquisition of hyperdiploidy or a translocation involving the immunoglobulin heavy chain locus. Chromosomal translocations found in myeloma patients include *t(11:14)(q13;q32)*, *t(4:14)(p16:q32)* and *t(4;16)*. Other chromosomal abnormalities include deletions of *13q14* and *17p13*. Malignant plasma cells express certain cluster differentiation glycoproteins, such as *CD38*, *CD56*, *CD138*, and *CD319*, while typically *CD19* and *CD45* negative. Abnormalities of oncogenes such as *MYC*, *NRAS*, *KRAS*, *FGFR3*, and *TP53* are associated with the disease process. Tumor cells secrete RANK ligand and interleukin-6 (osteoclast activating factors) as well as DKK1 and SOST (osteoblast inhibitory factors), a process which leads to bone resorption, further myeloma cell proliferation and immune suppression.

PATHOPHYSIOLOGY AND COMPLICATIONS

The disease consists of plasma and myeloma cell proliferation, immunoglobulin production, bone resorption at tumor sites, and bone marrow replacement. Resorption of bone leads to release of calcium and serum hypercalcemia. Skeletal-related events (SREs) are complications of MM that are typically related to bone metastases and can include fractures, spinal cord compression, and pain. Bone marrow replacement by tumorous cells leads to anemia, leukopenia, thrombocytopenia, and eventually a decrease in plasma immunoglobulins. Pneumonia and pyelonephritis commonly develop due to hypogammaglobulinemia. During the early to middle stages of disease, increased plasma viscosity contributes to altered platelet function, excessive bleeding, renal impairment, and neuropathy. Renal failure results from tubular damage caused by excretion of light chains (of immunoglobulin) or by glomerular deposition of amyloid, hyperuricemia, recurrent pyelonephritis, or local infiltration of tumor cells. Infections, such as pneumonia and pyelonephritism, are common because of diffuse hypogammaglobulinemia that is caused by decreased production of normal antibodies. Infection is a primary cause of death followed by renal failure in patients with MM.

CLINICAL PRESENTATION

Most patients develop signs and symptoms of MM due to plasma cell infiltration into bone or other organs and the first symptom is often persistent bone pain. The sites most commonly affected are along the spine, ribs, and sternum. Anemia is accompanied by weakness, weight loss, and recurrent infection. Headache and peripheral neuropathy are associated with hypercalcemia. Tumor destruction of bone may cause pathologic fracture. A prominent radiographic feature of MM is are multiple "punched-out" lesions or mottled areas, which represent areas of tumor that appear in the spine, ribs, and cortical regions

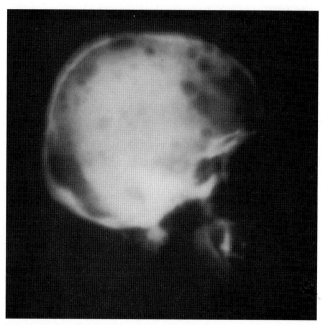

FIG. 23.11 Multiple myeloma. Punched-out lytic lesions in the skull containing malignant plasma cells.

of the skull (Fig. 23.11). Osteolytic lesions of the jaw occur in up to 30% of patients. Amyloid deposition is seen in various soft tissues (e.g., heart, liver, nervous system).

Laboratory and Diagnostic Findings

Features of MM include osteolytic bone lesions, elevated serum calcium, increased immunoglobulins in the blood, abnormal immunoglobulin light chains (Bence–Jones proteins) in the urine, anemia (normocytic and normochromic), neutropenia, and thrombocytopenia. Diagnostic criteria for MM and related conditions, as outlined by the International Myeloma Working Group, is presented in Tables 23.8 and 23.9.

MEDICAL MANAGEMENT

The International Staging System is a commonly used system for staging and prognosis of MM on the basis of serum β_2-microglobulin and serum albumin levels. This system has been updated to the Revised International Staging System, which includes information on the presence of high-risk genetic lesions either alone or in combination, or increased lactate dehydrogenase concentration (Table 23.10).

Treatment of patients with MM is shown in Table 23.11. Typically, treatment is chemotherapy followed by autologous stem cell transplant (ASCT). Transplant patients receive induction chemotherapy with a triplet regimen 3–4 months prior to stem cell collection. The preferred initial therapy for patients who are candidates for ASCT is bortezomib, lenalidomide, and dexamethasone (VRd). VRd is a well-tolerated regimen and

TABLE 23.8   Diagnostic Criteria for Multiple Myeloma.

Feature	Multiple Myeloma (MM)
Clonal bone marrow plasma cell infiltration	Greater than or equal to 10% or a biopsy-proven plasmacytoma
CRAB features	Hypercalcemia: serum calcium >1 mg/dL higher than the >11 mg/dL
	Renal insufficiency: creatinine clearance <40 mL per minute or serum creatinine >2 mg/dL
	Anemia: hemoglobin value of >2 g/dL below the lower limit of normal, <10 g/dL
	Bone lesions: one or more osteolytic lesions on skeletal radiography, computed tomography (CT), or positron emission tomography-CT (PET-CT)
Myeloma Defining Events* (MDE)	CRAB features
	Clonal bone marrow plasma cell percentage of greater than 60%
	An involved-to-uninvolved serum light-chain ratio of greater than 100
	Two or more focal lesions on MRI
	*If no end-organ damage, presence of one or more biomarkers is sufficient for diagnosis

Adapted from Kumar SK. et al. Multiple myeloma. *Nat Rev Dis Primers*. 2017;3:17046.

TABLE 23.9   Diagnostic Criteria for Monoclonal Gammopathy of Unknown Significance (MGUS) and Smoldering Multiple Myeloma (SMM)

Feature	MGUS	SMM
Serum monoclonal protein levels	Less 3 g per dl and	Greater than or equal to 3 g per dl and/or
Clonal bone marrow plasma cell infiltration	<10%	10%–60%
Symptomatology	Absence of CRAB features	Absence of MDE or amyloidosis

Adapted from Kumar SK, et al. Multiple myeloma. *Nat Rev Dis Primers*. 2017;3:17046.

TABLE 23.10   International Staging System for Myeloma

Staging	Median Survival Time
I. International Staging System (Serum β$_2$-Microglobulin and Albumin)	
Stage I (serum β$_2$-microglobulin <3.5 mg/L and serum albumin >3.5 g/dL)	62 months
Stage II (neither stage I or III)	44 months
Stage III (serum β$_2$-microglobulin >5.5 mg/L)	29 months
II. Revised International Staging System (R-ISS)	
Stage 1	
All of the following: serum albumin ≥3.5 g/dL; serum beta-2-microglobulin <3.5 mg/L; no high risk cytogenetics; normal serum lactate dehydrogenase level	
Stage II: not fitting Stage I or III	
Stage III	
Both of the following: serum beta-2-microglobulin >5.5 mg/L; high risk cytogenetics [t(4;14), t(14;16), or del(17p)] or elevated serum lactate dehydrogenase level	

Adapted from: Rajkumar SV. Multiple myeloma: 2020 update on diagnosis, risk-stratification and management. *Am J Hematol*. 2020;95:548–567.

(Dara-VRd) may be used in high-risk patients. Those deemed ineligible for ASCT receive combination chemotherapy followed by maintenance therapy until disease progression unless there are significant adverse effects. Radiation therapy is used as palliative treatment, for example, in patients with painful bone lesions. Interventions are provided to manage anemia, prevent infection, and treat or prevent bone disease. Usually, anemia is controlled with recombinant erythropoietin. Intravenous immunoglobulins and antibiotics are given selectively to prevent infection. Antiresorptives are used to maintain bone strength and to reduce bone pain associated with this disease. Reported 5-year survival rates for MM, based on data up to 2016, range from 25% to 55%.

Oral Manifestations

Patients with MM may have jaw lesions, soft tissue plasmacytomas, and soft tissue deposits of amyloid. Bone and soft tissue lesions often are painful. Dental radiographs may show "punched-out" lesions or mottled areas that represent areas of tumor. These osteolytic lesions are more common in the posterior body of the mandible and may be associated with cortical plate expansion. Extramedullary plasmacytomas can occur in the oral cavity/oropharynx and typically arise from bone. Amyloid-like protein can deposit in the tongue, resulting in enlargement (macroglossia) and pain. Biopsy and special amyloid stains can be used for diagnosis. Medication-related osteonecrosis of the

associated with high overall and complete response rates. An alternative to VRd is daratumumab, lenalidomide, and dexamethasone (DRd) for patients with preexisting neuropathy or those who have intolerance to VRd. Daratumumab added to the standard VRd regimen

TABLE 23.11	Common Treatments for Multiple Myeloma	
Type of Therapy	**Agent(s) or Technique(s)**	**Complications**
Traditional chemotherapy	Melphalan Cyclophosphamide Doxorubicin Bendamustine	Hair loss Mouth sores (ulceration) Loss of appetite Nausea and vomiting Low blood counts Increased risk of infection Bleeding and bruising Tiredness
Corticosteroids	Dexamethasone Prednisone	Increased blood sugar Increased appetite Problems sleeping Infection (weakened immune system)
Immunomodulating agents	Thalidomide Lenalidomide Pomalidomide	Sleepiness Tiredness Nerve damage Infection (decrease in WBCs) Bleeding (decrease in platelets)
Proteasome inhibitors	Bortezomib Carfilzomib Ixazomib	Nausea and vomiting Tiredness Diarrhea or constipation Bleeding and bruising Decreased appetite Fever Peripheral neuropathy
Monoclonal antibodies	Elotuzumab Daratumumab Isatuximab	Diarrhea or constipation Tiredness Peripheral neuropathy Fever Decreased appetite Cough Upper respiratory infection
Antiresorptives	Pamidronate Zoledronic acid Denosumab	Osteonecrosis of the jaws
Stem cell transplantation	Autologous	Infection
Radiation therapy (for bone lesions that do not respond to drugs for pain relief)		
Surgery (relieve spinal cord compression, placement of rods for long bone support)		

Adapted from: Rajkumar SV. Multiple myeloma: 2020 update on diagnosis, risk-stratification and management. *Am J Hematol.* 2020;95:548–567; van de Donk NWCJ, Pawlyn C, Yong KL. Multiple myeloma. *Lancet.* 2021;397:410–427.

jaw (MRONJ) is a potentially serious complication of antiresorptive agents commonly used in the management of MM. MRONJ is characterized by areas of exposed and necrotic bone more commonly observed in the mandible, which may or may not be symptomatic. The reader is referred to Chapter 26 for more information related to this condition.

DENTAL MANAGEMENT

Medical Considerations

Identification. A thorough assessment for evidence of WBC disorders is essential in all patients who present for dental treatment. Clinical recognition of such disorders is critical because patients with leukemia or lymphoma may be at high risk for life-threatening outcomes if the disease is not detected before dental treatment is started. Patients with leukemia whose disease has not been diagnosed may experience serious bleeding complications after surgical procedures, may have altered healing of surgical wounds, and are prone to postsurgical infection. Thus, it is important for the dentist to attempt to identify these patients through history and clinical examination before starting any treatment.

Comprehensive evaluation requires a consistent approach by which important medical, historical, and clinical information is obtained from the patient. Specific questions regarding blood disorders and cancer in family members, weight loss, fever, swollen or enlarged lymph nodes, and bleeding tendencies should be asked. In addition, the dentist should emphasize the importance of routine annual physical examinations that will provide hematologic assessment for potential abnormalities.

Examination of the head, neck, and mouth should include a thorough inspection of the oropharynx, head, and cervical and supraclavicular lymph nodes. The dentist should be cognizant that an enlarged nontender supraclavicular node is suggestive of malignancy. Cranial nerve examination is important for identifying abnormalities suggestive of invasive neoplasms. Panoramic images also provide insight into potential osteolytic lesions associated with WBC disorders (see Fig. 23.8).

A patient who displays classic signs or symptoms of leukemia, lymphoma, or MM should be promptly referred directly to a physician for appropriate laboratory tests or biopsy of soft tissue and osseous lesions. Screening laboratory tests include a CBC with differential (total and differential WBC counts, hemoglobin, hematocrit, platelet count) and a smear for cell morphologic study. If screening tests are ordered by the dentist and one or more results are abnormal, the patient should be promptly referred for medical evaluation and treatment.

Treatment Planning Modifications

Dental management of patients in whom a WBC disorder is diagnosed requires consideration of the three phases of medical therapy: (1) pretreatment assessment and preparation of the patient; (2) oral health care during medical therapy; and (3) posttreatment management, including long-term considerations and possible remission.

Pretreatment Evaluation and Considerations. Through consultation with the patient's physician, the dentist must be aware of the specific diagnosis, severity of the disorder, type of treatment selected for the patient, and whether the WBC disorder can be effectively managed. Full knowledge of this information is required for effective decision-making regarding dental treatment. For patients in whom leukemia or lymphoma has been recently diagnosed, the dentist should become involved early during the treatment planning stages of cancer therapy. Guidance regarding the health of the oral cavity and jaws can help prevent severe oral complications (i.e., infection). Accordingly, pretreatment assessment should include a thorough extraoral and intraoral examination, panoramic film, and review of blood laboratory findings, with the overall goal of minimizing or eliminating active or potential oral disease before the start of chemotherapy. Radiographic assessment for retained root tips, impacted teeth, and osseous disease is important.

Pretreatment care should include oral hygiene instructions that emphasize the importance of meticulous plaque removal. Caries and infection should be eliminated, if possible, before initiation of chemotherapy, and treatment should be directed first toward acute needs (e.g., periapical disease, large carious lesions treated before small lesions). If pulpal disease is present, the dentist may recommend root canal therapy or extraction of teeth before chemotherapy. Oral hygiene procedures should be emphasized, including using fluoride gels, encouraging a noncariogenic diet, eliminating mucosal and periodontal disease, eliminating sources of mucosal injury, and protecting the salivary glands if head and neck irradiation is planned. Extraction should be considered if periodontal pocket depths are greater than 5 mm, periapical inflammation is present, the tooth is nonfunctional or partially erupted (as with third molars), or if one or more teeth have a questionable prognosis.

Recommendations for extraction in patients before chemotherapy (or radiation therapy to the head and neck) include scheduling a minimum of 2 weeks between the time of extraction and initiation of therapy and attaining primary closure. If invasive procedures are planned and the platelet count is less than 50,000/μL, platelet transfusion prior to treatment should be discussed with the patient's physician. It is important to note that in many cases of acute leukemia, chemotherapy is initiated within a few days of diagnosis, so dental treatment may have to be provided promptly before the patient becomes neutropenic as a result of chemotherapy.

There is a lack of evidence-based literature regarding antimicrobial prophylaxis for neutropenic patients (ANC <1000 cells/uL) undergoing dental procedures. It is recommended that dentists consult with the patient's physician to discuss proposed dental procedures, need for antibiotic prophylaxis, appropriate choice of antimicrobial and dosing regimen in patients with neutropenia.

Medical Complications. Patients who are undergoing chemotherapy, radiotherapy, or allo HCT are susceptible to many oral complications, including mucositis, neutropenia, infection, excessive bleeding, GVHD, and alterations in growth and development in pediatric patients treated at a young age.

Mucositis. Patients with leukemia, lymphoma, or MM may develop mucositis as a result of treatment (see Chapter 26 for more detail about this condition).

Neutropenia and Infection. Patients may present with neutropenia alone, neutropenia combined with leukemia or lymphoma, or neutropenia that results from medical treatment (chemotherapy or drug induced) (Fig. 23.12). Patients who have neutropenia are unable to provide a protective response against oral microbes. Accordingly, these patients develop acute gingival inflammation and mucosal ulcerations. Chronic neutropenia contributes to severe destruction of the periodontium with loss of attachment when oral hygiene is less than optimal. Periodontal therapy that includes instruction on oral hygiene, frequent scaling, and antimicrobial therapy can reduce the adverse effects associated with this disorder.

Oral infection is less of a problem in patients with chronic leukemia than in those with acute leukemia because the cells are more mature and functional in chronic leukemia. However, in the later stages of both CML and CLL, infection can become a serious complication. Splenectomy because of massive splenomegaly may also increase the risk of infection.

Signs of infection often are masked in patients with leukemia and less frequently with lymphoma and MM due to neutropenia. The swelling and erythema usually

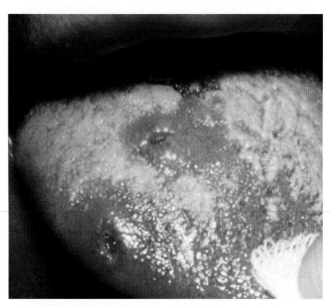

FIG. 23.12 Oral ulcers caused by neutropenia.

associated with oral infection are often less distinctive. In these patients, severe infection can occur with minimal clinical signs, which can make clinical diagnosis more difficult. Infections often develop in the presence of neutropenia as the result of invasion by unusual oral pathogens such as *Pseudomonas* spp., *Klebsiella* spp., *Proteus* spp., *Escherichia coli*, or *Enterobacter* spp. Often, these infections present as oral ulcerations. When oral infection develops in such patients, a specimen of exudate should be sent for culture, diagnosis, and antibiotic sensitivity testing. If a bacterial infection is suspected, amoxicillin–clavulanic acid should be considered. If the clinical course shows little or no improvement in several days, laboratory findings should be used to select a more appropriate antimicrobial agent and referral to a physician should be considered.

A common opportunistic infection is acute pseudomembranous candidiasis. When this complication occurs, the patient should be treated with one of the antifungal medications listed in Appendix C. Infrequently, unusual oral fungal infections (e.g., aspergillosis, and mucormycosis) occur, or fungal septicemia may originate from the oral cavity. These patients require potent systemic antifungal agents, such as voriconazole.

Another common infection in this patient population is recurrent herpes simplex virus (HSV) infection. Herpetic lesions tend to be larger and take longer to heal than in patients without leukemia. To prevent recurrence, antiviral therapy (e.g., acyclovir) is prescribed to HSV antibody–positive patients who are undergoing chemotherapy. In patients in whom HSV infection develops, the diagnosis can be made rapidly using PCR. Immunocompromised patients also are susceptible to varicella-zoster and cytomegalovirus infections, and lesions in the oral cavity attributed to these viruses have been reported.

Bleeding. Small or large areas of submucosal hemorrhage may be found in the patients with leukemia (see Fig. 23.2A). These lesions result from minor trauma (e.g., tongue biting) and are related to thrombocytopenia. Patients with acute leukemia and primarily in AML also may report spontaneous and severe gingival bleeding that is aggravated by poor oral hygiene. Enlarged and boggy gingiva (Fig. 23.13) bleeds easily, especially if significant thrombocytopenia is present. The dentist should make efforts to improve oral hygiene and should use local measures to control bleeding. A gelatin sponge with thrombin or microfibrillar collagen can be placed over the area, or an oral antifibrinolytic rinse may be used. If local measures fail, medical help will be needed and may involve platelet transfusion. Platelet counts ideally should be at least 50,000/µL before proceeding with invasive dental procedures. In addition, if patients are skilled at flossing without traumatizing soft tissues, it is reasonable to continue this practice throughout their treatment.

Graft-Versus-Host Disease. Patients with leukemia and lymphoma may develop GVHD as a result of allogeneic

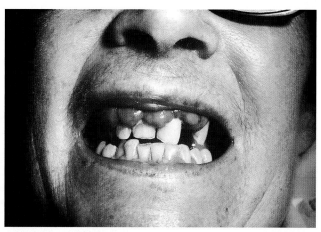

FIG. 23.13 Leukemic gingival enlargement in a patient who has acute myeloid leukemia. Enlargement is caused by leukemic infiltrations in the gingival tissue. (From Hoffbrand AV, Pettit JE. *Color Atlas of Clinical Hematology.* 4th ed. London: Mosby; 2010.)

HCT. The reader is referred to Chapter 26 for more information on this topic.

Adverse Drug Effects. A small number of patients describe paresthesias that result from leukemic infiltration of the peripheral nerves or as a result of chemotherapy (vincristine). An adverse effect of cyclosporine use in BMT patients is gingival overgrowth. Pigmentation of the hard palate has been associated with imatinib.

Growth and Development. Chemotherapy during childhood can affect growth and development of the teeth and facial bones. This effect is not observed in adults. Restricted growth of the jaws leads to micrognathia, retrognathia, or malocclusion. Damage to the teeth that occurs at the time of chemotherapy can manifest as shortened or blunted roots, dilacerations, calcification abnormalities, pulp enlargement, microdontia, and hypodontia.

Medication-Related Osteonecrosis of the Jaw. Medication-related osteonecrosis of the jaw is a significant complication of long-term antiresorptive therapy for patients with MM (see Chapter 26 for more information).

Management of Patients in Remission. Patients who have WBC disorders and are in a state of remission can receive most indicated dental treatment (Box 23.2). Dental treatment planning for patients with advanced disease and a limited prognosis should be considered appropriately.

If invasive (e.g., scaling) or surgical procedures are planned for a patient who has a WBC disorder that is considered medically stable, platelet count should be obtained prior to the procedure to ensure an adequate number of platelets are present. If the platelet count is low, the procedure should be delayed until the patient's physician is consulted. In patients whose disease is stable but who are still thrombocytopenic, platelet replacement by the physician can be instituted if a dental procedure must be done. Dental management of the patient receiving radiation or chemotherapy is discussed further in Chapter 26.

In HL, the spleen may be involved and surgically removed. Subsequently, the patient is at risk for bacterial infection. Risk for such infection is greatest during the first 6 months after splenectomy. While antibiotic prophylaxis has been suggested for invasive procedures during the first 6 months after splenectomy, the benefit of antibiotic prophylaxis for invasive dental procedures in these patients or after 6 months has not been established.

Up to 80% of patients in whom MM is newly diagnosed present with osteopenia, osteolysis, and pathologic fractures. Patients who have MM may remain on antiresorptive therapy for years, and even if discontinued, remain at lifelong risk of developing MRONJ.

| BOX 23.2 | Checklist for Dental Management of Patients with White Blood Cell Disorders[a] |

PREOPERATIVE RISK ASSESSMENT

R
Recognize Risks
- Be **aware** of adverse events that may occur in the management of a patient who has a medical condition.

P
Patient Evaluation
- Review **medical history** and discuss relevant issues with the patient.
- Identify all **medications and drugs** being taken or supposed to be taken by the patient.
- **Examine** the patient for signs and symptoms of disease and obtain vital signs.
- Review or obtain recent **laboratory test** results or **images** required to assess risk.
- Obtain a **medical consultation** if the patient has a poorly controlled or undiagnosed problem or if the patient's health status is uncertain.

A

Analgesics	No issues. For MM patients with renal dysfunction: (1) use caution with acetaminophen, aspirin, and narcotics and (2) avoid NSAIDs.
Antibiotics	Antibiotic sensitivity testing should be done for oral infections; infections should be treated in a conservative manner with the indicated antibiotic, heat, and strong analgesics for pain. Chlorhexidine rinse may be helpful to promote healing of mucositis. Provide antifungal medications for oral candidiasis. Consult physician regarding need for antibiotics when invasive procedures are planned for patients who have an ANC of <1000 µL.
Anesthesia	Ensure profound local anesthesia. Epinephrine-containing local anesthetic can be used with minimal risk if limited to 0.036 mg epinephrine (two capsules containing 1:100,000 concentration) in patients with cardiac complications of radiation and/or chemotherapy. Higher doses may be tolerated, but the risk of

	complications increases with dose. Avoid the use of epinephrine in retraction cord.
Anxiety	No issues.

B

Bleeding	If the platelet count is less than 50,000/µL, platelet transfusion may be needed before certain invasive and surgical procedures. Confirm by medical consultation.
Blood pressure and vital sign monitoring	Obtain pretreatment vital signs. Monitor blood pressure and oxygen saturation.

C

Capacity to tolerate care Chair position	Nausea, vomiting, and fatigue can affect the ability of patients to tolerate care. For patients with MM who have macroglossia, avoid supine positioning to minimize risk of airway obstruction.

D

Devices	No issues.
Drugs	Patients on chemotherapy may complain of paresthesias; those receiving cyclosporine may develop gingival overgrowth. Patients may develop oral pigmentation secondary to chemotherapeutic agents.

E

Equipment	No issues.
Emergencies and urgent care	Be prepared to manage airway obstruction secondary to macroglossia with MM; also potential for excessive bleeding during invasive procedures if patient has concurrent thrombocytopenia

POSTOPERATIVE CARE

F
Follow-up care
- Follow-up evaluation during hospitalization to ensure oral health and minimize the discomfort of mucositis is recommended. After hospitalization, routine follow-up is recommended pending determination of medical stability in consultation with patient's physician.

[a]*Strength of recommendation taxonomy (SORT) Grade: C (see Preface for further explanation).*
ANC, absolute neutrophil count; *MM*, multiple myeloma; *NSAID*, nonsteroidal antiinflammatory drug.

BIBLIOGRAPHY

1. Albagoush SA, Azevedo AM. Multiple myeloma. In: *StatPearls*. Treasure Island (FL): StatPearls Publishing; 2021.

2. Appelbaum FR. The acute leukemias. In: Goldman L, Ausiello D, eds. *Cecil Medicine*. 23rd ed. Philadelphia, PA: Saunders; 2008:1390–1396.

3. Kumar V, Abbas A, Aster J. Diseases of white blood cells, lymph nodes, spleen and thymus. In: Kumar V, Abbas A, Aster J, eds. *Robbins and Cotran Pathologic Basis of Disease*. 10th ed. Philadelphia: Elsevier; 2021:583–633.

4. Aster JC, Fleming M. Introduction to hematologic malignancies. In: Aster JC, Bunn HF, eds. *Pathophysiology of Blood Disorders*. 2nd ed. New York: McGraw Hill Education; 2017:1–12.

5. Bagby G. Leukopenia and leukocytosis. In: Goldman L, Ausiello D, eds. *Cecil Medicine*. 23rd ed. Philadelphia, PA: Saunders; 2008:1252–1263.

6. Barosi G, Boccadoro M, Cavo M, et al. Management of multiple myeloma and related disorders: guidelines from the Italian Society of Hematology (SIE), Italian Society of Experimental Hematology (SIES) and Italian Group for Bone Marrow Transplantation (GITMO). *Haematologica*. 2004;89:717–741.

7. Baz R, Bolwell B. Multiple myeloma. In: Carey WD, ed. *Current Clinical Medicine 2009—Cleveland Clinic*. Philadelphia: Elsevier Saunders; 2009:647–654.

8. Bejar R, Steensma DP. Recent developments in myelodysplastic syndromes. *Blood*. 2014;124:2793–2803.

9. Bhatia R, Radich J. Chronic myeloid leukemia. In: Hoffman R, Benz E, Shattil S, et al., eds. *Hematology: Basic Principles and Practice*. 5th ed. Philadelphia, PA: Churchill Livingstone; 2009:1109–1124.

10. Bierman P, Armitage J. Non-Hodgkin's lymphoma. In: Goldman L, Schafer A, eds. *Goldman's Cecil Medicine*. 24th ed. Philadelphia: Saunders Elsevier; 2012:1218–1228.

11. Blum W, Bloomfield CD. Acute myeloid leukemia. In: Jameson J, Fauci S, Kasper D, Hauser S, Longo D, Loscalzo J, eds. *Harrison's Principles of Internal Medicine, 20e*. 20e. New York: McGraw Hill; 2018:1–21.

12. Brice P, de Kerviler E, Friedberg JW. Classical hodgkin lymphoma. *Lancet*. 2021;398:1518–1527.

13. Burkitt DP. The discovery of Burkitt's lymphoma. *Cancer*. 1983;51:1777–1786.

14. Casulo C, Friedberg JW. Burkitt lymphoma—a rare but challenging lymphoma. *Best Pract Res Clin Haematol*. 2018;31:279–284.

15. Choi DK, Schmidt ML. Chemotherapy in children with head and neck cancers: perspectives and review of current therapies. *Oral Maxillofac Surg Clin N Am*. 2016;28:127–138.

16. Connors J. Hodgkin's lymphoma. In: Goldman L, Ausiello D, eds. *Cecil Medicine*. 23rd ed. Philadelphia: Elsevier Saunders; 2008:1420–1425.

17. Dechartres A, Chevret S, Lambert J, et al. Inclusion of patients with acute leukemia in clinical trials: a prospective multicenter survey of 1066 cases. *Ann Oncol*. 2011;22:224–233.

18. Dentistry AAoP. Guideline on dental management of pediatric patients receiving chemotherapy, hematopoietic cell transplantation, and/or radiation. *Pediatr Dent*. 2013;35:E185–E193.

19. Smith K, Chiu A, Parikh R, Yahalom J, Younes A. Hodgkin lymphoma: clinical manifestations, staging and therapy. In: Hoffman R, Benz E, Silberstein L, et al., eds. *Hematology: Basic Principles and Practice*. 7th ed. Philadelphia: Elsevier; 2018:1212–1229.

20. Dunleavy K, Wilson W. Diagnosis and treatment of non-Hodgkin lymphoma. In: Hoffman R, Benz E, Shattil S, et al., eds. *Hematology: Basic Principles and Practice*. 5th ed. Philadelphia, PA: Churchill Livingstone; 2009:1293–1301.

21. Ferri FF. Leukemia, acute. In: Ferri FF, ed. *Ferri's Clinical Advisor*. Philadelphia, PA: Elsevier (Saunders); 2015:688–701.

22. Ferri FF. Leukemia, chronic. In: Ferri FF, ed. *Ferri's Clinical Advisor*. 13th ed. Philadelphia, PA: Elsevier (Saunders); 2015:694–700.

23. Ferri FF. Lymphoma, non-Hodgkin. In: Ferri FF, ed. *Ferri's Clinical Advisor*. 13th ed. Philadelphia, PA: Elsevier (Saunders); 2015:715–720.

24. Ferri FF. Multiple myeloma. In: Ferri FF, ed. *Ferri's Clinical Advisor*. 13th ed. Philadelphia, PA: Elsevier (Saunders); 2015:783–790.

25. Filleul O, Crompot E, Saussez S. Bisphosphonate-induced osteonecrosis of the jaw: a review of 2,400 patient cases. *J Cancer Res Clin Oncol*. 2010;136:1117–1124.

26. Gribben J. Clinical manifestations, staging, and treatment of indolent non-Hodgkin lymphoma. In: Hoffman R, Benz E, Shattil S, et al., eds. *Hematology: Basic Principles and Practice*. 5th ed. Philadelphia, PA: Churchill Livingstone; 2009:1281–1292.

27. Hallek M, Shanafelt TD, Eichhorst B. Chronic lymphocytic leukaemia. *Lancet*. 2018;391:1524–1537.

28. Helby J, Bojesen SE, Nielsen SF, et al. IgE and risk of cancer in 37,747 individuals from the general population. *Ann Oncol*. 2015;26:1784–1790.

29. Hoelzer D. Acute lymphoid leukemia. In: Jameson J, Fauci A, Kasper D, Hauser S, Longo D, Loscalzo J, eds. *Harrison's Principles of Internal Medicine, 20e*. New York: McGraw Hill; 2018:1–13.

30. Jacobson CA, Longo DL. Hodgkin's lymphoma. In: Jameson J, Fauci A, Kasper D, Hauser S, Longo D, Loscalzo J, eds. *Harrison's Principles of Internal Medicine, 20e*. New York: McGraw Hill; 2018:1–7.

31. Jacobson CA, Longo DL. Non-Hodgkin's lymphoma. In: Jameson J, Fauci A, Kasper D, Hauser S, Longo D, Loscalzo J, eds. *Harrison's Principles of Internal Medicine, 20e*. New York: McGraw Hill; 2018:1–22.

32. Kantarjian H, Cortes J. Chronic myeloid leukemia. In: Jameson J, Fauci A, Kasper D, Hauser S, Longo D, Loscalzo J, eds. *Harrison's Principles of Internal Medicine, 20e*. New York: McGraw Hill; 2018:1–18.

33. Kantarjian H, Shah NP, Hochhaus A, et al. Dasatinib versus imatinib in newly diagnosed chronic-phase chronic myeloid leukemia. *N Engl J Med*. 2010;362:2260–2270.

34. Kasamon YL, Swinnen LJ. Treatment advances in adult Burkitt lymphoma and leukemia. *Curr Opin Oncol*. 2004;16:429–435.

35. Kinane D. Blood and lymphoreticular disorders. *Periodontology*. 2000;21:84–93.

36. Leukemia & Lymphoma Society. *Updated Data on Blood Cancers. Facts 2020-2021*; 2021. https://www.lls.org. Accessed November 15, 2021.

37. Leukemia & Lymphoma Society. *Acute Promyelocytic Leukemia Facts*; 2021. https://www.lls.org. Accessed November 15, 2021.

38. Lewis WD, Lilly S, Jones KL. Lymphoma: diagnosis and treatment. *Am Fam Physician.* 2020;101:34−41.

39. Awan F, Byrd J. Chronic lymphocytic leukemia. In: Hoffman R, Benz E, Silberstein L, et al., eds. *Hematology: Basic Principles and Practice.* 7th ed. Philadelphia: Elsevier; 2018:1244−1264.

40. Lipton A. Bone continuum of cancer. *Am J Clin Oncol.* 2010;33(3 suppl):S1−S7.

41. Malard F, Mohty M. Acute lymphoblastic leukaemia. *Lancet.* 2020;395:1146−1162.

42. Mattsson U, Halbritter S, Mörner Serikoff E, et al. Oral pigmentation in the hard palate associated with imatinib mesylate therapy: a report of three cases. *Oral Surg Oral Med Oral Pathol Oral Radiol Endod.* 2011;111:e12−e16.

43. Migliorati CA, Siegel MA, Elting LS. Bisphosphonate-associated osteonecrosis: a long-term complication of bisphosphonate treatment. *Lancet Oncol.* 2006;7:508−514.

44. Miller K, Pihan G. Clinical manifestations of acute myeloid leukemia. In: Hoffman R, Furie B, McGlave P, et al., eds. *Hematology: Basic Principles and Practice.* 5th ed. Philadelphia, PA: Churchill Livingstone; 2009:933−964.

45. Munshi NC, Longo DL, Anderson KC. Plasma cell disorders. In: Jameson J, Fauci A, Kasper D, Hauser S, Longo D, Loscalzo J, eds. *Harrison's Principles of Internal Medicine, 20e.* New York: McGraw Hill; 2018:1−19.

46. Neville BW. Hematologic disorders. In: Neville BW, Dam DD, Allen CM, et al., eds. *Oral and Maxillofacial Pathology.* 3rd ed. St. Louis: Elsevier Saunders; 2009:571−612.

47. Pau M, Beham-Schmid C, Zemann W, et al. Intraoral granulocytic sarcoma: a case report and review of the literature. *J Oral Maxillofac Surg.* 2010;68:2569−2574.

48. Piris MA, Medeiros LJ, Chang KC. Hodgkin lymphoma: a review of pathological features and recent advances in pathogenesis. *Pathology.* 2020;52:154−165.

49. Quesenberry P. Hematopoiesis and hematopoietic growth factors. In: Goldman L, Ausiello D, eds. *Cecil Medicine.* 23rd ed. Philadelphia, PA: Saunders; 2008:1165−1172.

50. Dinner S, Gurbuxani S, Jain N, Stock W, et al. Acute lymphoblastic leukemia in adults. In: Hoffman R, Benz E, Silberstein L, et al., eds. *Hematology: Basic Principles and Practice.* 7th ed. Philadelphia: Elsevier; 2018:1029−1054.e2.

51. Rajkumar SV, Kyle RA. Plasma cell disorders. In: Goldman L, Ausiello D, eds. *Cecil Medicine.* 23rd ed. Philadelphia: Elsevier Saunders; 2008:1426−1436.

52. Rajkumar SV. Multiple myeloma: 2020 update on diagnosis, risk-stratification and management. *Am J Hematol.* 2020;95:548−567.

53. Raut A, Huryn J, Pollack A, et al. Unusual gingival presentation of post-transplantation lymphoproliferative disorder: a case report and review of the literature. *Oral Surg Oral Med Oral Pathol Oral Radiol Endod.* 2000;90:436−441.

54. Sampaio MM, Santos MLC, Marques HS, et al. Chronic myeloid leukemia-from the Philadelphia chromosome to specific target drugs: a literature review. *World J Clin Oncol.* 2021;12:69−94.

55. Sandlund J, Link M. Malignant lymphomas in childhood. In: Hoffman R, Benz E, Shattil S, et al., eds. *Hematology: Basic Principles and Practice.* 5th ed. Philadelphia, PA: Churchill Livingstone; 2009:1303−1317.

56. Sankar V, Villa A. Hematologic diseases. In: Glick M, Greenberg MS, Lockhart PB, Challacombe SJ, eds. *Burket's Oral Medicine.* 13th ed. Hoboken: John Wiley & Sons, Inc.; 2021:627−664.

57. Short NJ, Rytting ME, Cortes JE. Acute myeloid leukaemia. *Lancet.* 2018;392:593−606.

58. Traer E, Deininger MW. How much and how long: tyrosine kinase inhibitor therapy in chronic myeloid leukemia. *Clin Lymphoma, Myeloma & Leukemia.* 2010;10(suppl 1):S20−S26.

59. Tricot G. Multiple myeloma. In: Hoffman R, ed. *Hematology: Basic Principles and Practice.* 5th ed. Philadelphia: Churchill Livingstone, Elsevier; 2009:1387−1412.

60. van de Donk NWCJ, Pawlyn C, Yong KL. Multiple myeloma. *Lancet.* 2021;397:410−427.

61. Walter C, Al-Nawas B, Frickhofen N, et al. Prevalence of bisphosphonate associated osteonecrosis of the jaws in multiple myeloma patients. *Head Face Med.* 2010;6:11.

62. Woyach JA, Byrd JC. Chronic lymphocytic leukemia. In: Jameson J, Fauci A, Kasper D, Hauser S, Longo D, Loscalzo J, eds. *Harrison's Principles of Internal Medicine, 20e.* New York: McGraw Hill; 2018:1−13.

63. Yee KW, O'Brien SM. Chronic lymphocytic leukemia: diagnosis and treatment. *Mayo Clin Proc.* 2006;81:1105−1129.

64. Zenz T, Frohling S, Mertens D, et al. Moving from prognostic to predictive factors in chronic lymphocytic leukaemia (CLL). *Best Pract Res Clin Haematol.* 2010;23:71−84.

Acquired Bleeding Disorders

Bleeding disorders are conditions that alter the ability of blood vessels, platelets, and/or coagulation factors to achieve hemostasis. Acquired bleeding disorders may occur as the result of diseases, drugs, or cancer treatments in which vascular wall integrity, platelet production or function, or coagulation factor production or activity are impaired. Many procedures that are performed in dentistry may cause bleeding, and under normal circumstances, these procedures can be performed with little clinical risk; however, in patients with acquired bleeding disorders, such procedures may be associated with serious outcomes unless the dental practitioner identifies the potential problem before initiation of treatment. This chapter presents an overview of the physiologic mechanisms involved in hemostasis, along with the epidemiology and pathophysiology of acquired bleeding disorders, and considerations for the dental management of these patients. It is estimated that in a dental practice of 2000 adults, about 100–150 patients have an acquired bleeding disorder.

EPIDEMIOLOGY

An estimated 8 million Americans are taking medications that alter hemostasis including patients on continuous antiplatelet or anticoagulation therapy to prevent/treat thromboembolic events including stroke, myocardial infarction, venous thromboembolism, or for the complications of atrial fibrillation, cardiac valve or percutaneously placed coronary stents, and other conditions. The prevalence of immune thrombocytopenia purpura, the most common type of acquired thrombocytopenia, is about 10 in 100,000 people. Other populations with acquired bleeding disorders include patients with liver

and kidney diseases (covered in Chapters 10 and 12, respectively), patients with certain types of cancer (e.g., leukemia), or undergoing chemotherapy for cancer (covered in Chapters 23 and 26, respectively). Other acquired bleeding disorders are rarely encountered in dental practice (see classification of acquired bleeding disorders in Box 24.1).

ETIOLOGY

Normal hemostasis is the result of a complex and highly regulated cascade of interactions. Pathologic perturbations in one or more of these interactions may result in bleeding. Bleeding disorders have diverse etiologies based on three categories: acquired vascular, platelet, or coagulation disorders (Box 24.1).

Pathophysiology

An appreciation of the pathophysiology underlying acquired bleeding disorders requires an understanding of normal hemostasis. Hemostasis involves an elaborately controlled balance between anticoagulant and procoagulant activity. The hemostatic system precisely responds to varying degrees of tissue injury (i.e., superficial wounds affecting smaller vessels, to severe and deep injuries affecting larger vessels). The degree of such tissue injury will dictate the blend of three overlapping mechanisms, namely vasoconstriction, formation of a platelet plug, and activation of the coagulation pathway leading to a fibrin clot. One additional mechanism occurs after hemostasis, i.e., fibrinolysis (Box 24.2).

Vascular wall integrity is critical for maintaining the fluidity of blood. The innermost layer, the vascular intima, is lined with a metabolically active endothelial cells

BOX 24.1 Classification of Acquired Bleeding Disorders

Vascular Disorders
Palpable noninflammatory vascular purpuras
    Dysproteinemias
    Thrombotic
    Embolic
    Arthropod bites
Palpable and nonpalpable inflammatory vascular purpuras
    Pyoderma gangrenosum
    Sweet syndrome
    Behçet disease
    Serum sickness
    Henoch—Schönlein purpura
    Infections
    Erythema multiforme
    Cutaneous polyarteritis nodosum
    Paraneoplastic vasculitis
    Drug-induced vasculitis
    Antineutrophilic cytoplasmic antibody—associated vasculitides
Nonpalpable inflammatory vascular purpuras
    Increased transmural pressure gradient and trauma
    Drug reactions
    Coagulation disorders
    Decreased vessel integrity without trauma
1. Senile purpura
2. Excess glucocorticoid (Cushing syndrome, glucocorticoid treatment)
3. Scurvy—vitamin C deficiency
4. Systemic amyloidosis
    Waldenström hypergammaglobulinemic purpura

Acquired Platelet Disorders
Acquired thrombocytopenia
Pseudo (spurious) thrombocytopenia
    Antibody-induced platelet aggregation
    Platelet satellitism
    Antiphospholipid antibodies
    Glycoprotein IIb/IIIa antagonists

Thrombocytopenia resulting from impaired platelet production
Acquired bone marrow disorders
  1. Nutritional deficiencies and alcohol-induced thrombocytopenia
  2. Clonal hematologic diseases (myelodysplastic syndrome, leukemias, myeloma, lymphoma, paroxysmal nocturnal hemoglobinuria)
  3. Aplastic anemia
  4. Marrow metastasis by solid tumors
  5. Marrow infiltration by infectious agents (e.g., HIV, tuberculosis, brucellosis)
  6. Hemophagocytosis
  7. Immune thrombocytopenia
  8. Drug-induced thrombocytopenia
  9. Pregnancy-related thrombocytopenia
Thrombocytopenia resulting from increased platelet destruction
  Immune thrombocytopenia (ITP)
1. Autoimmune thrombocytopenia (primary and secondary ITP)
2. Alloimmune thrombocytopenia
    Thrombotic microangiopathies (thrombotic thrombocytopenic purpura, hemolytic uremic syndrome)
    Disseminated intravascular coagulopathy
    Pregnancy-related thrombocytopenia
    Hemangiomas (Kasabach—Merritt phenomenon)

Drug-induced immune thrombocytopenia (quinidine, heparin, abciximab)
    Artificial surfaces (hemodialysis, cardiopulmonary bypass, extracorporeal membrane oxygenation)
Thrombocytopenia resulting from abnormal distribution of the platelets
    Hypersplenism
    Hypothermia
    Massive blood transfusions
    Excessive fluid infusions
Miscellaneous causes
    Cyclic thrombocytopenia, acquired pure megakaryocytic thrombocytopenia

Acquired Qualitative Platelet Disorders
Drugs that affect platelet function
    Aspirin and other nonsteroidal antiinflammatory drugs
    $P2Y_{12}$ antagonists
    PAR1 thrombin receptor antagonist
    Glycoprotein IIb/IIIa receptor antagonists
    Drugs that increase platelet cyclic adenosine monophosphate
    Antibiotics
    Anticoagulants and fibrinolytic agents
    Cardiovascular drugs (nitrates and calcium antagonists [at high doses])
    Volume expanders
    Psychotropic agents
    Anesthetics
    Oncologic drugs
Hematologic disorders associated with abnormal platelet function
    Chronic myeloproliferative neoplasms
    Leukemias and myelodysplastic syndromes
    Dysproteinemias
    Acquired von Willebrand disease
Systemic disorders associated with abnormal platelet function
    Uremia
    Antiplatelet antibodies
    Cardiopulmonary bypass
    Chronic liver disease
    Disseminated intravascular coagulation
    HIV Infection

Acquired Coagulation Disorders
Anticoagulation drugs
    Heparin
    Low-molecular-weight heparins
    Synthetic heparin
    Warfarin
    Direct thrombin inhibitors
Fibrinolytic drugs
    Alteplase
    Reteplase
    Tenecteplase
Trauma-induced coagulopathy
Liver disease
Chronic renal failure
Vitamin K—associated disorders
    Vitamin K deficiency
Autoantifactor VIII inhibitor and acquired hemophilia
Acquired von Willebrand disease
Disseminated intravascular coagulation

Adapted from Alexandrescu DT, Marcel Levi M. The vascular purpuras; Kaushansky K. Thrombocytopenia; Levi M. Acquired qualitative platelet disorders. In: Kaushansky K, Prchal JT, Burns LJ, et al., eds. *Williams Hematology, 10e.* McGraw Hill; 2021. Fritsma GA. Hemorrhagic disorders and their laboratory assessment. In: Keohane EM, Otto CN, Walenga JM, eds. *Rodak's Hematology, Clinical Principles and Applications.* 6th ed. St. Louis: Saunders, Elsevier; 2020.

BOX 24.2 Normal Control of Bleeding

1. Vascular phase:
   a. Vasoconstriction occurs in area of injury, and increase in extravascular pressure.
   b. Begins immediately after injury.
2. Platelet phase:
   a. Platelets and vessel wall become "sticky" and adhere.
   b. Activation and aggregation of platelets results in formation of a mechanical plug and scaffold for coagulation.
   c. Begins seconds after injury.
3. Coagulation phase:
   a. The initiation of coagulation occurs at the site of injury via the tissue factor pathway (extrinsic pathway).
   b. Propagation of coagulation via the tissue factor pathway then activates the intrinsic pathway which more strongly activates factor X to form thrombin.
   c. Final coagulation to produce the fibrin clots occurs through the common pathway.
   d. Takes place more slowly than other phases.
4. Fibrinolytic phase:
   a. Release of plasminogen which is converted to plasmin on the clot.
   b. Plasmin cleaves and dissolves the fibrin into fibrin degradation products.

that under normal conditions has vasodilatory, antiplatelet, and anticoagulant properties. Endothelial cells produce nitric oxide, which leads to vasodilation, and prostacyclin, which inhibits platelets. They also produce and express heparan sulfate, thrombomodulin, and endothelial protein C receptor (EPCR), which collectively inhibit thrombin formation. Finally, they produce tissue factor pathway inhibitor (TFPI), which is potent anticoagulant of the tissue factor pathway (also known as the extrinsic pathway). Most importantly, the endothelial cell layer acts as a barrier to the exposure of the blood to deeper subendothelial structures that have strong procoagulant properties.

Immediately following tissue injury, there is vasoconstriction of larger vessels (i.e., arteries and arterioles) and an increase of extravascular pressure from the blood escaping cut vessels. This pressure aids in collapsing the adjacent capillaries and veins, facilitating a number of proplatelet (primary hemostasis) and procoagulant (secondary hemostasis) mechanisms, the latter of which is more important for larger vessel injuries where a stronger clot is required.

Platelets are cellular fragments from the cytoplasm of megakaryocytes that last 8–12 days in the circulation. About 30% of platelets are sequestered in the microvasculature or spleen and serve as a functional reserve. Aged or nonviable platelets are removed and destroyed by the

spleen and liver. Box 24.3 summarizes the functions of platelets.

The steps in platelet plug formation include adhesion, activation, aggregation, and secretion. Following injury, exposure of blood to subendothelial connective tissue (i.e., collagen) promotes initial platelet adhesion particularly in low flow areas. Such injury causes endothelial cells to synthesize and secrete von Willebrand factor (vWF), which promotes platelet adhesion particularly in high flow injury sites. Endothelial cells also express adhesion molecules (i.e., P-selectin, intercellular adhesion molecules (ICAMs), and platelet endothelial adhesion molecules (PEAMs)), which further effect initial communication with blood components (i.e., white blood cells and platelets). Platelet surface glycoproteins Ia/IIa (GPIa/IIa) and VI (GPVI) bind to collagen in the injured vessel wall, and glycoproteins Ib (GPIb), IX (GPIX), and V (GPV) bind to vWF. These adhesion mechanisms lead to platelet activation leading to expression of other glycoproteins on the surface of the platelets (GPIIb/IIIa), which in turn allow binding of fibrinogen, vWF, and other binding proteins. Subsequently, these activated platelets secrete granules containing a number of procoagulants including adenosine diphosphate (ADP), serotonin, Ca^{2+}, β-thromboglobulin, factor V, factor XI, fibrinogen, vWF, protein S, platelet factor 4, and platelet-derived growth factor, all of which further stimulate platelet aggregation. ADP and Ca^{2+} activate phospholipase A_2, which converts membrane phospholipids into arachidonic acid. Cyclo-oxygenase then converts the arachidonic acid to prostaglandin G_2 and H_2. Thromboxane synthetase then converts these prostaglandins into thromboxane A_2, which mediates the release of Ca^{2+}, a strong promoter of further aggregation. The activated platelet surface is ideally suited for the coagulation pathways to occur resulting in the formation of a fibrin-clot.

The coagulation pathways are depicted in Fig. 24.1. For coagulation to work there must be sufficient production of thrombin, which catalyzes the final step in the formation of the clot, the conversion of fibrinogen to fibrin (Figs. 24.2 and 24.3). Thrombin is generated via two interconnected pathways, the "tissue factor" pathway (traditionally referred to as the extrinsic pathway) and the "intrinsic" pathway. These two pathways flow into a "common" pathway. There are numerous coagulation factors involved (see Table 24.1), and many are proenzyme zymogens (serine proteases) that become activated in a cascade manner—that is, one factor becomes activated, and it in turn activates another, and so forth in an ordered sequence. A factor that has been activated is denoted with an "a" suffix (i.e., factor VIIa).

BOX 24.3   Platelet Functions and Activation

1. Plasma membrane receptors:
   a. Glycoprotein Ia/IIa and VI binds to collagen in the injured vessel wall.
   b. Glycoproteins Ib, V, and IX bind to von Willebrand factor, which attaches to subendothelial tissue.
   c. Glycoproteins IIb and IIIa attach to fibrinogen, vWF, or other binding proteins.
2. Platelets contain three types of secretory granules:
   a. Lysosomes.
   b. Alpha granules—contain platelet factor 4; β-thromboglobulin; and several growth factors, including platelet-derived growth factor (PDGF), endothelial cell growth factor (PD-ECGF), and transforming growth factor-β (TGF-β); also several hemostatic proteins: fibrinogen, factor V, and von Willebrand factor.
   c. Dense bodies (electron-dense organelles)—contain ATP, ADP, calcium, and serotonin.
3. Platelets provide a surface for activation of soluble coagulation factors:
   a. Activated platelets expose specific receptors that bind factors Xa and Va, thus increasing their local concentration, thereby accelerating prothrombin activation.
   b. Factor X also is activated by factors IXa and VIII on the surface of the platelet.
4. Platelets contain a membrane phospholipase C:
   a. When activated, it forms diglyceride.
   b. Diglyceride is converted to arachidonic acid by diglyceride lipase.
   c. Arachidonic acid is a substrate for prostaglandin synthetase (COX).
   d. COX formation is inhibited by aspirin and NSAIDs.
   e. The prostaglandin endoperoxide PGG_2 is required for ADP-induced aggregation and release, as is thromboxane A_2. The formation of both of these agents is dependent on COX.
5. The functions of platelets include:
   a. Nurturing endothelial cells.
   b. Endothelial and smooth muscle regeneration.
   c. Formation of a platelet plug for initial control of bleeding.
   d. Stabilization of the platelet plug.

ADP, adenosine diphosphate; *ATP,* adenosine triphosphate; *COX,* cyclooxygenase; *NSAID,* nonsteroidal antiinflammatory drug.

Adapted from McMillan R. Hemorrhagic disorders: abnormalities of platelet and vascular function. In: Goldman L, Ausiello D, eds. *Cecil Medicine.* 23rd ed. Philadelphia: Saunders; 2008 and Baz R, Mekhail T. Disorders of platelet function and number. In: Carey WD, et al., eds. *Current Clinical Medicine 2009—Cleveland Clinic.* Philadelphia: Saunders; 2009.

The extrinsic pathway is initially triggered by the binding of factor VII to tissue factor expressed at the site of injury, followed by activation of factors IX and X to cleave prothrombin and generate a small amount of thrombin. This initiates coagulation by activating platelets, factors V, VIII, and XI, and initiates fibrin production. The propagation phase to generate the remaining thrombin required for clot formation ensues on the surface of the aggregated platelets: Factors Va and VIIIa bind to platelets and serve as receptors for IXa and Xa. In the intrinsic pathway, IXa binds to its cofactor VIIIa which activates circulating factor X. This "intrinsic" pathway can activate factor X at 50–100 times the rate of the extrinsic pathway. More factor IXa is also generated via XIa. Activation of the intrinsic pathway may also be mediated by a "contact factor complex" mediated by factor XII, Fitzgerald factor (HMWK), and Fletcher factor (pre-K) (HMWK:pre-K:factor XIIa) precipitated by exposure of blood to foreign materials (e.g., stents). The extrinsic and intrinsic pathways converge into the "common pathway." Factor Va binds Xa to form prothrombinase which generates the remaining thrombin needed to form the clot. Factor XIII further stabilizes the fibrin clot. The time from injury to a fibrin-stabilized clot is about 9–18 min.

Factors II (prothrombin), VII, IX, and X (and the regulatory proteins limiting clot propagation: protein C, protein S, and protein Z) are part of the prothrombin group and dependent on vitamin K, which catalyzes an important posttranslational step in their synthesis, γ-carboxylation of amino-terminal glutamic acids. Vitamin K is present in green leafy vegetables and is also generated by intestinal bacteria *Bacteroides fragilis* and *Escherichia coli.* Without vitamin K, these factors cannot bind to Ca^{2+} and this prevents formation of the membrane-bound complexes. This is the basis for the mechanism of action of the anticoagulant warfarin, which is a vitamin K antagonist.

Built-in negative feedback mechanisms help prevent clot formation in the healthy uninjured state and clot propagation beyond the injured area. A number of anticoagulants mediate this process, principally tissue factor pathway inhibitor (TFPI), antithrombin (AT), and activated protein C (APC). TFPI is produced by endothelial cells and inactivates Xa. Following coagulation initiation, AT binds and neutralizes serine proteases (thrombin, IXa, Xa, XIa, XIIa, pre-K, and plasmin). Its activity is greatly enhanced by heparin (produced de novo or from heparan sulfate by endothelial cells). In conjunction with protein S, APC neutralizes Va and VIIIa. Other anticoagulants include protein Z protease inhibitor (ZPI), protein C inhibitor, α-1 antitrypsin, α-2 macroglobulin, α-2 antiplasmin, and plasminogen activator inhibitor-1.

The fibrinolytic system begins to mobilize as the clot forms in order to prevent coagulation propagation away from the site of injury. Fibrinolysis is important for dissolving the clot after it has served its function in hemostasis (Box 24.4). The fibrinolytic system involves plasminogen, a proenzyme for the enzyme plasmin, which is produced in the liver, and various plasminogen activators and inhibitors of plasmin. Circulating plasminogen binds to fibrin but requires tissue plasminogen activator (tPA) to activate the conversion of plasminogen

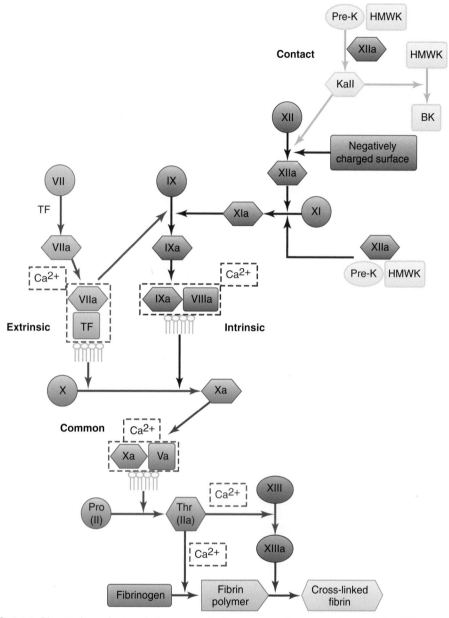

FIG. 24.1 Plasma-based coagulation cascade. The coagulation cascade consists of the contact system (simplified here) and the intrinsic, extrinsic, and common pathways. In the intrinsic pathway (*red*), the contact factors XII, prekallikrein (pre-K), and high-molecular-weight kininogen (HMWK) are activated and proceed to activate factors XI, IX, VIII, X, and V and prothrombin, which converts fibrinogen to fibrin. In the extrinsic pathway (*green*), tissue factor (TF) activates factor VII, which activates factors X, V, and prothrombin, cleaving fibrinogen to fibrin. Both the intrinsic and extrinsic pathways converge with the activation of factor X, so factors X, V, prothrombin, and fibrinogen are called the common pathway (*blue*). *Dashed* boxes indicate the coagulation factor complexes that assemble on phospholipid (*yellow* symbol). These pathways are the basis of clinical coagulation laboratory tests. Thr, Thrombin. (From Keohane EM, Otto CN, Walenga JM, eds. *Rodak's Hematology, Clinical Principles and Applications*. 6th ed. St. Louis: Saunders, Elsevier; 2020:626–649.)

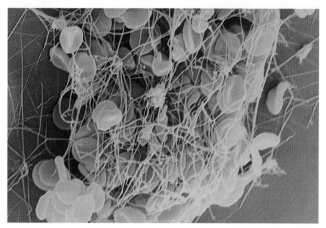

FIG. 24.2 A blood clot or thrombus, showing blood cells trapped by fibrin strands (scanning electron microscope photograph). (From Stevens ML. *Fundamentals of Clinical Hematology.* Philadelphia: WB Saunders; 1997.)

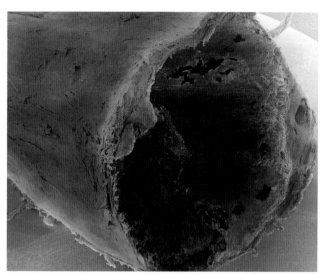

FIG. 24.3 A colored scanning electron micrograph of a blood clot or thrombus inside the coronary artery of a human heart. (Reprinted with permission of P. M. Motta, G. Macchiarelli, S. A. Nottola/Photo Researchers, Inc.)

TABLE 24.1	Blood Coagulation Components	
Factor	**Deficiency**	**Function**
Factor II (prothrombin)	Acquired—common	Protease zymogen
Factor X	Acquired—common	Protease zymogen
Factor IX	Acquired—common	Protease zymogen
Factor VII	Acquired—common	Protease zymogen
Factor VIII	Acquired—rare	Cofactor
Factor V	Acquired—rare	Cofactor
Factor XI	Acquired—common	Protease zymogen
Factor I (fibrinogen)	Acquired—common	Structural
von Willebrand factor	Acquired—rare	Adhesion

From McVey JH. Coagulation factors. In: Young NS, Gerson SL, High KA, eds. *Clinical Hematology.* St. Louis: Elsevier; 2006.

BOX 24.4 Fibrin-Lysing (Fibrinolytic) System

1. Activation of coagulation also activates fibrinolysis.
2. Active enzyme: plasmin.
3. Plasminogen activated to plasmin:
   a. Tissue-type plasminogen activator (t-PA).
   b. Prourokinase (scu-PA).
   c. Urokinase (u-PA), streptokinase.
4. t-PA:
   a. t-PA is produced by endothelial cells.
   b. It is released by injury.
   c. It activates plasminogen bound to fibrin.
   d. Circulating plasminogen is not activated.
   e. t-PA will dissolve clot, not cause systemic fibrinolysis.
5. Action of plasmin:
   a. Plasmin splits large pieces of alpha and beta polypeptides from fibrin.
   b. It splits small pieces of gamma chains.
   c. First product is X monomer.
   d. Each X monomer splits into one E fragment and two D fragments.
   e. Split products are called fibrin split products (FSPs) and fibrin degradation products (FDPs).
6. Action of fibrin degradation products:
   a. Increase vascular permeability.
   b. Interfere with thrombin-induced fibrin formation.

Data from Lijnen HR, Collen D. Molecular and cellular basis of fibrinolysis. In: Hoffman R, et al., eds. *Hematology: Basic Principles and Practice.* Philadelphia: Churchill Livingstone; 2009 and Kessler CM. Hemorrhagic disorders: coagulation factor deficiencies. In: Goldman L, Ausiello D, eds. *Cecil Textbook of Medicine.* 23rd ed. Philadelphia: Saunders; 2008.

to plasmin. tPA is the primary endogenous activator of the fibrinolysis system. It is released by endothelial cells at the site of injury and also binds to fibrin. The effect of plasmin on fibrin is to split off large pieces that are then broken up into smaller and smaller segments. The final smaller pieces are called *split products*, also referred to as *fibrin degradation products* (FDPs). FDPs further promote binding of plasminogen and tPA and augment fibrinolysis. Circulating antiplasmin factors rapidly destroy free plasmin but are relatively ineffective against plasmin that is bound to fibrin and therefore does not interfere with the initial formation of a clot.

CLINICAL PRESENTATION

Signs and Symptoms

Signs associated with acquired bleeding disorders may be mucocutaneous or involve deeper structures. Acquired bleeding disorders affecting platelet formation (i.e., primary hemostasis) may lead to an immediate clinical bleeding problem after an invasive dental procedure or surgery. However, for some surgical procedures where primary hemostatic mechanisms alone are insufficient to stop bleeding and secondary hemostasis (i.e.,

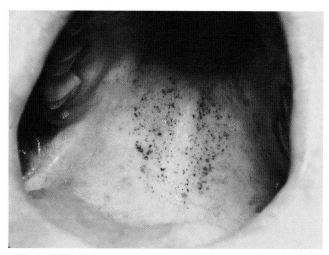

FIG. 24.4 Palatal petechiae in a patient with leukemia. (From Hoffbrand AV. *Color Atlas of Clinical Hematology.* 3rd ed. St. Louis: Mosby; 2000.)

coagulation) is abnormal, the bleeding problem may not appear until several hours or longer after the surgical procedure. If the coagulation defect is severe, this slow loss of blood can, in some cases, continue for days. Even with this "trivial" rate, significant loss of blood may occur (0.5 mL/min or about 2 units of blood/day).

Petechiae (Fig. 24.4), purpura, or ecchymosis (Fig. 24.5) are the mucocutaneous signs most commonly observed in patients with acquired thrombocytopenia, qualitative platelet disorders (i.e., primary hemostatic disorders), or acquired vascular disorders (see Box 24.1). Other signs include spontaneous or prolonged gingival bleeding, epistaxis, hematemesis, hematuria, or hematochezia, or profuse menstrual bleeding. Bleeding within deeper structures such as joints (hemarthrosis) or other compartments or prolonged or delayed bleeding following surgical procedures such as dental extractions may be indicative of an acquired coagulopathy (i.e., secondary hemostatic disorder). Bleeding involving

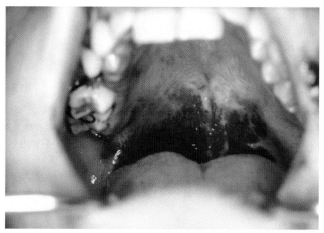

FIG. 24.5 Ecchymoses on the mucosa of the hard and soft palate in a patient with chronic liver disease.

deeper structures or organs may lead to specific functional changes (e.g., headache, confusion, or seizures). Severe or chronic bleeding may result in anemia with features of pallor and fatigue.

Laboratory and Diagnostic Findings

Several tests are available to screen patients for bleeding disorders and to help identify the specific defect. In general, screening is performed when a patient reveals a history of a bleeding problem (or a family history of a bleeding problem), or when signs or symptoms of bleeding disorders are discovered during a visit.

Tests recommended for use in the initial screening for possible acquired bleeding disorders include complete blood count, activated partial thromboplastin time (aPTT), prothrombin time (PT), and thrombin time (TT) (also known as thrombin clotting time) (Fig. 24.6). Patients with positive screening test results should be evaluated further, typically by a hematologist, to identify the specific disorder. As an important component of the complete blood count, the platelet count (normal range: 150,000 to 450,000/μL of blood) provides insight as to risk of bleeding. For example, patients with a platelet count of between 50,000 and 100,000/μL manifest excessive bleeding only with severe trauma. Patients with counts below 50,000/μL may bleed excessively with minor trauma. Patients with platelet counts below 20,000/μL may experience spontaneous bleeding. The hematocrit, hemoglobin, reticulocyte count, and white blood cell count may be useful to identify anemia due to blood loss, or to screen for underlying myeloproliferative cancers.

The partial thromboplastin time (PTT) is the best single screening test for coagulation disorders, and is used to evaluate the intrinsic system (factors VIII, IX, XI, and XII) and the common pathways (factors V and X, prothrombin (Factor II), and fibrinogen). A phospholipid platelet substitute is added to the patient's blood to initiate the coagulation process via the intrinsic pathway. When a contact activator such as kaolin is added, the test is referred to as *activated PTT* (aPTT). In general, a normal aPTT ranges from 25 to 35 s. Results in excess of 35 s are considered abnormal or prolonged.

The prothrombin time (PT) is used to evaluate the extrinsic pathway (factor VII) and the common pathway (factors V and X, prothrombin, and fibrinogen). For this test, tissue thromboplastin is added to the test sample to serve as the activating agent. In general, the normal range is 11–15 s. When the test is used to evaluate the level of anticoagulation in patients taking warfarin, the international normalized ratio (INR) format is recommended. INR is a method that standardizes PT assays.

The thrombin time (TT, or thrombin clotting time) is the time taken to convert fibrinogen in the blood to insoluble fibrin. This test bypasses the intrinsic, extrinsic, and most of the common pathways. Thrombin is added to the patient's blood sample as the activating agent. Generally, the normal range for the TT is 9–13 s, and

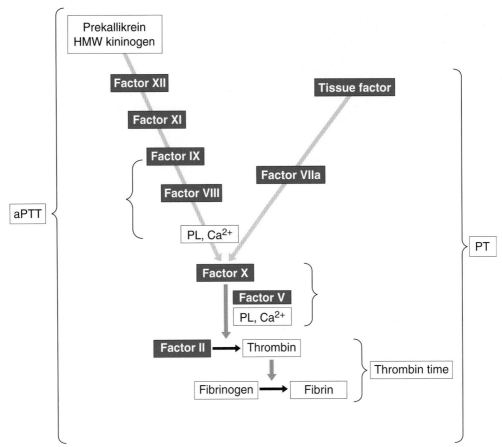

FIG. 24.6 Coagulation cascade indicating the intrinsic pathway measured by activated partial thromboplastin time (aPTT); the extrinsic pathway measured by prothrombin time (PT); and the conversion of fibrinogen to fibrin, which is measured by thrombin time (TT). Other proteins—prekallikrein and high-molecular-weight (HMW) kininogen—participate in the contact activation phase but are not considered coagulation factors. Ca^{2+}, calcium; *PL*, phospholipid. (From Rick ME. Coagulation testing. In: Young NS, Gerson SL, High KA, eds. *Clinical Hematology*. St. Louis: Mosby; 2006.)

results in excess of 16–18 s are considered abnormal or prolonged.

When one or more of the screening tests yield an abnormal result, additional tests may be indicated to pinpoint the specific defect of the bleeding disorder. The platelet count is very effective for identifying patients with thrombocytopenia, but it is not effective for identifying patients with qualitative platelet disorders. Bleeding time is now an obsolete test for platelet function and has been replaced with platelet aggregometry comprising a number of sophisticated tests to assess platelet adhesion, aggregation, and secretion. Testing may use different agonists such as thrombin, ADP, epinephrine, collagen, arachidonic acid, and ristocetin to activate platelets and determine the functional defects.

Some acquired coagulation disorders can produce prolonged aPTT but with normal PT. These include unfractionated heparin therapy, lupus anticoagulant antibodies, and antibodies to other coagulation factors (e.g., factors VIII and IX). Heparin-induced prolongation of aPTT is typically very high (i.e., 60–100 s). Tests for autoimmune acquired coagulopathies include PTT "mixing" studies to indicate the possible presence of autoantibodies, and then confirmatory tests for specific antibodies. Acquired coagulopathies with prolonged PT along with normal aPTT and platelets suggest a factor VII deficiency associated with liver disease, vitamin K deficiency, or disseminated intravascular coagulation (DIC). The PT also will be prolonged in patients taking warfarin, although the INR is used for this patient population. Obtaining factor V and VII levels can help differentiate liver disease (assays for both factors V and VII will be reduced) from vitamin K deficiency (only the factor VII assay will be reduced). When both the aPTT and PT test results are both prolonged, an acquired common pathway factor deficiency is usually indicated. Often, multiple factors are found to be deficient.

The TT will be prolonged in patients taking unfractionated heparin and direct thrombin inhibitors (e.g., dabigatran). It will also be prolonged when fibrinogen levels are low due to liver disease, in which case fibrinogen assays can be performed. If these are normal, then tests for fibrinolysis are performed to assess fibrin degradation products (FDPs) such as D-dimers. Fibrinolysis due to acquired plasminogen deficiencies (i.e., secondary to DIC or other systemic diseases such as leukemia) can be assessed by plasminogen assays.

Patients with vascular abnormalities (Box 24.1) that can cause clinical bleeding may not be identified by screening tests. In most cases, the diagnosis must be based on history and clinical findings.

MEDICAL MANAGEMENT

In this section, the identification and management of patients with acquired bleeding disorders is considered. A large proportion of patients with acquired bleeding disorders have a history or risk factors for a variety of hypercoagulable diseases with an increased risk for emboli or thrombus formation for which they have been prescribed antithrombotic agents (i.e., antiplatelet, anticoagulant, or profibrinolytic agents). A minority of patients have other acquired disorders that increase their risk for bleeding (Box 24.1). Focus will be placed on acquired bleeding disorders due to the use of antithrombotic agents, and other selected disorders of importance to the dentist.

Antiplatelet Therapy

Platelets are an important contributor to arterial thrombi or emboli; hence antiplatelet treatment may be indicated for a number of conditions, including the primary or secondary prevention of vascular events (i.e., coronary, cerebral, or peripheral vascular events), and others. Antiplatelet therapy has been reported to reduce the overall mortality rate from arterial vascular disease by 15% and to reduce nonfatal vascular complications by 30%. There are numerous actionable pathways influencing platelet adhesion, aggregation, or secretion. Antiplatelet drugs include aspirin, dipyrimadole, $P2Y_{12}$ receptor antagonists, PDE inhibitors, glycoprotein (GpIIb/IIIa) receptor antagonists, and PAR1 receptor antagonists. These drugs may be used as single agents or in combination (e.g., dual antiplatelet therapy), or in conjunction with anticoagulant drugs. The antiplatelet drugs are summarized in Table 24.2, and their mechanism of action is depicted in Fig. 24.7.

Aspirin is the least expensive, most widely used, and most studied antiplatelet drug. It exerts its action by irreversibly inhibiting COX-1 in platelets, preventing synthesis of thromboxane A_2, and impairing platelet secretion and aggregation. Upon discontinuation, aspirin's activity lasts for the life of the platelet,

TABLE 24.2 Antithrombotic Drugs

Agent	Mechanism of Action	Significant Adverse Effects	Metabolism and Relevant Major Drug Interactions	Reversal
Antiplatelet agents				
Aspirin (oral)	Irreversible inhibition of COX 1 and 2	GI ulceration/bleeding, hypersensitivity reaction (angioedema, urticaria, bronchoconstriction).	Substrate of CYP2C9 (minor). NSAIDs, such as ibuprofen may reduce efficacy of aspirin, and increase risk for GI ulceration/bleeding.	Following discontinuation, normal platelet function returns after 7—10 days. OR Platelet transfusions.
Dipyridamole (oral)	Prevents breakdown of cAMP	Headache, dizziness, exacerbation of angina.	None reported.	Following discontinuation, normal platelet function returns after 1 day.
Cilostazol (oral)	Phosphodiesterase-3 inhibitor	Arrhythmias, leukopenia.	Substrate of CYP2C19 and CYP3A4 (major); CYP1A2 and CYP2D6 (minor). Inhibits CYP3A4 (weak). Erythromycin and azole antifungals may increase cilostazol levels.	Following discontinuation, normal platelet function returns after 4 days.
Clopidogrel (oral)	$P2Y_{12}$/ADP inhibitor (irreversible)	Bleeding, thrombotic thrombocytopenic purpura, hypersensitivity reactions (angioedema, urticaria, maculopapular rash).	Substrate of CYP219 (major) and CYP3A4 (minor). Fluconazole may reduce clopidogrel levels.	Following discontinuation, normal platelet function returns within 7—10 days. OR Platelet transfusion.
Prasugrel (oral)	P2Y12/ADP inhibitor (irreversible)	Bleeding, thrombotic thrombocytopenic purpura, hypersensitivity reactions (angioedema, urticaria, maculopapular rash).	Substrate of CYP2B6 and CYP3A4 (minor). NSAIDs, such as ibuprofen increase risk of bleeding.	Following discontinuation, normal platelet. Function returns within 7—10 days. OR Platelet transfusion.

Continued

TABLE 24.2   Antithrombotic Drugs—cont'd

Agent	Mechanism of Action	Significant Adverse Effects	Metabolism and Relevant Major Drug Interactions	Reversal
Ticagrelor (oral)	$P2Y_{12}$/ADP inhibitor (reversible)	Bleeding, bradyarrhythmias, hyperuricemia, dyspnea, central sleep apnea, thrombocytopenic purpura.	Substrate of CYP3A4 (major). Itraconazole and voriconazole may increase ticagrelor levels.	After discontinuation, normal platelet function returns within 3–5 days. OR Consider aminocaproic acid, tranexamic acid, recombinant factor VIIa.
Cangrelor (administered iv)	$P2Y_{12}$/ADP inhibitor (reversible)	Bleeding, hypersensitivity reactions (angioedema, urticaria, maculopapular rash).	None reported.	After discontinuation, normal platelet function returns within 3–5 days. OR Consider aminocaproic acid, tranexamic acid, recombinant factor VIIa.
Ticlopidine	$P2Y_{12}$/ADP inhibitor (irreversible)	Thrombotic thrombocytopenia purpura, neutropenia, aplastic anemia.	Inhibits CYP1A2 CYP2B6, CYP2C19, and CYP2D6 (weak).	After discontinuation, normal platelet function returns within 7–10 days.
Tirofiban (administered iv)	Glycoprotein IIb/IIIa inhibitor (nonpeptide)	Bleeding, thrombocytopenia.	None reported.	After discontinuation, normal platelet function returns within 4–8 h.
Abciximab (administered iv)	Glycoprotein IIb/IIIa inhibitor (monoclonal antibody)	Bleeding, thrombocytopenia, hypersensitivity reactions (including anaphylaxis).	None reported.	After discontinuation, normal platelet function returns within 2 days.
Eptifibatide (administered iv)	Glycoprotein IIb/IIIa (fibrinogen receptor) inhibitor (peptide)	Bleeding, thrombocytopenia, hypersensitivity reactions (including anaphylaxis).	None reported.	After discontinuation, normal platelet function returns within 4–8 h.
Vorapaxar (oral)	PAR1 receptor antagonist	Bleeding.	Substrate of CYP3A4 (major); CYP2J2 (minor). NSAIDs, such as ibuprofen increase risk of bleeding. Clarithromycin may increase vorapaxar levels.	After discontinuation, normal platelet function takes >4 weeks to return.
Anticoagulants				
Heparin (administered iv or sc)	Standard heparin. Potentiates action of antithrombin III.	Bleeding, heparin resistance, hyperkalemia, hypersensitivity reactions, osteoporosis, thrombocytopenia.	None reported.	After discontinuation, normal coagulation function returns within 4–8 h. OR Protamine.
Dalteparin (administered sc)	Low molecular weight heparin. Potentiates action of antithrombin III.	Bleeding, hyperkalemia, thrombocytopenia.	None reported. NSAIDs, such as ibuprofen increase risk of bleeding.	Ciraparantag (under investigation).
Enoxaparin (administered iv or sc)	Low molecular weight heparin. Potentiates action of antithrombin III	Bleeding, hyperkalemia, thrombocytopenia.	None reported. NSAIDs, such as ibuprofen increase risk of bleeding.	Ciraparantag. OR Andexanet alfa (iv recombinant modified human factor Xa decoy protein).
Tinzaparin (administered sc)	Low molecular weight heparin. Potentiates action of antithrombin III	Bleeding, hyperkalemia, thrombocytopenia.	None reported. NSAIDs, such as ibuprofen increase risk of bleeding.	Ciraparantag.
Fondaparinux (administered iv or sc)	Synthetic heparin. Antithrombin III-mediated selective inhibition of factor Xa	Bleeding, thrombocytopenia.	None reported. NSAIDs, such as ibuprofen increase risk of bleeding.	

Warfarin (oral)	Vitamin K antagonist	Bleeding, acute renal injury, hypersensitivity reaction, calciphylaxis, gangrene, atheroemboli.	Substrate of CYP1A2 (minor), 3A4 (minor), 2C9 (major), and 2C19 (minor). Vitamin K-containing foods and alcohol will decrease warfarin levels. Vitamin E will increase warfarin levels. Amoxicillin, macrolides, metronidazole, and azole antifungals may increase warfarin levels. Carbamazepine may reduce warfarin levels. NSAIDs, such as ibuprofen increase risk of bleeding.	Vitamin K (iv). OR Prothrombin complex concentrates (iv) OR Fresh frozen plasma (iv).
Dabigatran (oral)	DOAC: Factor IIa inhibitor	Bleeding, thromboembolic events (upon premature discontinuation), GI signs and symptoms.	Substrate of P-glycoprotein/ABCB1 (major). Cyclosporine may increase dabigatran levels. Carbamazepine may reduce dabigatran levels. NSAIDs, such as ibuprofen increase risk of bleeding.	Idarucizumab (iv) is a reversal agent. OR Prothrombin complex concentrates (iv).
Rivaroxaban (oral)	DOAC: Factor Xa inhibitor	Bleeding.	Substrate of BCRP/ABCG2, CYP2J2 (minor), CYP3A4 (major), P-glycoprotein/ABCB1 (minor). Carbamazepine may reduce rivaroxaban levels. Azole antifungals, may increase rivaroxaban levels. NSAIDs, such as ibuprofen increase risk of bleeding.	Andexanet alfa (iv recombinant modified human factor Xa decoy protein). OR Prothrombin complex concentrates.
Apixaban (oral)	DOAC: Factor Xa inhibitor	Bleeding.	Substrate of BCRP/ABCG2, CYP3A4 (major), CYP1A2, CYP2C19, CYP2C8, CYP2C9 (minor), P-glycoprotein/ABCB1 (minor). Carbamazepine may reduce apixban levels. Azole antifungals, may increase rivaroxaban levels. NSAIDs, such as ibuprofen increase risk of bleeding.	Andexanet alfa (iv recombinant modified human factor Xa decoy protein). OR Prothrombin complex concentrates.
Edoxaban (oral)	DOAC: Factor Xa inhibitor	Bleeding.	Substrate of P-glycoprotein/ABCB1 (major). Cyclosporine, macrolides, and azole antifungals may increase edoxaban levels. Carbamazepine may reduce edoxaban levels. NSAIDs, such as ibuprofen increase risk of bleeding.	Andexanet alfa (iv recombinant modified human factor Xa decoy protein). OR Prothrombin complex concentrates.
Betrixaban (oral)	DOAC: Factor Xa inhibitor	Bleeding.	Substrate of P-glycoprotein/ABCB1 (major). Cyclosporine, macrolides, and azole antifungals may increase betrixaban levels. Carbamazepine may reduce betrixaban levels. NSAIDs, such as ibuprofen increase risk of bleeding.	None reported.
Desirudin (administered iv)	Direct thrombin inhibitor	Hypersensitivity reactions (anaphylaxis), bleeding.	None reported. NSAIDs, such as ibuprofen, and corticosteroids increase risk of bleeding.	None reported.
Argatroban (administered iv)	Direct thrombin inhibitor	Hypersensitivity reactions, bleeding.	None reported.	None reported.
Bivalirudin (administered iv)	Direct thrombin inhibitor	Hypersensitivity reactions (anaphylaxis), bleeding.	None reported.	None reported.

ADP, adenosine diphosphate; *cAMP,* cyclic adenosine monophosphate; *COX,* cyclo-oxygenase; *CYP,* cytochrome P450 enzyme system; *DOAC,* direct oral anticoagulant; *GI,* gastrointestinal; *iv,* intravenously; *NSAID,* nonsteroidal antiinflammatory drug; *sc,* subcutaneously.

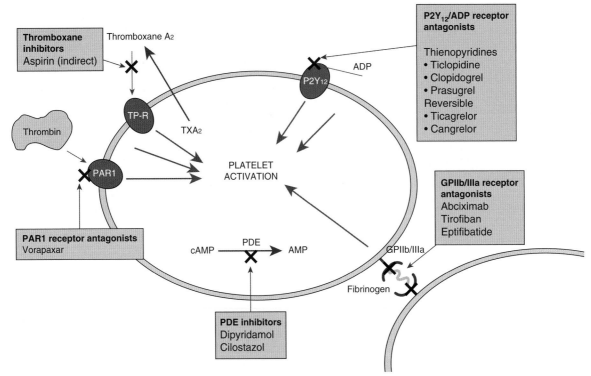

FIG. 24.7 Site of action of antiplatelet drugs. Aspirin inhibits thromboxane A$_2$ (TXA$_2$) synthesis by irreversibly acetylating cyclooxygenase-1 (COX-1). Dipyrimadole and cilostazol are phosphodiesterase inhibitors. Ticlopidine, clopidogrel, prasugrel, ticagrelor, and cangrelor block the P2Y$_{12}$, a key adenosine diphosphate (ADP) receptor on the platelet surface. Abciximab, eptifibatide, and tirofiban inhibit the final common pathway of platelet aggregation by blocking fibrinogen binding to activated glycoprotein (GP) IIb/IIIa.

approximately 7–10 days. Dipyridamole increases cyclic adenosine monophosphate, which inhibits ADP. The P2Y$_{12}$ receptor antagonists (which binds to ADP at the surface of the platelets) include ticlopidine, clopidogrel, and prasugrel, which irreversibly inhibit P2Y$_{12}$; cangrelor and ticagrelor reversibly inhibit P2Y$_{12}$ (with the advantage that the antiplatelet effect is reversed in 3–5 days following discontinuation). During platelet activation, glycoprotein IIb/IIIa receptors bind fibrinogen and VWF allowing for platelet aggregation. Abciximab, a monoclonal antibody; and the small molecule inhibitors, eptifibatide and tirofiban, block the glycoprotein IIb/IIIa receptors. Vorapaxar blocks one of the platelet receptors for thrombin, PAR-1, thereby inhibiting thrombin-mediated platelet aggregation. Compared to aspirin the newer agents are more potent, and therefore the risk for serious bleeding is increased. Many of these antiplatelet agents are prescribed dually (often in combination with aspirin), further increasing risk.

Anticoagulant Therapy

Important indications for anticoagulant therapy include the prevention and treatment of arterial and venous thromboembolism, and the prevention of stroke in patients with atrial fibrillation. Venous thromboembolism usually occurs in otherwise normal vessel walls and the

two most common types are deep vein thrombosis (DVT) followed by pulmonary emboli (PE). The anticoagulants prescribed for these disorders include heparin and it's derivatives, vitamin K antagonists, and direct oral anticoagulants (DOACs). The anticoagulant drugs are summarized in Table 24.2, and their mechanism of action is depicted in Fig. 24.8.

Standard heparin consists of an unfractionated heterogeneous mixture of polysaccharide chains with a mean molecular weight of 12,000–16,000. Heparin itself is not an anticoagulant, but rather it is a catalyst for the formation of plasma antithrombin III (ATIII). It inhibits factor Xa and thrombin equally. Treatment with standard heparin usually consists of an IV infusion in a hospital setting and requires monitoring with aPTT. Standard heparin has a half-life of 1–2 h.

Low-molecular-weight heparin (LMWH) is prepared by depolymerization of unfractionated heparin chains, yielding heparin fragments with a mean molecular weight of 4000–6000. LMWH preparations have greater activity against factor Xa than thrombin. LMWHs exhibit less binding to plasma proteins, endothelial cells, and macrophages than is seen with standard heparin. Thus, they have better bioavailability when administered subcutaneously, demonstrate a longer half-life (2–4 h), and offer more predictable anticoagulant effects. LMWHs are

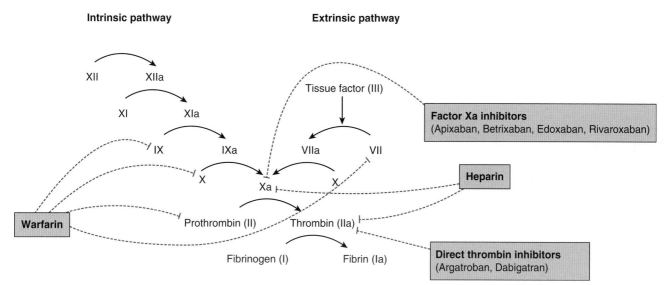

FIG. 24.8 Site of action of anticoagulant drugs. (From https://upload.wikimedia.org/wikipedia/commons/f/f4/Coagulation_Cascade_and_Major_Classes_of_Anticoagulants.png.)

administered subcutaneously in the abdomen. The dosage is based on body weight, and no laboratory monitoring is needed. Treatment with LMWHs may also be provided on an outpatient basis. LMWH preparations that are used commonly in North America for the treatment of VTE include dalteparin, enoxaparin, and tinzaparin. Their anti-Xa—to—thrombin ratio ranges from 1.9 for tinzaparin to 3.8 for enoxaparin. Two synthetic heparin analogues are available for anticoagulant use, fondaparinux and idraparinux, and these agents have a very long half-life (17 and 80 h, respectively) and are administered subcutaneously.

The vitamin K antagonists (i.e., warfarin) inhibit the biosynthesis of vitamin K–dependent coagulation proteins (factors VII, IX, and X and prothrombin). Warfarin is named after the patent holder, Wisconsin Alumni Research Foundation. Therapeutic anticoagulation with warfarin takes 4–5 days. INR is used to monitor patients on warfarin therapy. Reliance on the INR (INR = [PTR]^{ISI}; PTR = prothrombin time ratio; ISI = international sensitivity index for the thromboplastin used) allows better comparison of PT values among different laboratories and minimizes the risk of bleeding caused by artificially low PT values. The recommended INR goal for a patient on low-intensity warfarin therapy is 2.5, with a range of 2.0–3.0. The INR goal for a patient on high-intensity anticoagulation therapy (i.e., those with mechanical heart valves) is 3.0, with a range of 2.5–3.5.

DOACs include direct thrombin inhibitors (dabigatran) and factor Xa inhibitors (rivaroxaban, apixaban, edoxaban, and betrixaban). The first orally administered DOAC, dabigatran, gained US Food and Drug Administration approval in 2010 for use to prevent stroke in patients with atrial fibrillation. Its approval led to the replacement of warfarin as the standard anticoagulant with the main advantages that INR monitoring is not needed, and it is not affected by foods. Subsequently, the

newer class of direct factor Xa inhibitors was approved in the United States: rivaroxaban in 2011, apixaban, and edoxaban in 2014, and betrixaban in 2017.

Other anticoagulants include the parenteral direct thrombin inhibitors lepirudin, desirudin, argatroban, and bivalirudin. They all have very short half-lives (only several hours) and are used in hospital settings.

Other Acquired Bleeding Disorders

Acquired thrombocytopenias and qualitative platelet disorders other than those secondary to antiplatelet therapy are less common and may include disorders suppressing ability for the bone marrow to produce platelets (e.g., drug-induced marrow suppression, nutritional deficiencies, or alcohol use), disorders destroying circulating platelets (e.g., immune thrombocytopenia purpura, drug-induced immune-thrombocytopenia, thrombotic thrombocytopenia purpura), or disorders affecting platelet function. Decompensated liver and end-stage renal diseases may be associated with complications of bleeding affecting primary and/or secondary hemostasis and are covered in Chapters 10 and 12, respectively.

Disseminated intravascular coagulation is an acquired bleeding disorder that results when both primary and secondary hemostasis is activated in all or a major part of the vascular system. Despite widespread fibrin production, the major clinical problem is bleeding, not thrombosis. DIC may be caused by obstetric complications, infection, injuries and burns, antigen-antibody complexes, sepsis and septic shock, acidosis, and cancer. Clinical manifestations of DIC include severe bleeding from small wounds; purpura; and spontaneous bleeding from the nose, gums, gastrointestinal tract, or urinary tract (Fig. 24.9). Screening tests are abnormal (i.e., increased aPTT and PT, and decrease in platelets) although these can be variable. Increased FDP titers in

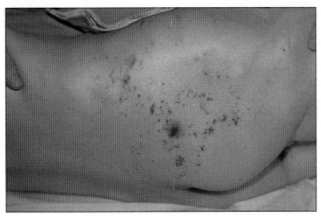

FIG. 24.9 Disseminated intravascular coagulation resulting from staphylococcal septicemia in a 56-year-old man. Note the characteristic skin hemorrhage, ranging in extent from small purpuric lesions to larger ecchymoses. The patient had non–insulin-dependent (type 2) diabetes, and the septicemia originated with an untreated large boil on his thigh. (From Forbes CD, Jackson WF. *Color Atlas and Text of Clinical Medicine*. 3rd ed. Edinburgh: Mosby; 2003.)

conjunction with a prolonged PT are generally more sensitive measures than abnormalities of the aPTT and platelet count. The most difficult differential diagnosis of DIC occurs in patients who have coexisting liver disease (which also can demonstrate increased aPTT/PT and a decrease in platelets).

DENTAL MANAGEMENT

The dentist should use these four methods to assess risk of a potential bleeding problem.

- A thorough history
- Physical examination
- Screening clinical laboratory tests
- Observation of excessive bleeding following an invasive procedure (Box 24.5)

History

The history provides the basis for identifying dental patients with abnormal hemostasis. Patients can be poor historians, therefore dentists must go beyond the typical screening questions listed on standard intake medical history forms. The history should include questions on the following topics:

1. *Presence of bleeding problems in relatives (see Chapter 25 on congenital bleeding disorders).*
2. *Excessive bleeding after operations/surgical procedures or dental procedures.*

All dental patients should be questioned about excessive bleeding after major or minor operations. The number of patients who have had an appendectomy, a

---

BOX 24.5   Clinical Recognition of the Patient Who Is a "Bleeder"

1. History
   a. Bleeding problems in relatives
   b. Bleeding problems after operations and tooth extractions
   c. Bleeding problems after trauma (e.g., cuts, scrapes)
   d. Medications that may cause bleeding problems:
      (1) Aspirin
      (2) Anticoagulants
      (3) Long-term antibiotic therapy
      (4) Certain herbal preparations
   e. Presence of illnesses that may be associated with bleeding problems:
      (1) Leukemia
      (2) Liver disease
      (3) Hemophilia
      (4) Congenital heart disease
      (5) Renal disease—uremia
   f. Spontaneous bleeding from nose, mouth, ears
2. Examination findings
   a. Jaundice, pallor
   b. Spider angiomas
   c. Ecchymoses
   d. Petechiae
   e. Oral ulcers
   f. Hyperplastic gingival tissues
   g. Hemarthrosis
3. Screening laboratory tests
   a. PT
   b. aPTT
   c. TT
   d. Platelet count
4. Surgical procedure—excessive bleeding after surgery may be first clue to underlying bleeding problem

aPTT, activated partial thromboplastin time; *PT*, prothrombin time; *TT*, thrombin time.

---

tonsillectomy, periodontal procedures (surgery or root scaling), or tooth extraction is large. Usually, the extraction of molar teeth is more traumatic than the extraction of incisors. A patient who reports prolonged or delayed bleeding following tooth extraction or other dental procedures should be asked whether the bleeding occurred at home, and if it was necessary to return to the dentist or hospital for treatment. Absence of a history of a significant acquired bleeding problem does not mean that the patient is free of such problem in the future. In those patients who report postoperative bleeding, it is important to establish the onset and length of prolonged bleeding. If further treatment was rendered, the dentist should attempt to establish what type of treatment was provided, and the need for hospitalization or transfusion. The patient should be asked about visits to other doctors or previous hospitalizations for bleeding problems, transfusions, any pertinent laboratory tests, or documented history of diseases associated with bleeding (e.g., liver, kidney, anemia, thrombocytopenia, cancer) or diseases for which a patient has been prescribed antithrombotic drugs).

3. *Excessive bleeding after injury or trauma.*

All dental patients should be asked whether they have experienced any trauma, and if so, whether excessive bleeding ensued. The more severe the trauma (knife wounds, automobile accidents), the more likely it is that the presence of an underlying bleeding disorder will be exposed. Small cuts in patients with coagulation disorders may not cause excessive bleeding initially because the vascular and platelet phases may be sufficient to control blood loss even if a defect in coagulation is present. However, small cuts in patients with platelet or vascular disorders usually result in excessive bleeding.

4. *Current use of antithrombotic drugs, or other drugs linked to bleeding.*

All dental patients should be asked whether they are currently taking one or more antithrombotic drugs. If the patient is receiving one of these drugs, and the indication, dosing, or effect on hemostasis is unclear in the context of the dental treatment plan, the dentist should contact the patient's physician. Patients also may be taking other drugs or foods linked to bleeding (e.g., recent treatment with a broad-spectrum antibiotic, excessive use of alcohol), as these can increase the risk for excessive postoperative bleeding. Some herbal preparations, vitamin supplements (see Appendix E) or some over-the-counter medications (i.e., aspirin) may cause excessive bleeding.

5. *Past and present illness or other diseases associated with bleeding.*

Assessment of past and current illnesses should identify a history of thrombocytopenia, liver disease, chronic renal disease, cancer, and whether the patient has received or is currently receiving cancer treatment (particularly chemotherapy that can reduce platelet production), which can affect hemostasis.

6. *Occurrence of spontaneous bleeding.*

All dental patients should be asked about a history of spontaneous bleeding related to an underlying platelet disorder, including gingival/oral, nasal, urinary, rectal/gastrointestinal, pulmonary, and, in women, vaginal/uterine bleeding. If spontaneous bleeding has occurred, the frequency, amount of blood lost, and steps that were necessary to control it should be determined. A history of gingival bleeding is common and related to local factors related to gingivitis or periodontal disease, therefore it is important to determine whether the bleeding occurs spontaneously.

Physical Examination

The dentist should inspect the exposed skin and oral mucosae for signs including petechiae, purpura, ecchymoses, spider angiomata, telangiectasias, jaundice, pallor, and cyanosis. When any of these signs are identified and cannot be explained by the history or other clinical findings, the patient should be referred for medical evaluation.

Screening Laboratory Tests

The dentist may order screening tests: complete blood count, aPTT, PT, and TT (Box 24.6). Abnormal test results should be discussed with the patient and their physician.

Preprocedural Evaluation of Hemostasis

Routine presurgical screening is not needed to rule out potential bleeding disorders in patients with a negative history and clinical findings who are scheduled for low-risk dental or surgical procedures from which bleeding is anticipated. There are no validated thresholds allowing for a perfect stratification of low vs. high risk for bleeding. Low-risk procedures are generally considered to include local anesthetic infiltrations and blocks, restorative, endodontic, or prosthodontic procedures, <3 uncomplicated dental extractions, implant placement, periodontal surgery, biopsy procedures, and subgingival scaling/root planning. High-risk procedures include major surgery typically performed by specialists, such as oral and maxillofacial or head and neck surgeons, and include complicated and multiple extractions with flaps, orthognathic surgery, oncologic resection, and reconstructive

---

BOX 24.6 **Screening Laboratory Tests for Detection of a Potential "Bleeder"**

1. PT—activated by tissue thromboplastin:
   a. Tests extrinsic and common pathways.
   b. Control should be run.
   c. Normal PT is 11–15 s, depending on laboratory.
   d. Control must be in normal range.
2. aPTT—initiated by phospholipid platelet substitute and activated by addition of contact activator (kaolin):
   a. Tests intrinsic and common pathways.
   b. Control should be run.
   c. Normal aPTT is 25–35 s, depending on laboratory.
   d. Control must be in normal range.
3. TT—activated by thrombin:
   a. Tests ability to form initial clot from fibrinogen.
   b. Controls should be run.
   c. Normal TT is 9–13 s.
4. Platelet count:
   a. Tests platelet phase for adequate number of platelets.
   b. Normal count is 140,000–400,000/μL.
   c. Clinical bleeding problem can occur if count is less than 50,000/μL.

aPTT, activated partial thromboplastin time; *PT*, prothrombin time; *TT*, thrombin time.

surgery. It is recommended that patients with a negative history of bleeding be screened prior to major surgery.

Irrespective of procedural risk for bleeding, patients with a positive history of bleeding should be referred to their physician or a hematologist for screening and peri-surgical testing.

Considerations for Patients on Antithrombotic Agents

Antiplatelet Therapy. There is an increased risk of thromboembolic events from discontinuing antiplatelet agents, and the risk of thromboembolism outweighs the risk for bleeding for most dental procedures. Risk is highest in patients who have recently undergone the following procedures: percutaneous coronary intervention, bare-metal stenting, or coronary artery bypass grafting (<3 months); acute coronary syndrome or myocardial infarction (<6 months); or drug-eluting stenting (<12 months). The medical history and procedural risk of bleeding should be taken into consideration, and consultation with the patient's physician is prudent.

Expert consensus supports the recommendation that patients who take single- or dual-antiplatelet drugs be maintained on their medication(s) for low-risk dental procedures/surgery. The importance of local hemostatic techniques cannot be overstated. In the case of high-risk procedures (i.e., major surgery) where significant bleeding is anticipated, a careful risk assessment should be made with input from the patient's physician, and a decision made to defer elective surgery until antiplatelet therapy is adjusted or briefly discontinued. Antiplatelet agents are active 1 h following resumption, hence bridging strategies are not indicated for antiplatelet therapies. Also, platelet transfusions are rarely required for these patients.

Nonsteroidal antiinflammatory drugs can also inhibit platelet aggregation. They inhibit COX reversibly, and the duration of their action depends on the specific drug dose given, the serum level, and drug half-life. NSAIDs should be avoided as analgesics and antiinflammatory agents in patients who take antiplatelet drugs.

Anticoagulant Therapy. There is also an increased risk of thromboembolic events in patients who discontinue anticoagulant therapy. Clinical practice guidelines for the management of patients taking anticoagulants vary based upon both the risk for thromboembolic events if discontinued and the degree of bleeding anticipated by the procedure. Such guidelines universally support the continuation of oral anticoagulation therapy (i.e., warfarin or DOACs) for minor dental/surgical procedures at low risk for causing bleeding.

Warfarin requires regular monitoring by INR to ensure that the patient is within the therapeutic window for anticoagulation, typically an INR of 2–3.5 depending on the indication (Table 24.3). Before performing any procedure generating bleeding the dentist should

TABLE 24.3	Recommended Therapeutic Range for Warfarin Therapy

INR 2.0–3.0 With a Target of 2.5

Prophylaxis of venous thrombosis (high-risk surgery)
Treatment of venous thrombosis
Treatment of PE
Prevention of systemic embolism
Tissue heart valves in aortic or mitral position for first 3 months
Tissue heart valves with history of PE
Tissue heart valves with atrial fibrillation
Acute MI
Atrial fibrillation
Valvular heart disease
Mitral valve prolapse with history of atrial fibrillation or embolism

INR 2.5–3.5 With a Target of 3.0

Mechanical prosthetic heart valves
Prevention of recurrent MI
Treatment of thrombosis associated with antiphospholipid antibodies

INR, International normalized ratio; *MI*, myocardial infarction; *PE*, pulmonary embolism.
Data from Hirsh J, Schulman S. Antithrombotic therapy. In: Goldman L, Ausiello D, eds. *Cecil Textbook of Medicine.* 23rd ed. Philadelphia: Saunders; 2008; Begelman SM. Venous thromboembolism. In: Carey WD, et al., eds. *Current Clinical Medicine 2009—Cleveland Clinic.* Philadelphia: Saunders; 2009; and Lim W, et al. Venous thromboembolism. In: Hoffman R, et al., eds. *Hematology: Basic Principles and Practice.* 5th ed. Philadelphia: Churchill Livingstone; 2009.

ascertain whether the patient is within this therapeutic window by obtaining a preoperative INR, ideally ordered within 72 h before the procedure. When the INR is 3.5 or less, minor procedures can be performed with local hemostatic measures alone. A preoperative INR outside of the window may require the warfarin to be adjusted by the physician, which once adjusted usually will take 3–5 days for any effective recalibration of the INR to occur. In emergencies, warfarin can be reversed with vitamin K, prothrombin complex concentrates, or fresh frozen plasma.

Warfarin levels are sensitive to the intake of foods high in vitamin K (i.e., green leafy vegetables), which can decrease levels. In contrast, some drugs can increase warfarin levels by potentially reducing the intestinal absorption of vitamin K (e.g., clindamycin and amoxicillin), or by inhibiting it's metabolism (i.e., metronidazole, azole antifungals, and carbamazepine).

Testing and monitoring parameters for the DOAC drugs have not yet been established. Dilute thrombin time (dTT), and ecarin-clotting time (ECT) may be used to assess dabigatran levels, although these tests are not commercially available. Antifactor Xa assays may be used to assess levels of rivaroxaban, apixaban, edoxaban, and betrixaban, although such assays are hampered by the turnaround time to generate the results (3–5 days).

DOAC drugs have potential drug interactions. Emergency reversal of DOACs may be possible following infusion of prothrombin complex concentrates. Three reversal agents for DOACs have been identified (Table 24.2). Idarucizumab, a reversal agent for dabigatran, received FDA approved in 2015. Andexanet alfa, a reversal agent for the factor Xa inhibitors (and also LMWH and fondaparinux which indirectly inhibit factor Xa) was FDA approved for rivaroxaban and apixaban in 2018. Ciraparantag binds to and reverses direct Xa inhibitors, direct thrombin inhibitors, and unfractionated and low-molecular-weight heparin (LMWH).

Guidelines and expert opinion vary in terms of major surgical procedures with some advocating protocols for the discontinuation of anticoagulants, while others strictly supporting the continuation of anticoagulants irrespective of surgical complexity/risk for bleeding. It is always prudent to discuss risk stratification with the patient's physician. If the physician recommends temporary discontinuation of anticoagulant therapy, there are strategies to mitigate the risk of thromboembolic events following discontinuation, particularly in high-risk patients (e.g., those with mechanical valves, or a recent (<3 months) venous thromboembolism). Heparin bridging can reduce the risk for thromboembolic event in such high-risk patients taking warfarin. Low-molecular-weight heparin has largely replaced standard heparin for this purpose (LMWH has a lower risk for heparin-associated thrombocytopenia). Warfarin therapy is typically discontinued 5 days before surgery and a series of 1 mg/kg subcutaneous enoxaparin injections every 12 h (at 9 a.m. and 9 p.m.) on an outpatient basis are given, starting 3 days before the surgery (Fig. 24.10). Following discontinuation of warfarin, the INR is allowed to normalize, and enoxaparin provides anticoagulation. The last enoxaparin injection is given at 9 p.m. on the evening before surgery. The INR should be checked on the morning of surgery and, if within normal values, the surgery can be performed. Enoxaparin injections are started again on the evening after the surgery; oral warfarin therapy is also restarted that evening. After 3 days, the postoperative enoxaparin injections are stopped. Patients taking warfarin who are at a lower risk for a thromboembolic event do not require bridging. The predictable and short half-life of DOAC agents abrogates the need for bridging, and if discontinued by the physician, patients are typically instructed to discontinue the agent 12–48 h before surgery and resume the day after surgery (Box 24.7).

Most patients undergoing treatment with standard heparin are hospitalized. Dental emergencies in these patients during hospitalization should be treated as conservatively as possible, with avoidance of invasive procedures, if possible. Patients treated with hemodialysis are given heparin. The half-life of heparin is only 1–2 h; thus, if patients wait until the day after dialysis, they can receive invasive dental treatment (see Chapter 12). However, dentists may see patients who are being treated on an outpatient basis with LMWHs. These agents are used in patients with recent total hip or knee replacement and those being treated on an outpatient basis for venous thromboembolism (VTE). Elective surgical procedures can be delayed until the patient is taken off the LMWH or synthetic heparin, which, in most cases, will occur within 3–6 months. If an invasive procedure must be performed, the dentist has several options. First, consult with the patient's physician regarding the need for and the type of surgery. The half-life of the LMWHs and fondaparinux is less than 1 day. Thus, the physician could suggest that the drug be stopped and the surgery be performed within 1–2 days. The other option is to continue the heparin treatment, proceed with the surgery, and control bleeding with local measures. In some cases, protamine may be given to reverse anticoagulation in heparinized patients, however it is not as effective in patients taking LMWH.

Vascular Disorders. In patients with autoimmune disease, infectious disease, structural malformation of vessels, scurvy, steroid therapy, small vessel vasculitis, or deposits of paraproteins, alterations of the vessel wall can result in excessive bleeding after surgical procedures. No reliable screening tests can detect those patients who will be bleeders. The dentist must rely on the medical history (questions related to excessive bleeding problems), clinical findings, and consultation with the patient's physician to identify these patients.

Other Diseases. Patients with history of liver disease, end-stage renal disease/renal dialysis, and acquired thrombocytopenia/qualitative platelet disorders may be at risk for bleeding. Patients with a history of jaundice or heavy alcohol use may have significant liver disease. Most coagulation factors are produced in the liver; therefore, if enough liver damage has occurred, the patient could have a serious bleeding problem because of defects in both primary and/or secondary hemostasis. Alcohol also can have a direct effect on hemostasis by

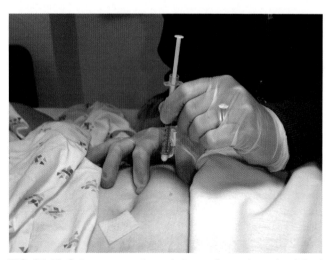

FIG. 24.10 Subcutaneous heparin is used to reduce the risk of deep vein thrombosis in medical and surgical procedures. (From Potter PA, Perry AG, Stockert P. *Basic Nursing.* 7th ed. St. Louis: Mosby; 2011.)

| BOX 24.7 | **Dental Management Considerations in Patients Taking Antithrombotic Agents**[a] |

PREOPERATIVE RISK ASSESSMENT
- Review medical, surgical, and dental history to determine why the patient is taking antithrombotic therapy; the current dosage; history of previous bleeding events.
- Discuss relevant issues with the patient in the context of the procedure(s) planned.
- Examine the patient for signs and symptoms of bleeding disorders and obtain vital signs.
- Review recent laboratory test results (if applicable).
- Confirm patient has a primary care provider (or hematologist).
- Obtain medical consultation to discuss risk for bleeding in the context of the procedure(s) planned. Any adjustments in antithrombotic therapy should be handled by the patient's physician.
- Order preoperative laboratory tests, if applicable.
- Low risk dental procedures can be performed without special precautions.

A

Analgesics	Avoid aspirin, aspirin-containing compounds, and other NSAIDs. Acetaminophen with or without codeine is suggested for most patients.
Antibiotics	Antibiotics such as clindamycin or amoxicillin may alter normal flora altering the absorption of Vitamin K and increase warfarin levels. Other antibiotics, such as metronidazole and macrolides can interact via the cytochrome P450 system with warfarin and some DOACs causing an increase in the levels of these agents.
Anesthesia	Use of local anesthetics with vasoconstrictors to control bleeding must be used judiciously in patients with cardiac issues.

B

Bleeding	Excessive bleeding is expected for all patients taking antithrombotic agents. The risk for bleeding for patients on antiplatelet agents cannot be measured. Patients taking two or more antiplatelet agents or combination antiplatelet/anticoagulant

agents are at a higher risk for bleeding. In patients taking warfarin, excessive bleeding after invasive dental procedures depends on the level of the patient's INR. If the INR is greater than 3.5, significant bleeding may occur after invasive dental and surgical procedures. These procedures can be performed with little risk of significant bleeding if the INR is between 2.0 and 3.5. In patients taking DOACs, the potential for bleeding is less than for warfarin.

Breathing	No issues.
Blood pressure	Elevated blood pressure complicates hemostasis.

C

Chair position	No issues.
Cardiovascular	Determine reason for antithrombotic therapy; if for cardiac reason, take appropriate management actions.

D

Devices	No issues.
Drugs	Avoid prescription of all drugs that may further increase the risk bleeding (i.e., NSAIDs), or interact to increase or reduce blood levels of antithrombotic agents. Drug interactions with antibiotics, azole antifungals, corticosteroids, cyclosporine, and carbemazepine are possible and should be checked before prescribing.

E

Equipment	Have needed armamentarium to manage hemostasis.
Emergencies	Excessive bleeding may occur after invasive dental procedures or surgery, and local measures may be required to control the bleeding (see Table 24.6).

F **Postoperative Care**

Follow-up	Patients should be contacted or examined within 24—48 h after surgical procedures to determine that excessive bleeding or infection is not occurring.

[a]Strength of recommendation taxonomy (SORT) Grade: C (see Preface for further explanation).
INR, international normalized ratio [INR = (PTR)[ISI]]; *ISI*, international sensitivity index (based on sensitivity of thromboplastin used in PT); *PT*, prothrombin time; *PTR*, prothrombin time ratio.

interfering with platelet function. If both the PT/INR and the platelet count are normal, surgery can be performed on liver disease patients with little risk of a postoperative bleeding problem. Liver disease patients with an INR > 2.5 are at high risk for bleeding. If results of both tests are abnormal, then the dentist should consult with the patient's physician regarding stabilization of the patient's bleeding status before surgery (see Chapter 10). Management of patients with end-stage renal disease and those on renal dialysis is covered in Chapter 12.

Patients with severe thrombocytopenia may require hospitalization and special precautions. A hematologist

should be involved with the diagnosis, presurgical assessment, preparation, and postsurgical management of these patients. There are no evidence-based guidelines for the risk stratification and dental management of patients with thrombocytopenia. Expert opinion suggests that most minor noninvasive dental procedures can be performed in patients with platelet counts above 30,000/μL. If the platelet count is below this level, such procedures should be delayed. For urgent or emergency dental needs, platelet replacement may be indicated. If the platelet count is above 50,000/μL, minor invasive procedures, such as uncomplicated extractions, can be performed. For more advanced surgery, the platelet count should be at least 80,000–100,000/μL. Patients with platelet counts below these levels routinely undergo platelet replacement before the planned procedures, although there is limited evidence to support this practice. Platelet transfusions are either those prepared from multiple pooled donor whole blood through centrifugation, or by apheresis to provide continuous centrifugation of blood donated by a single donor, thereby reducing the risk of infection. These products must be used within several days or cryopreserved for future use. Patients can develop severe alloimmune reactions to platelets. Some patients may fail to respond to platelet replacement therapy due to "platelet transfusion refractoriness" that can occur on an immune or a nonimmune basis. The need for platelet transfusions can be reduced through the use of local measures, by using topical platelet concentrates, desmopressin, or the antifibrinolytic agents epsilon aminocaproic acid or tranexamic acid to control bleeding. Eltrombopag, a thrombopoietin receptor agonist, also has been advocated to raise platelets in patients with chronic thrombocytopenia.

Local Measures for Postoperative Bleeding. There are no evidence-based guidelines for postoperative local hemostatic techniques. In most cases, the application of firm and consistent mechanical compression with gauze for several minutes will suffice. The use of vasoconstrictive agents, hemostatic agents, electrocautery, and the placement of sutures may be used when pressure alone is insufficient. Vasoconstrictive agents, such as epinephrine-containing local anesthetic agents, should be used judiciously in cardiac patients. If excessive postoperative bleeding occurs after an extraction, local hemostatic agents, such as absorbable gelatin sponges, gelatin-thrombin products, oxidized-cellulose, microfibrillar collagen, fibrin glue, or recombinant thrombin powder may be placed in the socket to control bleeding, ideally with primary closure.

The antifibrinolytic agents, tranexamic acid (TXA) and epsilon aminocaproic acid (EACA) block the binding of plasminogen to fibrin. These agents are commercially available (or extemporaneously prepared) as mouthwashes, or given intravenously or orally. Gauze used for compression soaked with TXA solution has also been advocated. There is moderate-level evidence to support that TXA mouthwashes (5%–10% solutions) have a beneficial effect on reducing postoperative bleeding when delivered postoperatively following minor oral surgery/dental extractions in patients taking antithrombotic agents. However, the superiority of TXA mouthwashes over standard local hemostatic techniques has not been demonstrated. The use of EACA formulations or oral/intravenous tranexamic has not been adequately studied in this population.

Patients should be provided clear postoperative instructions and extra gauze for managing bleeding that occurs at home. These include head elevation, gauze compression, and reducing any activities that might dislodge the clot. Vasoconstrictive agents such as ice or a moistened bag of black tea, which contain tannins, may be recommended. Follow-up communication with this patient population within 24–48 h of the procedure is strongly advised.

Treatment Planning Modifications

With proper preparation, most indicated dental treatment can be provided safely for patients with acquired bleeding disorders. Patients with bleeding problems related to diseases that may be in the terminal phase (i.e., end-stage liver or kidney diseases, or cancer) or at high risk for thromboembolism should be treated conservatively with input from their physicians. Careful surgical technique along with local hemostatic measures is important. In general, aspirin and other NSAIDs should not be prescribed for pain relief in those who have acquired bleeding disorders (e.g., those who take antiplatelet or anticoagulant drugs). Instead acetaminophen with or without codeine/hydrocodone may be used, with proper consideration for limiting the dose and duration of opioid use.

Oral Manifestations

Patients with acquired bleeding disorders may experience spontaneous gingival bleeding, or unanticipated bleeding during minor dental procedures. The oral mucosae may show petechiae, ecchymoses, or hematomas. Patients with jaundice or pallor may have underlying systemic diseases with acquired bleeding disorders (e.g., liver disease, or a myeloproliferative cancer).

BIBLIOGRAPHY

1. Barnes GD, Lucas E, Alexander GC, et al. National trends in ambulatory oral anticoagulant use. *Am J Med.* 2015;128(12):1300–5.e2.
2. Walenga JM. Normal hemostasis. In: Keohane EM, Otto CN, Walenga JM, eds. *Rodak's Hematology, Clinical Principles and Applications.* 6th ed. Elsevier; 2020:626–649. Accessed December 31, 2021.
3. Furie B, Furie BC. Mechanisms of thrombus formation. *N Engl J Med.* 2008;359(9):938–949.
4. Smith SA, Travers RJ, Morrissey JH. How it all starts: initiation of the clotting cascade. *Crit Rev Biochem Mol Biol.* 2015;50(4):326–336.
5. Italiano JE, Whiteheart SW, Bray PF, et al. Platelet morphology, biochemistry, and function. In: Kaushansky K, Prchal JT, Burns LJ, et al., eds. *Williams Hematology, 10e.* McGraw Hill; 2021. Accessed December 31, 2021.
6. DeChristopher PJ, Jeske WP. Thrombocytopenia and thrombocytosis. In: Keohane EM, Otto CN, Walenga JM, eds. *Rodak's Hematology, Clinical Principles and Applications.* 6th ed. Elsevier; 2020:696–719. Accessed December 31, 2021.
7. Little JW, Miller CS, Henry RG, et al. Antithrombotic agents: implications in dentistry. *Oral Surg Oral Med Oral Pathol Oral Radiol Endod.* 2002;93(5):544–551.

8. Levi M, Kaushansky K. Classification, clinical manifestations, and evaluation of disorders of hemostasis. In: Kaushansky K, Prchal JT, Burns LJ, et al., eds. *Williams Hematology, 10e.* McGraw Hill; 2021. Accessed December 31, 2021.

9. Thachil J. Antiplatelet therapy—a summary for the general physicians. *Clin Med (Lond).* 2016;16(2):152−160.

10. Fritsma GA. Antithrombotic therapies and their laboratory assessment. In: Keohane EM, Otto CN, Walenga JM, eds. *Rodak's Hematology, Clinical Principles and Applications.* 6th ed. St. Louis: Saunders, Elsevier; 2020:756−764. Accessed December 31, 2021.

11. Hogg K, Weitz JI. Blood coagulation and anticoagulant, fibrinolytic, and antiplatelet drugs. In: Brunton LL, Hilal-Dandan R, Knollmann BC, eds. *Goodman & Gilman's: The Pharmacological Basis of Therapeutics, 13e.* McGraw Hill; 2017. Accessed December 31, 2021.

12. Douketis JD, Spyropoulos AC, Spencer FA, et al. Perioperative management of antithrombotic therapy: antithrombotic therapy and prevention of thrombosis, 9th ed: American College of Chest Physicians evidence-based clinical practice guidelines. *Chest.* 2012;141(2 Suppl):e326S−e350S. Erratum in: *Chest.* 2012 Apr;141(4):1129.

13. Ortel TL, Neumann I, Ageno W, et al. American Society of Hematology 2020 guidelines for management of venous thromboembolism: treatment of deep vein thrombosis and pulmonary embolism. *Blood Adv.* 2020;4(19):4693−4738.

14. Hornor MA, Duane TM, Ehlers AP, et al. American College of Surgeons' guidelines for the perioperative management of antithrombotic medication. *J Am Coll Surg.* 2018;227(5):521−536.e1.

15. Ansell J, Hirsh J, Dalen J, et al. Managing oral anticoagulant therapy. *Chest.* 2001;119(1 suppl):22S−38S.

16. Samuelson BT, Cuker A, Siegal DM, et al. Laboratory assessment of the anticoagulant activity of direct oral anticoagulants: a systematic review. *Chest.* 2017;151(1):127−138.

17. Mahmood H, Siddique I, McKechnie A. Antiplatelet drugs: a review of pharmacology and the perioperative management of patients in oral and maxillofacial surgery. *Ann R Coll Surg Engl.* 2020;102(1):9−13.

18. Brennan MT, Shariff G, Kent ML, et al. Relationship between bleeding time test and postextraction bleeding in a healthy control population. *Oral Surg Oral Med Oral Pathol Oral Radiol Endod.* 2002;94(4):439−443.

19. Hu TY, Vaidya VR, Asirvatham SJ. Reversing anticoagulant effects of novel oral anticoagulants: role of ciraparantag, andexanet alfa, and idarucizumab. *Vasc Health Risk Manag.* 2016;12:35−44.

20. Buhatem Medeiros F, Pepe Medeiros de Rezende N, Bertoldi Franco J, et al. Quantification of bleeding during dental extraction in patients on dual antiplatelet therapy. *Int J Oral Maxillofac Surg.* 2017;46(9):1151−1157.

21. Tabrizi R, Khaheshi I, Hoseinzadeh A, et al. Do antiplatelet drugs increase the risk of bleeding after dental implant surgery? A case-and-crossover study. *J Oral Maxillofac Surg.* 2018;76(10):2092−2096.

22. Tang M, Yu C, Hu P, et al. Risk factors for bleeding after dental extractions in patients over 60 years of age who are taking antiplatelet drugs. *Br J Oral Maxillofac Surg.* 2018;56(9):854−858.

23. Bajkin BV, Wahl MJ, Miller CS. Dental implant surgery and risk of bleeding in patients on antithrombotic medications: a review of the literature. *Oral Surg Oral Med Oral Pathol Oral Radiol.* 2020;130(5):522−532.

24. Cocero N, Bezzi M, Martini S, et al. Oral surgical treatment of patients with chronic liver disease: assessments of bleeding and its relationship with thrombocytopenia and blood coagulation parameters. *J Oral Maxillofac Surg.* 2017;75(1):28−34.

25. Medina JB, Andrade NS, de Paula Eduardo F, et al. Bleeding during and after dental extractions in patients with liver cirrhosis. *Int J Oral Maxillofac Surg.* 2018;47(12):1543−1549.

26. Lusk KA, Snoga JL, Benitez RM, et al. Management of direct-acting oral anticoagulants surrounding dental procedures with low-to-moderate risk of bleeding. *J Pharm Pract.* 2018;31(2):202−207.

27. Vargas M, Marra A, Perrone A, et al. Bleeding management in patients on new oral anticoagulants. *Minerva Anestesiol.* 2016;82(8):884−894.

28. Nathwani S, Wanis C. Novel oral anticoagulants and exodontia: the evidence. *Br Dent J.* 2017;222(8):623−628.

29. Rocha AL, Oliveira SR, Souza AF, et al. Bleeding assessment in oral surgery: a cohort study comparing individuals on anticoagulant therapy and a non-anticoagulated group. *J Craniomaxillofac Surg.* 2019;47(5):798−804.

30. Wahl M. Dental surgery in anticoagulated patients. *Arch Intern Med.* 1998;158:1610−1616.

31. Wahl MJ, Pinto A, Kilham J, Lalla RV. Dental surgery in anticoagulated patients—stop the interruption. *Oral Surg Oral Med Oral Pathol Oral Radiol.* 2015;119(2):136−157.

32. Wahl MJ. The mythology of anticoagulation therapy interruption for dental surgery. *J Am Dent Assoc.* 2018;149(1):e1−e10.

33. Bajkin B, Popovic S, Selakovic S. Randomized, prospective trial comparing bridging therapy using low-molecular-weight heparin with maintenance of oral anticoagulation during extraction of teeth. *J Oral Maxillofac Surg.* 2009;67:990−995.

34. Johnson-Leong C, Rada RE. The use of low-molecular-weight heparins in outpatient oral surgery for patients receiving anticoagulation therapy. *J Am Dent Assoc.* 2002;133(8):1083−1087.

35. Karasneh J, Christoforou J, Walker JS, et al. World Workshop on Oral Medicine VII: platelet count and platelet transfusion for invasive dental procedures in thrombocytopenic patients: a systematic review. *Oral Dis.* 2019;25(Suppl 1):174−181.

36. Engelen ET, Schutgens RE, Mauser-Bunschoten EP, et al. Antifibrinolytic therapy for preventing oral bleeding in people on anticoagulants undergoing minor oral surgery or dental extractions. *Cochrane Database Syst Rev.* 2018;7(7):CD012293.

37. Kumbargere Nagraj S, Prashanti E, et al. Interventions for treating post-extraction bleeding. *Cochrane Database Syst Rev.* 2018;3(3):CD011930.

38. Ockerman A, Vanassche T, Garip M, et al. Tranexamic acid for the prevention and treatment of bleeding in surgery, trauma and bleeding disorders: a narrative review. *Thromb J.* 2021;19(1):54.

39. Flanagan D. Tranexamic acid tamponade to control postoperative surgical hemorrhage. *J Oral Implantol.* 2015;41(3):e82−e89.

25

Congenital Bleeding and Hypercoagulable Disorders

KEY POINTS

- Invasive dental procedures may cause prolonged postoperative bleeding in patients with congenital bleeding conditions.

  ⊘These conditions include hereditary hemorrhagic telangiectasia (Osler–Weber–Rendu syndrome), von Willebrand disease, Bernard–Soulier disease, Glanzmann thrombasthenia, hemophilia A, hemophilia

- B (Christmas disease), and congenital hypercoagulability disorders.
- Dental providers must be able to properly assess these patients and implement adequate measures that will control intraoperative and postoperative bleeding.
- Prolonged postoperative bleeding from dental procedures may result in severe hemorrhage and death.

Inherited (congenital) bleeding disorders involve a deficiency of one of the coagulation factors, abnormal construction of platelets, deficiency of von Willebrand factor, or malformation of vessels (Box 25.1). They are not as prevalent as acquired bleeding disorders. Inherited hypercoagulability disorders increase the risk for thromboembolism caused by a genetic deficiency of an antithrombotic factor or increasing a prothrombotic factor.

EPIDEMIOLOGY

In a typical dental practice of 2000 patients, at most 10–20 patients will have a congenital bleeding disorder. The most common inherited bleeding disorder is von Willebrand disease, which affects about 1% of the US population. The disease is usually inherited as an autosomal dominant trait.

Hemophilia A (Factor VIII deficiency) is the most common of the inherited coagulation disorders. It occurs in about 1 of every 5000 male births. More than 20,000 individuals in the United States have hemophilia A, and worldwide about 400,000 patients have severe hemophilia. Because of its genetic mode of transfer, certain areas of the United States contain higher concentrations of people with hemophilia.

Hemophilia B (Christmas disease, factor IX deficiency) is found in about 1 of every 30,000 male births. About 80% of all genetic coagulation disorders are hemophilia A, 13% are hemophilia B, and 6% are factor XI deficiency.

Bernard–Soulier disease and Glanzmann thrombasthenia are rare inherited platelet disorders. Hereditary hemorrhagic telangiectasia (HHT) is a rare (1:8000 to 1:50,000) vascular disorder. Ehlers–Danlos disease, osteogenesis imperfecta, pseudoxanthoma elasticum, and

Marfan syndrome are rare hereditary connective tissue disorders that may be associated with bleeding problems but are not covered in this chapter.

An inherited hypercoagulable state has been reported in more than 60% of patients presenting with idiopathic venothromboembolism.

ETIOLOGY

Patients may be born with a deficiency of one of the factors needed for blood coagulation; for example, factor VIII deficiency as in hemophilia A or factor IX deficiency as in hemophilia B. Congenital deficiencies of the other coagulation factors have been reported but are rare (Table 25.1). When congenital deficiency of a coagulation factor occurs, only a single factor is affected.

In von Willebrand disease, the primary problem involves defects in von Willebrand factor (vWF), which are needed to attach platelets to damaged vascular wall tissues and to carry factor VIII in circulation. In the most severe form of the disease, bleeding occurs as a consequence of lack of platelet adhesion and deficiency of factor VIII.

Bernard–Soulier disease is a disorder of platelet adhesion to vWF caused by a lack of glycoprotein (GP) Ib on the platelet membrane. These platelets are unable to bind to vWF and thus are unable to adhere to the subendothelium.

Glanzmann thrombasthenia is a disorder of platelet aggregation due to abnormality of the platelet membrane complex GP IIb/IIIa that allows platelets to adhere to the subendothelium but not to fibrinogen.

Hereditary hemorrhagic telangiectasia is a disorder consisting of multiple telangiectatic lesions involving the skin and mucous membranes. Bleeding occurs because of inherent mechanical fragility of the affected vessels.

BOX 25.1 Classification of Congenital Bleeding and Thrombotic Disorders

Nonthrombocytopenic Purpuras
Vascular Wall Alterations
Hereditary hemorrhagic telangiectasia

Disorders of Platelet Function
von Willebrand disease (may have secondary factor VIII deficiency)
Bernard–Soulier disease[a]
Glanzmann thrombasthenia
Others

Thrombocytopenic Purpuras
Gray platelet syndrome
May–Hegglin anomaly
Hereditary thrombocytopenia, deafness, and renal disease
Fechtner syndrome
Alport syndrome
Sebastian platelet syndrome
Others

Disorders of Coagulation
Hemophilia A (factor VIII deficiency)
Hemophilia B (factor IX deficiency)
Other coagulation factor deficiencies

Hypercoagulable States
Antithrombin III deficiency
Protein C deficiency
Protein S deficiency
Factor V Leiden mutation
Prothrombin G2021A mutation
Hyperhomocysteinemia

[a]Bernard–Soulier disease also has been classified as a thrombocytopenic disorder.

TABLE 25.1 Blood Coagulation Components

Factor	Description	Function
Factor II (prothrombin)	Congenital—rare	Protease zymogen
Factor X	Congenital—rare	Protease zymogen
Factor IX	Congenital—rare	Protease zymogen
Factor VII	Congenital—very rare	Protease zymogen
Factor VIII	Congenital—more common	Cofactor
Factor V	Congenital—rare	Cofactor
Factor XI	Congenital—rare	Protease zymogen
Factor XII	Deficiency reported but does not cause bleeding; aPTT will be prolonged	Protease zymogen
Factor I (fibrinogen)	Congenital—rare	Structural
von Willebrand factor	Congenital—most common	Adhesion
Tissue factor	Not applicable	Cofactor initiator
Factor XIII	Congenital—rare; will cause bleeding, but aPTT and PT will be normal	Fibrin stabilization
High-molecular-weight kininogen	Deficiency does not cause bleeding; will prolong aPTT	Coenzyme
Prekallikrein	Deficiency does not cause bleeding; will prolong aPTT	Coenzyme

aPTT, activated partial thromboplastin time; *PT*, prothrombin time.
Data from McVey JH. Coagulation factors. In: Young NS, Gerson SL, High KA, eds. *Clinical Hematology.* St. Louis: Mosby; 2006.

Pathophysiology and Complications

The three sequential phases of hemostasis for controlling bleeding are vascular, platelet, and coagulation. This chapter addresses each of these phases separately.

The vascular and platelet phases are referred to as primary hemostasis, and the coagulation phase is secondary hemostasis. The coagulation phase is followed by the fibrinolytic phase, during which the clot is dissolved. These hemostatic mechanisms are discussed in detail in Chapter 24 regarding acquired bleeding disorders. Complications from any type of bleeding disorder can include intestinal bleeding, hemarthrosis/joint complications, risk for blood borne disease/HIV, and others.

CLINICAL PRESENTATION

The most common objective findings in patients with genetic coagulation disorders are ecchymoses, hemarthrosis, and dissecting hematomas (Figs. 25.1 and 25.2). The signs seen most commonly in patients with abnormal

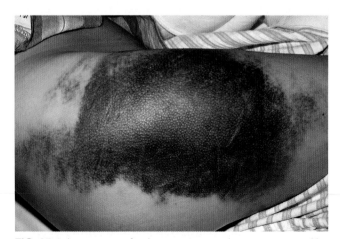

FIG. 25.1 Large area of subcutaneous ecchymoses caused by trauma in a patient with hemophilia. (From Hoffbrand AV, Pettit JE. *Color Atlas of Clinical Hematology.* 4th ed. London: Mosby; 2010.)

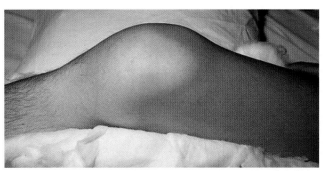

FIG. 25.2 Acute hemarthrosis of the knee is a common complication of hemophilia. It may be confused with acute infection unless the patient's coagulation disorder is known because the knee is hot, red, swollen, and painful. (From Forbes CD, Jackson WF. *Color Atlas and Text of Clinical Medicine.* 3rd ed. London: Mosby; 2003.)

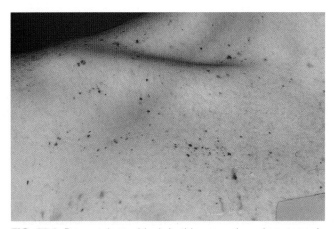

FIG. 25.3 Purpura (petechiae), in this case, thrombocytopenia purpura. The patient was a 15-year-old boy. (From Forbes CD, Jackson WF: *Color atlas and text of clinical medicine,* ed 3, London, 2003, Mosby.)

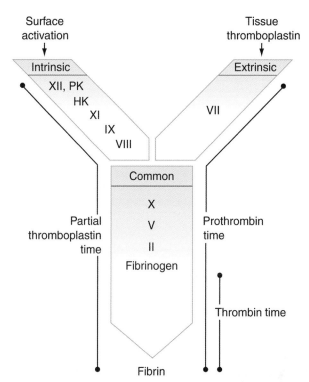

FIG. 25.4 Organization of the coagulation system based on current screening assays. The intrinsic coagulation system consists of the protein factors XII, XI, IX, and VIII; prekallikrein (PK); and high-molecular-weight kininogen (HK). The extrinsic coagulation system consists of tissue factor and factor VII. The common pathway of the coagulation system consists of factors X, V, and II and fibrinogen (I). The activated partial thromboplastin time requires the presence of every protein except tissue factor and factor VII. The prothrombin time requires tissue factor; factors VII, X, V, and II; and fibrinogen. The thrombin clotting time only tests the integrity of fibrinogen. (From McPherson RA, Pincus MR, eds. *Henry's Clinical Diagnosis and Management by Laboratory Methods.* 22nd ed. London: Saunders; 2012.)

platelets or thrombocytopenia are petechiae and ecchymoses (Fig. 25.3). The signs seen most commonly in patients with vascular defects are petechiae and bleeding from the skin or mucous membrane.

Laboratory and Diagnostic Findings

Three tests are recommended for use in initial screening for possible bleeding disorders: activated partial thromboplastin time (aPTT), prothrombin time (PT), and platelet count (Fig. 25.4).

Patients with positive results on screening tests should be evaluated further so that the specific deficiency can be identified and the presence of inhibitors ruled out. A hematologist orders these tests, establishes a diagnosis that is based on the additional testing, and makes recommendations for treatment of the patient who is found to have a significant bleeding problem. The screening laboratory tests are discussed in detail in Chapter 24.

In patients with prolonged aPTT, PT, and TT, the defect involves the last stage of the common pathway, which is the activation of fibrinogen to form fibrin to stabilize the clot. The plasma level of fibrinogen is determined, and if it is within normal limits, then tests for fibrinolysis are performed. These tests, which detect the presence of fibrinogen, fibrin degradation products, or both, consist of staphylococcal clumping assay, agglutination of latex particles coated with antifibrinogen antibody, and euglobulin clot lysis time.

MEDICAL MANAGEMENT

Emphasis is placed on identification of patients with a potential bleeding problem and management of these patients if surgical procedures are needed.

Table 25.2 summarizes the nature of the defects and the medical treatment available for excessive bleeding in patients with the disorders covered in this section. Tables 25.3 and 25.4 list commercial products that are available to treat bleeding problems in these disorders. These products generally work by replacing a coagulation factor or elevating the level of a specific factor in the blood.

TABLE 25.2 Medical Treatment of Congenital Bleeding Disorders

Condition	Defect	Medical Management
Hereditary hemorrhagic telangiectasia	Multiple telangiectasias with mechanical fragility of the abnormal vessels	Laser Surgery Estrogen Estrogen plus progesterone Thalidomide
von Willebrand disease	Deficiency or defect in vWF causing poor platelet adhesion and in some cases deficiency of factor VIII	Desmopressin Aminocaproic acid Factor VIII replacement that retains vWF
Hemophilia A	Deficiency or defect in factor VIII	Desmopressin Aminocaproic acid Factor VIII
	Some patients develop antibodies (inhibitors) to factor VIII	Porcine factor VIII, PCC, aPCC, factor VIIa, and/or steroids for patients with inhibitors
Hemophilia B	Deficiency or defect in factor IX	Desmopressin Aminocaproic acid Factor IX
	Development of antibodies (inhibitors) to factor IX is much less common than with hemophilia A	PCC, aPCC, factor VIIa,[a] and/or steroids for patients with inhibitors
Bernard—Soulier disease	Genetic defect in platelet membrane, absence of GP Ib causes disorder in platelet adhesion	Platelet transfusion Desmopressin Factor VIIa
Glanzmann thrombasthenia	Genetic defect in platelet membrane, absence of GP IIb/IIIa	Platelet transfusion Desmopressin Factor VIIa

[a]Factor VIIa is activated factor VII.

aPCCs, activated prothrombin complex concentrates; *GP*, glycoprotein; *PCCs*, prothrombin complex concentrates; *vWF*, von Willebrand factor.

TABLE 25.3 Food and Drug Administration–Approved Clotting Concentrates for Hemophilia A and B

Preparation With Virucidal Technique(s)	Type (Manufacturer)	Specific Activity (IU/mg Protein)
Ultrapure Recombinant Factor VIII		
Immunoaffinity; ion exchange chromatography	Recombinate (Baxter)	>4000
Ion exchange chromatography, nanofiltration	Refacto (Wyeth)	11,200–15,000
Ion exchange chromatography, ultrafiltration	Kogenate FS (Bayer)	>4000
No human or animal protein used in culture; immunoaffinity and ion exchange chromatography	Advate (Baxter)	>4000–10,000
Ultrapure Human Plasma Factor VIII		
Chromatography and pasteurization	Monoclate P (ZLB Behring)	>3000
Chromatography and solvent detergent	Hemofil M (Baxter)	>3000
High-Purity Human Plasma Factor VIII		
Chromatography, solvent detergent, dry heating	Alphanate SD (Grifols) vWF	50–>400
Solvent detergent, dry heating	Koate-DVI (Bayer) vWF	50–100
Pasteurization (heating in solution)	Humate-P (ZLB-Behring) vWF	1–10
Porcine Plasma-Derived Factor VIII		
Solvent detergent viral attenuation	Hyate-C (Ibsen/Biomeasure)	>50
Ultrapure Recombinant Factor IX		
Affinity chromatography and ultrafiltration	BeneFix (Wyeth)	>200
Very highly purified plasma factor IX		
Chromatography and solvent detergent	AlphaNine SD (Grifols)	>200
Monoclonal antibody ultrafiltration	Mononine (ZLB-Behring)	>160

Continued

Low-Purity Plasma Factor IX Complex		
Solvent detergent	Profilnine SD (Grifols)	<50
Vapor heat	Bebulin VH (Baxter)	<50
Activated Plasma Factor IX Complex Concentrate (Used Primarily for Patients With Alloantibody and Autoantibody Factor VIII and IX Inhibitor)		
Vapor heat	FEIBA VH (Baxter)	<50
Recombinate Factor VIIA (Indicated for Patients With Alloantibody and Autoantibody Factor VIII and IX Inhibitors)		
Affinity chromatography, solvent detergent	NovoSeven (Novo Nordis)	50,000

vWF, von Willebrand factor.
Data from Kessler CM. Hemorrhagic disorders: coagulation factor deficiencies. In: Goldman L, Ausiello D, eds. *Cecil Medicine.* 23rd ed. Philadelphia: Saunders; 2008.

TABLE 25.4 Food and Drug Administration–Approved Coagulation Proteins and Replacement Therapies Available in the United States

Deficiency	Inheritance	Prevalence	Minimum Hemostatic Level	Replacement Source(s)
Factor I			50–100 mg	Cryoprecipitate/FFP
Afibrinogenemia	Autosomal R	Rare; <300 families		
Dysfibrogenemia	Autosomal D or R	Rare; >variants		
Factor II (prothrombin)	Autosomal D or R	Rare; 25 kindreds	30% normal	FFP, factor IX complex
Factor V (labile factor)	Autosomal R	1/1 million births	25% normal	FFP
Factor VII	Autosomal R	1/500,000 births	25% normal	Recombinant factor VIIa
Factor VIII (antihemo-philic factor)	X-linked R	1/5000 births	25%–30% for minor bleeds, 50% for serious bleeds, 80% –100% for surgery or life-threatening bleeds	Factor VIII concentrates
von Willebrand disease				
Types 1 and 2	Autosomal D	1% prevalence	>50% vWF	Desmopressin
Type 3	Autosomal R	1/1 million births	>50% vWF	Factor VIII concentrate with vWF
Factor IX (Christmas factor)	X-linked R	1/30,000 births	25%–50% normal	Factor IX complex concentrates
Factor X (Stuart–Prower factor)	Autosomal R	1/500,000 births	10%–25% normal	FFP or factor IX complex concentrates
Factor XI (hemophilia C)	Autosomal D, severe type R	4% Ashkenazi Jews; 1/1 million in general population	20%–40% normal	FFP or factor IX concentrate
Factor XII (Hageman factor)	Autosomal R	Not available	No treatment necessary	
Factor XIII (fibrin-stabilizing factor)	Autosomal R	1/3 million births	5% of normal	FFP, cryoprecipitate or virus-attenuated factor XIII concentrate

D, dominant; *FFP*, fresh-frozen plasma; *R*, recessive; *vWF*, von Willebrand factor.
From Kessler CM. Hemorrhagic disorders: coagulation factor deficiencies. In: Goldman L, Ausiello D, eds. *Cecil Medicine.* 23rd ed. Philadelphia: Saunders; 2008.

Vascular Defects—Hereditary Hemorrhagic Telangiectasia

Hereditary hemorrhagic telangiectasia, also referred to as Osler–Weber–Rendu syndrome, is a rare autosomal dominant disorder that is characterized by multiple telangiectatic lesions involving the skin, mucous membranes, and viscera. One form of the disorder, characterized by a high frequency of symptomatic pulmonary arteriovenous malformations and cerebral abscesses, has been identified. Causative genes *ENG* and *ACVRL1* encode putative receptors for transforming growth factor-beta (TGF-β) superfamily that play a critical role for proper development of the blood vessels.

Pathophysiology and Complications

Telangiectasias consist of focal dilation of postcapillary venules with connections to dilated arterioles, initially through capillaries and later directly. Perivascular mononuclear cell infiltrates also are observed. The vessels of HHT show a discontinuous endothelium and an incomplete smooth muscle cell layer. The surrounding stroma lacks elastin. Thus, the bleeding tendencies are thought to be because of mechanical fragility of the abnormal vessels. Lesions usually appear in affected persons by the age of 40 years, and they increase in number with age.

Clinical Findings. On clinical examination, venous lakes and papular, punctate, mat-like, and linear telangiectasias appear on all areas of the skin and mucous membranes, with a predominance of lesions on and under the tongue and on the face, lips, perioral region, nasal mucosa, fingertips, toes, and trunk. Recurrent epistaxis is a common finding and symptoms tend to worsen with age. Thus, the severity of the disorder often can be gauged by the age at which the nosebleeds begin, with the most severely affected patients experiencing recurrent epistaxis during childhood. Cutaneous changes usually begin at puberty and progress throughout life. Bleeding can occur in virtually every organ, with GI, oral, and urogenital sites most commonly affected (Fig. 25.5). In the GI tract, the stomach and duodenum are more frequent sites of bleeding than is the colon. Other features may include hepatic and splenic arteriovenous shunts, as well as intracranial, aortic, and splenic aneurysms. Pulmonary arteriovenous fistulas are associated with oxygen desaturation, hemoptysis, hemothorax, brain abscess, and cerebral ischemia caused by paradoxical emboli. Cirrhosis of the liver has been reported in some families.

Laboratory and Diagnostic Findings

The diagnosis is based on clinical (Curacao) criteria; there are no reliable laboratory tests to determine the tendency for bleeding to occur in affected persons. Clinical findings and a history of bleeding problems are the only effective means to identify patients at risk.

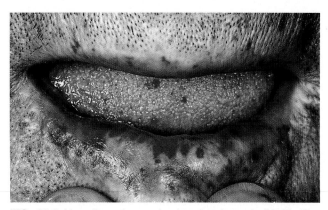

FIG. 25.5 Hereditary hemorrhagic telangiectasia (HHT). The diagnosis usually is clear from a careful clinical examination, although the telangiectases are not always as obvious, as in this patient with multiple lesions on the face, lip, and tongue. (From Forbes CD, Jackson WF. *Color Atlas and Text of Clinical Medicine*. 3rd ed. London: Mosby; 2003.)

MEDICAL MANAGEMENT

Therapy for HHT remains complicated consisting of laser treatment for cutaneous lesions; split-thickness skin grafting, embolization of arteriovenous communications, or hormonal therapy (estrogen or estrogens plus progesterone) for epistaxis; pulmonary resection or embolization for pulmonary arteriovenous malformations; and hormonal therapy and laser coagulation for GI lesions. Estrogen or progesterone treatment has been advised, but benefit has not been demonstrated in a placebo-controlled randomized trial. Treatment with thalidomide can reduce the severity and frequency of nosebleeds (epistaxis). One of the most promising treatments for HHT is bevacizumab (Avastin) given intravenously. Other drugs that block blood vessel growth are pazopanib (Votrient) and pomalidomide (Pomalyst).

The antifibrinolytic agents aminocaproic acid and tranexamic acid have been reported to be beneficial in controlling hemorrhage, but negative results with antifibrinolytic therapy also have been reported. Improvement in lesions has been reported in cases using an antagonist to vascular endothelial growth factor and sirolimus and aspirin. Patients with GI bleeding should receive supplemental iron and folate; red blood cell transfusions and parenteral iron may be required in some patients.

Platelet Disorders
von Willebrand Disease

vWF serves as a carrier protein for Factor VIII and helps with platelet aggregation and adhesion of platelets to damaged endothelium. In von Willebrand disease, affected patients experience platelet dysfunction. This disease is caused by an inherited gene mutation on chromosome 12 (see Fig. 25.6). These gene mutations result in either a deficiency in or qualitatively defective vWF. vWF is produced by megakaryocytes and endothelial cells. vWF is synthesized as a single monomer that polymerizes into huge complexes, which are needed to carry (bind) factor VIII and to allow platelets to adhere to surfaces. Unbound factor VIII is destroyed in the circulation.

The disease has several variants, depending on the severity of genetic expression (Table 25.5). Most of the variants are transmitted as autosomal dominant traits (types 1 and 2). These variants tend to result in mild to moderate clinical bleeding problems. Type 1 is the most common form of von Willebrand disease and accounts for about 70%−80% of cases. The greater the deficiency of vWF in type 1 disease, the more likely it is that signs and symptoms of hemophilia A will be found. Type 2A is responsible for 15%−20% of cases. Type 3, which is rare, is transmitted as an autosomal recessive trait that leads to severe deficiency of vWF and FVIII. Variants of von Willebrand disease with a significant reduction in

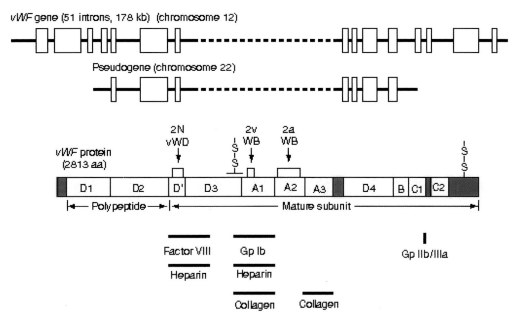

FIG. 25.6 The structure of the von Willebrand factor (vWF) gene and protein. The structures of the vWF gene and pseudogene are indicated schematically at the *top* of the figure. The corresponding protein also is depicted, including the homologous repeat domain structure. The localization within vWF of point mutations associated with von Willebrand disease (vWD) variants also is indicated. *AA*, amino acids; *GP*, glycoprotein. (From Hoffman R, Furie B, McGlave P, et al., eds. *Hematology: Basic Principles and Practice.* 5th ed. Philadelphia: Churchill Livingstone; 2009.)

TABLE 25.5   **Multimeric Patterns of von Willebrand Disease and Laboratory Diagnosis by Type**

Type	Multimeric Pattern	Ristocetin Cofactor Activity	Factor VIII Activity	High-Molecular-Weight vWF Multimers	Ristocetin-Induced Platelet Aggregation
1 (classic)	Uniform reduced in all	Mildly decreased	Moderately decreased	Normal	Mildly decreased or normal
2A	Reduced in large and intermediate multimers	Moderately decreased	Mildly decreased or normal	Moderately decreased	Mildly decreased
2B	Reduced in large multimers	Moderately decreased	Mildly decreased or normal	Mildly decreased	Increased
2M	Mildly decreased or normal	Mildly decreased	Mildly decreased or normal	Normal	Mildly decreased
2N	Normal	Normal	Moderately decreased	Normal	Normal
3	Absent	Markedly decreased	Markedly decreased	Markedly decreased or absent	Markedly decreased

vWF, von Willebrand factor.
Data from Kessler CM. Hemorrhagic disorders: coagulation factor deficiencies. In: Goldman L, Ausiello D, eds. *Cecil Medicine.* 23rd ed. Philadelphia: Saunders; 2008:1301–1313 and Baz R, Mekhail T. Disorders of platelet function and number. In: Carey WD, et al., eds. *Current Clinical Medicine 2009*—Cleveland Clinic. Philadelphia: Saunders; 2009.

vWF or with a vWF that is unable to bind factor VIII may show signs and symptoms of hemophilia A, in addition to those associated with defective platelet adhesion. In mild cases, bleeding occurs only after surgery or trauma. In the more severe cases—type 2N and type 3—spontaneous epistaxis or oral mucosal bleeding may be noted.

Clinical Presentation

Signs and Symptoms. Mild variants of von Willebrand disease are characterized by a history of cutaneous and mucosal bleeding because platelet adhesion is lacking. In the more severe forms of the disease, in which factor VIII levels are low, hemarthroses and dissecting intramuscular

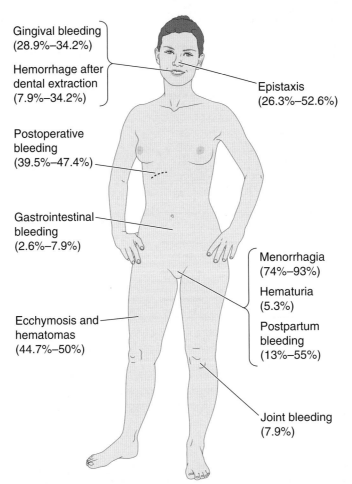

Gingival bleeding
(28.9%–34.2%)

Hemorrhage after
dental extraction
(7.9%–34.2%)

Epistaxis
(26.3%–52.6%)

Postoperative
bleeding
(39.5%–47.4%)

Gastrointestinal
bleeding
(2.6%–7.9%)

Menorrhagia
(74%–93%)

Hematuria
(5.3%)

Postpartum
bleeding
(13%–55%)

Ecchymosis and
hematomas
(44.7%–50%)

Joint bleeding
(7.9%)

FIG. 25.7 Clinical bleeding symptoms by type and frequency in patients with type 1 von Willebrand disease. (From Armstrong E, Konkle BA. von Willebrand disease. In: Young NS, Gerson SL, High KA, eds. *Clinical Hematology*. St. Louis: Mosby; 2006.)

hematomas are part of the clinical picture. Petechiae are rare in patients with vWD. However, GI bleeding, epistaxis, and menorrhagia are very common. Fig. 25.7 shows the sites and frequency of bleeding in patients with type 1 von Willebrand disease. Serious bleeding can occur in these patients after trauma or surgical procedures. Patients with more severe forms of the disease may describe a family history of bleeding and report having had problems with bleeding after injury or surgery. Patients with mild forms of the disease may have a negative history for bleeding problems.

Laboratory and Diagnostic Findings. The diagnosis of vWD requires laboratory investigation. Screening laboratory tests may show prolonged aPTT, normal or slightly reduced platelet count, normal PT, and normal TT. Additional laboratory tests are needed to establish the diagnosis and type of von Willebrand disease. These consist of ristocetin cofactor activity, ristocetin-induced platelet aggregation, immunoassay of vWF, multimeric analysis of vWF, and specific assays for factor VIII.

Medical Management. Treatment depends on the type of von Willebrand disease diagnosed. Available treatment options include cryoprecipitate, factor VIII concentrates that retain HMW vWF multimers (Humate-P, Koate HS),

and desmopressin (1-deamino-8-D-arginine vasopressin [DDAVP]). Before desmopressin is given, the patient must be tested for response to the agent as some patients are nonresponsive. Desmopressin can be given parenterally or by nasal spray 1 h before surgery. With parenteral administration, the dose of desmopressin is 0.3 µg/kg of body weight, with a maximum dose of 20–24 µg. The nasal spray, Stimate, contains 1.5 mg/mL of desmopressin and is given at a dose of 300 mg/kg. Usually, one dose is sufficient. If a second dose is needed, it is given 8–24 h after the first dose. Desmopressin should be used with caution in older patients with cardiovascular disease because of the potential risk of drug-induced thrombosis.

Patients with type 1 von Willebrand disease (type I vWD) are the best candidates for desmopressin therapy. Desmopressin treatment must not be started without previous testing to determine which variant form of von Willebrand disease is involved. It is not effective for type 3 and most variants of type 2 von Willebrand disease. These patients are treated with factor VIII replacement that retains the HMW (high molecular weight) vWF multimers (Humate-P or Koate HS). In patients with type 2 variants with qualitative defects in vWF, Humate-P or

Koate HS supplies functional HMW vWF and factor VIII for those with decreased levels. In patients with type 3 von Willebrand disease, these replacement agents supply deficient materials, vWF, and factor VIII. Affected women are often given oral contraceptive agents to suppress menses and avoid excessive physiologic loss of blood.

Other Hereditary Platelet Function Disorders

The two most common hereditary platelet function disorders (HPFDs), Bernard–Soulier syndrome and Glanzmann thrombasthenia, are discussed in this chapter as examples of platelet function disorders. Other HPFDs include an abnormal alpha granule formation as in the gray platelet syndrome (with marrow myelofibrosis), and of organelle biogenesis in the Hermansky–Pudlak and Chédiak–Higashi syndromes where platelet dense body defects are linked to abnormalities of other lysosome-like organelles including melanosomes. Finally, defects involving surface receptors (P2Y[12], TPα) needed for activating stimuli, of proteins essential for signaling pathways (including Wiskott–Aldrich syndrome), and of platelet-derived procoagulant activity (Scott syndrome) can result in HPFDs.

Hereditary thrombocytopenia (HT) is very rare. Several conditions are classified as HT. These include Fechtner syndrome, Alport syndrome, Sebastian platelet syndrome, and a syndrome consisting of HT, deafness, and renal disease. Owing to the rarity of these conditions, they are not covered in this book, and readers are referred to standard hematology textbooks for more information regarding these disorders.

Bernard–Soulier Syndrome. Bernard–Soulier syndrome represents one of the more common hereditary disorders of platelet adhesion. In this disease, the platelets are large and defective and unable to interact with vWF. In some cases, the platelet count is decreased and hence the tendency of some authors to classify the syndrome as an HT disorder. The disease is caused by mutations in genes controlling the expression of the platelet GP Ib/IX-V complex. It is characterized by qualitative and quantitative defects of GP Ib of the platelet membrane. GP Ib appears to function as a receptor for vWF.

Clinical Presentation. Classic clinical findings in Bernard–Soulier syndrome include epistaxis, easy bruising, mucous membrane bleeding, perioperative bleeding, and menorrhagia. Ecchymosis and gingival and GI bleeding may occur. Bleeding may be intermittent and unpredictable.

Laboratory and Diagnostic Findings. Laboratory testing for the platelet-type bleeding disorders hinges on an adequate assessment by history and physical examination. Patients with a lifelong history of platelet-type bleeding symptoms and perhaps a positive family history of bleeding are appropriate for testing. For patients thought to have an inherited disorder, testing for von Willebrand disease should be done initially

because approximately 1% of the population has the disorder. The complete von Willebrand disease panel (factor VIII coagulant activity, vWf antigen, ristocetin cofactor activity) should be performed because many patients have abnormalities of only one particular panel component. If the results of these studies are normal, platelet aggregation testing should be performed, ensuring that no antiplatelet medications have been ingested at least 1 week before testing.

Platelet morphology can easily be evaluated to screen for two uncommon qualitative platelet disorders: Bernard–Soulier syndrome (associated with giant platelets) and gray platelet syndrome, a subtype of storage pool disorder in which platelet granulation is morphologically abnormal by light microscopy. The lack of well-standardized test systems continue to make the diagnosis of platelet defects cumbersome for practicing clinicians. Patient history and description of clinical bleeding symptoms are essential. Exclusion of von Willebrand disease, platelet count, and investigation of blood smears may provide a tentative diagnosis. Light transmission aggregometry is still considered the "gold standard" modality for assessing platelet function. In summary, laboratory tests show a low platelet count, large platelets, faulty platelet adhesion, and poor aggregation with ristocetin.

Medical Management. Treatment of patients with Bernard–Soulier syndrome generally is supportive, with platelet transfusions when absolutely necessary and avoidance of antiplatelet medications. Recombinant activated factor VII and desmopressin have been used to shorten bleeding times; however, their effectiveness varies from patient to patient.

Glanzmann Thrombasthenia. Glanzmann thrombasthenia (GT) is a rare autosomal recessive disease of platelet dysfunction characterized by a deficiency or defect of the fibrinogen receptor (GP IIb/IIIa) on the platelet surface. The GP IIb/IIIa receptor has an essential function in the adhesion and aggregation of platelets. In GT, platelets can adhere to the subendothelium by means of vWF but cannot bind fibrinogen and aggregation does not occur. Bleeding in this condition is very unpredictable.

Glanzmann thrombasthenia occurs in high frequency in certain ethnic populations with an increased incidence of consanguinity such as in Indians, Iranians, Iraqi Jews, Palestinian and Jordanian Arabs, and a few others.

Clinical Presentation. The recurrent features of GT are epistaxis, easy bruising, oral and gingival hemorrhage, GI bleeding, perioperative bleeding, hemarthrosis, and menorrhagia. Bleeding may be intermittent and unpredictable. Patients often experience bleeding from minor cuts and trauma.

Laboratory and Diagnostic Findings. Laboratory diagnostic testing for GT is the same as described for Bernard–Soulier syndrome.

Medical Management. Lifestyle advice and patient education programs, local measures, antifibrinolytic agents, hormone treatment, platelet transfusions, and recombinant activated factor VII are used to control bleeding. Activated factor VII at a dose of 80–120 µg/kg has been reported to be effective in controlling bleeding after tonsillectomy and severe epistaxis refractory to platelet transfusion.

Coagulation Disorders
Hemophilia A

The hemostatic abnormality in hemophilia A is caused by a deficiency or a defect of factor VIII. Factor VIII circulates in plasma bound to vWF.

Hemophilia A is inherited as an X-linked recessive trait; meaning 50% of male offspring will have the disease, and women serve as carriers. The defective gene is located on the X chromosome (*F8* gene). Severity of bleeding varies greatly; however, within a given affected family, the clinical severity of the disorder is relatively consistent (e.g., affected relatives have similar phenotypes of severity). Because of the high mutation rate of the responsible gene, a negative family history is of limited value in excluding the possibility of a diagnosis of hemophilia A.

The assay of factor VIII activity can be used to identify female carriers of the trait. About 35% of carriers will show a decrease in factor VIII (≈50% of normal factor VIII levels). Immunoassays for vWF can greatly improve the detection rate among carriers of hemophilia A. Polymorphic DNA probes are capable of detecting 90% of affected families and 96% or more of carriers.

Normal homeostasis requires at least 30% factor VIII activity. Symptomatic patients usually have factor VIII levels below 5%. Those with factor VIII levels between 5% and 30% have a mild form of the disease (~40% of patients with hemophilia A). Patients with levels between 1% and 5% have moderate disease (~40% of patients), and severe forms of the disease occur when the level is less than 1% of normal (~20% of patients).

Clinical Presentation. Most affected patients are males who will demonstrate various aspects of bleeding; albeit hemophilia A can rarely manifest in women. Severe hemophilia A is associated with extensive bleeding after trivial injuries. However, the most characteristic bleeding manifestations associated with hemophilia A are hemarthrosis, which often develop without significant trauma (Fig. 25.8).

The frequency and severity of bleeding problems in patients with hemophilia are generally related to the blood level of factor VIII. Patients with *severe hemophilia* (<1% of factor VIII) may experience severe, spontaneous bleeding, with common findings including hemarthrosis, ecchymoses, soft tissue hematomas (Figs. 25.9 and 25.10), and gastrointestinal and genitourinary bleeding. Spontaneous bleeding from the mouth, gingivae, lips, tongue, and nose may occur in these patients. Those with *moderate hemophilia* (1%–5% of factor VIII) exhibit

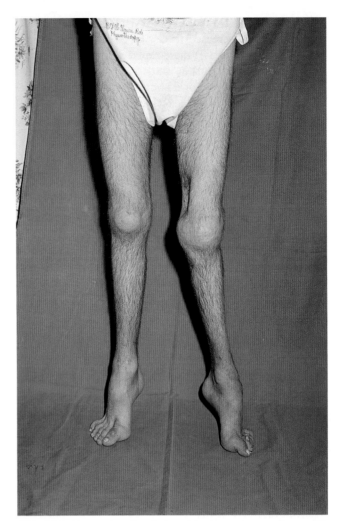

FIG. 25.8 Hemarthrosis of the right knee in a patient with hemophilia. (From Hoffbrand AV. *Color Atlas of Clinical Hematology*. 3rd ed. St. Louis: Mosby; 2000.)

moderate bleeding with minimal trauma or surgery. Hemarthrosis and soft tissue hematomas occur less often. Persons with *mild hemophilia* (5%–30% of factor VIII) may experience mild bleeding after major trauma or surgery. Hemarthrosis and soft tissue hematomas are seldom found in these patients.

Patients with hemophilia usually do not bleed abnormally from small cuts such as razor nicks. After larger injuries, however, bleeding out of proportion to the extent of injury is common. This bleeding may be massive and life-threatening or it may persist as a slow, continuous oozing for days, weeks, or months. The onset of excessive bleeding usually is delayed; at the time of surgery or injury, hemostasis appears to be normal, but bleeding of sudden onset and serious proportions may develop several hours or even several days later.

Laboratory and Diagnostic Findings. Screening tests that show prolonged aPTT, normal PT, and normal platelet count (except in some cases of von Willebrand disease) indicate a problem in the intrinsic pathway. The next step is to mix (mixing tests) the patient's blood with

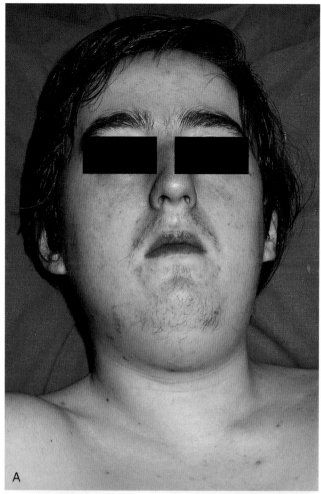

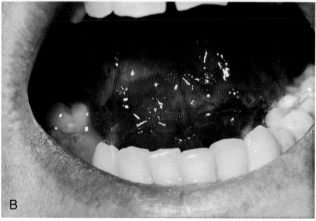

FIG. 25.9 A) The swelling in the submandibular region in a patient with hemophilia was caused by bleeding after intraoral trauma. **(B)** The floor of the mouth has been elevated because of the bleeding. (From Hoffbrand AV. *Color Atlas of Clinical Hematology.* 3rd ed. St. Louis: Mosby; 2000.)

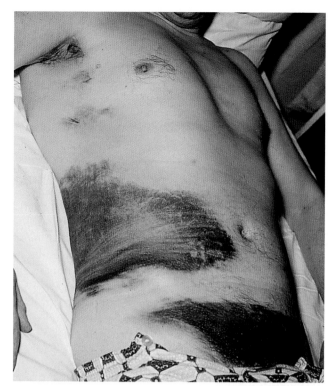

FIG. 25.10 Massive hematomas in a patient with hemophilia. In the absence of major trauma, hematomas of this size always indicate a severe coagulation abnormality. (From Forbes CD, Jackson WF. *Color Atlas and Text of Clinical Medicine.* 3rd ed. London: Mosby; 2003.)

Medical Management. Important nonpharmacologic aspects in the management of patients with hemophilia include patient education regarding the disease with the promotion of exercises such as swimming and avoidance of contact sports, avoidance of aspirin and other nonsteroidal antiinflammatory drugs (NSAIDs), orthopedic evaluation and physical therapy evaluation in patients with joint involvement, and hepatitis vaccination.

The long-term survival of patients with hemophilia has been greatly affected by contamination of donated blood with human immunodeficiency virus (HIV) and hepatitis C virus (HCV). Despite the advent of virally safe blood products and blood treatment programs, nearly 70% of patients with hemophilia are HIV seropositive. Survival is of normal expectancy in HIV-negative persons with mild disease. Intracranial bleeds are the second most common cause of death in patients with hemophilia after acquired immunodeficiency syndrome (AIDS) in HIV-infected persons. Intracranial bleeds are fatal in 30% of patients, occur in 10% of affected individuals, and are generally the result of trauma. By contrast, the lifetime risk of death from intracranial hemorrhage is 2%–8%. The anti-HIV protease inhibitors result in prolonged HIV disease survival among this group of patients. With the exception of HIV and HCV infection, life expectancy is related to the severity of hemophilia, and the mortality rate is four to six times higher for severe disease than for

a sample of pooled plasma and repeat the aPTT. If this test result is normal, then the specific missing factor is identified by specific assays. If the mixing test result is abnormal, tests for inhibitor activity (antibodies to the factor) are performed.

mild to moderate disease. The mortality rate among patients with inhibitors is much greater than among those without inhibitors.

The aim of long-term treatment is to prevent spontaneous bleeding and excessive bleeding during any surgical intervention. Prophylaxis with recombinant factor VIII can prevent joint damage. Implantation of genetically altered fibroblasts that produce factor VIII is safe and well tolerated.

Reversal and prevention of acute bleeding in hemophilia A and B are based on adequate replacement of deficient or missing factor protein. The choice of the product for replacement therapy is guided by availability, capacity, concerns, and cost. Recombinant factors cost two to three times as much as plasma-derived factors, and the limited capacity to produce recombinant factors often results in periods of shortage. In the United States, 60% of patients with severe hemophilia use recombinant products.

Factor VIII concentrates are effective in controlling spontaneous and traumatic hemorrhage in severe hemophilia. Alloantibodies (inhibitors) that neutralize factor VIII clotting function occur in nearly 30% of patients with severe hemophilia A after exposure to factor VIII. Recombinant activated VII is useful to stop spontaneous hemorrhages and prevent excessive bleeding during surgery many patients with inhibitors.

Replacement Factors. Factor VIII replacement guidelines for the control of bleeding from trauma or surgical procedures in patients with severe hemophilia are as follows. For minor spontaneous bleeding or minor traumatic bleeding, 25%−30% replacement of factor VIII is required. For treatment or prevention of severe bleeding during procedures such as major dental surgery or maintenance replacement therapy after major surgery, 50% replacement or greater is needed. Treatment of life-threatening bleeding and limb-threatening bleeding during major surgery requires 80%−100% replacement of factor VIII.

The choice of which type of factor concentrate should be used is based on specific findings from the patient's management history and infectious disease exposure (see Table 25.3). The efficacy of replacement preparations, whether recombinant or plasma derived, is the same. Recombinant factor VIII concentrates are recommended for all patients with no history of factor concentrate treatment, for those who have received concentrates but who are HCV and HIV seronegative, and after surgery or trauma for those with mild or moderate hemophilia that does not respond sufficiently to desmopressin therapy. Plasma-derived concentrates are recommended for patients who are HCV and HIV seropositive.

Patients With Hemophilia Without Inhibitors. All types of general surgical procedures can be performed in patients with hemophilia A who do not have inducible inhibitors of factor VIII (inhibitors are antibodies to factor VIII that result from previous contact with factor VIII replacement). The expected rate of postoperative bleeding

problems is 6%−23%; with orthopedic surgery on the knee, this rate increases to 40%. Patients with mild deficiency of factor VIII can undergo surgical procedures if desmopressin (1-deamino-8-D-arginine [DDAVP], also called vasopressin) is used alone or in combination with ε-aminocaproic acid. Desmopressin, which transiently increases the factor VIII level, can be given parenterally at a dose of 0.3 mg/kg or at an intranasal dose of 300 mg/kg. A second dose can be given if needed 8−24 h after the first dose.

Aminocaproic acid is a potent antifibrinolytic agent that can inhibit plasminogen activators present in oral secretions and stabilize clot formation in tissue. Patients with more severe anti−hemophilic factor (AHF) deficiency require factor VIII replacement. Aminocaproic acid also is given to patients who are receiving factor replacement. Aspirin, aspirin-containing drugs, and other NSAIDs that impair platelet function and may cause severe bleeding must be avoided. Factor VIIa, a recombinant product, is now used in some patients with severe hemophilia A with inducible inhibitors.

Patients With Hemophilia With Inhibitors. A complication that poses great difficulties in the management of patients with hemophilia is the appearance of factor VIII inhibitors. These inhibitors are usually immunoglobulin G (IgG) antibodies to factor VIII. Factor VIII inhibitors (antibodies) develop in patients who have received multiple factor VIII replacement therapy. About 5%−10% of patients with hemophilia have factor VIII inhibitors. The increasing use of factor VIII concentrates increases the risk for development of factor VIII inhibitors; 20%−30% of severe hemophiliac patients are affected. About 40% of patients with hemophilia with inhibitors are *low responders*. Patients with hemophilia whose inhibitor levels rise with additional contact with factor VIII concentrates are called *high responders*; this situation is found in about 60% of patients with hemophilia with inhibitors. Medical management of patients with hemophilia is determined by low or high responder status.

Low responders with minor bleeding can be treated with human factor VIII concentrates. The dosage for these patients is larger than for those without inhibitors. Activated prothrombin complex concentrates may be used if needed in this group of patients. Porcine factor VIII also can be used if low levels of cross-reactivity with this agent occur. For surgical or invasive procedures in low responders, any of these treatments may be used.

High responders often are difficult to manage. Recombinant activated factor VIIa (NovoSeven) is the recommended treatment for these patients.

Hemophilia B

In hemophilia B (Christmas disease) occurs when factor IX is deficient or defective. It is inherited as an X-linked recessive trait (*F9* gene), thus males are primarily affected; however, factor IX levels below 10% have been reported in a few women. Severe disease, in which affected patients have less than 1% of normal amounts of factor IX, is less common than in hemophilia A. Clinical manifestations of the two disorders are identical. Screening laboratory test results are similar for both diseases. Specific factor assays for factor IX establish the diagnosis. Purified and recombinant factor IX products (see Table 25.3) are used for the treatment of minor and major bleeding.

Other Genetic Clotting Factor Deficiencies

Congenital deficiency of prothrombin occurs rarely. Factor V deficiency also is rare; only about 1 case per 1 million people is reported. Factor VII deficiency is inherited as an autosomal recessive trait and therefore affects males and females equally with an incidence of about 1 in 500,000. Factor X deficiency also affects about 1 in 500,000 persons. Factor XI deficiency most often occurs in Ashkenazi Jews but also is seen in other populations. Subjects with a deficiency of factor XII, prekallikrein, or high-molecular-weight kininogen do not have clinical bleeding problems but do have prolonged aPTT. Deficiency of factor XIII is exceedingly rare (~100 clinical cases reported) but potentially very serious; PT and aPTT test results are normal in these patients.

Factor XIII deficiency, α_2 plasmin inhibitor deficiency, and plasminogen activator inhibitor-1 deficiency (major inhibitor of plasminogen activators) are three known diseases associated with defects in the coagulation system; however, they do not affect PT, aPTT, or TT. Patients with a strong clinical history of bleeding and normal coagulation test results (PT, aPTT, and TT) require additional testing, such as the use of 5M urea.

Congenital Hypercoagulability. Many patients with venous thromboembolism have an inherited basis for hypercoagulability. The initial episode of venous thromboembolism usually occurs in early adulthood, but onset may be at any time from early childhood to old age. Arterial thrombosis is unusual in patients with inherited hypercoagulable states. Primary hypercoagulable states result from a deficiency of antithrombotic factors (antithrombin III, protein C or protein S) or increased prothrombotic factors (factor Va [activated protein C resistance, factor V Leiden]: prothrombin [prothrombin G20210A mutation]; factors VII, XI, IX, VIII; von Willebrand factor; fibrinogen; and hyperhomocysteinemia) (Fig. 25.11).

Inherited quantitative or qualitative deficiency of antithrombin III leads to increased fibrin accumulation and a lifelong propensity to thrombosis. Antithrombin is the major physiologic inhibitor of thrombin and other activated coagulation factors; therefore, its deficiency leads to unregulated protease activity and fibrin formation. The frequency of asymptomatic heterozygous antithrombin deficiency in the general population may be 1 in 350. Most of the affected persons have clinically silent mutations and never have thrombotic manifestations. The frequency of symptomatic antithrombin deficiency in

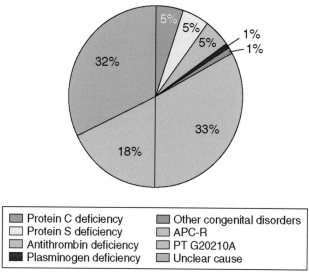

FIG. 25.11 Results of testing for congenital hypercoagulable states projected for patients who had experienced idiopathic deep venous thrombosis. *APC-R,* activated protein C resistance; *PT G20210A,* prothrombin G20210A mutation. (From Deitcher SR. Hypercoagulable states. In: Carey WD, et al., eds. *Cleveland Clinic's Current Clinical Medicine.* 2nd ed. Philadelphia: Saunders; 2010.)

the general population has been estimated to be between 1 in 2000 and 1 in 5000. Among all patients seen with venous thromboembolism, antithrombin deficiency is detected in only about 1%.

Protein C deficiency leads to unregulated fibrin generation because of impaired inactivation of factors Va and VIIIa two essential cofactors in the coagulation cascade. The prevalence of heterozygous protein C deficiency in the general population is about 1 in 200–500. Protein C deficiency is found in 3%–4% of all patients with venous thromboembolism.

Protein S is the principal cofactor of activated protein C (APC), and its deficiency mimics that of protein C in causing loss of regulation of fibrin generation by impaired inactivation of factors VIIIa and Va. The prevalence of protein S deficiency in the general population is unknown. Its frequency in all patients evaluated for venous thromboembolism (2%–3%) is comparable to that of protein C deficiency.

The *factor V Leiden* mutation (activated protein C resistance) is frequent (3%–7%) in white populations and far less prevalent in black and Asian populations. In various studies, activated protein C resistance was found in a wide range of frequencies (10%–64%) among patients with venous thromboembolism.

A mutation (substitution of G for A at nucleotide 20210) of the prothrombin gene has been associated with elevated plasma levels of prothrombin and an increased risk for venous thrombosis. The allele frequency for this gain-of-function mutation is 1%–6% in white populations, but it is much less prevalent in other racial groups. The *prothrombin G20210A mutation* is found in 6%–8% of all patients with venous thromboembolism.

The laboratory diagnosis of primary hypercoagulable states requires testing for each of the disorders individually because no general screening test is available to determine whether a patient may have such a condition.

Dental Management

Patient Identification. The four methods by which the dentist can identify the patient who may have a bleeding problem are a good history, careful physical examination, screening laboratory tests, and occurrence of excessive bleeding after a surgical or invasive dental procedure.

History and Symptoms. Patients with severe coagulation disorders may have dramatic abnormal bleeding histories but often do not volunteer this information unless asked. A history of spontaneous hemarthroses and muscle hemorrhages is highly suggestive of severe hemophilia. By contrast, epistaxis, gingival bleeding, and menorrhagia are common in patients with thrombocytopenia, platelet disorders, or von Willebrand disease. Several hemorrhagic symptoms are more specific for certain disorders—for example, a history of prolonged bleeding after extraction of teeth is more suggestive of von Willebrand disease or platelet disorders than of hemophilia. Patients with a history of bruising and bleeding but with normal results on coagulation tests and normal platelet counts may be afflicted with vascular disorders such as HHT, Cushing disease, scurvy, Ehlers–Danlos syndrome, or other similar conditions.

The history should include questions on six topics: bleeding problems in relatives; excessive bleeding after operations, surgical procedures, and tooth extractions; excessive bleeding after trauma; use of drugs for prevention of coagulation or chronic pain; past and present illness; and occurrence of spontaneous bleeding (e.g., nosebleeds).

Bleeding Problems in Relatives.

Male offspring of parents with a family history of hemophilia are at risk for the disease. Hemophilia is very rare in females but can occur when a man with hemophilia marries a female carrier and they have female children, half of whom will have hemophilia. Children of a parent with von Willebrand disease type 1 also are at risk; about 33% of them will inherit the disorder. Children of parents with a hereditary disorder of connective tissue or HHT are at risk for a bleeding disorder. In rare cases of a family history of disorders of platelet function, such as Bernard–Soulier syndrome or Glanzmann thrombasthenia, the bleeding disorder may be passed to offspring.

The most meaningful data are reported as a recent negative or positive history of excessive bleeding after a major hemostatic challenge. With a negative history, the patient is not a bleeder. By contrast, the patient with a positive history is a bleeder. A negative history of bleeding after minor insults in a patient with a mild bleeding diathesis does not rule out a problem with more severe surgical or traumatic events. Thus, the more recent and severe the surgical or traumatic event, the more accurate it will be in revealing the presence of a bleeding disorder.

Physical Examination.

The dentist should inspect the exposed skin and mucosa of the oral cavity and pharynx of the patient for signs that might indicate a possible bleeding disorder. Signs include petechiae, ecchymoses, spider angiomas, telangiectasias, jaundice, pallor, and cyanosis (possible thrombocytopenia). When any of these signs are found by the dentist and cannot be explained by the history or other clinical findings, the patient should be referred for medical evaluation.

Screening Laboratory Tests.

The dentist can use four clinical laboratory tests to screen patients for congenital bleeding disorders: platelet count, aPTT, PT, and TT. The platelet count is ordered to screen for thrombocytopenia. The aPTT test is used to measure the status of the intrinsic and common pathways of coagulation. This test reflects the ability of blood remaining within vessels in the area of injury to coagulate. It will be prolonged in coagulation disorders affecting the intrinsic and common pathways (hemophilia, liver disease) and in cases of excessive fibrinolysis.

If indeed prolonged beyond the normal range, the results of these screening tests direct the hematologist to the possible source of a bleeding disorder and allow for the selection of more specific tests to identify the nature of the defect.

Medical Considerations. Oral surgical procedures may need to be delayed on a patient who is suspected of having a bleeding problem. Such a patient should be screened by the dentist through appropriate history and clinical laboratory tests, and/or referred to a physician/hematologist for screening. After consultation with the patient's physician/hematologist and after appropriate preparations have been made to avoid excessive bleeding, surgery may be performed.

Management of the Patient With a Serious Bleeding Disorder. Before any invasive dental treatment is performed for a patient with a bleeding disorder, the dentist must consult with the patient's physician to determine the severity of the disorder and the need for special preparations for dental treatment. Patients with significant bleeding disorders are at increased risk for spontaneous gingival bleeding or excessive bleeding after minor trauma to the oral tissues. The risk of such problems is greater if surgical procedures are performed without special preparations. Hemophilia A and von Willebrand disease are presented here to demonstrate how patients with a serious bleeding disorder can be managed to avoid significant bleeding complications.

Hemophilia. When a patient with hemophilia A (factor VIII deficiency) (or with a clinical history suggestive of the disorder) presents for dental treatment, consultation with a hematologist is essential. The hematologist first establishes the diagnosis and determines the degree of factor VIII deficiency, whether any factor VIII inhibitors are present, if the patient is a low or a high responder, and whether hospitalization will be needed. The type of therapy is selected (Box 25.2; see also Table 25.3), and the hematologist may make recommendations regarding the appropriate agents to use.

Patients with severe hemophilia A exhibit signs and symptoms at a very early age. It is important that preventive dentistry practices be initiated early and maintained through adulthood for all patients with hemophilia. Dental caries and periodontal disease should be minimized in these patients. The use of fluorides and fissure sealants and dietary recommendations regarding refined carbohydrate restriction are important for minimizing tooth loss. Toothbrushing, flossing, and regular

dental visits are important for prevention of caries and periodontal disease, which should be treated when detected. Through maintenance of good oral hygiene and dental repair, the need for dental procedures requiring factor VIII replacement can be minimized.

In general, block anesthesia, lingual infiltrations, or injections into the floor of the mouth and intramuscular injections must be avoided unless appropriate replacement factors have been used in patients with moderate to severe factor VIII deficiency. Complex restorative procedures usually require replacement therapy.

Infiltration anesthesia and intraligamentary injections usually can be given without replacement therapy. Simple restorative procedures often can be performed without replacement therapy, as can endodontic treatment of nonvital teeth; however, overinstrumentation and

---

BOX 25.2 | Checklist for Dental Management of Patients With Patients With a Bleeding Disorder[a]

PREOPERATIVE RISK ASSESSMENT
- Evaluate and determine whether a bleeding disorder exists.
- Obtain medical consultation if undiagnosed, poorly controlled, or if uncertain. signs.
- Screen patients with bleeding history or clinical signs of a bleeding disorders with PT, aPTT, TT, and platelet count.
- Review recent laboratory test results to assess risk.

A

Analgesics	Avoid aspirin, aspirin-containing compounds, and other NSAIDs; acetaminophen with or without codeine is suggested for most patients.
Antibiotics	No issues.
Anesthesia	Avoid block anesthetic injections in patients not on desmopressin, aminocaproic acid, or factor concentrates.
Anxiety	No issues.
Allergy	Patients placed on factor VIII replacement need to be observed for signs and symptoms of allergy.

B

Bleeding	These patients are at great risk of bleeding from invasive dental procedures. Special precautions must be taken before invasive procedures. Patients with mild to moderate hemophilia can be managed using desmopressin and aminocaproic acid for many dental procedures. Factor VIII replacement is needed for patients with more severe hemophilia. Patients who are low responders for inhibitors (antibody response to factor VIII) require higher doses of factor VIII. Patients who are high responders are most difficult to manage and require activated factor VII, porcine factor VIII, steroids, or other special preparations such as prothrombin complex concentrates or activated prothrombin complex concentrations.

Breathing	No issues.
Blood pressure	No issues.

C

Chair position	No issues.
Cardiovascular	No issues.
Consultation	The patient's hematologist must be consulted before any invasive dental procedures are performed. The severity of disease must be established. The presence of inhibitors and level of response to factor VIII need to be determined. Determine if the patient can be managed with desmopressin and aminocaproic acid. Establish the type and dosage of factor replacement needed for invasive dental procedures or surgery. Determine if the patient can be managed in the dental office or will require hospitalization.

D

Devices	Splints may be constructed before multiple extractions or surgical procedures in patients with severe hemophilia.
Drugs	Avoid all drugs that may cause bleeding, such as aspirin and other NSAIDs, certain herbal medications, and over-the-counter drugs containing aspirin.

E

Equipment	No issues.
Emergencies	Excessive bleeding may occur after invasive dental procedures or surgery. Systemic and local means may be required to control the bleeding (see Tables 25.3 and 25.6).

POSTOPERATIVE CARE
F

Follow-up	Patients should be seen and examined for signs of bleeding within 24—48 h after surgical procedures.

NSAID, nonsteroidal antiinflammatory drug; *PT*, prothrombin time; *PTT*, partial thromboplastin time; *TT*, thrombin time.
[a]Strength of recommendation taxonomy (SORT) Grade: C (see Preface for further explanation).

overfilling must be avoided. Intracanal injection of a local anesthetic along with epinephrine will help to control bleeding.

Orthodontic treatment can be provided to patients with hemophilia, but sharp edges on appliances must be avoided. Sharp edges can injure the mucosa, causing significant bleeding in patients with severe to moderate hemophilia.

Periodontal surgery, root planing, extractions, dentoalveolar surgery, soft tissue surgery, and complex oral surgery usually require factor replacement in patients with moderate to severe factor VIII deficiency. When mucoperiosteal flaps are required in the mandibular region, the buccal or labial approach is preferred in order to minimize bleeding. Also, the buccal approach is recommended for surgical removal of mandibular third molars. Trauma to mandibular lingual tissues increases the risk of bleeding, which can lead to airway obstruction. Mandibular acrylic splints are not used as often as they were in the past because of problems with tissue trauma and infection. If local bleeding occurs, one or more of the procedures listed in Table 25.6 can be used to control it.

Conservative periodontal procedures, including polishing with a prophy cup and supragingival calculus removal, often can be performed without replacement therapy as long as injury to the gingival tissues is avoided. Patients with mild factor VIII deficiency who lack inhibitors often can be managed in the dental office for less invasive procedures such as scaling, soft tissue surgery, and extractions without factor VIII replacement; desmopressin and aminocaproic acid or tranexamic acid may be used if needed. Patients with moderate factor VIII deficiency without inhibitors may require factor VIII replacement for less invasive dental procedures. Patients with moderate hemophilia and no inhibitors will require factor VIII replacement for major oral surgery. Patients with severe hemophilia will require factor VIII replacement for all invasive dental treatments. One or more of the local procedures listed in Table 25.6 can be used as adjuncts to aid in the control of bleeding.

Tranexamic acid can be administered orally, intravenously, or as a mouth wash to control hemorrhage during or after tooth extraction. The oral form (Lysteda oral tablets, Ferring Pharmaceuticals, Saint-Prex, Switzerland) is approved by the US Food and Drug Administration for use in patients with heavy menstrual bleeding. Lysteda comes in 500 mg tablets, 25 mg/kg, and is given just before the surgery and then three to four times per day as needed. The dentist can request the pharmacy to prepare a 5% solution of tranexamic acid to be used as a mouthwash. The patient is instructed to take 5 mL of the solution and hold in the mouth for 2 min and then spit it out. The first dose should be taken just before the procedure and repeated four times per day as needed.

An intravenous form of tranexamic acid, Cyklokapron (IV) (Pfizer, New York), has been approved for use in the United States. It is given (10 mg/kg) just before the

surgical procedure and then three times per day as needed. It is supplied in 100-mg vials. Care must be taken with use of this drug because of the risk for thrombotic events, particularly in older patients and with long-term use.

Aminocaproic acid (Amicar) is an antifibrinolytic agent used to treat serious bleeding conditions, especially when the bleeding occurs after dental surgery. Amicar is typically given before oral surgery by tablet or solution to prevent serious bleeding for patients with bleeding problems in order to reduce complications. Dosing for adults—5 grams (g) or four teaspoonfuls as a single dose for the first hour, followed by 1 g or one teaspoonful every hour for 8 h or until bleeding has been controlled. Amicar must be given on a fixed schedule.

Patients with hemophilia with inhibitors who are low responders usually will require factor VIII replacement for any invasive dental procedure. Human, porcine, or ultrapure factor VIII replacements may be used, depending on the clinical situation. Patients with hemophilia who are high responders require factor VIIa concentrate for all invasive dental procedures.

Patients with hemophilia who have undergone invasive dental procedures should be seen within 24–48 h by the dentist to check on control of bleeding. If bleeding is occurring, the hematologist may have to give additional factor VIII replacement concentrates, or the dentist may need to apply one or more of the local procedures listed in Table 25.6. Patients who have received factor VIII replacements also must be examined within 24–48 h after surgery for any evidence of an allergic reaction to the concentrates and to determine whether the wound is healing without complications.

Before oral surgery, the dentist can make splints so that mechanical displacement of the clot in wounds healing by secondary intention is prevented. Care should be taken in the construction of the splints so that pressure is not placed on soft tissues; such pressure could lead to tissue injury, bleeding, and infection. All extraction sites should be packed with microfibrillar collagen, and the wound should be closed with sutures for primary healing whenever possible. Endodontic procedures should be performed, rather than extractions, whenever possible because the risk for serious bleeding is lessened by this approach.

In many instances, the patient must be hospitalized for dental surgical procedures. This decision should be made according to the procedure planned and in consultation with the patient's hematologist. Patients who have a mild to moderate form of hemophilia without inhibitors can be managed on an outpatient basis with the use of desmopressin, aminocaproic acid, or tranexamic acid, or with replacement therapy plus aminocaproic acid. Box 25.2 reviews the roles and functions of the hematologist and the dentist in managing patients with hemophilia. Postoperative pain control usually can be obtained with the use of acetaminophen with or without codeine (see Box 25.2).

TABLE 25.6   Topical Hemostatic Agents Used to Control Bleeding

Product	Company or Manufacturer	Description	Indications and Features
Gauze		2 × 2-inch sterile gauze pads; placed over the wound, with pressure applied by patient (by closing jaws or with fingers)	Bleeding immediately after extractions or minor surgical procedures
Gelfoam	Pharmacia & Upjohn	Absorbable gelatin sponge made from purified gelatin solution; absorbs in 3–5 days	Useful for most patients taking an antithrombotic agent; helpful to place topical thrombin on Gelfoam; for extensive or invasive surgery, can be placed inside a splint
HemCon Dental Dressing	HemCon Medical Technologies	10- × 12-mm or 1- × 3-inch dressing; place on wound (best if some blood is present, helps stick dressing to the wound); made of chitosan from shellfish	Can be used on extraction sites and oral wounds; can be used in patients taking anticoagulants
Cellulose			
Surgicel Oxycel	Johnson & Johnson Becton Dickinson	Oxidized regenerated cellulose; exerts physical effect rather than physiologic; swells on contact with blood with resulting pressure adding to hemostasis; thrombin is ineffective with these agents because of inactivation as a result of pH factors	After 24–48 h, it becomes gelatinous; can be left in place or removed; useful to control bleeding when other agents ineffective
Collagen			
Instat	Johnson & Johnson	Absorbable collagen made from purified and lyophilized bovine dermal collagen; can be cut or shaped; adheres to bleeding surfaces when wet but does not stick to instruments, gloves, or gauze sponges	Mild to moderate bleeding usually controlled in 2–5 min; more expensive than Gelfoam
Avitene Helistat	MedChem Products Marion Merrell Dow	Microfibrillar collagen hemostat: dry, sterile, fibrous, water insoluble HCl acid salt—purified bovine corium collagen: MCH attracts platelets and triggers aggregation in fibrous mass	Thrombin ineffective with these agents because of inactivation as a result of pH factors; moderate to severe bleeding
Colla-Cote, Tape, Plug	Zimmer Dental	Absorbable collagen dressings from bovine sources; can be sutured into place, used under stents or dentures or alone; fully resorbed in 10–14 days	Shaped according to intended use: "cote" $3/4$ × 1.5 inch, tape 1 × 3 inch, plug $3/8$ × $3/4$ inch; all are superior hemostats for moderate to severe bleeding
Thrombin			
Thrombostat Thrombinar Thrombogen	Parke-Davis Jones Medical Johnson & Johnson—Merck	Topical thrombin—directly converts fibrinogen to fibrin; derived from bovine sources	One 5000-unit vial dissolved in 5 mL of saline can clot equal amount of blood in <1 s; useful in severe bleeding.
Tranexamic acid Lysteda (tablets) Cyklokapron (IV)	Xanodyne Pfizer	Tranexamic acid works as a competitive inhibitor of plasminogen activation; used as a mouth wash (5%), taken orally as a tablet, or given IV	Useful in the short term for preventing hemorrhage after dental extractions
Amicar Tablets (500 mg) Syrup (1.25 g/ 5 mL) IV (250 mg/mL)	Wyeth-Ayerst	ε-Aminocaproic acid works as a competitive inhibitor of plasminogen activation; most often used as a mouth wash; can be taken orally or by IV	Useful in the short term to prevent bleeding
Histocryl	B. Braun	Active ingredient is N-butyl 2-cyanoacrylate, serves as a glue to protect surgical wounds	Useful in the short term to prevent bleeding
Beriplast	Behring Werke	Fibrin/tissue glue	Not available in the United States

IV, intravenous; *MCH*, mean corpuscular hemoglobin (hemoglobin content of red blood cells).

von Willebrand Disease. Surgical procedures can be performed in patients with mild von Willebrand disease (type 1 and some type 2 variants) with the use of desmopressin, tranexamic acid, or aminocaproic acid (also known as epsilon-aminocaproic acid, EACA). Patients with more severe types of von Willebrand disease require factor VIII concentrates such as Humate-P that retain vWF multimers to replace the missing vWF and factor VIII. A study by Federici and colleagues reported the results of bleeding complications in 63 consecutive patients with von Willebrand disease. In this study where all patients had extractions or periodontal surgery, bleeding was controlled in 97% of the patients with the use of local measures combined with tranexamic acid, fibrin glue, and desmopressin. In all cases, tranexamic acid was given before and for 7 days after surgery and the desmopressin was administered systemically. The investigators concluded that tranexamic acid, fibrin glue, and desmopressin can prevent bleeding complications in the vast majority of patients with von Willebrand disease (84%). Thus, surgery can be safely performed by providing adequate and timely hemostasis during and after the procedure in patients with von Willebrand disease. Box 25.2 reviews the roles and functions of the hematologist and dentist in the management of patients with von Willebrand disease.

Treatment Planning Modifications. With proper preparation, most indicated dental treatment can be provided for patients with mild to moderate bleeding problems; however, those with severe bleeding disorders may require hospitalization. Patients with congenital coagulation defects must be encouraged to improve and maintain good oral hygiene. Aspirin and other NSAIDs should be avoided for pain relief in patients who have known bleeding disorders or who are receiving anticoagulant medication. Medications that contain aspirin include Anacin, Synalgos-DC, Fiorinal, Bufferin, Alka-Seltzer, Empirin with Codeine, and Excedrin. Also, herbal medications that may be associated with excessive bleeding are to be avoided (see Appendix E).

Oral Manifestations. Patients with congenital bleeding disorders may experience spontaneous gingival bleeding. Oral tissues (e.g., soft palate, tongue, buccal mucosa) may show ecchymoses and petechiae. Bleeding occurring after the extraction of teeth may be the first evidence of mild coagulation disorders such as hemophilia A, hemophilia B, or von Willebrand disease variants with factor VIII deficiency (Fig. 25.12). Spontaneous gingival bleeding and petechiae usually are found in patients with genetic platelet disorders or HHT. Hemarthrosis of the temporomandibular joint is a rare finding in patients with genetic coagulation disorders.

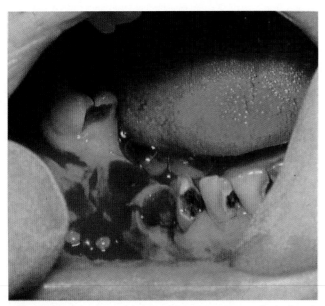

FIG. 25.12 Severe hemorrhage after dental extraction often is the first clue to more minor degrees of coagulation disorder and is a common presentation in patients with hemophilia A, hemophilia B, and von Willebrand disease. (From Forbes CD, Jackson WF. *Color Atlas and Text of Clinical Medicine.* 3rd ed. London: Mosby; 2003.)

BIBLIOGRAPHY

1. Arruda V, High KA. Coagulation disorders. Boyce JA, Austen KF. Allergies, anaphylaxis and systemic mastocytosis. In: Jameson J, Fauci AS, Kasper DL, et al., eds. *Harrison's™ Principles of Internal Medicine.* 20th ed. McGraw-Hill Publishers; 2018. Copyright © 2018. Volume 1 eBook ISBN 978-1-259-64400-9; MHID 1-259-64400-6; Volume 2 eBook ISBN 978-1-259-64402-3; MHID 1-259-64402.

2. Bennett JS. Hereditary disorders of platelet function. Boyce JA, Austen KF. Allergies, anaphylaxis and systemic mastocytosis. In: Jameson J, Fauci AS, Kasper DL, et al., eds. *Harrison's™ Principles of Internal Medicine.* 20th ed. McGraw-Hill Publishers; 2018. Copyright © 2018.

3. Bauer KA. Hypercoagulable states. In: Hoffman R, Furie B, McGlave P, eds. *Hematology: Basic Principles and Practice.* 5th ed. Philadelphia: Churchill Livingstone, Elsevier; 2009:2021−2042.

4. Coller BS, Schneiderman PI. Boyce JA, Austen KF. Allergies, anaphylaxis and systemic mastocytosis. In: Jameson J, Fauci AS, Kasper DL, et al., eds. *Harrison's™ Principles of Internal Medicine.* 20th ed. McGraw-Hill Publishers; 2018. Copyright © 2018. Volume 1 eBook ISBN 978-1-259-64400-9; MHID 1-259-64400-6; Volume 2 eBook ISBN 978-1-259-64402-3; MHID 1-259-64402.

5. Kessler CM. Hemorrhagic disorders: coagulation factor deficiencies. In: Goldman L, Ausiello D, eds. *Cecil Textbook of Medicine.* Philadelphia: Saunders; 2004:1069−1078.

6. Konkle BA. Disorders of platelets and vessel wall. Boyce JA, Austen KF. Allergies, anaphylaxis and systemic mastocytosis. In: Jameson J, Fauci AS, Kasper DL, et al., eds. *Harrison's™ Principles of Internal Medicine.* 20th ed. McGraw-Hill Publishers; 2018. Copyright © 2018. Volume 1 eBook ISBN 978-1-259-64400-9; MHID 1-259-64400-6; Volume 2 eBook ISBN 978-1-259-64402-3; MHID 1-259-64402.

7. McVey JH. Coagulation factors. In: Young NS, Gerson SL, High KA, eds. *Clinical Hematology*. St. Louis: Elsevier - Mosby; 2006:103–123.

8. Nichols WL. von Willebrand disease and hemorrhagic abnormalities of platelet and vascular function. Boyce JA, Austen KF. Allergies, anaphylaxis and systemic mastocytosis. In: Jameson J, Fauci AS, Kasper DL, et al., eds. *Harrison's^TM Principles of Internal Medicine*. 20th ed. McGraw-Hill Publishers; 2018. Copyright © 2018. Volume 1 eBook ISBN 978-1-259-64400-9; MHID 1-259-64400-6; Volume 2 eBook ISBN 978-1-259-64402-3; MHID 1-259-64402.

9. Ragni MV, Kessler CM, Lozier JN. Clinical aspects and therapy of hemophilia. In: Hoffman R, Furie B, McGlave P, eds. *Hematology: Basic Principles and Practice*. 5th ed. Philadelphia: Churchill Livingstone, Elsevier; 2009: 1911–1930. Volume 1 eBook ISBN 978-1-259-64400-9; MHID 1-259-64400-6; Volume 2 eBook ISBN 978-1-259-64402-3; MHID 1-259-64402-.

10. Windyga J, Dolan G, Altisent C, et al. Practical aspects of DDAVP use in patients with von Willebrand disease undergoing invasive procedures: a European survey. *Haemophilia*. 2016;22(1):110–120.

26

Cancer and Oral Care of Patients With Cancer

KEY POINTS

- Dentists should obtain a thorough medical history for patients with cancer that includes the diagnosis, stage, past and current therapies, complications, and overall prognosis.
- Dentists must perform a risk assessment for dental treatment, including review of relevant lab values and past and current therapies, to assess for risk of
- complications such as bleeding, infection, compromised healing and jaw osteonecrosis, and drug interactions.
- Dentists should perform an oral cancer screening during exams and can play an active role in risk reduction through promotion of smoking cessation, regular exercise, and eating a healthy diet.

Cancer is a heterogeneous disease that affects all ages that is characterized by unregulated cellular growth and proliferation and tissue destruction. Cancers arising in the oral cavity and head and neck region may be detected by dentists during routine examination. Treatment of cancer is associated with a variety of oral health–related complications that can lead to significant morbidity and interfere with the delivery of cancer care. Dental clearance protocols are indicated prior to certain cancer therapies due to high risk of infection and impaired healing. Dentists play an important role in the management of the cancer patient from diagnosis through survivorship and must understand how to assess risk and provide safe and appropriate dental care.

EPIDEMIOLOGY

A total of 1,762,450 new cancer cases and 606,880 cancer deaths were projected to occur in the United States in 2019 (Fig. 26.1). Among men, cancers of the prostate, lung and bronchus, and colon and rectum account for more than 50% of all newly diagnosed cancers. In women, the most common cancers are breast, lung, colon, and uterine. Over 10,000 children in the United States under the age of 15 will be diagnosed with cancer in 2021, with the most common cancers being leukemia, brain and spinal cord tumors, neuroblastoma, Wilms tumor, lymphoma (including both Hodgkin and non-Hodgkin), rhabdomyosarcoma, retinoblastoma, and bone cancer (including osteosarcoma and Ewing sarcoma).

The death rate from all cancers combined has decreased slightly in the past 10 years (Fig. 26.2). As with many diseases, ethnic and racial disparities exist; for example, African American men and women have 40% and 18% higher death rates from all cancers combined than do white men and women, respectively. Minority populations also are more likely than whites to be diagnosed with advanced-stage disease. These higher rates likely relate to

social, economic, and historical disparities and differences in environment, personal behavior, and habits. When deaths are aggregated by age, cancer has surpassed heart disease as the leading cause of death in those younger than age 85, and after accidents, cancer is the second leading cause of death in children ages 1–14. Globally, cancer is the second leading cause of death, responsible for approximately 10 million deaths per year, with about 70% occurring in low- and middle-income countries. Despite this, the population of cancer survivors in the United States continues to grow (Fig. 26.3). In a typical dental practice with 2000 patients, approximately 100 patients would be expected to have an active or past diagnosis of cancer.

ETIOLOGY

Carcinogenesis is a highly complex multistep process that involves the accumulation of mutations, epigenetic alterations, and the loss of regulatory control over cell division, differentiation, apoptosis, and adhesion (Fig. 26.4). Mutations can arise de novo as well as from exposure to hazardous chemicals and pathogens that lead to activation of oncogenes, inactivation of tumor suppressor genes, and chromosomal abnormalities (translocations, deletions, insertions). Infection with oncogenic viruses such as high-risk HPV strains (HPV16, HPV18) leads to integration of viral genetic material into the host DNA that inactivate tumor suppressor genes leading to carcinogenesis. The tumor microenvironment also has been shown to be actively involved in the development and progression of cancer. Both immunosuppression and chronic inflammation increase the risk of cancer. Patients with cancer are at an increased risk for developing additional cancers, and some cancer therapies are associated with high risk of secondary malignancies. Some chronic inflammatory diseases are associated with increased risk of cancer. Numerous syndromes

Estimated New Cases

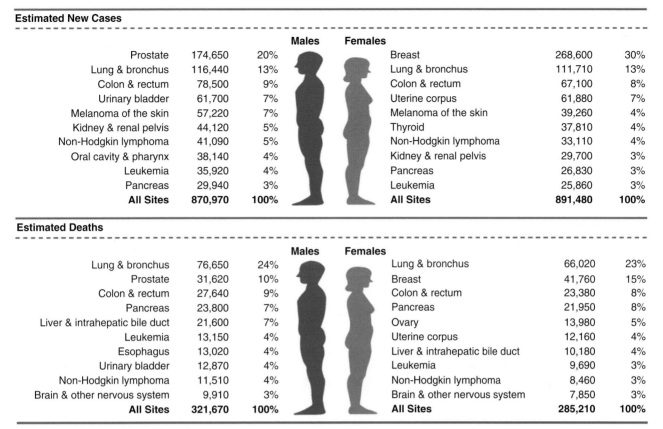

	Males				Females		
Prostate	174,650	20%		Breast	268,600	30%
Lung & bronchus	116,440	13%		Lung & bronchus	111,710	13%
Colon & rectum	78,500	9%		Colon & rectum	67,100	8%
Urinary bladder	61,700	7%		Uterine corpus	61,880	7%
Melanoma of the skin	57,220	7%		Melanoma of the skin	39,260	4%
Kidney & renal pelvis	44,120	5%		Thyroid	37,810	4%
Non-Hodgkin lymphoma	41,090	5%		Non-Hodgkin lymphoma	33,110	4%
Oral cavity & pharynx	38,140	4%		Kidney & renal pelvis	29,700	3%
Leukemia	35,920	4%		Pancreas	26,830	3%
Pancreas	29,940	3%		Leukemia	25,860	3%
All Sites	**870,970**	**100%**		**All Sites**	**891,480**	**100%**

Estimated Deaths

	Males				Females		
Lung & bronchus	76,650	24%		Lung & bronchus	66,020	23%
Prostate	31,620	10%		Breast	41,760	15%
Colon & rectum	27,640	9%		Colon & rectum	23,380	8%
Pancreas	23,800	7%		Pancreas	21,950	8%
Liver & intrahepatic bile duct	21,600	7%		Ovary	13,980	5%
Leukemia	13,150	4%		Uterine corpus	12,160	4%
Esophagus	13,020	4%		Liver & intrahepatic bile duct	10,180	4%
Urinary bladder	12,870	4%		Leukemia	9,690	3%
Non-Hodgkin lymphoma	11,510	4%		Non-Hodgkin lymphoma	8,460	3%
Brain & other nervous system	9,910	3%		Brain & other nervous system	7,850	3%
All Sites	**321,670**	**100%**		**All Sites**	**285,210**	**100%**

FIG. 26.1 Ten leading cancer types for the estimated new cancer cases and deaths by sex, United States, 2019. Estimates are rounded to the nearest 10 and exclude basal cell and squamous cell skin cancers and in situ carcinoma except urinary bladder. Ranking is based on modeled projections and may differ from the most recent observed data. (Reproduced from Siegel RL, Miller KD, Jemal A. Cancer statistics, 2019. *CA Cancer J Clin.* 2019;69:7—34.)

predispose to cancer (e.g., Cowden syndrome, PTEN mutation; Fanconi anemia, FANCA, B, C mutations). The aggregation of cancer in a family can be due to genetic (e.g., inheritance of genes that predispose to cancer) or epigenetic causes (e.g., common exposure to carcinogenic agents or lifestyle).

Cytogenetic studies of various leukemias have established four cardinal attributes of genetic change in cancer: (1) specific or nonrandom chromosomal changes may characterize individual cancer types; (2) tumor genomes are genetically unstable and subject to continuing change, a feature recognized as genomic instability; (3) all cells in a given tumor trace back to a single progenitor cell and therefore are clonal; and (4) tumor progression is often associated with additional alterations in subpopulations of tumor cells that lead to clonal diversity and evolution. Chromosomal and genomic instability occurs due to several mechanisms including gain of an entire chromosome (aneuploidy) or a region of it (duplication), loss of an entire chromosome (monosomy) or a region of it (deletion), translocation or inversion (rearrangement), and amplification.

Globally, around one-third of deaths from cancer are collectively due to tobacco use (overall the most important risk factor for cancer), high body mass index, alcohol use, low fruit and vegetable intake, and lack of physical activity. Infections (e.g., hepatitis and HPV) are responsible for approximately 30% of cancer cases in low- and lower-middle-income countries.

Cancer control efforts focus on the reduction or elimination of factors known to be associated with cancer. Recommendations from the American Cancer Society are to minimize exposure to tobacco smoke and to environmental and occupational carcinogens (e.g., asbestos fibers, arsenic compounds, chromium compounds, pesticides), decrease intake of fat and exposure to ultraviolet (UV) light, moderate the intake of alcohol, obtain an adequate intake of dietary fiber and antioxidants (vitamins C and E, selenium), perform moderate levels of physical activity, and utilize preventive screenings.

Pathophysiology and Complications

Cancer is characterized by uncontrolled growth and spread of aberrant neoplastic cells. There are universal cellular abnormalities and "mechanisms" of malignancy that have been collectively described as the "hallmarks of cancer"; these include (1) sustaining proliferative signaling, (2) evading growth suppressors, (3) resisting

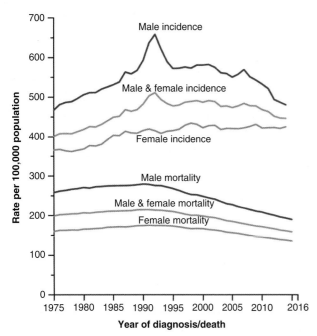

FIG. 26.2 Trends in cancer incidence (1975–2015) and mortality rates (1975–2016) by sex, United States. Rates are age adjusted to the 2000 US standard population. Incidence rates also are adjusted for delays in reporting. (Reproduced from Siegel RL, Miller KD, Jemal A. Cancer statistics, 2019. *CA Cancer J Clin.* 2019;69:7–34.)

cell death, (4) enabling replicative immortality, (5) inducing angiogenesis, (6) abnormal metabolic pathways, (7) evading the immune system, and (8) activating invasion and metastasis (Fig. 26.5). Cancerous cells invade and destroy tissues through direct extension and spread to distant sites by metastasis through blood, lymph, or serosal (intraabdominal) surfaces (Fig. 26.6). Direct complications of cancer are largely related to the type of cancer, primary site of the cancer, invasive properties, and/or site(s) of metastasis.

Metastases can develop anywhere throughout the body; however, bones, liver, lungs, and brain are most frequently affected. Progressive disease leads to end-organ failure, obstructions, pathologic bleeds, and death. Bone metastases are common with advanced solid cancers (e.g., lung, prostate, breast) and multiple myeloma, and are associated with pain and pathological fractures; these complications are referred to as *skeletal-related events* and are associated with a high degree of morbidity (Fig. 26.7).

In addition to direct cancer-related complications described above, cancer patients are at risk for developing various short- and long-term treatment-related complications that are summarized in Medical Management.

CLINICAL PRESENTATION

Screening

Screening for cancer can identify disease in asymptomatic individuals, potentially improving survival outcomes through earlier diagnosis and treatment before the cancer has had the ability to spread and metastasize. Screening

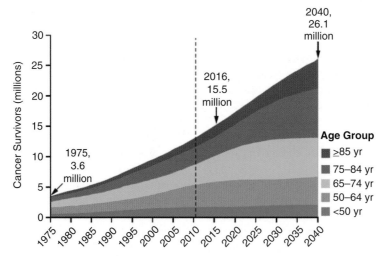

FIG. 26.3 Changing demographic characteristics of cancer survivors in the United States. Shown is the number of cancer survivors according to age group, starting in 1975, when there were 3.6 million cancer survivors, and projected to 2040, with an estimated 26.1 million survivors. The vertical broken line at 2011 indicates the year when the first baby boomers (a population born between 1946 and 1964) turned 65 years old. (From *Statistics and Graphs*, National Institute of Health (NIH) National Cancer Institute. https://nam11.safelinks.protection.outlook.com/?url=https%3A%2F%2Fcancercontrol.cancer.gov%2Focs%2Fstatistics&data=05%7C01%7CK.Madhavan%40elsevier.com%7C4940bcd5ebe74cc06bdd08dada4baff8%7C9274ee3f94254109a27f9fb15c10675d%7C0%7C0%7C638062315890027612%7CUnknown%7CTWFpbGZsb3d8eyJWIjoiMC4wLjAwMDAiLCJQIjoiV2luMzIiLCJBTiI6Ik1haWwiLCJXVCI6Mn0%3D%7C3000%7C%7C%7C&sdata=wLSmMkc8EkdSsaiCq0e%2FjPQuoafFpaTH2LXF3Vfnay4%3D&reserved=0 https://cancercontrol.cancer.gov/ocs/statistics.)

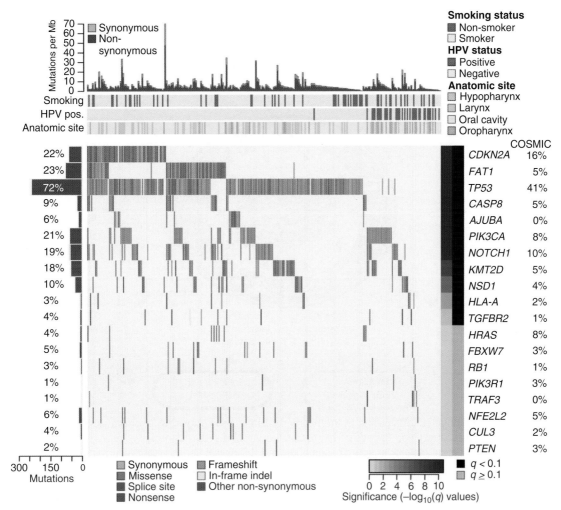

FIG. 26.4 Significantly mutated genes in head and neck squamous cell carcinoma. Genes (rows) with significantly mutated genes (identified using the MutSigCV algorithim; q < 0.1) ordered by q value; additional genes with trends toward significance are also shown. Samples (columns, n = 279) are arranged to emphasize mutual exclusivity among mutations. *Left,* mutation percentage in TCGA. *Right,* mutation percentage in COSMIC ("upper aerodigestive tract" tissue). *Top,* overall number of mutations per megabase. Color coding indicates mutation type. *TCGAs,* The Cancer Genome Atlas. (Reproduced from Lawrence, M. et al. Comprehensive genomic characterization of head and neck squamous cell carcinomas. *Nature.* 2015;517:576–582.)

for cancer can be generalized to the general population, based on age, sex, and other risk factors (e.g., smoking), or be highly individualized due to family history or genetic predisposition. The American Cancer Society provides routinely updated cancer screening guidelines for the most common cancers based on the recommendations of the US Preventive Services Task Force (Table 26.1).

Solid cancers often manifest as a palpable mass that increases in size over time. Initial features can include a change in surface color, a lump, ulceration, an enlarged lymph node, or altered organ function. Symptoms can include pain and paresthesia but may also be vague and nonspecific, contributing to delays in diagnosis. Other nonspecific features include fevers, night sweats, and unexplained weight change.

Staging

The American Joint Committee on Cancer provides an evidence-based guide for cancer staging that is used to establish standards in the field, determine prognosis, and help guide management. Most solid cancers are staged according to the TNM system: tumor size (T), locoregional lymph node involvement (N), and presence of distant metastases (M) (Box 26.1). In general, Stage 1 disease is localized and confined to the organ of origin. Stage 2 disease is regional, affecting nearby structures (e.g., spread to regional lymph nodes with head and neck cancer; Fig. 26.8). Stage 3 disease extends beyond the regional site, crossing several tissue planes, and Stage 4 disease is widely disseminated. The patient's prognosis

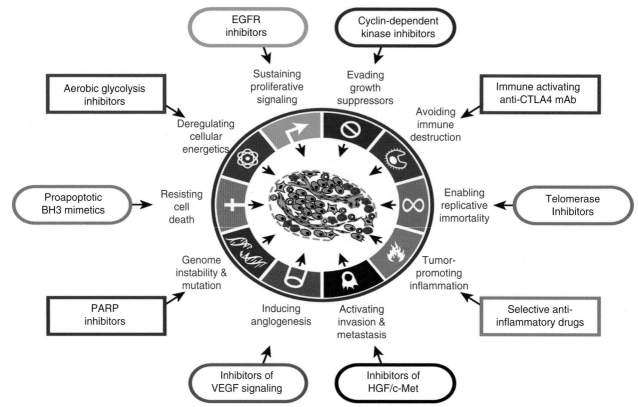

FIG. 26.5 Therapeutic targeting of the hallmarks of cancer. Drugs that interfere with each of the acquired capabilities necessary for tumor growth and progression have been developed and are in clinical trials or in some cases approved for clinical use in treating certain forms of human cancer. Additionally, the investigational drugs are being developed to target each of the enabling characteristics and emerging hallmarks depicted in Figure 26.3, which also hold promise as cancer therapeutics. The drugs listed are but illustrative examples; there is a deep pipeline of candidate drugs with different molecular targets and modes of action in development for most of these hallmarks. (Reproduced from Hanahan D, Weinberg RA. Hallmarks of cancer: the next generation. *Cell.* March 4, 2011;144(5):646–674.)

depends in large part on the stage of disease at the time of diagnosis, with worse survival outcomes associated with more advanced stages. For example, the overall 5-year survival rate for floor of mouth squamous cell carcinoma (a high-risk site) is 51%. When this type of cancer is localized without lymph node spread survival rises to 76%, but survival decreases to 20% when there is distant spread.

Laboratory and Diagnostic Findings

The diagnosis of cancer is dependent on examination of a representative sample of tissue taken from the tumor. Tissue can be obtained by cytologic smears, needle biopsy, or incisional or excisional biopsy. Biopsy specimens are analyzed for characteristic histopathologic findings as well as molecular features (e.g., immunostaining, in situ hybridization, chromosomal analysis, flow cytometry, oncogene panels) that help establish or refine the cancer diagnosis and determine potential susceptibility to targeted therapies. Tumors expressing certain markers, for example EGFR+ lung cancer, or HER2+ breast cancer, may be treated with "targeted" anticancer therapies and may be associated with better outcomes than tumors that

do not express these markers (Box 26.2). Serum tumor markers such as carcinoembryonic antigen (CEA) for colorectal carcinoma, cancer antigen 15-3 (CA 15-3) or CEA in breast cancer, and CA 125 for ovarian cancer have low sensitivity for the detection of early-stage cancers but are useful in monitoring disease progression and response to therapy. With the advent of immune checkpoint inhibitors, testing for programmed death ligand 1 (PD-L1) positivity can help determine whether a patient is likely to benefit from immunotherapy.

Cancer imaging is used to determine the size, location, and position of the tumor, as well as to evaluate for the presence of local and distant metastases. Plain film radiographs are used for screening for solid cancers, for example of the breast and lungs (Fig. 26.9). Both CT (best for imaging hard tissue) and MRI (best for imaging soft tissue) provide important diagnostic information as well as essential details for surgical planning (e.g., proximity to major vessels). Nuclear medicine imaging with positron emission tomography (PET) uses the radioactive molecule ^{18}F fluorodeoxyglucose (FDG-PET) to delineate the extent of cancer for surgical and radiation

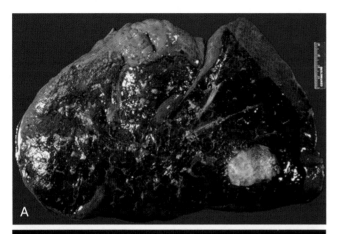

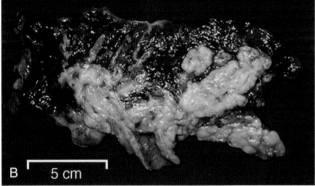

FIG. 26.6 **(A and B)** Large cell undifferentiated carcinoma infiltrating the entire lung shown in cross-section. (Reproduced from Klatt ED. *Robbins and Cotran Atlas of Pathology.* 2nd ed. Philadelphia: Saunders; 2010.)

planning, to screen for distant metastases, and to assess response to treatment (Fig. 26.10). PET and CT are frequently acquired together (PET-CT) so that the PET findings can be precisely localized. The National Comprehensive Cancer Network provides detailed diagnostic work-up guidelines for the most common cancers (www.nccn.org).

Medical Management

Cancer therapy is a continuously evolving field driven by parallel and frequently bidirectional advances from the lab and clinic. The goal of cancer therapy is curative, however, this is not always possible, and disease control with long-term remission, while minimizing complications and optimizing quality of life, can in many situations be considered a very good outcome. Disease status is monitored according to disease- and protocol-specific intervals, often with PET-CT imaging, or in the case of hematologic malignancies, blood and marrow sampling. Therapeutic modalities include surgery, radiation therapy, chemotherapy, targeted therapy, immune checkpoint inhibitor therapy, and cellular therapies (i.e., hematopoietic cell transplantation and chimeric antigen receptor T-cell therapy). Some cancers do not initially require treatment and are monitored only.

Cancer is managed according to evidence-based guidelines, such as those provided by the National Comprehensive Cancer Network (https://www.nccn.org/professionals/physician_gls/default.aspx), that are based on the results of large national and international

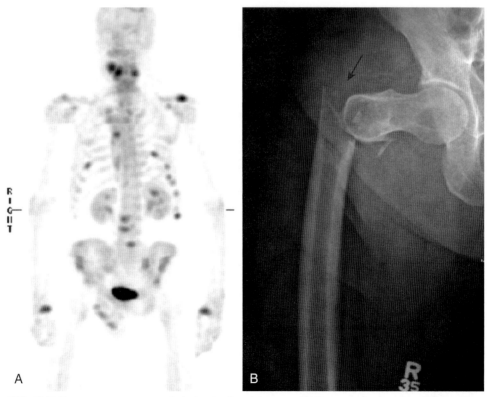

FIG. 26.7 Bone metastases and skeletal related events. (A) Bone scan showing diffuse bone metastases; (B) X-ray film showing a pathological fracture through an osteolytic lesion (*arrowed*). (Reproduced from Wilkinson AN, et al. *BMJ.* 2008; 337.)

TABLE 26.1   American Cancer Society Recommendations for the Early Detection of Cancer in Average-Risk, Asymptomatic People[a]

Cancer Site	Population	Test or Procedure	Recommendation
Breast	Women aged 40–54 years	Mammography	Women should undergo regular screening mammography starting at age 45 years; women aged 45–54 years should be screened annually; women should have the opportunity to begin annual screening between the ages of 40 and 44 years.
	Women aged ≥55 years	Mammography	Women aged ≥55 years should transition to biennial screening or have the opportunity to continue screening annually; women should continue screening mammography as long as their overall health is good and they have a life expectancy of 10 years or longer.
Cervix	Women, aged 21–29 years	Pap test	Cervical cancer screening should begin at age 21 years; for women aged 21–29 years, screening should be done every 3 years with conventional or liquid-based Pap tests.
	Women, aged 30–65 years	Pap test and HPV DNA test	For women aged 30–65 years, screening should be done every 5 years with both the HPV test and the Pap test (preferred), or every 3 years with the Pap test alone (acceptable).
	Women aged >65 years	Pap test and HPV DNA test	Women aged >65 years who have had ≥3 consecutive negative Pap tests or ≥2 consecutive negative HPV and Pap tests within the last 10 years, with the most recent test occurring in the last 5 years, should stop cervical cancer screening.
	Women who have had a total hysterectomy		Women who have had a total hysterectomy should stop cervical cancer screening.
Colorectal	Men and women, aged 45–75 years, for all tests listed	Fecal immunochemical test (FIT) [annual], or high-sensitivity guaiac-based fecal occult blood test (HSgFOBT) [annual], or multi-target stool DNA test (mt-sDNA), [every 3 years per manufacturer's recommendation], or colonoscopy [every 10 years], or CT colonography (CTC) [every 5 years], or flexible sigmoidoscopy (FS) [every 5 years]	Adults aged 45 years and older should undergo regular screening with either a high-sensitivity stool-based test or a structural (visual) exam, depending on patient preference and test availability. As part of the screening process, all positive results on noncolonoscopy screening tests should be followed up with timely colonoscopy. Adults in good health with a life expectancy of greater than 10 years should continue screening through the age of 75 years.
	Men and women aged 76–85 years		Screening decisions should be individualized, based on patient preferences, life expectancy, health status, and prior screening history. If a decision is made to continue screening patient should be offered options as listed above.
	Men and women over age 85 years		Individuals should be discouraged from continuing screening.
Endometrial	Women, at menopause		At the time of menopause, women should be informed about risks and symptoms of endometrial cancer and strongly encouraged to report any unexpected bleeding or spotting to their physicians.
Lung	Current or former smokers aged 55–74 years in good health with at least a 30-pack-year history of smoking	Low-dose helical CT	Annual screening in adults who • Currently smoke or have quit within the past 15 years; *and* • Have at least a 30 pack-year smoking history; *and* • Receive evidence-based smoking cessation counseling, if they are current smokers; *and* • Have undergone a process of informed/shared decision-making that included information about the potential benefits, limitations, and harms of screening with low-dose CT; *and*

			• Have access to a high-volume, high quality lung cancer screening and treatment center
Prostate	Men, aged ≥50 years	Prostate-specific antigen test (PSA) with or without digital rectal examination (DRE)	Men who have at least a 10-years life expectancy should have an opportunity to make an informed decision with their health care provider about whether to be screened for prostate cancer after receiving information about the potential benefits, risks, and uncertainties associated with prostate cancer screening; prostate cancer screening should not occur without an informed decision-making process.

aFor previous guidelines that are unchanged, see Supporting Table 1.
From Smith RA, et al. Cancer screening in the United States, 2018: a review of current American Cancer Society guidelines and current issues in cancer screening. *CA Cancer J Clin*. July–August 2018;68:297–316. https://acsjournals.onlinelibrary.wiley.com/doi/full/10.3322/caac.21446#caac21446-tbl-0002.

randomized controlled trials. Patient comorbidities as well as age, prognosis, and personal preferences may factor into treatment decisions. A cancer patient's "performance status," or their ability to perform activities of daily living, is often included in physician assessments and indicates eligibility criteria for clinical trials and guides standard treatment recommendations (Fig. 26.11). Patients who have a worse performance status tend to have more difficulty tolerating rigorous cancer treatments. In advanced cases when treatment is no longer effective or appropriate and death is imminent, patients may be transitioned to hospice care, with the intent of maintaining comfort and ensuring a respectable end of life.

Supportive care is an essential aspect of cancer therapy that improves quality of life and contributes indirectly and directly to improved survival outcomes. This encompasses various therapies provided for prevention and/or management of cancer- or treatment-related complications, which do not directly treat the cancer. Management of oral complications of cancer therapies (see Dental Management) is considered a component of supportive care. Cancer patients are routinely assessed for treatment-related toxicities, most commonly using the National Cancer Institute's Common Terminology Criteria for Adverse Events (CTCAE; https://ctep.cancer.gov/protocoldevelopment/electronic_applications/docs/CTCAE_v5_Quick_Reference_5x7.pdf). The CTCAE grades each toxicity according to a 1–5 scale, with 1 generally being no symptoms/impact, and 5 being death. Two very important and common complications are infections due to neutropenia and pathological bone fractures due to metastases. Both the chemotherapy regimen as well as the cancer type (e.g., hematologic malignancies), in addition to other patient-related factors, affect the risk of developing febrile neutropenia or sepsis (Box 26.3). The American Society for Clinical Oncology

provides guidelines for the prophylactic or therapeutic use of hematopoietic colony-stimulating factors (e.g., filgrastim, Neupogen; pegfilgrastim, Neulasta), which help prevent or reduce the duration and severity of neutropenia by stimulating white blood cell production. Antiresorptive agents, including nitrogen-containing bisphosphonates (most commonly zoledronic acid) and denosumab, are used in patients with metastatic bone disease (including multiple myeloma) to prevent pathologic fractures (Fig. 26.12).

Cancer survivorship, as defined by the National Cancer Institute, focuses on the health and well-being of a person with cancer from the time of diagnosis until the end of life. After completion of cancer therapy, patients require careful monitoring for recurrence and secondary cancers, screening for treatment-related complications, and promotion of psychological and physical health and well-being. Disease-specific guidelines for the follow-up of cancer survivors are provided by various professional oncology organizations (e.g., American Society of Clinical Oncology, National Comprehensive Cancer Center Network, American Cancer Society, Children's Oncology Group; Box 26.4). Pediatric cancer survivors, especially those patients treated with chemotherapy and radiation therapy at very young ages, are at risk for a wide range of medical complications and late effects including growth and development abnormalities (Box 26.5).

Surgery. Surgery is indicated for solid cancers when anatomy permits or if the cancer is limited in size, and without known distant metastases; this can be a primary therapy or combined with adjuvant postsurgical chemotherapy and/or radiation therapy. Tumors are fully removed with margins of normal tissue; frozen pathology sections of freshly resected tumor tissue may be examined peri-procedurally to help with surgical decision making. Regional lymph nodes are often removed as part of

BOX 26.1   Staging of Cancers of Lip, Oral Cavity, and p16 Negative Oropharynx

Overall stage is determined after the cancer is assigned a letter or number to describe tumor (T), node (N), and metastasis (M) categories.

Tis, N0, M0 (Stage 0)
Cancer within epithelium (top layer of cells lining oral cavity and oropharynx). Also called carcinoma in situ (Tis). No spread to lymph nodes (N0) or distant sites (M0).

T1, N0, M0 (Stage I)
Cancer is ≤ 2 cm. No growth into nearby tissues (T1). No spread to lymph nodes (N0) or distant sites (M0).

T2, N0, M0 (Stage II)
Cancer is 2- ≤ 4 larger cm. No growth into nearby tissues (T2). No spread to nearby lymph nodes (N0) or distant sites (M0).

T3, N0, M0 (Stage III)
Cancer > 4 cm (T3). For oropharynx cancers, T3 also includes tumors that grow into the epiglottis. No spread to nearby lymph nodes (N0) or to distant sites (M0).

T1, T2, or T3, N1, M0 (Stage III)
Cancer any size, may be found in nearby structures if oropharynx cancer (T1-T3) *and* has spread to 1 lymph node on same side as primary tumor. No growth outside of the lymph node and the lymph node is no larger than 3 cm (N1). No spread to distant sites (M0).

T4a, N0, or N1, M0 (Stage IVA)
Cancer can be any size. Known as moderately advanced local disease (T4a). Cancer is growing into nearby structures:
- For lip cancers: nearby bone, the inferior alveolar nerve, the floor of the mouth, or the skin of the chin or nose (T4a)
- For oral cavity cancers: jaw or face bones, deep muscle of the tongue, facial skin, or the maxillary sinus (T4a)
- For oropharyngeal cancers: the larynx, the tongue muscle, or bones such as medial pterygoid, the hard palate, or the jaw (T4a).
    And either of the following: no spread to nearby lymph nodes (N0); spread to 1 lymph node on the same side as primary tumor, but no growth outside of lymph node and lymph node is no larger than 3 cm (N1).
    It has not spread to distant sites (M0).

T1, T2, T3 or T4a. N2, M0 (Stage IVA)
Cancer any size, may have grown into nearby structures (T0-T4a). No spread to distant organs (M0). Spread to one of the following: one lymph node on same side as primary tumor, but not grown outside of the lymph node and the lymph node is between 3 cm and 6 cm (approx. 2 ½ inches) (N2a); *or* spread to more than 1 lymph node on same side as primary tumor, but not grown outside any lymph nodes and none are larger than 6 cm (N2b); *or* spread to 1 or more lymph nodes either on opposite side of primary tumor or both sides of neck, but not grown outside any the lymph nodes and none are larger than 6 cm (N2c).

Any T, N3, M0 (Stage IVB)
Cancer any size, may have grown into nearby soft tissues or structures (Any T) *and* any of the following: spread to 1 lymph node that's larger than 6 cm but has not grown outside of lymph node (N3a); *or* spread to 1 lymph node that's larger than 3 cm and clearly grown outside lymph node (N3b); *or* spread to more than 1 lymph node on the same side, the opposite side, or both sides of the primary cancer with growth outside of lymph node(s) (N3b); *or* spread to 1 lymph node on the opposite side of the primary cancer that's 3 cm or smaller and has grown outside of the lymph node (N3b). No spread to distant organs (M0).

T4b, Any N, M0 (Stage IVB)
Cancer any size, grown into nearby structures such as the base of the skull or other nearby bones, or surrounding the carotid artery—known as *very advanced local disease* (T4b). Might or might not have spread to nearby lymph nodes (Any N). No spread to distant organs (M0).

Any T, Any N, M1 (Stage IVC)
Cancer any size, may be found in nearby soft tissues or structures (Any T) *and* it might or might not have spread to nearby lymph nodes (Any N). It has spread to distant sites such as the lungs (M1).

2 cm = about ¾ inch; 3 cm = about 1¼; 4 cm = about 1½

Data from Dirven R, et al: Tumor thickness versus depth of invasion—Analysis of the 8th edition American Joint Committee on Cancer Stage for oral cancer, *Oral Oncology.* 2017;Vol. 74;30—33; Kato MG, et al: Update on oral and oropharyngeal cancer staging—International perspectives, *World J Otorhinolaryngol Head Neck Surg.* Mar 2020;6(1); 66—75; American Cancer Society, *Oral Cavity and* Oropharyngeal Cancer Stages, 2022, American Cancer Society, Inc.

cancer surgery to assess for localized spread. Advances in reconstructive surgery using free flap tissue grafts has contributed to significantly improved functional and cosmetic outcomes, especially in the head and neck region. Complications are anatomically dependent but may include deficits and disabilities. In the head and neck region, these may include anatomic defects, trismus, lymphedema, difficulty speaking, eating, and swallowing, motor and sensory nerve deficits, and chronic neuropathic pain.

Radiation Therapy. Radiation therapy leads to cell death by damaging cancer cell DNA and is used when surgery alone is insufficient or contraindicated, or for cancers that are radiosensitive. Most cancers that are treated with radiation therapy are treated with external beam radiation therapy, delivered in fractions, typically 5 days in a row with 2 days off for the weekend, for up to 6–7 weeks. Cancers that are located near critical anatomical structures and organs (e.g., head and neck, prostate) are treated with intensity modulated radiation therapy, a more sophisticated three-dimensional technique that allows for a precision approach to focusing the most intense dose to the tumor and relatively sparing unaffected tissues. Proton therapy is another technique that can reduce the amount of radiation damage to healthy tissue near a tumor and is being increasingly used in cancers located in particularly complex areas such as the head and neck and prostate. Internally delivered radiation therapies include brachytherapy, an implanted device that emits very localized radiation to a tumor, and radioactive iodine therapy for treatment of thyroid cancer. Complications of radiation, like surgery, are location specific. In the head and neck these include dermatitis, mucositis, salivary gland hypofunction, hypogeusia/dysgeusia, soft tissue and bone necrosis, trismus, and secondary malignancy.

Chemotherapy. Chemotherapy, as single agents or in combinations, is used for the management of many different cancers by broadly targeting rapidly dividing cancer cells through disruption of DNA replication and the cell cycle. Chemotherapy can be a primary curative therapy (single or multiple combined or sequenced agents), or be provided as a neoadjuvant therapy (prior to surgery or radiation), adjuvant therapy (to destroy any remaining cancer after surgery/radiation), as a radiosensitizer during concurrent radiation therapy, or to treat recurrent or metastatic cancer. The most commonly used chemotherapy agents are classified as alkylating agents (cause DNA damage), plant alkaloids (disrupt cell division), antitumor antibiotics (disrupt cell cycle), antimetabolites (interrupt cell cycle, block cell division), and topoisomerase inhibitors (inhibit cell division) (Fig. 26.13). Chemotherapy may be delivered topically for some skin cancers (e.g., topical 5-fluorouracil) and intraperitoneally (typically during surgical procedure), but in most cases is given systemically as an infusion or as an oral agent. While specific toxicities are associated with specific classes of therapies, many are common to several chemotherapy agents and include bone marrow toxicity (leading to anemia, leukopenia, neutropenia, and thrombocytopenia), as well as gastrointestinal toxicity (characterized by nausea and vomiting, diarrhea, and mucositis) (Fig. 26.14).

Targeted Therapy. Targeted cancer therapies include small molecule inhibitors and monoclonal antibodies that block the growth and spread of cancer by interfering with specific receptors, molecules, and pathways that are involved in the growth, progression, and spread of cancer (Fig. 26.15). These therapies have revolutionized the management of some cancers leading to in some cases drastically improved outcomes (e.g., chronic myelogenous leukemia and the targeted agent imatinib; Fig. 26.16). Tumor testing may be necessary to determine whether a targeted therapy is likely to be effective (Box 26.2). Classes of targeted therapies include hormone therapies, signal transduction inhibitors, gene expression modulators, apoptosis inducers, angiogenesis inhibitors, and toxin delivery molecules (antibody–drug conjugates) (Table 26.2). Toxicities are class-specific and distinct from traditional chemotherapy agents.

Immune Checkpoint Inhibitor Therapy. The immune system has built in "checkpoints" that help prevent overreactive T-cell responses, and some cancers evade immune detection through these pathways. Immune checkpoint inhibitors block the checkpoint proteins from binding with their partner proteins, thereby preventing the "off" signal from being sent, allowing the T cells to kill cancer cells (Fig. 26.17). Immune checkpoint inhibitors target cytotoxic T-lymphocyte antigen 4 (CTLA-4), programmed death receptor-1 (PD-1), and programmed death-ligand 1 (PD-L1). These agents are used alone or in combination (i.e., anti-CTLA-4 and anti-PD-1/PD-L1), or in combination with other chemotherapy or targeted therapies. While responses are variable, long-term remissions are possible. Immunotherapy-related adverse events are distinct from toxicities associated with traditional chemotherapy and targeted therapies, presenting with features typical of autoimmune and rheumatologic conditions. Management of irAEs may require systemic immunosuppressive therapy as well as interrupting or discontinuing immune checkpoint inhibitor therapy.

Cellular Therapy. Cellular therapies include allogeneic hematopoietic cell transplantation (see Chapter 21) and chimeric antigen receptor T-cell therapy (CAR T-cell therapy). With CAR T-cell therapy, autologous T-cells are collected and modified in the laboratory to produce

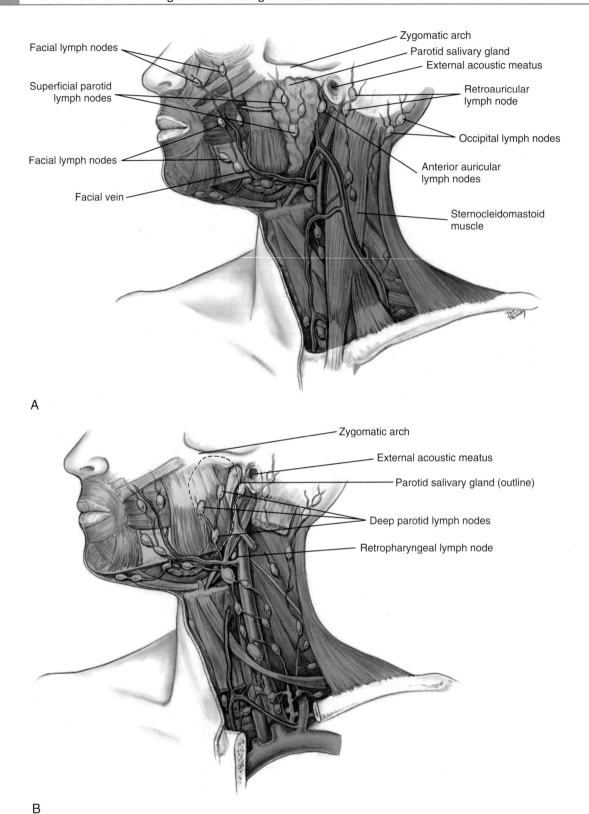

Facial lymph nodes

Superficial parotid
lymph nodes

Facial lymph nodes

Facial vein

Zygomatic arch
Parotid salivary gland
External acoustic meatus

Retroauricular
lymph node

Occipital lymph nodes

Anterior auricular
lymph nodes

Sternocleidomastoid
muscle

A

Zygomatic arch

External acoustic meatus

Parotid salivary gland (outline)

Deep parotid lymph nodes

Retropharyngeal lymph node

B

FIG. 26.8 Regional lymph node anatomy. (Reproduced from Fehrenbach MJ, Herring SW. *Illustrated Anatomy of the Head and Neck.* 4th ed. St. Louis: Saunders; 2012.)

special structures called chimeric antigen receptors (CARs) on their surface that target tumor antigens when reinfused into the patient (Fig. 26.18). CAR T-cell therapy is approved for young patients who have relapsed or refractory acute lymphoblastic leukemia and adults who have aggressive non-Hodgkin lymphoma.

BOX 26.2   Tumor Markers That Are in Common Use, Mainly to Determine Treatment or to Help Make a Diagnosis of Cancer

Tumor Marker	Cancer Type	What's Analyzed	How Used
ALK gene rearrangements and overexpression	Non–small cell lung cancer and anaplastic large cell lymphoma	Tumor	To help determine treatment and prognosis
Alpha-fetoprotein (AFP)	Liver cancer and germ cell tumors	Blood	To help diagnose liver cancer and follow response to treatment; to assess stage, prognosis, and response to treatment of germ cell tumors
B-cell immunoglobulin gene rearrangement	B-cell lymphoma	Blood, bone marrow, or tumor tissue	To help in diagnosis, to evaluate effectiveness of treatment, and to check for recurrence
Beta-2-microglobulin (B2M)	Multiple myeloma, chronic lymphocytic leukemia, and some lymphomas	Blood, urine, or cerebrospinal fluid	To determine prognosis and follow response to treatment
Beta-human chorionic gonadotropin (beta-hCG)	Choriocarcinoma and germ cell tumors	Urine or blood	To assess stage, prognosis, and response to treatment
Bladder tumor antigen (BTA)	Bladder cancer and cancer of the kidney or ureter	Urine	As surveillance with cytology and cystoscopy of patients already known to have bladder cancer
BRCA1 and BRCA2 gene mutations	Ovarian and breast cancers	Blood and/or tumor	To determine whether treatment with a particular type of targeted therapy is appropriate
BCR-ABL fusion gene (Philadelphia chromosome)	Chronic myeloid leukemia, acute lymphoblastic leukemia, and acute myelogenous leukemia	Blood or bone marrow	To confirm diagnosis, predict response to targeted therapy, determine whether treatment with a particular type of targeted therapy is appropriate, and monitor disease status
BRAF V600 mutations	Cutaneous melanoma, Erdheim–Chester disease, colorectal cancer, and non–small cell lung cancer	Tumor	To select patients who are most likely to benefit from treatment with certain targeted therapies
C-kit/CD117	Gastrointestinal stromal tumor, mucosal melanoma, acute myeloid leukemia, and mast cell disease	Tumor, blood, or bone marrow	To help in diagnosing and determining treatment
CA15-3/CA27.29	Breast cancer	Blood	To assess whether treatment is working or if the cancer has recurred
CA19-9	Pancreatic, gallbladder, bile duct, and gastric cancers	Blood	To assess whether treatment is working
CA-125	Ovarian cancer	Blood	To help in diagnosis, assessment of response to treatment, and evaluation of recurrence
CA 27.29	Breast cancer	Blood	To detect metastasis or recurrence
Calcitonin	Medullary thyroid cancer	Blood	To aid in diagnosis, check whether treatment is working, and assess recurrence
Carcinoembryonic antigen (CEA)	Colorectal cancer and some other cancers	Blood	To keep track of how well cancer treatments are working and check if cancer has come back or spread
CD20	Non-Hodgkin lymphoma	Blood	To determine whether treatment with a targeted therapy is appropriate
CD22	Hairy cell leukemia and B-cell neoplasms	Blood and bone marrow	To help in diagnosis

Continued

BOX 26.2   Tumor Markers That Are in Common Use, Mainly to Determine Treatment or to Help Make a Diagnosis of Cancer—cont'd

Tumor Marker	Cancer Type	What's Analyzed	How Used
CD25	Non-Hodgkin (T-cell) lymphoma	Blood	To determine whether treatment with a targeted therapy is appropriate
CD30	Mycosis fungoides and peripheral T-cell lymphoma	Tumor	To determine whether treatment with a targeted therapy is appropriate
CD33	Acute myeloid leukemia	Blood	To determine whether treatment with a targeted therapy is appropriate
Chromogranin A (CgA)	Neuroendocrine tumors	Blood	To help in diagnosis, assessment of treatment response, and evaluation of recurrence
Chromosome 17p deletion	Chronic lymphocytic leukemia	Blood	To determine whether treatment with a certain targeted therapy is appropriate
Chromosomes 3, 7, 17, and 9p21	Bladder cancer	Urine	To help in monitoring for tumor recurrence
Circulating tumor cells of epithelial origin (CELLSEARCH)	Metastatic breast, prostate, and colorectal cancers	Blood	To inform clinical decision making, and to assess prognosis
Cytokeratin fragment 21-1	Lung cancer	Blood	To help in monitoring for recurrence
Des-gamma-carboxy prothrombin (DCP)	Hepatocellular carcinoma	Blood	To monitor the effectiveness of treatment and to detect recurrence
DPD gene mutation	Breast, colorectal, gastric, and pancreatic cancers	Blood	To predict the risk of a toxic reaction to 5-fluorouracil therapy
EGFR gene mutation	Non–small cell lung cancer	Tumor	To help determine treatment and prognosis
Estrogen receptor (ER)/progesterone receptor (PR)	Breast cancer	Tumor	To determine whether treatment with hormone therapy and some targeted therapies is appropriate
FGFR2 and FGFR3 gene mutations	Bladder cancer	Tumor	To determine whether treatment with a certain targeted therapy is appropriate
Fibrin/fibrinogen	Bladder cancer	Urine	To monitor progression and response to treatment
FLT3 gene mutations	Acute myeloid leukemia	Blood	To determine whether treatment with certain targeted therapies is appropriate
Gastrin	Gastrin-producing tumor (gastrinoma)	Blood	To help in diagnosis, to monitor the effectiveness of treatment, and to detect recurrence
HE4	Ovarian cancer	Blood	To plan cancer treatment, assess disease progression, and monitor for recurrence
HER2/neu gene amplification or protein overexpression	Breast, ovarian, bladder, pancreatic, and stomach cancers	Tumor	To determine whether treatment with certain targeted therapies is appropriate
5-HIAA	Carcinoid tumors	Urine	To help in diagnosis and to monitor disease
IDH1 and IDH2 gene mutations	Acute myeloid leukemia	Bone marrow and blood	To determine whether treatment with certain targeted therapies is appropriate
Immunoglobulins	Multiple myeloma and Waldenström macroglobulinemia	Blood and urine	To help diagnose disease, assess response to treatment, and look for recurrence
JAK2 gene mutation	Certain types of leukemia	Blood and bone marrow	To help in diagnosis
KRAS gene mutation	Colorectal cancer and non–small cell lung cancer	Tumor	To determine whether treatment with a particular type of targeted therapy is appropriate
Lactate dehydrogenase	Germ cell tumors, lymphoma, leukemia, melanoma, and neuroblastoma	Blood	To assess stage, prognosis, and response to treatment

BOX 26.2 Tumor Markers That Are in Common Use, Mainly to Determine Treatment or to Help Make a Diagnosis of Cancer—cont'd

Microsatellite instability (MSI) and/or mismatch repair deficient (dMMR)	Colorectal cancer and other solid tumors	Tumor	To guide treatment and to identify those at high risk of certain cancer-predisposing syndromes
Neuron-specific enolase (NSE)	Small cell lung cancer and neuroblastoma	Blood	To help in diagnosis and to assess response to treatment
Nuclear matrix protein 22	Bladder cancer	Urine	To monitor response to treatment
PCA3 mRNA	Prostate cancer	Urine (collected after digital rectal exam)	To determine need for repeat biopsy after negative biopsy
PML/RARα fusion gene	Acute promyelocytic leukemia (APL)	Blood and bone marrow	To diagnose APL, to predict response to all-trans-retinoic acid or arsenic trioxide therapy, to assess effectiveness of therapy, to monitor minimal residual disease, and to predict early relapse
Prostatic acid phosphatase (PAP)	Metastatic prostate cancer	Blood	To help in diagnosing poorly differentiated carcinomas
Programmed death ligand 1 (PD-L1)	Non–small cell lung cancer, liver cancer, stomach cancer, gastroesophageal junction cancer, classical Hodgkin lymphoma, and other aggressive lymphoma subtypes	Tumor	To determine whether treatment with a particular type of targeted therapy is appropriate
Prostate-specific antigen (PSA)	Prostate cancer	Blood	To help in diagnosis, to assess response to treatment, and to look for recurrence
ROS1 gene rearrangement	Non–small cell lung cancer	Tumor	To determine whether treatment with a particular type of targeted therapy is appropriate
Soluble mesothelin–related peptides (SMRPs)	Mesothelioma	Blood	To monitor progression or recurrence
Somatostatin receptor	Neuroendocrine tumors affecting the pancreas or gastrointestinal tract (GEP-NETs)	Tumor (by diagnostic imaging)	To determine whether treatment with a particular type of targeted therapy is appropriate
T-cell receptor gene rearrangement	T-cell lymphoma	Bone marrow, tissue, body fluid, blood	To help in diagnosis; sometimes to detect and evaluate residual disease
Thiopurine S-methyltransferase (TPMT) enzyme activity or TPMT genetic test	Acute lymphoblastic leukemia	Blood and buccal (cheek) swab	To predict the risk of severe bone marrow toxicity (myelosuppression) with thiopurine treatment
Thyroglobulin	Thyroid cancer	Blood	To evaluate response to treatment and to look for recurrence
UGT1A1*28 variant homozygosity	Colorectal cancer	Blood and buccal (cheek) swab	To predict toxicity from irinotecan therapy
Urine catecholamines: VMA and HVA	Neuroblastoma	Urine	To help in diagnosis
Urokinase plasminogen activator (uPA) and plasminogen activator inhibitor (PAI-1)	Breast cancer	Tumor	To determine aggressiveness of cancer and guide treatment
FoundationOne CDx (F1CDx) genomic test	Any solid tumor	Tumor	As a companion diagnostic test to determine whether treatment with a particular type of targeted therapy is appropriate
5-Protein signature (OVA1)	Ovarian cancer	Blood	To preoperatively assess pelvic mass for suspected ovarian cancer
17-Gene signature (Oncotype DX GPS test)	Prostate cancer	Tumor	To predict the aggressiveness of prostate cancer and to help manage treatment

Continued

BOX 26.2 **Tumor Markers That Are in Common Use, Mainly to Determine Treatment or to Help Make a Diagnosis of Cancer—cont'd**

Tumor Marker	Cancer Type	What's Analyzed	How Used
21-Gene signature (Oncotype DX)	Breast cancer	Tumor	To evaluate risk of distant recurrence and to help plan treatment
46-Gene signature (Prolaris)	Prostate cancer	Tumor	To predict the aggressiveness of prostate cancer and to help manage treatment
70-Gene signature (Mammaprint)	Breast cancer	Tumor	To evaluate risk of recurrence

This list does not include the many tumor markers that are tested by immunophenotyping and immunohistochemistry to help diagnose cancer and to distinguish between different types of cancer. Some tumor markers listed are targets for targeted therapy in multiple cancers but serve as tumor markers for only a subset of cancers. From *Tumor Markers in Common Use*. National Cancer Institute at the National Institutes of Health; 2021. https://www.cancer.gov/about-cancer/diagnosis-staging/diagnosis/tumor-markers-list.

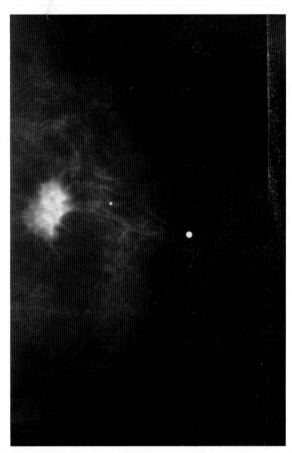

FIG. 26.9 Mammogram showing a radiodense area in the breast suggestive of a malignancy that should be recommended for biopsy. (Courtesy of A.R. Moore, Lexington, KY.)

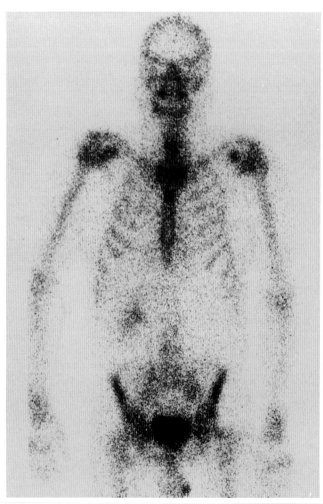

FIG. 26.10 Radionuclide scan showing increased uptake of technetium at sites of bony metastasis from prostate cancer. (Reproduced from Dale A. Miles, DDS, Fountain Hills, AZ.)

Potentially serious complications of CAR T-cell therapy include cytokine release syndrome and neurotoxicity. Cytokine release syndrome is characterized by flu-like symptoms with a high fever and/or chills; low blood pressure; difficulty breathing; or confusion. Neurological complications can include swelling, confusion, seizures, or severe headaches. No oral complications have been described associated with CAR T-cell therapy.

Performance status			
Karnofsky scale		**Zubrod scale**	
Normal, no evidence of disease	100	Normal activity	0
Able to perform normal activity with only minor symptoms	90		
Normal activity with effort, some symptoms	80	Symptomatic and ambulatory	1
Able to care for self but unable to do normal activities	70	Cares for self	
Requires occasional assistance, cares for most Needs	60	Ambulatory >50% of the time	2
Requires considerable assistance	50	Occasional assistance	
Disabled, requires special assistance	40	Ambulatory 50% of the time	3
Severely disabled	30	Nursing care needed	
Very sick, requires active supportive treatment	20	Bedridden	4
Moribund	10		
The scoring scale used may depend on patient population, disease, study goal and other criteria. Many definitions of the scale scoring do not match the standard.			

FIG. 26.11 Performance status scales for use in patients with cancer. (From U.S. Department of Health. National Institutes of Health (NIH): National Cancer Institute, Center for Biomedical Informatics & Information Technology.)

BOX 26.3 Patient Risk Factors for Febrile Neutropenia

In addition to chemotherapy regimen and type of malignancy, consider the following factors when estimating patient's overall risk of febrile neutropenia:

Age >65 years
  Advanced disease
Previous chemotherapy or radiation therapy
  Preexisting neutropenia or bone marrow involvement with tumor infection
  Open wounds or recent surgery
  Poor performance status or poor nutritional status
  Poor renal function
  Liver dysfunction, most notably elevated bilirubin
  Cardiovascular disease
  Multiple comorbid conditions
  HIV infection

From Smith TJ, Bohlke K, Lyman GH, et al. *J Clin Oncol.* 2015;333199–333212.

Allogeneic hematopoietic cell transplantation and the significant complication of chronic graft-versus-host disease are reviewed in detail in Chapter 21.

DENTAL MANAGEMENT

Dentists play an important part in the management of patients with cancer (Box 26.6). A primary role is early recognition of the disease. Accordingly, dentists must take a consistent approach for ascertaining pertinent medical, historical, and clinical information from the patient. The dentist should question the patient carefully for signs and symptoms of cancer, particularly those in the head and neck region. Questions regarding overall health, exercise, diet, tobacco and alcohol use, and cancer in family members are important and permit a global assessment of cancer risk in the patient. A basic review of systems may also identify report of symptoms that should be further evaluated by a patient's primary care physician. The dentist can also discuss the importance of having a primary care physician and the benefits of cancer screening of organ systems (e.g., breast, colon, rectum, cervix, mouth, ovary, prostate, and skin) and its impact on survival.

A head and neck and intraoral visual/tactile soft tissue examination should be performed on each patient to assess for signs of malignancy (Box 26.7). Suspicious skin lesions should be referred for further evaluation (Fig. 26.19). Patients with lymph nodes that are enlarged, hard, and/or fixed are malignant until proven otherwise and should be referred to a head and neck oncologic surgeon for further evaluation. Intraoral lesions clinically suspicious for cancer (e.g., erythroplakia, erythroleukoplakia, ulceration with induration, mass) and those that fail to heal within 14 days despite alleviating measures should be biopsied (Fig. 26.20). Level of suspicion should be elevated in patients with risk factors for and in those previously treated for head and neck cancer.

Treatment Planning Modifications

Dental treatment planning for a patient with cancer begins with obtaining a history of the cancer diagnosis,

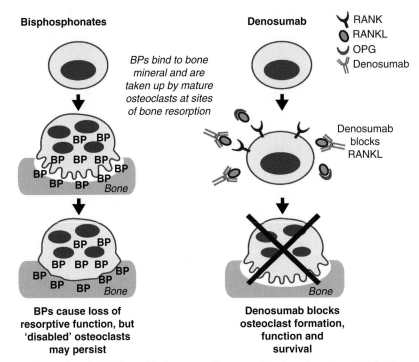

FIG. 26.12 Osteoclast inhibition with denosumab versus bisphosphonates (BPs). (Reproduced from Baron R, Ferrari S, Russell RG. Denosumab and bisphosphonates: different mechanisms of action and effects. *Bone.* April 1, 2011;48(4):677–692.)

stage, previously received, ongoing and planned therapies, any significant complications, and overall performance status. Risk assessment is primarily focused on the stage of therapy and risk for developing infection, mucositis, and jaw osteonecrosis. Patients should be educated regarding common and potential anticipated oral toxicities. Planning involves (1) pretreatment evaluation and preparation of the patient; (2) oral health care during cancer therapy; and (3) posttreatment management of the patient, including long-term considerations.

Pretreatment Evaluation and Considerations

A pretreatment oral evaluation is recommended for most cancer patients before the initiation of cancer therapy (Box 26.8). This is performed to identify the following risks: (1) odontogenic infection that may exacerbate during cancer therapy due to anticipated immunosuppression and neutropenia, (2) teeth or restorations with sharp edges that may increase the risk of developing mucositis, and (3) nonsalvageable teeth or teeth with poor long-term prognosis in patients who are scheduled to receive radiation therapy to the head and neck or to initiate antiresorptive therapy. The evaluation should include a thorough clinical and radiographic examination and review of any relevant laboratory studies (e.g., platelet count). Edentulous regions should be surveyed to rule out impacted teeth, retained root tips, and latent osseous disease. A panoramic image may be

sufficient unless unable to assess for caries or periapical disease. It is best for all dental care to be completed at least 1–2 weeks prior to initiation of cancer therapy whenever possible.

Oral Care During Cancer Therapy

Dentists can play an important role in management of acute oral complications that may arise during cancer therapy. Patients should maintain good oral hygiene throughout their treatment, including brushing and flossing. While most dental care can be deferred during active therapy, emergencies arise and must be managed. Furthermore, some cancer patients may remain on extended courses of chemotherapy. Patients who are neutropenic or thrombocytopenic should not undergo invasive dental procedures without special precautions and careful coordination with the oncology team. In general, dental procedures can be performed if the granulocyte count is greater than 2000/mm³, the platelet count is greater than 50,000/μm, and the patient is able to tolerate dental care (see Box 26.2 and Chapter 25). For outpatient care, general dental care is generally safe after chemotherapy when blood counts are recovering (e.g., day 14–17), prior to the next chemotherapy cycle. If urgent care is needed and the platelet count is below 50,000/mm³, consultation with the patient's oncologist is required. Platelet transfusion may be indicated if invasive dental procedures are to be performed. Localized

BOX 26.4   The American Cancer Society Head and Neck Cancer Survivorship Care Guideline Recommendations

Target population: Adult posttreatment head and neck cancer (HNC) survivors

Target audience: Primary care clinicians, medical oncologists, and other clinicians caring for HNC survivors

Methods: An expert panel was convened to develop clinical practice guideline recommendations based on a systematic review of the medical literature

ACS key recommendations for HNC survivorship care

Surveillance for HNC recurrence

History and physical

Recommendation 1.1. It is recommended that primary care clinicians: (a) should individualize clinical follow-up care provided to HNC survivors based on age, specific diagnosis, and treatment protocol as recommended by the treating oncology team (LOE = 2A); (b) should conduct a detailed cancer-related history and physical examination every 1–3 months for the first y after primary treatment, every 2–6 months in the second y, every 4 –8 months in years 3–5, and annually after 5 years (LOE - = 2A);[10] (c) should confirm continued follow-up with otolaryngologist or HNC specialist for HN-focused examination (LOE = 2A).

Surveillance education

Recommendation 1.2. It is recommended that primary care clinicians: (a) should educate and counsel all HNC survivors about the signs and symptoms of local recurrence. (LOE = 0); (b) should refer HNC survivors to an HNC specialist if signs and symptoms of local recurrence are present (LOE = 0).

Screening and early detection of second primary cancers (SPCs)

Recommendation 2.1. It is recommended that primary care clinicians: (a) should screen HNC survivors for other cancers as they would for patients in the general population by adhering to the ACS Early Detection Recommendations (cancer.org/professionals; LOE = 0); (b) should screen HNC survivors for lung cancer according to ASCO or NCCN[14] recommendations for annual lung cancer screening with LDCT for high-risk patients based on smoking history (LOE = 2A); (c) should screen HNC survivors for another HN and esophageal cancer as they would for patients of increased risk (LOE = 0, IIA).

Assessment and management of physical and psychosocial long-term and late effects of HNC and its treatment

Recommendation 3.1. It is recommended that primary care clinicians should assess for long-term and late effects of HNC and its treatment at each follow-up visit (LOE = 0).

Spinal accessory nerve (SAN) palsy

Recommendation 3.2. It is recommended that primary care clinicians should refer HNC survivors with SAN palsy occurring postradical neck dissection to a rehabilitation specialist to improve range of motion and ability to perform daily tasks (LOE = IA).

Cervical dystonia/muscle spasms/neuropathies

Recommendation 3.3. It is recommended that primary care clinicians: (a) should assess HNC survivors for cervical dystonia, which is characterized by painful dystonic spasms of the cervical muscles and can be caused by neck dissection, radiation, or both (LOE = 0); (b) should refer HNC survivors to a rehabilitation specialist for comprehensive

neuromusculoskeletal management if cervical dystonia or neuropathy is found (LOE = 0); (c) should prescribe nerve-stabilizing agents, such as pregabalin, gabapentin, and duloxetine, or refer to a specialist for botulinum toxin type A injections into the affected muscles for pain management and spasm control as indicated (LOE = 0, IIA).

Shoulder dysfunction

Recommendation 3.4. It is recommended that primary care clinicians: (a) should conduct baseline assessment of HNC survivor shoulder function posttreatment for strength, range of motion, and impingement signs, and continue to assess as follow-up for ongoing complications or worsening condition (LOE = IIA); (b) should refer HNC survivors to a rehabilitation specialist for improvement to pain, disability, and range of motion where shoulder morbidity exists (LOE = IA).

Trismus

Recommendation 3.5. It is recommended that primary care clinicians: (a) should refer HNC survivors to rehabilitation specialists and dental professionals to prevent trismus and to treat trismus as soon as it is diagnosed (LOE = 0); (b) should prescribe nerve-stabilizing agents to combat pain and spasms, which may also ease physical therapy and stretching devices (LOE = IIA).

Dysphagia/aspiration/stricture

Recommendation 3.6. It is recommended that primary care clinicians: (a) should refer HNC survivors presenting with complaints of dysphagia, postprandial cough, unexplained weight loss, and/or pneumonia to an experienced speech-language pathologist for instrumental evaluation of swallowing function to assess and manage dysphagia and possible aspiration (LOE = IIA); (b) should recognize potential for psychosocial barriers to swallowing recovery and refer HNC survivors to an appropriate clinician if barriers are present (LOE = IIA); (c) should refer to a speech-language pathologist for videofluoroscopy as the first-line test for HNC survivors with suspected stricture due to the high degree of coexisting physiologic dysphagia (LOE = IIA); (d) should refer HNC survivors with stricture to a gastroenterologist or HN surgeon for esophageal dilation (LOE = IIA).

Gastroesophageal reflux disease (GERD)

Recommendation 3.7. It is recommended that primary care clinicians: (a) should monitor HNC survivors for developing or worsening GERD, as it prevents healing of irradiated tissues and is associated with increased risk of HNC recurrence or SPCs (LOE = IIA); (b) should counsel HNC survivors on an increased risk of esophageal cancer and the associated symptoms (LOE = IIA); (c) should recommend PPIs or antacids, sleeping with a wedge pillow or 3-inch blocks under the head of the bed, not eating or drinking fluids for 3 h before bedtime, tobacco cessation, and avoidance of alcohol (LOE = IIA); (d) should refer HNC survivors to a gastroenterologist if symptoms are not relieved by treatments listed in 3.7c (LOE = IIA).

Lymphedema

Recommendation 3.8. It is recommended that primary care clinicians: (a) should assess HNC survivors for lymphedema using the NCI CTCAE v.4.03, or referral for endoscopic evaluation of mucosal edema of the oropharynx and larynx, tape measurements, sonography, or external photographs

Continued

(LOE = IIA); (b) should refer HNC survivors to a rehabilitation specialist for treatment consisting of MLD and, if tolerated, compressive bandaging (LOE = IIA).

Fatigue

Recommendation 3.9. It is recommended that primary care clinicians: (a) should assess for fatigue and treat any causative factors for fatigue, including anemia, thyroid dysfunction, and cardiac dysfunction (LOE = 0); (b) should offer treatment or referral for factors that may impact fatigue (e.g., mood disorders, sleep disturbance, pain, etc) for those who do not have an otherwise identifiable cause of fatigue (LOE = I); (c) should counsel HNC survivors to engage in regular physical activity and refer for CBT as appropriate (LOE = I).

Altered or loss of taste

Recommendation 3.10. It is recommended that primary care clinicians should refer HNC survivors with altered or loss of taste to a registered dietitian for dietary counseling and assistance in additional seasoning of food, avoiding unpleasant food, and expanding dietary options (LOE = IIA).

Hearing loss, vertigo, vestibular neuropathy

Recommendation 3.11. It is recommended that primary care clinicians should refer HNC survivors to appropriate specialists (i.e., audiologists) for loss of hearing, vertigo, or vestibular neuropathy related to treatment (LOE = IIA).

Sleep disturbance/sleep apnea

Recommendation 3.12. It is recommended that primary care clinicians: (a) should screen HNC survivors for sleep disturbance by asking HNC survivors and partners about snoring and symptoms of sleep apnea (LOE = 0); (b) should refer HNC survivors to a sleep specialist for a sleep study (polysomnogram) if sleep apnea is suspected (LOE = 0); (c) should manage sleep disturbance similar to patients in the general population (LOE = 0); (d) should recommend nasal decongestants, nasal strips, and sleeping in the propped up position to reduce snoring and mouth breathing; room cool-mist humidifiers can aid sleep as well by keeping the airway moist (LOE = 0); (e) should refer to a dental professional to test the fit of dentures to ensure proper fit and counsel HNC survivors to remove dentures at night to avoid irritation (LOE = 0).

Speech/voice

Recommendation 3.13. It is recommended that primary care clinicians: (a) should assess HNC survivors for speech disturbance (LOE = 0); (b) should refer HNC survivors to an experienced speech-language pathologist if communication disorder exists (LOEs = IA, IIA).

Hypothyroidism

Recommendation 3.14. It is recommended that primary care clinicians should evaluate HNC survivor thyroid function by measuring TSH every 6–12 months (LOE = III).

Oral and dental surveillance

Recommendation 3.15. It is recommended that primary care clinicians: (a) should counsel HNC survivors to maintain close follow-up with the dental professional and reiterate that proper preventive care can help reduce caries and gingival disease (LOE = IA); (b) should counsel HNC survivors to avoid tobacco, alcohol (including mouthwash containing alcohol), spicy or abrasive foods, extreme temperature liquids, sugar-containing chewing gum or sugary soft drinks, and acidic or citric liquids (LOE = 0); (c) should refer HNC survivors to a dental professional specializing in the care of oncology patients (LOE = 0).

Caries

Recommendation 3.16. It is recommended that primary care clinicians: (a) should counsel HNC survivors to seek regular professional dental care for routine examination and cleaning and immediate attention to any intraoral changes that may occur (LOE = 0); (b) should counsel HNC survivors to minimize intake of sticky and/or sugar-containing food and drink to minimize risk of caries (LOE = 0); (c) should counsel HNC survivors on dental prophylaxis, including brushing with remineralizing toothpaste, the use of dental floss, and fluoride use (prescription 1.1% sodium fluoride toothpaste as a dentifrice or in customized delivery trays; LOE = IA, 0).

Periodontitis

Recommendation 3.17. It is recommended that primary care clinicians: (a) should refer HNC survivors to a dentist or periodontist for thorough evaluation (LOE = 0); (b) should counsel HNC survivors to seek regular treatment from and follow recommendations of a qualified dental professional and reinforce that proper examination of the gingival attachment is a normal part of ongoing dental care (LOE = 0).

Xerostomia

Recommendation 3.18. It is recommended that primary care clinicians: (a) should encourage use of alcohol-free rinses if an HNC survivor requires mouth rinses (LOE = 0); (b) should counsel HNC survivors to consume a low sucrose diet and to avoid caffeine, spicy and highly acidic foods, and tobacco (LOE = 0); (c) should encourage HNC survivors to avoid dehydration by drinking fluoridated tap water, but explain that consumption of water will not eliminate xerostomia (LOE = 0).

Osteonecrosis

Recommendation 3.19. It is recommended that primary care clinicians: (a) should monitor HNC survivors for swelling of the jaw and/or jaw pain, indicating possible osteonecrosis (LOE = 0); (b) should administer conservative treatment protocols, such as broad-spectrum antibiotics and daily saline or aqueous chlorhexidine gluconate irrigations, for early stage lesions.(LOE = 0); (c) should refer to an HN surgeon for consideration of hyperbaric oxygen therapy for early and intermediate lesions, for debridement of necrotic bone while undergoing conservative management, or for external mandible bony exposure through the skin (LOE = 0).

Oral infections/candidiasis

Recommendation 3.20. It is recommended that primary care clinicians: (a) should refer HNC survivors to a qualified dental professional for treatment and management of complicated oral conditions and infections (LOE = 0); (b) should consider systemic fluconazole and/or localized therapy of clotrimazole troches to treat oral fungal infections (LOE = 0).

Body and self-image

Recommendation 3.21. It is recommended that primary care clinicians: (a) should assess HNC survivors for body and self-image concerns (LOE = IIA); (b) should refer for psychosocial care as indicated (LOE = IA).

BOX 26.4   The American Cancer Society Head and Neck Cancer Survivorship Care Guideline Recommendations—cont'd

Distress/depression/anxiety

Recommendation 3.22. It is recommended that primary care clinicians: (a) should assess HNC survivors for distress/depression and/or anxiety periodically (3 months posttreatment and at least annually), ideally using a validated screening tool (LOE = I); (b) should offer in-office counseling and/or pharmacotherapy and/or refer to appropriate psycho-oncology and mental health resources as clinically indicated if signs of distress, depression, or anxiety are present (LOE = I); (c) should refer HNC survivors to mental health specialists for specific QoL concerns, such as to social workers for issues like financial and employment challenges or to addiction specialists for substance abuse (LOE = I).

Health promotion

Information

Recommendation 4.1. It is recommended that primary care clinicians: (a) should assess the information needs of the HNC survivor related to HNC and its treatment, side effects, other health concerns, and available support services (LOE = 0); (b) should provide or refer HNC survivors to appropriate resources to meet identified needs (LOE = 0).

Healthy weight

Recommendation 4.2. It is recommended that primary care clinicians: (a) should counsel HNC survivors to achieve and maintain a healthy weight (LOE = III); (b) should counsel HNC survivors on nutrition strategies to maintain a healthy weight for those at risk for cachexia (LOE = 0); (c) should counsel HNC survivors if overweight or obese to limit consumption of high-calorie foods and beverages and increase physical activity to promote and maintain weight loss (LOE = IA).

Physical activity

Recommendation 4.3. It is recommended that primary care clinicians should counsel HNC survivors to engage in regular physical activity consistent with the ACS guideline, and specifically: (a) should avoid inactivity and return to normal daily activities as soon as possible after diagnosis (LOE = III); (b) should aim for at least 150 min of moderate or 75 min of vigorous aerobic exercise per week (LOE = I, IA); (c) should include strength training exercises at least 2 days/week (LOE = IA).

Nutrition

Recommendation 4.4. It is recommended that primary care clinicians: (a) should counsel HNC survivors to achieve a dietary pattern that is high in vegetables, fruits, and whole grains, low in saturated fats, sufficient in dietary fiber, and avoids alcohol consumption (LOE = IA, III); (b) should refer HNC survivors with nutrition-related challenges (e.g., swallowing problems that impact nutrient intake) to a registered dietician or other specialist (LOE = 0).

Tobacco cessation

Recommendation 4.5. It is recommended that primary care clinicians should counsel HNC survivors to avoid tobacco products and offer or refer patients to cessation counseling and resources (LOE = I).

Personal oral health

Recommendation 4.6. It is recommended that primary care clinicians: (a) should counsel HNC survivors to maintain regular dental care, including frequent visits to dental professionals, early interventions for dental complications, and meticulous oral hygiene (LOE = 0); (b) should test fit dentures to ensure proper fit and counsel HNC survivors to remove them at night to avoid irritation (LOE = 0); (c) should counsel HNC survivors that nasal strips can reduce snoring and mouth-breathing and that room humidifiers and nasal saline sprays can aid sleep as well (LOE = 0); (d) should train HNC survivors to do at-home HN self-evaluations and be instructed to report any suspicions or concerns immediately (LOE = 0).

Care coordination and practice implications

Survivorship care plan

Recommendation 5.1. It is recommended that primary care clinicians should consult with the oncology team and obtain a treatment summary and survivorship care plan (LOE = 0, III).

Communication with other providers

Recommendation 5.2. It is recommended that primary care clinicians: (a) should maintain communication with the oncology team throughout diagnosis, treatment, and posttreatment care to ensure care is evidence-based and well-coordinated (LOE = 0); (b) should refer HNC survivors to a dentist to provide diagnosis and treatment of dental caries, periodontal disease, and other intraoral conditions, including mucositis and oral infections, and communicate with the dentist on follow-up recommendations and patient education (LOE = 0); (c) should maintain communication with specialists referred to for management of comorbidities, symptoms, and long-term and late effects (LOEs = 0).

Inclusion of caregivers

Recommendation 5.3. It is recommended that primary care clinicians should encourage the inclusion of caregivers, spouses, or partners in usual HNC survivorship care and support (LOE = 0).

Level of Evidence Criteria

I Metaanalyses of RCTs

IA RCT of HNC survivors

IB RCT based on cancer survivors across multiple cancer sites

IC RCT not based on cancer survivors but on general population experiencing a specific long-term or late effect (e.g., managing fatigue, etc.)

IIA Non-RCTs based on HNC survivors

IIB Non-RCTs based on cancer survivors across multiple sites

IIC Non-RCTs not based on cancer survivors but on general population experiencing a specific long-term or late effect (e.g., managing fatigue, etc)

III Case–control study or prospective cohort study

0 Expert opinion, observational study (excluding case-control and prospective cohort studies), clinical practice, literature review, or pilot study

2A NCCN Category 2A: Based upon lower-level evidence, there is uniform NCCN consensus that the intervention is appropriate

HNC, indicates head and neck cancer; *NCCN*, National Comprehensive Cancer Network; *RCTs*, randomized controlled trials.

BOX 26.5   Late Effects and High-Risk Features of Childhood Cancer and Its Treatment

Body System	LATE EFFECTS	Exposure	Selected High-Risk Factors	At-Risk Diagnostic Groups[a]
Neurocognitive	Neurocognitive deficits Functional deficits in: executive function sustained attention memory Processing speed Visual-motor integration Learning deficits diminished IQ behavioral change	Chemotherapy: • Methotrexate Radiation impacting brain: • Cranial • Ear/infratemporal • Total body irradiation (TBI)	• Age <3 years at time of treatment • Female sex • Supratentorial tumor • Premorbid or family history of learning or attention problems • Radiation doses >24 Gy • Whole brain irradiation	Acute lymphoblastic leukemia Brain tumor Sarcoma (head and neck or osteosarcoma)
Neurosensory	Hearing loss, sensorineural Hearing loss, conductive Tympanosclerosis Otosclerosis Eustachian tube dysfunction Visual impairment Cataracts Lacrimal duct atrophy Xerophthalmia Retinopathy Glaucoma Peripheral neuropathy, sensory	Chemotherapy: • Cisplatin • Carboplatin Radiation impacting hearing: • Cranial • Infratemporal • Nasopharyngeal radiation impacting hearing: • Cranial • Infratemporal • Nasopharyngeal Chemotherapy: • Busulfan • Glucocorticoids radiation impacting eye: • Cranial • Orbital/eye • TBI Chemotherapy: • Vincristine • Vinblastine • Cisplatin • Carboplatin	• Higher cisplatin dose (360 mg/m²) • Higher radiation dose impacting ear (>30 Gy) • Concurrent radiation and cisplatin • Higher radiation dose impacting ear (>30 Gy) • Higher radiation dose impacting eye (>15 Gy for cataracts; >45 Gy for retinopathy and visual impairment) • Higher cisplatin dose (≥300 mg/m²)	Brain tumor Germ cell tumor Sarcoma (head and neck) Neuroblastoma Hepatoblastoma Brain tumor Sarcoma (head and neck) Brain tumor Acute lymphoblastic leukemia Retinoblastoma Rhabdomyosarcoma (orbital) Allogeneic HSCT Acute lymphoblastic leukemia Brain tumor Hodgkin's lymphoma Germ cell tumor Non-Hodgkin's lymphoma Sarcoma Neuroblastoma Wilms' tumor Carcinoma
Neuromotor	Peripheral neuropathy, motor	Chemotherapy: • Vincristine • Vinblastine		Acute lymphoblastic leukemia Hodgkin's lymphoma Non-Hodgkin's lymphoma Sarcoma Brain tumor Neuroblastoma Wilms' tumor
Endocrine	GH deficiency Precocious puberty Obesity Hypothyroidism, central Gonadotropin deficiency Adrenal insufficiency, central Hypothyroidism, primary	Radiation impacting HPA: • Cranial • Orbital/eye • Ear/infratemporal • Nasopharyngeal • TBI • Neck, mantle irradiation	• Females • Radiation dose to HPA >18 Gy • Females • Younger age (<4 years) • Radiation dose to HPA >18 Gy • Radiation dose to thyroid >20 Gy	Acute lymphoblastic leukemia Sarcoma (facial) Carcinoma (nasopharyngeal) Acute lymphoblastic leukemia Brain tumor Sarcoma (facial) Carcinoma (nasopharyngeal) Hodgkin's lymphoma

BOX 26.5   Late Effects and High-Risk Features of Childhood Cancer and Its Treatment—cont'd

Reproductive	Gonadal dysfunction delayed or arrested Puberty Premature menopause (females) Germ cell dysfunction/failure Infertility	Chemotherapy alkylating: • Busulfan • Carmustine (BCNU) • Chlorambucil • Cyclophosphamide • Ifosfamide • Lomustine (CCNU) • Mechlorethamine • Melphalan • Procarbazine Radiation impacting reproductive system: • Whole abdomen (females) • Pelvic • Lumbar/sacral spine (females) • Testicular (males) • TBI	Higher alkylating agent dose Alkylating agent conditioning for HSCT Radiation dose $\geq$ 15 Gy in prepubertal girls Radiation dose $\geq$ 10 Gy in pubertal girls For germ cell failure in males, any pelvic irradiation For androgen insufficiency, gonadal irradiation, $\geq$20 −30 Gy in males	Acute lymphoblastic leukemia, high risk Brain tumor Hodgkin's lymphoma, advanced/ unfavourable Non-Hodgkin's lymphoma, advanced/unfavourable Sarcoma Neuroblastoma Wilms' tumor, advanced autologous or allogeneic HSCT
Cardiac	Cardiomyopathy Arrhythmias Cardiomyopathy Arrhythmias Pericardial fibrosis Valvular disease Myocardial infarction Atherosclerotic heart disease	Chemotherapy • Daunorubicin • Doxorubicin • Idarubicin Radiation impacting heart: • Chest • Mantle • Mediastinum • Axilla • Spine • Upper abdomen	• Female sex • Age <5 years at time of treatment • Higher doses of chemotherapy ($\geq$300 mg/m^2) • Higher doses of cardiac radiation ($\geq$30 Gy) • Combined modality therapy with cardiotoxic chemotherapy and irradiation	Hodgkin's lymphoma Leukemia Non-Hodgkin's lymphoma Sarcoma Wilms' tumor Neuroblastoma
Pulmonary	Pulmonary fibrosis Interstitial pneumonitis Restrictive lung disease Obstructive lung disease	Chemotherapy • Bleomycin • Busulfan • Carmustine (BCNU) • Lomustine (CCNU) radiation impacting lungs: • Mantle • Mediastinum • Whole lung • TBI	• Higher doses of chemotherapy • Combined modality therapy with pulmonary toxic chemotherapy and irradiation	Brain tumor Germ cell tumor Hodgkin's lymphoma Sarcoma (chest wall or intrathoracic) autologous or allogeneic HCST
Gastrointestinal	Chronic enterocolitis Strictures Bowel obstruction	Radiation impacting GI tract ($\geq$30 Gy) Abdominal surgery	• Higher radiation dose to bowel ($\geq$45 Gy) • Combined modality therapy with abdominal irradiation and radiomimetic chemotherapy (dactinomycin or anthracyclines) • Combined modality therapy with abdominal surgery and irradiation	Sarcoma (retroperitoneal or pelvic primary)
Hepatic	Hepatic fibrosis Cirrhosis	Radiation impacting liver	• Higher radiation dose or treatment volume (20 −30 Gy to entire liver or $\geq$40 Gy to at least 1/3 of liver)	Sarcoma Neuroblastoma

Continued

BOX 26.5   Late Effects and High-Risk Features of Childhood Cancer and Its Treatment—cont'd

Body System	LATE EFFECTS	Exposure	Selected High-Risk Factors	At-Risk Diagnostic Groups[a]
Renal	Renal insufficiency Hypertension Glomerular injury Tubular injury	Chemotherapy • Ifosfamide • Cisplatin • Carboplatin Radiation impacting kidneys: • Whole abdomen • Upper abdominal fields • TBI	Higher ifosfamide dose ($\geq$60 g/m^2) Higher cisplatin dose ($\geq$200 mg/m^2) Renal radiation dose $\geq$15 Gy Combined modality therapy with above agents	Brain tumor Germ cell tumor Sarcoma Wilms' tumor Neuroblastoma Hepatoblastoma Carcinoma Autologous or allogeneic HSCT

[a]Based on contemporary treatment protocols.
From Kurt BA, Armstrong GT, Cash DK, et al. Primary care management of the childhood cancer survivor. *J Pediatr*. April 2008;152(4):458–466. Late effects and high-risk features of childhood cancer and its treatment.

measures include but are not limited to postoperative topical therapy using thrombin, microfibrillar collagen, suturing, and application of pressure (see Chapter 24).

Mucositis. Mucositis is defined as inflammation of the oral mucosa and is a common toxicity associated with chemotherapy and head and neck radiation therapy. The inflammation and ulceration of the oral mucosa results from both direct and indirect cytotoxic effects of therapies on rapidly dividing oral epithelium. Mucositis rates are highest in the settings of dose-intensive chemotherapy regimens (e.g., induction regimens for acute leukemia, hematopoietic cell transplantation) and head and neck chemoradiation therapy. Mucositis can be a dose-limiting toxicity, leading to dose interruptions, reductions, or discontinuation depending on severity and impact. Mucositis develops 7–14 days after chemotherapy, and after 2–3 weeks of radiation therapy, and generally subsides within weeks after completion of therapy (Fig. 26.21).

Mucosal erythema is followed by painful ulcerations that frequently affect the lateral tongue and buccal mucosa, generally sparing keratinized sites. The condition may be sufficiently painful to require a soft or liquid diet, or, in severe cases, intravenous or even total parenteral nutrition to maintain adequate hydration and nutrition. Symptoms can be managed with use of bland mouth rinses (e.g., mix 1/4 teaspoon of baking soda and 1/8 teaspoon of salt in 1 cup of warm water), saline or saline-based topical devices (e.g., Caphosol, a supersaturated calcium phosphate solution), as well as topical anesthetic formulations (see Appendix 3); however, systemic analgesics, including opioids, may be indicated. The Multinational Association of Supportive Care in Cancer and the International Association of Oral Oncology (MASCC/ISOO) provides evidence-based guidelines for prevention and management of mucositis are available for several very specific clinical indications and interventions (Box 26.9).

Oral mucositis is also associated with targeted therapies and immune checkpoint inhibitor therapies. The class of targeted therapy with greatest risk of mucositis is the mTOR inhibitors, which are associated with painful small oral ulcerations that resemble aphthous stomatitis and are distinct from mucositis associated with traditional chemotherapy agents (Fig. 26.22). Topical steroid therapy with dexamethasone solution is effective for both prevention and management of this toxicity. Oral mucosal immune-related adverse events (irAEs) include lichenoid/ lichen planus-like inflammation, erythema multiforme-like inflammation, and, rarely, oral lesions of bullous or mucous membrane pemphigoid (Fig. 26.23). Sjögren syndrome-like disease, characterized by abrupt onset of oral dryness, also has been well described. These irAEs may be limited to the oral cavity or may be associated with cutaneous, rheumatologic, or other systemic toxicities. Oral irAEs can be effectively managed with topical steroid therapy for mucosal inflammation, and supportive care measures for xerostomia, including prescription sialogogue therapy; however, depending on severity and impact, including extraoral irAEs, systemic steroids or other immunomodulatory therapy may be indicated.

Infections. During cancer therapy patients are prone to secondary infections due to both immunosuppression and salivary gland dysfunction. The most common oral infection is candidiasis (most frequently caused by *Candida albicans*), which is opportunistic and develops due to both immunosuppression (common with chemotherapy and some targeted therapies, as well as with use of intraoral topical steroids) as well as salivary gland hypofunction. Symptoms variably include pain, burning, taste alterations, and intolerance to foods and drinks. The most common presentation is *pseudomembranous* candidiasis, characterized by white plaques that are easily scraped off, leaving behind tiny petechial hemorrhages (Fig. 26.24). The *erythematous,* or atrophic form, may

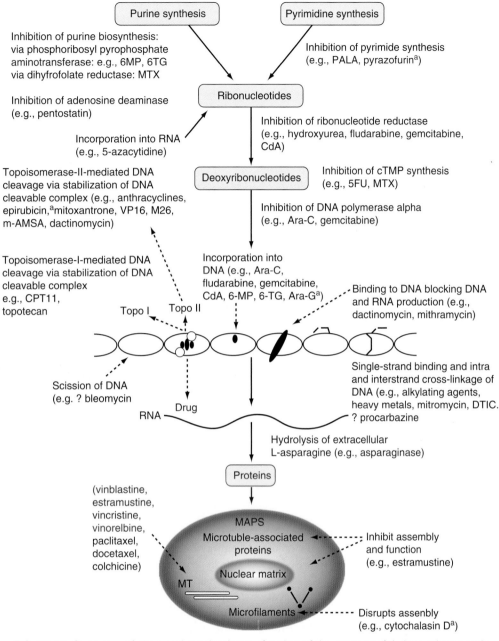

FIG. 26.13 Overview of sites and mechanisms of action of the most useful chemotherapeutic agents. (Reproduced from MGlave P, et al. *Hematology: Basic Principles and Practice.* 5th ed. St Louis: Elsevier; 2009.)

present more subtly, manifesting as red patches accompanied by a burning sensation. Antifungal therapy (topical and systemic) is effective for management of candidiasis, as well as prophylaxis in case of highly immunosuppressive chemotherapy regimens (e.g., allogeneic hematopoietic cell transplantation), or in cases of recurrent infections during or following cancer therapy (see Appendix C).

Recrudescent herpes simplex virus infections can develop during chemotherapy and other cancer therapies due to immunosuppression and stress. These irregular and painful ulcerations most frequently affect the lips and tongue but can affect any intraoral site and tend to be more extensive and take longer to heal than in non-immunocompromised patients (Fig. 26.25). Diagnosis can be confirmed by PCR, direct fluorescent antibody test, culture, and cytology; only culture can be evaluated for antiviral resistance and drug susceptibility. Management requires systemic antiviral therapy with acyclovir or valacyclovir (Appendix C). Antiviral susceptibility testing should be considered for patients with unresolving infections despite antiviral therapy. Acyclovir prophylaxis is given to seropositive patients prior to highly immunosuppressive cancer therapy regimens (e.g., allogeneic hematopoietic cell transplantation); furthermore,

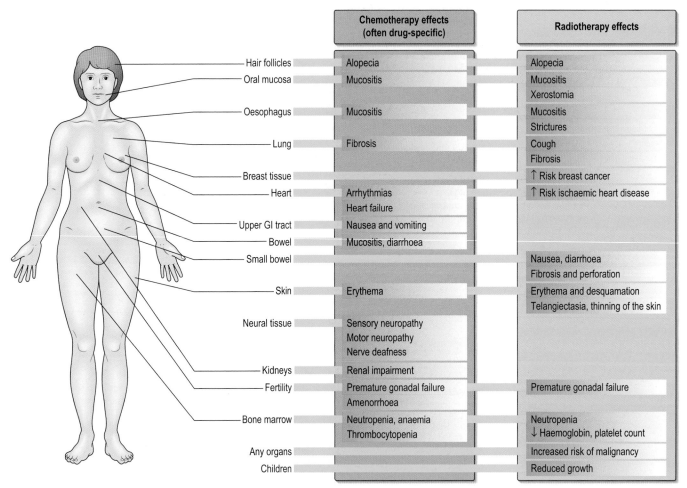

FIG. 26.14 Side effects of chemotherapy and radio-therapy—acute (in *pink*) and dlate (in *blue*). (Reproduced from Peate I. *Alexander's Nursing Practice: Hospital and Home.* 5th ed. London: Elsevier Ltd; 2020.)

prophylaxis should be considered following an episode of recrudescence, especially if cancer therapy will be ongoing.

Odontogenic infections may not present with typical signs of swelling, erythema, and purulence in immuno-suppressed cancer patients. Fever or pain may be the only presenting features. Odontogenic infections require prompt management with antibiotics and definitive care (e.g., extraction of infected tooth). Patients with jaw osteonecrosis may also present with bacterial infection characterized by mixed oral flora (see Jaw Osteonecrosis below).

Bleeding. Cancer patients who undergo high-dose chemotherapy, or who have bone marrow involvement because of disease (e.g., leukemia), are susceptible to thrombocytopenia and risk of oral bleeding. Gingival bleeding and submucosal hemorrhage can occur as a result of minor trauma (e.g., tongue biting, toothbrushing, swallowing) when the platelet count drops below 50,000 (and especially below 20,000) cells/mm³. Common clinical findings include palatal petechiae, purpura on the lateral margin of the tongue, and gingival bleeding or oozing. Gingival hemorrhage is

aggravated by poor oral hygiene. When gingival tissues bleed easily, the patient should begin using softer cleansing devices such as sponge Toothettes and avoid use of dental floss. In case of uncontrolled gingival bleeding, local measures, such as application of pressure with a gelatin sponge with thrombin or microfibrillar collagen placed over the area or use of gauze soaked in an oral antifibrinolytic solution (e.g., aminocaproic acid [Amicar] syrup 250 mg/mL). Platelet transfusion may be necessary if local measures fail (see Chapter 24).

Neural and Chemosensory Changes. Patients receiving radiation therapy to the head and neck often experience a diminished sense of taste, likely related to damage to the taste receptors. Patients receiving chemotherapy may complain of a bitter taste in the mouth, unpleasant odors, and aversions to certain foods, which may impact diet, nutrition, and weight. These changes are typically temporary and resolve weeks to months after completion of therapy.

Neurotoxicity is a side effect of chemotherapeutic agents, particularly vincristine and vinblastine (see Fig. 26.14). Although this complication more commonly arises in the peripheral nerves affecting the hands and

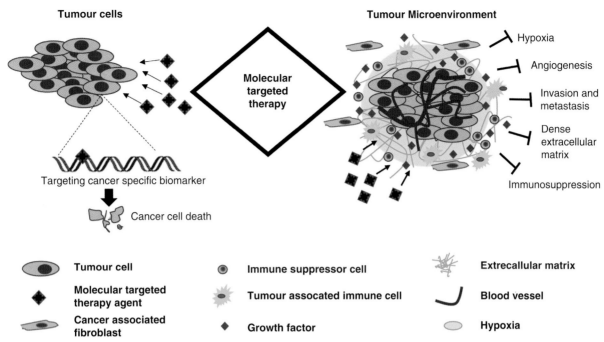

FIG. 26.15 Overview of molecular targeted therapy mechanism. Molecular targeted therapy on cancer focuses on targeting specific cancer-associated molecules that are highly expressed in cancer cells or by modulating the tumor microenvironment related to tumor vasculature, metastasis, or hypoxia. (Reproduced from Lee YT, Tan YJ, Oon CE. Molecular targeted therapy: treating cancer with specificity. *Eur J Pharmacol.* September 5, 2018;834:188–196.)

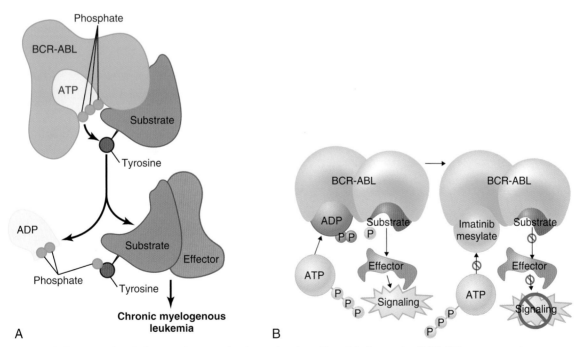

FIG. 26.16 Imatinib mesylate mechanism of action. *Panel A* shows the BCR-ABL oncoprotein with a molecule of adenosine triphosphate (ATP) in the kinase pocket. The substrate is activated by the phosphorylation of one of its tyrosine residues. It can then activate other downstream effector molecules. When imatinib occupies the kinase pocket (*Panel B*), the action of BCR-ABL is inhibited, preventing phosphorylation of its substrate. ADP denotes adenosine diphosphate. (From Rogers JL: McCance & Huether's Pathophysiology: The Biologic Basis for Diseases in Adults and Children, ed 9, Elsevier, 2023, St. Louis.)

TABLE 26.2   FDA-Approved Targeted Therapies for Cancer (2010–2019)

Drugs	Target	Drug Type	FDA-Approved Indication	Toxicities, Adverse Effects, Precautions	Unique Monitoring
Acute Myelogenous Leukemia					
Enasidenib (Idhifa), ivosidenib (Tibsovo)	IDH1/2	Small molecule inhibitors	Newly diagnosed and relapsed/refractory IDH1/2+ acute myelogenous leukemia	Edema, hepatotoxicity, prolonged QTc	Alkaline phosphatase, ALT, AST, CBC, chemistry, CK, ECG, total bilirubin
Gilteritinib (Xospata), midostaurin (Rydapt)	FLT3	Small molecule inhibitors	Newly diagnosed and relapsed/refractory FLT3+ acute myelogenous leukemia	Hepatotoxicity, prolonged QTc, rash, vomiting	Alkaline phosphatase, ALT, AST, CBC, chemistry, ECG, total bilirubin
Anaplastic Thyroid Cancer					
Dabrafenib (Tafinlar) plus trametinib (Mekinist)	*BRAF* and MEK	Small molecule inhibitors	Locally advanced or metastatic with V600E mutation	Colitis, cutaneous squamous cell cancers, fever, heart failure, hepatotoxicity, hyperglycemia, rash, thrombosis	Alkaline phosphatase, ALT, AST, blood glucose, ECG, electrolytes, renal function, skin examination, total bilirubin
Bladder Cancer					
Erdafitinib (Balversa)	FGFR2/3	Small molecule inhibitor	Metastatic or locally advanced FGFR2/3 alterations	Central serous retinopathy, hand-foot syndrome, hyperphosphatemia, onycholysis	Eye examination, phosphate
Breast Cancer					
Ado-trastuzumab emtansine (Kadcyla)	HER2	Antibody–drug conjugate	Early stage HER2+ with residual disease after neoadjuvant treatment; metastatic HER2+	Cardiotoxicity, hepatotoxicity, interstitial lung disease, neuropathy	Alkaline phosphatase, ALT, AST, CBC, ECG, total bilirubin
Alpelisib (Piqray)	PIK3CA	Small molecule inhibitor	PIK3CA-mutated metastatic	Dermatologic (Stevens–Johnson syndrome), hyperglycemia, severe diarrhea	A1C, blood glucose
Atezolizumab (Tecentriq)	PD-L1	Immunotherapy	PD-L1–positive metastatic triple negative breast cancer, in combination with chemotherapy	Colitis, endocrinopathies, hepatitis, myocarditis, pneumonitis, rash	Alkaline phosphatase, ALT, AST, blood glucose, renal function, total bilirubin, TSH
Fam-trastuzumab deruxtecan (Enhertu)	HER2	Antibody–drug conjugate	Metastatic HER2+	Cardiotoxicity, hematologic, interstitial lung disease (9%)	CBC, echocardiography
Olaparib (Lynparza), talazoparib (Talzenna)	Poly- (adenosine diphosphate-ribose) polymerase	Small molecule inhibitors	Breast cancer gene–mutated metastatic	Hematologic, increased mean corpuscular volume, pneumonitis, rare acute myelogenous leukemia	CBC, renal function
Pertuzumab (Perjeta)	HER2	Monoclonal antibody	Metastatic, neoadjuvant, and adjuvant HER2+	Cardiotoxicity, diarrhea	Echocardiography

TABLE 26.2   FDA-Approved Targeted Therapies for Cancer (2010–2019)—cont'd

Chronic Lymphocytic Leukemia

Ibrutinib (Imbruvica)	BTK	Small molecule inhibitor	Chronic lymphocytic leukemia with 17p deletion	Atrial fibrillation, diarrhea, edema, hemorrhage	Alkaline phosphatase, ALT, AST, CBC, renal function, total bilirubin
Venetoclax (Venclexta)	BCL2	Small molecule inhibitor	Chronic lymphocytic leukemia with 17p deletion	Severe pancytopenia, tumor lysis syndrome	CBC, electrolytes, renal function; may require hospitalization for tumor lysis syndrome monitoring

Chronic Myelogenous Leukemia

Bosutinib (Bosulif), dasatinib (Sprycel), nilotinib (Tasigna), ponatinib (Iclusig)	*BCR-ABL*	Small molecule inhibitors	Initial treatment: dasatinib, nilotinib, bosutinib; second-line treatment or T315I mutation: ponatinib	Arterial thrombotic events (ponatinib), diarrhea (bosutinib), edema, effusions (dasatinib), heart failure (all), hematologic, pancreatitis, prolonged QTc (nilotinib)	Alkaline phosphatase, ALT, AST, blood pressure, CBC, chemistry, ECG, glucose, lipid profile, total bilirubin; provide low-dose aspirin with ponatinib

Colorectal Cancer

Cetuximab (Erbitux)	EGFR	Monoclonal antibody	Metastatic without mutation in *RAS*	Acneiform rash, hypomagnesemia	Electrolytes

Gastroesophageal Cancer

Trastuzumab (Herceptin)	HER2	Monoclonal antibody	Metastatic with HER2 overexpression	Cardiotoxicity	Echocardiography

Gastrointestinal Stromal Tumor

Imatinib (Gleevec)	c-KIT	Small molecule inhibitor	Adjuvant following complete resection of c-KIT positive gastrointestinal stromal tumor	Edema, heart failure, hematologic	Alkaline phosphatase, ALT, AST, CBC, electrolytes, renal function, total bilirubin

Lung Cancer (Adenocarcinoma)

Afatinib (Gilotrif), dacomitinib (Vizimpro), erlotinib (Tarceva), gefitinib (Iressa), osimertinib (Tagrisso)	EGFR	Small molecule inhibitors	Metastatic, EGFR exon 19 deletion or exon 21 (L858R) substitution	Diarrhea, hepatotoxicity, prolonged QTc, rash, trichiasis	Alkaline phosphatase, ALT, AST, ECG, electrolytes, renal function, total bilirubin
Alectinib (Alecensa), brigatinib (Alunbrig), ceritinib (Zykadia), crizotinib (Xalkori), lorlatinib (Lorbrena)	Anaplastic lymphoma kinase	Small molecule inhibitors	Metastatic, anaplastic lymphoma kinase fusion	Bradycardia, hepatotoxicity, nausea, ocular toxicity, QT prolongation, vomiting	Alkaline phosphatase, ALT, AST, CBC, renal function, total bilirubin

Continued

TABLE 26.2 FDA-Approved Targeted Therapies for Cancer (2010–2019)—cont'd

Drugs	Target	Drug Type	FDA-Approved Indication	Toxicities, Adverse Effects, Precautions	Unique Monitoring
Crizotinib, entrectinib (Rozlytrek)	ROS1	Small molecule inhibitors	Metastatic, ROS1 positive	Entrectinib: cardiotoxicity, cognitive impairment, fractures, hepatotoxicity, ocular toxicity	Alkaline phosphatase, ALT, AST, ECG, echocardiography, electrolytes, total bilirubin
Dabrafenib	BRAF	Small molecule inhibitors	Metastatic, BRAF V600E mutation	Cutaneous squamous cell cancer, colitis, fever, heart failure, hepatotoxicity, hyperglycemia, rash, thrombosis	Alkaline phosphatase, ALT, AST, blood glucose, echocardiography, skin examination, total bilirubin
Melanoma					
Binimetinib (Mektovi), cobimetinib (Cotellic), dabrafenib, encorafenib (Braftovi), trametinib, vemurafenib (Zelboraf)	BRAF + MEK	Small molecule inhibitors	Metastatic, V600E, V600K mutation (all) Adjuvant (dabrafenib + trametinib)	BRAF inhibitors: alopecia, arthralgia, diarrhea, fatigue, nausea, rash MEK inhibitors: diarrhea, rash, retinopathy	Alkaline phosphatase, ALT, AST, blood glucose, echocardiography, skin examination, total bilirubin
Mismatch Repair Deficient Solid Tumors					
Ipilimumab (Yervoy), nivolumab (Opdivo), pembrolizumab (Keytruda)	PD-1 or CTLA-4	Immunotherapies	Metastatic mismatch repair-deficient solid tumor	Adrenal insufficiency, colitis, myocarditis (rare but morbid), pneumonitis, rash, thyroiditis	Alkaline phosphatase, ALT, AST, blood glucose, renal function, total bilirubin, TSH
Neurotrophin Receptor Kinase Fusion Solid Tumors					
Entrectinib, larotrectinib (Vitrakvi)	Neurotrophin receptor kinase	Small molecule inhibitors	Metastatic solid tumors with neurotrophin receptor kinase fusion protein	Cardiotoxicity, cognitive impairment, fractures, hepatotoxicity, ocular toxicity	Alkaline phosphatase, ALT, AST, ECG, echocardiography, total bilirubin
Ovarian					
Niraparib (Zejula), olaparib, rucaparib (Rubraca)	Poly- (adenosine diphosphate-ribose) polymerase	Small molecule inhibitors	Advanced or metastatic ovarian cancer with breast cancer gene mutation	Myelodysplastic syndrome, pancytopenia CBC	CBC

ALT, alanine transaminase; *AST*, aspartate transaminase; *BCL2*, B-cell leukemia/lymphoma 2; *BCR-ABL*, a fusion gene when pieces of chromosomes 9 and 22 break off and trade places; *BRAF*, B-raf proto-oncogene; *BTK*, Bruton tyrosine kinase; *c-KIT*, gene encoding tyrosine-protein kinase KIT; *CBC*, complete blood count; *CK*, creatine kinase; *CTLA-4*, cytotoxic T-lymphocyte–associated protein 4; *ECG*, electrocardiography; *EGFR*, epidermal growth factor receptor; *FDA*, U.S. Food and Drug Administration; *FGFR2/3*, fibroblast growth factor receptor 2/3; *FLT3*, fms-like tyrosine kinase 3; *HER2*, human epi-dermal growth factor receptor 2; *IDH1/2*, isocitrate dehydrogenase 1/2; *MEK*, MAP kinase-ERK kinase; *PD-1*, programmed cell death protein 1; *PD-L1*, programmed cell death ligand 1; *PIK3CA*, phosphatidylinositol-4,5-bisphosphate 3-kinase catalytic subunit alpha; *ROS1*, receptor tyrosine kinase encoded by gene *ROS1*; *TSH*, thyroid-stimulating hormone.
Adapted from Smith C, Prasad V. *Am Fam Physician*. 2021;103(3):155–163. From Smith CEP, Prasad V. Targeted cancer therapies. *Am Fam Physician*. February 1, 2021;103(3):155–163. PMID: 33507053.

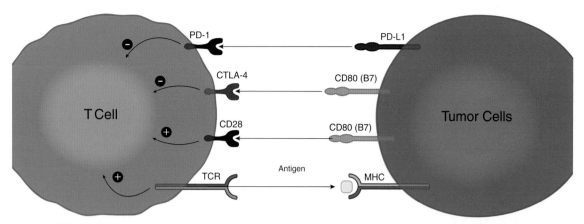

FIG. 26.17 Immune-checkpoint inhibitors. Immune-checkpoint inhibitors PD-1/PD-L1 and CTLA-4/CD80 receptor are responsible for inhibition or decreased stimulation of T cells. PD-1 and CTLA-4 inhibitor blockade is accomplished by monoclonal antibodies (PD-1: nivolumab and pembrolizumab; CTLA-4: ipilimumab), resulting in proliferation and increased T-cell response against tumor cells. (Reproduced from Winn HR. *Youmans & Winn Neurological Surgery*. 8th ed. St louis: Elsevier; 2023.)

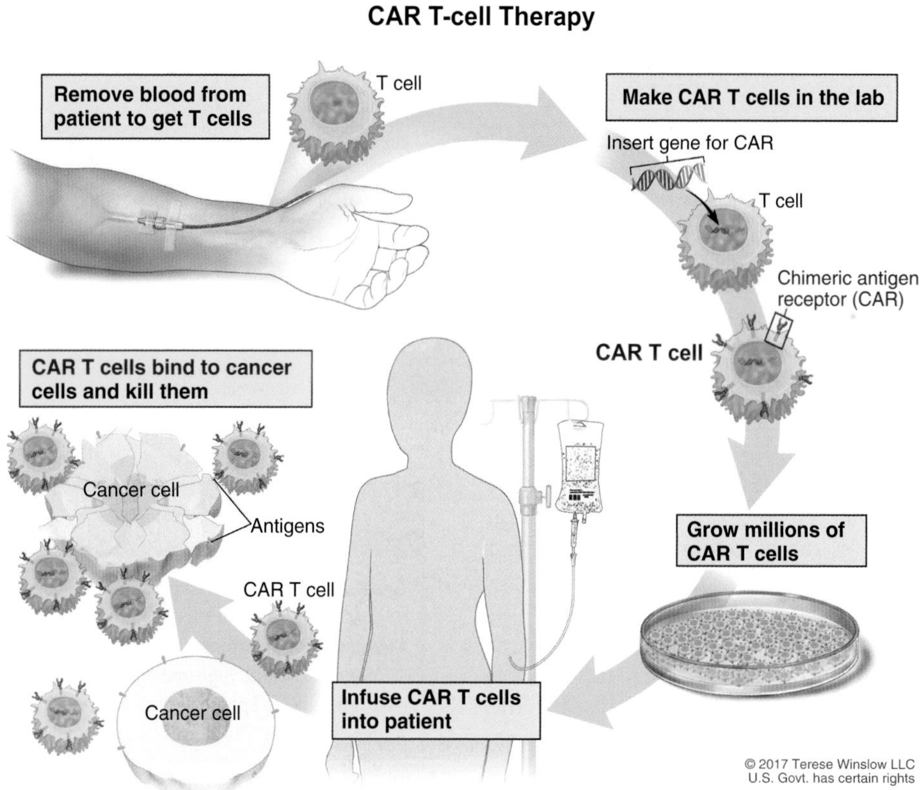

CAR T-cell Therapy

Remove blood from patient to get T cells

T cell

Make CAR T cells in the lab

Insert gene for CAR

T cell

Chimeric antigen receptor (CAR)

CAR T cell

CAR T cells bind to cancer cells and kill them

Cancer cell

Antigens

CAR T cell

Cancer cell

Grow millions of CAR T cells

Infuse CAR T cells into patient

© 2017 Terese Winslow LLC
U.S. Govt. has certain rights

FIG. 26.18 CAR T-cell therapy. A type of treatment in which a patient's T cells (a type of immune cell) are changed in the laboratory so they will bind to cancer cells and kill them. Blood from a vein in the patient's arm flows through a tube to an apheresis machine (not shown), which removes the white blood cells, including the T cells, and sends the rest of the blood back to the patient. Then, the gene for a special receptor called a chimeric antigen receptor (CAR) is inserted into the T cells in the laboratory. Millions of the CAR T cells are grown in the laboratory and then given to the patient by infusion. The CAR T cells are able to bind to an antigen on the cancer cells and kill them. (https://www.cancer.gov/publications/dictionaries/cancer-terms/def/car-t-cell-therapy.)

BOX 26.6 Checklist for Dental Management of Cancer Patients

PREOPERATIVE RISK ASSESSMENT

R

Recognize Risks

- Be **aware** of adverse events that may occur in the management of a cancer patient
  - Infection
  - Bleeding
  - Jaw osteonecrosis
  - Oral mucosal toxicities
  - Salivary gland hypofunction
  - Neuropathic pain and chemosensory disorders

P

Patient Evaluation

- Review **cancer history** and discuss relevant issues with the patient.
- Identify all **cancer treatments and supportive care measures** that are planned or that have been received.
- **Examine** the patient for signs and symptoms of disease and obtain vital signs.
- Review or obtain recent **laboratory test results** or **imaging studies** required to assess risk.
- Obtain a **medical consultation** if the patient's health status is uncertain.

A	
Antibiotics	No standard-of-care indication for antibiotic prophylaxis prior to invasive procedures. Postprocedural antibiotics should be considered in patients who are neutropenic (ANC < 1000 cells/uL), and in patients who are at risk for jaw osteonecrosis.
Analgesics	N/A
Anesthesia	N/A
Anxiety	N/A

B	
Bleeding	Patients receiving dose-intensive chemotherapy may be thrombocytopenic; platelet count should be reviewed prior to invasive procedures. Patients with hematologic malignancies may be thrombocytopenic. Platelet transfusion should be considered prior to invasive procedures when the platelet count is <50,000 cells/uL.
Breathing	N/A
Blood pressure	N/A

C	
Capacity to tolerate care	Cancer patients who are actively undergoing therapy may experience fatigue and malaise.

D	
Drugs	Patients treated with antiresorptive therapies, and to a lesser extent antiangiogenic therapies, are at risk for developing osteonecrosis of the jaw.
Devices	N/A

E	
Equipment	N/A
Emergencies	N/A

POSTOPERATIVE CARE

F

Follow-up care

Patients who are at risk for developing jaw osteonecrosis should be followed carefully for healing after performing invasive surgical procedures.

---

feet, patients treated with these agents may experience symptoms affecting the lips or tongue (e.g., tingling, numbness, burning), or rarely odontogenic pain that mimics irreversible pulpitis.

Post–Cancer Treatment Management

As is the case prior to and during cancer treatment, it is essential to understand the patient's overall disease and performance status, their prognosis, and any risk factors for developing oral complications. For patients in remission with good long-term prognosis, most dental treatment plans do not require modification unless related to specific risk factors. For patients with poor prognosis and limited life expectancy, dental treatment should be limited in scope to ensuring comfort, basic oral function, and absence of infection. Pediatric cancer survivors may develop dental (e.g., microdontia, hypodontia, root abnormalities) and skeletal abnormalities (e.g., delayed growth) that require multidisciplinary specialty care. At all dental follow-up visits, cancer patients require thorough extraoral and intraoral examination to

BOX 26.7 Clinical Features of Cancers of the Oral Cavity, Head, and Neck

Basal cell carcinoma: Slightly raised lesion with rolled waxy border and central ulceration on sun-exposed surface.

Squamous cell carcinoma: Irregular red-white lesion; ulcer; or fungating mass. High-risk sites include the lateral tongue, floor of the mouth, lip.

Kaposi sarcoma: Purple plaques or nodules of the palate, gingiva, or face.

Melanoma: Brown or black enlarging plaque on skin or palate with irregular features.

Mucoepidermoid carcinoma: Dome-shaped swelling with central ulceration of palate, retromolar region, or lytic osseous lesion.

Leukemia: Gingival enlargement, and bleeding, skin pallor, small hemorrhages of the skin and mucous membranes, and bruising.

Lymphoma: Enlarged, nonpainful lymph nodes, palatal or pharyngeal swellings, retromolar ulcerations

Advanced breast, prostate, and renal cancer: Lytic and opaque osseous metastases in the mandible, lip/mental nerve paresthesia.

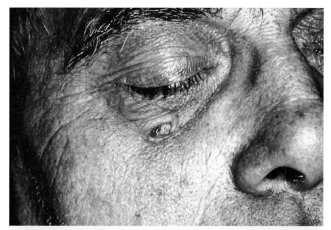

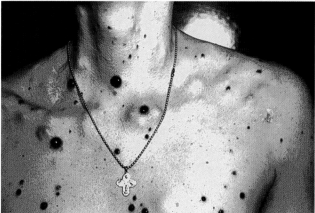

FIG. 26.19 Skin cancers. (A) Basal cell carcinoma manifesting as a facial lesion in a dental patient; (B) Malignant melanoma of the chest. The arms, face, and neck are readily visible surfaces that can be examined by the dentist.

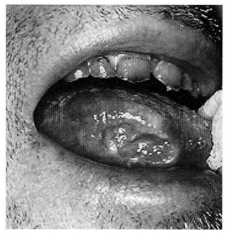

FIG. 26.20 Irregular deep ulceration of the ventrolateral tongue with associated leukoplakia. Biopsy demonstrated invasive squamous cell carcinoma.

screen for recurrent/metastatic disease as well as new primary disease. In addition to risk for malignancy, cancer survivors may be at risk for a spectrum of late complications (e.g., salivary gland hypofunction, jaw

---

BOX 26.8 Guidelines for Dental Screening and Clearance Prior to Initiation of Cancer Therapy

Patient Evaluation
- Collect a detailed **cancer history**
- Obtain dental radiographs
- Perform a comprehensive soft and hard tissue **clinical examination**
- Develop a treatment plan
  - Remove sources of trauma
  - Definitive management of odontogenic infections
  - Periodontal care, stabilization
  - Home hygiene, diet

Indications for Dental Extraction
- Broken-down, nonrestorable tooth
- Periodontal pocket depths ≥6 mm, excessive mobility, purulence on probing
- Radiographic evidence of periapical inflammation[a]
- Partially erupted third molars with history of pericoronitis
- Teeth otherwise considered to have poor prognosis
- Extractions should be completed:
  - at least 7 days before initiation of chemotherapy
  - at least 2 weeks prior to initiation of radiation therapy or antiresorptive therapy

Management Considerations
- No universal indications for antibiotic prophylaxis before invasive dental procedures in neutropenic patients (ANC < 1000 cells/μL). Antibiotic prophylaxis is not indicated for cancer patients with an indwelling catheter (Hickman catheter or port).
- Postprocedural antibiotics should be considered in neutropenic patients.
- Platelet transfusion should be considered in patients with platelet count <50,000/μL.
- Removable prosthodontic appliances should not be used during head and neck radiation or high dose chemotherapy. Orthodontic bands should be removed before initiation of therapy.
- Management of carious teeth that are asymptomatic, at low risk for infection, and otherwise restorable can be deferred until after completion of cancer therapy.
- Management of head and neck cancer patients who are treated surgically should include coordination with a maxillofacial prosthodontist.

[a]Exception is an asymptomatic endodontically treated tooth with stable but persistent periapical radiolucency.

---

osteonecrosis) that can impact on oral health and oral health–related quality of life.

Hyposalivation and Its Sequelae. Long-term salivary gland hypofunction is an almost universal complication after radiation therapy to the head and neck, especially when the parotid glands receive at least 26 Gy. This complication also may occur in patients who have received radioactive iodine therapy for thyroid cancer

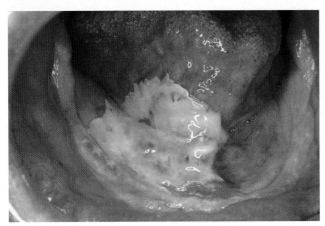

FIG. 26.21 Extensive mucositis that developed from the effects of radiation on the oral mucosa. (Reproduced from Neville BW, et al. *Oral and Maxillofacial Pathology.* 3rd ed. St. Louis: Saunders; 2009.)

(see Chapter 16), patients with chronic GVHD after allogeneic hematopoietic cell transplantation (see Chapter 21), and patients who were treated with immune checkpoint inhibitors. Saliva is reduced in volume and altered in consistency, pH, buffering and remineralization capacity, and concentration of immunoglobulin and other antimicrobial proteins. The consistency may be mucinous, thick, sticky, and ropy, and examination often demonstrates notably dry and often atrophic appearing oral mucosa (see Fig. 26.26).

Extreme difficulty in lubricating and masticating food (sticking to the tongue or hard palate) and difficulty swallowing food (dysphagia) are common. Additionally, lack of or altered taste perception (hypogeusia or dysgeusia) and altered tolerance for acidic foods (e.g., citrus fruits, acetic acid/vinegar) may occur in the absence of adequate saliva. As a result, nutritional intake may be impaired.

Infectious complications of salivary gland hypofunction include dental caries and recurrent oral candidiasis. Dental caries frequently present at the cervical, interproximal, and incisal surfaces (Fig. 26.27). Patients should be educated regarding limiting sugar intake and maintaining good oral hygiene practices and be provided with fluoride both in-office (e.g., fluoride varnish) and for home use (prescription fluoride toothpaste or gel, see Appendix C). Recurrent oral candidiasis can be managed with prophylactic antifungal therapy (see Appendix C).

Patients should be encouraged to drink plenty of water and fluids and to avoid diuretics such as coffee or tea and alcohol. Use of sugar-free gum or candy throughout the day can help stimulate salivary flow and keep the mouth feeling moist. Over-the-counter dry mouth relief products include rinses, gels, and saliva substitutes. Prescription sialogogue therapy with the muscarinic cholinergic agonists pilocarpine (Salagen) and cevimeline (Evoxac) can be effective in increasing salivary output and improving symptoms of xerostomia (see Appendix C).

Trismus. Head and neck cancer surgery, radiation therapy to the head and neck, or the combination are risk factors for developing trismus. Another infrequent cause of trismus is in patients with chronic GVHD who develop soft tissue sclerodermatous changes. In addition to difficulty eating and maintaining adequate oral hygiene due to limited mouth opening, trismus may be associated with pain and spasms. Management requires long-term physical therapy with passive jaw-stretching exercises using various devices and appliances, including a simple approach of slowly increasing the number of tongue blades that can be stacked in the mouth at least three times a day for 10-minute intervals; advanced cases may need to be addressed by a professional physical therapist. Jaw opening therapy should be approached with caution in patients who have received radiation therapy to the mandible due to risk of pathologic fracture. Dentists must be particularly attentive to diagnosis and management of dental caries in patients with trismus. Fluoride should be applied in-office and prescribed for home use.

Jaw Osteonecrosis. Osteonecrosis of the jaw (ONJ) can develop after radiation therapy to the head and neck (*osteoradionecrosis*) or after treatment with antiresorptive therapies, or rarely antiangiogenic targeted therapies (*medication-related osteonecrosis of the jaw—MRONJ*) (Fig. 26.28). Osteoradionecrosis results from radiation-induced changes (hypocellularity, hypovascularity, and ischemia) in the jaws. MRONJ results from an imbalance in bone homeostasis due to osteoclast inhibition. Jaw osteonecrosis is characterized by exposed necrotic bone, or necrotic bone that can be probed through a fistula, that has been present for at least 8 weeks. ONJ can develop spontaneously, or may develop after dental extraction, or in the setting of chronic dental infection (e.g., periodontal disease), or following trauma, or from the pressure of denture wearing. Secondary soft tissue infection is common and the most frequent cause of symptoms; advanced infection may lead to an extraoral fistula. Other causes of symptoms include impingement of the inferior alveolar nerve and pathologic fracture. Risk for development of this complication is greatest in posterior mandibular sites and in patients who have received radiation doses in excess of 6500 cGy to the jaw, those with higher cumulative doses of antiresorptive therapy, smokers, and those who have undergone a traumatic (e.g., extraction) procedure in the presence of local anesthetic containing epinephrine. The American Association of Oral and Maxillofacial Surgeons guidelines for staging and managing MRONJ can be applied to all cancer patients with jaw osteonecrosis (Box 26.10).

If the dentist is unsure of the amount of radiation received and invasive procedures are planned, the

BOX 26.9   MASCC/ISOO Clinical Practice Guidelines for the Management of Mucositis Secondary to Cancer Therapy

Multinational Association of Supportive Care in Cancer and International Society of Oral Oncology
Clinical Practice Guidelines for Oral Mucositis

Section	LoE	Guideline Statement
BOC	III	• The panel suggests that implementation of *multiagent combination* oral care protocols is beneficial for the prevention of OM during CT.
	III	• The panel suggests that implementation of *multiagent combination* oral care protocols is beneficial for the prevention of OM during H&N RT.
	III	• The panel suggests that implementation of *multiagent combination* oral care protocols is beneficial for the prevention of OM during HSCT.
	III	• No guideline was possible regarding the use of *professional oral care* for the prevention of OM in patients with hematologic, solid, or H&N cancers because of limited and inconsistent data. An expert opinion complements this guideline: although there was insufficient evidence to support the use of professional oral care for OM prevention, the panel is of the opinion that dental evaluation and treatment as indicated before cancer therapy are desirable to reduce risk for local and systemic infections from odontogenic sources.
	III	• No guideline was possible regarding the use of *patient education* for the prevention of OM in patients with hematologic cancer during HSCT or CT because of limited and inconsistent data. An expert opinion complements this guideline: the panel is of the opinion that educating patients about the benefits of BOC strategies is still appropriate because this may improve self-management and adherence to the recommended oral care protocol during cancer treatment.
	III	• No guideline was possible regarding the *use of saline or sodium bicarbonate* rinses in the prevention or treatment of OM in patients undergoing cancer therapy because of limited data. An expert opinion complements this guideline: despite the limited data available for both saline and sodium bicarbonate, the panel recognizes that these are inert, bland rinses that increase oral clearance, which may be helpful for maintaining oral hygiene and improving patient comfort.
	III	• The panel suggests that *CHX* not be used in the prevention of OM in patients undergoing H&N RT.
Antiinflammatory agents	I	• The panel recommends *benzydamine* mouthwash for the prevention of OM in patients with H&N cancer receiving a moderate dose RT ($<$50 Gy).
	II	• The panel suggests the use of *benzydamine* mouthwash for the prevention of OM in patients with H&N cancer who receive RT-CT.
PBM	I	• The panel recommends the use of intraoral *PBM* therapy using low-level laser therapy for the prevention of OM in adult patients receiving HSCT conditioned with high-dose CT, with or without TBI, using one of the selected protocols listed in Table 26.2.
	II	• The panel recommends the use of intraoral *PBM* therapy using low-level laser therapy for prevention of OM in adults receiving RT to the H&N (without CT) (Table 26.2); safety considerations unique to patients with oral cancer should be considered.
	I	• The panel recommends the use of intraoral *PBM* therapy using low-level laser therapy for the prevention of OM in adults receiving RT-CT for H&N cancer (Table 26.2); safety considerations unique to patients with oral cancer should be considered.
		• For all PBM guidelines, it is recommended that the specific PTPs of the selected protocol will be followed for optimal therapy.
Cryotherapy	II	• The panel recommends using oral *cryotherapy* to prevent OM in patients undergoing autologous HSCT when the conditioning includes high-dose melphalan.
	II	• The panel recommends using 30 min of oral *cryotherapy* to prevent OM in patients receiving bolus 5-FU CT during the infusion of the CT.
Antimicrobials, coating agents, anesthetics, and analgesics	III	• Topical *morphine* 0.2% mouthwash is suggested for the treatment of OM-associated pain in patients with H&N cancer who receive RT-CT.
	II	• *Sucralfate* (combined topical and systemic) is not recommended for the prevention of OM-associated pain in patients with H&N cancer who receive RT.
	II	• *Sucralfate* (combined topical and systemic) is not recommended for the treatment of OM-associated pain in patients with H&N cancer who receive RT.
	II	• *Sucralfate* (combined topical and systemic) is not recommended for the treatment of OM-associated pain in patients with solid cancer who receive CT.

Continued

BOX 26.9		MASCC/ISOO Clinical Practice Guidelines for the Management of Mucositis Secondary to Cancer Therapy—cont'd
Growth factors and cytokines	I	• The use of *KGF-1* intravenously is recommended for the prevention of OM in patients with hematologic cancer undergoing autologous HSCT with a conditioning regimen that includes high-dose CT and TBI.
	II	• The evidence suggests that topical *GM-CSF* should not be used for the prevention of OM in patients undergoing HSCT.
Natural and miscellaneous	I	• The panel recommends against the use of *glutamine* (parenteral) for the prevention of OM in patients undergoing HSCT.
	II	• The panel suggests oral *glutamine* for the prevention of OM in patients with H&N cancer who receive receiving RT-CT. The suggestion is with caution because of the higher mortality rate seen in patients undergoing HSCT who receive parenteral glutamine.
	II	• *Honey* is suggested for the prevention of OM in patients with H&N cancer who receive treatment with either RT or RT-CT.
	III	• *Chewing gum* is not suggested for the prevention of OM in pediatric patients with hematological or solid cancer who receive CT.

Abbreviations: *5-FU*, 5-fluorouracil; *BOC*, basic oral care; *CHX*, chlorhexidine; *CT*, chemotherapy; *GM-CSF*, granulocyte-macrophage colony-stimulating factor; *Gy*, grays; *H&N*, head and neck; *HSCT*, hematopoietic stem-cell transplantation; *KGF-1*, keratinocyte growth factor 1; *LoE*, level of evidence; *OM*, oral mucositis; *PBM*, photobiomodulation; *PTPs*, photobiomodulation therapy parameters; *RT*, radiotherapy; *TBI*, total body irradiation.

From Elad S, Cheng KKF, Lalla RV, et al.; Mucositis Guidelines Leadership Group of the Multinational Association of Supportive Care in Cancer and International Society of Oral Oncology (MASCC/ISOO). MASCC/ISOO clinical practice guidelines for the management of mucositis secondary to cancer therapy. *Cancer.* October 1, 2020;126(19):4423–4431.

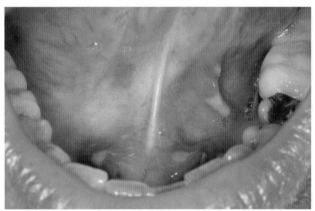

FIG. 26.22 mTOR inhibitor–associated oral mucositis with aphthous-like characteristics. (Reproduced from Sonis S, et al. Preliminary characterization of oral lesions associated with inhibitors of mammalian target of rapamycin in cancer patients. *Cancer.* January 1, 2010;116(1):210–215.)

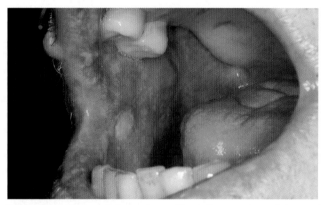

FIG. 26.23 Diffuse lichen planus-like inflammation of the oral mucosa in a cancer patient receiving an immune checkpoint inhibitor.

radiation oncologist should be contacted to determine the total dose to the head and neck region before dental care is initiated. Clinicians should be aware that risk of osteoradionecrosis increases with increasing dose to the jaws (e.g., 7500 cGy is associated with greater risk than 6500 cGy). Duration and cumulative dose of anti-resorptive therapy are similarly associated with higher risk of MRONJ. Patients determined to be at risk should be provided with the appropriate preventive measures. Protocols to reduce the risk of jaw osteonecrosis include selection of endodontic therapy over extraction, atraumatic surgical technique (if surgery is necessary), and

prophylactic antibiotics beginning the day of surgery and continuing during the week of healing (penicillin VK for 7 days). There is low level evidence to support the use of (i) local anesthetic without epinephrine, or (ii) hyperbaric oxygen therapy before invasive procedures in patients at risk for ORN. Hyperbaric oxygen therapy involves sequential daily "dives" under 2 atmospheres of oxygen pressure in a chamber and is not without risks (e.g., middle ear injury, myopia, seizures).

When jaw osteonecrosis occurs, conservative management is usually effective in controlling symptoms and stabilizing the condition (Box 26.10). The exposed bone should be brushed well, and patients should rinse with chlorhexidine twice a day. Bony sequestrum, if present,

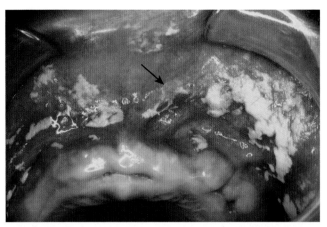

FIG. 26.24 Oral candidiasis (pseudomembranous form) in a patient undergoing chemotherapy. *Arrow* indicates lesions of pseudomembranous candidiasis. (Reproduced from Allen CM, Blozis GG. Oral mucosal lesions. In: Cummings CW, et al., eds. *Otolaryngology: Head and Neck Surgery.* 3rd ed. St. Louis: Mosby; 1998.)

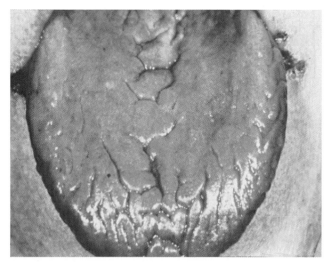

FIG. 26.26 Severe xerostomia that developed from the effects of radiation on the oral mucosa. Note the angular cheilitis.

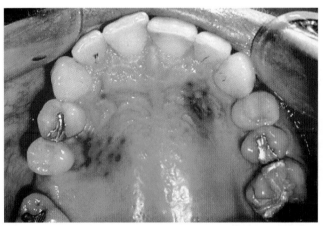

FIG. 26.25 Recurrent herpes simplex virus infection manifesting as a large ulcer on the palate of a patient undergoing chemotherapy.

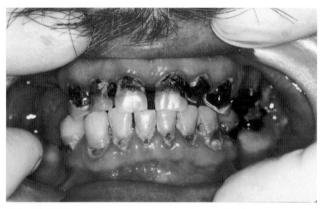

FIG. 26.27 Extensive cervical caries in a patient who received radiotherapy. (Reproduced from R. Gorlin, Minneapolis, MN.)

should be removed to allow for epithelialization. Debridement procedures may reduce secondary infection and improve symptoms. If swelling and suppuration are present, broad-spectrum antibiotics are indicated. Pathologic fractures must be managed with a surgeon, although all fractures do not require surgery. Cases that do not respond to conservative measures may require surgical resection of involved bone. For the management of ORN specifically, there is low level evidence supporting the use of hyperbaric oxygen treatment (60- to 90-min dives, 5 days per week, for a total of 20–30 dives) as well as the combination of pentoxifylline and tocopherol.

Neuropathic Pain and Chemosensory Changes

While relatively uncommon, cancer patients may experience long-term persistent orofacial neuropathic pain and taste changes. Regardless of the primary treatment

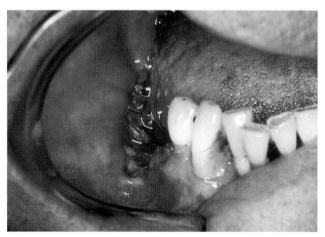

FIG. 26.28 Osteoradionecrosis. Exposed necrotic bone is evident in the posterior mandible edentulous ridge of a patient who previously received radiation therapy to the head and neck region.

BOX 26.10   The American Association of Oral and Maxillofacial Surgeons Staging and Management of Jaw Osteonecrosis in Cancer Patients

Staging of Medication-Related Osteonecrosis of the Jaw[a]	Treatment Strategies[b]
At risk—no apparent necrotic bone in patients who have been treated with oral or intravenous bisphosphonates	No treatment indicated
	Patient education
Stage 0—no clinical evidence of necrotic bone but nonspecific clinical findings, radiographic changes, and symptoms	systemic management, including use of pain medication and antibiotics
	Antibacterial mouth rinse
Stage 1—exposed and necrotic bone or fistulas that probes to bone in patients who are asymptomatic and have no evidence of infection	clinical follow-up on a quarterly basis
	Patient education and review of indications for continued bisphosphonate therapy
Stage 2—exposed and necrotic bone or fistulas that probes to bone associated with infection as evidenced by pain and erythema in the region of exposed bone with or without purulent drainage	symptomatic treatment with oral antibiotics oral antibacterial mouth rinse
	Pain control
	Debridement to relieve soft tissue irritation and infection control
Stage 3—exposed and necrotic bone or a fistula that probes to bone in patients with pain, infection, and ≥1 of the following: exposed and necrotic bone extending beyond the region of alveolar bone (i.e., inferior border and ramus in mandible, maxillary sinus, and zygoma in maxilla) resulting in pathologic fracture, extraoral fistula, oral antral or oral nasal communication, or osteolysis extending to inferior border of the mandible or sinus floor	Antibacterial mouth rinse
	Antibiotic therapy and pain control
	surgical debridement or resection for longer-term palliation of infection and pain

[a]Exposed or probeable bone in the maxillofacial region without resolution for longer than 8 weeks in patients treated with an antiresorptive or an antiangiogenic agent who have not received radiation therapy to the jaws.

[b]Regardless of disease stage, mobile segments of bony sequestrum should be removed without exposing uninvolved bone. Extraction of symptomatic teeth within exposed necrotic bone should be considered because it is unlikely that extraction will exacerbate the established necrotic process.

These guidelines can be applied to patients with mediation-related osteonecrosis of the jaw as well as patients with osteoradionecrosis. Ruggiero SL, Dodson TB, Fantasia J, et al.; American Association of Oral and Maxillofacial Surgeons. American Association of Oral and Maxillofacial Surgeons position paper on medication-related osteonecrosis of the jaw—2014 update. *J Oral Maxillofac Surg*. 2014;72:1938–1956.

---

modality (e.g., surgery vs. radiation therapy), head and neck cancer patients may develop chronic neuropathic symptoms at the site of treatment. While symptoms can vary, the most common description is intense burning, often exacerbated with movement and function. Rarely, patients with a history of previously severe and extensive ulcerations (e.g., mucositis, GVHD), as well as patients with history of severe herpes simplex virus recrudescence, develop postinflammatory dysesthesias, typically characterized by burning but sometimes also causing diminished or altered taste. Persistent dysgeusia or hypogeusia can occur after radiation therapy. Management is challenging, but patients may benefit from topical and systemic anticonvulsant medications.

BIBLIOGRAPHY

1. CDC. *Human Papillomavirus (HPV) and Cancer*; 2021. https://www.cdc.gov/cancer/hpv/index.htm.
2. Chaturvedi AK, Engels EA, Pfeiffer RM, et al. Human papillomavirus and rising oropharyngeal cancer incidence in the United States. *J Clin Oncol*. November 10, 2011;29(32):4294–4301.
3. Ferlay J, Ervik M, Lam F, et al. *Global Cancer Observatory: Cancer Today*. Lyon: International Agency for Research on Cancer; 2020. https://gco.iarc.fr/today. Accessed February 2021.
4. Freymiller EG, Sung EC, Friedlander AH. Detection of radiation-induced cervical atheromas by panoramic radiography. *Oral Oncol*. 2000;36:175–180.
5. Hanahan D, Weinberg RA. Hallmarks of cancer: the next generation. *Cell*. March 4, 2011;144(5):646–674.
6. Kurt BA, Armstrong GT, Cash DK, et al. Primary care management of the childhood cancer survivor. *J Pediatr*. April 2008;152(4):458–466.
7. Lawrence M, Sougnez C, Lichtenstein L, et al. Comprehensive genomic characterization of head and neck squamous cell carcinomas. *Nature*. 2015;517:576–582.
8. LeVeque FG, Montgomery M, Potter D, et al. A multicenter, randomized, double-blind, placebo-controlled, dose-titration study of oral pilocarpine for treatment of radiation-induced xerostomia in head and neck cancer patients. *J Clin Oncol*. 1995;114:1141–1149.
9. Lydiatt WM, Patel SG, O'Sullivan B, et al. Head and neck cancers-major changes in the American Joint Committee on cancer eighth edition cancer staging manual. *CA Cancer J Clin*. March 2017;67(2):122–137.

10. Rhodus NL, Kerr AR, Patel K. Oral cancer: leukoplakia and squamous cell carcinoma. In: Sollectio TS, ed. *Lesions Oral. Dental Clinics of North America.* Vol 57. 2014:143–156. Issue 3, ISBN-978-0-323-28995-5, [Chapter 6].

11. Ruggiero SL, Dodson TB, Fantasia J, et al. American Association of Oral and Maxillofacial Surgeons. American Association of Oral and Maxillofacial Surgeons position paper on medication-related osteonecrosis of the jaw—2014 update. *J Oral Maxillofac Surg.* October 2014;72(10):1938–1956. https://doi.org/10.1016/j.joms. 2014.04.031. Epub 2014 May 5. Erratum in: J Oral Maxillofac Surg. 2015 Jul;73(7):1440. Erratum in: J Oral Maxillofac Surg. 2015 Sep;73(9):1879.

12. Shapiro CL. Cancer survivorship. *N Engl J Med.* 2018;379:2438–2450.

13. Siegel RL, Miller KD, Jemal A. Cancer statistics, 2019. *CA Cancer J Clin.* 2019;69:7–34.

14. Smith C, Prasad V. Targeted cancer therapies. *Am Fam Physician.* 2021;103(3):155–163.

15. Smith RA, Andrews K, Brooks D, et al. Cancer screening in the United States, 2016: a review of current American Cancer Society guidelines and current issues in cancer screening. *CA Cancer J Clin.* March–April 2016;66(2):96–114.

16. Wilkinson AN, Viola R, Brundage MD. Managing skeletal related events resulting from bone metastases. *BMJ.* November 3, 2008;337:a2041.

27

Neurologic Disorders

Neurologic disorders are common in the general population, and dental patients will regularly present with these conditions. Several diseases affecting the nervous system are of clinical significance in dental practice and vary in severity and consequences. The focus of this chapter is on five common and significant neurologic diseases—**stroke, Parkinson disease, Alzheimer disease, epilepsy,** and **multiple sclerosis (MS)**. Also discussed are cerebrospinal fluid (CSF) shunts because of the assumed risk of bacterial seeding after an invasive dental procedure in patients with such shunts.

STROKE (CEREBROVASCULAR ACCIDENT)

Definition

Stroke is a generic term used to refer to a cerebrovascular accident (CVA)—a serious and often fatal neurologic event caused by sudden interruption of oxygenated blood to the brain. The associated ischemic injury results in focal necrosis of brain tissue, which may be fatal depending on the extent of damage. Even if a stroke is not fatal, the survivor often is debilitated in motor function, speech, or cognition to varying degrees. The scope and health impact of stroke are reflected in the fact that stroke is the leading cause of serious, long-term disability in the United States.

Epidemiology

Stroke is one of the most significant health problems in the United States and is the fifth leading cause of death, with more than 140,000 Americans dying of stroke

annually. Each year in the United States, about 800,000 people experience new or recurrent stroke. Three of four of these (600,000) are new strokes. This figure translates to the occurrence of one stroke about every 4 min; 75% of persons survive their stroke. An estimated 6.6 million Americans have had a stroke with an overall prevalence of approximately 2.6%.

Cerebrovascular disease is the primary factor associated with stroke. Atherosclerosis and cardiac pathosis [myocardial infarction (MI), atrial fibrillation] increase the risk of thrombotic and embolic strokes, and hypertension is the most important risk factor for ischemic and hemorrhagic stroke. The incidence of stroke increases directly to the degree of elevation of systolic and diastolic arterial blood pressure above threshold values. Evidence indicates that control of hypertension prevents strokes with an approximate 30%–40% reduction in stroke risk with blood pressure reduction. Heart failure, diabetes, and additional factors that increase the risk for stroke are listed in Box 27.1. Increased risk for hemorrhagic stroke also occurs with age and use of phenylpropanolamine, an α-adrenergic agonist.

Approximately 7%–10% of men and 5%–7% of women older than 65 years of age have asymptomatic carotid stenosis of greater than 50%. Epidemiologic studies suggest that the rate of unheralded stroke evolving ipsilateral to a stenosis is about 1%–2% annually.

Nonvalvular atrial fibrillation carries a 3%–5% annual risk for stroke, with the risk becoming even higher in the presence of advanced age, previous transient ischemic attack (TIA) or stroke, hypertension, impaired left ventricular function, and diabetes mellitus.

BOX 27.1 Risk Factors for Stroke

Hypertension[a]
Congestive heart failure
Diabetes mellitus
History of TIAs or previous CVA[a]
Age older than 75 years[a]
Hypercholesterolemia
Coronary atherosclerosis
Smoking tobacco

[a]The risk of stroke increases by a factor of 1.5 for each of these conditions. With the combination of several factors, the risk obviously becomes much greater.

CVA, cerebrovascular accident (stroke); *TIA*, transient ischemic attack.

Individuals who have a TIA and survive the initial high-risk period have a 10-year stroke risk of approximately 20% and a combined 10-year stroke, MI, or vascular death risk of 43% (4% per year). Stroke risk in smokers is almost double that in nonsmokers, but the risk becomes essentially identical to that in nonsmokers by 2–5 years after tobacco cessation. The relative risk for stroke is two to six times greater for patients with Type 1 diabetes. African Americans are at 38% greater risk for a first stroke with a similar greater risk of death compared to whites. Also, 40,000 more women than men have a stroke each year. Risk of stroke increases with age; however, approximately 28% of people who have a stroke are younger than 65 years of age. There are nearly 5 million stroke survivors living in the United States, and an average dental practice of 2000 adult patients will include about 31 patients who have had or will experience a stroke.

Pathophysiology and Complications. Stroke is caused by the interruption of blood supply and oxygen to the brain as a result of ischemia or hemorrhage. The most common type is ischemic stroke induced by thrombosis (in up to 75%–80% of cases) of a cerebral vessel. Ischemic stroke also can result from occlusion of a cerebral blood vessel by distant emboli. Hemorrhage causes about 15%–20% of all strokes and carries a 1-year mortality rate greater than 60%. Hemorrhage can be intracerebral or subarachanoid.

Pathologic changes associated with stroke result from infarction or hemorrhage. Cerebral infarctions are most commonly attributed to atherosclerotic thrombi or emboli of cardiac origin. The extent of an infarction is determined by a number of factors, including the site of the occlusion, size of the occluded vessel, duration of the occlusion, and collateral circulation. The production and circulation of proinflammatory cytokines, the occurrence of clotting factors, and arterial inflammation contribute to platelet aggregation. Neurologic abnormalities result from free radical accumulation, inflammation, mitochondrial and DNA damage, and apoptosis of the region supplied by the damaged artery.

The most common cause of intracerebral hemorrhage is hypertensive atherosclerosis, which results in microaneurysms of the arterioles (Fig. 27.1). Vessels within the

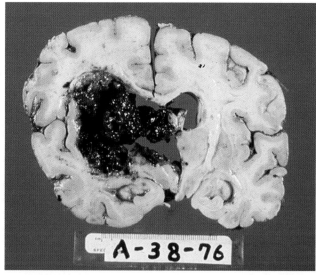

FIG. 27.1 Cerebral infarction in a patient who had chronic hypertension.

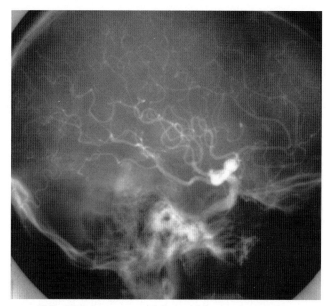

FIG. 27.2 Aneurysm of the middle cerebral artery.

circle of Willis often are affected (Fig. 27.2). Rupture of these microaneurysms within brain tissue leads to extravasation of blood, which displaces brain tissue, causing an increase in intracranial volume until resultant tissue compression halts bleeding. The most common cause of subarachnoid hemorrhage (SAH) is rupture of a saccular aneurysm at the bifurcation of a major cerebral artery.

The most serious outcome of stroke is death, which occurs in 8% of those who experience ischemic strokes and 38%–47% of those with hemorrhagic strokes within 1 month of the event. Overall, about 23% of patients die within 1 year. Mortality rates are directly related to type of stroke, with 80% of patients dying after an intracerebral hemorrhage, 50% after an SAH, and 30% after occlusion of a major vessel by a thrombus. Death from stroke may not be immediate (sudden death) but rather may occur hours, days, or even weeks after the initial stroke episode.

If the victim survives, it is highly likely that a neurologic deficit or disability of varying degree and duration will remain. Of those who survive the stroke, 10% recover with no impairment, 50% have a mild residual disability, 15%–30% are disabled and require special services, and 10%–20% require institutionalization. Approximately 50% of those who survive the acute period (the first 6 months) are alive 7 years later.

The type of residual deficit that results from a stroke is directly dependent on the size and location of the infarct or hemorrhage. Deficits include unilateral paralysis, numbness, sensory impairment, dysphasia, blindness, diplopia, dizziness, and dysarthria. Return of function is unpredictable and usually takes place slowly, over several months. Even with improvement, patients frequently are left with some permanent residual disability, such as difficulty in walking, using the hands, performing skilled acts, or speaking. Dementia also may be an outcome.

Clinical Presentation

Familiarity with the warning signs and symptoms of stroke can lead to appropriate action that may be life-saving. Signs of stroke include hemiplegia; temporary loss of speech or trouble in speaking or understanding speech; temporary dimness or loss of vision, particularly in one eye (may be confused with migraine); unexplained dizziness; unsteadiness; or a sudden fall.

TIA is defined as an acute, short-duration, focal neurologic deficit, typically lasting less than 1 h, without evidence of infarction on brain imaging. Approximately 20% of all strokes are heralded by a TIA; the short-term risk of stroke after TIA is 10% at 90 days, with the highest risk being in the first 24 h; 80% of all strokes following TIA are preventable. Within 1 year of a TIA, 12% of patients die.

Clinical manifestations that remain after a stroke vary in accordance with the site and size of residual brain deficits; these include language disorders, hemiplegia, and paresis; the latter is a form of paralysis that is associated with loss of sensory function and memory and weakened motor power. Box 27.2 presents the different behavioral manifestations of right- versus left-sided brain damage. Of note, in most patients with stroke, the intellect remains intact; however, massive left-sided stroke has been associated with cognitive decline.

Laboratory and Diagnostic Findings. Patients suspected of having had a stroke usually undergo a variety of laboratory tests and diagnostic imaging procedures to rule out conditions that can produce neurologic alterations, such as diabetes mellitus, uremia, abscess, tumor, acute alcoholism, drug poisoning, and extradural hemorrhage. Such investigations often include urinalysis, blood sugar level, complete blood count, erythrocyte sedimentation rate, serologic tests for syphilis, blood cholesterol and lipid levels, chest radiographs, and electrocardiography (ECG). Various abnormalities may be revealed by the test results, depending on the type and severity of stroke and its causative factors. A lumbar puncture may be used to check for blood or protein in the CSF and for altered CSF pressure, which would be suggestive of SAH. Doppler blood flow studies, EEG, cerebral angiography, computed tomography (CT) (Fig. 27.3), and magnetic resonance imaging (MRI, including diffusion and perfusion studies of the brain) are important for determining the extent and location of arterial injury.

Medical Management

The first aspect of stroke management is prevention. This is accomplished by identifying specific risk factors (e.g., hypertension, diabetes, atherosclerosis, cigarette smoking) and attempting to reduce or eliminate as many of these as possible. Blood pressure–lowering (see Chapter 3), antiplatelet (see Chapter 24), and statin therapies are primary stroke prevention methods. Carotid endarterectomy is a secondary stroke prevention method. The benefit of lowering blood pressure is evident in the

BOX 27.2	Manifestations of Right-Sided Versus Left-Sided Brain Damage
Right-Sided Brain Damage	**Left-Sided Brain Damage**
• Paralyzed left side	• Paralyzed right side
• Spatial-perceptual deficits	• Language and speech problems
• Impaired thought process	• Decreased auditory memory (inability to remember long instructions)
• Quick, impulsive behavior	
• Inability to use mirror	
• Difficulty performing tasks (toothbrushing)	• Slow, cautious, disorganized behavior
• Memory deficits—for events or people, generalized	• Memory deficits—language based
• Neglect of left side	• Anxiety

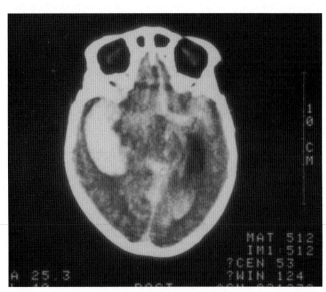

FIG. 27.3 Computed tomography scan of the brain demonstrating a cerebrovascular accident (stroke) lesion that extended from the midbrain to the temporal lobe.

fact that a reduction of systolic blood pressure by 10 mm Hg is associated with a one-third reduction in risk for stroke. Regimens of aspirin, ticlopidine, or extended-release dipyridamole are accepted preventive therapies for ischemic stroke in patients who have experienced TIAs or who have had a stroke. Aspirin dosed at 81–325 mg daily reduced the risk of stroke by preventing emboli. Likewise, surgical intervention through endarterectomy reduces the risk by about 1% per year, such that one stroke is prevented for every 20 patients who undergo surgery over a 5-year period.

Treatment for stroke generally has three components. The immediate task is to sustain life during the period immediately after the stroke. This is done by means of life support measures and transport to a hospital. The second task involves emergency efforts to prevent further thrombosis or hemorrhage and to attempt to lyse the clot in cases of thrombosis or embolism. Recanalization of occluded vessel (reperfusion of ischemic tissue that can be saved, known as the penumbra), optimization of collateral flow, and avoidance of secondary brain injury are the core principals of acute stroke care. Thrombolysis with intravenous tissue plasminogen activator (t-PA) can improve reperfusion, minimize infarction, and reduce disability. The American Heart Association and American Stroke Association advisory statement recommends administration of t-PA within 3–4.5 h after stroke onset. Advanced perfusion imaging techniques now enable identification of patients who may benefit from treatment of ischemic stroke up to 24 h after, utilizing catheter-based mechanical thrombectomies for large cerebral occlusions where brain tissue can be still be rescued.

After the initial period, efforts to stabilize the patient continue with anticoagulant medications such as heparin, coumarin, aspirin, and dipyridamole combined with aspirin (Aggrenox) in cases of thrombosis or embolism. Whereas heparin is administered intravenously during acute episodes, coumarin, dipyridamole, aspirin, subcutaneous low-molecular-weight heparin, or platelet receptor antagonists (clopidogrel, abciximab, ticlopidine) are used for prolonged periods to reduce risk of thrombosis (e.g., deep vein thrombosis). Newer oral anticoagulants are Factor Xa inhibitors and direct thrombin inhibitors. Factor Xa inhibitors interrupt the clotting cascade through inhibition of clotting factor Xa, resulting in decreased production of thrombin and disruption of platelet aggregation, and include apixiban, rivaroxaban, and edoxaban. Dabigatran is a direct thrombin inhibitor that blocks the conversion of fibrinogen to fibrin and consequently thrombi formation. Corticosteroids may be used acutely after a stroke to lessen the cerebral edema that accompanies cerebral infarction and can markedly reduce the likelihood of complications. Surgical intervention may be indicated for removal of a superficial hematoma or management of a vascular obstruction. The latter usually is accomplished by thromboendarterectomy or bypass grafts in the neck or thorax. Diazepam,

phenytoin, and other anticonvulsants are prescribed in the management of seizures that may accompany the postoperative course of stroke.

If the patient survives, the third and final task consists of institution of preventive therapy, administration of medications that reduce the risk of another stroke (statins and antihypertensive drugs), and initiation of rehabilitation. Rehabilitation generally is accomplished by intense physical, occupational, and speech therapy (if indicated). Although marked improvement is common, many patients are left with some degree of permanent deficit.

Dental Management

Dentists can play a role as educators in stroke prevention and identification of stroke-prone patients. Patients with a history or clinical evidence of hypertension, congestive heart failure, diabetes mellitus, previous stroke or TIA, and advancing age are predisposed to stroke, as well as to MI. Concurrency of these factors increases level of risk (Box 27.1). The dentist should assess patient risk, encourage persons with risk factors to seek medical care, and eliminate or control all possible risk factors (see Box 27.3).

Assessment of risk helps in the decision-making process regarding the timing and type of dental care to be provided. For example, the risk of stroke is greater in a patient who has had a previous stroke or TIA than in a person who has not had either. Prior history of TIA or stroke increases the risk of a future or second stroke, with the highest risk during the first 90 days. A comparative retrospective study examining complications of invasive dental treatment following acute stroke found no evidence to support the historical intuitive guideline to defer elective dental treatment for 6 months following a stroke or for a patient with active TIAs. Patients who are medically stable (e.g., absence of clinical symptoms) can receive routine dental care. If not medically stable, consultation with a physician is advised (Box 27.3).

Patients who take coumarin are at risk for increased bleeding. The status of coumarin anticoagulation is monitored by assessment of the international normalized ratio (INR). An INR level of 3.5 or less rarely requires dose modification before routine dental and minor oral surgical treatment. If the INR is greater than 3.5, the patient may be at risk for more substantial bleeding, and the physician should be consulted regarding modification of the anticoagulant dosage. In such cases, a reduction in dose of the anticoagulant is recommended over interruption of anticoagulation therapy because the risk for significant adverse outcomes is minimized by this approach (see Chapter 24). Also, metronidazole and tetracycline may increase the INR by inhibiting the metabolism of warfarin (Coumadin); therefore, concurrent use of these drugs should be avoided. Dose modification or interruption of antiplatelet agents, Xa inhibitors and direct thrombin inhibitors are typically not warranted for patients undergoing minor invasive dental

BOX 27.3	Checklist for Dental Management of Patients With Stroke[a]

PREOPERATIVE RISK ASSESSMENT

R: Recognize Risks
- Be **aware** of adverse events that may occur in the management of a patient who has a medical condition.

P: Patient Evaluation
- Review **medical history** and discuss relevant issues with the patient.
- Identify all **medications and drugs** being taken or supposed to be taken by the patient.
- **Examine** the patient for signs and symptoms of disease and obtain vital signs.
- Review or obtain recent **laboratory test** results or **images** required to assess risk.
- Obtain a **medical consultation** if the patient has a poorly controlled or undiagnosed problem or if the patient's health status is uncertain.

A

Analgesics	Use of acetaminophen as pain reliever is recommended; avoid the use of ASA and other NSAIDs (including for postoperative pain) because of increased risk of bleeding.
Anesthesia	Good pain control should be achieved during the procedure, but the dose of epinephrine should be limited to two carpules; no epinephrine-containing retraction cord should be used.
Antibiotics	Avoid use of metronidazole and tetracyclines in patients taking warfarin (Coumadin) because of its decreased metabolism.
Anxiety	No issues.

B

Bleeding	Patients taking an anticoagulant or on antiplatelet therapy are at increased risk for bleeding: • Aspirin ± dipyridamole (Aggrenox), clopidogrel (Plavix), abciximab (ReoPro), or ticlopidine (Ticlid). • Apixiban (Eliquis), rivaroxaban (Xarelto), edoxaban (Savaysa) or dabigatran (Pradaxa). • Coumarin—pretreatment INR ≤3.5. Higher levels require consultation with physician for dose modification. • Heparin, intravenous—use palliative emergency dental care only, or 6–12 h before surgery, discontinue heparin and start another anticoagulant (e.g., warfarin [Coumadin]) with

physician's approval. Then restart heparin after clot forms (6 h later). Heparin, subcutaneous (low molecular weight)—generally, no changes required. Use measures that minimize hemorrhage (atraumatic surgery, pressure, Gelfoam, suturing) as needed. Have available nonadrenergic hemostatic agents and devices (stents, electrocautery unit). Additional steps should be taken to achieve hemostasis in patients on an anticoagulant or antiplatelet therapy.

Blood pressure and vital sign monitoring	Obtain pretreatment vital signs. Monitor blood pressure and oxygen saturation.

C

Capacity to tolerate care	Patients with active, symptomatic disease may defer elective dental treatment until condition(s) are stable.
Chair position	Deficits from a previous stroke may warrant assistance for patient transfer to the chair, effective oral evacuation and airway management, and rigorous oral hygiene measures delivered by a health care provider.

D

Devices	No issues.
Drugs	Use minimum amount of anesthetic containing a vasoconstrictor. Avoid use of epinephrine-impregnated retraction cord. Also avoid the use of metronidazole and tetracyclines in patients taking warfarin (Coumadin) because these agents cause decreased warfarin metabolism.

E

Emergencies and urgent care	Appointments should be short and stress free, with good anesthesia achieved using nitrous oxide –oxygen. Monitoring of blood pressure and oxygen saturation is indicated throughout the procedure. Recognize signs and symptoms of a stroke, provide emergency care, and activate EMS system as needed.
Equipment	No issues.

POSTOPERATIVE CARE

F

Follow-up care	Schedule appointments as indicated. Shorter appointments may be necessary.

[a]*Strength of recommendation taxonomy (SORT) Grade: C (see Preface for further explanation).*
ASA, aspirin; EMSs, emergency medical services; INR, international normalized ratio; NSAIDs, nonsteroid antiinflammatory drugs.

procedures (e.g., <3 extractions), as local measures, such as suture placement and use of gelatin sponges, are usually effective in managing bleeding. Aspirin should be avoided for management of postoperative dental pain, which is better managed with acetaminophen (see Box 27.3).

Patients whom have recently undergone a stroke (>90 days) may be safely and effectively managed in the dental clinic without complications as long as the patient is carefully identified and monitored according to his or her status. Management of stroke-prone patients or patients with a history of stroke includes the use of short, midmorning appointments with minimization of stress and anxiety. Nitrous oxide–oxygen may be given if good oxygenation is maintained at all times. Assisted transfer to the dental chair may be needed. And, it is important not to overestimate the patient's abilities, especially because good verbalization skills may mask a surprising lack of self-awareness regarding the extent of paresis that is present, reflecting a "neglect" syndrome. Dental providers should move slowly around the patient and should speak clearly, with the mask off, while facing the patient. Effective communication techniques are listed in Box 27.4.

Blood pressure should be monitored to ensure good control. Pulse oximeter monitoring is indicated to ensure that oxygenation is adequate. Pain control is important; therefore, adequate anesthesia is essential. A local anesthetic with 1:100,000 or 1:200,000 epinephrine may be used in judicious amounts (4 mL or less). Gingival retraction cord impregnated with epinephrine should not be used.

A patient who develops signs or symptoms of a stroke in the dental office should receive oxygen, and the emergency medical services (EMS) system should be activated. Transport to a medical facility should not be delayed (minutes count in the treatment of patients with acute stroke). For ischemic stroke, thrombolytic agents should be administered within 3–4.5 h if they are to be maximally effective in reestablishing arterial flow. The phrase "time is brain" emphasizes the urgency of the situation. Finally, the dental staff should recognize that patients who have had a stroke typically experience feelings of grief, loss, and depression and should be treated with compassion.

Technical modifications may be required for patients with residual physical deficits who have difficulty in practicing adequate oral hygiene. For these patients, extensive bridgework is typically not an ideal choice. However, fixed prostheses may be more desirable than removable ones because of difficulties associated with daily placement and removal. Individualized treatment plans are important. All restorations should be placed with ease of cleansability in mind. Hygiene often is facilitated by an electric toothbrush, a large-handled toothbrush, or a water irrigation device. Flossing aids should be prescribed, and family members and personal care providers should be instructed on how and when these services should be provided. Frequent professional prophylaxis and the provision of topical fluoride and chlorhexidine are advisable.

Oral Manifestations. A patient experiencing a stroke event may demonstrate slurred speech, weak muscles, or difficulty swallowing. After a stroke, complete loss of or difficulty in speech, unilateral paralysis of the orofacial musculature, and loss of sensory stimuli of oral tissues may occur. The tongue may be flaccid, with multiple folds, and may deviate on extrusion. Dysphagia is common, along with difficulty in managing liquids and solids. Patients with right-sided brain damage may neglect the left side. Thus, food and debris may accumulate around the teeth, beneath the tongue, or in alveolar folds. Patients may need to learn to clean their teeth or dentures with only one hand, or they may require assistance to maintain oral hygiene; otherwise, caries, periodontal disease, and halitosis occur commonly.

Calcified atherosclerotic plaques have been demonstrated on panoramic films in the carotid arteries of older patients and patients with diabetes (Fig. 27.4). This radiographic feature indicates a risk for stroke and warrants referral to the patient's physician for evaluation. Also of note, severe periodontal bone loss is associated with carotid artery plaques and increased risk for stroke. However, the exact causative relationship

---

BOX 27.4 Effective Communication Techniques for Patients Who Have Had a Stroke

- Face the patient.
- Use a slower, more deliberate, less complex pattern of speech.
- Communicate at eye level.
- Be positive.
- Ask "yes-or-no" questions—be simple and brief.
- Give frequent, accurate, and immediate feedback.
- Use simple drawings to explain procedures.
- Do not underestimate or overestimate abilities.
- Do not raise voice or use baby talk.
- Do not wear a mask when talking to the patient.
- Communicate also with significant other or personal care provider.

Data adapted from Ostuni E. Stroke and the dental patient. *J Am Dent Assoc.* 1994;125:721–727 and Robbins MR. Neurologic diseases in special care patients. *Dent Clin N Am.* 2016;60:707–735.

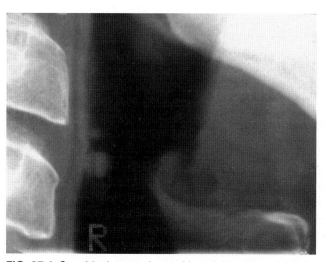

FIG. 27.4 Carotid atheroma in an older adult patient at risk for stroke. The calcification usually is located near cervical vertebrae 3 and 4, generally at a 45-degree angle from the angle of the mandible.

between periodontal disease and stroke remains to be defined.

PARKINSON DISEASE

General Description

Parkinson disease (PD) is a progressive neurodegenerative disorder of neurons that produce dopamine. Loss of these neurons results in characteristic motor disturbances—resting tremor, muscular control and rigidity, movement, bradykinesia, and postural instability. Dopaminergic neurons are found in the nigrostriatal pathway of the brain. Approximately 60%–80% of the dopamine in these neurons must be depleted before symptoms of the disease emerge. This disease is chronic and progressive, and there is no cure.

Epidemiology

Parkinson disease is the second most common neurodegenerative disorder after Alzheimer disease (AD); it occurs in 8–19 per 100,000 people in the United States, with more than 1 million currently affected. PD occurs in 2% of persons older than 65 years and 5% in persons older than 85 years. Each year, this disease is diagnosed in 60,000 persons. Men are 1.5 times more likely to be affected by PD than women. In keeping with current US demographics, a three- to fourfold increase in PD frequency is predicted over the next 50 years. PD has a peak age at onset between 55 and 66 years, but a particular form of the disease can strike teenagers. An average dental practice of 2000 adult patients is predicted to include about 4 patients who have PD.

Pathophysiology and Complications. PD is caused by depletion of dopaminergic neurons, which are manufactured in the substantia nigra (Fig. 27.5) and released in the caudate nucleus and putamen (the nigrostriatal pathway).

The etiology of PD is believed to be a variable combination of genetic and environmental factors and both autosomal dominant and recessive genes can cause PD. The protein α-synuclein, the chief constituent of the hallmark cytoplasmic inclusion, known as the Lewy body, is critical in the pathogenesis of PD. Damaged neurons display neuronal cytoskeleton changes, including eosinophilic intraneuronal inclusion (Lewy) bodies and Lewy neurites in their neuronal processes. Inclusion bodies contain compacted aggregates of presynaptic protein α-synuclein. Abnormal aggregation of the protein, either from mutations in the α-synuclein gene or occurring as a result of excessive production of the normal protein caused by gene duplications or triplications, is associated with various disease phenotypes. Other causes include stroke, brain tumor, and head injury (e.g., boxing) that damage cells in the nigrostriatal pathway. Exposure to manganese (in miners and welders), mercury, carbon disulfide, certain agricultural

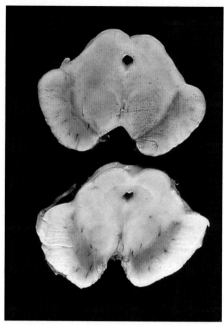

FIG. 27.5 Parkinson disease. Normal pigmentation of dopaminergic neurons in the substantia nigrans of a healthy patient (*top*) in contrast with depleted and depigmented dopaminergic neurons of the substantia nigrans in a patient who has PD (*bottom*).

herbicides (rotenone), and street heroin contaminated with a meperidine analogue (1-methyl-4-phenyl-1,2,3,6-tetrahydropyridine) can be neurotoxic, giving rise to PD symptoms. Also, neuroleptic drugs (phenothiazines, butyrophenones) may cause parkinsonian symptoms and rigidity.

PD is thought to be caused by environmental and genetic factors that trigger failure in proteasome-mediated protein turnover in susceptible neurons, resulting in accumulation of toxic proteins. This toxicity leads to degeneration and loss of pigmented neurons, primarily those of the substantia nigra, and destructive lesions in the circuitry to the limbic system, motor system, and centers that regulate autonomic functions. The course of the disease is complicated by degeneration of other regions in the brain such as the cholinergic nucleus basalis, which can result in depression.

Clinical Presentation

PD can be divided into three stages: (1) preclinical phase, where neurodegeneration has begun but the patient is asymptomatic; (2) prodromal phase, where symptoms are present but are insufficient to make the diagnosis; and (3) clinical phase, where symptoms are recognizable and meet the criteria for PD. Major clinical manifestations of PD are resting tremor (that is attenuated during activity), muscle rigidity, slow movement (bradykinesia, shuffling gait), and facial impassiveness (mask of PD) (Fig. 27.6). The tremor, which is rhythmic and fine and best seen in the extremity at rest, produces a "pill-rolling rest tremor" and handwriting changes. Cogwheel-type rigidity

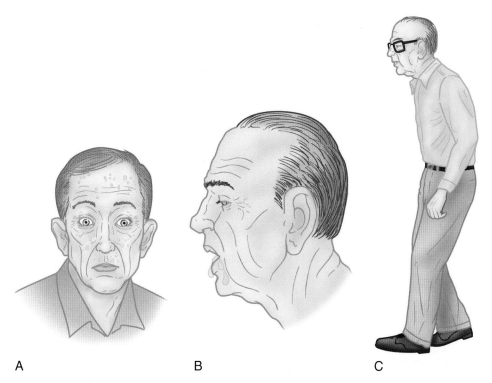

FIG. 27.6 Characteristic features of Parkinson disease. (**A**) Masklike appearance, stare, and excessive sweating. (**B**) Drooling with excessive saliva. (**C**) Parkinsonian gait with rapid, short, shuffling steps and reduced arm swinging. (From Seidel HM, Stewart RW, Ball JW. *Mosby's Guide to Physical Examination.* 7th ed. St. Louis: Mosby; 2011.)

(decreased arm swing with walking and foot dragging), stooped posture, unsteadiness, imbalance (gait instability), and falls are common features. In addition, pain (musculoskeletal, sensory [burning, numbness, tingling], or akathisia-motor restlessness, such as restless leg syndrome), orthostatic hypotension, and bowel and bladder dysfunction occur in approximately 50% of patients. Cognitive impairment of memory and concentration occurs to a variable degree, depending on the extent of destruction of the cortical–basal ganglia–thalamic neural loops. Mood disturbances (depression, dysthymia, apathy, anxiety), insomnia, and fatigue occur in approximately 40% of patients; dementia occurs in approximately 25%. Psychosis, related to dopaminergic medications, occurs in approximately 20% of patients.

Laboratory and Diagnostic Findings. No diagnostic tests are available to detect PD, therefore, diagnosis requires a thorough history, clinical examination, and specific tests and imaging procedures to rule out diseases that can produce similar clinical manifestations, such as Wilson disease, arteriosclerotic pseudoparkinsonism, multiple stem atrophy, and progressive supranuclear palsy.

Medical Management

The goal of PD therapy is to increase dopamine levels in the brain. As no optimal drug treatment is available for

PD, each person is managed on an individual basis with a variety of drugs. The six classes of drugs used to manage the symptoms of PD are shown in Table 27.1. Drug therapy generally is not initiated until lifestyle impairment such as slowness or imbalance occurs. Drug selection is based on anticipated adverse effects and complications, and therapy is initiated at the lowest effective dose.

The mainstay of treatment for advanced PD is carbidopa–levodopa (Sinemet), an immediate precursor of the neurotransmitter dopamine. Use of this agent generally is reserved for later in the course of the disease because its activity wanes after about 5–10 years, and when given over the long term, it produces complicating adverse effects (dyskinesia—involuntary rapid, flowing movements of limbs, trunk, or head). Management of progressive disease requires a careful balance between the beneficial effects of Sinemet or controlled-release levodopa (Sinemet CR) and the use of adjunctive medications such as (1) dopamine agonists and (2) catechol-O-methyltransferase (COMT) inhibitors (entacapone) used to diminish motor fluctuations, as well as (3) serotonin reuptake inhibitors used to manage depression and (4) acetylcholinesterase inhibitors given for dementia. Dosage adjustments are required when dyskinesias, immobility, psychosis, or other adverse effects occur. Physical therapy is important for providing patients with

TABLE 27.1   Drugs Used in the Management of Parkinson Disease

Drug or Class	Reason Used	Adverse Effects	Dental Treatment Considerations
Anticholinergic	Blocks the effect of another brain neurotransmitter (acetylcholine) to rebalance its levels with dopamine		Dry mouth
Trihexyphenidyl HCl (Artane)		Sedation, urinary retention, constipation	Dry mouth
Benztropine mesylate (Cogentin)			
Dopamine precursor	Provides a drug that is metabolized into dopamine (dopamine replacement)		
Levodopa		Orthostatic hypotension	Oropharyngeal pain
Carbidopa-levodopa (Sinemet CR)		Dyskinesia, fatigue, headache, anxiety, confusion, insomnia, orthostatic hypotension	If choreiform movements, dyskinesias, or tremors are present, sedation techniques may be required to perform dentistry; caution on getting up from the dental chair
Dopamine agonist	Mimics the action of dopamine		
Bromocriptine mesylate (Parlodel)[a]		Dopaminergic effects: psychosis (hallucinations, delusions), orthostatic hypotension, dyskinesia, nausea	Caution on getting up from the dental chair
Pramipexole (Mirapex)			Mirapex adversely interacts with erythromycin; dry mouth, dysphagia
Ropinirole HCl (Requip)		Orthostatic hypotension	Xerostomia, dysphagia, caution on getting up from the dental chair
Catechol-O-methyltransferase (COMT) inhibitor[b]	Used along with levodopa; this medication blocks the enzyme COMT to prevent levodopa breakdown in the intestine, thus allowing more of levodopa to reach the brain		
Tolcapone (Tasmar)[a,b] Entacapone (Comtan)		Potentiate levodopa effects: dyskinesia, psychosis, or orthostatic hypotension; nausea and diarrhea, abnormal taste	Caution with use of vasoconstrictors Monitor vital signs during and after administration of first capsule; limit dose to two capsules containing 1:100,000 epinephrine (36 µg) or less, depending on vital signs and patient response; aspirate to avoid intravascular injection
Monoamine oxidase B inhibitor[b]	Prevents metabolism of dopamine within the brain		
Selegiline[b]		Dizziness, orthostatic hypotension, nausea	Select adrenergic agents (i.e., amphetamine, pseudoephedrine, tyramine) may cause increased pressor response. However, this does not appear to occur with epinephrine or levonordefrin
Glutamate antagonists	Weak NMDA receptor noncompetitive antagonist—exact mechanism unknown		
Amantadine		Sedation, urinary retention, peripheral edema, nausea, constipation, confusion	Dry mouth

[a]May cause significant hepatic toxicity.
[b]Also has adverse vasoconstrictive properties.

safe methods for rising from a chair, walking around a room, navigating stairs, and combating immobility and contractures.

If symptoms progress despite drug therapy, surgery is an alternative for patients with PD. Deep brain stimulation of subthalamic nuclei, thalamotomy, or pallidotomy is the most common surgical procedure for PD and is reserved for patients with advanced disease and severe disabling or intractable tremor.

Dental Management

The dentist can play an important role in recognizing the features of PD and making a referral to a physician for evaluation of persons who exhibit features of the disease. After the diagnosis has been made, concerns in dental management are twofold: (1) minimizing the adverse outcomes of muscle rigidity and tremor and (2) avoiding drug interactions (Box 27.5).

Because the muscular defect and tremor can contribute to poor oral hygiene, the dentist should assess the patient's ability to maintain adequate oral hygiene by demonstration. For patients unable to provide adequate home care, alternative solutions should be provided, such as the introduction of the Collis curve toothbrush, mechanical toothbrushes, assisted brushing, or chlorhexidine rinses.

Drug interactions of concern in dentistry are outlined in Table 27.1. Although adverse interactions have not been reported between COMT inhibitors (tolcapone [Tasmar], entacapone [Comtan]) and epinephrine at dosages typically used in dentistry, they can potentially interact, and it is advisable to limit the dose of epinephrine to two carpules containing 1:100,000 epinephrine (36 µg) in patients who take COMT inhibitors. Erythromycin should not be given to patients who take the dopamine agonist pramipexole (Mirapex). The clinician

---

BOX 27.5	Dental Management Considerations in Patients With Parkinson Disease[a]

PREOPERATIVE RISK ASSESSMENT

R: Recognize Risks
- Be **aware** of adverse events that may occur in the management of a patient who has a medical condition.

P: Patient Evaluation
- Review **medical history** and discuss relevant issues with the patient.
- Identify all **medications and drugs** being taken or supposed to be taken by the patient.
- **Examine** the patient for signs and symptoms of disease and obtain vital signs.
- Review or obtain recent **laboratory test** results or **images** required to assess risk.
- Obtain a **medical consultation** if the patient has a poorly controlled or undiagnosed problem or if the patient's health status is uncertain.

A	
Analgesics	Clinicians should provide good pain control.
Antibiotics	No issues.
Anesthesia	Obtain adequate anesthesia to reduce stress, which may worsen the movement disturbance. Epinephrine (1:100,000) in local anesthetics generally is well tolerated.
Anxiety	Patients with untreated or poorly controlled disease may experience exaggerated trembling and involuntary shaking movements and appear very anxious and stressed. Use of special anxiety and stress reduction techniques may be indicated.

B	
Bleeding	No issues.
Blood pressure and vital sign monitoring	Obtain pretreatment vital signs. Monitor blood pressure as dopamine can cause hypotension.

C	
Capacity to tolerate care	Well-controlled Parkinson disease poses no issues for capacity to tolerate care.
Chair position	No issues if the patient is under good medical management; with symptoms of impending syncope, however, a supine position may not be tolerated. The patient taking dopamine may experience hypotension, warranting precautions with getting seated or on arising. The chair may need adjustment for adequate support to help reduce unnecessary movement or to stabilize the patient in a comfortable position.

D	
Devices	No issues.
Drugs	These patients typically take anticholinergic and dopamine agonist drugs, which may have adverse effects, including sedation, drowsiness, slow mentation, fatigue, confusion, and dizziness (see Table 27.1).

E	
Equipment	No issues.
Emergencies and urgent care	Tremors most commonly are self-limited, but rarely the movement disturbance may be severe enough to interrupt dental treatment or to necessitate cessation of treatment.

POSTOPERATIVE CARE

F	
Follow-up care	Routine follow-up is recommended. In patients who have undergone surgery or other complex dental procedures, a follow-up call within the next day or two is advisable to check on clinical status.

[a]Strength of recommendation taxonomy (SORT) Grade: C (see Preface for further explanation).

should be aware that antiparkinsonian drugs can be central nervous system (CNS) depressants and a dentally prescribed sedative may have an additive effect.

Orthostatic hypotension and rigidity are common in patients who have PD. Orthostatic hypotension is an adverse effect associated with COMT inhibitors. To reduce the risk of a fall from the dental chair, the patient should be assisted to and from the chair. At the end of the appointment, the chair should be inclined slowly to allow for re-equilibration.

The treatment plan for the patient with PD may require modification based on the patient's ability to maintain adequate oral hygiene. When communicating the treatment plan and other advice, the dentist should directly face the patient. This provides effective communication with a person who has the potential for cognitive impairment (see Box 27.5).

Patients should receive dental care during the time of day at which their medication has maximum effect (generally, 2–3 h after taking it). The presence of tremors or choreiform movements may warrant use of stabilization techniques and / or sedation procedures.

Oral Complications and Manifestations. PD is associated with staring, drooling, and decreased frequency of blinking and swallowing. Muscle rigidity makes repetitive muscle movement and maintenance of good oral hygiene difficult. By contrast, the drugs used to manage the disease (anticholinergics, dopaminergics, amantadine, and L-dopa) often result in xerostomia, nausea, and tardive dyskinesia. Dental recall visits should be more frequent for this population, and specific measures (specialized toothbrushes, e.g., Collis curve toothbrush, mechanical brushes) should be devised to maintain adequate oral hygiene. If the patient is experiencing xerostomia, dysphagia and poor denture retention are likely to result. Salivary substitutes are beneficial in alleviating symptoms. Topical fluoride should be considered for use in dentate patients with xerostomia to prevent root caries. Personal care providers should be educated about their role in assisting and maintaining the oral hygiene of these patients.

DEMENTIA AND ALZHEIMER DISEASE
General Description

Dementia is as an acquired deterioration in cognitive abilities that impairs the successful performance of activities of daily living. It is characterized as a slow, progressive, chronic decline in intellectual abilities that includes impairment in memory, abstract thinking, and judgment. It is primarily a disease of aging; 1% of cases appear by age 60 years, and more than 40% of cases occur by age 85 years. Overall, the course of dementia is chronic in 65% of cases, partially treatable in 25% of cases, and reversible in only 10% of cases. The most common causes of dementia are AD, vascular dementia,

and dementia caused by PD. Other causes include hepatic encephalopathy, acid–base and electrolyte disturbances, hypoglycemia, head trauma, thyroid disease (involving either low or high levels of hormone), uremia, primary or metastatic brain lesions, acquired immunodeficiency syndrome (AIDS), trauma, syphilis, MS, stroke, and drugs. A small subset of dementias, such as Creutzfeldt–Jakob disease, may have a very rapid onset with a clinical course of less than 1 year.

Because of its relatively high prevalence, AD serves as the prototype for discussion of dementia in this chapter. This disease, which was first described by Alois Alzheimer in 1907, predominantly affects older adults. However, the process may occur in younger adults as well.

Epidemiology

The prevalence of dementia increases with age and worldwide there are nearly 50 million cases of dementia with approximately 8 million new cases each year. The global prevalence of dementia has been predicted to quadruple by the year 2050. Among persons older than 65 years of age, the prevalence is about 7%. From age 70 years on, the prevalence doubles every 5 years. By age 85 years, more than 40% of persons will have developed AD. Approximately 8 million people in the United States experience dementia, and approximately 70% of these cases are of the Alzheimer type. Women are at greater risk (3 : 2 female-to-male ratio) for developing the disease; therefore, almost 70% of all patients with AD are women, primarily because women live longer than men. Older African Americans and Hispanics are more likely than older whites to have Alzheimer and other dementias. An average dental practice of 2000 adult patients is predicted to include about 20 patients who experience AD.

Pathophysiology and Complications. The exact cause of AD is unknown but appears to involve the loss of cholinergic neurons. Unidentified factors trigger the deposition of beta-amyloid plaques that initiate an inflammatory response, oxidative damage, progressive neuritic injury, and loss of cortical neurons. As a result, levels of neurotransmitters important for learning and memory decrease. Genetic predisposition contributes to fewer than 20% of all cases. In these cases, the disease appears to be inherited by way of the apolipoprotein E4 (ApoE4) allele located on chromosome 19. Three other chromosomes have been implicated to a lesser degree in the transmission of AD—an amyloid precursor gene on chromosome 21, a presenilin-1 gene on chromosome 14, and a presenilin-2 gene on chromosome 1. As chromosome 21 contains a gene that expresses a cleavage product of the amyloid precursor protein, adults with trisomy 21 (Down syndrome) consistently develop neuropathologic hallmarks of AD if they survive beyond the age of 40 years. Risk factors for AD include age, family history of dementia, and the presence of both ApoE4 alleles.

AD is characterized by beta-amyloid plaques and neuroinflammation that results in neurofibrillary tangles and loss of cortical neurons. The process begins in the hippocampus and the entorhinal cortex. Over time, it spreads to specific regions of the brain (temporal, parietal, and frontal lobes) that are important for learning and memory. Affected neurons make up part of the cholinergic system and use acetylcholine and glutamate as their primary neurotransmitters. These neurotransmitters are intimately involved in cognition. Progressive destruction of the neurons leads to atrophy of the cerebral cortex and enlargement of the ventricles. Motor, visual, and somatosensory portions of the cerebral cortex typically are spared. Resultant cognitive defects and associated memory loss cause significant impairment in social and occupational functioning.

Clinical Presentation

Updated clinical criteria recognize three stages of AD: (1) preclinical AD; (2) mild cognitive impairment due to AD; and (3) dementia due to AD. Preclinical AD occurs before changes in cognition and everyday activities are observed and is primarily used for research purposes. Cognitive impairment due to AD is characterized by mild changes in memory and other cognitive abilities that are noticeable to patients and families, but are not sufficient to interfere with day-to-day activities. Dementia due to AD is characterized by changes in two or more aspects of cognition and behavior that interfere with the ability to function in everyday life. First signs of AD are loss of recent memory, orientation, or language or a change in personality (apathy) or behavior. Slowly, cognitive problems at the early stage begin to interfere with daily activities such as keeping track of finances, following instructions on the job, driving, shopping, and housekeeping. The signs and symptoms of dementia can be seen in Table 27.2. Some patients remain unaware of these developing problems; others are aware of them and become frustrated and anxious. With disease progression, the patient is unable to work, is easily lost and confused, and requires daily supervision. Patients may become lost while taking walks or driving. Social etiquette, routine conversation, and superficial conversation may be maintained for variable periods. Language may be impaired, especially comprehension and naming of objects. Motor skills such as eating, dressing, or solving simple puzzles are eventually lost. Patients are unable to do simple calculations or to tell time. Loss of inhibitions and belligerence may occur, and nighttime wandering may become a problem with some patients. Anxiety and depression become more of a problem as the disease progresses. In advanced stages of AD, patients may become rigid, mute, incontinent, and bedridden, often requiring a nursing facility. Generalized seizures may occur. Death usually results from malnutrition, secondary infection, or heart disease. The typical duration of AD is 5–15 years. However, the course of the

illness can range from 1 to 20 years. Some patients exhibit a progressive course; others may have prolonged plateaus without major deterioration.

Laboratory and Diagnostic Findings. Although the definitive diagnosis of AD can be made only by brain biopsy or at autopsy, the clinical diagnosis of AD can be made on the basis of patient history and clinical findings. Criteria for making this diagnosis include (1) progressive functional decline and dementia established by clinical examination and mental status testing, (2) the presence of at least two cognitive deficits, (3) normal level of consciousness at presentation, (4) onset between the ages of 40 and 90 years, and (5) absence of any other condition that could account for the deficits. The battery of tests useful in ruling out other correctable causes of dementia include a complete blood count, electrolyte panel, screening metabolic panel, thyroid function tests, determination of vitamin B_{12} and folate levels, tests for syphilis and human immunodeficiency virus (HIV) antibodies, urinalysis, CSF analysis, EEG, ECG, chest radiograph, and noncontrast CT scan or MRI of the brain.

At autopsy, characteristic macroscopic changes include cerebral cortical atrophy and ventricular enlargement. Microscopic features include neurofibrillary tangles, neuritic plaques that contain beta-amyloid, and accumulation of beta-amyloid in the walls of cerebral vessels (amyloid angiopathy). On a biochemical level, a

---

TABLE 27.2 Signs and Symptoms of Dementia by Stage

Dementia affects each person in a different way, depending upon the impact of the disease and the person's personality before becoming ill. The signs and symptoms linked to dementia can be understood in three stages.

Early stage: The early stage of dementia is often overlooked because the onset is gradual. Common symptoms include
- Forgetfulness
- Losing track of the time
- Becoming lost in familiar places

Middle stage: As dementia progresses to the middle stage, the signs and symptoms become clearer and more restricting. These include
- Becoming forgetful of recent events and people's names
- Becoming lost at home
- Having increasing difficulty with communication
- Needing help with personal care
- Experiencing behavior changes, including wandering and repeated questioning

Late stage: The late stage of dementia is one of near total dependence and inactivity. Memory disturbances are serious, and the physical signs and symptoms become more obvious. Symptoms include
- Becoming unaware of the time and place
- Having difficulty recognizing relatives and friends
- Having an increasing need for assisted self-care
- Having difficulty walking
- Experiencing behavior changes that may escalate and include aggression

deficiency of acetylcholine and its associated enzymes has been confirmed.

Medical Management

There is no cure for AD, and management remains difficult. Standard medications used in the treatment of mild to moderate disease have been the cholinesterase inhibitors. These drugs—donepezil (Aricept), rivastigmine (Exelon), galantamine (Razadyne)—increase acetylcholine levels in the brain by inhibiting hydrolysis of cholinesterase (Table 27.3). Clinical trials indicate that these agents perform better than placebo but have limited effectiveness in preventing disease progression and in reversing memory deficits. Fewer than 50% of patients appear to benefit from these medications. Common adverse effects of the cholinesterase inhibitors include gastrointestinal disturbance and headache.

To slow the progression of disease, vitamin E may be considered as an additional medication. Studies have shown that vitamin E and selegiline (two antioxidants) each can delay the development of dementia in patients with AD.

Memantine, a noncompetitive N-methyl-D-aspartate (NMDA) receptor antagonist believed to protect neurons from glutamate-mediated excitotoxicity, is used for treatment of moderate to severe AD. Studies suggest that it may preserve or improve memory and learning, and when given with the cholinesterase inhibitors appears to produce additive beneficial effects. Memantine-related adverse effects are mild and include headache and

confusion. Memantine combined with donepezil (Namzaric) is approved to treat moderate to severe AD.

Noncognitive symptoms of AD are manageable. Although efforts are made to use nonpharmacologic approaches to manage symptoms such as anxiety, depression, irritability, and sleep disturbances, medications inevitably are generally required. Antidepressants, sedative–hypnotics, and antipsychiatric agents are used with varying degrees of success. A small percentage of patients experience seizures, which are treated with standard anticonvulsant agents. Nursing home care often is provided during the latter stages of the disease.

Dental Management

Dental management requires knowledge of the stage of disease, medications taken, and cognitive abilities of the patient (Box 27.6). Patients with mild to moderate disease generally maintain normal systemic organ function and can receive routine dental treatment. As the disease progresses, antipsychotics, antidepressants, and anxiolytics frequently are used to manage behavioral disturbances. These medications (see Table 27.3) contribute to xerostomia with increased risk for dental caries.

Patients should be monitored when a new medication is started. Any unusual symptoms should be reported to the prescribing doctor. It is important to follow the physician's instructions for taking any medication, including vitamins and herbal supplements. Also, any additions to or changes in medications should be cleared beforehand with the patient's physician.

TABLE 27.3 Drugs Used in the Management of Alzheimer Disease

Drug	Reason Used	Common Side Effects	Dental Treatment Considerations
Memantine (Namenda)	NMDA antagonist prescribed to treat symptoms of moderate to severe Alzheimer disease Blocks the toxic effects associated with excess glutamate and regulates glutamate activation	Dizziness, headache, constipation, confusion	Patient positioning due to possible dizziness.
Galantamine (Razadyne)	Cholinesterase inhibitor prescribed to treat symptoms of mild to moderate Alzheimer disease Prevents the breakdown of acetylcholine and stimulates nicotinic receptors to release more acetylcholine in the brain	Nausea, vomiting, diarrhea, weight loss, loss of appetite	Possible sialorrhea. Avoid use of clarithromycin, erythromycin and ketoconazole as it can impair metabolism of galantamine. Caution with NSAIDs as they may increase risk of GI irritation and/or bleeding with concomitant use.
Rivastigmine (Exelon)	Cholinesterase inhibitor prescribed to treat symptoms of mild to moderate Alzheimer disease Prevents the breakdown of acetylcholine and butyrylcholine (a brain chemical similar to acetylcholine) in the brain	Nausea, vomiting, diarrhea, weight loss, loss of appetite, muscle weakness	Possible sialorrhea. Avoid use of clarithromycin, erythromycin and ketoconazole as it can impair metabolism of galantamine. Caution with NSAIDs as they may increase risk of GI irritation and/or bleeding with concomitant use.
Donepezil (Aricept)	Cholinesterase inhibitor prescribed to treat symptoms of mild to moderate, and moderate to severe Alzheimer disease Prevents the breakdown of acetylcholine in the brain	Nausea, vomiting, diarrhea	Possible sialorrhea. Avoid use of clarithromycin, erythromycin and ketoconazole as it can impair metabolism of galantamine. Caution with NSAIDs as they may increase risk of GI irritation and/or bleeding with concomitant use.

BOX 27.6	Dental Management Considerations in Patients With Alzheimer Disease or Other Dementias[a]

PREOPERATIVE RISK ASSESSMENT

R: Recognize Risks
- Be **aware** of adverse events that may occur in the management of a patient who has a medical condition.

P: Patient Evaluation
- Review **medical history** and discuss relevant issues with the patient.
- Identify all **medications and drugs** being taken or supposed to be taken by the patient.
- **Examine** the patient for signs and symptoms of disease and obtain vital signs.
- Review or obtain recent **laboratory test** results or **images** required to assess risk.
- Obtain a **medical consultation** if the patient has a poorly controlled or undiagnosed problem or if the patient's health status is uncertain.

A

Analgesics	Avoid NSAIDs in patients using cholinesterase inhibitors due to risk of GI irritation and/or bleeding.
Antibiotics	No issues.
Anesthesia	Local anesthesia obtained with epinephrine (1:100,000) in local anesthetics generally is not associated with any problems.
Anxiety	Patients with untreated or poorly controlled disease may experience difficulty in understanding commands or instructions and appear very anxious or stressed. Use of special anxiety or stress reduction techniques may be indicated.

B

Bleeding	No issues.
Blood pressure and vital sign monitoring	Obtain pretreatment vital signs. Monitor blood pressure as some medications may cause hypotension.

C

Capacity to tolerate care	Well-controlled Alzheimer disease poses no issues for capacity to tolerate care; however, this may change with advancing disease.
Chair position	This usually is not a problem if the patient is under good medical management: With symptoms of impending syncope, however, a supine position may not be tolerated. The chair may need adjustment to address patients' concerns or fears. Caution in patients using galantamine as it may cause dizziness.

D

Devices	No issues.
Drugs	These patients typically take anticholinergic and dopamine agonist drugs, which may have adverse effects, including sedation, drowsiness, slow mentation, fatigue, confusion, and dizziness (see Table 27.3).

E

Equipment	No issues.
Emergencies and urgent care	Most commonly, cognitive problems are self-limited, but rarely the patient's condition may progress acutely to warrant interruption of dental treatment or to necessitate cessation of treatment.

POSTOPERATIVE CARE

F

Follow-up care	Routine follow-up is recommended. In patients who have undergone surgery or other complex dental procedures, a follow-up call within the next day or two is advisable to check on clinical status.

[a]Strength of recommendation taxonomy (SORT) Grade: C (see Preface for further explanation).
GI, gastrointestinal; *NSAIDs*, nonsteroid antiinflammatory drugs.

Patients with AD are best managed with use of an understanding and empathetic approach. The dental team should communicate a positive, hopeful attitude regarding maintenance of the patient's oral health to both the patient and family members (see Box 27.6). The dental team should determine whether the patient is legally able to make rational decisions and should be discussed with the patient and family. Treatment planning often involves input and permission from a family member so that appropriate decisions can be made. Before initiation of any procedure, the patient's attention should be engaged, and the dentist should explain what is going to happen. The dentist should communicate using short words and sentences and should repeat instructions and explanations. Nonverbal communication can be very

helpful. Facial expression and body posture of the dentist should show support—cues that the patient is understood and that the dentist is attentive to the patient's well-being. Positive nonverbal communication includes direct eye contact, smiling, touching the patient on the arm, and so forth. Patients with AD should be placed on an aggressive preventive dentistry program, including 3-month recall, oral examination, prophylaxis, fluoride gel application, oral hygiene education, and adjustment of prostheses.

In a patient with mild dementia, good oral health should be maintained because of the progressive nature of the disease. Subsequent care should concentrate on preventing dental disease as dementia progresses. A patient with moderate dementia may not be as amenable to dental treatment as in earlier stages of the disease. In such cases, treatment consists of maintaining dental status and minimizing deterioration. Complex dental procedures should be performed, if at all, before the disease has reached the moderate to advanced stage.

Patients with advanced dementia often are anxious, hostile, and uncooperative in the dental office and very difficult to treat. These patients are best served with short appointments and noncomplex procedures; use of sedation may be required for more complex and tedious procedures. Sedative medication should be selected in consultation with the patient's physician. Chloral hydrate and benzodiazepines can be used to provide the level of sedation required for performance of routine dental procedures.

In advanced cases, removable prosthetic devices may have to be taken from the patient because of the danger of self-injury. All treatment should be provided with the knowledge that these patients have memory loss, lack of drive, and slowed thinking. Their ability to maintain proper daily oral hygiene can become severely compromised. Thus, the caregiver should be intimately involved in the provision of daily oral hygiene as the disease advances.

Oral Manifestations. Patients with moderate to severe AD may not have an interest in caring for themselves, and they may lack the ability to do so. Hence, their oral hygiene is poor, and dental problems are increased. Most of the medications used to treat psychiatric disorders contribute to increased dental problems in such patients because hyposalivation is one of their primary adverse effects. Patients with AD have a greater incidence of dry mouth, mucosal lesions, candidiasis, plaque and calculus buildup, periodontal disease, and smooth surface (root) and coronal caries, along with an increased risk for aspiration pneumonia.

These patients often sustain oral injuries from falls and ulcerations of the tongue, cheeks, and alveolar mucosa as the result of accidents with forks or spoons or with mastication, attrition and abrasion of teeth, missing teeth, and migration of teeth. Edentulous patients with dementia may misplace or lose their dentures and at times may even attempt to wear the upper denture on the lower arch and vice versa.

Antipsychotic drugs sometimes taken by these patients can cause agranulocytosis, leukopenia, or thrombocytopenia. Additional adverse effects of antipsychotic agents include muscular problems such as dystonia, dyskinesia, and tardive dyskinesia in the oral and facial regions.

EPILEPSY
General Description
The term *epilepsy* includes disorders or syndromes with widely variable pathophysiologic findings, clinical manifestations, treatments, and outcomes. Epilepsy is not a specific diagnosis but rather a chronic disorder of the brain characterized by a disposition toward recurrent unprovoked seizures and by the neurobiological, cognitive, psychological, and social consequences of this condition. Seizures may be convulsive (i.e., accompanied by motor manifestations) or may occur with other changes in neurologic function (i.e., sensory, cognitive, and emotional).

Seizures are characterized by discrete episodes, which tend to be recurrent and often are unprovoked, in which movement, sensation, behavior, perception, and consciousness are disturbed. Symptoms are produced by excessive temporary neuronal discharging, which may result from intracranial or extracranial causes.

Although seizures are required for the diagnosis of epilepsy, not all seizures imply presence of epilepsy. Seizures may occur during many medical or neurologic illnesses, including stress, sleep deprivation, fever, alcohol or drug withdrawal, and syncope. In 2017, the International League Against Epilepsy (ILAE) revised the classification system of seizures and epilepsy (Box 27.7). The original seizure classification was based on clinical behaviors and electroencephalographic changes, however, the revised classification takes into account other variables, such as focal or generalized onset, genetics, age at onset, and pathophysiologic mechanisms of disease. Discussion in this section is limited to generalized tonic-clonic seizures because these represent the most severe expression of epilepsy that dentists are likely to encounter.

Epidemiology
Epilepsy is the most common chronic neurologic condition. It affects people of all ages, with a peak incidence in childhood and old age. In the United States, the incidence of all types of epilepsy is approximately 48 cases per 100,000 population with approximately 150,000 cases per year. Cases of epilepsy vary by age: 60–70 per

---

BOX 27.7   International League Against Epilepsy 2017 Classification of Seizure Types

I. Focal
- Aware/Impaired Awareness
- Motor Onset/Nonmotor Onset
- Focal to Bilateral Tonic Clonic

II. Generalized
- Motor (Tonic-Clonic, Other Motor)
- Nonmotor (Absence)

III. Unknown
- Motor (Tonic-Clonic, Other Motor)
- Nonmotor
- Unclassified

Adapted from Sarmast ST, Abdullahi A, Jahan N. Current classification of seizures and epilepsies: scope, limitations and recommendations for future action. *Cureus*. September 20, 2020;12(9):e10549.

100,000 per year in young children (younger than 5 years of age), 45 per 100,000 in adolescents, and as low as 30 per 100,000 in the early adult years but rising through the sixth and seventh decades of life reaching as high as 150–200 per 100,000 in persons older than 75 years. Cerebrovascular disease is the most common factor underlying seizures occurring in older adults. The incidence in males is higher at every age. Estimates of the prevalence of epilepsy range from 4.7 to 6.9 per 1000, but its prevalence is much higher in less developed countries for all age groups.

Approximately 10% of the population will have at least one seizure in their lifetimes, and 2%–4% will experience recurrent seizures at some point. The overall incidence of seizures is 1%. Seizures are most common during childhood, with as many as 4% of children experiencing at least one seizure during the first 15 years of life. While most children outgrow the disorder, about 4 in 1000 children do not outgrow the disorder and will require medical care. In a typical dental practice of 2000 patients, 3 or 4 can be expected to have a seizure disorder.

Pathophysiology and Complications. Six etiologic categories now exist for seizures: (1) structural, (2) genetic, (3) infectious, (4) metabolic, (5) immune, and (6) unknown; prior terms, such as symptomatic and cryptogenic, are no longer used. Structural implies a structural lesion on neuroimaging in combination with EEG data, suggesting that the lesion is the cause of the seizure. Causes include stroke, trauma, or tumor. Genetic implies the existence of known or presumed genetic mutation(s) where seizures are a known complication of the genetic disorder that is the result of the mutation(s). This etiology includes some of the well-known genetic epilepsy syndromes, such as juvenile myoclonic epilepsy, or may include an unknown mutation but obvious familial inheritance pattern. Infectious etiologies include neurocysticercosis, HIV, cytomegalovirus (CMV), cerebral toxoplasmosis, and prior meningitis or encephalitis. Metabolic etiologies are due to a metabolic disorder, with the core tenet being that a change in diet or supplementation may affect the disease course. An immune cause of seizures is defined either by a causal autoimmune disorder such as paraneoplastic syndrome or by an immune therapy used to treat the immunologic disease.

Seizures sometimes can be evoked by specific stimuli. Approximately 1 of 15 patients reports that seizures occurred after exposure to flickering lights, monotonous sounds, music, or a loud noise. Syncope and diminished oxygen supply to the brain also are known to trigger seizures. It is valuable for the dentist to know what factors have the potential to exacerbate a seizure in a particular patient, so that certain stimuli can be avoided.

The basic event underlying an epileptic seizure is an excessive focal neuronal discharge that spreads to thalamic and brainstem nuclei. The cause of this abnormal electrical activity is not precisely known, although a number of theories have been put forth. These include altered sodium channel function, altered neuronal membrane potentials, altered synaptic transmission, diminution of inhibitory neurons, increased neuronal excitability, and decreased electrical threshold for epileptic activity. During the seizure, blood becomes hypoxic, with consequent development of lactic acidosis.

Approximately 60%–80% of patients with epilepsy achieve complete control over their seizures within 5 years; the remainder achieve only partial or poor control. A significant problem in the medical management of epileptic patients is one of compliance (i.e., adherence to prescribed treatment regimens including medication). This problem is common to many chronic disorders, such as hypertension, because patients may have to take medication for the rest of their lives even though they remain asymptomatic. Evidence suggests that patients who have epilepsy from an early age have a higher incidence of future complications and die at an earlier age. Noncompliance may be a clinically important consideration in dental patients because it is associated with a higher risk of later complications that may lead to death. Complications of seizures include trauma (as a result of falls) to the head, neck, and mouth and aspiration pneumonia. Also, frequent and severe seizures are associated with altered mental function, dullness, confusion, argumentativeness, and increased risk of sudden death (about 1 in 75 persons in this group die annually).

A serious acute complication of epilepsy (especially the tonic-clonic type) is the occurrence of repeated seizures over a short time without a recovery period, called *generalized convulsive status epilepticus*. This condition most frequently is caused by abrupt withdrawal of anticonvulsant medication or an abused substance but may be triggered by infection, neoplasm, or trauma. Status epilepticus constitutes a medical emergency. Patients may become seriously hypoxic and acidotic during this event and sustain permanent brain damage or death. Patients with epilepsy also are at increased risk for sudden death and death due to accident.

Clinical Presentation

The clinical manifestations of generalized tonic-clonic convulsions are classic. An aura (a momentary sensory alteration that produces an unusual smell or visual disturbance) precedes the convulsion in one-third of patients. Irritability is another premonitory signal. After the aura warning, the patient emits a sudden "epileptic cry" (caused by spasm of the diaphragmatic muscles) and immediately loses consciousness. The tonic phase consists of generalized muscle rigidity, pupil dilation, rolling of the eyes upward or to the side, and loss of consciousness. Breathing may stop because of spasm of respiratory muscles. This phase is followed by clonic activity consisting of uncoordinated beating movements of the limbs and head, forcible jaw closing, and up and down head rocking. Urinary incontinence is common, but fecal incontinence is rare. The seizure (ictus) usually does not last longer than 60 s; thereafter, movement ceases and muscles relax, with a gradual return to consciousness, accompanied by stupor, headache, confusion, and mental dulling. Several hours of rest or sleep may be needed for the patient to regain full cognitive and physical abilities.

Laboratory and Diagnostic Findings. The diagnosis of epilepsy generally is based on the history of seizures and presence of abnormalities on the electroencephalogram (EEG). Seizures produce characteristic spike and sharp wave patterns on the EEG tracing. Serial recordings during sleep deprivation, which can induce seizures, may help to establish the diagnosis. Other diagnostic procedures that are useful for ruling out other causes of seizures include CT, MRI, single-photon emission computed tomography (SPECT), lumbar puncture, serum chemistry profiles, and toxicology screening.

Medical Management

The medical management of epilepsy usually is based on long-term drug therapy. Phenytoin (Dilantin), carbamazepine (Tegretol), and valproic acid are considered first-line agents for treatment of this disease. Several other drugs are available for control of generalized tonic-clonic seizures (Table 27.4). These drugs reduce the frequency of seizures by elevating the seizure threshold of motor cortex neurons, depressing abnormal cerebral electrical discharge, and limiting the spread of excitation from abnormal foci. Phenytoin and carbamazepine are efficient at blocking sodium or calcium channels of motor neurons. Many of the other antiepileptic drugs augment γ-aminobutyric acid (GABA), which inhibits glutamate activity—the major determinant of brain excitability. Adverse effects of phenytoin include anemia, ataxia, gingival overgrowth, cosmetic changes (coarsening of facial features, hirsutism, facial acne), lethargy, skin rash, and gastrointestinal disturbances. Phenobarbital, which

TABLE 27.4   Anticonvulsants Used in the Management of Generalized Tonic-Clonic Seizures

Drug	Trade Name(s)	Mechanism of Action	Dental Treatment Considerations
Drugs of Choice			
Phenytoin[a]	Dilantin	Blocks sodium channels	Gingival hyperplasia, increased incidence of microbial infection, delayed healing, gingival bleeding (leukopenia), osteoporosis, Stevens–Johnson syndrome
Carbamazepine[a]	Tegretol	Blocks sodium channels	Xerostomia, microbial infection, delayed healing, gingival bleeding (leukopenia and thrombocytopenia), ataxia, osteoporosis, Stevens–Johnson syndrome *Drug interactions:* propoxyphene, erythromycin
Valproic acid[a]	Depakene, Depakote	GABA augmentation and NMDA receptor	Excessive bleeding and petechiae, decreased platelet aggregation, increased incidence of microbial infection, delayed healing, drowsiness, gingival bleeding (leukopenia and thrombocytopenia), hepatotoxicity *Drug interactions:* aspirin and other NSAIDs
Lamotrigine[a]	Lamictal	Blocks sodium and calcium channels, reduces glutamate	Ataxia; may require help getting into and out of the dental chair; risk for development of Stevens–Johnson syndrome
Alternatives			
Clonazepam[a]	Klonopin	Augments inhibitory GABAergic system	*Drug interactions:* CNS depressants
Ethosuximide	Zarontin	Blocks sodium and calcium channels	Risk for development of Stevens–Johnson syndrome, blood dyscrasias
Felbamate	Felbatol	Blocks sodium channels, reduces glutamate	Risk for development of aplastic anemia, Stevens–Johnson syndrome
Gabapentin	Neurontin	Modulates calcium channel; augments GABAergic system	Dizziness
Oxcarbazepine	Trileptal	Blocks sodium channels	Liver enzyme induction but less than with carbamazepine
Phenobarbital[a]	Luminal	Blocks calcium channel; augments inhibitory GABAergic system	Sedation, liver enzyme induction *Drug interactions:* CNS depressants
Primidone[a]	Mysoline	Blocks calcium channel; augments inhibitory GABAergic system	Ataxia, vertigo—increased risk of falls
Topiramate	Topamax	Blocks sodium channels; augments inhibitory GABAergic system	Impaired cognition
Vigabatrin	Sabril	Augments inhibitory GABAergic system	*Drug interactions:* CNS depressants

[a]Preexisting liver disease can exacerbate adverse effects associated with antiepileptics. Drugs of choice for absence (petit mal) seizures: ethosuximide (Zarontin), valproate, lamotrigine, or clonazepam. Drugs of choice for status epilepticus: lorazepam 4–8 mg, diazepam 10 mg, intravenously.
CNS, central nervous system; *GABA*, γ-aminobutyric acid; *NMDA*, N-methyl-D-aspartate; *NSAID*, nonsteroidal antiinflammatory drug.

is considered a second-line drug, can induce hepatic microsomal enzymes that promote the metabolism of concurrently used drugs. Several antiseizure medications (see Table 27.4) may cause drowsiness, sedation, ataxia, weight gain, cognitive impairment, and hypersensitivity reactions. Adverse effects are more common at the start of therapy, when drugs are administered rapidly or at high dose. For these reasons, and to facilitate compliance, single-drug therapy and a slow increase in dose are recommended. The use of combination therapy is often necessary for seizure control. Discontinuation of pharmacologic therapy is considered when seizure control has been achieved. The following patient characteristics yield the greatest chance of remaining seizure free after discontinuation of drug therapy: (1) complete medical control of seizures for 1−5 years; (2) single seizure type; (3) normal neurologic examination, including intelligence; and (4) a normal EEG.

Approximately 30% of patients are resistant to all medical therapies. Surgical procedures may be indicated for these patients, including limited removal of the hippocampus and amygdala, temporal lobectomy, or hemispherectomy. Those patients who are not candidates for brain surgery may benefit from vagus nerve stimulation (VNS), whereby a subcutaneous pulse generator is implanted in the left chest wall and delivers electrical signals to the left vagus nerve through a bipolar lead. The stimulated vagus nerve provides direct projection to regions in the brain potentially responsible for the seizure and is associated with an increased seizure threshold.

Dental Management

The first step in the management of an epileptic dental patient is identification of the patient as having the disorder (Box 27.8). This is accomplished by the medical history and by discussion with the patient or family members. After a patient with epilepsy has been identified, the dental practitioner must inquire about the seizure history, including the type of seizures, age at onset, cause (if known), current and regular use of medications, frequency of physician visits, quality of seizure control, frequency of seizures, date of last seizure, and any known precipitating factors. In addition, a history of previous injuries associated with seizures and their treatment may be helpful.

Fortunately, most patients with epilepsy are able to attain good control of their seizures with anticonvulsant drugs and are therefore able to receive normal routine dental care. In some instances, however, the history may reveal a degree of seizure activity that suggests noncompliance or a severe seizure disorder that does not respond to anticonvulsants. For these patients, a consultation with the physician is advised before dental treatment is rendered. A patient with poorly controlled disease may require additional anticonvulsant or sedative medication, as directed by the physician.

Patients who take anticonvulsants may suffer from the toxic effects of these drugs, and the dentist should be aware of these manifestations. In addition to the more common adverse effects (see Table 27.4), allergy may be seen occasionally as a rash, erythema multiforme, or Stevens−Johnson syndrome. Phenytoin, carbamazepine, and valproic acid can cause bone marrow suppression, leukopenia, and thrombocytopenia, resulting in an increased incidence of microbial infection, delayed healing, and gingival and postoperative bleeding. Valproic acid can decrease platelet aggregation, leading to spontaneous hemorrhage and petechiae. Patients taking these medications may require laboratory evaluation prior to dental treatment, including a complete blood count with differential, to assess white blood cell and platelet counts, and coagulation studies to assess clotting ability. If a patient is severely neutropenic (ANC < 500) due to medication side effect, consider antibiotic prophylaxis prior to invasive dental treatment. Patients on long-term carbamazepine should have serum blood levels evaluated prior to initiating dental treatment, as insufficient doses may result in inadequate seizure control and excessive doses have been associated with hepatotoxicity.

Propoxyphene and erythromycin should not be administered to patients who are taking carbamazepine because of interference with metabolism of carbamazepine, which could lead to toxic levels of the anticonvulsant drug. Aspirin and other nonsteroidal antiinflammatory drugs should not be administered to patients who are taking valproic acid because these agents can further decrease platelet aggregation, leading to hemorrhagic episodes. No contraindication has been identified to the use of local anesthetics in proper amounts in these patients. Patients who have a VNS device implanted in the chest do not need antibiotic prophylaxis before undergoing invasive dental procedures.

Despite consistent use of appropriate preventive measures by both the dentist and patient, the possibility always exists that patients with epilepsy may experience a generalized tonic-clonic convulsion in the dental office. The dentist and office staff members should anticipate and be prepared for such events. Preventive measures include knowing the patient's history, scheduling the patient at a time within a few hours of taking the anticonvulsant medication, using a mouth prop, removing dentures, and discussing with the patient the urgency of mentioning an aura as soon as it is sensed. The clinician also should be aware that irritability often is a symptom of impending seizure, whereas calming music has been shown to suppress seizure brain activity in patients with epilepsy and thus might be used as a palliative approach for these patients. With a premonitory stage of sufficient duration, 0.5−2 mg of lorazepam can be given sublingually, or diazepam 2−10 mg can be given intravenously.

BOX 27.8   Dental Management Considerations in Patients With Seizure Disorders[a]

PREOPERATIVE RISK ASSESSMENT

R: Recognize Risks
- Be **aware** of adverse events that may occur in the management of a patient who has a medical condition.

P: Patient Evaluation
- Review **medical history** and discuss relevant issues with the patient.
- Identify all **medications and drugs** being taken or supposed to be taken by the patient.
- **Examine** the patient for signs and symptoms of disease and obtain vital signs.
- Review or obtain recent **laboratory test** results or **images** required to assess risk.
- Obtain a **medical consultation** if the patient has a poorly controlled or undiagnosed problem or if the patient's health status is uncertain.

A	
Analgesics	Clinicians should provide good pain control to avoid stress, which may precipitate a seizure.
Antibiotics	Generally, there is no indication for antibiotic prophylaxis. If a patient is severely neutropenic (ANC < 500) due to medication side effect, consider antibiotic prophylaxis prior to invasive dental treatment.
Anesthesia	Obtain adequate anesthesia to reduce stress as possible precipitant for a seizure. Epinephrine (1:100,000 and no more than two carpules) in local anesthetics generally is well tolerated.
Anxiety	Patients with untreated or poorly controlled seizure-associated disorders may appear very anxious and stressed, increasing the risk for a seizure. Use of special anxiety and stress reduction techniques may be indicated.
Allergy	Allergic skin changes (rash, erythema multiforme) may signify a reaction to antiepileptic medications.

B	
Bleeding	Bleeding tendency associated with valproic acid (Depakene) or carbamazepine (Tegretol) as the result of platelet interference.
Blood pressure and vital sign monitoring	Obtain pretreatment vital signs. Monitor blood pressure because it may significantly increase or decrease with onset of a seizure.

C	
Capacity to tolerate care	Well-controlled seizure disorders pose no issues for capacity to tolerate care.

Chair position	This usually is not a problem if the patient is under good medical management; with symptoms of impending syncope associated with cardiac stress or pulmonary congestion, however, a supine position may not be tolerated. In patients at risk for seizure, the chair back should be in supported supine position.

D	
Devices	No issues.
Drugs	These patients typically take anticonvulsant drugs, which may have adverse effects including drowsiness, depressed cognition, dizziness, others.

E	
Equipment	No issues.
Emergencies and urgent care	Be prepared for occurrence of a tonic–clonic seizure: • Placement of a ligated mouth prop at the beginning of the procedure may be considered. • The dental chair should be in supported supine position. During a seizure: • Clear the area. • Turn the patient to the side (to avoid aspiration). • Do not attempt to use a padded tongue blade. • Passively restrain. After a seizure: • Examine for traumatic injuries. • Discontinue treatment; arrange for patient transport. Most commonly seizures are self-limited, but rarely a seizure may progress to cardiac arrest, necessitating emergency medical treatment; call 911. A patient who is ambulatory and stable should seek urgent medical care. Ongoing vital signs must be monitored and cardiopulmonary resuscitation initiated if necessary; transport patient to emergency medical facilities.

F	
Follow-up care	Follow-up with the patient (and physician) is indicated after any seizure event in the dental office. In patients who have undergone surgery, a follow-up phone call within the next day or two is advised.

[a]Strength of recommendation taxonomy (SORT) Grade: C (see Preface for further explanation).
ANC, absolute neutrophil count.

If a patient has a seizure while in the dental chair, the primary task of management is to protect the patient and try to prevent injury. No attempt should be made to move the patient to the floor. Instead, the instruments and instrument tray should be cleared from the area, and the chair should be placed in a supported supine position (Fig. 27.7). The patient's airway should be maintained patent. No attempt should be made to restrain or hold

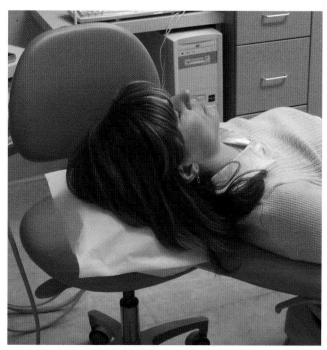

FIG. 27.7 Dental chair in the supine position with the back supported by the operator's or assistant's stool.

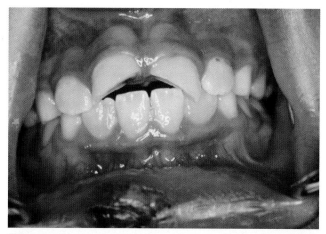

FIG. 27.8 Fracture of teeth and laceration of lower lip sustained during a tonic clonic seizure. (Courtesy of Gerald A. Ferretti, DDS, Lexington, KY.)

down the patient. Passive restraint should be used only to prevent injury that may result when the patient hits nearby objects or falls out of the chair.

If a mouth prop (e.g., a padded tongue blade between the teeth to prevent tongue biting) is used, it should be inserted at the beginning of the dental procedure (see Box 27.8). Trying to insert a mouth prop is not advised during the seizure because doing so may damage the patient's teeth or oral soft tissue and may be nearly impossible. An exception is the case in which the patient senses an impending seizure and can cooperate.

A tonic clonic seizure generally does not last longer than a few minutes. Afterward, the patient may fall into a deep sleep from which he or she cannot be aroused. Oxygen (100%), maintenance of a patent airway, and mouth suction should be provided during this phase. Alternatively, the patient can be turned to the side to control the airway and to minimize aspiration of secretions. Within a few minutes, the patient gradually regains consciousness but may be confused, disoriented, and embarrassed. Headache is a prominent feature during this period. If the patient does not respond within a few minutes, the seizure may be associated with a low serum glucose level, and delivery of glucose may be needed.

No further dental treatment should be attempted after a generalized tonic-clonic seizure, although examination for sustained injuries (e.g., lacerations, fractures) should be performed. In the event of avulsed or fractured teeth (Fig. 27.8) or a fractured appliance, an attempt should be made to locate the tooth or fragments to rule out aspiration. A chest radiograph may be required to locate a missing fragment or tooth.

In the event that a seizure becomes prolonged (status epilepticus) or is repeated, IV lorazepam (0.05–0.1 mg/kg) 4–8 mg, 10 mg of diazepam, or midazolam nasal spray 5 mg is generally effective in controlling it. Lorazepam is preferred by many experts because it is more efficacious and lasts longer than diazepam. Midazolam administered as a single-dose nasal spray results in effective seizure control and one spray into one nostril is indicated as a rescue medication. If seizures continue after 10 min, a second spray may be given into the other nostril. Oxygen and respiratory support should be provided because respiratory function may become depressed. If the seizure lasts longer than 15 min, the following protocol should be implemented: secure IV access, repeat lorazepam dosing, administer fosphenytoin, and activate the EMS system.

Edentulous spaces should be addressed if possible to prevent the tongue from being traumatized in these areas during a seizure. Generally, a fixed prosthesis or implant is preferable to a removable one as the removable prosthesis becomes dislodged more easily. For fixed prostheses, all-metal or zirconium units should be considered when possible to minimize the chance of fracture. When placing anterior castings, the dentist may wish to consider using three-quarter crowns or retentive nonporcelain facings.

Removable prostheses are nevertheless sometimes constructed for patients with epilepsy. Metallic palates and bases are preferable to all-acrylic ones. If acrylic is used, it should be reinforced with wire mesh.

Oral Manifestations. The most significant oral complication seen in patients with epilepsy is gingival overgrowth, which is most commonly associated with phenytoin (Fig. 27.9). The incidence of phenytoin-induced gingival overgrowth in patients with epilepsy ranges from 0% to 100%, with an average rate of approximately 42%. A greater tendency to develop gingival overgrowth occurs in youngsters than in

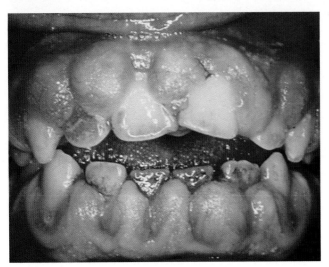

FIG. 27.9 Phenytoin-induced gingival overgrowth. (Courtesy of H. Abrams, Lexington, KY.)

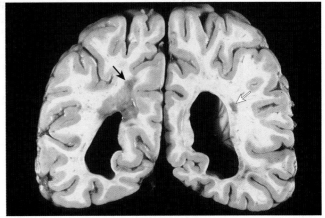

FIG. 27.10 Multiple sclerosis. Large periventricular "demyelinated plaque" (*dark region* above left ventricle, *black arrow*) and smaller "demyelinated plaque" (*white arrow*) lateral to the right ventricle, shown in a coronal section of the brain of a patient who had multiple sclerosis. (Courtesy of Daron G. Davis, MD, Lexington, KY.)

adults. The anterior labial surfaces of the maxillary and mandibular gingivae are most commonly and severely affected.

Meticulous oral hygiene is important for preventing overgrowth and significantly decreasing its severity. Good home care must always be combined with the removal of irritants, such as overhanging restorations and calculus. Frequently, gingival overgrowth can interfere with function or appearance, and surgical reduction may become necessary.

Traumatic injuries such as broken teeth, tongue lacerations, and lip scars also are common in patients who experience generalized tonic-clonic seizures. Stomatitis, erythema multiforme, and Stevens–Johnson syndrome are rare adverse effects associated with the use of phenytoin, valproic acid, lamotrigine, phenobarbital, and carbamazepine. These complications are more common during the first 8 weeks of treatment.

MULTIPLE SCLEROSIS

General Description

Multiple sclerosis is a common autoimmune disease of the nervous system and characterized pathologically by inflammation, axonal injury, and demyelination of the CNS. MS typically manifests in young adults with episodic neurologic dysfunction, and 85% of patients present with relapsing and remitting symptoms. Demyelinated regions are generally limited to the white matter of the CNS and are randomly located and multiple (Fig. 27.10). The peripheral nervous system is not affected.

Epidemiology

Multiple sclerosis is second only to head trauma as the leading cause of neurologic disability in early to middle adulthood. Approximately 900,000 people in the United States and up to 3 million worldwide have the disease, for a prevalence rate of about 1.5 cases per 1000 persons with increasing incidence. The disease typically manifests between the ages of 20–40 years and affects women nearly three times as often as men. MS prevalence is historically highest in temperate regions of the world (i.e., Northern and Southern latitudes), and is infrequently seen along the Equator, however, the concept that MS prevalence increases with increasing distance from the equator has been disproved. Dentists who manage 2000 adult patients can expect to have about 3 patients in their practice in whom this condition has been diagnosed.

Pathophysiology and Complications. The cause of MS remains unknown and the most widely accepted theory is that MS is an inflammatory autoimmune disorder caused by autoreactive lymphocytes resulting in demyelination of axons in the CNS. Epidemiologic evidence supports the role of an environmental exposure in MS and two common infectious agents to be implicated in the pathogenesis of this disease are Epstein–Barr virus and human herpesvirus 6. Other viruses that have been implicated in the pathogenesis of MS include measles, mumps, rubella, *Chlamydia pneumoniae*, parainfluenza, vaccinia, and human T-lymphotropic virus 1. Genetic susceptibility to MS exists with the major histocompatibility complex (MHC) on chromosome 6p21 (*HLA-DRB1* gene) identified as one genetic determinant for MS. The MHC encodes the genes for the human leukocyte antigen (HLA) system, and susceptibility to MS lies with the class II alleles, particularly the class II haplotypes DR15, DQ6, and Dw2.

Demyelination of MS occurs in scattered white matter regions in the brain. Areas of myelin loss range in size from 1 mm to several centimeters in diameter. Affected regions show inflammatory demyelination and axonal damage with accumulation of macrophages, T lymphocytes, and plasma cells. The acute MS lesion is accompanied by generation of inflammatory cytokines and antimyelin immunoglobulins that influence macrophages to attack myelin, resulting in tissue destruction, swelling, and breakdown of the blood–brain barrier. Demyelinated disease areas or "plaques" show impairment in axonal conduction and the most commonly affected regions are the optic nerve, periventricular cerebral white matter, and cervical spinal cord.

A significant complication of axonal damage associated with MS is that progressive disease will eventually cause patients to require ambulatory assistance. Historically, 80% of MS patients reached this level of functional disability within 25 years of disease onset. Continued muscle atrophy can lead to restriction to a wheelchair or a bed, thus increasing the chances for development of pneumonia. The risk of ischemic stroke in patients with MS is significantly higher than normal. In a 60-year longitudinal study of MS patients, a median reduction in life expectancy of 7 years and an almost threefold increase in mortality rate in MS was observed compared with the matched general population.

Clinical Presentation

Clinical manifestations vary according to which region of the CNS is involved (motor or sensory region) and what degree of disruption occurs in the myelin sheath. Disturbances in visual function (sometimes resulting in blindness) and abnormal eye movements (nystagmus and double vision) are the most common presenting manifestations. Motor disturbances that affect walking and use of the hands (incoordination, spasticity, difficulty in walking, loss of balance and vertigo, coordination or weakness, tremor or paralysis of a limb) and that cause bowel and bladder incontinence; spastic paresis of skeletal muscles (imprecise speech or tremor); and sensory disturbances, including loss of touch, pain, temperature, and proprioception (numbness, pins and needles sensations) are common. The classic Lhermitte sign is described as sensory shock that runs up and down the spine, which is typically brought on by neck flexion. Fatigue is a major symptom and worsening fatigue occurs in the afternoon. Patients with MS often experience Uhthoff's symptom, which is an exacerbation of neurologic symptoms in response to an elevation of the body's core temperature and is seen in response to increased physical activity. Symptoms exacerbated by heat (e.g., hot baths, sun exposure) and dehydration generally emerge over a few days before stabilizing and subside a few weeks later. Problems with concentration also occur.

The course of MS is unpredictable and depends on the frequency of attacks and the extent of recovery. Categories used to describe the disease are relapsing (occurs in 90% of patients) and progressive (primary and secondary) (Table 27.5). Recovery in most cases is temporary

TABLE 27.5	Clinical Categories of Multiple Sclerosis
Clinical Category	**Key Clinical Features**
Relapsing MS (RMSs)	• Discrete attacks of neurologic dysfunction • Attacks evolve over days to weeks • Substantial to complete recovery between attacks
Secondary progressive MS (SPMSs)	• Always starts as RMS • Deterioration in function not associated with acute attacks • Greater amount of fixed neurologic dysfunction compared to RMS
Primary progressive MS (PPMSs)	• Steady decline in neurologic function since diagnosis • No attacks • Diagnosed later than RMS (approx. 40 years of age)

because remyelination is only transient. Repeated attacks can cause permanent physical damage; however, intellectual function remains intact. Depression and emotional instability are features that commonly accompany this disease.

Laboratory and Diagnostic Findings. The diagnosis of MS usually is made on the basis of information derived from the history, clinical examination, CSF analysis, MRI and sensory evoked potential studies. CSF-specific oligoclonal bands are found in 95% of patients, which indicate evidence of chronic autoimmune dysfunction. MRI scans typically reveal multiple hypodense demyelinated regions (plaques) in white matter, usually near the ventricles (see Fig. 27.10), brainstem cerebellum, and optic nerves. Myelin destruction causes slowing of conduction velocity. The conduction response to visual stimuli (visual evoked potential) or to somatosensory evoked stimuli usually is delayed and altered in amplitude.

Recent formulations of the diagnostic criteria for MS begin with an initial clinical presentation typical for an MS attack known as the McDonald criteria. These are relatively complex criteria, but essentially rely on the presence of at least one distinct monophasic clinical episode lasting greater than 24 h, which is then supported by confirmation of at least two distinct objective correlating findings, either on MRI imaging, evoked potentials, optical imaging, or the presence of CSF-specific oligoclonal bands. These criteria require evidence of more than one distinct lesion occurring at different times (time and space), as the differential diagnosis of a single monophasic attack is broad and includes CNS vascular events, neoplasm, and infections.

Medical Management

Management of MS can be divided into three categories: (1) treatment of acute attacks; (2) disease-modifying

TABLE 27.6   Drugs Used in the Management of Multiple Sclerosis

Drug	Dental Management Considerations	Local Anesthetic or Vasoconstrictor
Primary Drugs		
Interferon beta-1a (Avonex, Rebif) injection	Transient flulike symptoms, anemia uncommon; may increase anticoagulant effects of warfarin	No information to suggest that any special precautions are required
Interferon beta-1b (Betaseron) injection	Transient flulike symptoms, anemia uncommon	No information to suggest that any special precautions are required
Natalizumab, ustekinumab, rituximab	Transient flulike symptoms, anemia uncommon, lymphoma	
Alternatives		
Glatiramer acetate (Copaxone) injection	Ulcerative stomatitis, lymphadenopathy, and salivary gland enlargement	No information to suggest that any special precautions are required
Mitoxantrone (Novantrone) infusion	Leukopenia, risk for cardiac complications and leukemia, mucositis, and stomatitis	No information to suggest that any special precautions are required

therapies; and (3) symptomatic therapy (Table 27.6). Corticosteroids are used to manage both initial attacks and acute exacerbations of MS and high-dose corticosteroids have been shown to hasten recovery. Intravenous methylprednisolone is typically administered at a dose between 500 and 1000 mg/day for 3–5 days to reduce the severity and length of an attack.

A number of disease-modifying agents have been approved for the treatment of MS over the past two decades that have shown various benefits to patients by decreasing relapse rate, clinical disease progression, and imaging-based progression. The choice of drugs is made based on the progression of disease, side effects, risk of complications, type of administration, patient preference, and response rate. Disease-modifying agents include subcutaneously injectable interferon (IFN)-β1a, IFN-β1b (cytokines that modulate immune responsiveness), and glatiramer acetate (mimics MBP). Fingolimod (inhibits T-cell migration), teriflunomide (inhibitor of pyrimidine synthesis), dimethyl fumarate (activates nuclear factor erythroid 2-related factor), cladribine (purine antimetabolite agent), and siponiod (sphingosine 1-phosphate receptor modulator) are oral agents approved for the treatment of MS. Mitoxantrone (Novantrone) is a chemotherapeutic agent administered intravenously that is effective in reducing neurologic disability and frequency of clinical relapses in patients with MS. Natalizumab (binds α-4 integrin), ocrelizumab (anti-CD 20), and alemtuzumab (binds CD52 surface proteins) are monoclonal antibodies administered intravenously.

The complications of MS require management with several drugs. Spasticity is managed with antispastic drugs such as baclofen (a GABA agonist), benzodiazepines (GABA receptor activators), dantrolene (modifier of calcium release in muscle fibers), and tizanidine (Zanaflex) (an α2-adrenergic agonist). An implantable pump for intrathecal administration of baclofen sometimes is used. Poor bladder control is managed with anticholinergics such as oxybutynin (Ditropan) or tolterodine tartrate (Detrol). Fatigue is managed with dedicated rest periods,

exercise, and amantadine (Symmetrel) or modafinil. Paroxysmal events respond to carbamazepine, phenytoin, gabapentin, and pergolide. Serotonin reuptake inhibitors (e.g., fluoxetine [Prozac]) and tricyclic antidepressants (TCAs) are used to manage the depression that accompanies MS in about half the patients. Associated conditions (e.g., trigeminal neuralgia, headache, optic neuritis) often are managed by appropriate health care providers.

Dental Management

The dentist can play an important role in directing the patient with clinical findings suggestive of MS to the appropriate health care provider for definitive diagnosis. Reports of abnormal facial pain (mimicking trigeminal neuralgia), numbness of an extremity, visual disturbance, or muscle weakness are suggestive of MS. The disease should be suspected if onset is progressive over several days, the patient is between 20 and 35 years of age, and afternoon fatigue is a feature. If MS is suspected, oral health care professionals should carefully evaluate cranial nerve function. If cranial nerve abnormalities are detected upon examination and any of the above symptoms are observed, the individual should be referred to a neurologist for further evaluation.

Patients experiencing a relapse are medically unstable to receive routine dental care due to possible airway compromise and limited mobility. Emergency dental care can be provided but may be affected by the medications taken by these patients. In particular, corticosteroids are immunosuppressive, and preprocedural supplementation may be required (see Chapter 15). The physician should be consulted before emergency dental care is provided to these patients.

The optimal time for dental treatment of patients with MS is during periods of remission. The dental care plan should take into consideration the potential effects on oral health of the medications used in management of MS. In particular, the anticholinergics (oxybutynin, tolterodine tartrate) and TCAs can cause a dry or burning mouth, which may require the use of salivary substitutes for relief. If additional relief is needed, the use of pilocarpine or cevimeline (see Appendix C) should be discussed with the physician. Several of the medications used in the treatment of patients with MS are immunosuppressants, thus placing patients at risk for opportunistic and community-acquired infections and for the development of cancers.

Treatment planning changes are dictated by levels of motor impairment and fatigue. Patients with stable disease and little motor spasticity or weakness can receive routine dental care. Patients with advanced disease may require help in transferring to and from the dental chair, may have difficulty maintaining oral hygiene, and may be poor candidates for reconstructive and prosthetic procedures. As fatigue is often worse in the afternoon, short morning appointments are advised. MS patients with significant dysfunction and/or who are medically unstable may require dental treatment in an operating room under general anesthesia due to the inability to undergo treatment in an outpatient setting.

Oral Manifestations. Oral manifestations of MS are reported to occur in 2%−3% of affected persons. These features may serve as the presenting symptoms of MS. The most common features include dysarthria, paresthesia, numbness of the orofacial structures, and trigeminal neuralgia. Dysarthria produces slow, irregular speech with unusual separation of syllables of words, referred to as *scanning speech*. During an attack, the patient may experience facial paresthesia, and muscles of facial expression (especially the periorbital) can undulate in a wavelike motion. The term *myokymia* is used to describe these unusual muscle movements, which have been said to feel like a "bag of worms" on palpation. Referral to a physician is advised if the condition has not been diagnosed.

Trigeminal neuralgia may be an initial manifestation of MS in up to 5% of cases. Features of MS-related TGN include the possible absence of trigger zones and continuous pain with lower intensity. Patients with MS may also demonstrate neuropathy of the maxillary (V2) and mandibular branches (V3) of the trigeminal nerve, which may include burning, tingling, and/or reduced sensation. Relief of trigeminal neuralgia and neuropathic pain can be obtained with the use of carbamazepine, oxcarbazepine, clonazepam, amitriptyline, or surgery.

Cerebrospinal Fluid Shunts

Within the spectrum of neurologic disorders is the condition known as *hydrocephalus*, characterized by an increasing accumulation of CSF within the cerebral ventricles. Management of hydrocephalus often requires placement of a shunt within cerebral ventricles and peripheral cavities to reduce increased CSF pressure. Several types of shunts are used to reduce fluid pressure; ventriculoperitoneal, ventriculoatrial, ventriculopleural, and lumboperitoneal are the most common types. In the United States, around 75,000 CSF shunts are placed each year.

With respect to dentistry, the most significant concern is the risk of CSF shunt infection. Overall, shunt infection rates range from about 5% to 15%, with most infections resulting from wound contamination. Almost 70% of infections are caused by skin flora, i.e., staphylococcal organisms. CSF shunt infections usually occur within 1 month after implantation. The infection rate is higher for ventriculoperitoneal shunts than for ventriculoatrial shunts. However, other types of complications include thromboemboli, severe complications of infection, and shunt malfunctions.

Cerebrospinal fluid shunts do not appear to increase the risk for infection produced by hematogenous seeding of bacteria after dental procedures. Thus, the American Heart Association has issued a statement indicating that antibiotic prophylaxis is not recommended for patients with CSF shunts who are undergoing dental procedures.

BIBLIOGRAPHY

1. Buchbender M, Schlee N, Kesting MR, et al. A prospective comparative study to assess the risk of postoperative bleeding after dental surgery while on medication with direct oral anticoagulants, antiplatelet agents, or vitamin K antagonists. *BMC Oral Health*. 2021;21:504.
2. Prat A. Special issue on molecular basis of multiple sclerosis. *Biochim Biophys Acta*. 2011;1812:131.
3. Albers GW, Bates VE, Clark WM, et al. Intravenous tissue-type plasminogen activator for treatment of acute stroke. *JAMA*. 2000;283:1145−1150.
4. Aoki N. Lumboperitoneal shunt: clinical implications, complications, and comparison with ventriculoperitoneal shunt. *Neurosurgery*. 1990;26:998−1003.
5. Ardekian L, Gaspar R, Peled M, Brener B, Laufer D. Does low-dose aspirin therapy complicate oral surgical procedures? *J Am Dent Assoc*. 2000;131:331−335.
6. Baddour LM, Bettmann MA, Bolger AF, et al. AHA. Nonvalvular cardiovascular device related infections. *Circulation*. 2003;108:2015−2031.
7. Bähr M. Special issue on multiple sclerosis. *Exp Neurol*. 2010;225:1.
8. Ballard C, Gauthier S, Corbett A, Brayne C, Aarsland D, Jones E. Alzheimer's disease. *Lancet*. 2011;377:1019−1031.
9. Bermel RA, Cohen JA. Multiple sclerosis: advances in understanding pathogenesis and emergence of oral treatment options. *Lancet Neurol*. 2011;10:4−5.
10. Blinder D, Manor Y, Martinowitz U, Taicher S, Hashomer T, et al. Dental extractions in patients maintained on continued oral anticoagulant: comparison of local hemostatic modalities. *Oral Surg Oral Med Oral Pathol Oral Radiol Endod*. 1999;88:137−140.
11. Budson AE, Solomon PR. New criteria for Alzheimer disease and mild cognitive impairment: implications for the practicing clinician. *Neurologist*. 2012;18:356−363.
12. Calvet D, Touze E, Oppenheim C, et al. DWI lesions and TIA etiology improve the prediction of stroke after TIA. *Stroke*. 2009;40:187−192.
13. Camfield C, Camfield P. Management guidelines for children with idiopathic generalized epilepsy. *Epilepsia*. 2005;46(suppl 9):112−116.

14. CDC. Vital signs: awareness and treatment of uncontrolled hypertension among adults—United States, 2003–2010. *MMWR Morb Mortal Wkly Rep*. 2012;61: 703–709.

15. Chandratheva A, Mehta Z, Geraghty OC, et al. Population-based study of risk and predictors of stroke in the first few hours after a TIA. *Neurology*. 2009;72: 1941–1947.

16. Chern JJ, Macias CG, Jea A, Curry D, Luerssen T, Whitehead W. Effectiveness of a clinical pathway for patients with cerebrospinal fluid shunt malfunction. *J Neurosurg Pediatr*. 2010;6:318–324.

17. Cree BA, Hauser SL. Multiple sclerosis. In: Jameson J, et al., eds. *Harrison's Principles of Internal Medicine, 20e*. New York: McGraw Hill; 2018:1–27.

18. Cummings JL. Alzheimer's disease. *N Engl J Med*. 2004; 351:56–67.

19. Danhauer SC, Miller CS, Rhodus NL, Carlson CR, et al. Impact of criteria-based diagnosis of burning mouth syndrome on treatment outcome. *J Orofac Pain*. 2002;16: 305–311.

20. Del Zoppo GJ, Saver JL, Jauch EC, Adams Jr HP. American Heart Association Stroke Council. Expansion of the time window for treatment of acute ischemic stroke with intravenous tissue plasminogen activator: a science advisory from the American Heart Association/American Stroke Association. *Stroke*. 2009;40:2945–2948.

21. Elad S, Zadik Y, Kaufman E, et al. A new management approach for dental treatment after a cerebrovascular event: a comparative retrospective study. *Oral Surg Oral Med Oral Pathol Oral Radiol Endod*. 2010;110: 145–150.

22. Fatahzadeh M, Glick M. Stroke: epidemiology, classification, risk factors, complications, diagnosis, prevention, and medical and dental management. *Oral Surg Oral Med Oral Pathol Oral Radiol Endod*. 2006;102:180–191.

23. Feigin V, Norrving B, Sudlow CLM, Sacco RL. Updated criteria for population-based stroke and transient ischemic attack incidence studies for the 21st century. *Stroke*. 2018; 49:2248–2255.

24. Fisher RS, Cross JH, French JA, et al. Operational classification of seizure types by the international League against epilepsy: position paper of the ILAE commission for classification and terminology. *Epilepsia*. 2017;58: 522–530.

25. Ford PJ, Amazaki K, Seymour GJ. Cardiovascular and oral disease interactions: what is the evidence? *Prim Dent Care*. 2007;14:59–66.

26. Fox EJ. Management of worsening multiple sclerosis with mitoxantrone: a review. *Clin Therapeut*. 2006;28: 461–474.

27. Fox RJ, Bethoux F, Goldman MD, Cohen JA. Multiple sclerosis: advances in understanding, diagnosing, and treating the underlying disease. *Cleve Clin J Med*. 2006; 73:91–102.

28. Franco V, Crema F, Iudice A, Zaccara G, Grillo E. Novel treatment options for epilepsy: focus on perampanel. *Pharmacol Res*. 2013;70:35–40.

29. Freedman MS. Present and emerging therapies for multiple sclerosis. *Continuum*. 2013;19:968–991.

30. Friedlander AH. Calcified carotid artery atheromas. *J Am Dent Assoc*. 2007;138:1191–1192.

31. Friedlander AH, Mahler M, Norman KM, Ettinger RL. Parkinson disease: systemic and orofacial manifestations, medical and dental management. *J Am Dent Assoc*. 2009; 140:658–669.

32. Furlan A, Higashida R, Wechsler L, et al. Intra-arterial prourokinase for acute ischemic stroke. *JAMA*. 1999; 282:2003–2011.

33. Gardner P, Leipzig TJ, Sadigh M. Infections of cerebrovascular shunts. *Curr Clin Top Infect Dis*. 1989;9: 185–214.

34. Giovannoni G, Cutter GR, Lunemann J, et al. Infectious causes of multiple sclerosis. *Lancet Neurol*. 2006;5: 887–894.

35. Go AS, Mozaffarian D, Roger VL, et al. Heart disease and stroke statistics—2013 update: a report from the American Heart Association. *Circulation*. 2013;127:e6–e245.

36. Go AS, Mozaffarian D, Roger VL, et al. Executive summary: heart disease and stroke statistics—2014 update: a report from the American Heart Association. *Circulation*. 2014;129:399–410.

37. Godazandeh K, Martinez Sosa S, Wu J, Zakrzewska JM. Trigeminal neuralgia: comparison of characteristics and impact in patients with or without multiple sclerosis. *Mult Scler Relat Disord*. 2019;34:41–46.

38. Grau-López L, Sierra S, Martínez-Cáceres E, Ramo-Tello C. Analysis of the pain in multiple sclerosis patients. *Neurologia*. 2011;26:208–213.

39. Greenwood RS. Adverse effects of antiepileptic drugs. *Epilepsia*. 2000;41(suppl 2):S42–S52.

40. Grover S, Rhodus NL. Parkinson's disease: dental treatment considerations. *NW Dent*. 2011;90:13–19.

41. Guerrini R. Epilepsy in children. *Lancet*. 2006;367: 499–524.

42. Haacke EM. Chronic cerebral spinal venous insufficiency in multiple sclerosis. *Expert Rev Neurother*. 2011;11:5–9.

43. Hacke W, Kaste M, Bluhmki E, et al. Thrombolysis with alteplase 3 to 4.5 hours after acute ischemic stroke. *N Engl J Med*. 2008;359:1317–1329.

44. Hall MJ, Levant S, DeFrances CJ. *Hospitalization for Stroke in U.S. Hospitals, 1989–2009 [PDF-322K]*. NCHS Data Brief, No. 95. Hyattsville, MD: National Center for Health Statistics; 2012.

45. Hallet M, Litvan I. Evaluation of surgery for Parkinson's disease. *Neurol Res*. 1999;53:1910–1921.

46. Henry RG, Smith BJ. Managing older patients who have neurologic disease: Alzheimer disease and cerebrovascular accident. *Dent Clin N Am*. 2009;53:269–294, ix.

47. Hirsch E, Graybiel AM, Agid YA. Melanized dopaminergic neurons are differentially susceptible to degeneration in Parkinson's disease. *Nature*. 1988;334:345–348.

48. Hu Z, Ou Y, Duan K, Jiang X. Inflammation: a bridge between postoperative cognitive dysfunction and Alzheimer's disease. *Med Hypotheses*. 2010;74:722–724.

49. Jeske AH, Suchko GD, ADA Council on Scientific Affairs and Division of Science, et al. Lack of a scientific basis for routine discontinuation of oral anticoagulation therapy before dental treatment. *J Am Dent Assoc*. 2003;134: 1492–1497.

50. Johnson-Leong C, Rada RE. The use of low-molecular-weight heparins in outpatient oral surgery for patients receiving anticoagulation therapy. *J Am Dent Assoc*. 2002;133:1083–1087.

51. Khaja A. Acute ischemic stroke management: administration of thrombolytics, neuroprotectants, and general principles of medical management. *Neurol Clin.* 2008;26:943–961.

52. Kieseier BC, Jeffery DR. Chemotherapeutics in the treatment of multiple sclerosis. *Ther Adv Neurol Disord.* 2010;3:277–291.

53. Koch-Henriksen N, Sorensen PS. The changing demographic pattern of multiple sclerosis epidemiology. *Lancet Neurol.* 2010;9:520–532.

54. Konecny P, Elfmark M, Urbanek K. Facial paresis after stroke and its impact on patients' facial movement and mental status. *J Rehabil Med.* 2011;43:73–75.

55. Kordower JH, Emborg ME, Bloch J, et al. Neurogeneration prevented by lentiviral vector. *Science.* 2000;290:767–773.

56. Levin EC, Acharya NK, Sedeyn JC, et al. Neuronal expression of vimentin in the Alzheimer's disease brain may be part of a generalized dendritic damage-response mechanism. *Brain Res.* 2009;1298:194–207.

57. Lewandowski L, Osmola K, Grodzki J. Dyskinesias of the tongue and other face structures. *Ann Acad Med Stetin.* 2006;52(suppl 3):61–63.

58. Lin R, Charlesworth J, van der Mei I, Taylor BV. The genetics of multiple sclerosis. *Practical Neurol.* 2012;12:279–288.

59. Lowenstein D. Seizures and epilepsy. In: Jameson J, et al., eds. *Harrison's Principles of Internal Medicine, 20e.* New York: McGraw Hill; 2018:1–36.

60. Lunde HMB, Assmus J, Myhr KM, Bø L, Grytten N. Survival and cause of death in multiple sclerosis: a 60-year longitudinal population study. *J Neurol Neurosurg Psychiatry.* 2017;88:621–625.

61. Lundkvist B, Koskinen LO, Birgander R, Eklund A, Malm J, et al. Cerebrospinal fluid dynamics and long-term survival of the Strata valve in idiopathic normal pressure hydrocephalus. *Acta Neurol Scand.* 2011;124:115–121.

62. Marler JR, Tilley BC, Lu M, et al. Early stroke treatment associated with better outcome: the NINDS rt-PA stroke study. *Neurology.* 2000;55:1649–1655.

63. Masood F, Wild RC, Jenkins J, Radfar L. Presence of carotid artery calcification on panoramic radiographs of patients with chronic diseases. *Gen Dent.* 2009;57:39–44.

64. Miller DM, Weinstock-Guttman B, Bethoux F, et al. A meta-analysis of methylprednisolone in recovery from multiple sclerosis exacerbations. *Mult Scler.* 2000;6:267–273.

65. Minassian C, D'Aiuto F, Hingorani AD, Smeeth L, et al. Invasive dental treatment and risk for vascular events: a self-controlled case series. *Ann Intern Med.* 2010;153:499–506.

66. Mollaoğlu M, Fertelli TK, Tuncay FÖ. Disability in elderly patients with chronic neurological illness: stroke, multiple sclerosis and epilepsy. *Arch Gerontol Geriatr.* 2011;53:e227–e231.

67. Morris JC, Ernesto C, Schafer K, et al. Clinical dementia rating training and reliability in multicenter studies. *Neurology.* 2012;48:1508–1510.

68. Motl RW, McAuley E, Sandroff BM, Hubbard EA. Descriptive epidemiology of multiple sclerosis. *Acta Neurol Scand.* 2015;131:422–425.

69. Mozaffarian D, Benjamin EJ, Go AS, et al. Heart disease and stroke statistics—2015 update: a report from the American Heart Association. *Circulation.* 2015;131:e29–e322.

70. Mupparapu M, Kim IH. Calcified carotid artery atheroma and stroke: a systematic review. *J Am Dent Assoc.* 2007;138:483–492.

71. Nogueira RG, Jadhav AP, Haussen DC, et al. Thrombectomy 6 to 24 hours after stroke with a mismatch between deficit and infarct. *N Engl J Med.* 2018;378:11–21.

72. Olanow CW, Klein C, Schapira AHV. Parkinson's disease. In: Jameson J, et al., eds. *Harrison's Principles of Internal Medicine, 20e.* New York: McGraw Hill; 2018:1–24.

73. Ovbiagele B, Goldstein LB, Higashida RT, et al. Forecasting the future of stroke in the United States: a policy statement from the American heart association and American stroke association. *Stroke.* 2013;44:2361–2375.

74. Parkinson's Foundation. Statistics. https://www.parkinson.org/Understanding-Parkinsons/Statistics. Accessed September 27, 2021.

75. Paulsen AH, Lundar T, Lindegaard KF. Twenty-year outcome in young adults with childhood hydrocephalus: assessment of surgical outcome, work participation, and health-related quality of life. *J Neurosurg Pediatr.* 2010;6:527–535.

76. Popova NF, Kamchatnov PR, Riabukhina OV, et al. Omaron in the complex treatment of patients with multiple sclerosis. *Zh Nevrol Psikhiatr Im S S Korsakova.* 2010;110:17–20.

77. Purroy F, Jimenez Caballero PE, Gorospe A, et al. Prediction of early stroke recurrence in transient ischemic attack patients from the PROMAPA study: a comparison of prognostic risk scores. *Cerebrovasc Dis.* 2012;33:182–189.

78. Rae-Grant A, Day GS, Marrie RA, et al. Practice guideline recommendations summary: disease-modifying therapies for adults with multiple sclerosis: report of the Guideline Development, Dissemination, and Implementation Subcommittee of the American Academy of Neurology. *Neurology.* 2018;90:777–788.

79. Rae-Grant A, Day GS, Marrie RA, et al. Comprehensive systematic review summary: disease-modifying therapies for adults with multiple sclerosis: report of the Guideline Development, Dissemination, and Implementation Subcommittee of the American Academy of Neurology. *Neurology.* 2018;90:789–800.

80. Ravina B, Elm J, Camicioli R, et al. The course of depressive symptoms in early Parkinson's disease. *Mov Disord.* 2009;24:1306–1311.

81. Ravina B, Marder K, Fernandez HH, et al. Diagnostic criteria for psychosis in Parkinson's disease: report of an NINDS, NIMH work group. *Mov Disord.* 2007;22:1061–1068.

82. Reich DS, Lucchinetti CF, Calabresi PA. Multiple sclerosis. *N Engl J Med.* 2018;378:169–180.

83. Reitz C, Mayeux R. Alzheimer disease: epidemiology, diagnostic criteria, risk factors and biomarkers. *Biochem Pharmacol.* 2014;88:640–651.

84. Rejnefelt I, Andersson P, Renvert S. Oral health status in individuals with dementia living in special facilities. *Int J Dent Hyg.* 2006;4:67–71.

85. Rhodus NL, Carlson CR, Miller CS. Burning mouth (syndrome) disorder. *Quintessence Int.* 2003;34:587−593.

86. Riley CS, Tullman MJ. Multiple sclerosis. In: Rowland LP, Pedley TA, eds. *Merritt's Neurology.* 12th ed. Philadelphia, PA: Lippincott, Williams, & Wilkins; 2010:903−918.

87. Rothwell PM, Giles MF, Chandratheva A, et al. Effect of urgent treatment of transient ischaemic attack and minor stroke on early recurrent stroke (EXPRESS study): a prospective population-based sequential comparison. *Lancet.* 2007;370:1432−1442.

88. Rothwell PM, Warlow CP. Timing of TIAs preceding stroke: time window for prevention is very short. *Neurology.* 2005;64:817−820.

89. Sacco D, Frost DE. Dental management of patients with stroke or Alzheimer's disease. *Dent Clin N Am.* 2006;50:625−633, viii.

90. Sacco RL, Foulkes MA, Mohr JP, et al. Determinants of early recurrence of cerebral infarction. The Stroke Data Bank. *Stroke.* 1989;20:983−989.

91. Sarmast ST, Abdullahi AM, Jahan N. Current classification of seizures and epilepsies: scope, Limitations and recommendations for future action. *Cureus.* 2020;12:e10549.

92. Scheffer IE, Berkovic S, Capovilla G, et al. ILAE classification of the epilepsies: position paper of the ILAE Commission for Classification and Terminology. *Epilepsia.* 2017;58:512−521.

93. Seely WW, Miller BL. Alzheimer's disease. In: Jameson J, Fauci A, Kasper D, Hauser S, Longo D, Loscalzo J, eds. *Harrison's Principles of Internal Medicine, 20e.* New York: McGraw Hill; 2018:1−12.

94. Shobha N, Bhatia R, Barber PA. Dental procedures and stroke: a case of vertebral artery dissection. *J Can Dent Assoc.* 2010;76:a82.

95. Sillanpaa M, Shinnar S. Long-term mortality in childhood-onset epilepsy. *N Engl J Med.* 2010;363:2522−2529.

96. Sloka S, Silva C, Pryse-Phillips W, et al. A quantitative analysis of suspected environmental causes of MS. *Can J Neurol Sci.* 2011;38:98−105.

97. Smith WS, Claiborne Johnston S, Claude Hempill III J. Cerebrovascular diseases. In: Jameson J, Fauci A, Kasper D, Hauser S, Longo D, Loscalzo J, eds. *Harrison's Principles of Internal Medicine, 20e.* New York: McGraw Hill; 2018:1−21.

98. Smith WS, Claiborne Johnston S, Claude Hempill III J. Ischemic stroke. In: Jameson J, Fauci A, Kasper D, Hauser S, Longo D, Loscalzo J, eds. *Harrison's Principles of Internal Medicine, 20e.* New York: McGraw Hill; 2018:1−25.

99. Smith WS, Claiborne Johnston S, Claude Hempill III J. Intracranial hemorrhage. In: Jameson J, Fauci A, Kasper D, Hauser S, Longo D, Loscalzo J, eds. *Harrison's Principles of Internal Medicine, 20e.* New York: McGraw Hill; 2018:1−12.

100. Sormani M, Bonzano L, Roccatagliata L, De Stefano N. Magnetic resonance imaging as surrogate for clinical endpoints in multiple sclerosis: data on novel oral drugs. *Mult Scler J.* 2011;17:630−633.

101. Souslova T, Marple TC, Spiekerman AM, Mohammed AA. Personalized medicine in Alzheimer's disease and depression. *Contemp Clin Trials.* 2013;36:616−623.

102. Sperling MR, Feldman H, Kinman J, Liporace JD, O'Connor MJ. Seizure control and mortality in epilepsy. *Ann Neurol.* 1999;46:45−50.

103. Tecoma ES, Iragui VJ. Vagus nerve stimulation use and effect in epilepsy: what have we learned? *Epilepsy Behav.* 2006;8:127−136.

104. Thompson AJ, Banwell BL, Barkhof F, et al. Diagnosis of multiple sclerosis: 2017 revisions of the McDonald criteria. *Lancet Neurol.* 2018;17:162−173.

105. Thompson AJ, Baranzini SE, Geurts J, Hemmer B, Ciccarelli O. Multiple sclerosis. *Lancet.* 2018;391:1622−1636.

106. Tseng CH, Huang WS, Lin CK, Chang YJ. Increased risk of ischemic stroke among patients with multiple sclerosis. *Eur J Neurol.* 2015;22:500−506.

107. Vangen-Lonne AM, Wilsgaard T, Johnsen SH, et al. Declining incidence of ischemic stroke: what is the impact of changing risk factors? The Tromso study 1995 to 2012. *Stroke.* 2017;48:544−550.

108. Vargas DL, Tyor WR. Update on disease-modifying therapies for multiple sclerosis. *J Invest Med.* 2017;65:883−891.

109. Wahl MJ. Myths of dental surgery in patients receiving anticoagulant therapy. *J Am Dent Assoc.* 2000;131:77−81.

110. Walker ML. Shunt survival. *J Neurosurg Pediatr.* 2010;6:526.

111. Walters KJ, Meador A, Galdo JA, Ciarrocca K. A pharmacotherapy review of the novel, oral antithrombotics. *Spec Care Dent.* 2017;37:62−70.

112. Weiner HL. Multiple sclerosis is an inflammatory T-cell-mediated autoimmune disease. *Arch Neurol.* 2004;61:1613−1615.

113. Wilkinson DG, Francis PT, Schwam E, Payne-Parrish J. Cholinesterase inhibitors used in the treatment of Alzheimer's disease: the relationship between pharmacological effects and clinical efficacy. *Drugs Aging.* 2004;21:453−478.

114. Wolf PA, D'Agostino RB, Belanger AJ, Kannel WB. Probability of stroke: a risk profile from the Framingham Study. *Stroke.* 1991;22:312−318.

115. Yokota O, Tsuchiya K, Uchihara T, et al. Lewy body variant of Alzheimer's disease or cerebral type Lewy body disease? Two autopsy cases of presenile onset with minimal involvement of the brainstem. *Neuropathology.* 2007;27:21−35.

116. Yoshida H, Terada S, Ishizu H, et al. An autopsy case of Creutzfeldt−Jakob disease with a V180I mutation of the PrP gene and Alzheimer-type pathology. *Neuropathology.* 2010;30:159−164.

117. Zakrzewska JM, Wu J, Brathwaite TS. A systematic review of the management of trigeminal neuralgia in patients with multiple sclerosis. *World Neurosurg.* 2018;111:291−306.

118. Zesiewicz TA. Parkinson disease. *Continuum.* 2019;25:896−918.

Psychiatric Disorders

1. Psychiatric disorders are common in the general population, with anxiety and depression each affecting approximately 5% of adults in the United States; patients visiting a dentist may be undiagnosed or may be diagnosed but suboptimally managed.
2. Patients with certain psychiatric disorders may be less attentive to their oral hygiene and at an increased risk for dental disease.
3. Medications used to manage psychiatric disorders may be associated with hyposalivation, xerostomia, and other orofacial side effects.
4. Patients with certain psychiatric disorders may present with oral findings related to habitual behaviors, stress, and self-injury.

Approximately one-third of the population in the United States will have at least one psychiatric disorder during their lifetime, and 20%–30% of adults in the United States will experience one or more psychiatric disorders during a 1-year period (Table 28.1). The American Psychiatric Association published the fifth edition of the *Diagnostic and Statistical Manual of Mental Disorders* (DSM-5) in 2013. It includes detailed descriptions of, and

TABLE 28.1 Important Psychiatric Syndromes and Disorders

Syndrome	Main Symptoms and Signs	May Occur as Part of These Disorders
Neurocognitive	Deficits in intellectual functions (e.g., level of consciousness, orientation, attention, memory, language, praxis, visuospatial, executive functions)	Neurocognitive disorders Intellectual disability (if onset in childhood)
Mood: depressive	Lowered mood, anhedonia, negativistic thoughts, neurovegetative symptoms	Neurocognitive disorders Mood disorders (bipolar or depressive) (primary or secondary) Psychotic disorders (schizoaffective disorder)
Mood: manic	Elevated or irritable mood, grandiosity, goal-directed hyperactivity with increased energy, pressured speech, decreased sleep need	Neurocognitive disorders Bipolar disorder (primary or secondary) Psychotic disorders (schizoaffective disorder)
Anxiety	All include anxious mood and associated physiologic symptoms (e.g., palpitations, tremors, diaphoresis); may include various types of dysfunctional thoughts (e.g., catastrophic fears, obsessions, flashbacks) and behavior (e.g., compulsions, avoidance behavior)	Neurocognitive disorders Mood disorders (bipolar or depressive) (primary or secondary) Psychotic disorders (primary or secondary) Trauma- and stressor-related disorders Anxiety disorders (primary or secondary) Obsessive-compulsive and related disorders
Psychotic	Impairments in reality testing: delusions, hallucinations, thought process derailments	Neurocognitive disorders Mood disorders (bipolar or depressive) (primary or secondary) Psychotic disorders
Somatic symptom syndromes	Somatic symptoms with associated distressing thoughts, feelings, or behaviors	Mood disorders (bipolar or depressive) (primary or secondary) Anxiety disorders (primary or secondary) Obsessive-compulsive and related disorders Trauma- and stressor-related disorders Somatic symptom disorders
Personality pathology	Enduring patterns of dysfunctional emotional regulation, thought patterns, interpersonal behavior, impulse regulation	Neurocognitive disorders (dementia) Personality change due to another medical condition Personality disorders

From Lyness JM: *Author Summary of American Psychiatric Association categories and criteria.* In Goldman L, Schafer A: Goldman-Cecil Medicine, ed 26, Elsevier, 2020, St. Louis.

the most current diagnostic criteria for, neurodevelopmental disorders, schizophrenia spectrum and other psychotic disorders, bipolar and related disorders, depressive disorders, anxiety disorders, feeding and eating disorders, sleep–wake disorders, substance-related disorders, addictive disorders, and other topics. It should be noted that psychiatric disorders do not always fit neatly within the boundaries of a single diagnosis, and some symptom domains (e.g., depression and anxiety) involve multiple diagnostic categories and may reflect common underlying vulnerabilities for other disorders.

Psychiatric disorders can influence and impact oral health and dental care in several ways, including behavioral and patient management considerations, potential for medication side effects and interactions, and oral manifestations of disease. The dentist must have a broad understanding and recognition of psychiatric disorders, how these disorders are managed, and the potential impact on oral health and delivery of oral health care. While this chapter does not provide an exhaustive overview of all conditions described in DSM-5, the most important and relevant conditions related to oral health and the practice of dentistry are reviewed.

NEURODEVELOPMENTAL DISORDERS

The neurodevelopmental disorders consist of a group of conditions with onset in the developmental period, often clinically evident in early childhood, that are characterized by developmental deficits that produce impairments of personal, social, intellectual, or occupational functioning. The developmental deficits are wide ranging from very specific limitations of learning or control of executive functions to global impairments of social skills or intelligence. This section focuses on autism spectrum disorder (ASD) and attention deficit/hyperactivity disorder (ADHD), common neurodevelopmental psychiatric disorders that are frequently encountered in the general population and in dental practices.

Epidemiology and Etiology

Autism Spectrum Disorder. The overall prevalence of ASD in Europe, Asia, and the United States ranges from 1 in 40 to 1 in 500. While the prevalence of ASD has increased over time (especially since the late 1990s), epidemiologic evidence suggests that this can largely be attributable to changes in case definition and increased awareness of the diagnosis. The male-to-female ratio is between three and four to one, although it is thought that ASD may be underdiagnosed in females. Siblings of affected patients are at increased risk for being diagnosed with ASD. There are various neurodevelopmental conditions (e.g., intellectual disability, attention deficit hyperactivity disorder, epilepsy) and genetic syndromes (e.g., tuberous sclerosis complex, Fragile X syndrome) that are associated with ASD.

The pathoetiology of ASD is incompletely understood and likely multifactorial and complex. While family history suggests a genetic basis, it is presumed that interactions between multiple genes as well as epigenetic factors and exposure to environmental modifiers contribute to the development and variable expression of ASD. Certain brain abnormalities (structural, chemical) have been identified and are believed to be contributing factors. Advanced parental age has also been associated with increased risk of ASD being diagnosed.

Attention Deficit/Hyperactivity Disorder. The reported prevalence of ADHD in children is estimated to be approximately 7.2% based on international studies and is more common in boys than girls (male to female ratio 4:1 for the predominantly hyperactive type and 2:1 for the predominantly inattentive type). In adults, the reported prevalence in the United States is 4.4% and 3.4% internationally. While ADHD can be initially diagnosed in adulthood, most patients are diagnosed during childhood, and most children who are diagnosed with ADHD continue to meet criteria for the disorder as adults. There is an increased risk of ADHD in first-degree relatives of patients with ADHD, and twin studies indicate a high degree of heritability. Comorbid psychiatric conditions are common and include mood disorders, anxiety, learning disabilities, and, in adults, substance use disorders.

The pathoetiology of ADHD is similarly incompletely understood. Functional brain imaging studies, animal studies, and response to medications with noradrenergic activity (e.g., methylphenidate) all suggest a genetic imbalance of catecholamine metabolism in the cerebral cortex. Structural brain imaging demonstrates significant abnormalities in many areas (e.g., smaller prefrontal cortical volumes, reduced thickness of the anterior cingulate cortex, and cortical thinning in bilateral superior frontal brain regions). Further, abnormalities have been noted in the caudate, putamen, and globus pallidus (subcortical structures that are part of the neural circuitry underlying motor control, executive functions, inhibition of behavior, and the modulation of reward pathways). As noradrenaline and dopamine activity influence behavior and cognition through fronto-striato-cerebellar circuitry, hypoactivity of these neurotransmitters appear to largely mediate the clinical features of ADHD.

Clinical Presentation and Medical Management

Autism Spectrum Disorder. The DSM-5 characterizes ASD as persistent deficits in social communication and interaction (e.g., deficits in social reciprocity; nonverbal communicative behaviors; and skills in developing, maintaining, and understanding relationships), and restricted, repetitive patterns of behavior, interests, or activities. These features must be present in early development; however, because symptoms may not be evident until social demands exceed limited capacities, there is no specified age threshold for "early development". Features that may be evident within the first 2 years of life include speech/language delays, failure to make eye contact, and limited interest in socializing. Children may achieve early developmental milestones, but then subsequently plateau or regress. Older toddlers and preschool-aged children often display speech/language delays and lack of interest in socializing, and may display restricted interests and marked resistance to change.

Persons who have ASD demonstrate limited and/or atypical social attention behaviors with respect to frequency, duration, and/or complexity. Examples include limited social interaction with siblings/peers, lack of typical social play interactions, lack of response to another's bid for social interaction, and inappropriate social interactions with respect to space and communication. Children with ASD have difficulty interpreting nonverbal communication (e.g., facial expressions, gestures) and have impaired pragmatic language skills, further complicating the ability to communicate with others effectively.

Management of ASD is complex and requires an individualized, comprehensive, and multidisciplinary approach. Intervention is most effective when started as early as possible. In addition to the patient's physician, involvement of other specialties may include psychology, speech and language, occupational therapy, audiology, and social work. While psychiatric medications may be indicated for management of certain aspects of a given patient's condition (e.g., anxiety, self-injury), these medications alone are not sufficient and must be used in conjunction and coordination with behavioral and environmental interventions. Children with ASD may wander off, in search of an enjoyable pursuit, or to escape something bothersome, potentially putting them at risk for accidents and injuries (e.g., accidental drowning, traffic-related injury). While prognosis is highly variable, features that are associated with less favorable long-term outcomes include lack of joint attention (coordination of attention with another person) by age 4, lack of functional speech by age 5, and intelligence quotient less than 70, seizures or other comorbidities.

Attention Deficit/Hyperactivity Disorder. ADHD is characterized by two categories of core symptoms: *hyperactivity/impulsivity* and *inattention*. Hyperactive and impulsive symptoms (e.g., excessive fidgeting, difficulty remaining seated, restlessness, excessive talking, interruption) are typically evident by age 4 and peak in severity around age 7−8, after which hyperactivity tends to subside but impulsivity persists. The inattentive subtype is characterized by reduced ability to focus attention (e.g., lack of attention to detail, careless mistakes, difficulty organizing and following through with things, easy distraction, forgetfulness) and may not be evident until age 8 or 9. As ADHD tends to continue into adulthood, characteristics in adults include problems with organization, prioritization, focus, forgetfulness, and time management and being able to follow through and complete tasks.

Management of ADHD requires a multifaceted approach that may include any of the following: behavioral therapy, medication, school-based programs, and psychologic interventions. Target goals, for example improved relationships or school performance, should be realistic, achievable, and measurable. Behavioral interventions include environmental modifications designed to change behavior through rewards rather than punishment. Examples include maintaining a daily schedule, minimizing distractions, setting goals, and rewarding positive behaviors.

First-line pharmacologic therapy begins with stimulants which effectively increase norepinephrine and dopamine levels at the central nervous system synapses. These include methylphenidate, a sympathomimetic stimulant that in part works through blocking reuptake of norepinephrine and dopamine, and amphetamines (e.g., dextroamphetamine). In addition to risk of various side effects with stimulants (e.g., decreased appetite, poor growth, mood lability), medication diversion and misuse, especially in adolescents and adults, is a common problem. Selective norepinephrine reuptake inhibitors, such as atomoxetine, can also be used as an alternative to methylphenidate. For patients who do not respond adequately to stimulants or selective norepinephrine reuptake inhibitors, or who experience unacceptable side effects, other medications, such as alpha-2-adrenergic agonists (e.g., guanfacine, clonidine), may be considered, although these agents are generally less effective and have sedative properties.

SCHIZOPHRENIA SPECTRUM AND OTHER PSYCHOTIC DISORDERS

Schizophrenia spectrum and other psychotic disorders are defined by abnormalities in one or more of the following domains: delusions, hallucinations, disorganized thinking (speech), grossly disorganized or abnormal motor behavior (including catatonia), and negative symptoms (characterized broadly as absence or lack of normal mental function involving thinking, behavior, and perception). This section primarily focuses on the diagnosis of schizophrenia.

Epidemiology and Etiology

The lifetime prevalence rate for schizophrenic disorders is about 1%−1.5% (across all cultures and both genders), and onset usually is during adolescence or early adulthood. Evidence for a genetic relationship has come from family, twin, and adoption studies; however, over 80% of patients do not have a parent or a sibling with the disease.

The predominant biologic hypothesis for a neurophysiologic defect in schizophrenia is the dopamine hypothesis, in which the symptoms of schizophrenia are caused in part by a disturbance in dopamine-mediated neuronal pathways in the brain. Drugs, medical illness, stressful psychosocial events, viral infection, and family situations characterized by conflicting and self-contradictory forms of communication have been reported to precipitate schizophrenia in susceptible people.

Clinical Presentation and Medical Management

Schizophrenia is a heterogeneous clinical syndrome characterized by a range of cognitive, behavioral, and emotional dysfunctions but with no single symptom being pathognomonic of the disorder. Schizophrenia can be diagnosed in patients who have two or more of the following symptoms for at least 1 month: hallucinations, delusions, disorganized speech, grossly disorganized or catatonic behavior, or negative symptoms such as affective flattening, alogia (poverty of speech, lack of additional unprompted content), or avolition (lack of desire, drive, or motivation). In addition, the patient's social or occupational functioning must have deteriorated.

Patients with schizophrenia show psychotic symptoms consisting of delusions, hallucinations, incoherence, catatonic behavior, or flat or grossly inappropriate affect. Delusions and hallucinations are referred to as "positive" symptoms, and withdrawal and reduction of affective expression are referred to as "negative" symptoms. Patients with schizophrenic disorders show deterioration in their level of functioning at work and in social relations, and in self-care. They often are confused, depressed, withdrawn, anxious, and without emotion. Physically, they may grimace and pace about, or they may be rigid and catatonic.

In schizophrenia, two types of thought disturbances are observed: formal thought disorder and disorder of thought content. *Formal thought disorders* affect relationships and associations among the words used to express thought. Thoughts may be strung together by incidental associations, or they may be completely unrelated. *Disorders of thought content* involve the development of delusions, which are fixed ideas that are based on incorrect perceptions of reality. Delusions, which commonly are paranoid or persecutory, also may be bizarre, somatic, grandiose, or referential (as to events that the patient believes have special significance). Perceptual disturbances in patients with schizophrenia include auditory, visual, tactile, olfactory, and gustatory hallucinations.

The most common emotional change in schizophrenia is a general "blunting" or "flattening" of affect. The patient seems to be emotionally detached or distant, may appear wooden and robot-like, and may lack warmth or spontaneity. Paranoid patients may feel frightened or enraged in response to a perceived threat or a delusion of persecution and may be very hostile and guarded to any perceived slight. Drug and alcohol abuse disorder is common.

The long-term course of illness is variable. About 25% of patients experience full remission of symptoms. Another 25% have mild residual symptoms. The remaining 50% continue to have moderate to severe symptoms.

First-line medical management for schizophrenia includes antipsychotic medications (e.g., haloperidol, risperidone, aripriprazole) with the goals of minimizing symptoms and functional impairments (Table 28.2). These medications block the dopamine receptor (first-generation antipsychotics) or are serotonin–dopamine antagonists (second-generation antipsychotics). Patient education is essential to promote adherence to medication regimens, with emphasis on common side effects of antipsychotics (e.g., extrapyramidal symptoms, tardive dyskinesia, sedation, dry mouth) and the increased risk of recurrence of symptoms due to premature discontinuation of medications. In addition to pharmacological treatment, psychosocial interventions include cognitive remediation and social skills training, cognitive-behavioral therapy, and family-based interventions. Regular follow-up and disease monitoring are essential.

Bipolar and Related Disorders

Bipolar and related disorders are separated from the depressive disorders in DSM-5 and include several disorders, with bipolar I disorder representing the modern understanding of the classic manic-depressive disorder and the primary focus of this section. Fig. 28.1A shows the normal variation in moods in otherwise healthy individuals.

Epidemiology and Etiology

Epidemiological studies demonstrate a lifetime prevalence of around 1% for bipolar I disorder in the general population. The mean age of onset of bipolar I disorder is in the early twenties. Socioeconomic variables and other social determinants of health do not appear to have a significant influence on rates of bipolar disease. Twin studies demonstrating monozygotic concordance of between 40% and 70%, and a lifetime risk of bipolar disease in first-degree relatives of 5%–10% point to the influence of genetics. Both childhood maltreatment and trauma as well as history of substance misuse and abuse are associated with an increased risk of developing bipolar disease. Comorbidities, including both psychiatric and nonpsychiatric medical conditions, are common.

Clinical Presentation and Medical Management

Bipolar I disorder consists of recurrences of mania and major depression or mixed states that occur at different time points or a mixture of symptoms that occur at the same time (see Fig. 28.1B). The essential feature of a manic episode is a distinct period during which the affected person's mood is elevated and expansive or irritable. Associated symptoms of the manic syndrome include inflated self-esteem, grandiosity, a decreased need

TABLE 28.2 Antipsychotic Agents

Name	Usual PO Daily Dose, mg	Side Effects	Sedation	Comments
First-Generation Antipsychotics				
Low Potency				
Chlorpromazine (Thorazine)	100–1000	Anticholinergic effects; orthostasis; photosensitivity; cholestasis; QT prolongation	+++	EPSEs usually not prominent; can cause anticholinergic delirium in elderly patients
Thioridazine (Mellaril)	100–600			
Mid Potency				
Trifluoperazine (Stelazine)	2–50	Fewer anticholinergic side effects	++	Well tolerated by most patients
Perphenazine (Trilafon)	4–64	Fewer EPSEs than with higher potency agents	++	
Loxapine (Loxitane)	30–100	Frequent EPSEs	++	
Molindone (Moban)	30–100	Frequent EPSEs	0	Little weight gain
High Potency				
Haloperidol (Haldol)	5–20	No anticholinergic side effects; EPSEs often prominent	0/+	Often prescribed in doses that are too high; long-acting injectable forms of haloperidol and fluphenazine available
Fluphenazine (Prolixin)	1–20	Frequent EPSEs	0/+	
Thiothixene (Navane)	2–50	Frequent EPSEs	0/+	
Second-Generation Antipsychotics				
Clozapine (Clozaril)	150–600	Agranulocytosis (1%); weight gain; seizures; drooling; hyperthermia	++	Requires weekly WBC count for first 6 months, then biweekly if stable
Risperidone (Risperdal)	2–8	Orthostasis	+	Requires slow titration; EPSEs observed with doses >6 mg qd
Olanzapine (Zyprexa)	10–30	Weight gain	++	Mild prolactin elevation
Quetiapine (Seroquel)	350–800	Sedation; weight gain; anxiety	+++	Bid dosing
Ziprasidone (Geodon)	120–200	Orthostatic hypotension	+/++	Minimal weight gain; increases QT interval
Aripiprazole (Abilify)	10–30	Nausea, anxiety, insomnia	0/+	Mixed agonist/antagonist; ER available
Paliperidone (Invega)	3–12	Restlessness, EPS, increased prolactin, headache	+	Active metabolite of risperidone
Iloperidone (Fanapt)	12–24	Dizziness, hypotension	0/+	Requires dose titration; long-acting injectable available
Asenapine (Saphris)	10–20	Dizziness, anxiety, EPS, minimal weight gain	++	Sublingual tablets; bid dosing
Lurasidone (Latuda)	40–80	Nausea, EPS	++	Uses CYP3A4
Brexpiprazole (Rexulti)	1–4	Anxiety, dizziness, fatigue	++	CYP3A4 and 2D6 interactions
Pimavanserin (Nuplazid)	34	Edema, confusion, sedation	++	Approved for Parkinson's disease psychosis
Cariprazine (Vraylar)	1.5–6	EPS, vomiting	++	Preferential D3 receptor affinity

EPS, extrapyramidal symptoms; *WBC*, white blood cell.
Psychiatric medications. In: Jameson J, Fauci AS, Kasper DL, et al., eds. *Harrison's Manual of Medicine, 20e.* McGraw Hill; Accessed August 3, 2021.

for sleep, excessive speech, flight of ideas, distractibility, psychomotor agitation, and excessive involvement in pleasurable activities. During a manic episode, the mood often is described as euphoric, cheerful, or "high." Speech often is loud, rapid, and difficult to interpret, and behavior may be intrusive and demanding. Poor judgment may lead to financial and legal problems. Drug and alcohol abuse also are common in this patient population.

The diagnosis of bipolar disorder is made as soon as the patient has one manic episode, even if the person has never had a depressive episode. Most patients who become manic eventually experience depression; however, about 10% of patients in whom bipolar disorder is diagnosed appear to have only manic episodes.

Men tend to have a greater number of manic episodes and more numerous depressive episodes than women. Untreated patients with bipolar disorder will experience a mean of nine affective episodes during their lifetime. The length of each cycle tends to decrease, although the number of cycles increases with age (Fig. 28.2). Each

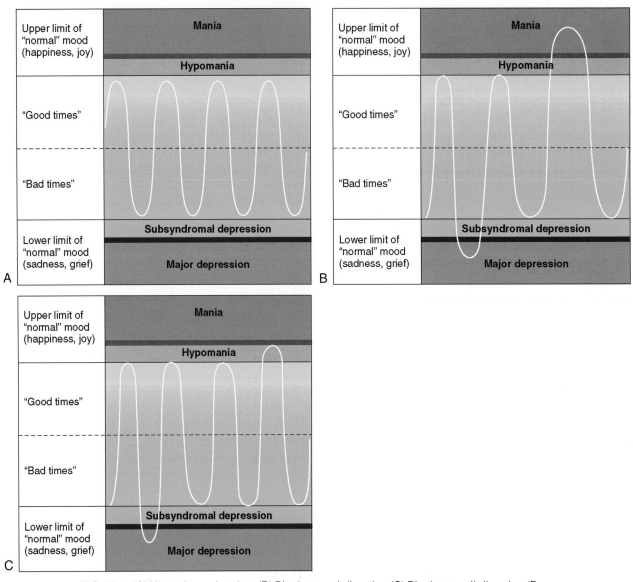

FIG. 28.1 (**A**) Normal mood cycles. (**B**) Bipolar type I disorder. (**C**) Bipolar type II disorder. (From Khalife S. Bipolar disorder. In: Carey WD, ed. *Current Clinical Medicine 2009—Cleveland Clinic*. 2nd ed. Philadelphia: Saunders; 2010.)

affective episode lasts about 8–9 months. In addition to other complications, patients with bipolar disease are at increased risk of death from suicide.

Management of bipolar disease includes pharmacotherapy and psychotherapy with the goal of reduction and/or resolution of mood symptoms and restored functioning. Hospitalization may be indicated in patients with suicidal ideation. The mainstays of drug therapy for bipolar disorders are the mood-stabilizing drugs, which generally act on both mania and depression (Table 28.3). Medications include lithium, valproic acid, or divalproex (valproate semisodium), lamotrigine, and carbamazepine. The most widely used mood stabilizer is lithium carbonate. Lithium is most helpful in patients with euphoric mania. When lithium is ineffective or when medical problems prevent its use, one of the anticonvulsants (valproic acid or divalproex, lamotrigine, or carbamazepine) with mood-stabilizing effects can be used. Electroconvulsive therapy is an effective antimanic treatment that may be used in cases of manic violence, delirium, or exhaustion, and is also appropriate for use with patients who do not respond adequately to medication.

DEPRESSIVE DISORDERS

The common feature of this group of disorders is the presence of a sad, empty, or irritable mood, accompanied by somatic and cognitive changes that significantly affect the individual's capacity to function. Major depressive disorder represents the classic condition in this group of disorders and is the focus of this section.

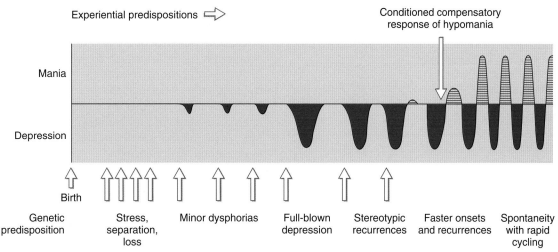

FIG. 28.2 Natural history of recurrent mood disorders: an integrated model. Genetic factors and early environmental stress may predispose to development of a mood disorder. Early episodes are likely to be precipitated by environmental stress; later episodes are more likely to occur closer together and spontaneously, without precipitants.

TABLE 28.3 Mood Stabilizers

Agent	Side Effects and Other Effects
Starting dose: 300 mg bid or tid Therapeutic blood level: 0.8–1.2 meq/L	Nausea/anorexia/diarrhea, fine tremor, thirst, polyuria, fatigue, weight gain, acne, folliculitis, neutrophilia, hypothyroidism Blood level is increased by thiazides, tetracyclines, and NSAIDs Blood level is decreased by bronchodilators, verapamil, and carbonic anhydrase inhibitors *Rare side effects:* Neurotoxicity, renal toxicity, hypercalcemia, ECG changes
Valproic Acid	**Common Side Effects**
Starting dose: 250 mg tid Therapeutic blood level: 50–125 µg/mL	Nausea/anorexia, weight gain, sedation, tremor, rash, alopecia Inhibits hepatic metabolism of other medications *Rare side effects:* pancreatitis, hepatotoxicity, Stevens–Johnson syndrome
Carbamazepine/Oxcarbazepine	**Common Side Effects**
Starting dose: 200 mg bid for carbamazepine, 150 mg bid for oxcarbazepine Therapeutic blood level: 4–12 µg/mL for carbamazepine	Nausea/anorexia, sedation, rash, dizziness/ataxia Carbamazepine, but not oxcarbazepine, induces hepatic metabolism of other medications *Rare side effects:* hyponatremia, agranulocytosis, Stevens–Johnson syndrome
Lamotrigine	**Common Side Effects**
Starting dose: 25 mg/day	Rash, dizziness, headache, tremor, sedation, nausea *Rare side effect:* Stevens–Johnson syndrome

ECG, electrocardiogram; *NSAIDs*, nonsteroidal antiinflammatory drugs.
Psychiatric medications. In: Jameson J, Fauci AS, Kasper DL, et al., eds. *Harrison's Manual of Medicine, 20e*. McGraw Hill; Accessed August 3, 2021.

Epidemiology and Etiology

About 5% of the adults in the United States have a clinically significant mood disorder, with women affected more frequently than men. Major depression may begin at any age, but the prevalence is highest among older adults followed by those 30–40 years of age, and rarely develops before puberty. Lifetime prevalence rates for major depressive disorders are 15%–20%. About one-third of depressed persons require hospitalization; 30%

follow a chronic course with residual symptoms and social impairment.

Several theories have been presented to explain the origin of mood disorders. Reduced brain concentrations of norepinephrine and serotonin (neurotransmitters) are believed to cause depression. In addition to neurotransmitters, the interactions between thyrotropin and thyroid-stimulating hormone as well as cortisol release by corticotropin-releasing factor and adrenocorticotropin

BOX 28.1   Risk Factors Associated With Suicide

- History of trauma or abuse as a child
- History of prior suicide attempts
- Alcohol and drug abuse
- Family history of suicide
- Economic loss
- Bereavement
- Serious illness; physical or chronic pain
- Social isolation
- Access to lethal means
- Recent release from inpatient psychiatric hospitalization

From Steele D: Keltner's Psychiatric Nursing, ed 9. Elsevier, 2023, St. Louis.

over a long period may be associated with the development of depression. This model suggests that depression is the result of a prolonged stress reaction.

Clinical Presentation and Medical Management

Patients with major depression are depressed most of the day, show a marked decrease in interest or pleasure in most activities, exhibit a marked gain or loss in weight, and have insomnia or hypersomnia. These symptoms must be present for at least 2 weeks before a diagnosis of major depression can be made. Up to 80% of persons who have had a major depressive episode will have at least one more depressive episode; 20% of these people will have a subsequent manic episode and are therefore reclassified as bipolar. An episode of major depression typically lasts 8−9 months if the patient is not treated.

An estimated 30,000 suicides occur each year in the United States; approximately 70% involve persons with major depression (Box 28.1). The physician must consider suicidal lethality in the management of patients with depression. In general, the risk for suicide is increased in association with the following factors: alcoholism, drug abuse, social isolation, elderly male status, terminal illness, and undiagnosed or untreated mental disorders (including major depression). Patients at greatest risk are those with a history of previous suicide attempts, drug or alcohol abuse, recent diagnosis of a serious condition, loss of a loved one, recent retirement, and those who live alone or lack adequate social support.

Management of major depressive disorder generally includes a combination of pharmacotherapy (Table 28.4) and psychotherapy (Table 28.5). The first-line medication for major depression is a single selective serotonin reuptake inhibitor (SSRI) such as citalopram. Venlafaxine (selective serotonin and norepinephrine reuptake inhibitor (SNRI)) and bupropion (norepinephrine-dopamine reuptake inhibitor (NDRI)) are second-line drugs that may be used in patients who fail to achieve remission with initial first-line therapy. Common side effects of antidepressant medications include diarrhea, nausea and vomiting, hyposalivation, sexual dysfunction, somnolence, and weight gain. The most commonly used psychotherapy methods include cognitive behavioral therapy (includes education, relaxation exercises, coping skills training, stress management, assertiveness training) and interpersonal psychotherapy (focuses on the individual's interpersonal life in four problem areas that include grief over loss, interpersonal disputes, role transitions, and interpersonal skill deficits).

ANXIETY DISORDERS

Anxiety is a natural response and a necessary warning adaptation in humans. Anxiety becomes a pathologic disorder when it is excessive and uncontrollable, requires no specific external stimulus, and results in physical and affective symptoms and changes in behavior and cognition. Anxiety disorders occur in two patterns[1]: chronic, generalized anxiety and[2] episodic, panic-like anxiety. Several related psychiatric disorders often coexist with anxiety disorders, including posttraumatic stress disorder, substance abuse disorder, and depression.

Anxiety is characterized by a feeling of impending disaster. The source of the problem usually is not apparent to persons with anxiety. The feeling is the same in anxious patients as that in patients with fear, but the latter are aware of what the problem is and why they are "fearful." Anxiety can be a purely psychological experience, with few somatic manifestations. Alternatively, it can be experienced as a purely physical phenomenon (e.g., tachycardia, palpitations, chest pain, indigestion, headaches) with no psychological distress other than concern about the physical symptoms. A *phobia* is defined as an irrational fear that interferes with normal behavior. Phobias are fears of specific objects, situations, or experiences. A *panic attack* consists of a sudden, unexpected, overwhelming feeling of terror with symptoms of dyspnea, palpitations, dizziness, faintness, trembling, sweating, choking, flushes or chills, numbness or tingling sensations, and chest pains.

Epidemiology and Etiology

Anxiety disorders constitute the most frequently encountered psychiatric condition in the general population. Simple phobia is the most common of the anxiety disorders (up to 25% of the population will experience a phobia); however, panic disorder (lifetime prevalence of 3.5%) is the most common anxiety disorder in people who seek medical treatment. Generalized anxiety disorder as well as posttraumatic stress disorder (PTSD) both have a lifetime prevalence of approximately 5%. Panic disorder, phobic disorders, and obsessive-compulsive disorders occur more frequently among first-degree relatives of affected persons than in the general population. Anxiety also is associated with mood disorders, schizophrenia, or personality disorders.

TABLE 28.4 Antidepressant Medications

Name	Usual Daily Dose, mg	Side Effects	Comments
SSRIs			
Fluoxetine (Prozac)	10–80	Headache; nausea and other GI effects; jitteriness; insomnia; sexual dysfunction; can affect plasma levels of other medicines (except sertraline); akathisia rare	Once-daily dosing, usually in the morning; fluoxetine has very long half-life; must not be combined with MAOIs
Sertraline (Zoloft)	50–200		
Paroxetine (Paxil)	20–60		
Fluvoxamine (Luvox)	100–300		
Citalopram (Celexa)	20–60		
Escitalopram (Lexapro)	10–30		
TCAs and Tetracyclics			
Amitriptyline (Elavil)	150–300	Anticholinergic (dry mouth, tachycardia, constipation, urinary retention, blurred vision); sweating; tremor; postural hypotension; cardiac conduction delay; sedation; weight gain	Once-daily dosing, usually qhs; blood levels of most TCAs available; can be lethal in overdose (lethal dose = 2 g); nortriptyline best tolerated, especially by elderly FDA approved for OCD
Nortriptyline (Pamelor)	50–200		
Imipramine (Tofranil)	150–300		
Desipramine (Norpramin)	150–300		
Doxepin (Sinequan)	150–300		
Clomipramine (Anafranil)	150–300		
Maprotiline (Ludiomil)	25–150		
Mixed Norepinephrine/Serotonin Reuptake Inhibitors (SNRI) and Receptor Blockers			
Venlafaxine (Effexor)	75–375	Nausea; dizziness; dry mouth; headaches; increased blood pressure; anxiety and insomnia	Bid-tid dosing (extended release available); lower potential for drug interactions than SSRIs; contraindicated with MAOIs
Desvenlafaxine (Pristiq)	50–400	Nausea, dizziness, insomnia	Primary metabolite of venlafaxine; no increased efficacy with higher dosing
Duloxetine (Cymbalta)	40–60	Nausea, dizziness, headache, insomnia, constipation	May have utility in treatment of neuropathic pain and stress incontinence
Mirtazapine (Remeron)	15–45	Somnolence, weight gain; neutropenia rare	Once-a-day dosing
Vilazodone (Viibryd)	40	Nausea, diarrhea, headache; dosage adjustment if given with CYP3A4 inhibitor/stimulator	Also 5-HT$_{1a}$ receptor partial agonist
Vortioxetine (Brintellix)	5–20	Nausea, diarrhea, sweating, headache; low incidence of sedation or weight gain	No specific p450 effects; 5-HT$_{3a}$ and 5-HT$_7$ receptor antagonist, 5-HT$_{1b}$ partial agonist, and 5-HT$_{1a}$ agonist
Levomilnacipran (Fetzima)	40–120	Nausea, constipation, sweating; rare increase in blood pressure/pulse	Most noradrenergic of SNRIs
Mixed-Action Drugs			
Bupropion (Wellbutrin)	250–450	Jitteriness; flushing; seizures in at-risk pts; anorexia; tachycardia; psychosis	Tid dosing, but sustained release also available; fewer sexual side effects than SSRIs or TCAs; may be useful for adult ADD
Trazodone (Desyrel)	200–600	Sedation; dry mouth; ventricular irritability; postural hypotension; priapism rare	Useful in low doses for sleep because of sedating effects with no anticholinergic side effects
Trazodone extended release (Oleptro)	150–375	Daytime somnolence, dizziness, nausea	
Amoxapine (Asendin)	200–600	Sexual dysfunction	Lethality in overdose; EPS possible
MAOIs			
Phenelzine (Nardil)	45–90	Insomnia; hypotension; edema; anorgasmia; weight gain; neuropathy; hypertensive crisis; toxic reactions with SSRIs; narcotics	May be more effective in pts with atypical features or treatment-refractory depression
Tranylcypromine (Parnate)	20–50		
Isocarboxazid (Marplan)	20–60		Less weight gain and hypotension than phenelzine
Transdermal selegiline (Emsam)	6–12	Local skin reaction hypertension	No dietary restrictions with 6-mg dose

ADD, attention deficit disorder; *EPS*, extrapyramidal symptoms; *FDA*, US Food and Drug Administration; *GI*, gastrointestinal; *MAOIs*, monoamine oxidase inhibitors; *OCD*, obsessive-compulsive disorder; *SSRIs*, selective serotonin reuptake inhibitors; *TCAs*, tricyclic antidepressants. Psychiatric medications. In: Jameson J, Fauci AS, Kasper DL, et al., eds. *Harrison's Manual of Medicine, 20e*. McGraw Hill; Accessed August 3, 2021.

TABLE 28.5   Psychotherapy Approaches for Management of Depression

Name of Psychotherapy	Approach
Cognitive psychotherapy	Identify and correct negativistic patterns of thinking
Interpersonal psychotherapy	Identify and work through role transitions or interpersonal losses, conflicts, or deficits
Problem-solving therapy	Identify and prioritize situational problems; plan and implement strategies to deal with top-priority problems
Psychodynamic psychotherapy	Use therapeutic relationship to maximize use of the healthiest defense mechanisms and coping strategies

From Lyness JM. Psychiatric disorders in medical practice. In: *Goldman-Cecil Medicine*, 26th ed. Elsevier; Accessed August 10, 2021. Author summary based on categories and criteria from American Psychiatric Association. *Diagnostic and Statistical Manual of Mental Disorders (DSM-5)*. 5th ed. Washington, DC: American Psychiatric Association; 2013.

Anxiety disorders may occur in persons who are under emotional stress, in those with certain systemic illnesses, or as a component of various psychiatric disorders. No single biologic or psychological cause of anxiety has been identified, and no single theory fully explains all anxiety disorders. The locus coeruleus, a brainstem structure that contains most of the noradrenergic neurons in the central nervous system (CNS), appears to be involved in panic attacks and anxiety. Panic and anxiety may be correlated with dysregulated firing of the locus coeruleus caused by input from multiple sources, including peripheral autonomic afferents, medullary afferents, and serotonergic fibers.

Clinical Presentation and Medical Management

Physiologic reactions to anxiety and to fear are the same and are mediated through the autonomic nervous system. Sympathetic and parasympathetic components may be involved. Signs and symptoms of anxiety caused by overactivation of the *sympathetic* nervous system include increased heart rate, sweating, dilated pupils, and muscle tension. Signs and symptoms of anxiety resulting from stimulation of the *parasympathetic* system include urinary frequency and episodic diarrhea. Some patients present with a persistent, diffuse form of anxiety characterized by signs and symptoms of motor tension, autonomic hyperactivity, and apprehension.

Generalized anxiety disorder is associated with significant disability and distress.

Phobias consist of three major groups: agoraphobia, social, and specific. Agoraphobia is a fear of having distressing or embarrassing symptoms on leaving home, and often accompanies panic disorder. Social phobias may be specific, such as fear of public speaking, or general, such as fear of being embarrassed when with people. Simple phobias include fear of snakes, heights, flying, darkness, and needles. The two phobias that may affect medical or dental care are needle phobia and claustrophobia, the latter during magnetic resonance imaging (MRI) or radiation therapy. Dental "phobia" is associated with extreme anxiety when attending a visit to the dentist. Previous frightening dental experiences are cited as the major cause. Patients may specifically fear the noise and vibration of the drill, the sight of the injection needle, and the act of sitting in the dental chair, and they may experience muscle tension, fast heart rate, accelerated breathing, sweating, or stomach cramps.

A person who has repeated panic attacks is described as having a *panic disorder*. Onset usually is between late adolescence and the mid-30s, but it may occur at any age. A key feature of panic is the adrenergic surge, which results in the fight-or-flight response. This response is an exaggerated sympathetic response. Panic attacks may be cued or uncued. An example of a cued attack is that occurring in a person who is fearful of flying. Many patients report that they are unaware of any life stressors preceding the onset of panic disorder; such attacks are classified as uncued. The major complication of repeated panic attacks is a restricted lifestyle adopted to avoid situations that might trigger an attack. Some patients develop agoraphobia, which can cause them to be housebound for years. Sudden loss of social supports or disruption of important interpersonal relationships appears to predispose the affected person to development of panic disorder.

Psychological, behavioral, and drug modalities are used to treat anxiety disorders. Psychological treatment involves psychotherapy, which, in general, is used in more severe cases. Behavioral treatment includes cognitive approaches (anxiety management, relaxation, and cognitive restructuring), biofeedback, hypnosis, relaxation imaging, desensitization, and flooding. Systemic desensitization (whereby the patient is gradually exposed to the feared situation) and flooding (by which the patient is exposed directly to the anxiety-provoking stimulus) are techniques used in the treatment of phobias. Drug treatment includes the use of tricyclic antidepressants (TCAs), selective serotonin reuptake inhibitors (SSRIs), monoamine oxidase (MAO) inhibitors, benzodiazepines, antihistamines, β-adrenergic receptor antagonists, and sedative-hypnotics (Table 28.6). Most patients benefit maximally from a combination of therapies such as cognitive therapy plus medication.

OBSESSIVE-COMPULSIVE AND RELATED DISORDERS

Obsessive-compulsive disorder (OCD) is characterized by recurrent intrusive thoughts, images, or urges

TABLE 28.6 Anxiolytic Medications

Name	Equivalent PO Dose, mg	Onset of Action	Half-Life, h	Comments
Benzodiazepines				
Diazepam (Valium)	5	Fast	20—70	Active metabolites; quite sedating
Flurazepam (Dalmane)	15	Fast	30—100	Flurazepam is a prodrug; metabolites are active; quite sedating
Triazolam (Halcion)	0.25	Intermediate	1.5—5	No active metabolites; can induce confusion and delirium, especially in elderly
Lorazepam (Ativan)	1	Intermediate	10—20	No active metabolites; direct hepatic glucuronide conjugation; quite sedating; FDA approved for anxiety with depression
Alprazolam (Xanax)	0.5	Intermediate	12—15	Active metabolites; not too sedating; FDA approved for panic disorder and anxiety with depression; tolerance and dependence develop easily; difficult to withdraw
Chlordiazepoxide (Librium)	10	Intermediate	5—30	Active metabolites; moderately sedating
Oxazepam (Serax)	15	Slow	5—15	No active metabolites; direct glucuronide conjugation; not too sedating
Temazepam (Restoril)	15	Slow	9—12	No active metabolites; moderately sedating
Clonazepam (Klonopin)	0.5	Slow	18—50	No active metabolites; moderately sedating; FDA approved for panic disorder
Clorazepate (Tranxene)	15	Fast	40—200	Low sedation; unreliable absorption
Nonbenzodiazepines				
Buspirone (BuSpar)	7.5	2 weeks	2—3	Active metabolites; tid dosing—usual daily dose 10—20 mg tid; nonsedating; no additive effects with alcohol; useful for controlling agitation in demented or brain-injured pts

FDA, US Food and Drug Administration.
Psychiatric medications. In: Jameson J, Fauci AS, Kasper DL, et al., eds. *Harrison's Manual of Medicine, 20e*. McGraw Hill; Accessed August 3, 2021.

(obsessions) that cause anxiety or distress (and that are not pleasurable), and by repetitive mental or behavioral acts (compulsions) that the individual feels driven to perform, either in relation to an obsession or according to rules that must be applied rigidly to achieve a sense of "completeness" (Box 28.2). Despite heterogeneity among patients with OCD, certain symptom dimensions are common including those of cleaning (contamination obsessions and cleaning compulsions); symmetry (symmetry obsessions and repeating, ordering, and counting compulsions); forbidden or taboo thoughts (e.g., aggressive, sexual, and religious obsessions and related compulsions); and harm (e.g., fears of harm to oneself or others and related checking compulsions).

Epidemiology and Etiology

Worldwide lifetime prevalence of OCD is approximately 1.0% in men and 1.5% in women, while approximately 2.3% of adults are affected in the United States. Comorbidity with anxiety and depression is common, and tic disorder may also be associated. Genetic and environmental factors, as well as abnormalities in the cortico-striato-thalamo-cortical (CSTC) circuits as well as other

neural circuits, appear to contribute to the development of OCD. New onset may occur following a traumatic event, or after a brain injury (e.g., traumatic brain injury, ischemic event).

Clinical Presentation and Medical Management

Obsessions are involuntary repetitive and persistent thoughts (e.g., of contamination), images (e.g., of violent or horrific scenes), or urges (e.g., to stab someone) that are not pleasurable and cause marked distress or anxiety. Compulsions (or rituals) are repetitive behaviors (e.g., washing, checking) or mental acts (e.g., counting, repeating words silently) that the individual feels driven to perform in relation to an obsession or according to rules that must be applied rigidly or to achieve a sense of "completeness." Avoidance behavior is common with OCD, and when severe can lead to significant dysfunction in daily living activities. OCD is associated with reduced quality of life as well as potentially high levels of social and occupational impairment. Lifetime suicidal ideation in patients with OCD is as high as 50%.

OCD can be effectively treated with serotonergic antidepressants as well as cognitive-behavioral therapy.

First-line pharmacotherapy is with an SSRI such as fluoxetine, fluvoxamine, sertraline, paroxetine, citalopram, and escitalopram.

Trauma- and Stressor-Related Disorders

Psychological distress following exposure to a traumatic or stressful event is normal and expected, but the nature of the response is highly variable. While many symptoms can be understood within an anxiety- or fear-based context, some individuals exhibit a distinct phenotype characterized by anhedonic and dysphoric symptoms, externalizing angry and aggressive symptoms, or dissociative symptoms. This group of disorders is closely related to anxiety disorders, obsessive-compulsive and related disorders, and dissociative disorders. This chapter focuses on acute stress disorder and posttraumatic stress disorder (PTSD).

Epidemiology and Etiology

Acute stress disorder is identified in less than 20% of individuals following traumatic events that do not involve interpersonal assault (e.g., motor vehicle accidents, mild traumatic brain injury), but with higher rates (i.e., 20%−50%) reported following interpersonal traumatic events (e.g., assault, rape, witnessing a mass shooting). Associated risk factors for acute stress disorder include history of a pretrauma psychiatric disorder, history of traumatic exposures prior to the recent exposure, female gender, trauma severity, neuroticism, and avoidance coping. The projected lifetime risk for PTSD at age 75 years is 8.7%, with a 12-month prevalence among US adults of 3.5%. Rates of PTSD are higher among veterans and others whose vocation increases the risk of traumatic exposure (e.g., police, firefighters, emergency medical personnel). The highest rates of PTSD (ranging from one-third to more than one-half of those exposed) occur in survivors of rape, military combat and captivity, and ethnically or politically motivated internment and genocide.

Clinical Presentation and Medical Management

Acute stress disorder develops after exposure of the patient to a traumatic event, and specific signs and symptoms resemble those of PTSD. In acute stress disorder, however, symptoms are of shorter duration (from 3 days to up to 1 month) and emerge more rapidly after the trauma (within hours to days). The symptomatic reaction is limited to the period during which the stressful event is occurring and its immediate aftermath. Patients with acute stress disorder typically present with frequent reexperiencing and anxiety in response to reminders of their recent trauma. Dissociative symptoms may lead to a flat or blunted affect (emotional or psychic numbing) and patients can appear to be in shock.

Cardinal features of PTSD include experience of a traumatic event (extreme trauma), intrusion symptoms (reexperiencing symptoms including nightmares and flashbacks), avoidance symptoms (avoidance of stimuli associated with the traumatic event, which can lead to impairment in daily life functioning), negative alterations in cognition or mood (depression, decreased pleasure, inability to connect with others), and arousal or reactivity changes (generalized irritability, reckless behavior, inability to concentrate, sleep disturbances). This can result in emotional numbing, diminished interest in everyday activities, and in extreme cases, detachment from others, leading to considerable social, occupational, and interpersonal dysfunction. While symptoms of PTSD usually begin within the first 3 months after the trauma, there may be a delay of months, or even years, before criteria for the diagnosis are met.

Treatment for acute stress disorder is oriented toward controlling and minimizing symptoms of acute stress responses and preventing their development into PTSD. Cognitive behavioral therapy (CBT) is generally the first-line intervention although medications (primarily benzodiazepines) may be considered. Management of PTSD includes trauma-focused psychotherapy (e.g., CBT), serotonin reuptake inhibitors (e.g., sertraline), or a combination of the two approaches, with the choice somewhat depending on patient preference. The US Food and Drug Administration has approved the SSRIs paroxetine and sertraline for the treatment of PTSD. In cases with comorbid psychiatric disorders or with especially severe symptoms of PTSD, a combination of psychotherapy and pharmacologic treatment is recommended as the first line of treatment. Co-occurring conditions such as substance abuse disorder or sleep disturbance also must be addressed as part of the management plan.

SOMATIC SYMPTOM AND RELATED DISORDERS

These disorders include somatic symptom disorder, illness anxiety disorder, conversion disorder (functional neurological symptom disorder), and factitious disorder, and are characterized by the prominence of somatic symptoms associated with significant distress and impairment (Table 28.7). Persons with somatoform disorders have physical complaints for which no general medical cause is present. Associated unconscious psychological factors contribute to the onset, exacerbation, or maintenance of physical symptoms, which may last for years.

Epidemiology and Etiology

The prevalence of somatoform disorders is around 5% and symptoms are more frequently reported in women. Comorbid anxiety or depression is common as well as recently experienced stressful life events. In this group of disorders, physical symptoms suggest a physical disorder for which no underlying physical basis can be found. Symptoms are linked to psychological factors. Somatization therefore is defined as the manifestation of psychological stress in somatic symptoms.

Clinical Presentation and Medical Management

Somatic Symptom Disorder. Somatization consists of multiple signs and symptoms and usually begins before the age of 30 years. Patients experience multiple, unexplained physical manifestations of illness or disease, which may include pain, diarrhea, bloating, vomiting, sexual dysfunction, blindness, deafness, weakness, paralysis, or coordination problems. Somatization disorder is a serious psychiatric illness. Many patients have concurrent anxiety, depression, or personality disorder.

Illness Anxiety Disorder. Illness anxiety disorder is characterized by excessive concern about having or

TABLE 28.7	Somatic Symptom and Related Disorders
Type	**Main Clinical Manifestations**
Somatic symptom disorder	Symptoms, a single symptom or multiple symptoms, together with excessive thoughts, feelings, or behaviors related to these symptoms; subsumes most of the former terms somatization disorder, pain disorder, undifferentiated somatoform disorder, and many with the former diagnosis of hypochondriasis
Illness anxiety disorder	Illness preoccupation and excessive health-related behaviors in the absence of or disproportionate to somatic symptoms; subsumes some patients with the former diagnosis of hypochondriasis
Conversion disorder (functional neurologic symptom disorder)	Neurologic somatoform symptoms (other than pain) with clinical evidence incompatible with recognized neurologic or general medical conditions (e.g., paralysis, blindness, dyscoordination, convulsion-like phenomena, memory or other neurocognitive complaints)
Psychological factors affecting other medical conditions	Psychological factors adversely affecting a (non–mental disorder) medical symptom or condition by worsening the course, interfering with treatment, adding to known health risks, or influencing underlying pathophysiology
Factitious disorder (commonly called Munchausen syndrome)	Falsification of physical or psychological signs or symptoms, with health- or help-seeking behaviors, in the absence of clear external rewards

From Lyness JM: *Author Summary of American Psychiatric Association categories and criteria.* In Goldman L, Schafer A: Goldman-Cecil Medicine, ed 26, Elsevier, 2020, St. Louis. Author summary based on categories and criteria from American Psychiatric Association. *Diagnostic and Statistical Manual of Mental Disorders (DSM-5).* 5th ed. Washington, DC: American Psychiatric Association; 2013.

developing a serious, undiagnosed medical disease. Illness anxiety preoccupations are heterogeneous and can focus on a specific diagnosis, a bodily function, normal variation in function, or vague somatic sensations. The condition is typically chronic, and the focus of concern may shift over time.

Conversion Disorder (Functional Neurological Symptom Disorder). Conversion disorder is a mono- or multisymptomatic somatoform disorder that affects the voluntary motor system or sensory functions. The patient may experience blindness, deafness, paralysis, or an inability to speak or to walk. Symptoms suggest a physical condition, but the cause is psychological. The diagnosis of conversion disorder should be based on the overall clinical picture and not on a single finding, with clear evidence of incompatibility with neurological disease. Onset may be associated with stress or trauma, either psychological or physical in nature.

Factitious Disorder. Factitious disorder is characterized by the falsification of medical or psychological signs and symptoms in oneself or others, with patients often seeking treatment for themselves or another following induction of injury or disease. Unlike with malingering behavior, factitious disorder occurs in the absence of obvious external incentives and rewards such as avoidance of responsibility or financial gain. However, individuals may be motivated by internal gains, such as a desire for attention or as a mechanism for coping with stress. Many affected persons also have other psychiatric disorders.

Treatment. Treatment of patients with somatic symptoms and related disorders is complex and often requires multiple therapeutic modalities, including psychotherapy for their interpersonal and psychological problems. Medication for the treatment of underlying depressive disorder also may be needed. Group therapy is beneficial in some cases.

FEEDING AND EATING DISORDERS

DSM-5 defines this group of disorders as being characterized by a persistent disturbance of eating or eating-related behavior that results in the altered consumption or absorption of food, and that significantly impairs physical health or psychosocial functioning. The two major eating disorders are anorexia nervosa and bulimia nervosa. *Anorexia nervosa* is characterized by three essential features that include (1) persistent energy intake restriction; (2) an intense fear of gaining weight or of becoming fat, or persistent behavior that interferes with weight gain; and (3) a disturbance in self-perceived weight or body shape. This is typically achieved through restriction of food intake, leading to weight loss and the medical sequelae of starvation (Fig. 28.3). *Bulimia nervosa* is also characterized by three essential features that include (1) recurrent episodes of binge eating (excessive food consumption within a discrete period of time accompanied by a sense of lack of control), (2) repeated inappropriate compensatory behaviors to prevent weight gain, and (3) self-evaluation that is unduly influenced by body shape and weight. Patients with bulimia are typically within the normal weight or overweight range, and attempts at restriction are interspersed with binge eating followed by various methods of trying to rid the body of food (e.g., induced vomiting, often by means of a finger or use of other instruments in the throat; laxatives; and diuretics).

Epidemiology and Etiology

The female to male ratio is approximately 10:1. Anorexia nervosa affects an estimated 1% of women between 12 and 25 years of age and is more common in white women and women from higher socioeconomic groups. The mean age at onset of anorexia nervosa is bimodal, with peaks at the ages of 14 and 18 years. Bulimia nervosa is more common than anorexia nervosa with a prevalence among women that ranges from 1.1% to 4.2%. The average age at onset for bulimia nervosa is about 20

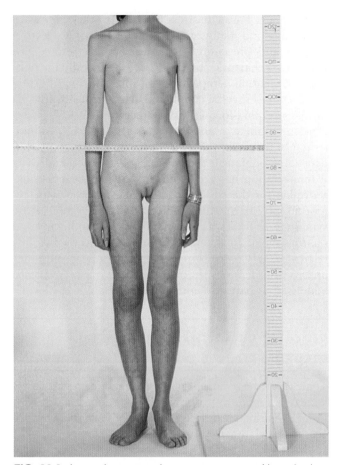

FIG. 28.3 Anorexia nervosa in a young woman. Note the low body weight and the preservation of breast tissue. (From Moshang T. *Pediatric Endocrinology: The Requisites in Pediatrics.* St. Louis: Mosby; 2005.)

years. In contrast with anorexia nervosa, bulimia nervosa occurs at about the same rate in higher and in lower socioeconomic groups but remains more common in white women than in women of ethnic minority groups.

The cause of eating disorders is unknown and appears to include genetic, cultural, and psychiatric factors. Genetic factors are recognized to contribute to the risk of development of anorexia nervosa, with a higher incidence in families with one affected member, and greater concordance in monozygotic twins compared with dizygotic twins. Cultural issues are important in the origin of eating disorders. The desire for health and slimness is a powerful force in modern society and may reinforce the fear of being overweight in patients with an eating disorder or may tip the borderline case into overt disease. Certain activities and occupations (e.g., modeling, skating, gymnastics, wrestling, track, ballet dancing) that emphasize body shape, weight, and appearance also may play a role in eating disorders.

Clinical Presentation and Medical Management

The diagnosis of an eating disorder is made on a clinical basis. The weight criterion for diagnosis of anorexia nervosa is 85% or less of expected ideal weight. An expressed intense fear of gaining weight or becoming fat, even when underweight, and a disturbance in body image complete the diagnostic triad. The diagnosis of bulimia nervosa is made with a history of binge eating without major weight gain, evidence of purging (induced vomiting or regular use of laxatives or diuretics), obsessive-compulsive behavior, and antisocial activity or self-mutilation.

Anorexia nervosa usually begins around puberty but may appear later, usually by the mid-20s. Despite severe weight loss, patients deny hunger, thinness, or fatigue. They often are physically active and participate in ritualized exercise. Amenorrhea usually accompanies or comes after weight loss, and constipation and cold intolerance are common. In advanced cases, bradycardia, hypothermia, and hypotension may occur. Little or no body fat is evident, and bony protrusions (e.g., at the hips or shoulder blades) are pronounced. Patients with anorexia nervosa are vulnerable to electrolyte imbalances that can lead to sudden death from ventricular tachyarrhythmias, with the risk of death becoming greater when weight declines to below 35% of ideal weight.

Patients with bulimia nervosa engage in episodic, compulsive ingestion of large amounts of food. They are aware that this eating is abnormal; they have a fear that they cannot stop eating and have feelings of depression at the completion of eating. Patients with bulimia also have a morbid fear of becoming fat. Secrecy about the eating–vomiting sequence is common. Bloating, constipation, esophagitis, abdominal pain, and nausea are common. Complications of bulimia include aspiration of vomitus, esophageal or gastric rupture, hypokalemia with cardiac arrhythmias, and pancreatitis. Painless bilateral parotid (and less frequently submandibular) gland swelling (sialadenosis) occurs in 10%–25% of patients secondary to repeated vomiting. The mechanism is not entirely clear but is likely related to repeated stimulation and gland hypertrophy. Erosion of the lingual enamel (perimyolysis) may also be detected secondary to repeated vomiting. Patients with bulimia nervosa have an overall better prognosis than those with anorexia nervosa.

Treatment of eating disorders is complex and involves an experienced interdisciplinary team that includes a mental health clinician, dietitian, and a general medical clinician. Medical evaluation may include complete blood count; electrolytes, renal function test, and liver function tests; calcium, magnesium, phosphate; cholesterol, lipids, amylase; thyroid function tests, urine analysis, electrocardiogram; and chest radiograph. The treatment of anorexia nervosa generally involves nutritional rehabilitation and psychotherapy. Patients with anorexia nervosa who are not medically stable require hospitalization. For patients with anorexia nervosa who are medically stable, treatment options usually include psychiatric inpatient hospitalization, partial hospital (day program), and

outpatient care; pharmacotherapy is not an initial or primary treatment for anorexia nervosa. Management for bulimia nervosa includes nutritional rehabilitation, psychotherapy, and pharmacotherapy, as well as monitoring patients for medical complications. Most patients with bulimia nervosa are treated as outpatients or in partial hospital programs, but hospitalization may be necessary for suicidal ideation or behavior, or uncontrolled purging.

Personality Disorders

DSM-5 defines a personality disorder as an enduring pattern of inner experience and behavior that deviates markedly from the expectations of the individual's culture, is pervasive and inflexible, has an onset in adolescence or early adulthood, is stable over time, and leads to distress or impairment. Personality disorders can be categorized into three clusters (odd/eccentric, dramatic/emotional/erratic, and anxious/fearful), although patients frequently present with co-occurring disorders from different clusters (Table 28.8).

Epidemiology and Etiology

It is estimated that up to 15% of adults in the United States have a personality disorder. The characteristics that define a personality disorder may not be considered problematic by the affected individual. There is high comorbidity with other psychiatric disorders.

Clinical Presentation and Medical Management

Behaviors and traits suggestive of personality disorders include frequent mood swings, angry outbursts, social anxiety sufficient to cause difficulty making friends, need to be the center of attention, feeling of being widely cheated or taken advantage of, difficulty delaying gratification, and externalizing and blaming the world for one's behaviors and feelings. Patients often feel that there is nothing wrong with their behavior (ego-syntonic symptoms). Individuals with a personality disorder can present challenges to the doctor–patient relationship due to patient distrust, irritability, poor or inappropriate communication skills, dependency, or excessive demands. Problematic behaviors can include late night phone calls, angry outbursts, repeated visits, or being otherwise noncompliant with recommended treatment. Personality disorders are important risk factors for a variety of risky behaviors and adverse outcomes, including injury from altercations and accidents due to impulsive and reckless behavior; suicide attempts; high-risk sexual behavior; comorbid anxiety mood, and/or substance use disorder.

First-line therapy, once a patient accepts the diagnosis, is psychotherapy, with medication used as an adjunctive treatment. Depending on a given patient's needs, interventions may include individual and group therapy, self-education, specialized substance use disorder treatment, partial hospitalization, or brief hospitalization during times of crises.

TABLE 28.8 Types of Personality Disorders

DISORDER	DEFINING CHARACTERISTICS
CLUSTER A: ODD/ECCENTRIC	
Paranoid personality disorder	Distrust of others, conviction that others will harm or deceive
Schizoid personality disorder	Detachment from social relationships, limited expression of emotions
Schizotypal personality disorder	Discomfort with close relationships, distorted thinking and perceptions, eccentric behavior
CLUSTER B: DRAMATIC/EMOTIONAL/ERRATIC	
Borderline personality disorder	Instability in interpersonal relationships, poor self-image, impulsive behavior, frequent and intense anger, excessive fear of abandonment
Antisocial personality disorder	Substantial disregard and violation for the safety and rights of self and others; unremorseful, deceptive, and often aggressive
Narcissistic personality disorder	Unrealistic sense of self and arrogance, need for admiration and praise, lack of empathy
Histrionic personality disorder	Attention seeking, dramatic behavior and speech, rapidly shifting emotions, easily influenced
CLUSTER C: ANXIOUS/FEARFUL	
Avoidant personality disorder	Social inhibition, feeling inadequate, oversensitivity to criticism, preoccupied with rejection and negative views from others
Dependent personality disorder	Extreme dependence on others, continuous need to be taken care of, fearing being unable to take care of self often resulting in submissive and insecure behavior, difficulty making decisions
Obsessive-compulsive personality disorder*	Preoccupation with details, order, and rules, excessive need for perfection, a strong desire to be in control of people, tasks and situations, unable to delegate tasks

*Obsessive-compulsive personality disorder is not the same as the anxiety disorder, obsessive-compulsive disorder.

Data from *Personality Disorders*, Mayo Clinic, https://www.mayoclinic.org; *What are Personality Disorders?*, American Psychiatric Association, https://www.psychiatry.org; and Goldman L, Schafer A: *Goldman-Cecil Medicine*, ed 26, Elsevier, 2020, St. Louis.

Dental Management

Most patients with psychiatric diseases who are clinically stable and able to cooperate can safely receive routine and emergency dental care without specific precautions. There may however be situations in which patients have conditions which are not well-controlled and where routine dental care should be deferred until a more appropriate time and setting. There also may be situations, such as when managing patients with neurodevelopmental disorders, where modifications are necessary to provide safe and effective dental care. Medical consultation is suggested to establish the patient's current status, ascertain the medications the

patient is taking, identify complications that may be present, and confirm dental medications and doses that will minimize possible drug interactions.

Medical Considerations

While diagnosis of psychiatric disease can be a complex process, dentists should recognize signs and symptoms of undiagnosed or poorly controlled psychiatric conditions. Patients with *severe depression* may experience significant impairment of all personal hygiene, including a total lack of oral hygiene. Patients with severe depression must be referred for medical evaluation and treatment, if not already actively receiving care. The dentist should ask whether the severely depressed patient has had any thoughts about suicide. Studies have shown that questions about suicide do not prompt the act in these patients. Patients who state they have had these thoughts must be referred for immediate medical care.

For patients with *schizophrenia*, it is recommended to consult with the patient's physician before initiating dental treatment to establish the patient's current status, medications the patient is taking, and the ability of the patient to give valid consent for treatment. Routine dental treatment of the patient should not be attempted unless the patient is under medical management. An attendant or family member should accompany the patient to maximize comfort and familiarity. Morning appointments may be preferred. Confrontation and an authoritative attitude on the part of the dentist should be avoided. If the standard approach does not allow for proper dental management, the dentist should consider sedation, which should be provided in consultation with the patient's physician.

Anxiety related to dental treatment is common. The origin of this anxiety may lie in negative personal dental experiences or in cognitive perceptions of what the dental visit will be like. By obtaining a comprehensive dental history (including negative dental experiences and the patient's perception of dental treatment) and observing the patient for signs of anxiety, the dentist can identify patients who may need additional supportive care during dental treatment. Potential behaviors and indicators include being overly alert, rapid heart rate, restlessness, checking certain portions of clothing, and rapid and disconnected speech. In interactions with the patient, the dentist should convey an appropriate level of personal interest, using consistent verbal and nonverbal communication skills. The dentist can begin by mentioning that the patient appears anxious and then invite the patient to talk about relevant feelings and fears. If a patient remains anxious, the dentist may elect to use various anxiety-reducing modalities to better manage the dental treatment.

Patients with *bulimia nervosa* may present with a pattern of tooth erosion (perimylolysis) that is consistent with habitual regurgitation of stomach contents; this may be the first indication of the presence of an eating

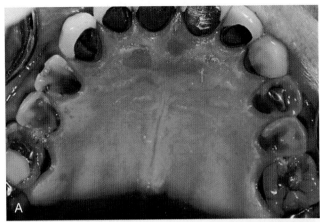

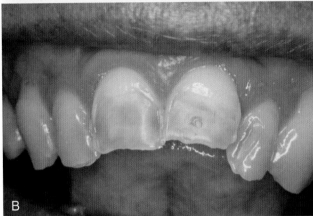

FIG. 28.4 (A) Lingual erosion of enamel in a patient with bulimia caused by regurgitation of stomach contents. **(B)** Labial erosion of enamel in a patient who habitually sucked on citrus products.

disorder (see Fig. 28.4). The erosive pattern involves the lingual surfaces of the teeth, primarily the maxillary teeth because the tongue protects the mandibular teeth. Erosion also can affect the occlusal surfaces of molar and premolar teeth, where the process can be accelerated by attrition.

Patients with *anorexia nervosa* may be difficult to identify. Young patients who appear to be anorexic should be approached delicately about the weight loss. If the initial examination and history reveal no evidence of serious medical disease such as cancer or diabetes mellitus, the possibility of self-starvation should be discussed with the patient. When young patients are involved, parents must be informed. Every attempt should be made to refer patients to a physician for evaluation and treatment.

Drug Interactions and Adverse Effects

Stimulants. The stimulants used in management of ADHD (e.g., methylphenidate, amphetamine, dextroamphetamine) can cause xerostomia, dysgeusia, and bruxism, as well as elevated blood pressure and heart rate. It is important to obtain good local anesthesia to avoid unnecessary pain and potential for endogenous catecholamine release.

Tricyclic Antidepressants. Many of the tricyclic antidepressants (TCAs) can cause hypotension, orthostatic hypotension, tachycardia, and cardiac arrhythmia (Table 28.4). When sedatives, hypnotics, barbiturates, and narcotics are used together with the heterocyclic antidepressants, severe respiratory depression may result. If these agents must be used, the dosage should be reduced. Small amounts of epinephrine (1:100,000) can be used in patients who are taking tricyclic antidepressants if the dentist aspirates before injecting; injects the anesthetic solution slowly; and, in general, uses no more than two cartridges. Other, more concentrated forms of epinephrine should be avoided.

Monoamine Oxidase Inhibitors. Patients who are taking MAO inhibitors can receive small amounts of epinephrine in local anesthetics. Other forms of epinephrine (retraction cord, topical for control of bleeding) are best avoided. Phenylephrine must not be used in patients who are taking MAO inhibitors. MAO inhibitors may interact with sedatives, narcotics, non-narcotic analgesics, antihistamines, and atropine to prolong and intensify their effects on the CNS (Table 28.4).

Antipsychotic Drugs. Several important drug interactions may occur in patients who are taking antipsychotic drugs (first-generation agents especially, Table 28.3). Anticonvulsants such as phenobarbital decrease the effectiveness of the antipsychotics. TCAs can result in increased plasma concentrations of either agent, which can result in clinical symptoms due to either agent. Thus, extreme care is indicated with use of sedatives, hypnotics, antihistamines, and opioids in patients who are taking neuroleptic agents, which will increase the respiratory depressant effects of these drugs. This potentiation can be dangerous, particularly in patients with compromised respiratory function. If these types of drugs must be used, the dosage must be reduced. The dentist should always consult with the patient's physician or check a drug interaction resource before using these agents.

Epinephrine must be used with caution in patients who are receiving an antipsychotic medication due to a theoretical risk of developing a severe hypotensive episode (due to the combination of α-adrenergic inhibition by antipsychotics that can result in decreased peripheral resistance, and β2-adrenergic mediated vasodilatory effects due to epinephrine). Small amounts of epinephrine (1:100,000) can be used if the dentist aspirates before injecting; injects the anesthetic solution slowly; and, in general, uses no more than two cartridges. Use of epinephrine-impregnated retraction cord or as a topically applied agent for control of bleeding should be avoided.

With older patients who are taking antipsychotic drugs, several important problems arise in terms of drug usage. Serum albumin levels decrease with age; hence, there may be a higher percentage of the drug in an unbound state. This free drug increases the risk for toxic reactions. In addition, older patients may have marginal

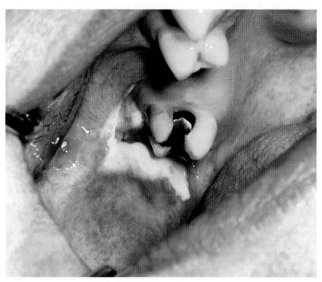

FIG. 28.5 Agranulocytosis. The dentist should be aware that agranulocytosis may be associated with the drugs used to treat psychoses. (From Sapp JP, Eversole LR, Wysocki GP. *Contemporary oral and Maxillofacial Pathology.* 2nd ed. St. Louis: Mosby; 2004.)

liver function; hence, drugs metabolized by the liver may remain in the circulation for longer periods and in increased concentrations.

Antipsychotic drugs may cause agranulocytosis, leukopenia, or thrombocytopenia, which rarely may be associated with oral findings (Fig. 28.5).

Benzodiazepines. The potential for clinically significant drug interactions between benzodiazepines—the mainstay of treatment for anxiety—and barbiturates, opioids, psychotropic agents (medications that affect brain chemistry/function), cimetidine, and erythromycin is well recognized (Table 28.6). In general, these agents potentiate the CNS depressant effects of benzodiazepines. Regarding the concomitant use of these agents and benzodiazepines, two situations are of clinical concern in dental treatment:

- Barbiturates (very rarely used in dentistry) and opioids used for dental sedation or pain control must be administered with caution and in decreased dosages in patients who are taking a benzodiazepine for an anxiety disorder.
- The dentist may prescribe a benzodiazepine for sedation to control dental treatment–related anxiety, but care must be taken with use of these drugs in patients receiving psychotropic agents for a psychiatric disorder.

The dentist should consult with the patient's physician before using these drug combinations, and the dosage of benzodiazepines may be reduced to avoid overdepression of the CNS.

Treatment Planning Considerations

The goals of treatment planning for patients with psychiatric disorders are to maintain oral health, comfort, and function and to prevent and control oral disease (Box 28.3). Without an aggressive approach to prevention, many of these patients will be susceptible to dental caries and periodontal disease. Susceptibility to such diseases increases because of the adverse effect of hyposalivation, which is associated with most of these medications, and the fact that some of the psychiatric conditions for which these patients are being treated are associated with reduced interest in performing or impaired ability to perform oral hygiene procedures. Also, many of these patients consume a diet containing foods or drinks that increase the risk for dental disease, and have an increased prevalence of tobacco smoking, alcohol, and drug use that contribute to risk for periodontal disease and oral cancer.

The dental team should communicate to the patient and family members a positive, hopeful attitude toward maintenance of the patient's oral health. The dental team should discuss with the patient and close relative or spouse whether the patient is legally able to make rational decisions. Under circumstances where a patient cannot make a rational decision, informed consent from a guardian is advised.

The dental treatment plan should include dietary and nutritional counseling and an individualized daily oral hygiene regimen, commensurate with the patient's perceived risk and ability to comply. The treatment plan must be realistic in terms of the patient's psychiatric disorder and physical status and must be sufficiently dynamic and flexible to account for changes in the acuity or severity of the psychiatric disorder and in the patient's physical status. The dentist must be particularly cautious when considering medications to be used in providing dental treatment to the patient. Some agents should be avoided, whereas others may require a modification in the usual dosage.

Patients with neurodevelopmental disorders can pose unique challenges to the dental team. Management of children and younger patients with ASD requires a family-centered approach and parent concerns must not be discredited. Patient behavior and ability to cooperate in the dental setting is the most important barrier affecting access to care in this patient population. The dental office can be an overwhelming environment due to sounds, lighting, wall decorations, and various objects and textures; minimizing stimulation and using the same dental operatory for each visit can be very helpful. Behavior guidance techniques can be effective in providing a calm and nonthreatening experience for the patient. These include use of social stories (visual or spoken) prior to the visit to prepare the child for what is involved in the dental visit, positive reinforcement, tell-show-do technique, distraction methods, nonverbal communication skills, and voice control. Additional

P: PATIENT EVALUATION AND RISK ASSESSMENT (SEE BOX 1.1)

- Evaluate and determine whether psychiatric disorder exists.
- Obtain medical consultation if patient's condition is poorly controlled, if signs and symptoms point to undiagnosed condition, or if diagnosis is uncertain.
- Engage with parents/caregivers of patients with neurodevelopmental disorders.

POTENTIAL ISSUES AND FACTORS OF CONCERN

A

Analgesics	Avoid sedative agents or use in reduced dosage (see drugs) in patients taking antidepressant or antipsychotic drugs. The control of postoperative pain is extremely important in anxious patients. In accordance with the procedure performed, the dentist should select the most appropriate drug for pain control (NSAIDs, salicylates, acetaminophen, and others).
Anesthesia	Use of epinephrine should be limited in patients taking antidepressants or antipsychotic drugs because hypertensive reaction (with antidepressants) or hypotensive reaction (with antipsychotics) can occur. Limit to two cartridges of 1:100,000 epinephrine (also avoid more concentrated forms of epinephrine in retraction cord or used to control bleeding). In patients with anxiety, oral sedation may be provided the night before and just before the dental appointment with a fast-acting benzodiazepine (alprazolam, 0.5-mg tablet; diazepam, 2-, 5-, or 10-mg tablet; or triazolam, 0.125- or 0.25-mg tablet). For more anxious patients, inhalation sedation with nitrous oxide, intramuscular sedation (midazolam, promethazine, or meperidine), or IV sedation (diazepam, midazolam, or fentanyl) can be considered.
Antibiotics	No specific considerations.
Anxiety	For patients with anxiety: establish effective communication; maintain an open and honest demeanor with appropriate level of genuine personal revelation; be consistent in verbal and nonverbal components of communication; provide explanations of procedures with short "question-and-answer" breaks to address the patient's concerns; and finally, if discomfort is anticipated, reassure the patient that all possible measures for a "pain-free" procedure will be used. If the patient appears overly anxious, confirmation of or attentiveness to this distress may be helpful (e.g., "You seem tense today—would you like to talk about it?" If yes, "Would you like something that would help with your anxiety?"). During the procedure, it is important to signal the patient when any discomfort may be expected and to let the patient know that things are going well. Advise the patient beforehand of what usually occurs after the procedure, what drugs and measures will be prescribed to minimize any discomfort, and any activities or medications to be avoided. Describe

B

	any complications that could occur, such as pain, bleeding, infection, or allergic reactions to any medications that may have been prescribed. Instruct the patient to contact the dental office if any complication occurs or, in the event of severe bleeding or allergic reaction, to go to the nearest hospital emergency department.
Bleeding	Thrombocytopenia and leukopenia may occur as side effects of medications used to treat patients with psychiatric disorders.
Breathing	No issues.
Blood pressure	Check blood pressure because hypertension (e.g., stimulants) and hypotension may occur as result of some medications (antidepressant and antipsychotic drugs).

C

Cardiovascular	No issues generally. Patients experiencing a panic attack may think that they are having a heart attack.
Chair position	Patients taking TCAs or MAO inhibitors may be prone to postural hypotension with sudden changes in chair position. Support patient getting out of the dental chair.
Consultation	Patient's physician should be consulted to confirm medications and the status of control of the disorder. Elective dental treatment may have to be deferred for patients with severe symptoms of mania, depression, or schizophrenia until the condition is better controlled. Confirm the need to adjust the dosage of drugs required in management of the patient's dental problems. If severe xerostomia is found, request the physician to change medication if possible. Refer patients found to have chronic extramedullary movement complications related to antipsychotic medications. With severe anxiety associated with any of the anxiety states such as PTSD or panic disorder, the patient's physician should be consulted regarding any special management considerations.

D

Devices	No issues.
Drugs	Avoid or use in reduced dosage sedatives, hypnotics, and narcotic agents in patients taking antidepressants or antipsychotic drugs. Avoid NSAIDs, tetracycline, and metronidazole in patients taking lithium because lithium toxicity may occur. Also, diazepam should be avoided with lithium because hypothermia may occur. Some psychiatric drugs may cause xerostomia.

E

Emergencies	Patients who make comments about suicidal thoughts should be referred for psychiatric care.
Equipment	No issues.

F

Follow-up	Ensure that patient is seeking routine follow-up for the psychiatric condition.

[a]Strength of recommendation taxonomy (SORT) Grade: C (see Preface for further explanation).
MAO, monoamine oxidase; *NSAID*, nonsteroidal antiinflammatory drug; *TCA*, tricyclic antidepressant.

measures that may be indicated include active and passive protective stabilization, sedation (e.g., benzodiazepines, nitrous oxide), and general anesthesia.

While patients with the inattentive subtype of ADHD do not typically pose challenges, those with the hyperactive/impulsive phenotype can be very difficult to manage in the dental setting. Patients are restless, fidgety, talkative, and have difficulty staying still and focusing on instructions. As behavior can be dependent on medication dosing throughout the day, it is important to know what medications the patient is taking and to schedule the dental visit accordingly. Techniques that can be particularly helpful when managing patients with ADHD include positive reinforcement, taking frequent but limited breaks, and engaging parents who can often provide invaluable insight and helpful hints.

Patients with PTSD may experience significant dental anxiety. These patients require a calm and patient approach to ensure that their anxiety can be controlled during dental care. In addition to careful patient management, the use of benzodiazepines prior to the visit, as well as periprocedural nitrous oxide, can help to reduce anxiety.

In patients with bulimia, complex restorative procedures should not be planned until the gorging and vomiting cycle has been broken. The diet of some patients with bulimia is rich in carbohydrates and carbonated liquids, which can lead to extensive dental caries and additional erosion of the teeth, especially in patients with poor oral hygiene. The dentist should provide instruction on toothbrushing, use of dental floss, and application of topical fluoride. After induced vomiting, patients should not immediately brush their teeth but rather be instructed to rinse with a basic solution such as sodium bicarbonate, or to sip milk or consume dairy products to buffer acidity in the oral cavity. Tooth sensitivity can be managed with the use of desensitizing toothpastes, fluoride applications, and other desensitizing agents. When the patient's overall health status is stable, restoration of teeth with severe erosion can begin. The dentist and the patient must be aware, however, that relapse is common and that complex restorations may fail with recurrence of chronic vomiting. With use of resin composite and adhesive systems, restoration can be achieved with minimal dental preparation and with less expense than fixed prosthodontics. However, patients with extensive erosion may require comprehensive prosthodontic rehabilitation.

Oral Complications and Manifestations

Patients who are taking antipsychotic agents may develop muscular problems (dystonia, dyskinesia, or tardive dyskinesia) in the oral and facial regions. A dyskinesia ("tardive" refers to delayed onset medication side effect) is characterized by atypical, repetitive, uncontrolled movements, often of the muscles of mastication or facial expression muscles. Some patients with dyskinesia may be susceptible to repeated soft tissue injury (e.g., traumatic ulcers of the oral mucosa), and provision of dental care can be challenging. Dystonias are less common in this setting and are characterized by involuntary muscle contractions that result in repetitive twisting or otherwise uncontrolled movements. If the

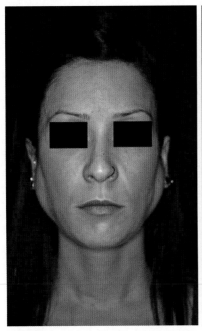
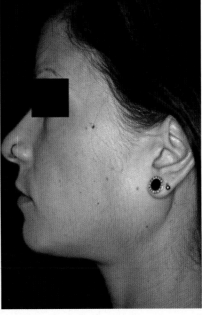

FIG. 28.6 Sialadenosis in a 34-year-old female patient with a long-standing history of bulimia nervosa. (Reproduced from Garcia Garcia B, Dean Ferrer A, Diaz Jimenez N, et al. Bilateral parotid sialadenosis associated with long-standing bulimia: a case report and literature review. *J Maxillofac Oral Surg.* June 2018;17(2):117–121.)

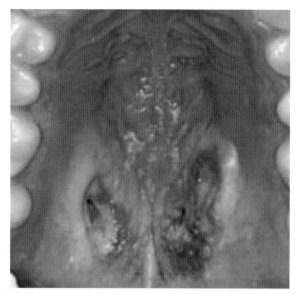

FIG. 28.7 Necrotizing sialometaplasia of the *right* and *left* hard palate in a 22-year-old female with bulimia nervosa. (Reproduced from Janner SF, Suter VG, Altermatt HJ, Reichart PA, Bornstein MM. Bilateral necrotizing sialometaplasia of the hard palate in a patient with bulimia: a case report and review of the literature. *Quintessence Int.* 2014;45(5):431–437. https://doi.org/10.3290/j.qi.a31543. PMID: 24634907.)

dentist observes such initial symptoms of dysfunction, the patient should be referred to the primary care physician, psychiatrist, or appropriate specialist.

Patients with psychiatric disorders may engage in painful self-injurious behavior. Acts of orofacial mutilation such as eye gouging, pushing sharp objects into the ear canal, lip/cheek/tongue biting, burning of oral tissues with the tip of a cigarette, mucosal injury with a sharp or blunt object, and gingival mutilation and self-extraction of teeth have been described.

In addition to severe erosion of the lingual and occlusal surfaces of the teeth in patients with bulimia nervosa, patients may develop sialadenosis, or painless enlargement of the parotid glands (Fig. 28.6). Sialadenosis also is reported in patients with anorexia nervosa. Patients with bulimia nervosa, presumably due to digital manipulation/injury to the palatal mucosa, are also at risk for developing necrotizing sialometaplasia, an otherwise very rare ulcerative condition that can be mistaken for squamous cell carcinoma (Fig. 28.7).

Patients with orofacial *somatic symptoms* may describe burning tongue, coated or swollen tongue, numbness of soft tissue, tingling sensations of oral tissues, and pain in the orofacial region. Similarly, patients with PTSD also may present with various orofacial pain

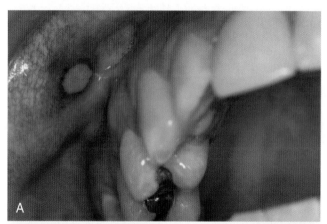

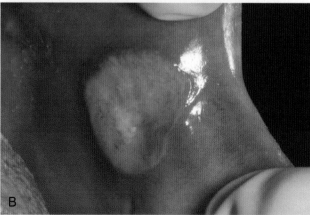

FIG. 28.8 (**A**) A single minor aphthous ulceration of the anterior buccal mucosa. (**B**) A large major aphthous ulceration of the left anterior buccal mucosa. (From Neville BW, Damm DD, Allen CM, Bouquot J. *Oral and Maxillofacial Pathology.* 3rd ed. Philadelphia: Saunders; 2009.)

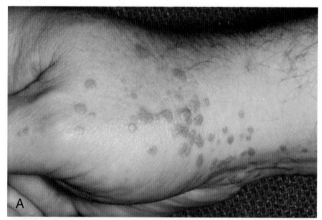

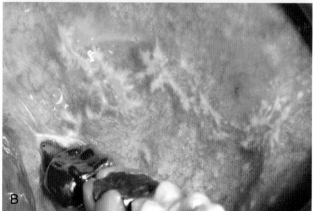

FIG. 28.9 (**A**) Lichen planus on the skin of the wrist. (**B**) Lichen planus on the buccal mucosa. (From Neville BW, Damm DD, Allen CM, Bouquot J. *Oral and Maxillofacial Pathology.* 3rd ed. Philadelphia: Saunders; 2009.)

conditions. It may be difficult if not impossible to differentiate somatic symptoms from neuropathic symptoms characteristic of oral dysesthesia (e.g., burning mouth syndrome/disorder) and persistent idiopathic facial pain. Dental treatment should not be provided unless a dental cause can be found and diagnosed to avoid needless extractions, root canal treatments, and other unnecessary or even potentially harmful procedures. A series of short appointments should be scheduled to reexamine the patient for possible signs of disease, to discuss symptoms, and to provide reassurance that tissue changes/dental pathologies are not clinically evident. Patients with a severe somatoform disorder should be referred to a psychiatrist; however, after a patient has been referred, the dentist should be willing to remain involved in the patient's care. The patient may need to be reexamined and the psychiatrist consulted regarding the findings. If patients feel that the dentist only wants to "get rid of them," the suggestion of referral will not be helpful or effective.

Certain oral medicine and orofacial pain conditions may be influenced and/or exacerbated by stress. Recurrent aphthous stomatitis (Fig. 28.8) and oral lichen planus (Fig. 28.9) can become more severe during periods of intense and prolonged stress. Similarly, stress can at least in part be a primary contributing factor to developing and/or exacerbating temporomandibularsorders.

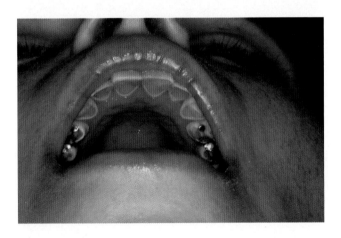

BIBLIOGRAPHY

1. Association AP. *Diagnostic and Statistical Manual of Mental Disorders (DSM-5TM)*. 5th ed. Arlington, VA: American Psychiatric Publishing; 2013:1–947.
2. Larry Jameson J. Harrison's Manual of Medicine. In: Jameson J, Fauci AS, Kasper DL, et al., eds. *Harrison's Principles of Internal Medicine*. McGraw Hill; 2018:20e.
3. Goldman L, Schafer AI, eds. *Goldman-Cecil Medicine*. 26th ed. Philadelphia, PA: Elsevier; 2020.
4. Schiffer RB. Psychiatric disorders in medical practice. In: Goldman L, Ausiello D, eds. *Cecil Textbook of Medicine*. Philadelphia Saunders; 2004:2212–2222.
5. Cleare A. Unipolar depression. In: Wright P, Stern J, Phelan M, eds. *Core Psychiatry*. 2nd ed. Edinburgh: Elsevier; 2005:271–295.
6. Reus VI. Mental disorders. In: Fauci AS, ed. *Harrison's Principles of Internal Medicine*. 17th ed. New York: McGraw-Hill; 2008:2710–2723.
7. Schiffer RB. Psychiatric disorders in medical practice. In: Goldman L, Ausiello D, eds. *Cecil Medicine*. 23rd ed. Philadelphia: Saunders Elsevier; 2008:2628–2638.
8. Shah A, Tovey E. Psychiatry of old age. In: Wright P, Stern J, Phelan M, eds. *Core Psychiatry*. 2nd ed. Edinburgh: Elsevier; 2005:481–493.
9. Giglio JA, Laskin DM. Prevalence of psychiatric disorders in a group of adult patients seeking general dental care. *Quintessence Int.* 2010;41(5):433–437.
10. Khalife S. Bipolar disorder. In: Carey WD, ed. *Current Clinical Medicine 2009*. Cleveland Clinic Philadelphia: Saunders Elsevier; 2009:1007–1012.
11. Tesar GE. Recognition and treatment of depression. In: Carey WD, ed. *Current Clinical Medicine 2009—Cleveland Clinic*. Cleveland Clinic Philadelphia: Saunders Elsevier; 2009:997–1006.
12. Scherger JE, Baustian GH, O'Hanlon KM, et al. *Bipolar Disorders*. Elsevier; 2006. http://www.firstconsult.com/bipolardisorders. Accessed March 29, 2006.
13. Rush AJ, Trivedi MH, Wisniewski SR, et al. Bupropion-SR, sertraline, or venlafaxine-XR after failure of SSRIs for depression. *N Engl J Med.* 2006;354(12):1231–1242.
14. Healy D. *Psychiatric Drugs Explained*. 5th ed. St. Louis: Churchill Livingstone Elsevier; 2009.
15. Srinath S. Suicide and deliberate self-harm. In: Wright P, Stern J, Phelan M, eds. *Core Psychiatry*. 2nd ed. Edinburgh: Elsevier; 2005:319–335.
16. Wright P, Perahia D. Psychopharmacology. In: Wright P, Stern J, Phelan M, eds. *Core Psychiatry*. 2nd ed. Edinburgh: Elsevier; 2005:579–611.
17. Russakoff LM. Psychopharmacology. In: Cutler JL, Marcus ER, eds. *Saunders Text and Review Series: Psychiatry*. Philadelphia: W.B. Saunders Company; 1999: 308–331.
18. Little JW. Dental implications of mood disorders. *Gen Dent.* 2004;52(5):442–450.
19. Goldberg RJ. *Practical Guide to the Care of the Psychiatric Patient*. St Louis: Mosby; 1995.
20. Friedlander AH, Marder SR. The psychopathology, medical management and dental implications of schizophrenia. *J Am Dent Assoc.* 2002;133(5):603–610. quiz 24-5.
21. Scully C, Cawson RA. *Medical Problems in Dentistry*. 5th ed. Edinburgh: Elsevier (Churchill Livingstone); 2005.
22. Friedlander AH, Brill NQ. Dental management of patients with schizophrenia. *Spec Care Dent.* 1986;6(5):217–219.
23. Stiefel DJ, Truelove EL, Menard TW, et al. A comparison of oral health of persons with and without chronic mental illness in community settings. *Spec Care Dent.* 1990; 10(1):6–12.
24. Metzger ED, Levine JM, McArdle CR, et al. Salivary gland enlargement and elevated serum amylase in bulimia nervosa. *Biol Psychiatry.* 1999;45(11):1520–1522.
25. Fichter MM, Quadflieg N. Mortality in eating disorders—results of a large prospective clinical longitudinal study. *Int J Eat Disord.* 2016;49(4):391–401.

26. Duarte C, Ferreira C, Pinto-Gouveia J. At the core of eating disorders: overvaluation, social rank, self-criticism and shame in anorexia, bulimia and binge eating disorder. *Compr Psychiatry*. 2016;66:123–131.

27. Armfield JM. Towards a better understanding of dental anxiety and fear: cognitions vs. experiences. *Eur J Oral Sci*. 2010;118(3):259–264.

28. van Wijk AJ, Hoogstraten J. Anxiety and pain during dental injections. *J Dent*. 2009;37(9):700–704.

29. Little JW. Eating disorders. *Oral Surg Oral Med Oral Pathol Oral Radiol Endod*. 2002;93(2):138–144.

30. Milosevic A, Brodie DA, Slade PD. Dental erosion, oral hygiene, and nutrition in eating disorders. *Int J Eat Disord*. 1997;21(2):195–199.

31. Spreafico RC. Composite resin rehabilitation of eroded dentition in a bulimic patient: a case report. *Eur J Esthetic Dent*. 2010;5(1):28–48.

32. Garcia Garcia B, Dean Ferrer A, Diaz Jimenez N, et al. Bilateral parotid sialadenosis associated with long-standing bulimia: a case report and literature review. *J Maxillofac Oral Surg*. 2018;17(2):117–121.

33. Janner SF, Suter VG, Altermatt HJ, et al. Bilateral necrotizing sialometaplasia of the hard palate in a patient with bulimia: a case report and review of the literature. *Quintessence Int*. 2014;45(5):431–437.

34. Conviser JH, Fisher SD, Mitchell KB. Oral care behavior after purging in a sample of women with bulimia nervosa. *J Am Dent Assoc*. 2014;145(4):352–354.

35. Nelson TM, Sheller B, Friedman CS, Bernier R. Educational and therapeutic behavioral approaches to providing dental care for patients with Autism Spectrum Disorder. *Spec Care Dent*. 2015;35(3):105–113.

36. Gandhi RP, Klein U. Autism spectrum disorders: an update on oral health management. *J Evid Base Dent Pract*. June 2014;14(suppl):115–126.

37. Sujlana A, Dang R. Dental care for children with attention deficit hyperactivity disorder. *J Dent Child*. 2013;80(2):67–70.

38. Bassiouny MA, Tweddale E. Oral health considerations in anorexia and bulimia nervosa. 2. Multidisciplinary management and personalized dental care. *Gen Dent*. 2017;65(5):24–31.

29

Substance Use Disorders

KEY POINTS

- Alcohol use comprises the largest proportion of patients with substance use disorders.
- Patients with substance use disorders may be undiagnosed, untreated, medically unstable, and may present with signs and symptoms recognizable in a dental setting.
- Dental providers can play an important role by screening and assessing patients for substance use disorders, and referring patients for treatment.

- Given the critical healthcare issue surrounding the misuse of opioids, dentists must minimize the prescribing of opioids to patients, especially at a young age, and remain well versed in the guidelines for the prescription of opioids and the management of patients with opioid use disorders.

The Diagnostic and Statistical Manual of Mental Disorders, fifth edition (DSM-V), of the American Psychiatric Association, provides diagnostic criteria for substance use disorders. As an example, there are 11 criteria for alcohol use disorder (Table 29.1), and the greater the number of criteria, the greater the severity. Similar diagnostic criteria have been developed for other substance use disorders which encompass 10 classes of substances/disorders, namely alcohol (alcohol use disorder, AUD), caffeine; cannabis; hallucinogens; inhalants; opioids; sedatives, hypnotics, and anxiolytics; stimulants (amphetamine-type substances, cocaine, and other stimulants); tobacco; and other (or unknown) substances.

Substance use is an already large-scale and growing global public health problem. Substance use disorders have far-reaching effects on persons engaging in such activity, as well as their families and communities, with a consequent heavy impact on law enforcement, the judicial system, politics, and health care. Patients who suffer from substance use disorders may be unable to function in the workplace and have increased risk for being in hazardous situations and at an increased risk for numerous medical issues, overdoses, suicide, and death. It is inevitable that dental practitioners will encounter patients with a history of substance use disorders, and some practitioners themselves suffer from these disorders. This chapter discusses the effects of alcohol and illicit drug use as they pertain to dental management. Nicotine use disorder is discussed in Chapter 8. In a dental practice of 2000 patients, it can be expected that approximately 250 of them satisfy the criteria for a substance use disorder, of which at least 160 are attributed to alcohol.

EPIDEMIOLOGY

Illicit "street" drugs include cannabis/marijuana, opioids (e.g., heroin), stimulants (e.g., cocaine (including crack), and methamphetamine), hallucinogens, and inhalants (see Table 29.2). Legally prescribed opioids, sedative–hypnotics, some stimulants, and cannabis may be misused. Alcohol is legal but is subject to misuse when consumed inappropriately or in excessive amounts. Recreational cannabis is now legal in many US states (and countries) with many more headed in the same direction.

According to the 2020 National Survey on Drug Use and Health (NSDUH), 40.3 million people aged 12 or older (or 14.5%) had a SUD in the past year, including 28.3 million with alcohol use disorder (AUD), 18.4 million with an illicit drug use disorder, and 6.5 million with both alcohol use disorder and an illicit drug use disorder. An estimated 50.0% of Americans aged 12 or older (or 138.5 million people) were current alcohol users (i.e., used alcohol in the past month), and almost 45% and 13% of current users were classified as binge drinkers (consumption of five or more drinks on the same occasion) or heavy drinkers (for men, consuming more than 4 drinks on any day or more than 14 drinks per week, and for women, consuming more than 3 drinks on any day or more than 7 drinks per week, respectively). Binge alcohol use was highest among young adults aged 18–25 (31.4%). Nearly 95,000 people died from alcohol-related causes in 2019, making alcohol the fourth leading preventable cause of death in the United States. Only 7.2% of adults who needed treatment for AUD received it.

An estimated 21.4% of Americans 12 years of age and older are current illicit drug users (almost 60 million people), and illicit drug use also is highest among young adults 18–25 years of age. The drug with the highest use was cannabis (49.6 million people), related in part to legalization for recreational use in some states (Alaska, Arizona, California, Colorado, Connecticut, Illinois, Maine, Massachusetts, Michigan, Montana, Nevada, New Jersey, New Mexico, New York, Oregon, Vermont, Virginia, Washington, and the District of Columbia as of 2022). Other states have made cannabis use legal for

TABLE 29.1 Alcohol Use Disorder

Diagnostic Criteria

A. A problematic pattern of alcohol use leading to clinically significant impairment or distress, as manifested by at least two of the following, occurring within a 12-month period:

1. Alcohol is often taken in larger amounts or over a longer period than was intended.

2. There is a persistent desire or unsuccessful efforts to cut down or control alcohol use.

3. A great deal of time is spent in activities necessary to obtain alcohol, use alcohol, or recover from its effects.

4. Craving, or a strong desire or urge to use alcohol.

5. Recurrent alcohol use resulting in a failure to fulfill major role obligations at work, school, or home.

6. Continued alcohol use despite having persistent or recurrent social or interpersonal problems caused or exacerbated by the effects of alcohol.

7. Important social, occupational, or recreational activities are given up or reduced because of alcohol use.

8. Recurrent alcohol use in situations in which it is physically hazardous.

9. Alcohol use is continued despite knowledge of having a persistent or recurrent physical or psychological problem that is likely to have been caused or exacerbated by alcohol.

10. Tolerance, as defined by either of the following:

   a. A need for markedly increased amounts of alcohol to achieve intoxication or desired effect.

   b. A markedly diminished effect with continued use of the same amount of alcohol.

11. Withdrawal, as manifested by either of the following:

   a. The characteristic withdrawal syndrome for alcohol (refer to Criteria A and B of the criteria set for alcohol withdrawal).

   b. Alcohol (or a closely related substance, such as a benzodiazepine) is taken to relieve or avoid withdrawal symptoms.

Specify if:

In early remission: After full criteria for alcohol use disorder were previously met, none of the criteria for alcohol use disorder have been met for at least 3 months but for less than 12 months (with the exception that Criterion A4, "Craving, or a strong desire or urge to use alcohol," may be met).

In sustained remission: After full criteria for alcohol use disorder were previously met, none of the criteria for alcohol use disorder have been met at any time during a period of 12 months or longer (with the exception that Criterion A4, "Craving, or a strong desire or urge to use alcohol," may be met).

Specify if:

In a controlled environment: This additional specifier is used if the individual is in an environment where access to alcohol is restricted.

Code based on current severity: Note for ICD-10-CM codes: If an alcohol intoxication, alcohol withdrawal, or another alcohol-induced mental disorder is also present, do not use the codes below for alcohol use disorder. Instead, the comorbid alcohol use disorder is indicated in the 4th character of the alcohol-induced disorder code (see the coding note for alcohol intoxication, alcohol withdrawal, or a specific alcohol-induced mental disorder). For example, if there is comorbid alcohol intoxication and alcohol use disorder, only the alcohol intoxication code is given, with the 4th character indicating whether the comorbid alcohol use disorder is mild, moderate, or severe: F10.129 for mild alcohol use disorder with alcohol intoxication or F10.229 for a moderate or severe alcohol use disorder with alcohol intoxication.

Specify current severity:

305.00 (F10.10) Mild: Presence of 2–3 symptoms.

303.90 (F10.20) Moderate: Presence of 4–5 symptoms.

303.90 (F10.20) Severe: Presence of 6 or more symptoms.

Reprinted with permission from the Diagnostic and Statistical Manual of Mental Disorders: DSM5, 5th ed., pp. 490–491 (Copyright © 2013). American Psychiatric Association. All Rights Reserved.

medical purposes only. There were 9.5 million people aged 12 or older who misused opioids in the past year (9.3 million misused prescription opioids and 902,000 people used heroin). The use of prescription opioids (e.g., oxycodone or fentanyl) for nonmedical reasons remains one of the fastest growing dimensions of illicit drug use in the United States.

The CDC has reported that for the year ending in April 2021, there were 1.6 and 0.7 million current cocaine and methamphetamine users aged 12 or older, respectively (collectively <1% of the population).

There were more than 100,000 deaths related to illicit substance use, an almost 30% annual increase. Overdose from opioids contributed to 75,673 of these deaths. Deaths attributed to stimulants are also increasing.

ETIOLOGY

The neurobiology of substance addiction and dependence is complex and involves a unique set of variables.

Evidence suggests that early exposure to the drug (i.e., during adolescence) is a major risk factor. These substances disrupt the endogenous reward systems in the brain; most often by disrupting the dopamine circuits. Acute changes increase synaptic dopamine and disrupt circuits that mediate motivation and drive, conditioned learning, and inhibitory controls. This enhancement of synaptic dopamine is particularly rewarding for persons with abnormally low density of the D_2 dopamine receptor (D_2DR). The neural circuitry underlying drug seeking behavior is delineated in Fig. 29.1. Although dopamine is the primary neurotransmitter in substance use disorders and addiction, many other neurotransmitters are involved, depending on the drug (Fig. 29.2). Inherited genetic factors also are involved in addiction. Psychological factors such as depression, personality disorder, poor coping skills, and self-medication (to relieve emotional distress) appear to be involved in addictive behavior. Social factors that may be involved include interpersonal, cultural, and societal influences.

TABLE 29.2 Commonly Used Drugs

Drug	Street Names	How Administered	Adverse Effects
Cannabis			
Marijuana	420, Blunt, Bud, Doobie, Dope, Ganja, Grass, Green, Herb, Joint, Mary Jane, Pot, Reefer, Sinsemilla, Skunk, Smoke, Stinkweed, Trees, Weed, Boom, Gangster, Hash Hemp Concentrates: Budder, Crumble, Shatter, Wax In food: Edibles	Smoked, vaped, eaten	Short-term: euphoria; relaxation; slowed reaction time; distorted sensory perception; impaired balance and coordination; increased heart rate and appetite; impaired learning, memory; anxiety; panic attacks; psychosis Long-term: chronic cough, frequent respiratory infections; possible mental health decline; addiction Oral: xerostomia, increased rates of caries and periodontitis
Opioids			
Heroin	Brown sugar, Chiva Dope, H, Horse, Junk, Skag, Skunk, Smack, White Horse. With OTC night-time cold medicine: Cheese. With Marijuana: A-Bomb	Injected, smoked, snorted	Short-term: euphoria; itching; nausea; vomiting; analgesia; drowsiness; impaired coordination; dizziness; confusion; nausea; sedation slowed breathing and heart rate
Prescription opioids	**Codeine:** Captain Cody, Coties, Schoolboy, With soft drinks/candy: Lean, Sizzurp, Purple Drank. With hypnotic sedatives: Doors and Fours, Loads, Pancakes and Syrup **Fentanyl:** Blonde, Blue Diamond, Snowflake, Humid, Jackpot, Murder 8, Tango and Cash, TNT. With heroin: Birria **Hydocodone:** Vikes, Veeks, Idiot Pills, Scratch, 357s, Lemonade, Bananas, Dones, Droco, Lorries. With valium and vodka: Triple V **Morphine:** Dreamer, First Line, Joy Juice, Morpho, Miss Emma, Monkey, White Stuff, Mister Blue, Unkie **Oxycodone:** 30s, 40s, 512s, Oxy, Beans, Blues, Buttons, Cotton, Kickers, Killers, Percs, Roxy	Injected, smoked, snorted, swallowed	Long-term: collapsed veins; abscesses; endocarditis; constipation and stomach cramps; liver or kidney disease; miscarriage, low birth weight, neonatal abstinence syndrome; pneumonia; hepatitis, HIV; addiction; fatal overdose Oral: xerostomia, caries, tolerance to local anesthesia, hyperalgesia
Stimulants			
Cocaine	Blow, Bump, C, Coke, Crack, Dust, Flake, Nose Candy, Rock, Snow, Sneeze, Sniff, Toot, White Rock With heroin: Speedball	Snorted, smoked, injected, or applied to gingivae	Short-term: narrowed blood vessels; enlarged pupils; increased body temperature, heart rate, and blood pressure; headache; abdominal pain and nausea; euphoria; increased energy, alertness; insomnia, restlessness; anxiety; erratic and violent behavior, panic attacks, paranoia, psychosis; heart rhythm problems, heart attack; stroke, seizure, coma. insomnia; intense itching leading to skin sores from scratching (methamphetamine)
Prescription Amphetamines	**Amphetamine:** Addys, Bennies, Beans, Black Beauties, Crosses, Hearts, Ivy League Drug, Pep Pills, Speed, Uppers **Methylphenidate:** Diet Coke, JIF, Kiddie Coke, MPH, R-Ball, RPop, Skippy, Study Buddies, The Smart Drug, Vitamin R	Swallowed, snorted, smoked, injected	Long-term: loss of sense of smell, nosebleeds, nasal damage and trouble swallowing from snorting; infection and death of bowel tissue from decreased blood flow; poor nutrition and weight loss; anxiety, confusion, mood problems, hallucinations (methamphetamine), delusions
Methamphetamine	Crank, Chalk, Crystal, Dunk, Gak, Ice, Meth, Pookie, Quartz, Rocket Fuel, Scooby Snax, Speed, Trash With cocaine: Croak, Shabu With MDMA: Hugs and Kisses, Party and Play (P&P)	Swallowed, snorted, smoked, injected	Oral: xerostomia, caries, periodontal disease (in the case of methamphetamine use, referred to as "Meth mouth"), dental erosion, bruxism/attrition, palatal perforation (cocaine)

Continued

Sedatives			
Benzodiazepines	Benzos, Downers, Poles, Tranks, Totem Z-Bars, Vs, Yellow/Blue Zs, Zannies	Swallowed, snorted	Short-term: drowsiness, slurred speech, poor concentration, confusion, dizziness, problems with movement and memory, lowered blood pressure, slowed breathing
Barbiturates	Barbs, Dolls, Phennies, Red/BlueBirds, Tooties, Yellow Jackets, Yellows	Swallowed, injected	Long-term: unknown
			Oral: unknown
Club Drugs			
MDMA	Adam, E, X, XTC, Beans, Candy, Ebomb, Thizz, Love Drug, Molly, Rolls, Skittles, Sweets, Vitamin E or X	Swallowed, snorted, injected	MDMA—mild hallucinogenic effects; increased tactile sensitivity; empathic feelings; lowered inhibition; anxiety; chills; sweating; teeth clenching; muscle cramping or sleep disturbances; depression; impaired memory; hyperthermia; addiction
Flunitrazepam	Circles, Date Rape Drug, Forget-Me Pill, La Rocha, Mind Eraser, Pingus, R2, Rib, Variations of: Roaches, Roapies, Rochas Dos, Roofies, Rope, Rophies, Rowie, Ruffies	Swallowed, snorted	Flunitrazepam—sedation; muscle relaxation; confusion; memory loss; dizziness; impaired coordination/addiction
GHB	G, Gamma-oh, GEEB, Gina, Goop, Grievous Bodily Harm, Liquid Ecstasy, Liquid X, Scoop, Soap	Swallowed	GHB—drowsiness; nausea; headache; disorientation; loss of coordination; memory loss or unconsciousness; seizures; coma
			Oral: not reported
Dissociative Drugs			
Ketamine	Cat Valium, K, Lady K, Special K, Vitamin K	Injected, snorted, smoked	Feelings of being separate from one's body and environment; impaired motor function or anxiety; tremors; numbness; memory loss; nausea
PCP and analogues	Angel Dust, Embalming Fluid, Hog, Rocket Fuel, Sherms Mixed with marijuana: Zoom	Swallowed, smoked, injected	Ketamine—also analgesia; impaired memory; delirium; respiratory depression and arrest; death
			PCP and analogues—also analgesia; psychosis; aggression; violence; slurred speech; loss of coordination; hallucinations
			Oral: not reported
Hallucinogens			
LSD	Acid, blotter, cubes, microdot yellow sunshine, blue heaven	Swallowed, absorbed through oral mucosa	Hallucinations, altered perception of time, inability to tell fantasy from reality, panic, muscle relaxation or weakness, problems with movement, enlarged pupils, nausea, vomiting, drowsiness. High doses: increased body temperature, heart rate, blood pressure; loss of appetite; sweating; sleeplessness; numbness, dizziness, weakness, tremors; impulsive behavior; rapid shifts in emotions
Psilocybin	Little Smoke, Magic Mushrooms, Purple Passion, Sacred Mush, Sewage Fruit, Shrooms, Zoomers	Swallowed	
Mescaline	Buttons, cactus, mesc, peyote	Swallowed, smoked	LSD and psilocybin also can cause flashbacks (hallucinogen, persisting perception disorder)
			Oral: not reported

GHB, γ-hydroxybutyrate; *LSD*, lysergic acid diethylamide; *PCP*, phencyclidine.
Adapted from the National Institutes of Health, National Institute on Drug Abuse (website), http://www.drugabuse.gov/DrugPages/DrugsofAbuse. html. Accessed February 2022.

CLINICAL PRESENTATION AND MEDICAL MANAGEMENT

Substance use disorders occur when the person using the substance takes it in larger amounts or over a longer period than was originally intended. A great deal of time may be spent in activities needed to procure the substance, take it, or recover from its effects. The person retreats from important social, occupational, and recreational activities because of substance use. Marked tolerance to the substance may develop; therefore, progressively larger amounts are needed to achieve intoxication or to produce the desired effect. Affected individuals continue to take the substance despite persistent or recurrent social, psychological, and physical problems that result from its use. Withdrawal may occur when the person stops or reduces intake of the substance and withdrawal symptoms generally vary in accordance with the substance involved. Physiologic signs of withdrawal are common after prolonged use of alcohol, opioids, sedatives, hypnotics, and anxiolytics. Such signs are less obvious in withdrawal from cocaine, amphetamines, and cannabis.

Cannabis

Cannabis refers to products from the different Cannabis plant species. *Marijuana* refers to the products containing the psychoactive chemical Delta-9-tetrahydrocannabinol (THC) and is the most commonly used illicit drug in the world. Several different preparations of marijuana are available (Table 29.2), and these preparations vary in potency and quality. They usually are smoked or vaped, but can also be taken orally. With inhalation, peak effects occur within 20–30 min; with oral ingestion, peak effects occur within 2–3 h. Most users describe an altered sense of time and distance perception. Acute intoxication may result in anxiety and paranoid ideation. Tolerance and physical dependence can occur, but clinical presentation of these symptoms is not common. Marijuana use can destabilize patients whose schizophrenia is in remission. Social and occupational impairment occurs but is less severe than that seen with alcohol or stimulant use. Acute recreational marijuana use rarely requires medical treatment. Anxiety reactions may require treatment with benzodiazepines. In terms of legal medical use, cannabis's

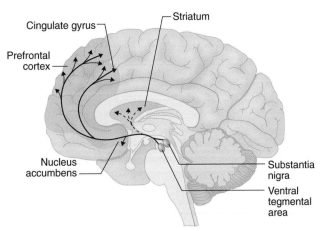

FIG. 29.1 Brain reward circuits. The major dopaminergic projections to the forebrain that underlie brain reward are shown superimposed on a diagram of the human brain: projection from the ventral tegmental area to the nucleus accumbens and prefrontal cerebral cortex. Also shown are projections from the substantia nigra to the dorsal striatum, which play a role in habit formation and in well-rehearsed motor behavior, such as drug seeking and drug administration. (From Hyman SE. Biology of addiction. In: Goldman L, Ausiello D, eds. *Cecil Medicine.* 23rd ed. Philadelphia: Saunders; 2008.)

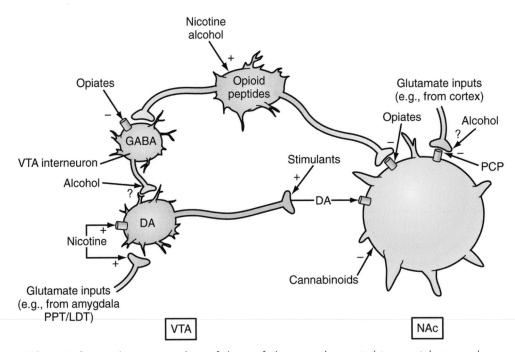

FIG. 29.2 Converging acute actions of drugs of abuse on the ventral tegmental area and nucleus accumbens. *DA,* dopamine; *GABA,* γ-aminobutyric acid; *LDT,* laterodorsal tegmentum; *NAc,* nucleus accumbens; *PCP,* phencyclidine; *PPT,* pedunculopontine tegmentum; *VTA,* ventral tegmental area. (From Renner JA, Ward EN. Drug addiction. In: Stern TA, et al., eds. *Massachusetts General Hospital Comprehensive Clinical Psychiatry.* Philadelphia: Mosby; 2008.)

action on cannabinoid receptors may be of benefit in reducing chronic pain, or nausea and vomiting associated with cancer chemotherapy; for increasing appetite; and for alleviating some types of seizures, and the symptoms of multiple sclerosis. Consumption of both marijuana and alcohol is more common among recreational users than medical users.

With the shifting legal landscape of cannabis, different methods of cannabis administration have important public health implications. How cannabis laws have influenced patterns of use such as vaping and edibles compared to smoking is unclear.

Opioids

The primary effects of the opioids and opiate-like drugs are to decrease pain perception, cause modest levels of sedation, and produce euphoria. Drugs in this category include those derived from the naturally occurring alkaloids morphine and codeine, semisynthetic drugs produced from morphine or thebaine molecules (e.g., hydrocodone, hydromorphone, heroin, and oxycodone), and synthetic opioids (e.g., meperidine, propoxyphene, diphenoxylate, fentanyl, buprenorphine, methadone, and pentazocine). Tolerance to any single opioid is likely to generalize to other drugs in the group.

Through direct effects on the central nervous system (CNS), opiates may produce nausea and vomiting, decreased pain perception, euphoria, and sedation. Additives in street drugs (i.e., opioids and other illicit drugs) can cause permanent damage to the nervous system, including peripheral neuropathy and CNS dysfunction. Users of such drugs may experience constipation, anorexia, and respiratory depression. Respiratory depression occurs as the result of a decreased response of the brainstem to carbon dioxide tension and can be significant in patients with compromised lung function.

Complications are common among those with opioid use disorder, especially when administered intravenously. Cardiovascular effects of opioids are mild. Orthostatic hypotension, probably caused by dilation of peripheral vessels, may occur. Intravenous (IV) use of these opioids (and other illicit drugs that are injected) involving the use of contaminated or shared needles when pathogens may be introduced can cause hepatitis B and C, HIV, and infective endocarditis. Infective endocarditis is unusual in that it predominantly affects the right side of the heart (the location of the tricuspid valve), with *Staphylococcus aureus* being the most common causative organism.

Dependence on opioids is seen in at least three groups of patients. The first group is the minority of patients with chronic pain syndromes who misuse prescribed drugs. The second group consists of physicians, dentists, nurses, and pharmacists who have easy access to the drugs. Members of the third and largest group procure opioids illicitly. When persistent opioid use has been established, the risk for overdose increases and such risk is greater with drugs such as fentanyl, which is 80–100

times more potent than morphine. IV overdose can rapidly lead to slow, shallow respirations; bradycardia; a drop in body temperature; and lack of responsiveness to external stimulation. Emergency treatment includes support of vital signs with the use of a respirator and administration of a reversal agent/opioid receptor antagonist such as naloxone by nasal spray (Narcan) (Figs. 29.3 and 29.4) or subcutaneous, intramuscular, or IV injection to reverse the effects of an opioid overdose. Any dental practice should consider having naloxone nasal spray available, but in particular in communities known to have high opioid use.

Withdrawal from opioids is an unpleasant but not life-threatening experience. Gastrointestinal upset, muscle cramps, rhinorrhea, and irritability are the prominent signs and symptoms. Treatment for opioid use disorder includes the use of medications in combination with counseling and behavioral therapies. Medications may include methadone (an opioid agonist), buprenorphine (a partial opioid agonist), naltrexone (an opioid antagonist given by long-acting injection), or combination buprenorphine/naloxone (Suboxone).

Cocaine

Cocaine is a stimulant with potent vasoconstrictor properties. After alcohol, it is the leading illicit substance in terms of frequency of emergency department (ED) visits, general hospital admissions, family violence, and other social problems. The drug produces physiologic and

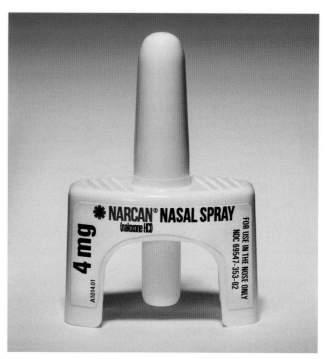

FIG. 29.3 Narcan device. (©2017 ADAPT Pharma, Inc. NARCAN is a registered trademark licensed to ADAPT Pharma Operations Limited. ADAPT Pharma, Inc. Radnor, PA. Adapt Pharma Inc. All rights reserved.)

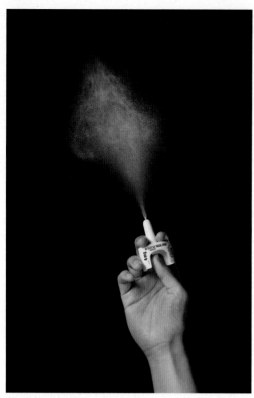

FIG. 29.4 Spray from a Narcan device. (©2017 ADAPT Pharma, Inc. NARCAN is a registered trademark licensed to ADAPT Pharma Operations Limited. ADAPT Pharma, Inc. Radnor, PA. Adapt Pharma Inc. All rights reserved.)

behavioral effects when administered orally, intranasally (snorting), topically on mucous membranes, intravenously, or by smoking. "Crack" cocaine, which is inhaled by "freebasing" or smoking, results in much higher blood levels of cocaine than those achievable by "snorting" and is particularly addictive. Cocaine has potent pharmacologic effects on dopamine, norepinephrine, and serotonin neurons in the CNS. Cocaine has an elimination half-life of 30 min to 1 h.

Cocaine intoxication produces a sense of well-being, a heightened awareness of sensory input, a decreased desire to sleep, restlessness, elation, grandiosity, agitation, and psychotic states (panic attack, paranoid ideation, delusions, and auditory and visual hallucinations). Acute users (people who are not addicted but have just recently taken the drug) experience intense euphoria often associated with increased sexual desire along with improved sexual function. These rewards often are followed by a moderate to severe post–cocaine use depression that provides a strong compulsion for further cocaine use. Physical findings in cocaine intoxication consist of tachycardia, cardiac arrhythmias, pupillary dilation, and elevated blood pressure. Affected persons may experience headache, as well as chills, nausea, and vomiting. Needle tracks (from "skin popping") may be found on the arms of injecting users of cocaine and heroin. Frequent,

chronic, or high-dose use of cocaine can produce anorexia and acute psychosis.

Cocaine overdose can be life-threatening. Myocardial infarction, arrhythmia, stroke, respiratory arrest, and symptoms consistent with neuroleptic malignant syndrome have been associated with cocaine use. Depression is common in cocaine addicts, particularly during periods of withdrawal.

Cocaine use disorder is treated using psychotherapy, behavioral therapy, and 12-step programs. Cocaine overdose constitutes a medical emergency requiring resuscitation in an intensive care unit. IV diazepam is effective for the control of seizures. Ventricular arrhythmias can be managed with IV propranolol. Cocaine users who inject the drug are also at increased risk for acquiring bloodborne pathogens.

Amphetamines

Amphetamine, methamphetamine, and related drugs are CNS stimulants. The primary action of these drugs is to increase synaptic dopamine by causing the release of dopamine stores into the synapse, which produces a dopamine "high" that is both more intense and longer lasting than that afforded by cocaine, and lasting anywhere from 8 to 24 h. Amphetamines are used clinically for weight loss and for treatment of attention deficit disorder, narcolepsy, and treatment-resistant depression. Many people develop dependence when they first use amphetamines for their appetite suppressant effects in an attempt at weight control. IV administration of amphetamine can lead to rapid development of dependence. Progressive tolerance is common in amphetamine dependence. Amphetamines result in similar complications to those occurring with cocaine.

Methamphetamine ("meth") is a potent synthetic form of amphetamine. It is highly addictive, and chronic use has been associated with psychotic symptoms. The biologic half-life of methamphetamine is much longer than that of cocaine. Symptoms of withdrawal from methamphetamine may be more intense than those associated with cocaine. Cessation after daily use may result in severe depression with suicidal ideation, hypersomnia, or sleeping difficulty.

Amphetamine analogues produce very similar signs and symptoms. Those associated with normal dosage include hyperalertness, euphoria, hyperactivity, and increased physical endurance. Higher doses of these drugs may be associated with dysphonia, headache, tachycardia, and confusion. When methamphetamine is introduced IV or by inhalation, a rapid, prolonged rush may result.

Medications that contain pseudoephedrine (over-the-counter [OTC] decongestants, such as Sudafed) can be used by illegal home laboratory operators to produce methamphetamine. As a result, many states passed laws to make it more difficult to purchase OTC medicines that contain pseudoephedrine.

Sedative–Hypnotics

The primary psychoactive substances used as sedatives and hypnotics are benzodiazepines (e.g., diazepam, lorazepam, or alprazolam) and, less commonly, barbiturates (e.g., phenobarbital, secobarbital). Sedatives, hypnotics, and anxiolytic drugs are frequently misused and are estimated to account for a third of emergency room visits.

The proportion of users of benzodiazepines who develop a substance use disorder is a function of dose, type, and duration of use. Longer use or higher dosage is more likely to lead to dependence; however, dependence also can occur when the drug is used in low doses for prolonged periods of time, as may be seen in clinical practice. Usage that lasts between 3 and 12 months leads to dependence in 10%–20% of users. The rate of dependency increases to 20%–45% when benzodiazepines are used for periods longer than a year. Benzodiazepines should be prescribed cautiously for dependence-prone persons with other risk factors for substance use disorder, in whom the use of these agents should be limited to no longer than 2 weeks when possible. Patients who are dependent on benzodiazepines are managed with gradual reduction in dose of the abused drug or by substitution of another long-acting sedative–hypnotic with gradual reduction in dosage.

Withdrawal symptoms produced by benzodiazepines are similar to those caused by withdrawal from alcohol. They can occur after several weeks or longer of moderate use of the drug. Signs and symptoms of withdrawal from benzodiazepines include nausea and vomiting, weakness, autonomic hyperactivity (tachycardia and sweating), anxiety, orthostatic hypotension, tremor, loss of appetite and weight loss, tinnitus, delirium with delusions, and hallucinations.

Alcohol

The behavioral and physiologic effects of alcohol depend on the amount of intake, its rate of increase in the blood, the presence of other drugs or medical problems, and the past experience with alcohol. Chronic use of heavy alcohol intake can result in clinically significant cognitive impairment (even when the person is sober), and the pattern displayed usually is one of intermittent relapse and remission. If the disease is allowed to progress untreated, many affected persons demonstrate other psychiatric problems (anxiety, antisocial behavior, and affective disorders), and some develop alcohol amnestic disorder and are unable to learn new material or to recall known material. Alcoholic blackouts may occur. In some patients, alcohol-induced dementia and severe personality changes develop.

Treatment of nondependent but at-risk problem drinkers may be accomplished by counseling, motivational techniques, and setting drinking limits below at-risk limits (e.g., less than one drink per day for women and two drinks per day for men). Treatment of alcohol use disorder can occur informally without professional assistance; however, the chances of a successful outcome are greater with an organized program based on professional help. The first step is complete withdrawal and abstinence from alcohol. Most often, this step can be accomplished on an outpatient basis, although for more severe dependence, inpatient treatment may be necessary. A thorough physical examination is performed to evaluate organ systems that could be impaired. This includes a search for evidence of liver failure, gastrointestinal bleeding, cardiac arrhythmia, and glucose or electrolyte imbalance. Major goals of medical management of alcohol withdrawal are to minimize the severity of withdrawal-related symptoms, to prevent specific withdrawal-related complications such as seizures and delirium tremens. Administration of a benzodiazepine, such as diazepam, in gradually decreasing doses to achieve downward titration of serum drug levels over a 3- to 5-day period, along with vitamin B supplements helps to alleviate alcohol withdrawal symptoms. Clonidine and carbamazepine are more recent additions to the pharmacotherapeutic management of withdrawal.

After treatment of withdrawal has been completed, the patient is educated about AUD. This aspect of management includes teaching the family and friends to stop protecting the patient from the problems caused by alcohol. Attempts are made to help the patient with AUD achieve and maintain a high level of motivation toward abstinence. Steps also are taken to help the patient with alcoholism readjust to life without alcohol and to reestablish a functional lifestyle. Relapse prevention may be accomplished using psychotherapeutic techniques (motivational enhancement techniques, "12-step program" facilitation, cognitive-behavioral coping skills), self-help groups (e.g., Alcoholics Anonymous [AA]), and pharmacotherapy. Three drugs are currently approved for the treatment of alcohol dependence: disulfiram, naltrexone, and acamprosate. Disulfiram inhibits aldehyde dehydrogenase causing accumulation of acetaldehyde blood levels and thus sweating, nausea, vomiting, and diarrhea when taken with ethanol. Naltrexone (an opioid antagonist) and acamprosate (an inhibitor of the γ-aminobutyric acid [GABA] system) may be used to decrease the amount of alcohol consumed or to shorten the period during which alcohol is used in cases of relapse.

DENTAL MANAGEMENT

Medical Considerations

The dentist should be aware that an opioid prescription written for dental pain can be the first exposure that disrupts brain circuitry leading to an opioid addiction. Thus, dentists need to be careful to minimize the prescribing of opioids to patients especially at a young age. Evidence indicates that an opioid prescription written for more than 3 days to an adolescent increases the risk of addiction by at least threefold. Moreover, opioids have not been shown to be more effective for managing post-operative pain associated with tooth extraction than nonsteroidal antiinflammatory drugs.

Dental providers should be on the alert for signs and symptoms that may indicate substance use disorders. Telltale cutaneous lesions often indicate parenteral use of drugs. Findings may include subcutaneous abscesses, cellulitis, thrombophlebitis, skin "tracks" (chronic inflammation from multiple injections), and infected lesions. Skin tracks usually appear as linear or bifurcated erythematous lesions, which may become indurated and hyperpigmented.

Opioids. Opioids users may try to obtain drugs from dentists by demanding pain medication for a dental problem (e.g., toothache) instead of problem-specific treatment. Likewise, pain medication may be requested (or demanded) after minor, nonsurgical procedures that typically would not be a cause of significant postoperative pain. The opioid user also may claim to be allergic to codeine or intolerant to nonsteroidal antiinflammatory drugs in an attempt to obtain a stronger drug such as hydrocodone or oxycodone. There are now laws in many states mandating annual continuing dental education on opioid use, enforcing electronic prescription of opioids to facilitate monitoring, and guidelines for prescribing opioids for acute pain (Box 29.1). Dentists must also be alert for

potential overdose in their community, indicating the potential need and use of naloxone on-site.

Marijuana. Chronic use of marijuana can lead to chronic bronchitis, airway obstruction, and poor oral health due to neglect and xerostomia. The autonomic effects of marijuana include tachycardia, reduced peripheral resistance, and, with large doses, orthostatic hypotension. Thus, marijuana use may be harmful to persons with ischemic heart disease or cardiac failure. Care should be taken in providing dental treatment to such patients, and if such an association is identified, dental treatment should be postponed until the patient is stable.

Cocaine. The danger of significant myocardial ischemia and cardiac arrhythmia is the primary concern in patients with cocaine intoxication. Patients who are "high" on cocaine should not receive any local anesthetic containing epinephrine for at least 6 h after the last administration of cocaine because cocaine potentiates the response of sympathomimetic amines. Use of epinephrine-impregnated retraction cord or local anesthetics containing epinephrine or levonordefrin should be avoided. Peak blood levels of cocaine occur within 30 min, and effects usually dissipate within 2 h. Before treating a patient who is participating in a cocaine treatment program, the dentist should consult the patient's physician regarding medications that the

---

BOX 29.1 Recommendations for Prescribing Opioids for Acute Pain in an Outpatient Dental Setting

1. Nonopioid therapies are effective for many common types of acute pain, including dental pain. Clinicians should only consider opioid therapy for acute pain if benefits are anticipated to outweigh risks to the patient (recommendation category: B, evidence type: 3).

   Systematic reviews of the literature suggest that NSAIDs alone or in combination with acetaminophen are more effective than opioids (alone or in combination with acetaminophen).[a]

   For short-term use NSAIDs and acetaminophen are associated with fewer adverse effects than opioids.[a]

   The number of patients needed to treat for benefit was lowest for ibuprofen in combination with acetaminophen (400 mg/1000 mg over 4–6 h vs. placebo).[b]

2. When starting opioid therapy for acute pain clinicians should prescribe immediate-release opioids instead of extended-release/long-acting (ER/LA) opioids (recommendation category: A, evidence type: 4).

3. When opioids are started for opioid-naive patients with acute pain, clinicians should prescribe the lowest dosage to achieve expected effects.

4. When opioids are needed for acute pain, clinicians should prescribe no greater quantity than needed for the expected duration of pain severe enough to require opioids (recommendation category: A, evidence type: 4).

5. When prescribing initial opioid therapy for acute pain clinicians should review the patient's history of controlled substance prescriptions using state prescription drug monitoring program (PDMP) data to determine whether the patient is receiving opioid dosages or combinations that put the patient at high risk for overdose (recommendation category: B, evidence type: 4).

6. Clinicians should use extreme caution when prescribing opioid pain medication and benzodiazepines concurrently and consider whether benefits outweigh risks of concurrent prescribing of opioids and other central nervous system depressants (recommendation category: B, evidence type: 3).

7. Clinicians should offer or arrange treatment with medication for patients with opioid use disorder (recommendation category: A, evidence type: 1).

[a]Chou R, Wagner J, Ahmed AY, et al. Treatments for Acute Pain: A Systematic Review. Comparative Effectiveness Review No. 240. (Prepared by the Pacific Northwest Evidence-based Practice Center under Contract No. 290-2015-00009-I.) AHRQ Publication No. 20(21)-EHC006. Rockville, MD: Agency for Healthcare Research and Quality; December 2020. https://doi.org/10.23970/AHRQEPCCER240.
[b]Moore PA, Ziegler KM, Lipman RD, et al. Benefits and harms associated with analgesic medications used in the management of acute dental pain: an overview of systematic reviews. *J Am Dent Assoc.* April 2018;149(4):256–265.
Adapted from 2022 draft CDC recommendations for prescribing opioids for outpatients with pain outside of sickle cell disease-related pain management, cancer pain treatment, palliative care, and end-of-life care. https://www.regulations.gov/document/CDC-2022-0024-0005. Accessed February 12, 2022.

patient may be taking and how best to manage procedure-related pain.

Methamphetamine. Significant myocardial ischemia, cardiac arrhythmia, hypertensive crisis, and stroke are the primary concerns in patients with methamphetamine intoxication. Peak blood levels occur within 30–60 min, and effects usually dissipate within 8 h; however, depending on the compound, the serum half-life of the various amphetamines can last up to 36 h. Patients who are "high" on methamphetamine should not receive dental treatment for at least 8 h after the last administration of the drug, and for maximum safety, dental treatment probably should not occur until at least 24 h after the last administration. Local anesthetics with epinephrine or levonordefrin must not be used during this period.

Alcohol. The dentist should assist patients may have alcohol use disorder. Of note, problems with alcohol transcend age, gender, and socioeconomic spectrum, and many patients are skilled at masquerading their dependence. A patient with suspected AUD can be appreciated during a carefully obtained history and examination. Noncompliance with appointments or instruction, exacerbation of anxieties and fears, failure to fulfill obligations, and emotional fluctuations may be indicators. A common scenario that should raise a red flag is that in which the patient presents for treatment with alcohol on their breath.

Screening for Substance Use Disorders. It has been shown that even brief advice or discussions in a clinical setting by a health care provider can have positive effects. The US Service Task Force recommends primary care screening of adults for substance use disorders (including alcohol and illicit drugs). Research indicates that brief interventions are more effective than no intervention and, in some cases, can be as effective as more extensive interventions. Similar to brief interventions for tobacco use, dentists can perform a simple screening and assessment for substance use, identify current/future oral and medical health issues, and discuss other difficulties expected if substance use continues. Assisting a patient into a treatment program requires that the dentist share concerns obtained from the screening assessment. Consultation with or referral to the patient's primary care provider (if the person has one) is advised. For those interested in learning more, the Substance Abuse and Mental Health Services Administration (SAMHSA) runs an initiative known as Screening, Brief Intervention, Referral, and Treatment (SBIRT).

When eliciting a patient history the dentist should obtain information from all adolescent and adult patients about the type, quantity, frequency, pattern of alcohol and illicit drug use, as well as consequences of their use, and family history of substance use disorders. A number of tools are available for screening and assessment of substance use (Table 29.3). The questioning should be done in an objective, nonjudgmental manner. Some tools are amenable to self-administration.

Treatment Planning Considerations

The goals of dental treatment for patients with substance use disorders are to maintain oral health, comfort, and function and to prevent and control oral disease. Without an aggressive approach to prevention, dental caries and periodontal disease may occur with increased frequency. Susceptibility to these problems stems from a reduced interest or inability to perform oral hygiene procedures. Also, in many of these patients, the diet typically is rich in foods and drinks that increase the risk for dental diseases.

The dental treatment plan should contain the following elements (see Box 29.2): (1) review of daily oral hygiene procedures; (2) convey to the patient a positive, hopeful attitude toward maintenance of the patient's oral health; (3) avoid complex dental procedures until the patient is in a stable condition in the context of the substance use disorder; and (4) careful selection of pain or anxiolytic medications. It is critical that appropriate pain and anxiolytic medication be provided to the patient; however, certain agents may have to be avoided, and others may require a reduction in their usual dosage. Consultation with the physician who is overseeing the management of the substance use disorder is advisable in order to discuss drug selection and administration. It also may be necessary to involve a third party, such as a "12-step program" sponsor, to monitor the taking of medication.

In addition to the above considerations, problems of major clinical importance in patients with alcoholic liver disease include bleeding tendencies and unpredictable metabolism of certain drugs (see Chapter 10).

Oral Complications and Manifestations

Patients with drug and alcohol abuse disorders tend to have more biofilm, calculus, caries, and gingival inflammation than is typical for patients without such disorders. These problems are related primarily to oral neglect rather than to any inherent property of the substance. Depending on the degree of neglect, the dentist should not provide extensive care until the patient demonstrates an interest in and ability to care for the dentition. With intraoral use of cocaine, gingival recession and erosion of the facial aspects of the maxillary teeth may result from persistent rubbing of the powder over these surfaces. Chronic intranasal use of cocaine can also lead to erosion of the nasal septum or floor of the nasal cavity, and in some cases palatal perforation. Chronic methamphetamine use often leads to consumption of sugary carbonated drinks that cause rampant caries. Chronic methamphetamine use also is associated with reports of a bad taste in the mouth, bruxism (grinding of the teeth),

TABLE 29.3   Substance Use Disorders Screening Instruments

THE TOBACCO, ALCOHOL, PRESCRIPTION MEDICATIONS, AND OTHER SUBSTANCE (TAPS) TOOL.

The TAPS Tool Part 1 is a 4-item screening for tobacco use, alcohol use, prescription medication misuse, and illicit substance use in the past year. Question 2 should be answered only by males and Question 3 only by females. Each of the four multiple-choice items has five possible responses to choose from. Patients who have a positive response to any question (except "Never") would then be invited to complete the TAPS Tool Part 2.

1. In the PAST 12 MONTHS, how often have you used any tobacco product (for example, cigarettes, e-cigarettes, cigars, pipes, or smokeless tobacco)?	Daily or almost daily	Weekly	Monthly	Less than monthly	Never
2. In the PAST 12 MONTHS, how often have you had 5 or more drinks containing alcohol in 1 day? One standard drink is about 1 small glass of wine (5 oz), 1 beer (12 oz), or 1 single shot of liquor. (Note: This question should only be answered by males).	Daily or almost daily	Weekly	Monthly	Less than monthly	Never
3. In the PAST 12 MONTHS, how often have you had 4 or more drinks containing alcohol in 1 day? One standard drink is about 1 small glass of wine (5 oz), 1 beer (12 oz), or 1 single shot of liquor. (Note: This question should only be answered by females).	Daily or almost daily	Weekly	Monthly	Less than monthly	Never
4. In the PAST 12 MONTHS, how often have you used any drugs including marijuana, cocaine or crack, heroin, methamphetamine (crystal meth), hallucinogens, ecstasy/MDMA?	Daily or almost daily	Weekly	Monthly	Less than monthly	Never
5. In the PAST 12 MONTHS, how often have you used any prescription medications just for the feeling, more than prescribed or that were not prescribed for you? Prescription medications that may be used this way include: Opiate pain relievers (for example, OxyContin, Vicodin, Percocet, Methadone) Medications for anxiety or sleeping (for example, Xanax, Ativan, Klonopin) Medications for ADHD (for example, Adderall or Ritalin)	Daily or almost daily	Weekly	Monthly	Less than monthly	Never

The TAPS Tool Part 2 is a brief assessment for tobacco, alcohol, and illicit substance use and prescription medication misuse in the PAST 3 MONTHS ONLY. Each of the following questions and subquestions has two possible answer choices—either yes or no.

1. In the PAST 3 MONTHS, did you smoke a cigarette containing tobacco? Yes No

   If "Yes," answer the following questions:

   a. In the PAST 3 MONTHS, did you usually smoke more than 10 cigarettes each day? Yes No

   b. In the PAST 3 MONTHS, did you usually smoke within 30 min after waking? Yes No

2. In the PAST 3 MONTHS, did you have a drink containing alcohol? Yes No

   If "Yes," answer the following questions:

   a. In the PAST 3 MONTHS, did you have 4 or more drinks containing alcohol in a day?* (Note: This question should only be answered by females). Yes No

   b. In the PAST 3 MONTHS, did you have 5 or more drinks containing alcohol in a day?* (Note: This question should only be answered by males). Yes No

   *One standard drink is about 1 small glass of wine (5 oz), 1 beer (12 oz), or 1 single shot of liquor.

   c. In the PAST 3 MONTHS, have you tried and failed to control, cut down or stop drinking? Yes No

   d. In the PAST 3 MONTHS, has anyone expressed concern about your drinking? Yes No

3. In the PAST 3 MONTHS, did you use marijuana (hash, weed)? Yes No

   If "Yes," answer the following questions:

   a. In the PAST 3 MONTHS, have you had a strong desire or urge to use marijuana at least once a week or more often? Yes No

   b. In the PAST 3 MONTHS, has anyone expressed concern about your use of marijuana? Yes No

4. In the PAST 3 MONTHS, did you use cocaine, crack, or methamphetamine (crystal meth)? Yes No

   If "Yes," answer the following questions:

   a. In the PAST 3 MONTHS, did you use cocaine, crack, or methamphetamine (crystal meth) at least once a week or more often? Yes No

   b. In the PAST 3 MONTHS, has anyone expressed concern about your use of cocaine, crack, or methamphetamine (crystal meth)? Yes No

5. In the PAST 3 MONTHS, did you use heroin? Yes No

   If "Yes," answer the following questions:

   a. In the PAST 3 MONTHS, have you tried and failed to control, cut down or stop using heroin? Yes No

   b. In the PAST 3 MONTHS, has anyone expressed concern about your use of heroin? Yes No

6. In the PAST 3 MONTHS, did you use a prescription opiate pain reliever (for example, Percocet, Vicodin) not as prescribed or that was not prescribed for you? Yes No

   If "Yes," answer the following questions:

   a. In the PAST 3 MONTHS, have you tried and failed to control, cut down or stop using an opiate pain reliever? Yes No

   b. In the PAST 3 MONTHS, has anyone expressed concern about your use of an opiate pain reliever? Yes No

Continued

7. In the PAST 3 MONTHS, did you use a medication for anxiety or sleep (for example, Xanax, Ativan, or Klonopin) not as prescribed or that was not pre-scribed for you? Yes No

If "Yes," answer the following questions:

a. In the PAST 3 MONTHS, have you had a strong desire or urge to use medications for anxiety or sleep at least once a week or more often? Yes No

b. In the PAST 3 MONTHS, has anyone expressed concern about your use of medication for anxiety or sleep? Yes No

8. In the PAST 3 MONTHS, did you use a medication for ADHD (for example, Adderall, Ritalin) not as prescribed or that was not prescribed for you? Yes No

If "Yes," answer the following questions:

a. In the PAST 3 MONTHS, did you use a medication for ADHD (for example, Adderall, Ritalin) at least once a week or more often? Yes No

b. In the PAST 3 MONTHS, has anyone expressed concern about your use of a medication for ADHD (for example, Adderall or Ritalin)? Yes No

9. In the PAST 3 MONTHS, did you use any other illegal or recreational drug (for example, ecstasy/molly, GHB, poppers, LSD, mushrooms, special K, bath salts, synthetic marijuana ("spice"),whip-its, etc.)? Yes No

If "Yes," answer the following questions:

In the PAST 3 MONTHS, what were the other drug(s) you used?

ALCOHOL USE DISORDERS IDENTIFICATION TEST (AUDIT) SELF-REPORT QUESTIONNAIRE

Patient: Because alcohol use can affect your health and can interfere with certain medications and treatments, it is important that we ask some questions about your use of alcohol. Your answers will remain confidential so please be honest. Circle the choice that best describes your answer to each question.

Questions	0	1	2	3	4	Score
1. How often do you have a drink containing alcohol?	Never	Monthly or less	2 to 4 times a month	2 to 3 times a week	4 or more times a week	
2. How many drinks containing alcohol do you have on a typical day when you are drinking?	1 or 2	3 or 4	5 or 6	7 to 9	10 or more	
3. How often do you have five or more drinks on one occasion?	Never	Less than monthly	Monthly	Weekly	Daily or almost daily	
4. How often during the past year have you found that you were not able to stop drinking once you had started?	Never	Less than monthly	Monthly	Weekly	Daily or almost daily	
5. How often during the past year have you failed to do what was normally expected of you because of drinking?	Never	Less than monthly	Monthly	Weekly	Daily or almost daily	
6. How often during the past year have you needed a first drink in the morning to get yourself going after a heavy drinking session?	Never	Less than monthly	Monthly	Weekly	Daily or almost daily	
7. How often during the past year have you had a feeling of guilt or remorse after drinking?	Never	Less than monthly	Monthly	Weekly	Daily or almost daily	
8. How often during the past year have you been unable to remember what happened the night before because of your drinking?	Never	Less than monthly	Monthly	Weekly	Daily or almost daily	
9. Have you or has someone else been injured because of your drinking?	No		Yes, but not in the last year		Yes, during the last year	
10. Has a relative, friend, doctor, or other health care worker been concerned about your drinking or suggested you cut down?	No		Yes, but not in the last year		Yes, during the last year	
					Total:	

and muscle trismus (jaw clenching). Neglect of personal oral hygiene and increased acidity from gastrointestinal regurgitation or vomiting also contribute to exaggerated caries and enamel erosion problems in persons who have a methamphetamine use disorder. The combination of these effects is referred to as "meth mouth" (Fig. 29.5). Meth users are "wired" and exhibit extremely high levels of energy and neuromuscular activity, often leading to parafunctional jaw activity and bruxism. Bruxism and

muscle trismus can compound the effects of periodontal disease. Patients who use ecstasy demonstrate bruxing activity during use of the drug.

A variety of oral abnormalities may be found in patients with alcohol abuse. Nutritional deficiencies can result in glossitis and loss of tongue papillae along with angular cheilitis, which is complicated by concomitant candidal infection. Vitamin K deficiency, disordered hemostasis, portal hypertension, jaundice, and splenomegaly (causing

BOX 29.2 | Dental Management Considerations in Patients With Substance Use Disorders

PREOPERATIVE RISK ASSESSMENT
- Evaluate to determine whether a substance use disorder is present.
- Obtain medical consultation if clinical signs and symptoms point to an undiagnosed problem or if the diagnosis is uncertain.

A

Antibiotics	No issues.
Analgesics	Avoid prescribing opioid analgesics. Clock-regulated use of NSAIDs with acetaminophen is generally recommended, though acetaminophen should be avoided in those with alcoholic liver disease. If needed, check the patient's physician and the state prescription drug monitoring program first, then prescribe an adequate-strength medication and only a limited number of doses (3 days maximum) with specific instructions, and no refills. It may be appropriate to have a third party monitor and dispense the medication. If the patient is taking medications for opioid use disorder (e.g., buprenorphine/naloxone [Suboxone]) and opioids are needed for acute pain, consult with patient's physician who is managing the substance use program.
Anesthesia	For a person who has a cocaine and methamphetamine use disorder, avoid the use of epinephrine for 24 h after the last dose of drug. Some patients may require additional anesthesia due to rapid drug metabolism.
Allergies	No issues.
Anxiety	If the patient requires an anxiolytic for treatment, contact the patient's physician to discuss options. Consider using a short-acting benzodiazepine and prescribe only enough for one appointment. Also consider intraoperative use of nitrous oxide–oxygen.

B

Bleeding	For patients with alcohol use disorder and cirrhosis, excessive bleeding secondary to liver disease is possible. Laboratory tests may be needed for confirmation.
Breathing	No issues.
Blood pressure	For a person who has a cocaine and methamphetamine use disorder, monitor blood pressure and pulse during appointment.

C

Chair position	No issues.
Cardiovascular	Persons who have a cocaine and methamphetamine use disorder are at increased risk for cardiac arrhythmias, myocardial infarction, and stroke.

D

Drugs	Epinephrine can potentiate the adverse cardiovascular effects of cocaine and amphetamines.
Devices	No issues.

E

Equipment	No issues.
Emergencies	For a person who has a cocaine and methamphetamine use disorder, cardiovascular emergencies are possible, especially with the use of epinephrine within 24 h of last drug use. Have naloxone (Narcan) available to reverse opioid overdose.

F

Follow-up	If narcotic analgesics are prescribed, the patient should be monitored to ensure proper drug use.

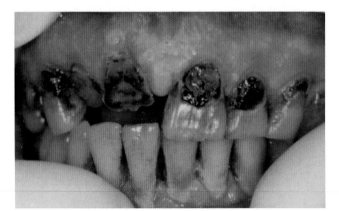

FIG. 29.5 "Meth mouth."

thrombocytopenia) can result in spontaneous gingival bleeding, mucosal ecchymoses, and petechiae. Other features include enlargement of the parotid glands (Fig. 29.6), spider angiomas (Fig. 29.7), and in some cases, rhinophyma (drinker's nose and face).

Alcohol and tobacco use are strong risk factors for the development of oral squamous cell carcinoma, and dentists must be diligent (as with all patients) in the detection of unexplained or suspicious soft tissue lesions (especially leukoplakia, erythroplakia, or ulceration) or a firm neck lymph node in patients with chronic alcoholism. High-risk sites for development of oral squamous cell carcinoma include the lateral border of the tongue and the floor of the mouth (see Chapter 26).

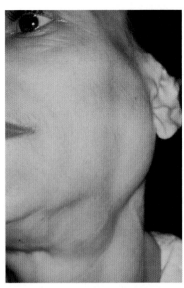

FIG. 29.6 Painless enlargement of the parotid glands associated with alcoholism. (Courtesy of Valerie Murrah, Chapel Hill, NC.)

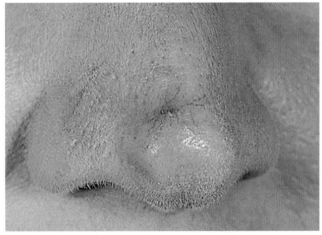

FIG. 29.7 Spider angiomas, which may be a sign of alcoholism. (From Seidel HM, et al. *Mosby's Guide to Physical Examination.* 6th ed. St. Louis: Mosby; 2006.)

BIBLIOGRAPHY

1. American Psychiatric Association. *Diagnostic and Statistical Manual of Mental Disorders.* 5th ed. Arlington, VA: American Psychiatric Association; 2013.
2. Weiss RD. Drug use and dependence. In: Goldman L, Ausiello D, eds. *Goldman-Cecil Medicine.* 24th ed. Philadelphia: Elsevier; 2012:153–159.
3. Hyman SE. Biology of addiction. In: Goldman L, Ausiello D, eds. *Goldman-Cecil Medicine.* 24th ed. Philadelphia: Elsevier; 2012:140–142.
4. O'Connor PG. Alcohol abuse and dependence. In: Goldman L, Ausiello D, eds. *Goldman-Cecil Medicine.* 24th ed. Philadelphia: Saunders Elsevier; 2012:146–153.
5. Puente D, Cabezas C, Rodriguez-Blanco T, et al. The role of gender in a smoking cessation intervention: a cluster randomized clinical trial. *BMC Publ Health.* 2011;11: 369.
6. Lipari RN, Kroutil LA, Pemberton MR. *Risk and Protective Factors and Initiation of Substance Use: Results from 2014 National Survey on Drug Use and Health.* 2015.
7. Smart RG. Effects of legal restraint on the use of drugs: a review of empirical studies. *Bull Narc.* 1976;28(1):55–65.
8. Pacula RL, Jacobson M, Maksabedian EJ. In the weeds: a baseline view of cannabis use among legalizing states and their neighbours. *Addiction.* 2016;111(6):973–980.
9. Peace MR, Stone JW, Poklis JL, et al. Analysis of a commercial marijuana e-cigarette formulation. *J Anal Toxicol.* 2016;40(5):374–378.
10. Rogers JS, Rehrer SJ, Hoot NR. Acetylfentanyl: an emerging drug of abuse. *J Emerg Med.* 2016;50(3):433–436.
11. Grant BF, Stinson FS, Dawson DA, et al. Prevalence and co-occurrence of substance use disorders and independent mood and anxiety disorders: results from the National Epidemiologic Survey on Alcohol and Related Conditions. *Arch Gen Psychiatr.* 2004;61(8):807–816.
12. National Institute on Alcohol and Alcoholism. *Helping Patients Who Drink too Much: A Clinician's Guide and Related Professional Support Resources.* Rockville, MD: U.S. Department of Health and Human Services; 2005.
13. Zawilska JB. Legal highs"—an emerging epidemic of novel psychoactive substances. *Int Rev Neurobiol.* 2015;120: 273–300.
14. Weiss RD. *Drugs of Abuse.* Philadelphia, PA: Elsevier (Saunders); 2016.
15. Wen H, Hockenberry JM, Cummings JR. The effect of medical marijuana laws on adolescent and adult use of marijuana, alcohol, and other substances. *J Health Econ.* 2015;42:64–80.
16. Borodovsky JT, Crosier BS, Lee DC, et al. Smoking, vaping, eating: is legalization impacting the way people use cannabis? *Int J Drug Pol.* 2016;36:141–147.
17. Cahill TJ, Prendergast BD. Infective endocarditis. *Lancet.* 2016;387(10021):882–893.
18. Leavitt SB. *Intransal Naloxone for at Home Opioid Rescue Practical Pain Management.* 2010(October):20–25.
19. Kanouse AB, Compton P. The epidemic of prescription opioid abuse, the subsequent rising prevalence of heroin use, and the federal response. *J Pain Palliat Care Pharmacother.* 2015;29(2):102–114.
20. Volkow ND, Fowler JS, Wang JS. The addicted brain: insights from imaging studies. *J Clin Invest.* 2003;111: 1444–1451.
21. Frauger E, Amaslidou D, Spadari M, et al. Patterns of methylphenidate use and assessment of its abuse among the general population and individuals with drug dependence. *Eur Addiction Res.* 2016;22(3):119–126.
22. Cho AK, Melega WP. Patterns of methamphetamine abuse and their consequences. *J Addict Dis.* 2002;21(1):21–34.
23. Winstock A. Psychoactive drug misuse. In: Wright P, Stern J, Phelan M, eds. *Core Psychiatry.* 2nd ed. Edinburgh: Elsevier; 2005:431–455.
24. Bockman CS, Abel PW. Drugs of abuse. In: Yagiella JA, Dowd FJ, Johnson BS, Mariotti AJ, Neidle EA, eds. *Pharmacology and Therapeutics for Dentistry.* St. Louis: Mosby Elsevier; 2011:799–813.

25. Albertson TE, Kenyon NJ, Morrissey B. Amphetamines and derivatives. In: Shannon MW, Borron SW, Burns MJ, eds. *Haddad and Winchester's Clinical Management of Poisoning and Drug Overdose*. Philadelphia: Saunders Elsevier; 2007.

26. Hamamoto DT, Rhodus NL. Methamphetamine abuse and dentistry. *Oral Dis*. 2009;15(1):27–37.

27. Little JW. Dental implications of mood disorders. *J Gen Dent*. 2004;52(5):442–450.

28. Lindroth JE, Herren MC, Falace DA. The management of acute dental pain in the recovering alcoholic. *Oral Surg Oral Med Oral Pathol Oral Radiol Endod*. 2003;95(4):432–436.

29. McCullough AJ, O'Shea RS, Dasarathy S. Diagnosis and management of alcoholic liver disease. *J Dig Dis*. 2011;12(4):257–262.

30. McNeely J, Wu L, Subramaniam G, et al. Performance of the tobacco, alcohol, prescription medication, and other substance use (TAPS) tool for substance use screening in primary care patients. *Ann Intern Med*. 2016;165:690–699.

31. Carter G, Yu Z, Aryana Bryan M, et al. Validation of the tobacco, alcohol, prescription medication, and other substance use (TAPS) tool with the WHO alcohol, smoking, and substance Involvement screening test (ASSIST). *Addict Behav*. March 2022;126:107178.

32. Le A, Palamar JJ. Oral health implications of increased cannabis use among older adults: another public health concern? *J Subst Use*. 2019;24(1):61–65.

33. Mattson CL, Tanz LJ, Quinn K, et al. Trends and geographic patterns in drug and synthetic opioid overdose deaths—United States, 2013-2019. *MMWR Morb Mortal Wkly Rep*. February 12, 2021;70(6):202–207.

34. Buresh M, Stern R, Rastegar D. Treatment of opioid use disorder in primary care. *BMJ*. May 19, 2021;373:n784.

35. US Preventive Services Task Force, Curry SJ, Krist AH, Owens DK, et al. Screening and behavioral counseling interventions to reduce unhealthy alcohol use in adolescents and adults: US preventive Services Task Force recommendation statement. *JAMA*. November 13, 2018;320(18):1899–1909.

36. Moore PA, Ziegler KM, Lipman RD, Aminoshariae A, Carrasco-Labra A, Mariotti A. Benefits and harms associated with analgesic medications used in the management of acute dental pain: an overview of systematic reviews. *J Am Dent Assoc*. April 2018;149(4):256–265. e3.

37. Chou R, Wagner J, Ahmed AY, et al. *Treatments for Acute Pain: A Systematic Review. Comparative Effectiveness Review No. 240. (Prepared by the Pacific Northwest Evidence-based Practice Center under Contract No. 290-2015-00009-I.) AHRQ Publication No. 20(21)-EHC006*. Rockville, MD: Agency for Healthcare Research and Quality; 2020.

38. Center for Behavioral Health Statistics and Quality. *Results from the 2020 National Survey on Drug Use and Health: Detailed Tables*. Rockville, MD: Substance Abuse and Mental Health Services Administration; 2021. Retrieved from https://www.samhsa.gov/data/.

Guide to Management of Common Medical Emergencies in the Dental Office*

GENERAL CONSIDERATIONS

The best management of a dental office medical emergency is prevention. Dental practitioners must be prepared to treat the seemingly well but chronically ill patient whose condition is managed by a variety of drugs. Prevention begins with the dental professional's awareness of the patient's medical condition at the outset of the dental visit. Knowledge of the type of condition, its severity, and the level of control provides a strong indicator of the patient's risk for experiencing a medical emergency. Proper assessment that includes review of the medical history, physical evaluation, and medical consultation gives the practitioner the opportunity to take measures that could prevent such emergencies. If an emergency does occur, an informed dentist will have a better idea of the type of medical problem the patient is experiencing. The dentist also must understand the pathophysiologic factors regulating disease processes and the pharmacodynamics of drug action and interaction.

Patients frequently experience physical reactions during treatment. Accordingly, considerable responsibility rests on the dentist first to recognize the signs and symptoms of the problem and then to respond to any emergency quickly, efficiently, and competently with adequate resuscitative procedures. Important precepts of good medical emergency management include (1) being well prepared, (2) having confidence in selected interventions, (3) having up-to-date emergency drugs close by, and (4) remaining calm in difficult circumstances. Health professionals are responsible for knowing and following techniques that are recognized to be up to date, safe, and efficient. An unfamiliar or unreliable maneuver should never be attempted. Dentists must be trained in providing basic life support (BLS) and in managing emergencies in the dental office. Advanced cardiac life support (ACLS) training to include intravenous (IV) drug administration may be useful in dental practices that more often encounter medically complex cases. Dental practitioners also should be aware of the changes in basic cardiopulmonary resuscitation (CPR) guidelines introduced in 2010 and 2017.

Although dentists should be prepared to provide resuscitation procedures in the dental setting, even more consideration should be directed at preventing such situations. Prevention begins with obtaining an adequate medical history of the patient, making an appropriate physical evaluation, and ensuring that both patient and environment are properly prepared before treatment begins. Sometimes a potentially catastrophic event may be prevented through recognition of physical conditions or limitations before treatment begins.

Management of emergencies must begin long before the point of occurrence. Preparation should include a designated plan of action and an adequate armamentarium to meet emergencies. To ensure an effective response, the actions of the dental team must be based on a thorough background in relevant subject matter, continued training and reinforcement, and carefully prepared and rehearsed emergency procedures in which each person has specific duties and responsibilities. This approach requires the availability of appropriate resuscitative equipment and drugs to permit the team to work together calmly and precisely. This teamwork must be based on knowledge, practice, sound judgment, and confidence. To this end, all members of the dental office (dentist, hygienist, assistant, receptionist) should be trained in and be able to perform BLS procedures properly, according to the American Heart Association guidelines, when needed. Also, every dental office should have a written plan that spells out specific duties for each member of the office staff, covering areas such as who

---

* Information from Malamed SF. *Medical Emergencies in the Dental Office*. 6th ed. St Louis: Mosby, 2007; Malamed SF. *Emergency Medicine in the Dental Office (DVD)*. Edmonds, WA: Health First Corporation, 2008, Joseph Massad Productions; 2005 American Hearth Association guidelines for cardiopulmonary resuscitation and emergency cardiovascular care. *Circulation*. 2005;112(suppl 24):IV1-2-3; Part 1: executive summary: 2010 American Heart Association guidelines for cardiopulmonary resuscitation and emergency cardiovascular care. *Circulation*. 2010;1222(suppl3):S640—S656; and Kleinman ME, et al. 2017 American Heart Association focused update on adult basic life support and cardiopulmonary resuscitation quality: an update to the American Heart Association guidelines for cardiopulmonary resuscitation an emergency cardiovascular care. *Circulation*. January 2, 2018;137(1): e7—e13. Epub 2017 Nov 6.

will activate the emergency medical services (EMS) system (i.e., call 911) and direct EMS to the location, start CPR, place an IV line, and administer drugs. A staff member should be designated to assist in necessary tasks during the emergency situation, such as getting and preparing drugs and recording every event and the time of each action.

Dental offices should have up-to-date emergency drugs, oxygen, a pulse oximeter, and an automated external defibrillator (AED). Electrocardiography is an elective adjunct modality for monitoring the patient's vital signs in dental practices where sedation is used.

GENERAL PRINCIPLES OF EMERGENCY CARE

Most life-threatening office emergencies occur in patients with preexisting systemic disease(s) and are caused by the patient's inability to withstand physical or emotional stress or the patient's reaction to drugs. Emergencies also can originate with a complication of a preexisting systemic disease. Cardiopulmonary systems can be involved, thereby necessitating some emergency supportive therapy.

Algorithms (i.e., standardized step-by-step procedures) are recommended to be performed during emergencies after the signs and symptoms of the condition are recognized. Most often when the patient becomes unconscious, the algorithm for medical emergencies follows the sequence P-A-B-C-D, where

P is for positioning,
A is for *airway,*
B is for *breathing,*
C is for *circulation,* and
D is for *definitive care* (e.g., diagnosis, drugs, and defibrillator and other equipment).

The American Heart Association recommends use of a slightly different algorithm for cardiac arrest, that is, P-C-A-B-D. If patient is unresponsive and has no pulse:
P: Positioning: Place patient in supine position and establish unresponsiveness (tap and shout). Evaluate for pulselessness. Call for help, activate EMS (call 911), and get defibrillator.

Circulation comes first (current BLS guidelines are that cardiac compressions are the most critical replacing the previous airway and rescue breathing first.)

C: Circulation and compressions: Health care provider should assess pulse (carotid) for no more than 10 s. If a pulse is not detected and the victim is not breathing and is unresponsive, promptly initiate chest compressions.

One operator: a rate of 100–120 compressions/min (depth of 2 inches)

Ventilation is no longer recommended in BLS; only the cardiac compressions are performed for a rate of 100–120 compressions/min. Continue compressions until spontaneous pulse returns.

NOTE: The importance of technique for chest compressions cannot be overemphasized; they must be hard, fast, and maximally effective, with minimal interruptions.

D: Defibrillator: Attach and use AED as soon as available (ideally within 3–5 min of collapse).

Our own contribution has been to add an E, for ensure proper patient response, and an F, for facilitate next steps in medical and dental care.

This appendix presents recommended management protocols, i.e., algorithms, that should be considered for use during various medical emergencies likely to be encountered in dental offices. There are some recommendations that should be applied only by those professionals with advanced training (ACLS).

Key Points

The following elements are essential to the successful treatment of medical emergencies:
1. Advance preparation and risk assessment
2. Quick recognition of signs and symptoms and early diagnosis of the underlying problem
3. Fast response time (4–6 min without oxygen leads to irreversible brain damage)
4. Systematic monitoring of the patient's well-being using an algorithm such as P-A-B-C-D-E-F or, for cardiac arrest, P-C-A-B-D-E-F

Pediatric basic life support algorithm for healthcare providers-2 or more rescuers

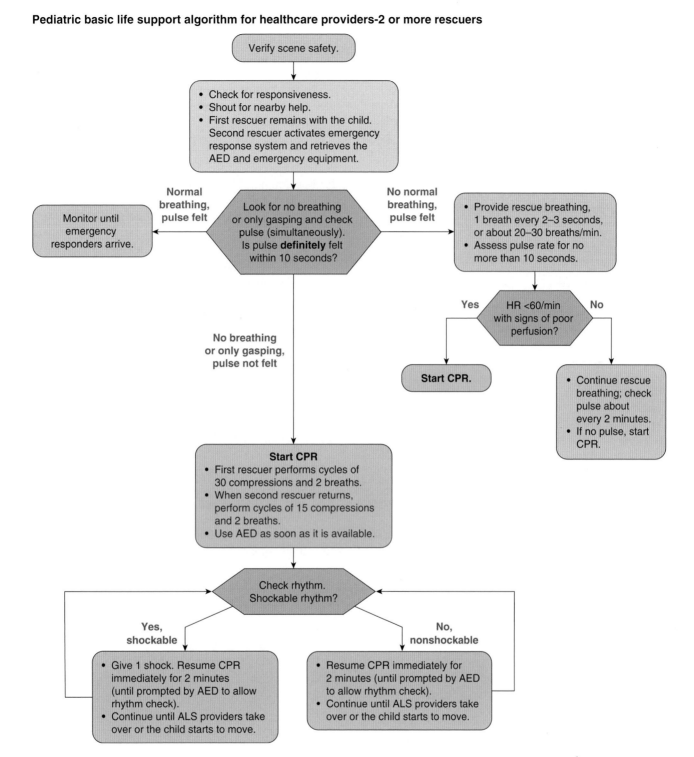

From CPR & First Aid Emergency Cardiovascular Care. *Algorithms.* American Heart Association; 2021. https://cpr.heart.org/en/resuscitation-science/cpr-and-ecc-guidelines/algorithms.

TYPES OF EMERGENCIES AND THEIR MANAGEMENT IN THE DENTAL OFFICE

Unconsciousness (Loss of Consciousness)

Syncope and Psychogenic Shock

Signs and Symptoms. Pallor, sweating, nausea, anxiety, pupillary dilation, yawning, decreased blood pressure, bradycardia (slow pulse), convulsive movements, unconsciousness.

Cause. Cerebral hypoxia (reduced blood flow to brain), sitting or standing stiff, anxiety.

Treatment.

P: Positioning: Place patient in supine position; lower head slightly and elevate legs (for pregnant women, roll on left side)—assess consciousness.

A: Airway: Ensure open airway.

B: Breathing: Check breathing—should be adequate.

C: Circulation: Check carotid pulse—should be adequate.

D: Dispense or administer:
- Oxygen at flow rate of 5–6 L/min
- Aromatic ammonia (e.g., Vaporole)—"smelling salts" (optional)
- Cold compresses applied to forehead

E: Ensure that vital signs, drug administration, and patient responses are properly monitored and recorded.

F: Facilitate next steps in medical and dental care depending upon patient's response and status and reassure patient.

Low Blood Pressure or Slow Pulse. For low blood pressure or pulse (systolic is less than previous diastolic), the following protocol is indicated:

Treatment: Low Blood Pressure.

P: Positioning: Place patient in supine position; lower head and raise legs.

A: Airway: Ensure open airway.

B: Breathing: Check breathing—should be adequate.

C: Circulation: Check pulse and ensure adequate circulation, which may be weak.

D: Dispense or administer:

Intravenous drip of 5% dextrose in lactated Ringer's solution (D5LR)

In *unresponsive patient:* a vasopressor drug such as phenylephrine 10 mg/mL (1 ampule), or epinephrine 0.3–0.5 mg given subcutaneously (SC) or intramuscularly (IM), or IV with ACLS training

E: Ensure vital signs, drug administration, and patient responses are properly monitored and recorded.

F: Facilitate next steps in medical and dental care depending upon patient's response and status and reassure patient.

Treatment: Slow Pulse (Less Than 60 beats/min), If Symptomatic.

P: Positioning: Place patient in supine position; lower head and raise arms and legs.

A: Airway: Ensure and maintain patent airway.

B: Breathing: Check breathing—should be adequate.

C: Circulation: Check—should be adequate in this situation.

D: Dispense or administer:
- Oxygen at flow rate of 5–6 L/min (if patient is hypoxemic)
- Atropine 0.5 mg IV (to increase heart rate). Repeat dose up to 3 mg; then consider use of additional vasopressors (dopamine or epinephrine).

E: Ensure that vital signs, drug administration, and patient responses are properly monitored and recorded.

F: Facilitate next steps in medical and dental care depending upon patient's response and status and reassure patient.

Cardiac Arrest

Signs and Symptoms. No pulse or blood pressure, sudden cessation of respiration (apnea), cyanosis, dilated pupils.

Cause. Abrupt interruption of blood supply and oxygen to the coronary arteries and heart muscle due to ischemia (clot).

Treatment. For unresponsive cardiac arrest victim (adult):

P: Positioning: Place patient in supine position and establish unresponsiveness (tap and shout). Call for help, activate EMS (call 911), and get defibrillator.

C: Circulation and compressions: Health care provider should assess pulse (carotid) for no more than 10 s. If a pulse is not detected and victim is not breathing and is unresponsive, promptly initiate chest compressions.

One operator: a rate of 100–120 compressions/min (depth of 2 inches)

Ventilation is no longer recommended in BLS; only the cardiac compressions are performed for a rate of 100–120 compressions/min. Continue compressions until spontaneous pulse returns.

NOTE: The importance of technique for chest compressions cannot be overemphasized; they must be hard, fast, and maximally effective, with minimal interruptions.

D: Defibrillator: Attach and use AED as soon as available (ideally within 3–5 min of collapse).
- Check rhythm and shock if indicated (repeated every 2 min).
- Resume CPR beginning with compressions immediately after each shock.

NOTE: With IV drugs: Start normal saline solution (with ACLS-trained rescuer).

- Epinephrine 1.0 mg 1:1000; repeat every 3–5 min as needed; can be given IM.
- Vasopressin 40 units can replace first or second dose of epinephrine.
- Amiodarone—*first dose:* 300 mg bolus; *second dose:* 150 mg

Other drugs used for treatment of cardiac arrest (with ACLS-trained rescuer)

- Lidocaine (antiarrhythmic agent)
- Calcium chloride (increases myocardial contractility)
- Morphine sulfate (for pain relief)
- Thrombolytic agents

E: Ensure that vital signs, drug administration, and patient responses are properly monitored and recorded.

F: Facilitate next steps in medical and dental care depending upon patient's response and status and reassure patient.

Hypoglycemia (Insulin Shock)

Signs and Symptoms. Hunger, weakness, trembling, tachycardia, pallor, sweating, paresthesias, uncooperative, mental confusion (headache), incoherent, uncooperative, belligerent, unconscious, tonic-clonic movements, hypotension, hypothermia, rapid thready pulse, coma.

Cause. Lack of blood glucose to the brain; (i.e., from taking insulin and not eating.)

Treatment.

P: Position:

In *conscious patient:* place in upright sitting position.

In *unconscious patient:* place in supine position.

A: Airway: Ensure open airway.

B: Breathing: Ensure that patient is breathing.

C: Circulation: Check pulse and confirm adequate circulation; pulse could be weak.

D: Dispense:

In *conscious patient:* Give a drink with high sugar content such as orange juice or a glucose paste (cake icing) applied to the buccal mucosa.

In *unconscious patient:* Activate EMS by calling 911; then administer:

- Oxygen at flow rate of 5–6 L/min
- Dextrose 5 lactated Ringer's solution (D5LR) IV: Run the IV drip as fast as possible.
- Alternatively, give glucagon 1 mg SC or IM (or IV) or epinephrine (for transient relief).

E: Ensure that vital signs, drug administration, and patient responses are properly monitored and recorded.

F: Facilitate next steps in medical and dental care depending upon patient's response and status which may include transport to hospital.

When patient regains consciousness, provide reassurance and information about what happened because the person is likely to have little memory of the incident.

Acute Adrenal Insufficiency

Signs and Symptoms. Altered consciousness, wet, clammy, confusion, weakness, fatigue, headache, pain in abdomen or legs, pigmented skin, nausea and vomiting, hypotension and syncope, coma.

Cause. Adrenal suppression (low adrenocorticotropic hormone) by exogenous steroids. The patient may be medicated with steroids or the cause may be primary or secondary malfunction of the adrenal cortex.

Treatment.

P: Positioning: Place patient in semireclined position and raise feet slightly; call for help.

A: Airway: Ensure open airway.

B: Breathing: Should be adequate (i.e., predicted to be adequate in this situation).

C: Circulation: Check pulse and confirm adequate circulation.

D: Dispense:

In conscious patient:

- Provide oxygen at flow rate of 5–6 L/min.
- Give hydrocortisone 100 mg or dexamethasone 4 mg (IV).

In unconscious patient:

- Place in supine position.
- Activate EMS by calling 911.
- Administer oxygen at flow rate of 5–6 L/min.
- Confirm diagnosis from review of medical history, signs, and symptoms.
- Then start IV administration of D5LR and run the IV drip as fast as possible.
- Also provide hydrocortisone 100 mg or dexamethasone 4 mg (IV).
- Give a vasopressor drug (e.g., epinephrine 1 : 1000, 0.5 mL).

E: Ensure vital signs, drug administration, and patient responses are properly monitored and recorded.

F: Facilitate or ensure next steps in medical care (transport to hospital); reassure patient.

Cerebrovascular Accident (Stroke)

Signs and Symptoms.

F — facial drooping

A — arm weakness

S — speech difficulties

T — time

Additionally, consider dizziness (patient may fall), vertigo and vision changes, nausea and vomiting, transient paresthesia, unilateral weakness or paralysis, headache, nausea, vomiting, convulsions, coma.

NOTE: Blood pressure and pulse generally are normal. Raised blood pressure and body temperature and lowered pulse and respiration indicate increased intracranial pressure.

Cause. Interruption of blood supply and oxygen to the brain occurring as a result of ischemia or hemorrhage.

Treatment.

P: Positioning: Place patient in reclined, semi-sitting position with the head elevated. Call for help and activate EMS (call 911).

A: Airway: Ensure that airway is open and maintained open.

B: Breathing: Ensure that breathing is adequate.

C: Circulation: Check pulse and confirm adequate circulation.

D: Dispense or administer:

- Use pulse oximeter to determine oxygenation.
- Administer oxygen at flow rate of 5–6 L/min, if needed.

E: Ensure vital signs, drug administration, and patient responses are properly monitored and recorded.

- Keep patient quiet and still.

F: Facilitate or ensure next steps in medical care (transport to hospital); reassure patients.

Convulsions (Seizure)

Signs and Symptoms. Aura (flash of light or sound, an unusual smell), mental confusion, excessive salivation, rolling back of eyes, loss of consciousness, tonic phase (contractions—clenching of teeth) followed by clonic phase (tremors, convulsive movements of extremities).

Causes. There are several potential causes of convulsions and seizures, including syncope, drug reactions (local anesthetic overdose), hypoglycemia, hyperventilation, cerebrovascular accident, and convulsive seizure disorder.

Treatment.

P: Positioning: Place patient in supine position; clear instruments and protect patient from injury (i.e., lightly restrain arms and legs from gross movements). Call for help.

After convulsion ceases:

A: Airway: Ensure that airway is open. Suction mouth along buccal surfaces of teeth if excessive secretions are making breathing difficult.
B: Breathing: Ensure that breathing is adequate.
C: Circulation: Check pulse and confirm adequate circulation.
D: Dispense or administer:
  • Oxygen at flow of 5–6 L/min

For status epilepticus (a seizure lasting more than 5 min):

• Activate EMS (call 911).
• For adult, give diazepam (Valium) 5–10 mg IV or intranasal lorazepam 2–8 mg *or* intranasal midazolam 5 mg, 1 spray per nostril (may not be readily available; ask pharmacist)

If convulsions persist for 5 min after treating, repeat with one-half dose.

E: Ensure that vital signs, drug administration, and patient responses are properly monitored and recorded.
  • Place patient in the 'recovery position'.
  • Support respiration (seizure may precipitate respiratory arrest).
F: Facilitate or ensure next steps in medical care (transport to hospital, if needed), and reassure patient.

Local Anesthesia Drug Toxicity

Signs and Symptoms. Confusion, talkative, restless, apprehensive state, excited manner, headache, lightheadedness, convulsions, increase in blood pressure and pulse rate. NOTE: Stimulation is followed by depression of the central nervous system.

Late features may include drowsiness, disorientation, convulsions followed by depression, drop in blood pressure, weak or rapid pulse or bradycardia, apnea,

unconsciousness, or death. NOTE: Lidocaine toxicity is documented to occasionally exhibit depression only, without the usual prodromal of the excitatory phase.

Causes. Excessive dose of local anesthetic or rapid absorption of local anesthetic or inadvertent IV injection or slow detoxification or elimination of drug.

Treatment.

P: Positioning: Place patient in comfortable position; convulsing or unconscious patient should be in supine position.

If patient is convulsing:

• Clear instruments and protect patient from injury.
• Call for help.

After convulsion ceases:

A: Airway: ensure airway is open.
B: Breathing: Ensure that breathing is adequate.
C: Circulation: Check pulse and confirm adequate circulation.
D: Dispense or administer:
  • Oxygen at flow rate of 5–6 L/min
  • If local anesthesia overdose results in seizure, a benzodiazepine (diazepam, lorazepam, or midazolam) as described in the seizure algorithm may be administered.
E: Ensure vital signs and drug administration are properly monitored and recorded; maintain blood pressure.
  - Place in recovery position, if a seizure occurred.
F: Facilitate or ensure next steps in medical care (provide supportive therapy):
  • Treat bradycardia (0.4 mg of atropine IV, with ACLS-trained rescuer*).
  • Transport to hospital.
  • Reassure patient.

NOTE: If patient becomes unconscious, maintain airway, administer BLS, and activate EMS (call 911).

Respiratory Difficulty

Hyperventilation

Signs and Symptoms. Rapid and shallow breathing, confusion, dizziness, paresthesias, cold hands, carpalpedal spasms; can progress to seizure.

Cause. Anxiety-hyperventilation-induced excessive loss of CO_2 from deep and rapid breathing; also respiratory alkalosis.

Treatment.

P: Positioning: Place patient in an upright position. Explain the problem and reassure the patient.
A: Airway: Maintain open airway by talking with patient.
B: Breathing: Instruct patient to be calm and breathe slowly into a paper bag or into the cupped hands over the nose and mouth (i.e., rebreathe carbon dioxide).

C: Circulation: No treatment required.

D: Dispense (i.e., provide) reassurance.

E: Ensure vital signs, drug administration, and patient responses are properly monitored and recorded.

F: Facilitate or ensure next steps in medical and dental care: Consider rescheduling appointment with anti-anxiety measures or presedation.

Aspiration of a Foreign Object

Signs and Symptoms. Coughing or gagging associated with a foreign object, inability to speak, possible cyanosis from airway obstruction, violent respiratory effort, suprasternal retraction, rapid pulse.

Cause. Foreign body in larynx or pharynx.

Treatment. With conscious victim:

P: Positioning: Keep the patient standing or sitting leaning forward. Ask: "Can you speak?" or "Are you choking?" Patient may indicate need for help by demonstrating the "universal choking sign"—clutching hands wrapping around the neck or nodding.

A: Airway: Open airway by placing arms around patient and applying Heimlich maneuver.

B: Breathing: Repeat maneuver until object is cleared and breathing is reestablished, or until patient becomes unconscious.

With unconscious or unresponsive victim:

P: Positioning: Place victim in supine position. Activate EMS (call 911); then initiate CPR in C-A-B sequence.

C: Circulation: Check pulse; begin CPR if no pulse is felt. Provide chest compressions in ratio of 30 per 2 ventilations. (NOTE: Chest compressions provide pressure to dislodge foreign object.)

A: Airway: Open airway by administering quick upward abdomen thrusts (up to 5).

B: Breathing: Check airway for breathing and attempt to ventilate. Each time the airway is opened, the rescuer should look for an object in the victim's mouth and remove it if found.
- Do not delay the 30 chest compressions for longer than 10 s while looking for object.
- Continue chest compressions and ventilation attempts until EMS unit arrives.

NOTE: If cricothyrotomy is necessary (i.e., rescuer is unable to ventilate for 4−5 min), refer to "Cricothyroid Membrane Puncture" procedure that follows.

After breathing has been reestablished:

D: Dispense or administer:
- Oxygen at flow rate of 5−6 L/min

E: Ensure vital signs, drug administration, and patient responses are properly monitored and recorded.

F: Facilitate or ensure next steps in medical care (maintain supine position and transport to hospital); reassure patient.

- Inform patient and request radiographs to locate foreign object or trauma to chest cavity is suspected, if needed (posterior-anterior chest view, lateral chest view, flat plane abdominal).

NOTE: If foreign object is in gastrointestinal tract, track with X-ray examination. Foreign object in trachea or lung requires removal using bronchoscopy or thoracotomy. If foreign object has occluded the airway, the Heimlich maneuver may be of benefit before initiation of a cricothyrotomy.

Cricothyroid Membrane Puncture. The approach to a patient with acute airway obstruction should consist of the following steps:

- Recognition of obstruction
- Use of nonsurgical maneuvers to relieve obstruction (i.e., back blows, Heimlich maneuver).
- Administration of mouth-to-mouth breathing to bypass obstruction or to diagnose obstruction
- Activation of EMS with 911 call
- Establishment of an emergency surgical airway (cricothyrotomy-if the clinician has advanced training) if Heimlich maneuver is unsuccessful

*Cricothyrotomy.

1. Place patient on back with neck hyperextended.
2. Ensure that chin and sternal notch are held in median plane.
3. Cut skin or puncture with very-large-bore needle over cricothyroid cartilage.
4. Insert cricothyrotomy cannula (Portex Mini-Trach II) or very-large-bore needle through skin over cricothyroid cartilage. Insert pointed end caudally to avoid damage to the vocal cords.

If cannula is not available:

a. Insert small scissors or hemostats through cricothyroid membrane and into the tracheal space, or use large (8-gauge) needle.
b. Expand instrument and dilate transversely.
c. Insert tube into trachea between beaks of dilating instrument.
d. Remove scissors or hemostats.
e. Tape tube into place.
f. Control bleeding.

5. Use positive pressure or enriched oxygen flow if patient is breathing independently.
6. Arrange for rapid transfer of patient to the hospital.

Bronchial Asthma

Signs and Symptoms. Sense of suffocation, pressure in chest, nonproductive cough, expiratory wheezes, prolonged expiratory phase, increased respiratory effort, chest distention, thick, stringy mucous sputum, cyanosis (in severe cases).

Causes. Can be induced by allergy, infection, exercise, anxiety leading to bronchial inflammation, bronchoconstriction, vascular permeability, occlusion of bronchioles by thick mucous plugs, and bronchospasm.

Treatment.

P: Positioning: Place patient in an upright comfortable position.

A: Airway: Ensure that airway is open by removing dental materials and listening to breath sounds.

B: Breathing: Encourage relaxed slow breathing.

C: Circulation and communication: generally, circulation is adequate if patient is conscious. Communicate with patient and staff to get a rapid bronchodilator for use. Calm the patient and the staff.

D: Dispense or administer:
- Two deep inhalations of fast-acting, β_2-agonist bronchodilator (e.g., albuterol mistometer)
- Repeat with two additional deep inhalations of bronchodilator if attack persists 5 min.
- Oxygen at flow rate of 5–6 L/min, if needed

E: Ensure that vital signs are properly monitored and recorded, including pulse oximeter.
- If attack persists after 4 puffs, activate EMS (call 911).

F: Facilitate next steps in medical care (transport to hospital); reassure patient.
- Maintain oxygen at flow rate of 5–6 L/min.
- With *unresponsive patient*: administer epinephrine 1: 1000 (0.3–0.5 mL IM); repeat every 20 min as needed.

If transport to hospital is pending:

- Give theophylline ethylenediamine (aminophylline) 250–500 mg IV slowly over a 10-min period.
- Administer hydrocortisone sodium succinate (Solu-Cortef), 100 mg IV.

NOTE: Because aminophylline may cause hypotension, it should be given with extreme caution to patients with asthma who are hypotensive.

Mild (Delayed Onset) Allergic Reaction

Signs and Symptoms. Mild pruritus (itching)—slow appearance; and mild urticaria (rash)—slow appearance.

It is necessary to address this situation because it could progress to anaphylaxis.

Cause. Overreaction to allergens such as drugs, pollens, or food in which mast cells degranulate and release histamine, often in skin or mucosa.

Treatment.

P: Positioning: Place patient in comfortable position (upright).

A: Airway: Ensure that airway is open by talking with patient.

B: Breathing: Ensure that breathing is adequate; use pulse oximeter—establish oxygenation level.

C: Circulation and communication: Should be adequate in this situation. Take blood pressure. There should be no tachycardia, hypotension, dizziness, dyspnea, or wheezing. Inform the patient that an antihistamine drug will be administered.

D: Dispense or administer:
- Diphenhydramine (Benadryl) 25–50 mg orally (PO) or IM (or IV if dentist has ACLS or advanced training).
- Repeat dose up to 50 mg every 6 h PO for 2 days if needed.

E: Ensure that vital signs, drug administration, and patient responses are properly monitored and recorded.

F: Facilitate or ensure next steps in medical care.
- In this case, allergy testing should be considered, and dentist should initiate discussion with physician to withdraw offending drug.

Severe (Immediate Onset) Allergic Reaction

Signs and Symptoms. Skin reactions—rapid appearance such as severe pruritus (itching of skin, throat, palate); severe urticaria (rash); swelling of lips, eyelids, cheeks, pharynx, and larynx (angioneurotic edema); and anaphylactic shock (cardiovascular—fall in blood pressure; respiratory—wheezing, choking, cyanosis, hoarseness; central nervous system—loss of consciousness, dilation of pupils).

Cause. Overreaction to allergens such as drugs, pollens, and food where mast cells degranulate and release histamine in cardiopulmonary system.

Treatment.

P: Positioning

With conscious patient: place in upright (most comfortable) position.

With unconscious patient: place in supine position and activate EMS (call 911).

A: Airway: Assess to ensure that airway is open.

B: Breathing: Ensure breathing is adequate by talking to and reassuring patient.

C: Circulation: No immediate requirement. Apply blood pressure cuff and pulse oximeter to assess circulation and oxygenation within 5 min.

D: Dispense or administer:
- Epinephrine 0.3–0.5 mg 1: 1000 SC, IM, or IV if dentist has ACLS training
- Oxygen maintained at flow rate of 5–6 L/min
- Repeat epinephrine 0.3–0.5 mg 1: 000 SC or IM every 5–10 min as needed.

E: Ensure that vital signs, drug administration, and patient responses are properly monitored and recorded.

NOTE: *Monitor blood pressure to ensure hypertension is not occurring.*

F: Facilitate or ensure next steps in medical care (transport to hospital); reassure patient.

If transport to hospital is pending:

- Give repeat doses of epinephrine 0.3–0.5 mg 1: 1000 IM every 5–10 min as needed.
- Also administer 25–50 mg diphenhydramine (Benadryl) when patient's life is no longer in danger.

If dentist has ACLS training and laryngeal edema is involved:

- Provide steroids—hydrocortisone sodium succinate (Solu-Cortef), 100 mg SC, IM, IV
- Perform CPR if patient stops breathing and has no pulse, include use of AED as needed.
- Perform cricothyrotomy if needed.

NOTE: Aminophylline may cause hypotension and should be used with extreme caution in patients with asthma who also are hypotensive.

Respiratory Arrest

Signs and Symptoms. Cessation of breathing, cyanosis.

Cause. Physical obstruction of airway (tongue or foreign object), drug-induced apnea.

Treatment.

P: Positioning: Place patient in supine position and activate EMS (call 911).

A: Airway: Maintain open airway, tilting the patient's head back as indicated.

B: Breathing: Respirations will be absent.
- Open mouth to see if foreign object is readily accessible; remove object if visible (in adult).
- If foreign object cannot be removed, perform Heimlich maneuver (abdominal thrusts) until object is removed or no pulse is detected. If no pulse is felt, initiate CPR (using the C-A-B sequence) and chest compressions in a ratio of 30 per 2 ventilations.
- When the airway is open, ventilate patient 12–15 times per minute.

C: Circulation: Support blood pressure through position of patient, parenteral fluids, and vasopressors.

D: Dispense or administer appropriate drug:

Use positive pressure or enriched oxygen flow if patient is breathing independently.

- or artificial respiration.

If apnea is secondary to sedative or benzodiazepine (e.g., diazepam) overdose: administer reversal agent:

- Flumazenil (0.2 mg IV over 15 s) if diazepam was used to sedate (with ACLS-trained rescuer); repeat 0.2 mg every minute up to 1 mg.

If apnea is secondary to narcotic or opioid overdose: administer reversal agent:

- 0.4 mg naloxone hydrochloride (Narcan) IV, IM, or SC plus oxygen
- Keep patient awake.

E: Ensure vital signs, drug administration, and patient responses are properly monitored and recorded.

F: Facilitate or ensure next steps in medical and dental care (transport to hospital, if necessary); reassure patient.

NOTE: Monitor patient carefully for the duration of action of reversal agent (e.g., naloxone), which may be less than that of the narcotic. No reversal agent exists for barbiturate overdose.

Chest Pain

Angina Pectoris

Signs and Symptoms. Substernal myocardial pain that can radiate to arms, neck, jaw, or abdomen; myocardial pain lasting less than 15 min and possibly radiating to the left shoulder; pain relieved by nitroglycerin; patient usually has a history of the condition.

NOTE: Vital signs are normal; no hypotension, sweating, or nausea occurs.

Cause. Blood supply to the cardiac muscle is insufficient for oxygen demand (atherosclerosis or coronary artery spasm). Angina episode may be precipitated by stress, anxiety, or physical activity.

Treatment.

P: Positioning: Place patient in sitting-up or semi-sitting-up (comfortable) position with head elevated.

A: Airway: Ensure open airway.

B: Breathing: Ensure that breathing is adequate.

C: Circulation and communication: Check pulse and communicate with patient and staff to get nitroglycerin.

D: Dispense or administer:
- Nitroglycerin 0.4-mg tablet sublingually or one or two metered spray doses (0.3–0.6 mg) of nitroglycerin sublingually
- Repeat 1 nitroglycerin tablet every 5 min up to a total of 3 tablets or 3 sprays in 15-min period.
- Oxygen at flow rate of 5–6 L/min
- If pain is not relieved with 3 doses of nitroglycerin, give one aspirin 325 mg and call 911.

E: Ensure that vital signs, drug administration, and patient responses are properly monitored and recorded.

F: Facilitate next steps in medical care (transport to hospital if needed); reassure patient.

NOTE: If any doubt exists about whether angina or myocardial infarction exists (i.e., pain continues, worsens, or subsides but then returns), activate EMS (call 911) or transport patient to hospital. After the nitroglycerin tablet container has been opened, the remaining tablets have a poor shelf life (30 days); a new supply should be stocked.

Myocardial Infarction

Signs and Symptoms. Development of chest pain, sometimes manifested as a crushing, squeezing, or heavy feeling, that is more severe than with angina, possibly radiating to the neck, shoulder, or jaw; lasting longer than 15 min; and not relieved by nitroglycerin tablets, in a conscious patient. Cyanotic, pale, or ashen appearance; weakness, cold sweat, nausea, vomiting, air hunger and sense of impending death; increased, irregular pulse beat of poor quality with palpitations, feeling of impending doom. These symptoms may vary between men and women, with women experiencing less severe, more gastrointestinal or fatigue-related symptoms.

Cause. Interruption of blood supply to the heart, most commonly caused by occlusion of coronary vessels. Anoxia, ischemia, and infarct are present.

Treatment. For adult victim who is conscious and responsive:

P: Positioning: Place patient in a comfortable position. Call for help and activate EMS (call 911).
A: Airway: Ensure open airway.
B: Breathing: Ensure that breathing is adequate by communicating with and reassuring patient.
C: Circulation: Evaluate vital signs
D: Dispense or administer:
  • Aspirin 325-mg tablet in conscious patient
  • Oxygen at flow rate of 5–6 L/min
E: Ensure vital signs, drug administration, and patient responses are properly monitored and recorded.
F: Facilitate or ensure next steps in medical and dental care (transport to hospital); reassure patient.

NOTE: Maintain patient in most comfortable position; this may not be the supine position because the air hunger may be associated with orthopnea.

• Administer nitrous oxide–oxygen (N_2O 30%, O_2 70%), if available.
• Alternatively, Demerol (50 mg IV) or morphine (10 mg IV) may be administered during a non-ST elevated MI and if the dentist has ACLS training.

The condition may progress to cardiac arrest.
With *unresponsive patient:* Initiate CPR, including use of AED.

Other Reactions

Extrapyramidal Reactions

Antipsychotic Drugs Producing Side Reactions. Phenothiazines (Compazine, Thorazine, Phenergan, Sparine, Stelazine, Trilafon, Mellaril); butyrophenones (Haldol, Innovar [general anesthetic]); thioxanthenes (Navane, Taractan).

Signs and Symptoms. Acute dystonic reaction (more frequent in young people and women): rapid onset, involuntary movement of tongue, muscles of mastication, and muscles of facial expression; neck muscles affected frequently (torticollis), arms and legs affected less frequently; akathisia (constant motion); parkinsonism, tardive dyskinesia (involving buccolinguomasticatory triad—sucking, smacking, chewing, fly-catching movements of tongue).

Cause. Adverse effects of drug.

Treatment.

P: Positioning: Place patient in semi-upright position.
A: Airway: Ensure open airway.
B: Breathing: Ensure that breathing is adequate by talking with and reassuring patient.
C: Circulation: Request blood pressure equipment or pulse oximeter to check circulation.
D: Dispense or administer:
  • Diphenhydramine HCl (Benadryl) 25–50 mg PO or IV if dentist has ACLS training
  • Oxygen at flow rate of 5–6 L/min
E: Ensure vital signs, drug administration, and patient responses are properly monitored and recorded.
F: Facilitate or ensure next steps in medical care (transport to hospital); reassure patient.

Response to Unknown Cause. When a likely cause for the patient's response cannot be identified, a period of observation is justified.

P: Positioning: Place patient in supine position and activate EMS (call 911).
A: Airway: Ensure open airway, support respiration, and administer oxygen.
B: Breathing: Ensure that breathing is adequate.
C: Circulation: Take blood pressure and use a pulse oximeter to check blood pressure, circulation and oxygenation.
D: Dispense or administer IV D5LR.
E: Ensure that vital signs, drug administration, and patient responses are properly monitored and recorded.
F: Facilitate or ensure next steps in medical and dental care:
  • Keep patient off all medication.
  • Reassure patient.
  • Transfer to hospital if patient's condition is serious.
  • Be prepared to do CPR and use the AED if needed.

Emergency Kit. Review contents, expiration date, and appearance of all drugs periodically (at least monthly). Ensure that kit contains the following:

1. Oxygen tank and setup (i.e., tank has sufficient oxygen in it for an emergency)
2. Blood pressure cuff
3. Stethoscope
4. Syringes (1, 5, 10, and 20 mL)
5. Lacrimal pocket mask
6. Disposable airway, nos. 2, 3, and 4
7. Butterfly needles, no. 3, 21 gauge
8. 22-gauge needles
9. IV tubing set, long no. 880-35
10. 250 mL dextrose, lactated Ringer's solution

11. Paper tape roll
12. Alcohol sponges
13. Drugs
    Atropine: 0.5 mg/1-mL ampule
    Aspirin: 325-mg tablets
    Benadryl (diphenhydramine): 50-mg tablets or 50 mg/1 mL syringe/22-gauge, 1-inch needle
    Aminophylline (theophylline ethylenediamine): 250 mg/1 mL syringe/22-gauge, 1-inch needle
    Hydrocortisone sodium succinate (Solu-Cortef): 100 mg/2 mL syringe/22-gauge, 1-inch needle
    Epinephrine 1: 1000
    - Twinject: two doses of 0.3 mg
    - EpiPen: auto-injector 0.3 mg
    - 1.0-mL ampules
    Glucagon: 1 mg/mL ampule
    Naloxone hydrochloride (Narcan): 0.4 mg/1-mL ampule/tuberculin syringe
    Nitroglycerin: 0.4-mg tabs (packed as 30/bottle) or pump spray (400 μg/spray)
    Phenylephrine: 10 mg/mL (two or three 1-mL ampules)
    Two ammonia inhalant buds (Vaporole)
    Orange juice, glucose paste, or dextrose 50%: 100 mL
    Diazepam (Valium): 5 mg/mL (Alternatively, stock lorazepam 2 mg/mL or midazolam 1 mg/mL; noting that midazolam comes in 5 mg per atomized nasal spray)
    Lidocaine 2%, 2-mL ampules
14. Curved cricothyrotomy cannula
15. Padded tongue blade
16. Pulse oximeter/ECG unit (medical resources)
17. AED (e.g., Cardiac Science, HeartSine, Medtronic Philips, Physio-Control, Survivalink, Zoll)

NOTE: Commercial medical emergency kits for dentistry are available from companies such as AED Superstore (Woodruff, WI), Banyan International (Abilene, TX), Dixie EMS Supply Co. (Franklin, TN), and HealthFirst (Mukilteo, WA).

Pediatric Drug Doses. Pediatric doses are presented on a weight basis, which can be simply multiplied based on the patient's weight. Although nomograms using weight, surface area, and other factors may be more accurate, use of the following method is suggested in an emergency situation.

1. Diphenhydramine HCl (Benadryl): 1—1.25 mg/kg, up to 50 mg maximum IV; then 1—1.25 mg/kg q6h PO or parenterally
2. Atropine sulfate: 0.01 mg/kg, up to 0.4 mg maximum, IV or SC
3. Theophylline ethylenediamine (aminophylline): 3—5 mg/kg IV slowly—20 mg/min maximum
4. Epinephrine (adrenaline) 1: 10000.05 mg to 0.3 mg maximum SC or IM (diluted to 1: 10,000 for IV administration)EpiPen Junior—autoinjector 0.15 mg
5. Ammonia inhalants (e.g., Vaporole): Same as for adults
6. Hydrocortisone sodium succinate: Adult dose IV—50 mg, 100 mg, and above
7. Naloxone HCl (Narcan): No pediatric doses clearly established; 0.01 mg/kg IV (preferably) every 2—3 min for two to three doses maximum
8. 50% dextrose injection: 0.5 mg/kg or 1 mL/kg
9. Diazepam (Valium): Dose not clearly established in patients younger than 12 years of age but in the range of 0.1—0.5 mg/kg for intractable seizures

Guidelines for Infection Control in Dental Health Care Settings

Principles of infection control require continuous evaluation of current infection control practices. This is necessary in dental practice because of new technologies, materials, equipment, and data. Dental patient care settings also may require specific strategies directed to preventing pathogen transmission among dental health care personnel (DHCP) and their patients.

The Centers for Disease Control and Prevention (CDC) published the *Guidelines for Infection Control in Dental Health-Care Settings—2003* for DHCP. The essential elements of this document still apply for dental practice. The CDC's evidence-based recommendations guide infection control practices in dental offices nationally and globally; provide direction for the public, DHCP, and policymakers; and influence technology development in the dental industry.

Recommended infection control practices are applicable to all settings in which dental treatment is provided, and will evolve with new evidence, improvements in technology, and the emergence of new infectious diseases. DHCP have important roles in recognizing the signs and symptoms of a number of infectious diseases and preventing the spread of such diseases. Dental offices that keep abreast of and follow new recommendations will strengthen safe dental practice, and a number of links are provided below. Patients and providers alike can be assured that oral health care can be delivered and received in a safe manner.

The COVID-19 (SARS-CoV-2) pandemic highlights the importance of respiratory viral infections. The clinical features of respiratory viral infections, the steps taken to control respiratory infections, and the role of vaccinations to control infectious diseases in the dental office are listed here.

CLASSIC FEATURES OF RESPIRATORY VIRAL INFECTIONS

- Fever
- Cough
- Sore throat
- Runny or stuffy nose
- Body aches
- Headache
- Chills
- Fatigue
- Sometimes diarrhea and vomiting

Control of Respiratory Infections

A hierarchy of control measures should be applied to prevent transmission of respiratory pathogens in all health care settings. To apply the hierarchy of control measures, facilities should take the following steps, ranked according to their likely effectiveness:

1. Elimination of potential exposures (e.g., deferral of treatment for ill patients and source control by masking persons who are coughing)
2. Engineering controls that reduce or eliminate exposure at the source without placing primary responsibility of implementation on individual employees
3. Administrative controls including sick leave policies and vaccination that depend on consistent implementation by management and employees
4. Personal protective equipment (PPE) for exposures that cannot otherwise be eliminated or controlled. PPE includes gloves, surgical face masks, respirators, protective eyewear, and protective clothing such as gowns.

COVID-19 Guidance for Dental Settings

https://www.cdc.gov/coronavirus/2019-ncov/hcp/dental-settings.html

Interim Infection Prevention and Control Recommendations for Healthcare Personnel During the Coronavirus Disease 2019 (COVID-19) Pandemic

https://www.cdc.gov/coronavirus/2019-ncov/hcp/infection-control-recommendations.html

This site is subject to updates.

Vaccination. Vaccination, an administrative control, is one of the most important interventions for preventing transmission of infectious diseases to health care personnel and their patients. More information on vaccinations is available in the CDC's *Vaccine Recommendations and Guidelines of ACIP* https://www.cdc.gov/vaccines/hcp/acip-recs/index.html https://www.cdc.gov/vaccines/schedules/index.html

Dental practitioners should note the following important links:

COVID-19 Guidance for Dental Settings https://www.cdc.gov/coronavirus/2019-ncov/hcp/dental-settings.html

Interim Infection Prevention and Control Recommendations for Healthcare Personnel During the Coronavirus Disease 2019 (COVID-19) Pandemic https://www.cdc.gov/coronavirus/2019-ncov/hcp/infection-control-recommendations.html

This site is subject to updates.

Prevention and Control of Seasonal Influenza with Vaccines https://www.cdc.gov/mmwr/volumes/70/rr/rr7005a1.htm

Dental practitioners should note the CDC recommendations concerning influenza vaccination of health care personnel in the United States.

CDC Health Advisory: Immediate Need for Healthcare Facilities to Review Procedures for Cleaning, Disinfecting, and Sterilizing Reusable Medical Devices https://emergency.cdc.gov/han/han00383.asp

INFECTION PREVENTION PRACTICES IN DENTAL SETTINGS

https://www.cdc.gov/oralhealth/infectioncontrol/pdf/safe-care2.pdf

HEPATITIS B FREQUENTLY ASKED QUESTIONS

These FAQs cover hepatitis B infections, vaccinations, chronic hepatitis B, serology, traveler's health, and more. http://www.cdc.gov/hepatitis/

Tuberculosis Infection Control Recommendations

The CDC's guidelines to prevent tuberculosis (TB) transmission in health care settings has changed because of the changing epidemiology of TB as well as dental practice techniques. Dental practitioners should review the CDC's TB infection control recommendations for dental settings and learn how these recommendations should be incorporated into an infection control program.

https://www.cdc.gov/mmwr/preview/mmwrhtml/rr5417a1.htm?s_cid=rr5417a1_e

Prevention of Methicillin-Resistant *Staphylococcus aureus* Transmission in Dental Health Care Settings

Methicillin-resistant *Staphylococcus aureus* (MRSA) is most often spread from patient to patient through the contaminated hands of health care professionals. The clinical utilization of Standard Precautions has been shown to be an effective strategy in preventing transmission. Learn more at CDC's About MRSA Skin Infections https://www.cdc.gov/mrsa/community/index.html

OTHER RELATED LINKS

CDC: Infection Prevention and Control Guidelines and Recommendations

http://www.cdc.gov/oralhealth/infectioncontrol/guidelines/index.htm

A slide set and accompanying speaker notes that provide an overview of many of the basic principles of infection control in the CDC's *Guidelines for Infection Control in Dental Health-Care Settings* can be downloaded as a PowerPoint presentation or viewed on the CDC's website.

Safety and Health Topics for Dentistry from the Occupational Safety and Health Administration (OSHA) (https://www.osha.gov/SLTC/dentistry/index.html)

National Institute for Occupational Safety and Health (NIOSH) http://www.cdc.gov/niosh/topics/bbp/

Organization for Safety, Asepsis and Prevention (http://www.osap.org/)

OSAP has produced a workbook that contains practical information to help health care professionals put the infection control recommendations into practice.

https://www.osap.org/from-policy-to-practice-osap-guide-to-the-cdc-guidelines-2019-edition

If Saliva Were Red: A Visual Lesson on Infection Control

The video training system, *If Saliva Were Red*, features an 8-minute DVD that uses dental professionals to highlight common infection control and safety flaws; the cross-contamination dental personnel would see if saliva were red; and how controlling contamination by using personal barrier protection, safe work practices, and effective infection control products reduces the risk of exposure.

American Dental Association (ADA) Infection Control Resources https://www.ada.org/resources/research/science-and-research-institute/oral-health-topics/infection-control-and-sterilization

CLINICAL IMPLICATIONS

The CDC *Guidelines for Infection Control in Dental Health Care Settings—2003* was a major update and revision of the CDC's *Recommended Infection Control Practices for Dentistry—1993*. As of 2022, these guidelines still apply (along with the previous updates on

H1N1 and TB). As the nation's disease prevention agency, the CDC develops a broad range of guidelines intended to improve the effect and effectiveness of public health interventions and to inform key audiences, most often clinicians, public health practitioners, and the public, about applicable findings.

Why are guidelines needed that are specific for dentistry? More than 600,000 DHCP work in the United States—approximately 200,000 dentists, 150,000 registered dental hygienists, 300,000 dental assistants, and 25,000 dental laboratory technicians. Many dentists are solo practitioners who work in outpatient, ambulatory care facilities. In these settings, no epidemiologists or other hospital infection control experts track possible health care–associated (i.e., nosocomial) infections or monitor and recommend safe practices. Instruments frequently used in dental practice generate spatter, mists, aerosols, or particulate matter. Unless precautions are taken, the possibility exists that patients and DHCP will be exposed to blood and other potentially pathogenic infectious material. Fortunately, by understanding certain principles of disease transmission and using infection control practices based on those principles, dental personnel can prevent disease transmission.

HISTORICAL MILESTONES

The CDC's first set of infection control recommendations for dentistry was published as an article in the *Morbidity and Mortality Weekly Report* in 1986. At that time, a position paper from the American Association of Public Health Dentistry commented on the state of dental infection control, noting: "Dental practitioners are virtually the only health care providers who routinely place an ungloved hand into a body cavity." Reports published from 1970 through 1987 described nine clusters of patients who were believed to be infected with hepatitis B virus (HBV) through treatment by an infected DHCP. However, since 1987, no transmission of HBV from dentist to patient has been reported, although cross-contamination from HBV-infected patients was reported in two reports from 2009 (a dental screening) and 2013 (an oral surgery office) and led to HBV infections among six patients (including two DHCPs). These statistics are likely linked to the widespread acceptance of the hepatitis B vaccine and adoption of standard (formerly universal) precautions, including routine glove use.

In early 1988, a published report described a dentist who was seropositive for human immunodeficiency virus (HIV) but had no admitted risk factors for HIV infection, which suggests the possibility of occupational transmission. In addition, during the early 1990s, the health care community was shaken when six cases of transmission from an HIV-infected dentist to his patients were reported. No additional reports have described HIV transmission from HIV-infected DHCP to patients, and

since the CDC began surveillance for occupationally acquired HIV, no cases of occupationally acquired HIV have been confirmed among DHCP.

In 1991, OSHA released the bloodborne pathogen standard that mandated certain practices for all dental offices. For example, employers must provide hepatitis B vaccine for their employees, and all employees must use appropriate PPE (e.g., gloves, protective eyewear, gowns). After OSHA published its standards, the CDC published Recommended Infection Control Practices for Dentistry in 1993. Those recommendations, which focused on preventing transmission of disease caused by bloodborne pathogens, were based primarily on health care precedent, theoretical rationale, and expert opinion. In contrast with OSHA (which is a regulatory agency), the CDC cannot mandate certain practices; it can only recommend. Nevertheless, many dental licensing boards have adopted the CDC's recommendations, or variations of them, as the infection control standard for dental practice in their states.

In 2003, the CDC updated and created major guidelines on specific topics such as hand hygiene, environmental infection control, *Mycobacterium tuberculosis*, disinfection and sterilization, prophylaxis after exposure to bloodborne pathogens, prevention of surgical site infection, immunization for health care workers, and infection control for health care personnel. Guidelines for Infection Control in Dental Health-Care Settings—2003. MMWR 52(No. RR-17): 39–48, 2003. See also http://www.cdc.gov/mmwr/pdf/rr/rr5217.pdf

These recommendations discuss portions of the numerous federal guidelines and regulatory mandates relevant to dentistry. The CDC also consolidated previous recommendations and added new ones specific to infection control in dental health care settings. The document emphasized the use of "standard precautions" (which replaces the term "universal precautions") for the prevention of exposure to and transmission not only of bloodborne pathogens but also of other pathogens encountered in oral health care settings. Although the guidelines focus mainly on practices in outpatient, ambulatory dental health care settings, the recommended infection control practices are applicable to all settings in which dental treatment is provided.

In the CDC recommendations, the term *DHCP* refers to all paid and unpaid personnel in dental health care who could experience occupational exposure to infectious materials, including body substances and contaminated supplies, equipment, environmental surfaces, water, or air. DHCP include dentists, dental hygienists, dental assistants, dental laboratory technicians (in-office and commercial), students and trainees, contract personnel, and other persons who are not directly involved in patient care but who could be exposed to infectious agents (such as administrative, clerical, housekeeping, maintenance, or volunteer personnel). The guidelines have two parts. The first part provides the background and scientific evidence on which recommendations are based. The second part lists the recommendations and explains the ranking system for the level of scientific evidence for each recommendation. Each recommendation is categorized on the basis of existing scientific data, theoretical rationale, and applicability. Rankings are based on the system used by the CDC and the Healthcare Infection Control Practices Advisory Committee to categorize recommendations:

- Category IA—*strongly recommended for implementation and strongly supported by well-designed experimental, clinical, or epidemiologic studies*
- Category IB—*strongly recommended for implementation and supported by experimental, clinical, or epidemiologic studies and a strong theoretical rationale*
- Category IC—*required for implementation as mandated by federal or state regulations or standards. When IC is used, a second rating can be included to provide the basis of existing scientific data, theoretical rationale, and applicability. Because of state differences, readers should not assume that the absence of a IC recommendation implies the absence of any state regulations.*
- Category II—*suggested for implementation and supported by suggestive clinical or epidemiologic studies or a theoretical rationale*
- Unresolved issue—*no recommendation. Insufficient evidence or no consensus regarding efficacy exists.*

Dental practitioners should note the following important links related infection control issues in dentistry:

COVID-19 Guidance for Dental Settings
https://www.cdc.gov/coronavirus/2019-ncov/hcp/dental-settings.html

Interim Infection Prevention and Control Recommendations for Healthcare Personnel During the Coronavirus Disease 2019 (COVID-19) Pandemic
https://www.cdc.gov/coronavirus/2019-ncov/hcp/infection-control-recommendations.html

This site is subject to updates.

Prevention and Control of Seasonal Influenza with Vaccines https://www.cdc.gov/mmwr/volumes/70/rr/rr7005a1.htm

Dental practitioners should note the CDC recommendations concerning influenza vaccination of health care personnel in the United States.

CDC Health Advisory: Immediate Need for Healthcare Facilities to Review Procedures for Cleaning, Disinfecting, and Sterilizing Reusable Medical Devices https://emergency.cdc.gov/han/han00383.asp

INFECTION PREVENTION PRACTICES IN DENTAL SETTINGS

https://www.cdc.gov/oralhealth/infectioncontrol/pdf/safe-care2.pdf

HEPATITIS B FREQUENTLY ASKED QUESTIONS

These FAQs cover hepatitis B infections, vaccinations, chronic hepatitis B, serology, traveler's health, and more. http://www.cdc.gov/hepatitis/

Tuberculosis Infection Control Recommendations

The CDC's guidelines to prevent TB transmission in health care settings has evolved because of the changing epidemiology of TB as well as dental practice techniques. Dental practitioners should review the CDC's TB infection control recommendations for dental settings and learn how these recommendations should be incorporated into an infection control program.

https://www.cdc.gov/mmwr/preview/mmwrhtml/rr5417a1.htm?s_cid=rr5417a1_e

Prevention of Methicillin-Resistant *Staphylococcus aureus* Transmission in Dental Health Care Settings

MRSA is most often spread from patient to patient through the contaminated hands of health care professionals. The clinical utilization of Standard Precautions has been shown to be an effective strategy in preventing transmission. Learn more at CDC's About MRSA Skin Infections https://www.cdc.gov/mrsa/community/index.html

OTHER RELATED LINKS

CDC: Infection Prevention and Control Guidelines and Recommendations

http://www.cdc.gov/oralhealth/infectioncontrol/guidelines/index.htm

A slide set and accompanying speaker notes that provide an overview of many of the basic principles of infection control in the CDC's *Guidelines for Infection Control in Dental Health-Care Settings* can be downloaded as a PowerPoint presentation or viewed on the CDC's website.

Safety and Health Topics for Dentistry from the Occupational Safety and Health Administration (OSHA) (https://www.osha.gov/SLTC/dentistry/index.html)

National Institute for Occupational Safety and Health (NIOSH) http://www.cdc.gov/niosh/topics/bbp/

Organization for Safety, Asepsis and Prevention (http://www.osap.org/)

OSAP has produced a workbook that contains practical information to help health care professionals put the infection control recommendations into practice.

https://www.osap.org/from-policy-to-practice-osap-guide-to-the-cdc-guidelines-2019-edition

If Saliva Were Red: A Visual Lesson on Infection Control

The video training system, *If Saliva Were Red*, features an 8-minute DVD that uses dental professionals to highlight common infection control and safety flaws; the cross-contamination dental personnel would see if saliva were red; and how controlling contamination by using personal barrier protection, safe work practices, and effective infection control products reduces the risk of exposure.

American Dental Association (ADA) Infection Control Resources https://www.ada.org/resources/research/science-and-research-institute/oral-health-topics/infection-control-and-sterilization

BIBLIOGRAPHY

1. Cleveland JL, Robison VA, Panlilio AL. Tuberculosis epidemiology, diagnosis and infection control recommendations for dental settings: an update on the centers for disease control and prevention guidelines. *J Am Dent Assoc.* 2009;140:1092−1099.

2. Jensen PA, et al. Guidelines for preventing the transmission of mycobacterium tuberculosis in health-care settings, 2005 *MMWR Recomm Rep.* 2005;54(RR-17):1−142.

3. Centers for Disease Control and Prevention. Guidelines for infection control in dental health-care settings—2003. *MMWR Morb Mortal Wkly Rep.* 2003;52(RR-17):1−66.

4. Centers for Disease Control and Prevention. Recommended infection control practices for dentistry. *MMWR Morb Mortal Wkly Rep.* 1993;41(RR-8):1−12.

5. Centers for Disease Control and Prevention. Recommended infection control practices for dentistry. *MMWR Morb Mortal Wkly Rep.* 1986;35:237−242.

6. Klein RS, et al. Low occupational risk of human immunodeficiency virus infection among dental professionals. *N Engl J Med.* 1988;318:86−90.

7. Ciesielski C, et al. Transmission of human immunodeficiency virus in a dental practice. *Ann Intern Med.* 1992;116:798−805.

8. Centers for Disease Control and Prevention. Epidemiologic notes and reports update: transmission of HIV infection during invasive dental procedures—Florida. *MMWR Morb Mortal Wkly Rep.* 1991;40:377−381.

9. Cleveland JL, Gray SK, Harte JA, Robison VA, Moorman AC, Gooch BF. Transmission of blood-borne pathogens in US dental health care settings: 2016 update. *J Am Dent Assoc.* 2016;147(9):729−738.

10. U.S. Department of Labor. Occupational Safety and Health Administration. 29 CFR Part 1910: occupational exposure to blood-borne pathogens; needlestick and other sharps injuries; final rule. *Fed Reg.* 2001;66:5317−5325.

Therapeutic Management of Common Oral Lesions*

This appendix is provided for clinicians as a guide to the management of common oral lesions encountered in dental practice. It is intended only as a reference and is based on correct diagnosis of the condition and background knowledge of how the recommended therapies can be properly used. This information is adapted from the American Academy of Oral Medicine (AAOM), which publishes a guide for clinicians (Siegel MA, Sollecito TP, Stoopler ET. *Clinician's Guide: Treatment of Common Oral Conditions*. Seattle, Washington: American Academy of Oral Medicine; 2018). We (all members of the AAOM) acknowledge our deep appreciation for the authorization to publish this information in this appendix.

This appendix is intended as a quick reference to the etiologic factors, clinical description, currently accepted therapeutic management, and patient education of common oral conditions. All recommended treatments were current and have been reported to be of clinical value at the time of publication. However, new medications are constantly made available to the clinician and therapeutic strategies evolve, as new knowledge becomes known. The prudent clinician is well advised to consider this when using this guide.

For many conditions described in this appendix, there is currently no cure, but there are treatment modalities that can relieve discomfort, shorten the clinical duration and frequency, and minimize recurrences. Some of the treatments recommended in this manuscript are considered as "off-label" use.

Clinicians are reminded that an accurate diagnosis is imperative for clinical success. Every effort should be made to determine the diagnosis prior to initiating treatment. Infection and malignancy must be ruled out. Where signs, symptoms, microscopic and other laboratory evidence do not support a definitive diagnosis, empirical treatment may be initiated and evaluated as a therapeutic trial. Further treatment can be determined by the patient's response. However, when healing of a lesion or when an expected response to treatment is not achieved within an expected period of time, a biopsy is recommended.

Patient management should be governed by the natural history of the oral condition and the fact that there is either a palliative, supportive, or curative treatment. Referral of patients should be made when the patient's problems are beyond the scope of the clinician.

All drugs in this appendix require a prescription, unless identified as over-the-counter (OTC) drugs. Please note that the Food and Drug Administration (FDA) has been active in recent years with allowing OTC status for drugs formerly available by prescription only. Be sure to check on the dosages of the newly released OTC drugs because they are usually of a different strength than those available by prescription.

The literature accompanying the prescription topical medications suggested in this guide may recommend "for external use only." The oral cavity is completely lined with keratinized or nonkeratinized squamous epithelium that is classified as ectoderm, an external body covering. It is therefore acceptable to use topical medications intraorally as recommended in this appendix, as they are not swallowed and have minimal systemic absorption.

Supportive Care

Management of oral mucosal conditions may require topical and/or systemic interventions. Therapy should address patient nutrition and hydration, oral discomfort, oral hygiene, management of secondary infection, identification of possible drug interactions, and local control of the disease process. Depending on the extent, severity, and location of oral lesions, consideration should be given to obtaining a consultation from a dentist who specializes in oral medicine, oral and maxillofacial pathology, or oral and maxillofacial surgery. When there is a question involving a medical condition, a physician should be consulted.

Symptomatic relief of painful conditions can be provided with topical preparations such as 2% viscous lidocaine hydrochloride or dyclonine hydrochloride

---

* From the American Academy of Oral Medicine (AAOM), which publishes a guide for clinicians (Siegel MA, Sollecito TP, Stoopler ET. *Clinician's Guide: Treatment of Common Oral Conditions*. Seattle, Washington: American Academy of Oral Medicine; 2018).

throat lozenges (OTC). Topical anesthetics can be used as a rinse in adults but should be applied with a cotton swab in a child so that the child does not swallow the medication. Swallowing these anesthetics is contraindicated, in part, because they may interfere with the patient's gag reflex. Symptomatic relief also can be obtained using diphenhydramine or sucralfate to coat ulcerated lesions. Diphenhydramine hydrochloride elixir can be mixed with equal parts of magnesium hydroxide or aluminum hydroxide, and is advised to be used as a rinse prior to meals. Alternatively, children's formula diphenhydramine hydrochloride elixir may be used for symptomatic relief, as it does not contain alcohol.

Mouth rinses containing a hydroalcoholic vehicle should be avoided because of the oral discomfort that will result from their use. The amount of oral discomfort experienced by patients with oral mucosal lesions varies and can often be controlled without the use of narcotic analgesics. Nonnarcotic analgesics are often helpful.

Meticulous oral hygiene is absolutely mandatory for these patients. Mucosal lesions contacting bacterial plaque present on the dentition are more likely to become secondarily infected. Patients should be seen by the dentist or hygienist for scaling and root planing, under local anesthesia when necessary, in all cases in which oral hygiene is suboptimal. Patients must be encouraged to brush and floss their teeth after meals in a gentle yet efficient manner. Placing a soft toothbrush under hot water to further soften the bristles may enhance this. Tartar control toothpastes containing calcium pyrophosphate should be avoided because of their irritating nature and reported involvement in circumoral dermatitis. Furthermore, peroxide-based bleaching agents may be associated with tooth sensitivity and irritation of soft tissues, particularly the gingiva.

HERPES SIMPLEX

Infection with herpes simplex virus (HSV) produces a disease that has a primary acute phase and a secondary or recurrent phase.

PRIMARY HERPETIC GINGIVOSTOMATITIS

Etiology

A transmissible infection with herpes simplex virus, usually type I, less commonly type II.

Clinical Description

Clear or yellowish vesicles develop intra- and extraorally. These rupture within hours and form shallow, painful ulcers that may bleed. The gingivae are often red, enlarged, and painful. The patient may have systemic signs and symptoms, including regional lymphadenitis, fever, and malaise. Usually, it is self-limiting, with resolution in 10–14 days.

Rationale for Treatment

Treatment should focus on early intervention with antiviral agents and relieving symptoms, preventing secondary infection, and supporting general health. Supportive therapy includes fluid maintenance, protein, vitamin and mineral food supplements, and rest. Systemic antiviral medications appear to be more effective if administered within the first 2 days of symptom onset. Topical steroid medications alone must be avoided because they tend to permit spread of the viral infection on mucous membranes, particularly ocular lesions. Patients should be cautioned to avoid touching the herpetic lesions and then touching the eye, genital, or other body areas because of the possibility of self-inoculation.

Topical Anesthetics and Coating Agents

Rx:

Diphenhydramine (Children's Benadryl) elixir 12.5 mg/ 5 mL (OTC) 4 oz mixed with Kaopectate or Maalox (OTC) 4 oz (to make a 50% mixture by volume).

Disp: 8 oz.

Sig: Rinse with 1 tbs (5 mL) every 2 h and spit out.

Rx:

Lidocaine (viscous) 2.0% or 1%.

Disp: 1-oz bottle.

Sig: Rinse with 1 teaspoonful for 2 min before each meal and spit out.

Rx:

Dyclonine HCl throat lozenges (Sucrets) (OTC).

Disp: 1 package.

Sig: Dissolve slowly in mouth every 2 h as necessary. Do not exceed 10 lozenges per day.

Could add Dyclonine HCl (Dyclone) 0.5% or 1%.

When topical anesthetics are used, patients should be cautioned concerning a reduced gag reflex and the need for caution while eating and drinking to avoid possible airway compromise. Allergies are rare but may occur.

Systemic Antiviral Therapy. Acyclovir oral capsules may relieve and decrease the duration of symptoms. Acyclovir oral capsules must be initiated during the viral prodromal stage or this therapy will be ineffective.

Rx:

Acyclovir (Zovirax) caps 200 mg.

Disp: 42 caps.

Sig: Take 2 caps three times daily for 7 days.

Rx:

Valacyclovir (Valtrex) caplets 500 mg.

Disp: 20 caplets.

Sig: Take 2 caplets twice a day for 7 days.

Rx:

Famciclovir (Famvir) (see CDC recommendations).

Nutritional Supplements.

Rx:

Meritene (protein, vitamin, and mineral food supplement) (OTC).

Disp: 1-lb can (plain vanilla, chocolate, and eggnog flavors).

Sig: Take 3 servings daily. Prepare as indicated on the label. Serve cold.

Rx:

Ensure Plus (protein, vitamin, and mineral food supplement) (OTC).

Disp: 20 cans.

Sig: Drink 3–5 cans in divided doses throughout the day as tolerated. Serve cold.

Analgesics

Rx:

Acetaminophen tablets 325 mg (OTC).

Sig: Take 2 tablets every 4 h as needed for pain and fever. Limit 3 g per 24 h.

For moderate to severe pain:

Acetaminophen 300 mg with codeine 30 mg (Tylenol #3).

Why no Disp:?? I suggest this number MAX: 10.

Sig: Take 1 or 2 tablets every 4 h for pain (requires Drug Enforcement Agency [DEA] number).

If the patient chooses to take only one tab of Tylenol No. 3 (30 mg of codeine), the patient should be instructed to take one regular-strength acetaminophen tab (Tylenol [OTC]) to ensure the administration of the recommended strength of acetaminophen.

RECURRENT (OROFACIAL) HERPES SIMPLEX

Etiology

Reactivation of the latent herpes simplex virus that resides in the sensory ganglion of the trigeminal nerve. Precipitating factors include fever, stress, exposure to sunlight, trauma, and hormonal alterations.

Clinical Description

*Intraoral**—single or small clusters of vesicles that quickly rupture, forming painful ulcers. Lesions usually occur on the keratinized tissue of the hard palate and gingiva at or near the sites of the original infection.

*Labialis**—clusters of vesicles on the lips that rupture within hours and then crust.

Rationale for Treatment

Treatment should be initiated as early as possible during the prodromal stage to reduce duration and symptoms of the lesion. Antiviral medications given prophylactically and therapeutically may be considered when episodes are frequent (greater than six per year). Recurrent herpetic episodes interfere with daily function and nutrition. The current recommendation from the Food and Drug Administration is that systemic acyclovir be used to treat oral herpes only for immunocompromised patients. Valacyclovir has been approved for the prevention and management of oral recurrent herpes simplex infections.

---

* In immunocompromised patients, HSV lesions can occur on any mucosal surface, may be resistant to healing, and may have atypical appearances.

Prevention

Rx:

PreSun 15 (or 30) sunscreen lotion (OTC).

Disp: 4 fl oz.

Sig: Apply to susceptible area 1 h before sun exposure and every hour thereafter.

Rx:

PreSun 15 (or 30) lip gel (OTC).

Disp: 15 oz.

Sig: Apply to lips 1 h before sun exposure and every hour thereafter.

Topical Antiviral Agents. Topical antiviral medications are most effective when initiated as early in the course of the episode as possible. Patients should be instructed to dab on the medication as soon as prodromal symptoms are felt. These medications should be dabbed on, not rubbed in, to minimize mechanical trauma to the lesions. Patients should be instructed to apply the antiviral agent with a cotton-tip applicator.

Rx:

Penciclovir (Denavir) cream 1%.

Disp: 2-g tube.

Sig: Dab on lesion every 2 h during waking hours for 4 days beginning when symptoms first occur.

Rx:

Docosanol (Abreva) cream (OTC).

Disp: 2-g tube.

Sig: Dab on lesion five times per day during waking hours for 4 days beginning when symptoms first occur.

Acyclovir. Acyclovir and hydrocortisone cream (Xerese)—please add

Systemic Antiviral Therapy. Systemic antiviral therapy is most effective when initiated as early in the course of the episode as possible. Patients should be instructed to take the systemic medication exactly as directed as soon as prodromal symptoms are felt. Total dosing is limited to 1 day.

Rx:

Valacyclovir (Valtrex) caplets 500 mg.

Disp: 40 caplets.

Sig: Take 4 caplets as soon as prodromal symptoms are recognized and then 4 caplets 12 h later; continue use for 3–5 days.

VARICELLA ZOSTER (SHINGLES)

Etiology

Herpes zoster (shingles) represents reactivation of VZV following previous infection with varicella (chickenpox). Precipitating factors include thermal, inflammatory, radiologic, and mechanical trauma, stress, as well as immunosuppression.

Clinical Description

Usually painful, segmental eruption of small vesicles that later rupture to form punctate or confluent ulcers that extend to the midline. Acute herpes zoster follows a portion of the trigeminal nerve distribution in approximately 20% of cases. It is rare in a young individual and found more commonly in the elderly patient.

Rationale for Treatment

Promptly initiate antiviral therapy to reduce the duration and symptoms of the lesions. Patients over 60 years of age are particularly prone to post herpetic neuralgia (PHN). In the absence of specific contraindications, consideration should be given to prescribing short-term, high-dose, corticosteroid prophylaxis for PHN in conjunction with oral antiviral therapy.

> *Rx:*
> Acyclovir (Zovirax) capsules 800 mg.
> *Disp:* 70 capsules
> *Sig:* Take 1 capsule five times daily for 14 days.
> *Rx:*
> Valacyclovir (Valtrex) HCl caplets 500 mg.
> *Disp:* 84 capsules.
> *Sig:* Take 2 capsules three times daily for 14 days.

RECURRENT APHTHOUS STOMATITIS

Etiology

An altered local immune response is the predisposing factor. Patients with frequent recurrences should be screened for diseases such as anemia, diabetes mellitus, vitamin deficiency, inflammatory bowel disease, and immunosuppression. Precipitating factors include stress, trauma, allergies, endocrine alterations, and dietary components, such as acidic foods and drinks, and foods that contain gluten. Inspect the oral cavity closely for sources of trauma.

Clinical Description

Minor aphthae (canker sore), <0.5 cm, small, shallow, painful ulceration covered by a gray membrane and surrounded by a narrow erythematous halo. They usually occur on nonkeratinized (moveable) oral mucosa. These lesions heal without scarring. Minor aphthae are the most form of recurrent aphthous stomatitis.

Major aphthae, >0.5 cm, large, painful ulcers. Major aphthae represent a more severe form of recurrent aphthous stomatitis that may last from 6 weeks to 3 months. Healing may result in mucosal scarring. These ulcerations may mimic other diseases, such as granulomatous or malignant lesions.

Herpetiform ulcers—crops of small, shallow, painful ulcers. They may occur anywhere on nonkeratinized oral mucosa and resemble recurrent intraoral herpes simplex clinically but are of unknown etiology.

Rationale for Treatment

Effective treatment involves barriers, chemical cauterization, topical or systemic corticosteroids, and immunosuppressant or combination therapy when indicated. Treatment should be initiated as early in the course of the lesions as possible. Identification and elimination of precipitating factors may serve to minimize recurrent episodes. Medications such as mycophenolate mofetil, pentoxiphylline, colchicine, and thalidomide are used to treat patients with severe, persistent recurrent aphthous ulcers (RAU) but should not be routinely used. Mixing topical steroid ointments with equal parts of Orabase B paste promotes adhesion and prolongs contact of the medication with the lesion being treated.

Topical Steroids. Therapies with steroids and immunomodulating drugs are presented to inform the clinician that such modalities are available. Because of the potential for adverse effects, close collaboration with the patient's physician is recommended when these medications are prescribed. These modalities may be beyond the scope of clinical experience of general dentists, and referral to a specialist in oral medicine or to an appropriate physician may be necessary.

> *Rx:*
> Dexamethasone (Decadron) elixir 0.5 mg/5 mL.
> *Disp:* 100 mL.
> *Sig:* Rinse with 1 teaspoon (5 mL) for 2 min four times daily and expectorate. Discontinue when lesions become asymptomatic.
> *Rx:*
> Triamcinolone acetonide (Kenalog) in Orabase 0.1%.
> *Disp:* 5-g tube.
> *Sig:* Coat the lesion with a thin film after each meal and at bedtime.

Other topical steroid preparations (cream, gel rinse, ointment) include the following:

Ultrapotent.
- Clobetasol propionate (Temovate) 0.05%
- Halobetasol propionate (Ultravate) 0.05%

Potent.
- Dexamethasone (Decadron) 0.5 mg/5 mL
- Fluocinonide (Lidex) 0.05%
- Fluticasone propionate (Cutivate) 0.05%

Intermediate.
- Betamethasone valerate (Valisone) 0.1%
- Triamcinolone acetonide (Kenalog) 0.1%
- Aclometasone dipropionate (Aclovate) 0.05%

Low.
- Hydrocortisone 1%
- Hydrocortisone probutate (Pandel) 0.1%

Prolonged use of topical steroids (greater than 2 weeks continuous use) may result in mucosal atrophy and secondary candidiasis and increase the potential of systemic absorption. Chronic use is discouraged. It may be necessary to prescribe antifungal therapy with steroids.

The oral cavity should be monitored for emergence of fungal infection for patients who are placed on therapy. Prophylactic antifungal therapy should be initiated in patients with a history of fungal infections with previous steroid administration (see "Candidiasis").

System Steroids and Immunosuppressants.

For severe cases:

Rx:

Dexamethasone (Decadron) elixir 0.5 mg/5 mL

Disp: 320 mL.

Sig: As directed not to exceed 2 continuous weeks.

Directions for using dexamethasone elixir:

Rinse for 1 min by the clock, four times daily, after meals and before bedtime. Do not drink or eat for 30 min after rinsing with dexamethasone elixir. Discontinue medication when lesions resolve.

- For 3 days, rinse with 1 tbsp (15 mL) four times daily and swallow. Then,
- For 3 days, rinse with 1 tsp (5 mL) four times daily and swallow. Then,
- For 3 days, rinse with 1 tsp (5 mL) four times daily and swallow every other time. Then,
- Rinse with 1 tsp (5 mL) four times daily and expectorate.

Rx:

Prednisone tablets 5 mg.

Disp: 40 tablets.

Sig: Take 5 tablets in the morning for 5 days; then take 5 tablets in the morning every other day until gone.

For very severe cases:

Rx:

Prednisone tablets 10 mg.

Disp: 26 tablets.

Sig: Take 4 tablets in the morning for 5 days; then decrease by 1 tablet on each successive day until gone.

Therapy with medications such as systemic steroids, immunosuppressants, and immunomodulators is presented to inform the clinician that such modalities have been reported effective for patients suffering from severe, persistent, recurrent aphthous stomatitis. Medications such as azathioprine, pentoxiphylline, levamisole, colchicine, dapsone, and thalidomide are used to treat patients with severe, persistent recurrent aphthous stomatitis but should not be routinely used because of the potential for side effects. Close monitoring and collaboration with the patient's physician is recommended when these medications are prescribed.

CANDIDIASIS

Etiology

Candida albicans is a yeast-like fungus. It is an opportunistic organism that tends to proliferate with the use of broad-spectrum antibiotics, corticosteroids, medications that reduce salivary flow, and cytotoxic agents. Conditions that contribute to this disease include xerostomia, uncontrolled diabetes mellitus, anemia, poor oral hygiene, prolonged use of prosthetic oral appliances, and suppression of the immune system, such as human immunodeficiency virus (HIV) infection, or as a side effect of many medications, including steroid inhalants. Antibiotics may shift the microflora and allow overgrowth of

Candida. Also high intake of sugar promotes fungal growth. It is important to determine predisposing factors prior to initiating therapy.

Clinical Description

This disease is characterized by soft, white, slightly elevated plaques that usually can be wiped away (pseudomembranous form), generalized erythematous sensitive areas (erythematous form), or confluent white areas that cannot be wiped away (hyperplastic form). Angular cheilitis, which is also described in this appendix, is frequently associated.

Rationale for Treatment

The rationale for the treatment of candidiasis is to reestablish a normal balance of oral flora and improve oral hygiene. The disinfection of all removable oral prostheses with antifungal denture-soaking solutions and the application of antifungal agents on the tissue-contacting surfaces is necessary to remove a potential source of fungal reinfection.

Medication should be continued for a few days after disappearance of clinical signs to prevent immediate recurrence. However, it is advisable to empirically treat candidiasis for a 10- to 14-day period. Identification and correction of contributing factors will minimize recurrence.

It is important that salivation be within normal limits. Many medications and systemic conditions, including immunosuppression, will decrease salivary flow, thereby predisposing the patient to candidiasis. Increasing oral moisture by using sugarless gum or candy, mouthrinses without alcohol, or sialogogues, such as pilocarpine or cevimeline, is often an important adjunctive measure when managing candidiasis (see Chapter, "Xerostomia [Reduced Salivary Flow and Dry Mouth]").

Topical Antifungal Agents

Rx:

Clotrimazole (Mycelex) troches 10 mg.

Disp: 70 troches.

Sig: Let 1 troche dissolve in mouth five times daily. Do not chew.

Rx:

Mycostatin pastilles 200,000 U.

Disp: 70 pastilles.

Sig: Let 1 pastille dissolve in mouth five times daily. Do not chew.

Rx:

Nystatin vaginal suppositories 100,000 U.

Disp: 40 suppositories.

Sig: Let 1 suppository dissolve in the mouth four times daily. Do not rinse for 30 min.

If there is concern about the sugar content of the mycostatin pastilles and clotrimazole troches, vaginal tabs/suppositories can be substituted (100–200 mg once or twice daily). Troches/pastilles may not be well tolerated when the patient has a dry mouth because of the inability to dissolve this dosage form. Consider a course of systemic antifungal therapy.

Rx:

Nystatin ointment.

Disp: 15 g tube.

Sig: Apply a thin coat to the inner surface of the denture and to the affected area after meals.

Rx:

Ketoconazole (Nizoral) cream 2%.

Disp: 15 g tube.

Sig: Apply a thin coat to the inner surface of the denture and to the affected area after meals.

Rx:

Clotrimazole (Gyne-Lotrimin, Mycelex-G vaginal cream 1% [OTC]).

Disp: One tube.

Sig: Apply a thin layer to the tissue side of the denture and/or to infected oral mucosa four times daily.

Rx:

Miconazole (Monistat 7) nitrate vaginal cream 2% (OTC).

Disp: One tube.

Sig: Apply thin layer to tissue side of denture and/or to infected oral mucosa four times daily.

Although some disagree with the use of vaginal creams intraorally, their efficacy has been observed clinically in selected cases where other topical antifungal agents have failed.

Creams and ointments are ideal for treating patients wearing complete or partial dentures. Application of an antifungal cream or ointment to the tissue-bearing surfaces of a denture serves to localize the medication to the affected soft tissues while simultaneously treating the denture. Patients must be reminded to remove their prostheses prior to going to bed. They should be instructed to apply the cream or ointment directly to the oral soft tissues at bedtime while cleaning their denture in a commercially available denture cleanser.

A few drops of nystatin oral suspension can be added to the water used for soaking acrylic prostheses. However, most commercially available denture cleansers have some degree of antifungal activity. Dentures may be soaked in a sodium hypochlorite solution (1 tsp of sodium hypochlorite in a denture cup of water) for 15 min and thoroughly rinsed for at least 2 min under running water (long-term soaking of dentures in even a mild bleach solution will fade the pigment in the denture acrylic). Chlorhexidine gluconate and Listerine both exhibit antifungal activity.

Rx:

Nystatin (Mycostatin, Nilstat) oral suspension 100,000 U/mL.

Disp: 240 mL.

Sig: Rinse with 5 mL four times daily for 3 min by the clock and expectorate.

Systemic Antifungal Agents. Fluconazole (Diflucan) is an effective and well-tolerated systemic drug for mucocutaneous and oropharyngeal candidiasis. It should be used with caution in patients with impaired liver function (a history of alcoholism or hepatitis). Diminishing response over time with fluconazole may indicate development of fungal resistance or the need to temporarily increase the medication dosage.

Rx:

Fluconazole (Diflucan) tablets 100 mg.

Disp: 15 tablets.

Sig: Take 2 tablets stat and then 1 tablet daily until gone.

Fluconazole is a potent inhibitor of cytochrome P-450 isoenzymes. These antifungal medications can significantly inhibit the hepatic metabolism of medications such as antihistamines, cholesterol-lowering medications, antihypertensive medications, warfarin compounds, and antiasthmatic medications that are primarily metabolized by this liver isoenzyme system. Toxic drug interactions have been reported with both ketaconazole and fluconazole; be sure to check appropriate pharmacology references. A new class of antifungal medications, Echinocandins, are available for IV administration to patients who are severely immunocompromised. Medications in the Echinocandin class include capsofungin, micafungin, and anidulafungin.

CHEILITIS AND CHEILOSIS

ANGULAR CHEILITIS AND CHEILOSIS

Etiology

Fissured lesions in the corners of the mouth are caused by a mixed infection of the microorganisms *Candida albicans*, staphylococci, and streptococci. Predisposing factors include excessive licking, drooling, a decrease in the intermaxillary space, anemia, vitamin deficiency immunosuppression, sugar consumption, and an extension of oral infections.

Clinical Description

Commissures may appear wrinkled, red, fissured, cracked, or crusted.

Rationale for Treatment

Identification and correction of predisposing factors, elimination of primary and secondary infections, eradication of inflammation.

Rx:

Nystatin–triamcinolone acetonide (Mycolog II, Mytrex) ointment.

Disp: 15 g tube.

Sig: Apply to affected area after meals and at bedtime.

Rx:

Polymyxin B/Bacitracin (Polysporin) ointment (OTC).

Disp: 15 g tube.

Sig: Apply to affected areas after meals and at bedtime.

Rx:

Clotrimazole—betamethasone dipropionate (Lotrisone) cream.

Disp: 15 g tube.

Sig: Apply to affected area after each meal and at bedtime.

Rx:

Hydrocortisone-iodoquinol (Vytone) cream 1%.

Disp: 15 g tube.

Sig: Apply to affected area after each meal and at bedtime.

Rx:

Ketoconazole (Nizoral) cream 2%.

Disp: 15 g tube.

Sig: Apply sparingly to corners of mouth after each meal and at bedtime.

Rx:

Clotrimazole (Gyne-Lotrimin, Mycelex-G) vaginal cream 1% (OTC).

Disp: One tube.

Sig: Apply sparingly to corners of mouth after each meal and at bedtime.

Rx:

Miconazole (Monistat 7) nitrate vaginal cream 2% (OTC).

Disp: One tube.

Sig: Apply sparingly to corners of mouth after each meal and at bedtime.

Vaginal creams may be used intraorally as their efficacy has been observed clinically in selected cases where other topical antifungal agents have failed.

ACTINIC CHEILITIS AND SOLAR CHEILOSIS

Etiology

Prolonged exposure to sunlight results in irreversible degenerative changes in the vermilion zone of the lips.

Clinical Description

The normal red translucent vermilion zone with regular vertical fissuring of a smooth surface is replaced by a white flat surface or an irregular scaly surface that may exhibit periodic ulceration.

Rationale for Treatment

Elimination of exposure to UV light. Educate patient regarding malignant potential because degenerative changes may progress to malignancy.

Rx:

PreSun 15 lip get (OTC).

Disp: 15 oz.

Sig: Apply to lips 1 hr before sun exposure and every hour thereafter.

Several OTC sunscreen preparations are available (e.g., PreSun 15 or PreSun 30 lotion and lip gel). For those patients allergic to PABA, non-PABA sunscreens should be suggested. For patients who have had a history of dysplasia or a lip malignancy, a zinc oxide or titanium dioxide product should be used. Many over-the-counter lip products contain sunscreen with SPF 15—SPF 50. Patients should be advised to use a sunscreen-containing lip protectant at all times when outdoors

When the lesion becomes scaly, leukoplakic or ulcerative, a biopsy is required to rule out dysplasia, carcinoma in situ, or squamous cell carcinoma.

GEOGRAPHIC TONGUE (BENIGN MIGRATORY GLOSSITIS; ERYTHEMA MIGRANS)

Etiology

The etiology is unknown, but has association with immunological hypersensitivity reaction. Since its histologic appearance is similar to psoriasis, some have associated it with psoriasis. This may be purely coincidental. Oral lesions should not be associated with psoriasis if there are no cutaneous signs of this disorder. It also has been associated with Reiter's syndrome and generalized atopy.

Clinical Description

A benign inflammatory condition caused by desquamation of superficial keratin and filiform papillae. It is characterized by both red, denuded, irregularly circinate-shaped patches of the tongue dorsum and lateral borders surrounded by a raised, white-yellow border.

Rationale for Treatment

Generally, no treatment is necessary because most patients are asymptomatic. When symptoms are present, they may be associated with secondary infection with *Candida albicans* (see "Candidosis, page 7"). Topical steroids, especially in combination with topical antifungal agents, have been used successfully to manage the condition. Patients must be told that this condition does not suggest a more serious disease and is not contagious. In most cases, biopsy is not indicated because of the pathognomonic clinical appearance. Some clinicians mix topical steroid ointments with equal parts of Orabase B paste to promote adhesion and prolong contact of the medication with the lesion being treated.

Rx:

Clotrimazole-betamethasone dipropionate (Lotrisone) cream.

Disp: 15-g tube.

Sig: Apply to affected area after each meal and at bedtime.

Rx:

Betamethasone valerate (Valisone) ointment 0.1%.

Disp: 15-g tube.

Sig: Apply to affected area after each meal and at bedtime.

Rx:

Nystatin ointment.

Disp: 15-g tube.

Sig: Apply to affected area after each meal and at bedtime.

XEROSTOMIA (REDUCED SALIVARY FLOW AND DRY MOUTH)

Etiology

Acute or chronic salivary flow alterations or xerostomia may result from drug therapy, mechanical blockage, dehydration, emotional stress, bacterial infection of the salivary glands, local surgery, avitaminosis, diabetes, anemia, connective tissue diseases, Sjögren's syndrome, radiation therapy, viral infections, and certain congenital disorders.

Clinical Description

The saliva may be ropey, with a film covering the teeth. The tissue may be dry, pale or red, and atrophic. The tongue may be devoid of papillae, atrophic, fissured, and inflamed. Multiple carious lesions may be present, especially at the gingival margin and on exposed root surfaces. The quantity and the quality of saliva may be altered.

Rationale for Treatment

Salivary stimulation or replacement therapy is used to keep the mouth moist, prevent caries and candidal infection, and provide palliative relief. For patients with removable dentures, the application of an artificial saliva or oral lubricant gel to the tissue contact surface of the denture reduces frictional trauma.

Xerostomia, reduced salivary flow, and dry mouth provide an excellent environment for the overgrowth of *Candida albicans*. The patient is likely to require treatment for candidiasis along with the treatment for dry mouth (see "Candidiasis"). In a dry oral environment, plaque control becomes more difficult. Meticulous oral hygiene is essential.

Saliva Substitutes

Rx:

Sodium carboxymethylcellulose 0.5% aqueous solution (OTC).

Disp: 8 fl oz.

Sig: Use as a rinse as frequently as needed. Generic carboxymethylcellulose solutions may be prepared by a pharmacist.

Plain water in a small plastic bottle is often used with success by many xerostomic patients.

COMMERCIAL SALIVA SUBSTITUTES (OTC)

- Glandosane
- Moi-Stir
- Mouth Kote
- Oasis
- Roxane Saliva Substitute
- Sage Moist Plus
- Salivart
- Ask your pharmacist

COMMERCIAL ORAL MOISTURIZING GELS (OTC)

- Laclede Oral Balance
- Sage Mouth Moisturizer

Relief from oral dryness and accompanying discomfort can be achieved conservatively by

- Sipping water frequently all day long
- Letting ice melt in the mouth
- Restricting caffeine and cola intake
- Avoiding mouth rinses, drinks, and medications containing alcohol
- Avoiding tobacco products
- Humidifying the sleeping area
- Coating the lips

Saliva Stimulants. The use of sugar-free gum, lemon drops, or mints is a conservative method to temporarily stimulate salivary flow in patients with medication xerostomia or with salivary gland dysfunction. Patients should be cautioned against using products that contain sugar or have a low pH.

Rx:

Biotene Dry Mouth Gum (OTC).

Disp: 1 package.

Sig: Chew as needed.

Owing to problems of abrasion of the mucosa under the denture and potential adhesion of the gum to the denture, use caution if the patient wears removable dentures.

Rx:

Pilocarpine HCl 5-mg tablets (Salagen).

Disp: 21 tablets.

Sig: Take 1 tab three times daily 30 min prior to meals.

Dose may be titrated to 2 tabs three times daily. Some recommend using 1 tab of pilocarpine four to five times daily.

Rx:

Cevimeline HCl (Evoxac) caps 30-mg.

Disp: 21 caps.

Sig: Take 1 cap three times daily.

Rx:

Pilocarpine HCL solution 1 mg/mL.

Disp: 100 mL.

Sig: Take 1 tsp (5 mL) four times daily.

Rx:

Bethanechol (Urecholine) tabs 25 mg.

Disp: 30 tabs.

Sig: Take 1 tab up to 5 times daily.

Cholinergic drugs should be prescribed in consultation with the physician-of record or specialist owing to significant side effects. The pilocarpine and cevimeline dosage should be adjusted to increase saliva while minimizing the adverse side effects (e.g., sweating, stomach upset). Patients should be warned that there is a wide range of sensitivity and that the adverse side effects may exceed the desired increased salivation; if this occurs, then the cholinergic drug should be discontinued. Pilocarpine and cevimeline should be avoided in a patient who has moderate-to-severe asthma/COPD, significant cardiovascular disease, gall bladder or urinary obstruction.

Caries Prevention

Rx:

Fluoride gel (see examples below).

Disp: 1 tube.

Sig: Place a 1-inch ribbon in a custom tray; apply for 5 min daily. Avoid rinsing or eating for 30 min following treatment.

Flouride Gels

0.4%Stannous Fluoride	1.1% Neutral or Acidulated Na Fluoride
Acclean Home Care gel	
Alpha-Dent	ControlRx
Gel-Kam	Denti-Care
Gel-Tin	FlurideX
Omnii Gel	FluoriSHIELD
Perfect Choice	NeutraCare
Plak Smacker	NeutraGard
Periocheck Oral Med	PreviDent gel
Stop	Pro-DenRx
Super-Dent	Topex
Take Home Care	

Rx:

PreviDent 1.1% gel.

Disp: 1 tube.

Sig: Place a 1-inch ribbon in a custom tray; apply for 5 min daily. Avoid rinsing or eating for 30 min following treatment.

Rx:

Thera-Flur-N 1.1% gel.

Disp: 1 tube.

Sig: Place a 1-inch ribbon on a toothbrush; brush for 2 min daily and expectorate. Avoid rinsing or eating for 30 min following treatment.

Rx:

Neutral NaF 1.1 % dental cream. PreviDent 5000 Plus toothpaste.

Disp: 1 tube.

Sig: Place a 1-inch ribbon on a toothbrush; brush for 2 min daily and expectorate. Avoid rinsing or eating for 30 min following treatment.

When the taste of acidulated fluoride gels is poorly tolerated or when there is etching of ceramic restorations, neutral pH sodium fluoride gel 1% (Thera-Flur-N, PreviDent) should be considered. FDA regulations have limited the size of bottles of fluoride owing to toxicity if ingested by infants. Since most preparations do not come in childproofed bottles, the sizes of topical fluoride preparations vary; 24 mL is approximately a 2-week supply for application to a full dentition in custom carriers.

ORAL LICHEN PLANUS

Etiology

It is postulated to be a chronic mucocutaneous autoimmune disorder with a genetic predisposition that may be initiated by a variety of factors, including emotional stress and hypersensitivity to drugs, dental products, or foods.

Clinical Description

Lichen planus varies in clinical appearance. Oral forms of this disorder include lacy white lines representing Wickham's striae (reticular), an erythematous form (atrophic), and an ulcerating form that is often accompanied by striae peripheral to the ulceration (ulcerative). The lesions are commonly found on the buccal mucosa, gingiva, and tongue but can be found on the lips and palate. Lichen planus lesions are chronic and may affect the skin. The dental and medical literature remains controversial as to whether certain forms of lichen planus transform into malignant neoplasia. Therefore, any persistent or refractory lesion(s) should be biopsied to establish a definitive diagnosis and to rule out a malignancy.

Rationale for Treatment

To provide oral comfort if the lesions are symptomatic. There is no known cure. Systemic and local relief with antiinflammatory and immunosuppressant agents is indicated. Identification of any dietary component, dental product, or medication (lichenoid drug reaction) should be undertaken to ensure against a hypersensitivity reaction. Therapies with steroids and immunomodulating drugs are presented to inform the clinician that such modalities are available. Because of the potential for side effects, close collaboration with the patient's physician is recommended when these medications are prescribed. These modalities may be beyond the scope of clinical experience of general dentists, and referral to a specialist in oral medicine or to an appropriate physician may be necessary.

Topical Steroids

Rx:

Fluocinonide (Lidex) gel 0.05%.

Disp: 30-g tube.

Sig: Coat the lesion with a thin film after each meal and at bedtime.

Rx:

Dexamethasone (Decadron) elixir 0.5 mg/5 mL.

Disp: 100 mL.

Sig: Rinse with 1 tsp (5 mL) for 2 min four times daily and spit out. Discontinue when lesions become asymptomatic.

Other topical steroid preparations (cream, gel, ointment) include the following:

Ultrapotent.
- Clobetasol propionate (Temovate) 0.05%
- Halobetasol propionate (Ultravate) 0.05%

Potent.
- Dexamethasone (Decadron) 0.5 mg/5 mL
- Fluocinonide (Lidex) 0.05%
- Fluticasone propionate (Cutivate) 0.05%

Intermediate.
- Betamethasone valerate (Valisone) 0.1%
- Alclometasone dipropionate (Aclovate) 0.05%
- Triamcinolone acetonide (Kenalog) 0.1%

Low.
- Hydrocortisone 1%
- Hydrocortisone probutate (Pandel) 0.1%

Mixing any of the above topical steroid ointments with equal parts of Orabase B paste promotes adhesion and prolongs contact of the medication with the lesion being treated.

Prolonged use of topical steroids (greater than 2 weeks continuous use) may result in mucosal atrophy and secondary candidosis and increase the potential of systemic absorption. It may be necessary to prescribe antifungal therapy with steroids. Therapy with topical steroids, once the lichen planus is under control, should be tapered to alternate-day therapy or less depending on disease control and tendency to recur.

Oral candidiasis may result from topical steroid therapy. The oral cavity should be monitored for emergence of fungal infection for patients who are placed on therapy. Prophylactic antifungal therapy should be initiated in patients with a history of fungal infections with previous steroid administration (see "Candidiasis"). Treatment of a secondary fungal infection with a systemic antifungal agent should be considered.

Systemic Steroids and Immunosuppressants

Rx:

Dexamethasone elixir 0.5 mg 5 mL.
Disp: 320 mL.
Sig: *As directed not to exceed 2 continuous weeks.*
Directions for using dexamethasone elixir:

Rinse for 1 min by the clock, four times daily, after meals and before bedtime. Do not drink or eat for 30 min after rinsing with dexamethasone elixir. Discontinue medication when lesions resolve.
- For 3 days, rinse with 1 tbsp (15 mL) four times daily and swallow. Then,
- For 3 days, rinse with 1 tsp (5 mL) four times daily and swallow. Then,
- For 3 days, rinse with 1 tsp (5 mL) four times daily and swallow every other time. Then,
- Rinse with 1 tsp (5 mL) four times daily and expectorate.

If oral discomfort recurs, the patient should return to the clinician for reevaluation.

Therapy with medications such as systemic steroids, immunosuppressants, and immunomodulators is presented to inform the clinician that such modalities have been reported effective for patients suffering from ulcerative lichen planus. Medications such as azathioprine, mycophenolate mofetil, tacrolimus, pimecrolimus, hydroxychloroquine-sulfate, acitretin, and cyclosporine are used to treat patients with severe persistent ulcerative lichen planus but should not be routinely used because of the potential for side effects. Close collaboration with the patient's physician is recommended when these medications are prescribed.

Topical tacrolimus, and to a lesser degree pimecrolimus, have been associated with neoplastic disease, such as lymphoma, and, therefore, should not be used indiscriminately for long periods of time. These medications are indicated for patients who cannot tolerate or are refractory to topical or systemic steroid therapy. All patients with lichen planus must be periodically followed for control of discomfort and to ensure against the very low risk of malignant transformation.

Rx:

Tacrolimus 0.1% ointment.
Disp: 30 tube.
Sig: Apply to affected site(s) twice daily as directed.

Rx:

Tacrolimus 0.03% ointment.
Disp: 30 tube.
Sig: Apply to affected site(s) twice daily as directed.

Rx:

Pimecrolimus 1.0% cream.
Disp: 30 tube.
Sig: Apply to affected site(s) twice daily as directed.

Rx:

Prednisone tabs 10 mg.
Disp: 26 tabs.
Sig: Take 4 tabs in the morning for 5 days and then decrease by 1 tab on each successive day.

Rx:

Prednisone tabs 5 mg.
Disp: 40 tabs.
Sig: Take 5 tabs in the morning for 5 days and then 5 tabs in the morning every other day until gone.

PEMPHIGUS AND MUCOUS MEMBRANE PEMPHIGOID

These are relatively uncommon conditions. They should be suspected when there are chronic, multiple oral ulcerations and a history of oral and skin blisters. Often, they occur only in the mouth. Diagnosis is based on the history and the histologic and immunofluorescent characteristics of a biopsy of the primary lesion.

Etiology

Both are autoimmune diseases with autoantibodies against antigens appearing in different portions of the epithelium (mucosa). In pemphigus, the antigens are within the epithelium (desmosomes), whereas in pemphigoid, the antigens are located at the base of the epithelium in the hemidesmosomes.

Clinical Characteristics

In pemphigus, the lesion may stay in one location for a long period of time with small flaccid bullae. The bullae may rupture, leaving an ulcer. Approximately 80–90% of the patients have oral lesions. In approximately two-thirds of patients, the oral manifestations are the first sign of the disease. All parts of the mouth may be involved. The bullae rupture almost immediately in the mouth but may stay intact for some time on the skin. One of the classic signs, Nikolsky's sign (blister formation induced with gentle rubbing of a normal, perilesional mucosal site), is positive in pemphigus but is not pathognomic because it may be observed in other disorders. Because the vesicle or bulla is intraepithelial, it is often filled with clear fluid. Histologically, there is a cleavage (Tzanck cells, acantholytic cells) within the spinous layer of the epithelium.

In pemphigoid, the cleavage or split is beneath the epithelium, resulting in bullae that are usually blood filled. Mucous membrane pemphigoid is often limited to the oral cavity, but some patients have ocular lesions (symblepharon, ankyloblepharon) that require evaluation by an ophthalmologist. The gingiva is the most common oral site involved. Pemphigoid may appear clinically as a red, nonulcerated gingival lesion. Patients should be queried with regard to ocular or pharyngeal involvement.

Rationale for Treatment

Since both pemphigus and pemphigoid are autoimmune disorders, the primary treatment is topical or systemic steroids or other immunomodulating drugs. Pemphigus requires the use of systemic medications. Custom trays may be used to localize topical steroid medications on the gingival tissues (occlusive therapy). Please see "Oral lichen planus" for topical medication recommendations. Because they can resemble other ulcerative-bullous diseases, a biopsy is necessary for a definitive diagnosis. Specimens should be submitted for light microscopic, immunofluorescent, and immunologic testing. Because of the potential serious nature, referral to specialists in oral medicine, dermatology, otorhinolaryngology, and ophthalmology must be considered. When ocular lesions are present, an ophthalmologist must be consulted immediately to prevent blindness.

Therapy with medications such as systemic steroids, immunosuppressants, and immunomodulators is presented to inform the clinician that such modalities have been reported effective for patients suffering from vesiculobullous disorders such as pemphigus vulgaris and mucous membrane pemphigoid. Therapies such as dapsone, methotrexate, mycophenolate mofetil, cyclosporine, niacinamide with tetracycline, rituximab and plasmapheresis are used to treat patients with vesiculobullous disorders such as pemphigus vulgaris and mucous membrane pemphigoid but should not be routinely used because of the potential for side effects. Close collaboration with the patient's physician is recommended when these medications are prescribed.

ORAL ERYTHEMA MULTIFORME

Etiology

Erythema multiforme is believed to be a hypersensitivity reaction most commonly due to medications and/or viruses (e.g. HSV-1). It may occur at any age. Drug reactions to medications such as penicillin and sulfonamides may play a role in some cases. It has been observed that a herpetic infection occurred immediately prior to the onset of clinical signs of erythema multiforme in a subset of patients.

Clinical Description

Signs of erythema multiforme include "blood-crusted" lips, "targetoid" or "bull's eye" skin lesions, and a nonspecific mucosal slough. The name multiforme is used because its appearance may take multiple different forms. Erythema multiforme as a skin disease occurs most frequently due to an allergic reaction. This condition may occur chronically or periodically in cycles.

Rationale for Treatment

Treatment is primarily antiinflammatory in nature. Steroids are initiated and then tapered. Due to the possible relationship of erythema multiforme with herpes simplex virus reactivation, suppressive antiviral therapy may be necessary in conjunction with steroid therapy. Patients should be carefully questioned about a previous history of recurrent herpetic infections as well as prodromal symptoms that might have preceded the onset of the erythema multiforme. Dosing must be titrated to specific situations.

Steroid Therapy

Rx:

Prednisone tablets 10 mg.

Disp: 100 tablets.

Sig: Take 6 tablets in the morning until lesions recede, then decrease by 1 tablet on each successive day. Do not exceed 14 days of therapy. If therapy exceeds 14 days, steroids should be tapered.

Suppressive Antiviral Therapy

Rx:
Acyclovir (Zovirax) 400-mg capsules.
Disp: Sufficient quantity.
Sig: Take 1 tablet two times daily.
Rx:
Valacyclovir (Valtrex) 500-mg capsules.
Disp: Sufficient quantity.
Sig: Take 1 tablet two times daily.

DENTURE SORE MOUTH

Etiology

Discomfort under oral prosthetic appliances may result from combinations of candidal infections, poor denture hygiene, an occlusive syndrome, and overextension or excessive movement of the appliance. This condition may be erroneously attributed to an allergy to denture material, which is a rare occurrence. This condition also may represent a pressure neuropathy owing to advanced mandibular alveolar resorption exposing the mental foramen. The retention and fit of the denture should be idealized, and mechanical irritation should be ruled out.

Clinical Description

The tissue covered by the appliance, especially one made of acrylic, is erythematous and smooth or granular. It may be either asymptomatic or associated with burning.

Rationale for Treatment

1. Institute appropriate antifungal medication (see "Candidiasis").
2. Improve oral and appliance hygiene. The patient may have to leave the appliance out for extended periods of time and should be instructed to leave the denture out overnight. The appliance should be soaked in a commercially available denture cleanser or soaked in a 1% sodium hypochlorite solution (1 tsp of sodium hypochlorite in a denture cup of water) for 15 min and thoroughly rinsed for at least 2 min under running water.
3. Reline, rebase, or fabricate a new appliance.
4. Apply an artificial saliva or oral lubricant gel, such as Laclede Oral Balance or Sage gel, to the tissue contact surface of the denture to reduce frictional trauma.

If all of the above fail to control symptoms, a biopsy or short trial of topical steroid therapy may be used to rule out contact mucositis (an allergic reaction to denture materials). If a therapeutic trial fails to resolve the condition, a biopsy should be performed to establish the diagnosis. If the patient's differential diagnosis includes any condition that may be premalignant or malignant, a biopsy should be immediately procured to determine the definitive diagnosis for the lesion.

BURNING MOUTH DISORDER

Etiology

Multiple conditions have been implicated in the causation of burning mouth disorder. Current literature favors neurogenic, vascular, and psychogenic etiologies. However, other conditions, such as hyposalivation, candidiasis, referred pain from the tongue musculature, parafunctional habits, chronic infections, use of ACE inhibitors, reflux of gastric acid, medications, blood dyscrasias, nutritional deficiencies, hormonal imbalances, and allergic and inflammatory disorders, need to be considered.

Clinical Description

Burning mouth disorder is characterized by the presence of oral burning symptoms and the absence of clinical signs.

Rationale for Treatment

To reduce discomfort by addressing possible causative factors.

Treatment

It is of the utmost importance to reassure the patient that this disorder is not infectious or contagious and does not progress to a premalignant or malignant condition. On the basis of history, physical evaluation, and specific laboratory studies, rule out all possible organic etiologies. Assessments should include tests for candidiasis, hyposalivation and blood studies that include CBC with differential, fasting glucose, iron, ferritin, folic acid and vitamin B_{12}, and a thyroid profile (thyroid-stimulating hormone, triiodothyronine, thyroxine).

Rx:
Diphenhydramine (Children's Benadryl) elixir 12.5 mg/ 5 mL (OTC).
Disp: 1 bottle.
Sig: Rinse with 1 teaspoon (5 mL) for 2 min before each meal and swallow.
Children's Benadryl is alcohol free.

When all other factors have been ruled out and burning mouth is considered psychogenic or idiopathic, then tricyclic antidepressants or benzodiazepines in low doses are used for their properties of analgesia and sedation and are frequently successful in reducing or eliminating the symptoms after several weeks or months. The dosage is adjusted according to patient reaction and clinical symptomatology. The following systemic therapies for burning mouth disorder may be best managed by appropriate specialist or the patient's physician due to the protracted nature of this therapy.

Rx:
Clonazepam (Klonopin) wafers 0.25 mg.
Disp: 60 wafers.

Sig: Dissolve slowly against the inside of the cheek and then swallow three times daily.

Rx:

Clonazepam (Klonopin) tabs 0.5 mg.

Disp: 100 tabs.

Sig: Take half to one tab three times daily and then adjust the dose after 3-day intervals. The patient should not be titrated to a dosage of greater than 2.0 mg daily.

Rx:

Amitriptyline (Elavil) tabs 25 mg.

Disp: 50 tabs.

Sig: Take 1 tab at bedtime for 1 week and then 2 tabs hs. Increase to 3 tabs hs after 2 weeks and maintain at that dosage or titrate as appropriate.

Rx:

Chlordiazepoxide (Librium) tabs 5 mg.

Disp: 50 tabs.

Sig: Take 1 or 2 tabs three times daily.

Rx:

Alprazolam (Xanax) tabs 0.25 mg.

Disp: 50 tabs.

Sig: Take 1 or 2 tabs three times daily.

Rx:

Diazepam (Valium) tabs 2 mg.

Disp: 50 tabs.

Sig: Take 1 or 2 tabs three times daily. The dosage should be adjusted according to the individual response of the patient. Anticipated side effects are dry mouth and morning drowsiness.

The rationale for the use of tricyclic antidepressant medications and other psychotropic drugs should be thoroughly explained to the patient, and the patient's physician should be made aware of the therapy. These medications have a potential for addiction and dependency.

Rx:

Tabasco sauce (capsaicin) (OTC).

Disp: 1 btl.

Sig: Place one part Tabasco sauce in 2–4 parts of water. Rinse with 1 tsp (5 mL) for 1 min four times daily and expectorate.

Rx:

Capsaicin (Zostrix) cream 0.025% (OTC).

Disp: 1 tube.

Sig: Apply sparingly to affected site(s) four times daily. Wash hands after each application and do not use near the eyes.

Topical capsaicin may serve to improve the burning sensation in some individuals. As with topical capsaicin, an increase in discomfort for a 2- to 3-week period should be anticipated.

CHAPPED OR CRACKED LIPS (CHEILOSIS)

Etiology

Alternate wetting and drying of the lip surface result in inflammation and possible secondary infection.

Clinical Description

The surface of the vermilion is rough and peeling and may be ulcerated with crusting.

Rationale for Treatment

To interrupt the irritating factors and allow healing. Pressing the lips together releases mucins from the minor salivary glands and aids in healing when performed repeatedly throughout the day.

Rx:

Oral Balance Moisturizing Gel (OTC).

Disp: 42 g tube.

Sig: Apply to lips whenever necessary.

Rx:

Nystatin–triamcinolone acetonide (Mycolog II, Mytrex) ointment.

Disp: 15 g tube.

Sig: Apply to lips after each meal and at bedtime.

Rx:

Betamethasone valerate (Valisone) ointment 0.1%.

Disp: 15-g tube.

Sig: Apply to the lips after each meal and at bedtime.

Rx:

Triamcinolone acetonide (Kenalog) 0.1%.

Disp: 15 g tube.

Sig: Apply to lips after meals and at bedtime.

Some suggest that three times daily application of these treatments is sufficient.

Prolonged use of corticosteroids (greater than 2 weeks) should be done cautiously to minimize the potential for side effects.

For maintenance, OTC lip care products such as Oral Balance, unflavored Chapstick, Vaseline, lanolin, or cocoa butter may be considered moisturizers. Avoid products containing desiccants, such as phenol or alcohol.

If the lesion(s) does not resolve with treatment, consider a biopsy to rule out dysplasia or malignant actinic changes.

GINGIVAL OVERGROWTH

Etiology

Antiepileptic medications such as phenytoin sodium (Dilantin), calcium channel blocking agents (e.g., nifedipine, diltiazem, verapamil), and cyclosporine are drugs known to predispose some patients to gingival overgrowth, especially those with poor oral hygiene practices. Poor oral hygiene, blood dyscrasias, and hereditary fibromatosis should be ruled out by clinical history, family history, and laboratory tests.

Clinical Description

The gingival tissues, especially in the anterior region, are dense, resilient, nontender, and enlarged but essentially of normal color.

Rationale for Treatment

Local factors such as plaque and calculus accumulation contribute to secondary inflammation and the collagen deposition/fibrotic process. This, in turn, further interferes with plaque control. Specific drugs tend to deplete serum folic acid levels, which may result in compromised tissue integrity.

Treatment.

- Meticulous plaque control.
- When possible, replace calcium channel blockers, cyclosporine, or other implicated medications in consultation with the patient's physician.
- Gingivoplasty or gingivectomy when indicated and only after oral hygiene is optimal.
- Test for serum folate level and supplement folic acid if necessary. When testing for serum folate level, it is judicious to also check for the vitamin B_{12} level because a vitamin B_{12} deficiency can be masked by the patient's use of folic acid supplement.

Rx:

Chlorhexidine gluconate (Peridex, PerioGard) oral rinse 0.12%.
Disp: 473 mL (16 oz).
Sig: Rinse with 15 mL twice for 30 s and spit out. Avoid rinsing or eating for 30 min following treatment. Rinse after breakfast and at bedtime.

TASTE AND SMELL DISORDERS (CHEMOSENSORY DISORDERS)

Etiology

Taste acuity may be affected by medications and by neurologic and physiologic changes. Complaints of taste loss should be differentiated from alterations in flavor perception, which is primarily derived from smell. Clinical examination and diagnostic procedures may identify potential etiologic factors such as nasal sinus disease (nasal polyps), viral infection, oral candidiasis, neoplasia, malnutrition, metabolic disturbances, chemical and physical trauma, drugs, and radiation sequelae. In some patients, anxiety or depression might be considered. Quantitative tests that assess salivary flow and the patient's ability to identify and discriminate odorants and taste stimuli may be useful. Laboratory studies for trace elements may be necessary to identify any existing deficiencies.

Rationale for Treatment

A reduction in salivary flow may concentrate electrolytes in the saliva, resulting in a salty or metallic taste (dysgeusia) (see "Xerostomia [Reduced Salivary Flow and Dry Mouth]"). Several medications, including angiotensin-converting enzyme inhibitors and lithium carbonate, are known to cause taste alterations. It may be prudent to contact the patient's physician to substitute these medications when practical. Oral hygiene must be optimal because patients may compensate for changes in taste or flavor acuity by overusing sugars. A deficiency of zinc, albeit rare, has been associated with a loss of taste (and smell) sensation. To prevent deficiency, the current recommended dietary allowance for zinc is 12–15 mg for adults. Additional zinc supplementation should be reserved for individuals with true deficiency states.

To ensure dietary allowance for Zinc

Rx:

Z-BEC tabs (OTC).
Disp: 60 tabs.
Sig: Take 1 tab daily with food or after meals.

Rx:

Zinc gluconate lozenges (OTC).
Disp: 48 lozenges.
Sig: Dissolve, by mouth, 1–2 lozenges daily.

MANAGEMENT OF PATIENTS RECEIVING ANTINEOPLASTIC AGENTS AND RADIATION THERAPY

Etiology

Head and neck radiation treatment of oral cancer can reduce saliva volume and alter composition when a major salivary gland is in the primary radiation field. Oral tissue delivery of multiple antimicrobial components of saliva, including histatins, lactoferrin, and lysozyme, is typically decreased. The balance of oral flora is then disrupted, allowing overgrowth of opportunistic organisms, such as *Candida albicans*. Advances over the past several years, including salivary gland protection during radiation dosing (via amifostine) and/or saliva stimulant (secretogogue) intervention (via pilocarpine hydrochloride or cevimeline), have helped reduce the morbidity associated with long-term salivary gland hypofunction in these patients.

Patients receiving anticholinergic medications during high-dose chemotherapy also may experience salivary compromise. However, glandular function tends to return to normal in the weeks following discontinuation of these medications.

Cytotoxic cancer therapy can impair normal, rapidly dividing cells, including those of the oral mucosa. This can result in painful, ulcerative oral mucositis with important clinical consequences. One drug, palifermin, is approved by the FDA for reducing the severity of oral mucositis in patients with hematologic malignancies who are receiving a bone marrow transplant. Other drugs for mucositis management are in development but are not FDA approved at this time for use outside a research environment. The information listed below is intended to assist the practicing dentist in the management of oncology patients once they are in an outpatient setting.

Clinical Description

The oral mucosa becomes red, inflamed, and/or ulcerated. The saliva may be viscous or absent.

Rationale for Treatment

The treatment of these patients is symptomatic and supportive and should be aimed at patient comfort and education, maintenance of proper nutrition and oral hygiene, and prevention of opportunistic infection. Frequent monitoring and close cooperation with the patient's physician are important.

All patients must have a preradiation therapy oral evaluation to eliminate any source of infection. Whenever possible, 14 days of oral healing time should be allowed prior to initiation of radiation therapy following oral surgical procedures. Oral hygiene is of paramount importance prior to, during, and after radiation therapy.

The oral discomfort may be relieved with topical anesthetics such as lidocaine HCl (Xylocaine) viscous, diphenhydramine elixir (Benadryl), and throat lozenges containing dyclonine HCl. Artificial salivas (e.g., Sage Moist Plus, Moi-Stir, Salivart) will reduce oral dryness. Mouth moisturizing gels such as Laclede Oral Balance Gel are helpful. Nystatin and clotrimazole preparations will control fungal overgrowth. Chlorhexidine rinses help control plaque and candidiasis. Fluorides are applied for caries control (dentifrices, gels, rinses).

A patient information sheet on this topic is presented in Box C.1, which can be reproduced as a patient handout.

Mouth Rinses (See, "Xerostomia [Reduced Salivary Flow and Dry Mouth]")

Rx:

Alkaline saline (salt/bicarbonate) mouthrinse.

Disp: Mix ½ tsp each of salt and baking soda in 16 oz of water.

Sig: Rinse with copious amounts at least five times daily.

Commercially available as Sage Salt and Soda Rinse.

Gingivitis Control

Rx:

Chlorhexidine gluconate (Peridex, PerioGard) 0.12%.

Disp: 473 mL (16 oz).

Sig: Rinse with 15 mL twice for 30 s and spit out. Avoid rinsing or eating for 30 min following treatment. Rinse after breakfast and at bedtime.

In patients suffering from low salivary flow, chlorhexidine gluconate should be used concurrently with artificial saliva to provide the needed protein-binding agent for efficacy and substantivity.

BOX C.1 Oral Care Patient Information Sheet

Listed here are general guidelines for oral care to be individualized by your doctor. Follow your doctor's advice or discuss any questions with your doctor if these guidelines differ from what you've been told or have heard.

A. Rinses

1. Rinse with warm, dilute solution of sodium bicarbonate (baking soda) or salt and bicarbonate every 2 h to bathe the tissues and control oral acidity. Take 2 teaspoonfuls of bicarbonate (or 1 teaspoonful of table salt plus 1 teaspoonful of bicarbonate) per quart of water.

2. If you are experiencing pain, rinse with 1 teaspoonful of elixir of Benadryl before each meal. Be careful when eating while your mouth is numb to avoid choking.

3. If your mouth is dry, sip cool water frequently (every 10 min) all day long. Allowing ice chips to melt in your mouth is comforting. Artificial salivas (e.g., Moi-Stir, Salivart, Xero-Lube, Orex) can be used as frequently as needed to make your mouth moist and "slick." Keep the lips lubricated with petrolatum or a lanolin-containing lip preparation. Commercial mouth rinses with alcohol and coffee, tea, and colas should be avoided as they tend to dry the mouth.

4. If an oral yeast infection develops, antifungal medications can be prescribed.

   a. Nystatin pastille,[a] let 1 dissolve in the mouth five times a day, or

   b. Let a 10-mg clotrimazole (Mycelex)[a] troche dissolve in the mouth five times a day.

B. Care of Teeth and Gums

1. Floss your teeth after each meal. Be careful not to cut your gums.

2. Brush your teeth after each meal. Use a soft, even-bristle brush and a bland toothpaste containing fluoride (e.g., Aim, Crest, Colgate). Brushing with a sodium bicarbonate—water paste also is helpful. Arm & Hammer Dental Care toothpaste and tooth powder are bicarbonate based. If a toothbrush is too irritating, cotton-tipped swabs (Q-Tips) or foam sticks (Toothettes) can provide some mechanical cleaning.

3. A pulsating water device (e.g., Waterpik) will remove loose debris. Use warm water with a half-teaspoonful of salt and baking soda and low pressure to prevent damage to tissue.

4. Have custom, flexible vinyl trays made by your dentist for use in self-applying fluoride gel to your teeth for 5 min once a day after brushing.

5. Rinse with an antiplaque solution (Peridex) (if prescribed by your dentist) two or three times a day when you cannot follow other oral hygiene procedures.

6. Follow any alternative oral hygiene instructions prescribed by your dentist.

C. Nutrition: Adequate intake of nutrition and fluid is very important for oral and general health. Use diet supplements (e.g., Carnation Breakfast Essentials, Meritene, Ensure). If your mouth is sore, a blender may be used to soften food.

D. Maintenance: Have your oral health status evaluated at regularly scheduled intervals by your dentist.

E. Supportive: A humidifier in the sleeping area will alleviate or reduce nighttime oral dryness. NOTE: The oral regimen for patients receiving chemotherapy and radiotherapy is outlined in Chapter 26 of this textbook. This regimen also is applicable to patients with acquired immunodeficiency syndrome (AIDS).

[a]Drugs that must be prescribed by your dentist or physician.

Caries Control. (See "Xerostomia. [Reduced Salivary Flow and Dry Mouth]")

Rx:

Neutral NaF gel (Thera-Flur-N) 1.1% or PreviDent 1.1%.

Disp: 1 tube.

Sig: Place 1-inch ribbon on toothbrush; brush for 2 min daily and expectorate. Avoid rinsing or eating for 30 min following treatment.

Topical Coating Agents and Anesthetics

Rx:

Sucralfate (Carafate) suspension 1 g/10 mL.
Disp: 420 mL (14 oz).
Sig: Rinse with 1 tbs (5 mL) every 2 h and spit out.

Rx:

Diphenhydramine (Children's Benadryl) elix 12.5 mg/5 mL (OTC) 4 oz mixed with Kaopectate or Maalox (OTC) 4 oz (to make a 50% mixture by volume).
Disp: 8 oz.
Sig: Rinse with 1 tbs (5 mL) every 2 h and spit out.

Rx:

Diphenhydramine (Children's Benadryl) elixir 12.5 mg/5 mL (OTC).
Disp: 4 oz btl.
Sig: Rinse with 1 tbs (5 mL) for 2 min before each meal and expectorate.

Rx:

Dyclonine HCl throat loz (Sucrets) (OTC).
Disp: 1 package.
Sig: Dissolve slowly in mouth every 2 h as necessary. Do not exceed 10 lozenges per day.

When topical anesthetics are used, patients should be cautioned concerning a reduced gag reflex and the need for caution while eating and drinking to avoid possible airway compromise.

ANTIFUNGAL AGENTS (See "Candidiasis")

SALIVA STIMULANTS (See "Xerostomia [Reduced Salivary Flow and Dry Mouth]")

BIBLIOGRAPHY

1. Al-Hashimi I, Schifter M, Lockhart PB, et al. Oral lichen planus and oral lichenoid lesions: diagnostic and therapeutic considerations. *Oral Surg Oral Med Oral Pathol Oral Radiol Endod.* 2008;103(Suppl):25−31.
2. Al-Johani KA, Fedele S, Porter SR. Erythema multiforme and related disorders. *Oral Surg Oral Med Oral Pathol Oral Radiol Endod.* 2008;103:642−654.
3. Akintoye SO, Greenberg MS. Recurrent aphthous stomatitis. *Dent Clin N Am.* 2014;58:281−297.
4. Atkinson JC, Fox PC. Sjögren's syndrome: oral and dental considerations. *J Am Dent Assoc.* 1993;124:74−86.
5. Bagan JV, Ramon C, Gonzalez L, et al. Preliminary investigation of the association of oral lichen planus and hepatitis C. *Oral Surg Oral Med Oral Pathol Oral Radiol Endod.* 1998;85:532−536.
6. Balasubramaniam R, Kuperstein AS, Stoopler ET. Update on oral herpes virus infections. *Dent Clin N Am.* 2014;58:265−280.
7. Berkhart NW, Burker EJ, Burkes EJ, et al. Assessing the characteristics of patients with oral lichen planus. *J Am Dent Assoc.* 1996;127:648−656.
8. Brown RS, Beaver WT, Bottomley WK. On the mechanism of drug-induced gingival hyperplasia. *J Oral Pathol Med.* 1991;20:201−209.
9. Brunet L, Miranda J, Farre M, et al. Gingival enlargement induced by drugs. *Drug Saf.* 1996;15:219−231.
10. Bukhari AF, Farag AM, Treister NS. Chronic oral lesions. *Dermatol Clin.* 2020;38:451−466.
11. Chainani-Wu N, Silverman Jr S, Lozada-Nur F, et al. Oral lichen planus: patient profile, disease progression and treatment responses. *J Am Dent Assoc.* 2001;132:901−909.
12. Chandrasekhar J, Liem AA, Cox NH, et al. Oxypentifylline in the management of recurrent aphthous oral ulcers. *Oral Surg Oral Med Oral Pathol Oral Radiol Endod.* 1999;87:564−567.
13. Chen A, Wai Y, Lee L, et al. Using the modified Schirmer test to measure mouth dryness. *J Am Dent Assoc.* 2005;136:164−170.
14. Ciarrocca KN, Greenberg MS. A retrospective study of the management of oral mucous membrane pemphigoid with dapsone. *Oral Surg Oral Med Oral Pathol Oral Radiol Endod.* 1999;88:159−163.
15. Cohen DM, Bhattacharyya I, Lydiatt WM. Recalcitrant oral ulcers caused by calcium channel blockers: diagnosis and treatment considerations. *J Am Dent Assoc.* 1999;130:1611−1618.
16. Dayan S, Simmons RK, Ahmed AR. Contemporary issues in the diagnosis of oral pemphigoid. *Oral Surg Oral Med Oral Pathol Oral Radiol Endod.* 1999;88:424−430.
17. De Rossi SS, Ciarrocca K. Oral lichen planus and lichenoid mucositis. *Dent Clin N Am.* 2014;58:299−313.
18. Eisen D. The clinical characteristics of intraoral herpes simplex virus infection in 52 immunocompetent patients. *Oral Surg Oral Med Oral Pathol Oral Radiol Endod.* 1998;86:432−437.
19. Eisen DE. The evaluation of cutaneous, genital, scalp, nail, esophageal and ocular involvement in patients with oral lichen planus. *Oral Surg Oral Med Oral Pathol Oral Radiol Endod.* 1999;88:431−436.
20. Epstein JB, Wan LS, Gorsky M, et al. Oral lichen planus: progress in understanding its malignant potential and the implications of clinical management. *Oral Surg Oral Med Oral Pathol Oral Radiol Endod.* 2003;96:32−37.
21. FDA Postmarket drug safety information for patients and providers. January 19, 2006. FDA approves updated labeling with boxed warning and medication guide for two eczema drugs, elidel and protopic. Available at: https://www.fda.gov/drugs/postmarket-drug-safety-information-patients-and-providers/fda-approves-updated-labeling-boxed-warning-and-medication-guide-two-eczema-drugs-elidel-and. Accessed March 10, 2021.
22. France K, Villa A. Acute oral lesions. *Dermatol Clin.* 2020;38:441−450.
23. Gonzales-Moles MA, Ruiz-Avila I, Rodriguez-Archilla A, et al. Treatment of severe erosive gingival lesions by topical application of clobetasol propionate in custom trays. *Oral*

Surg Oral Med Oral Pathol Oral Radiol Endod. 2003;95:688−692.

24. Gonzales-Moles MA, Morales P, Rodriguez-Archilla A, et al. Treatment of severe chronic oral erosive lesions with clobetasol propionate in aqueous solution. *Oral Surg Oral Med Oral Pathol Oral Radiol Endod.* 2002;93:264−270.

25. Gorsky M, Silverman Jr S, Chinn H. Clinical characteristics and management outcome in the burning mouth syndrome. *Oral Surg Oral Med Oral Pathol.* 1991;72:192−195.

26. Greenspan D. Xerostomia: diagnosis and management. *Oncology.* 1996;10(3 suppl):7−11.

27. Grisius MM. Salivary gland dysfunction: a review of systemic therapies. *Oral Surg Oral Med Oral Pathol Oral Radiol Endod.* 2001;92:156−162.

28. Grushka M, Epstein J, Mott P. An open-label, dose escalation pilot study of the effect of clonazepam in burning mouth syndrome. *Oral Surg Oral Med Oral Pathol Oral Radiol Endod.* 1998;86:557−561.

29. Henkin RI. Drug-induced taste and smell disorders. Incidence, mechanisms and management related primarily to treatment of sensory receptor dysfunction. *Drug Saf.* 1994;11:318−377.

30. Hersh EV, Moore PA. Drug interactions in dentistry. *J Am Dent Assoc.* 2004;135:298−311.

31. Heyneman CA. Zinc deficiency and taste disorder. *Ann Pharmacother.* 1996;30:186−187.

32. Ikebe K, Morii K, Kashiwagi J, et al. Impact of dry mouth on oral symptoms and function in removable denture wearers in Japan. *Oral Surg Oral Med Oral Pathol Oral Radiol Endod.* 2005;99:704−710.

33. Islam MN, Cohen DM, Ojha J, et al. Chronic ulcerative stomatitis: diagnostic and management challenges—four new cases and review of literature. *Oral Surg Oral Med Oral Pathol Oral Radiol Endod.* 2008;104:194−203.

34. Klein B, Thoppay JR, De Rossi SS, et al. Burning mouth syndrome. *Dermatol Clin.* 2020;38:477−483.

35. Kutcher MJ, Ludlow JB, Samuelson AD, et al. Evaluation of a bioadhesive device for the management of aphthous ulcers. *J Am Dent Assoc.* 2001;132:368−376.

36. Lalla RV, Saunders DP, Peterson DE. Chemotherapy or radiation-induced oral mucositis. *Dent Clin N Am.* 2014;58:341−349.

37. Lamey PJ, Lamb AB. Lip component of burning mouth syndrome. *Oral Surg Oral Med Oral Pathol Oral Radiol Endod.* 1994;78:590−593.

38. Lozada F, Silverman Jr S, Migliorati C. Adverse side effects associated with prednisone in the treatment of patients with oral inflammatory ulcerative diseases. *J Am Dent Assoc.* 1984;109:269−270.

39. Lozada-Nur F, Miranda C, Miliksi R. Double-blind clinical trial of 0.05% clobetasol propionate ointment in orabase and 0.05% fluocinonide ointment in orabase in the treatment of patients with oral vesiculoerosive diseases. *Oral Surg Oral Med Oral Pathol.* 1994;77:598−604.

40. Miller CS, Cunningham LL, Lindroth JE, et al. The efficacy of valacyclovir in preventing recurrent herpes simplex virus infections associated with dental procedures. *J Am Dent Assoc.* 2004;135:1311−1318.

41. Miller CS, Danaher RJ. Asymptomatic shedding of herpes simplex virus (HSV) in the oral cavity. *Oral Surg Oral Med Oral Pathol Oral Radiol Endod.* 2008;105:43−50.

42. Muzyka BC, Epifanio RN. Update on oral fungal infections. *Dent Clin N Am.* 2013;57:561−581.

43. Napeñas JJ, Brennan MT, Fox PC. Diagnosis and treatment of xerostomia (dry mouth). *Odontology.* 2009;97: 76−783.

44. Napeñas JJ, Rouleau TS. Oral complications of Sjögren's syndrome. *Oral Maxillofac Surg Clin N Am.* 2014;26:55−62.

45. Navazesh M. How can oral health care providers determine if patients have dry mouth? *J Am Dent Assoc.* 2003;134:613−620.

46. Navazesh M. Salivary gland hypofunction in elderly patients. *J Calif Dent Assoc.* 1994;22:62−68.

47. Ogura M, Morita M, Wantanabe T. A case controlled study on food intake of patients with recurrent aphthous stomatitis. *Oral Surg Oral Med Oral Pathol Oral Radiol Endod.* 2001;91:45−49.

48. Pajukoski, Meurman JH, Halonen P, et al. Prevalence of subjective dry mouth and burning mouth in hospitalized elderly patients and outpatients in relation to saliva, medication, and systemic diseases. *Oral Surg Oral Med Oral Pathol Oral Radiol Endod.* 2001;92:641−649.

49. Patton LL, Siegel MA, De Laat A. Management of burning mouth syndrome: systematic review and management recommendations. *Oral Surg Oral Med Oral Pathol Oral Radiol Endod.* 2007;103(suppl):39−44.

50. Pinto A, Lindemeyer RG, Sollecito TP. The PFAPA syndrome in oral medicine: differential diagnosis and treatment. *Oral Surg Oral Med Oral Pathol Oral Radiol Endod.* 2006;102:148−153.

51. Raborn GW, Chan KS, Grace M. Treatment modalities and medication recommended by health care professionals for treating recurrent herpes labialis. *J Am Dent Assoc.* 2004;135:48−54.

52. Samim F, Auluck A, Zed C, et al. Erythema multiforme: a review of epidemiology, pathogenesis, clinical features, and treatment. *Dent Clin N Am.* 2013;57:583−596.

53. Santoro FA, Stoopler ET, Werth VP. Pemphigus. *Dent Clin N Am.* 2013;57:597−610.

54. Shanti RM, Tanaka T, Stanton DC. Oral biopsy techniques. *Dermatol Clin.* 2020;38:421−427.

55. Sherrell W, Desai B, Sollecito TP. Dental considerations in patients with oral mucosal diseases. *Dermatol Clin.* 2020;38:535−541.

56. Ship JA, Grushka M, Lipton JA, et al. Burning mouth syndrome: an update. *J Am Dent Assoc.* 1995;126: 842−853.

57. Ship JA, Vissink A, Challacombe SJ. Use of prophylactic antifungals in the immunocompromised host. *Oral Surg Oral Med Oral Pathol Oral Radiol Endod.* 2008; 103(suppl):6−11.

58. Ship JA. Gustatory and olfactory considerations in general dental practice. *J Am Dent Assoc.* 1993;124:55−61.

59. Ship JA. Recurrent aphthous stomatitis. *Oral Surg Oral Med Oral Pathol Oral Radiol Endod.* 1996;81:141−147.

60. Siegel MA, Anhalt GJ. Direct immunofluorescence of detached gingival epithelium for diagnosis of cicatricial pemphigoid. *Oral Surg Oral Med Oral Pathol.* 1993;75: 296−302.

61. Siegel MA. Strategies for management of commonly encountered oral mucosal disorders. *J Calif Dent Assoc.* 1999;27:210−227.

62. Silverman Jr S, Gorsky M, Lozada-Nur F, et al. A prospective study of findings and management in 214 patients with oral lichen planus. *Oral Surg Oral Med Oral Pathol.* 1991;72:665–670.

63. Xu HH, Werth VP, Parisi E, et al. Mucous membrane pemphigoid. *Dent Clin N Am.* 2013;57:611–630.

64. Stoopler ET, Balasubramaniam R. Topical and systemic therapies for oral and perioral herpes simplex virus infections. *J Calif Dent Assoc.* 2013;41:259–262.

65. Stoopler ET, Greenberg MS. Update on herpes virus infection. *Dent Clin N Am.* 2003;47:517–532.

66. Stoopler ET, Sollecito TP. Oral mucosal diseases: evaluation and management. *Med Clin N Am.* 2014;98:1323–1352.

67. Su N, Ching V, Grushka M. Taste disorders: a review. *J Can Dent Assoc.* 2013;79:d86.

68. Suresh L, Kumar V. Significance of IgG4 in the diagnosis of mucous membrane pemphigoid. *Oral Surg Oral Med Oral Pathol Oral Radiol Endod.* 2008;104:359–362.

69. Telles DR, Karki N, Marshall MW. Oral fungal infections: diagnosis and management. *Dent Clin N Am.* 2017;61:319–349.

70. Turner MD, Jahangiri L, Ship JA. Hyposalivation, xerostomia and the complete denture: a systematic review. *J Am Dent Assoc.* 2008;139:146–150.

71. Turner MD, Ship JA. Dry mouth and its effects on the oral health of elderly people. *J Am Dent Assoc.* 2007;138(suppl):15–20.

72. van der Meij EH, Schepman KP, Smeele LE, et al. A review of the recent literature regarding malignant transformation of oral lichen planus. *Oral Surg Oral Med Oral Pathol Oral Radiol Endod.* 1999;88:307–310.

73. van der Meij EH, Schepman KP, van der Waal I. The possible premalignant character of oral lichen planus and oral lichenoid lesions: a prospective study. *Oral Surg Oral Med Oral Pathol Oral Radiol Endod.* 2003;96:164–171.

74. von Bültzingslöwen I, Sollecito TP, Fox PC, et al. Salivary dysfunction associated with systemic diseases: systematic review and clinical management recommendations. *Oral Surg Oral Med Oral Pathol Oral Radiol Endod.* 2008;103(suppl):57–65.

75. Woo SB, Challacombe SJ. Management of recurrent oral herpes simplex infections. *Oral Surg Oral Med Oral Pathol Oral Radiol Endod.* 2007;103(Suppl):S12.e1–S12.e18.

76. Woo S, Sonis ST. Recurrent aphthous ulcers: a review of diagnosis and treatment. *J Am Dent Assoc.* 1996;127:1202–1213.

77. Yuan A, Woo SB. Adverse drug events in the oral cavity. *Oral Surg Oral Med Oral Pathol Oral Radiol.* 2015;119:35–47.

Drug Interactions of Significance in Dentistry

Drug–drug interactions can result in adverse outcomes that range from mild to severe and possibly hospitalization or death. These interactions are due to alterations in drug absorption, bioavailability, protein binding, metabolism, receptor binding, and/or therapeutic action. The altered therapeutic action generally occurs as antagonism, potentiation (synergy), or unexpected drug effects. A drug is associated with increased risk of an adverse event when it displays one or more of the features shown in Table D.1, or is given in too large of a quantity.

TABLE D.1 Pharmacological Features of Drug–Drug Interactions

Pharmacological Feature Affects	Examples
Absorption	These drugs can alter the GI absorption of other drugs: alcohol, acidic fruit juices, certain antibiotics that affect GI flora, antacids, cimetidine, cholestyramine, epinephrine, MAOIs, mineral oil, tyramine (in beer, ripened cheese, red wine), proton pump inhibitors.
	Food–drug interactions and delayed absorption occurs when tetracycline is taken with iron supplements, magnesium-, aluminum-, or calcium-containing foods/products.
Bioavailability	Limited bioavailability with orally administered anticancer drugs, morphine, propanolol, nitroglycerin.
Protein Binding	These drugs are highly protein bound and can compete for plasma protein binding to other drugs: aspirin, NSAIDs, antidepressants, antipsychotics, methotrexate, phenytoin, quinidine, oral hypoglycemics, propranolol, tricyclic sedatives (barbiturates, benzodiazepines), warfarin.
Therapeutic Index	These drugs have a narrow therapeutic index and are at risk for reaching toxic blood levels: aminophylline, carbamazepine, clindamycin, clonidine, digoxin, disopyramide, oral contraceptives, guanethidine, isoproterenol inhalation, lithium, metaproterenol, minoxidil, oxytriphylline, phenytoin, primidone, procainamide, quinidine, theophylline, valproic acid, and orally administered anticancer drugs.
Metabolism	There are a number of drug-metabolizing enzyme systems that can be subdivided into phase 1 and phase 2 reactions. Phase 1 reactions include the cytochrome P450 (CYPs) system, flavin-containing mono-oxygenases (FMOs), or epoxide hydrolases (EHs). These reactions typically inactivate the drug or, in the case of a pro-drug, activate it. Phase 2 reactions include the UDP-glucuronosyltransferases (UGTs), glutathione-S-transferases (GSTs), N-acetyltransferases (NATs), methyltransferases (MTs), which facilitate the elimination of the drug. In addition there are important transport proteins, particularly in the intestine (i.e., p-glycoprotein/ABCB1 or BCRP/ABCG2 transporters), which can be induced or inhibited by drugs and cause drug interactions.
	In terms of CYPs, it should be recognized that they are responsible for most of the drug–drug interactions. CYPs can be inducers or inhibitors, which leads to a decrease or increase in it's own metabolism or that of coadministered drug(s). Importantly, providers should avoid prescribing a drug that is a substrate for a CYP when another co-administered drug is metabolized by the same CYP. Also, providers should be aware that some drugs can inhibit a CYP without being a substrate.
	Enzyme inducers (CYP3A4): anticonvulsants (carbamazepine, phenobarbital, phenytoin, sodium valproate), rifampin.
	Enzyme inhibitors: (CYP3A4 and CYP3A5): AZOLES (itraconazole, ketoconazole), diltiazem, MYCINS (clarithromycin, erythromycin, telithromycin) ritonavir, verapamil, grapefruit.
	(acetaldehyde dehydrogenase): metronidazole.
	(CYP2D6): Amiodarone, cimetidine, diphenhydramine, fluoxetine, paroxetine, quinidine, ritonavir, terbinafine.
	See Table 18.2 for drug interactions with antiretroviral drugs.
Receptor Binding	These drugs compete for receptor binding, and can influence target cell activity, including cognition: Alcohol, amantadine, antineoplastics, bromocriptine, cimetidine, clonidine, corticosteroids, diuretics, digitalis, hydralazine, isoniazid, meprobamate, methyldopa, metoprolol, opioids (codeine, hydrocodone, meperidine, oxycodone, methadone, fentanyl) indomethacin, phenylbutazone, levodopa, procainamide, sedatives (benzodiazepines, barbiturates).
Excretion Rate	A drug can alter the acidity of urine altering excretion:
	NSAIDs with lithium
	Metronidazole with lithium

GI, gastrointestinal; *NSAIDs*, nonsteroidal antiinflammatory drugs.

Patient factors also can be involved. Young persons who have low weight, the elderly, and medically compromised patients are more susceptible to drug–drug interactions and adverse drug effects. Dosing may need to be adjusted for these patients (Table D.2).

TABLE D.2   Drug Interactions of Significance in Dentistry by Category

Dental Drug	Interacting Drug	Medical Condition or Situation	Effect
Antibiotics			
Antibiotics	Oral contraceptives (birth control pills)	Contraception	Decreased effectiveness of oral contraceptives has been suggested for several antibiotic classes because of the potential for lowering plasma levels of the contraceptive drug. However, most well-designed studies do not show any reduction in estrogen serum levels in patients taking antibiotics (except rifampin). **RECOMMENDATION: Okay to use dental antibiotics**. Provide advice to patient about potential risk and for consideration of additional contraceptive measures.
Beta-Lactams (Penicillins, Cephalosporins)	Allopurinol (Lopurin, Zyloprim)	Gout	Incidence of minor allergic reactions to ampicillin is increased. Other penicillins have not been implicated. **RECOMMENDATION: Avoid ampicillin**.
	Beta-blockers (e.g., Tenormin, Lopressor, Inderal, Corgard)	Hypertension	Serum levels of atenolol are reduced after prolonged use of ampicillin. Anaphylactic reactions to penicillins or other drugs may be more severe in patients taking beta-blockers because of increased mediator release from mast cells. **RECOMMENDATION: Use ampicillin cautiously; advise patient of potential reaction**.
	Tetracyclines and other bacteriostatic antibiotics	Infection, acne, or periodontal disease	Effectiveness of penicillins and cephalosporins may be reduced by bacteriostatic agents. **RECOMMENDATION: Avoid interaction**.
Tetracyclines, Fluoroquinolones	Antacids	Dyspepsia, gastroesophageal reflux, peptic ulcer	Antacids, dairy products, and other agents containing divalent (calcium, iron, aluminum) and trivalent cations will chelate these antibiotics and limit their absorption. Doxycycline is least influenced by this interaction. **RECOMMENDATION: Avoid interaction**.
	Insulin	Diabetes mellitus	Doxycycline and oxytetracycline have been documented as enhancing the hypoglycemic effects of exogenously administered insulin. **RECOMMENDATION: Select a different antibiotic or increase carbohydrate intake**.
Doxycycline	Methotrexate	Immunosuppression	In patients taking high-dose methotrexate, interaction can lead to increased methotrexate concentrations, making toxicity likely. **RECOMMENDATION: Select different antibiotic**.

Metronidazole	Ethanol	Alcohol use or abuse	Co-administration will cause severe disulfiram-like re-actions are well documented. **RECOMMENDATION: Avoid interaction.**
	Lithium	Manic depression	Co-administration will inhibit renal excretion of lithium, leading to elevated or toxic levels of lithium. Lithium toxicity produces confusion, ataxia, and kidney damage. **RECOMMENDATION: Avoid interaction.**
MYCIN Antibiotics [Erythro-mycin, Clarithromycin], and AZOLE Antifungals [Ketoconazole, Flucona-zole, Itraconazole, Posaco-nazole, Vorixonazole] and Select Antiretrovirals [Dor-avirine, Elvitegravir, Rito-navir, see Table 18.2] are Metabolized by Inhibit CYP3A4 and CYP1A2, CYP29C	Antiretroviral drugs	HIV treatment	Co-administration can increase blood levels of antire-troviral drug.
	Benzodiazepines	Anxiety	Co-administration will delay metabolism of benzodi-azepine, increasing blood levels and the pharmaco-logic effects that can result in excessive sedation and irrational behavior. **RECOMMENDATION: Reduce dose of benzodiazepine or avoid interaction.**
	Buspirone	Depression	Co-administration will delay metabolism of buspir-one, increasing pharmacologic effect. **RECOMMENDATION: Avoid interaction.**
	Calcium channel blockers (e.g., Diltiazem [Cardizem], Verapamil [Calan], Amlodipine [Norvasc])	Hypertension	Co-administration will delay metabolism of calcium channel blockers, increasing the pharmacologic ef-fect, resulting in hypotension with use of macrolide antibiotics. **RECOMMENDATION: Avoid interaction.**
	Carbamazepine (Tegretol)	Seizure disorder	Co-administration will increase blood levels of carba-mazepine, leading to toxicity; symptoms include drowsiness, dizziness, nausea, headache, and blurred vision. Hospitalization has been required. **RECOMMENDATION: Avoid interaction.**
	Cisapride	Gastroesophageal reflux	Co-administration will delay metabolism of cisapride, increasing the pharmacologic effects and risk for cardiac arrhythmia and sudden death. **RECOMMENDATION: Avoid interaction.**
	Cyclosporine	Organ transplantation	Co-administration will enhance immunosuppression and nephrotoxicity. **RECOMMENDATION: Avoid interaction.**
	Disopyramide, Quinidine	Cardiac arrhythmias	Co-administration will inhibit CYP3A4 metabolism, resulting in large increases in antiarrhythmia drug that can lead to arrhythmias. **RECOMMENDATION: Avoid interaction.**
	Lovastatin, pravastatin, simva-statin, and other statins	Hyperlipidemia	Co-administration will increase plasma concentration of statin drugs; may result in muscle (eosinophilia) myalgia and rhabdomyolysis (muscle breakdown and pain) and acute renal failure. **RECOMMENDATION: Avoid interaction.**

Continued

TABLE D.2   Drug Interactions of Significance in Dentistry by Category—cont'd

Dental Drug	Interacting Drug	Medical Condition or Situation	Effect
	Pimozide	Antipsychotic, used to control motor tics	Co-administration may result in increased concentrations of pimozide and possibly prolongation of the QT interval. **RECOMMENDATION: Avoid interaction.**
	Prednisone, methylprednisolone	Autoimmune disorders, organ transplantation	Co-administration increases the risk of Cushing syndrome and immunosuppression. **RECOMMENDATION: Monitor patient and shorten duration of antibiotic administration if possible.**
	Theophylline (Theo-Dur)	Asthma	Erythromycins inhibit the metabolism of theophylline, leading to toxic serum levels (symptoms of toxicity: headache, nausea, vomiting, confusion, thirst, cardiac arrhythmias, and convulsions). Conversely, theophylline reduces serum levels of erythromycin. **RECOMMENDATION: Avoid prescribing erythromycin.**
Antibiotics (Especially Erythromycin, Clarithromycin, and Tetracycline)	Digoxin (Lanoxin)	Congestive heart failure	Co-administration alters GI flora and retards metabolism of digoxin in roughly 10% of patients, resulting in dangerously high digoxin serum levels that may persist for several weeks after discontinuation of antibiotic. Strongest documentation has been acquired for macrolide antibiotics and tetracycline. Patients should be cautioned to report any signs of digitalis toxicity (salivation, visual disturbances, and arrhythmias) during antibiotic therapy. **RECOMMENDATION: Safe in 90%; should have digoxin levels monitored during antimicrobial therapy.**
Antibiotics, Cephalosporins, Erythromycin, Clarithromycin, Metronidazole	Warfarin (Coumadin)	Atrial fibrillation, MI, recent (postoperative) major surgery, stroke prevention	Anticoagulant effect of warfarin may be increased by several antibiotic classes. Reduced synthesis of vitamin K by gut flora is a putative mechanism, but several antibiotics have antiplatelet and anticoagulant activity. Cephalosporins, macrolide antibiotics, and metronidazole have the most convincing documentation, monitor INR. **RECOMMENDATION: Penicillins, tetracyclines, and clindamycin are preferred choices but must be used cautiously.**
Analgesics			
Acetaminophen	Alcohol	Alcohol use and abuse	Co-administration increases the risk of liver toxicity, especially during fasting state or ≥4 g of acetaminophen per day. **RECOMMENDATION: Use lower dose of acetaminophen and encourage discontinuation of alcohol use. Limit dose when liver disease is present.**
Acetaminophen	Warfarin (Coumadin)	Atrial fibrillation, thrombosis	Data are somewhat conflicting: Increased risk of bleeding if acetaminophen is given at a dose of >2 g/day for >1 week. **RECOMMENDATION: Limit acetaminophen dosing and duration; monitor INR.**

Aspirin	Oral hypoglycemic (e.g., sulfonylureas: Glyburide, chlorpropamide, acetohexamide)	Diabetes type 2	Co-administration increases hypoglycemic effects. **RECOMMENDATION: Avoid interaction.**
Aspirin, other NSAIDs	Anticoagulants (Coumarin)	Atrial fibrillation, MI, recent (postoperative) surgery, clot prevention	Co-administration increases risk of bleeding (GI, oral). **RECOMMENDATION: Avoid interaction.**
Aspirin, other NSAIDs	Alcohol	Alcohol use and abuse	Co-administration will increases risk of GI bleeding. **RECOMMENDATION: Lower dose; encourage discontinuation of alcohol use.**
Aspirin	Diltiazem	Hypertension, angina	Co-administration will enhance antiplatelet activity of aspirin. **RECOMMENDATION: Monitor for risk of prolonged bleeding. Advise patient to notify physician or dentist if she or he experiences unusual bleeding or bruising.**
NSAIDs	Beta-blockers, ACE inhibitors, Alpha-blockers (doxazosin [Catapres], prazosin [Minipress]); or combined Alpha—Beta blockers (carvedilol [Coreg], labetalol [Normodyne])	Hypertension, recent MI	Co-administration decreases the antihypertensive effect. **RECOMMENDATION: Limit duration of NSAID dosage to about 4 days. Use acetaminophen products instead.**
NSAIDs	Lithium	Manic depression	Co-administration can produce symptoms of lithium toxicity, including nausea, vomiting, slurred speech, and mental confusion. **RECOMMENDATION: NSAIDs should not be prescribed to patients who take lithium. It can result in toxic levels of lithium; consider consulting with physician to reduce lithium dose.**
NSAIDs (Naproxen)	Alendronate	Osteoporosis, multiple myeloma	Co-administration increases risk for gastric ulcers. **RECOMMENDATION: Use acetaminophen products.**
NSAIDs	SSRIs (citalopram, fluoxetine, paroxetine, sertraline)	Depression	Co-administration increases risk of peptic ulcers. **RECOMMENDATION: Avoid long-term use of NSAIDs; use acetaminophen products instead.**
NSAIDs	Methotrexate (MTX)	Connective tissue disease, cancer therapy	Toxic level of methotrexate may accumulate. **RECOMMENDATION: Avoid interaction if the patient is taking high-dose MTX for cancer therapy. Low-dose MTX for arthritis is not a concern.**
Meperidine	MAO inhibitors (e.g., isocarboxazid, phenelzine)	Depressants (NOTE: MAO inhibitors often are last line of therapy)	Co-administration will may produce severe and potentially fatal adverse excitatory or depressive reactions. **RECOMMENDATION: Avoid interaction.**
Propoxyphene	Carbamazepine	Seizure, trigeminal neuralgia	Co-administration can significantly increase the plasma concentrations of carbamazepine. **RECOMMENDATION: Avoid interaction.**

Continued

TABLE D.2   Drug Interactions of Significance in Dentistry by Category—cont'd

Dental Drug	Interacting Drug	Medical Condition or Situation	Effect
Anesthetics			
Lidocaine	Bupivacaine		Additive effect of these two local anesthetics increases the risk of CNS toxicity. **RECOMMENDATION: Limit dose of each**.
Lidocaine	Tramadol		Co-administration will may rarely cause seizures. More likely in elderly, those with seizures, or if undergoing alcohol drug withdrawal. **RECOMMENDATION: Avoid interaction; limit dose**.
Mepivacaine	Meperidine (Demerol)		Sedation with opioids may increase risk of local anesthetic toxicity; especially in children. **RECOMMENDATION: Reduce anesthetic dose**.
Sedatives			
Barbiturates	Digoxin, theophylline, corticosteroids, oral anticoagulants (coumarin)	Congestive heart failure, asthma, autoimmune disease, atrial fibrillation	Barbiturates bind P-450 cytochrome system in liver and enhance the metabolism of many drugs, reducing the effect of the anticoagulant. **RECOMMENDATION: Generally avoid. If necessary, limit dose and observe for adverse effects**.
	Benzodiazepines, alcohol, antihistamines	Anxiety, alcohol use and abuse, seasonal allergies	Co-administration has additive sedation and respiratory depression effects. **RECOMMENDATION: Reduce dose and administer combination of sedatives with extreme caution**.
Benzodiazepines (BZDPs) (e.g., Alprazolam, Chlordiazepoxide, Diazepam, Triazolam)	Cimetidine, oral contraceptives, fluoxetine, isoniazid (INH), alcohol, azole antifungals (fluconazole, itraconazole, ketoconazole)	Peptic ulcer disease, depression, tuberculosis, alcohol use and abuse	Co-administration will delay metabolism of BZDP, increasing the systemic exposure and pharmacologic effects, can result in excessive sedation and adverse psychomotor effects. **RECOMMENDATION: Reduce dose of benzodiazepine or avoid interaction**.
	Digoxin (Lanoxin), phenytoin, theophylline (Theo-Dur)	Congestive heart failure, epilepsy, asthma	Serum concentrations of digoxin and phenytoin may be increased, resulting in toxicity. Antagonize sedative effects of benzodiazepine. **RECOMMENDATION: Avoid interaction**.
	Protease inhibitors (indinavir, nelfinavir)	HIV infection and AIDS	Co-administration will increase bioavailability and effects of benzodiazepines, especially triazolam and oral midazolam. **RECOMMENDATION: Avoid interaction**.

Vasoconstrictors

Epinephrine and Levonordephrine (Neo-Cobefrin)	Nonselective beta-blockers: propranolol (Inderal), nadolol (Corgard), penbutolol (Levatol), pindolol (Visken), sotalol (Betapace), timolol (Blocadren)	Angina pectoris, hypertension, glaucoma, migraine, headache, hyperthyroidism, panic syndromes	Unopposed effects—Increased blood pressure with secondary bradycardia. **RECOMMENDATION: Initial dose is one-half cartridge containing 1:100,000 epinephrine; aspirate to avoid intravascular injection, and inject slowly. Monitor vital signs; if no adverse cardiovascular changes occur, up to two cartridges containing a vasoconstrictor can be administered. Provide a 5-minute interval between the first and second cartridges, with continual monitoring. Avoid epinephrine-containing retraction cord and higher concentrations of epinephrine in the dental anesthetic.**
	Cocaine	Illicit use, topical anesthetic for mucous membrane procedures	Blocks reuptake of norepinephrine and intensifies postsynaptic response to epinephrine-like drugs. This potentiates the adrenergic effects on the heart, with the potential for a heart attack. **RECOMMENDATION: Recognize signs and symptoms of cocaine abuse; avoid use of vasoconstrictors in these patients until cocaine has been withheld for at least 24 hours.**
	Halothane	General anesthetic for surgical procedures	Stimulation of alpha and beta receptors, resulting in arrhythmia at doses that exceed 2 μg/kg. **RECOMMENDATION: Limit dose to remain below 2 μg/kg threshold; aspirate to avoid intravascular injection. Monitor vital signs. Avoid epinephrine-containing retraction cord and concentrations of epinephrine higher than 1:100,000.**
	Tricyclic antidepressants[a] (amitriptyline [Elavil], amoxapine, clomipramine [Anafranil], desipramine [Norpramin], doxepin [Sinequan], imipramine [Tofranil], nortriptyline [Pamelor], protriptyline [Vivactil], trimipramine [Surmontil])	Depression, severe anxiety, neuropathic pain, attention deficit disorder	Blocks reuptake of norepinephrine, resulting in unopposed effects—increased pressor response (increased BP, increased heart rate)—and potential cardiac arrhythmias; effect is greater with levonordefrin. **RECOMMENDATION: Avoid levonordefrin; limit dose to two cartridges containing 1:100,000 epinephrine (36 μg); aspirate to avoid intravascular injection. Monitor vital signs. Avoid epinephrine-containing retraction cord and higher concentrations of epinephrine in the dental anesthetic.**
	MAO inhibitors (isocarboxazid [Marplan], phenelzine [Nardil], tranylcypromine [Parnate])	Depression	Although no reports have documented the effects on BP or heart rate after dental procedures, the potential for increased pressor response is present. **RECOMMENDATION: Avoid levonordefrin; limit dose to two cartridges containing 1:100,000 epinephrine (36 μg); aspirate to avoid intravascular injection. Monitor vital signs. Avoid epinephrine-containing retraction cord and higher concentrations of epinephrine in the dental anesthetic.**

Continued

TABLE D.2 Drug Interactions of Significance in Dentistry by Category—cont'd

Dental Drug	Interacting Drug	Medical Condition or Situation	Effect
	Antipsychotics Some examples: chlorpromazine (Thorazine), trifluoperazine (Stelazine), clozapine (Clozaril), olanzapine (Zyprexa)	Schizophrenia	Decrease BP (hypotension). **RECOMMENDATION: Use only small amounts of epinephrine; limit dose to two cartridges containing 1:100,000 epinephrine (36 µg); aspirate to avoid intravascular injection. Monitor vital signs.**
	Peripheral adrenergic antagonists (reserpine [Serpasil], guanethidine [Ismelin], guanadrel [Hylorel])	Hypertension	Potential for increased sensitivity of adrenergic receptors to epinephrine and levonordefrin. **RECOMMENDATION: Administer cautiously. Monitor vital signs during and after administration of first cartridge. Limit dose to two cartridges containing 1:100,000 epinephrine (36 µg) or less, depending on vital signs and patient response. Aspirate to avoid intravascular injection. Avoid epinephrine-containing retraction cord and higher concentrations of epinephrine in the dental anesthetic.**
	Catechol-*O*-methyltransferase inhibitors (tolcapone [Tasmar], entacapone [Comtan])	Parkinson disease	Potential for increased sensitivity of adrenergic receptors to epinephrine and levonordefrin, resulting in increased heart rate, BP, and arrhythmias. **RECOMMENDATION: Administer cautiously. Monitor vital signs during and after administration of first cartridge. Limit dose to two cartridges containing 1:100,000 epinephrine (36 µg) or less, depending on vital signs and patient response. Aspirate to avoid intravascular injection. Avoid epinephrine-containing retraction cord and higher concentrations of epinephrine in the dental anesthetic.**

[a]Antidepressants, such as the selective serotonin reuptake inhibitors (SSRIs), do not interact with vasoconstrictors. However, antidepressants that block norepinephrine uptake (venlafaxine [Effexor], bupropion [Wellbutrin]) have the potential to interact with vasoconstrictors, resulting in pressor responses.

ACE, angiotensin-converting enzyme; *AIDS*, acquired immunodeficiency syndrome; *BP*, blood pressure; *CNS*, central nervous system; *GI*, gastrointestinal; *HIV*, human immunodeficiency virus; *INR*, international normalized ratio; *MAO*, monoamine oxidase; *MI*, myocardial infarction; *NSAID*, nonsteroidal antiinflammatory drugs.

Herbal Supplements Used in Complementary and Alternative Medicine of Potential Importance in Dentistry

Complementary and alternative medicine (CAM), also referred to as complementary and integrative medicine, encompasses medical therapies, interventions, and practices that are not generally considered to be components of standard Western medical care. These modalities may be referred to as being more "natural" or "holistic" compared with traditional Western medicine practices. While there can be some degree of overlap, the five primary categories of CAM include mind-body therapies (e.g., meditation, yoga), biologically based practices (e.g., vitamins, herbs, and botanicals), manipulative and body-based practices (e.g., deep massage, reflexology, acupuncture), biofield therapy (e.g., Reiki), and whole medical systems (e.g., Chinese traditional medicine, Ayurvedic medicine, homeopathic medicine). Many of these treatments are increasingly recognized for their health and wellness benefits and have been increasingly incorporated into traditional Western medicine, often blurring the distinction. There is also growing evidence based on randomized controlled trials to support the efficacy and health benefits of many of these therapies. Nearly half of Americans use and engage in CAM therapies, which are supported by an estimated $30 billion industry.

While most CAM therapies are considered safe and have little if any potential to interfere or interact with "conventional" medical care, several commonly used herbal and plant-based treatments have potential for significant drug interactions for which the dentist must be aware.

HERBAL MEDICINES

Herbal medicines are a subset of natural plant-based and botanical products or supplements (phytomedicines) that have been used by humans for thousands of years to treat and prevent a wide range of diseases and ailments. Several herbal remedies have been rigorously evaluated in placebo-controlled randomized controlled trials, and systematic reviews of these studies demonstrate that some of these supplements indeed demonstrate efficacy for certain conditions (Table E.1). For example, ginkgo biloba has been shown to be effective for the symptomatic treatment of dementia and intermittent claudication, and echinacea and zinc have demonstrated benefit for treatment of the common cold.

The FDA classifies herbal supplements as foods rather than drugs, and as such, they are not subject to the same testing, manufacturing, labeling standards, and regulations as medications. Further, the composition, quality, and purity of herbal supplements can vary greatly across and even sometimes within manufacturers. It is important for the dentist to include a section in the patient's medical history on taking herbal medications and OTC drugs.

The National Institutes of Health Office of Dietary Supplements maintains an excellent website (https://ods.od.nih.gov/factsheets/list-all/) with links to fact sheets for all of the commonly used supplements including vitamins, minerals, herbs, and botanicals and probiotics.

ADVERSE EFFECTS AND DRUG INTERACTIONS

While generally very safe, toxicity may be associated with the use of herbal supplements (Table E.2). If a plant contains constituents known to affect the bioavailability or pharmacokinetics of other drugs, clinically significant and potentially serious drug interactions may occur (Table E.3). Certain herbal supplements have the potential to interact with and affect proteins involved in drug absorption, distribution, metabolism, or excretion. These proteins include the cytochrome P450 enzymes (CYP enzymes), the uridine diphosphate-glucuronosyltransferase (UGT) conjugating enzymes, the adenosine triphosphate-binding cassette (ABC) drug uptake/efflux transporters, and the organic anion-transporting polypeptide (OATP) drug transporters. Of note, the six CYP enzymes (CYP1A2, CYP2C9, CYP2C19, CYP2D6, CYP2E1, and CYP3A4) account for the metabolism of approximately 80% of prescribed medications. For example, St. John's wort, commonly taken for symptoms of depression, induces the activity of CYP3A4, leading to diminished activity of drugs that are CYP3A4 substrates. Persons who take a prescription medicine, especially those with cardiac,

TABLE E.1   Commonly Used Herbal Supplements

Product	Indication
Kava	Anxiety
Artichoke	Hyperlipidemia
Feverfew	Women's health ailments, inflammatory diseases, migraine headaches
Garlic	Hypertension, hyperlipidemia
Ginger	Nausea and vomiting
Echinacea	Common cold
Ginkgo Biloba	Cerebral insufficiency and to prevent loss of cognitive function, tinnitus
Hawthorn	Heart failure
Horse Chestnut	Venous congestion
Saw Palmetto	Benign prostate enlargement
St. John's Wort	Depression

TABLE E.2   Natural Supplements With Potentially Serious Adverse Effects

Product	Effect
Aristolochia	Nephrotoxicity
	Carcinogenicity
Chaparral	Cholestatic hepatitis
Comfrey	Acute and chronic hepatitis
Digitalis Leaf	Arrhythmia
Ephedra	Hypertension
	Stroke
	Myocardial infarction
Germander	Acute and chronic hepatitis
Kava	Hepatitis
Khat	Tachycardia
	Psychosis
Kombucha	Hepatotoxicity
	Lactic acidosis
Mistletoe	Anaphylaxis
Skullcap	Seizures
	Acute and chronic hepatitis
St. John's Wort	Photosensitivity
	Possible hypertension with tyramine-containing foods

TABLE E.3   Selected Plant-Based Medicines That Potentiate or Interfere With Approved Drugs

Natural Medicine	Approved Drug
Ephedra	Theophylline (P)
	Antihypertensives (I)
	Corticosteroids (I)
Evening Primrose	Anticoagulants (P)
	Antiplatelet agents (P)
	Low-molecular-weight heparins (P)
	Anticonvulsants (I)
Garlic	Aspirin (P)
	Clopidogrel (P)
	Ticlopidine (P)
Ginkgo Biloba	Anticoagulants (P)
	Antiplatelet agents (P)
	Anticonvulsants (I)
Glucosamine	Diabetic agents (I)
Panax Ginseng	Anticoagulants (P)
	Diabetic agents (possible P)
	Nifedipine (P)
Saw Palmetto	Hormone replacement therapies (P)
Soy	Estrogenic drugs (P)
St. John's Wort	Antidepressants (P)
	HIV protease inhibitors (I)
	Cyclosporine (I)
Valerian	Sedatives (P)
Yohimbe	Antihypertensives (I)

I, interferes, reducing effect of drug; *P*, potentiates, increasing effect of drug.

diuretic, sedative, hypotensive, or other potentially dangerous properties, should consult with their physicians before taking an herbal supplement. With respect to medications typically prescribed by dentists (e.g., antibiotics, analgesics, topical steroids, etc.), caution should be taken when prescribing NSAIDs in patients who are taking herbal supplements due to possible risk of increased bleeding.

In addition to intrinsic toxicities related to herbal supplements, there is risk for adverse reactions related to product manufacturing, quality, and purity. While pharmaceutical agents must be produced under highly regulated and controlled measures, this does not extend to the herbal supplement industry. These adverse reactions may be due to accidental or deliberate contamination of the product. For example, lead, mercury, cadmium, pesticides, microorganisms, and fumigants have been found to contaminate some herbal products. Substitution of animal substances such as enzymes, hormones, or organ extracts has accounted for some of the toxic reactions to herbal products. Adulteration caused by the accidental or deliberate substitution of the original plant material by other plant species also has been reported to be a source of toxic reactions to herbal products.

BIBLIOGRAPHY

1. Abebe W. Review of herbal medications with the potential to cause bleeding: dental implications, and risk prediction and prevention avenues. *EPMA J.* 2019;10(1): 51−64. https://doi.org/10.1007/s13167-018-0158-2. PMID: 30984314.
2. Asher GN, Corbett AH, Hawke RL. Common herbal dietary supplement-drug interactions. *Am Fam Physician.* 2017; 96(2):101−107. PMID: 28762712.

3. Eisenberg DM, Davis RB, Ettner SL, et al. Trends in alternative medicine use in the United States, 1990–1997: results of a follow-up national survey. *JAMA*. 1998;280(18):1569–1575.

4. Micozzi M. *Fundamentals of Complementary and Alternative Medicine*. 5th ed. St. Louis: Saunders; 2015.

5. *National Center for Complementary and Integrative Health Washington D.C.* National Institutes of Health; 2021. https://www.nccih.nih.gov/.

6. *National Institutes of Health Office of Dietary Supplements Dietary Supplement Fact Sheets*; 2021. https://ods.od.nih.gov/factsheets/list-all/.

INDEX

Page numbers followed by "*f*" indicate figures, "*t*" indicate tables, and "*b*" indicate boxes.